Physician Practice Management

Essential Operational and Financial Knowledge

Second Edition

Lawrence F. Wolper, MBA, FACMPE

President

L. Wolper, Inc.

Morristown, NJ

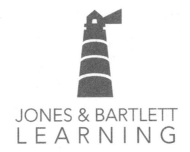

JONES & BARTLETT
LEARNING

World Headquarters
Jones & Bartlett Learning
5 Wall Street
Burlington, MA 01803
978-443-5000
info@jblearning.com
www.jblearning.com

Jones & Bartlett Learning books and products are available through most bookstores and online booksellers. To contact Jones & Bartlett Learning directly, call 800-832-0034, fax 978-443-8000, or visit our website, www.jblearning.com.

Substantial discounts on bulk quantities of Jones & Bartlett Learning publications are available to corporations, professional associations, and other qualified organizations. For details and specific discount information, contact the special sales department at Jones & Bartlett Learning via the above contact information or send an email to specialsales@jblearning.com.

Copyright © 2013 by Jones & Bartlett Learning, LLC, an Ascend Learning Company

All rights reserved. No part of the material protected by this copyright may be reproduced or utilized in any form, electronic or mechanical, including photocopying, recording, or by any information storage and retrieval system, without written permission from the copyright owner.

Physician Practice Management, Second Edition is an independent publication and has not been authorized, sponsored, or otherwise approved by the owners of the trademarks or service marks referenced in this product.

The authors, editor, and publisher have made every effort to provide accurate information. However, they are not responsible for errors, omissions, or for any outcomes related to the use of the contents of this book and take no responsibility for the use of the products and procedures described. Treatments and side effects described in this book may not be applicable to all people; likewise, some people may require a dose or experience a side effect that is not described herein. Drugs and medical devices are discussed that may have limited availability controlled by the Food and Drug Administration (FDA) for use only in a research study or clinical trial. Research, clinical practice, and government regulations often change the accepted standard in this field. When consideration is being given to use of any drug in the clinical setting, the health care provider or reader is responsible for determining FDA status of the drug, reading the package insert, and reviewing prescribing information for the most up-to-date recommendations on dose, precautions, and contraindications, and determining the appropriate usage for the product. This is especially important in the case of drugs that are new or seldom used.

Production Credits
Publisher: William Brottmiller
Acquisitions Editor: Katey Birtcher
Managing Editor: Maro Gartside
Associate Editor: Teresa Reilly
Editorial Assistant: Kayla Dos Santos
Associate Production Editor: Jill Morton
Production Assistant: Emma Krosschell
Marketing Manager: Grace Richards
Manufacturing and Inventory Control Supervisor: Amy Bacus
Composition: Cenveo Publisher Services
Cover Design: Scott Moden
Cover Image: © Loongar/Dreamstime.com
Printing and Binding: Courier Companies
Cover Printing: Courier Companies

Library of Congress Cataloging-in-Publication Data
Physician practice management : essential operational and financial knowledge / [edited by] Lawrence F. Wolper. — 2nd ed.
    p. ; cm.
  Includes bibliographical references and index.
  ISBN 978-0-7637-7101-0—ISBN 0-7637-7101-5
  I. Wolper, Lawrence F.
  [DNLM: 1. Practice Management, Medical—organization & administration. 2. Financial Management—organization & administration. 3. Group Practice--organization & administration. W 80]

  362.1068—dc23
                        2011046461

6048
Printed in the United States of America
16 15 14 13 12   10 9 8 7 6 5 4 3 2 1

To our darling Sophie,
a bright ray of sunshine every day.

Contents

Foreword

The U.S. healthcare system is in the process of its most significant change since the creation of Medicare and Medicaid in 1965. The passage of the Patient Protection and Affordable Care Act in 2010 initiated a series of changes in government programs that will change who has health insurance, how doctors and hospitals are paid, and how physicians relate to patients, hospitals, and insurance companies. Simultaneously with the federal health reform initiatives, commercial health insurance companies are on a parallel path to create care delivery programs that are designed to improve quality and reduce the total cost of care.

Whether change is due to federal legislation or a response to market forces, the healthcare system of the future will have a very different structure than what is observed today. In order to prepare for a transformed healthcare environment, medical practices and their leaders need a firm foundation. The second edition of *Physician Practice Management: Essential Operational and Financial Knowledge* was designed to provide the information that practice leaders will need now and in the future. Every critical aspect of practice is addressed in the text by authors who have attained national recognition for their expertise and knowledge.

In the midst of the changes underway in the healthcare system, the Medical Group Management Association (MGMA) and the American College of Medical Practice Executives (ACMPE) are in their own transformation. In October 2011, the respective memberships of the two organizations approved their merger into a new association effective January 1, 2012. The new association, MGMA-ACMPE, will be better positioned to serve our members and the industry in the rapidly changing healthcare marketplace. The MGMA-ACMPE vision to "be the foremost resource for members and their organizations in creating and improving systems that complement the delivery of affordable, quality patient care" shows our commitment to the needs of medical practices and their leaders.

The 21 chapters of the second edition of *Physician Practice Management: Essential Operational and Financial Knowledge* address the spectrum of management issues facing medical practices. The text is divided into three sections to concentrate similar topics for the reader's convenience. Each of these sections, Practice Operations and Functions, Monitoring and Controlling Physician Organizations, and Essential Knowledge for Contemporary Management, could stand alone as a definitive text; in combination, they make this text the most comprehensive source of practice management information available in a single document.

Section I, Practice Operations and Functions, provides a broad overview of health issues including the evolution of medicine and how healthcare is delivered in other countries. The section continues with chapters that address general practice operations, the organization of medical groups, physician leadership, nursing leadership, human resources management, and marketing. Six of the chapters in this section were in the *First Edition* and have received extensive updates, including the differences in the manner in which malpractice lawsuits are handled and the impact of these lawsuits in the United States. A new Chapter 7, Public Health and Private Physician Medical Practice Preparedness: Can We Be Medically Prepared for the Next Disaster?, replaces the chapter on bioterrorism in the first edition with information that discusses how a medical practice can prepare for and minimize the impact of natural or human-caused disasters.

Section II, Monitoring and Controlling Physician Organizations, addresses the controlling and management systems within the practice. This section has chapters that address governance, accounting, finance, benchmarking techniques, electronic health records, management information systems, and risk management that update the content of the first edition. It begins with a new chapter, Physician Practice: Organization, Management, and Operation, which introduces the section and provides a summary of information on practice governance and organizational structure.

The last section, Essential Knowledge for Contemporary Management, has six chapters that update the content of the *First Edition*. These chapters cover the laws and federal regulations that affect internal operations and external relationships. They also address how compensation plans can incentivize provider productivity and how facility design affects patient care and throughput. Two new chapters focus on the information that healthcare leaders need to structure physician employment contracts that comply with federal regulations.

Just as this text is the definitive reference for a medical practice or senior hospital executive, it also is the ideal reference for administrators seeking ACMPE certification or Fellowship. The certification test process is designed to verify and validate expertise and experience in medical practice management; administrators who pass the ACMPE certification examinations are recognized as having the unique knowledge and skill set for medical practice management. The extensive depth of content in the second edition of *Physician Practice Management: Essential Operational and Financial Knowledge* makes this text the ideal study guide for the ACMPE examinations because the chapters in this book cover the entire scope of the body of knowledge for medical practice management.

The chapter authors represent a cross-section of the most knowledgeable authorities in their fields. The authors come from academia, healthcare organizations, law firms, associations, architectural firms, and consulting organizations and bring a level of expertise that is unmatched in any other health management publication. The authors' academic and professional credentials are exemplary, with many holding dual professional degrees. Additionally, most of the authors have attained the highest level of certification and recognition in their respective fields. Among the medical practice executives who contributed to this text, nine are either Certified Medical Practice Executives or Fellows in the American College of Medical Practice Executives (ACMPE). Attaining Fellowship in the ACMPE is the highest credential in medical practice management.

The first edition of *Physician Practice Management: Essential Operational and Financial Knowledge* was published in 2005 and was quickly recognized as the authoritative text describing medical practice management. This second edition adds new information that keeps the publication current so it can continue to meet the demanding information needs of medical practice leaders. This text should be included on the bookshelf of every medical practice executive.

Susan Turney, MD, MS, FACP, FACMPE
President and Chief Executive Officer
MGMA-ACMPE
Englewood, Colorado

Acknowledgments

When the outlining of this book began, all authors, coauthors, and editors realized that we were entering a time of significant change in the healthcare industry. As stated in the foreword, it did not matter whether the change was being influenced by legislation or by other exogenous factors. Rapid and, at times, contentious change was occurring. The challenge was how to write and produce a text that would both be able to address these possible changes and be accurate and educational. The writing of the manuscripts was paced in such a way that the authors would have enough time to research and absorb possible changes, and to determine the degree to which they could or would affect their specific topical areas. Some authors' topics were likely to be dramatically affected, and others to a lesser degree. In retrospect it appears that the longer process time for the book has paid off.

There are 21 chapters in the second edition of this text, all written by authors with outstanding reputations in each of their respective areas of expertise. Most have terminal degrees in their fields, and nine are Fellows in the American College of Medical Practice Executives. There are new authors as well, such as Sheila Richmeier who wrote an outstanding chapter on nursing management and the changes that are, and will be, occurring in that area, and Neill Piland who coordinated, with his coauthors, a very robust chapter on disaster preparedness. The lead author of that chapter, Denise O'Farrell, has achieved excellence in threading many subtopics together into a critical chapter, and doing so in such a highly professional manner, while at the same time personally facing other life challenges. Other new authors are Richard Naegele and Kelly Ann VanDenHaute, who took a topic of quite some detail, tax-qualified retirement plans and fringe benefits, and made it easily understood and very much on point. Perhaps the most likely area to absorb major change now and in the future is information systems, and Margret Amatayakul wrote an exemplary chapter on this topic. Changes affecting this area can be encompassed in entire texts, but Margret has covered the subject well, and logically, in just one chapter. Dan Buscko and his coauthors also wrote an excellent chapter on medical malpractice, an area that may change in the future.

Special thanks to Bruce Johnson, who, with an extremely busy schedule, was able to complete two chapters, one with colleague Jennifer Weinfeld and one by himself. Peter Stergios and colleagues wrote a chapter on labor and employment law that is very interesting, and is one of those areas that is likely to sustain substantial change in the future.

Thanks to each of the authors who have published in previous editions of this book for their unhesitating willingness to, once again, go through the process. The accounting and budgeting chapter written by Steven Andes and Dave Gans, the chapter on financial management and reporting by Lee Ann Webster, and the one on practice benchmarking written by Elizabeth Woodcock, all updated, integrate with each other as if they were meant to be a small book on these interlocking topics. Continued thanks to Geraldine Amori for her chapter on risk management, and Mike Kelley and colleagues for their chapter exploring practice organization and finance.

Another area that is likely to continue to experience significant change, as MDs coalesce into large and super-large groups and hospitals continue to acquire practices, is facility design for large practices. The chapter on facility design, written by Richard Sprow and colleagues, is exemplary in exploring the architectural and design implications of the medical office of the future. As Medicare, Medicaid, and commercial insurers increase the intensity of fraud and abuse auditing, and Medicare in particular continues to recoup large sums of money for noncompliance, the chapter composed by Michael Costa and his colleagues is a must-read.

The remaining authors who are to be acknowledged are Grant Savage and his colleagues, who, once again, have raised the bar on their comparative analysis of, now, 12 countries. They also have expanded the analysis of these countries to include the manner in which malpractice lawsuits are adjudicated, whether there are limitations on malpractice monetary awards, and, in the case of the United States, how much is spent on malpractice awards. Stephen Wagner has written an excellent chapter on the organization and operations of medical groups. As the number of large medical groups continues to increase, whether they are independent or part of a system, physician leadership and "team" physician and lay leadership become more important.

In the 1990s, when large-scale physician acquisition by hospitals occurred, some believed that not enough time was expended in on-boarding physicians who had long practiced in small groups, and little time and attention were given by many organizations to accommodate the abrupt change from private practice to employed physician. They were now legally employees of hospitals, but the result, in retrospect, did not appear to be satisfactory or productive. Dr. Gary Kaplan, the chairman and CEO of Virginia Mason Health System, a very respected integrated system, has shared his experience about physician leadership in medical group practice.

The challenges in building a team approach to leadership and management, and the positive alignment of hospitals with physicians, is an addition to this book that is well worth reading. An award-winning book, *Transforming Health Care: Virginia Mason Medical Center's Pursuit of the Perfect Patient Experience*, by Charles Kenney, also is worth reading. It takes the reader through the ups and downs of creating an aligned system that works, the end product of which is a positive patient experience and keen attention to clinical outcomes.

Many hospitals currently may be making "oversights" similar to those in the 1990s, and in addition to the previously mentioned topic of physician leadership, the area of marketing also continues to be overlooked. Roberta Clarke, a professor, author, and leader in marketing healthcare, writes a comprehensive chapter that addresses good marketing in general, but how marketing is even more important in a changing industry. Branding an enlarging health system as a "system" is important, but creating a public identity for a large physician network or group also is important.

In 1910 Abraham Flexner wrote a book on medical education in the United States and Canada (*The Flexner Report*); to this day, many of the suggestions he made continue to influence hospitals and physicians. Many aspects of the book, sponsored by the Carnegie Foundation, also remain controversial. It stated, among many things, that the hospital was the doctor's workshop (much less so now with the emergence of very large independent groups with satellite offices that provide a wide range of services). Flexner's statement is likely to be the case in the future, regardless of the size and geographic reach of a system. Therefore, subordinating the identity of a large physician group or network that is owned by a health system may be underutilizing the marketing and public relations "capital" of the physicians. Dr. Clark provides a compelling argument for the importance of marketing in today's changing environment. It is perhaps even more important now than historically, because as systems expand in size, the consumer has greater difficulty in differentiating the centers of excellence among these organizations because without astute marketing they may sound like they all are excellent in all things . . . and logic suggests that this cannot be the case.

The last area that has evolved quickly in response to the speed of change in the industry is human resources management, and Michael O'Connell has produced a chapter that considers the new pressures on this critical function in a rapidly changing setting; as in the first edition, he does so in an easy-reading, yet detailed manner.

In summary, the authors of this text all are highly skilled, trained, and respected in their respective fields. Many have multiple academic degrees. Yet, in spite of the fact that they all are extremely busy, they took the time and effort to research, to speculate on the impact of changes in the industry, and to envision the impact of those changes on their own areas of specialization.

I thank all authors, coauthors, and editors for selflessly taking the time to work on this project. It is my hope that this text becomes one that is widely read for the knowledge and wisdom that it contains, and the contemporary healthcare issues that it addresses.

Lawrence F. Wolper
Managing Editor/Author

About the Managing Editor/Author

Lawrence F. Wolper, MBA, FACMPE, is president of L. Wolper, Inc., in Morristown, New Jersey. The firm is a full-service consulting organization specializing in all aspects of physician group practice, hospital alignment, revenue cycle assessment, and managed care. In addition, L. Wolper, Inc., has extensive experience in managing large physician group practices and ambulatory surgery centers in order to assist them in achieving strategic growth goals and to augment operational and financial efficiencies.

Mr. Wolper has more than 25 years of consulting and senior executive experience, and has been the advisor to, or managed, major group practices, faculty practice plans, ambulatory surgery centers, and integrated networks. Prior to founding his firm in 1987, he was a partner in KPMG, International, LLP, with New York area and national responsibility for physician practice and ambulatory care consulting. At that time, he was involved in the development of large group practices, faculty practice plans, and provider networks. Prior to his partnership in KPMG, he was a consulting partner with Ingram, Weitzman, Mertens & Co., a large regional healthcare accounting and consulting firm.

He has published more than 35 professional journal articles and 8 texts on a variety of subjects that are germane to physician and faculty practice, and to healthcare administration. His book *Health Care Administration: Principles, Practices, Structure, and Delivery, Second Edition*, won a prestigious national award as one of the top 250 texts in the health sciences industry. The text was recently released in its fifth edition, and remains one of the leading texts in the industry.

Mr. Wolper received an MBA in healthcare administration from Bernard M. Baruch College/Ricklin School of Business–Mount Sinai School of Medicine, and a BA in advertising/marketing from Hofstra University. He was a Robert Wood Johnson Foundation Fellow in HMO management at the Wharton School, University of Pennsylvania, and an Association of University Programs in Hospital Administration (AUPHA) Fellow studying the British National Health System at the Kings Fund College of Hospital Management in London, England.

He is a Fellow in the American College of Medical Practice Executives, and was an Associate Adjunct Professor in the Executive MPH Program at Columbia University, teaching a course on managed care and organized delivery systems.

Contributors

Margret Amatayakul, MBA, RHIA, CHPS, CPHIT,
   CPEHR, CPHIE, FHIMSS
President
Margret\A Consulting, LLC
Schaumburg, Illinois

Geraldine Amori, PhD, ARM, CPHRM, DFASHRM
Vice President, Education Center
Risk Management and Patient Safety Institute
Shelburne, Vermont

Stephen M. Andes, PhD, CPA
Research Assistant Professor, Division of Health Policy
   and Administration
University of Illinois School Public Health
Niles, Illinois

Keri D. Black, PhD, CFNP
Assistant Professor and Clinical Educator
University of New Mexico College of Nursing
Albuquerque, New Mexico

Christian F. Bormann, AIA, NCARB, LEED AP
Architect
Perkins & Will
New York, New York

Mohamed Bouras, MS
University of Missouri-Columbia
Columbia, Missouri

Julie M. Brightwell, BSN, JD, CPHRM
Director, Patient Safety Programs
The Doctors Company
Powell, Ohio

Dan Bucsko, MBA, MHA, FACHE, CMPE, CPHRM
Vice President
The Doctors Company
Vacaville, California

Roberta N. Clarke, MBA, DBA
Associate Professor, Health Care
   Management Program
Boston University
Weston, Massachusetts

Michael R. Costa, JD, MPH
Attorney, Greenberg Trauig, LLP
Boston, Massachusetts

Sonya Dufner, FASID
Director of Workplace
Perkins & Will
New York, New York

Steven Falcone, MD, MBA
Chief Operating Officer, UHealth Faculty Practice
University of Miami Miller School of Medicine
Miami, Florida

David N. Gans, MSHA, FACMPE
Vice President, Innovation and Research
Medical Group Management Association
Englewood, Colorado

Jason Harper, AIA, LEED AP
Associate Principal
Perkins & Will
New York, New York

Jennifer Itzkoff, JD
Associate
McCarter & English
Boston, Massachusetts

Bruce A. Johnson, JD, MPA
Shareholder
Polsinelli Shughart, PC
Denver, Colorado

Gary S. Kaplan, MD, FACMPE, FACP
Chairman and CEO
Virginia Mason Health System
Seattle, Washington

Michael J. Kelley, MBA, CMPE
Vice Chairman, University of Miami Medical Group
University of Miami Miller School of Medicine
Miami, Florida

John M. McKelway, JD
Partner
McCarter & English
Boston, Massachusetts

Chris Morrison, Esq
Attorney
Adventist Health System
Winter Park, Florida

Richard A. Naegele, BA, MA, JD
Wickens, Herzer, Panza, Cook & Batista Co.
Avon, Ohio

Richard D. Norwood, CPA, FHMA, MBA
Finance Director, Faculty Practice
University of Miami Miller School of Medicine
Miami, Florida

Michael A. O'Connell, MHA, FACHE, FACMPE
Vice President of Clinical Services
Marymount and Southpoint Hospitals
Solon, Ohio

Denise O'Farrell, MPH
Healthcare Liaison
Southeastern District Health Department
Pocatello, Idaho

Annette Phillipp, PhD, MPH
Research Assistant Professor, Institute of Rural Health
Idaho State University
Meridian, Idaho

Neill F. Piland, PhD
Research Professor, Director, Institute of Rural Health
Idaho State University
Pocatello, Idaho

Darrell Ranum, JD, CPHRM
Regional Vice President, Patient Safety
The Doctors Company
Columbus, Ohio

Leo van der Reis, MD
Director
Quincy Foundation for Medical Research
    University of Alabama at Birmingham
San Francisco, California

Sheila Richmeier, MS, RN, FACMPE
Owner and Consultant
Remedy Healthcare Consulting, LLC
Kansas City, Montana

John Rodenbeck, AIA, NCARB, LEED AP BD+C
Architect
Perkins & Will
New York, New York

Grant T. Savage, PhD, MBA, BA
Professor of Management
University of Alabama at Birmingham
Birmingham, Alabama

Stephen G. Schwartz, MD, MBA
Associate Professor of Clinical Ophthalmology
University of Miami Miller School of Medicine
Miami, Florida

Susan Shephard, MSN, CPHRM
Director, Patient Safety Education
The Doctors Company
Niceville, Florida

Howard L. Smith, PhD
Professor, Department of Management
College of Business and Economics,
    Boise State University
Boise, Idaho

Richard Sprow, AIA
Architect
Perkins & Will
New York, New York

Peter D. Stergios, JD
Partner
McCarter & English
New York, New York

Kelly Ann VanDenHaute, BS, JD
Attorney
Wickens, Herzer, Panza, Cook & Batista Co.
Avon, Ohio

Stephen L. Wagner, PhD, FACMPE
Vice President Medical Education and Research
Carolinas Healthcare System
Charlotte, North Carolina

Lee Ann H. Webster, MA, CPA, FACMPE
Pathology Associates of Alabama, PC
Birmingham, Alabama

Jennifer L. Weinfeld, JD
Counsel
Polsinelli Shughart, PC
Denver, Colorado

Elizabeth W. Woodcock, MBA, FACMPE, CPC
Principal
Woodcock & Associates
Atlanta, Georgia

Contributor Biographies

Chapter 1

Mohamed Bouras, MS, is a graduate student in health administration at the University of Missouri-Columbia. Mr. Bouras holds a Master of Science degree in agriculture and resource economics from the University of Connecticut. His research interests focus on medical groups' productivity, health information technology, and management of healthcare systems.

Leo van der Reis, MD, graduated with honors from the University of Chicago in 1954. His postgraduate training was in internal medicine and gastroenterology. In addition to the clinical practice of medicine, Dr. van der Reis has done extensive research and written on issues of healthcare policy. Dr. van der Reis is director of the Quincy Foundation for Medical Research–Charitable Trust and an adjunct professor in healthcare management and clinical professor of community and rural medicine at The University of Alabama.

Grant T. Savage, PhD, MBA, BA, is professor of management in the School of Business at the University of Alabama at Birmingham and holds joint appointments in the School of Medicine and School of Public Health. He codirects the Healthcare Leadership Academy for the UAB academic medical center, and is a founding series editor for *Advances in Health Care Management*, published by Emerald Group

Publishing. Dr. Savage has written extensively on healthcare management, communication, and negotiation issues, focusing primarily on stakeholder analysis and collaboration. He has coauthored six award-winning papers, and currently is engaged in healthcare research on employee and patient safety and on comparative international health management, as well as multisector research on stakeholder collaboration and economic development.

Chapter 2

Stephen L. Wagner, PhD, FACMPE, lives in Charlotte, North Carolina, and serves as the Vice President of Business Curriculum and Resident Development for the Carolinas Healthcare System, the third largest public healthcare system in the United States. He has been active in the field of healthcare as an executive, teacher, and researcher for more than 35 years.

Dr. Wagner currently teaches healthcare management in the Seton Hall University in the Master's of Health Administration program and serves as the Executive in Residence. He also teaches at University of North Carolina at Charlotte. Dr. Wagner holds a master's degree in healthcare fiscal management from The University of Wisconsin-Madison School of Business and a PhD from the University of Louisville College of Business in healthcare public policy analysis. Dr. Wagner's principal areas of emphasis are in medical practice administration, medical economics, community health, international medicine, new healthcare and educational technologies, and healthcare policy. His research has focused on outcome measurement for cardiovascular services, cardiovascular health, the use of Internet-based tools for patient self-management, and the development of healthcare systems in underserved communities, both domestic and international. Dr. Wagner has been involved in establishing medical practices and community services in St. Petersburg, Russia, and continues to work on healthcare service and cardiovascular issues in Charlotte.

Other publications include a book titled *Organizational Governance and Group Dynamics*, published by the MGMA as part of its American College of Medical Practice Executive Body of Knowledge Series (2006, revised 2008). More recently, Dr Wagner served as the coinvestigator of a study, "Effect of a Web-Based Self-Management Intervention on Patient Activation: A Randomized Controlled Trial." The study was presented at the HIMSS11 Annual Conference and an article of the same name is in press at the *Journal of Medical Internet Research*.

Dr. Wagner is a Fellow in the American College of Medical Practice Executives and has served as its examination committee chair.

Chapter 3

Gary S. Kaplan, MD, FACMPE, FACP, has served as chairman and CEO of the Virginia Mason Health System since 2000. He is a practicing internal medicine physician at Virginia Mason.

During Dr. Kaplan's tenure as chairman and CEO, Virginia Mason has received significant national and international recognition for its efforts to transform healthcare. Recent recognitions include:

- Virginia Mason was named the "Top Hospital of the Decade" for patient safety and quality by The Leapfrog Group, a distinction shared with only one other hospital.
- Virginia Mason received the highest overall score of any reporting hospital in the Pacific Northwest in the 2010 and 2011 surveys by The Leapfrog Group. In 2010, Virginia Mason also had the best safety ratings in Washington state for high-risk procedures, as well as the best overall patient safety ratings among all reporting hospitals.
- Virginia Mason is one of only 238 hospitals out of 6,000 nationwide to receive the 2011 HealthGrades Patient Safety Excellence Award.

- Virginia Mason was one of five hospitals honored with the 2011 American Hospital Association-McKesson Quest for Quality Prize, presented annually to honor leadership and innovation in quality improvement and safety.
- Virginia Mason was named a 2011 Distinguished Hospital for Clinical Excellence by HealthGrades, placing Virginia Mason among the top 5% of hospitals nationwide—the fourth time Virginia Mason had earned this honor.

Virginia Mason is considered to be the national leader in deploying the Toyota Production System to healthcare management—reducing the high costs of healthcare while improving quality, safety, and efficiency to deliver better, faster, and more affordable care.

In addition to caring for patients and serving as chairman and CEO, Dr. Kaplan is a clinical professor at the University of Washington and has been recognized for his service and contribution to many regional and national boards, including the Institute for Healthcare Improvement, the Medical Group Management Association, the National Patient Safety Foundation, the Greater Seattle Chamber of Commerce, the Washington Healthcare Forum, the Seattle Foundation, and Special Olympics of Washington.

Dr. Kaplan is a founding member of Health CEOs for Health Reform and has been recognized nationally for his healthcare leadership.

- *Modern Healthcare* ranked Dr. Kaplan thirty-third in its 2011 listing of the 100 Most Influential People in Healthcare.
- *Modern Physician* and *Modern Healthcare* ranked Dr. Kaplan twelfth in the 2011 listing of the 50 Most Influential Physician Executives.
- In 2011, *Becker's Hospital Review* listed Dr. Kaplan as one of the 13 Most Influential Patient Safety Advocates in the United States, and named him as one of 291 U.S. Health and Hospital Leaders to Know.

Some of Dr. Kaplan's other awards and distinctions include:

- The 2009 John M. Eisenberg Award from the National Quality Forum and The Joint Commission for Individual Achievement at the national level for his outstanding work and commitment to patient safety and quality.
- The Harry J. Harwick Lifetime Achievement Award for outstanding contributions to healthcare from the Medical Group Management Association and the American College of Medical Practice Executives.

Dr. Kaplan received his medical degree from the University of Michigan and is board certified in internal medicine. He is a Fellow of the American College of Physicians (FACP), the American College of Medical Practice Executives (FACMPE), and the American College of Physician Executives (FACPE).

Chapter 4

Sheila Richmeier, MS, RN, FACMPE, has established significant expertise in medical practice redesign with over 20 years of experience in healthcare. Key to her qualifications and success is her ability to objectively analyze situations and determine potential opportunities. Throughout her career, Sheila has managed clinical staff; provided oversight for business, financial, and clinical aspects of a medical office; and provided key insights in various consulting projects. Drawing upon diverse hospital, home health, and primary and specialty care experiences, Sheila provides practical efficiency solutions to medical offices. As a facilitator, Sheila has worked with primary care practices throughout the country to assist with the transformation to patient-centered medical homes. This work was a culmination of all her experiences and expertise in medical practice management and clinical operations. Successes include improvement in quality and clinical outcome analysis, and physician, staff, and patient satisfaction, along with improved efficiencies in financial and operational areas. Recently Sheila opened her own business, Remedy Healthcare Consulting, and provides services to both primary and specialist practices throughout the country.

Sheila is a registered nurse and a fellow in the American College of Medical Practice Executives with a master's degree in nursing administration from the University of Kansas. Sheila speaks on the national stage and has published numerous books, including *Leading Your Clinical Team: A Comprehensive Guide to Optimizing Productivity and Quality*, published by MGMA in July 2009, and *The New Healthcare Supervisor's Guide: The Secrets to Success*, published by MGMA in March 2010. She also authored *Fast Facts: Medical Office Nursing*, published by Springer Publishing in June 2010.

Chapter 5

Michael A. O'Connell, MHA, FACHE, FACMPE, is an experienced senior healthcare leader working at two of Cleveland Clinic's regional hospitals and medical groups in Cleveland, Ohio. He has been responsible for operations of medical practices, hospitals, and physician services including recruitment, retention, and development of employees and physicians. He has worked extensively to engage teams to accomplish great results in the areas of patient experience, employee engagement, operations, and process improvements. He has served on the local boards of the American College of Healthcare Executives (ACHE) and Medical Group Management Association (MGMA) and is a fellow in the ACHE and American College of Medical Practice Executives (ACMPE). He has made numerous national presentations and spoken on diverse topics such as human resources, healthcare operations, sustainability, and corporate compliance. He has authored a book for the MGMA on the body of knowledge review titled *Human Resource Management*. He also has worked extensively to mentor medical practice leaders to pursue their board certification in the ACMPE and presently serves as the ACMPE's Advancement Chair. He has a Bachelor of Science from University of Illinois, Urbana, and a Master of Health Administration from Saint Louis University, Saint Louis, Missouri.

Chapter 6

Roberta N. Clarke, MBA, DBA, is associate professor in Boston University's Health Care Management Program. She is vice chairman of the Board of the Academy for Educational Development, one of the largest human development agencies, and also a member of the Board of Trustees of the New England Organ Bank. Professor Clarke is the 1995 recipient of the American Marketing Association's prestigious Philip Kotler Award for Excellence in Health Care Marketing. She is former president of the Society for Health Care Planning and Marketing, at that time a national professional society of 3,500 members affiliated with the American Hospital Association. Dr. Clarke won the Health Care Marketer of the Year Award from the American College of Health Care Marketing in 1985, the first year it was awarded. She has been teaching healthcare marketing courses at Boston University's Health Care Management Program since January 1974. Professor Clarke has served on the editorial review board of the *Journal of Health Care Marketing* as well as other healthcare publications. With Philip Kotler, she coauthored *Marketing for Health Care Organizations*, considered to be the first and leading text in the field of healthcare marketing. She was the cofounder of Great Moves!, a pediatric weight management program affiliated with The Physicians of Children's Hospital Boston. She currently is the president and cofounder of Advance Medical, an expert second medical opinion service serving over 1.4 million people in the United States. Professor Clarke received her master's and doctorate from the Harvard Graduate School of Business Administration.

Chapter 7

Keri D. Black, PhD, CFNP, is an associate professor at the University of New Mexico College of Nursing and a family nurse practitioner in urgent care.

David N. Gans, MSHA, FACMPE, is the vice president of Innovation and Research at the Medical Group Management Association (MGMA). Mr. Gans administers research and development at the MGMA and its research affiliate, the MGMA Center for Research. In addition to his management responsibilities, he is an educational speaker, authors a monthly column in MGMA's journal, and serves as the association's staff resource on all areas of medical group practice management. The current research focus addresses the four issues of importance to medical practice executives: patient safety and quality; administrative simplification, cost efficiency, and the dissemination of best practices; information technology; and preparing for healthcare reform and a transformed health delivery system.

Mr. Gans received his Bachelor of Arts degree in government from the University of Notre Dame, a Master of Science degree in education from the University of Southern California, and a Master of Science degree in health administration from the University of Colorado. Mr. Gans is retired from the U.S. Army Medical Service Corps in the grade of Colonel, U.S. Army Reserve. He is a Certified Medical Practice Executive and a Fellow in the American College of Medical Practice Executives.

Denise O'Farrell, MPH, has a master's degree in public health from Idaho State University. Ms. O'Farrell is employed with the Southeastern District Health Department in the Public Health Preparedness Program. She is the emergency preparedness healthcare liaison, working with eight hospitals, community health centers, and emergency medical services agencies developing emergency preparedness and response plans in southeastern Idaho for the Assistant Secretary for Preparedness and Response's Hospital Preparedness Program. Ms. O'Farrell is also the coordinator for the Southeast Idaho Medical Reserve Corps unit.

Annette Phillipp, PhD, MPH, is a research assistant professor for the Institute of Rural Health at Idaho State University. Her professional and educational background is in health services research, health promotion, disease prevention, community health education, consumer health information, and outcomes research. Dr. Phillipp has significant research experience in emergency preparedness, specifically in the areas of health services and simulation-based training. Additional areas of research include the economics of injuries, human patient simulation integration within clinical education, and adolescent and childhood obesity. Dr. Phillipp is a member of several professional organizations and currently serves on the board of the Idaho Rural Health Association. Dr. Phillipp has presented research findings at national, state, and local meetings regarding emergency preparedness and curriculum development, community-based hospital discharge planning for persons with disabilities, and various health and wellness topics. Her publications have focused on emergency preparedness for office practices as well as wellness, health promotion and disease prevention interventions, services, and outcomes.

Neill F. Piland, PhD, is research professor and director at the Idaho State University (ISU) Institute of Rural Health. Prior to coming to ISU in 2002 he was director of the Medical Group Management Association (MGMA) Center for Research for 6 years, founding director of New Mexico's Lovelace Institute for Health and Population Research for 13 years, and assistant director of the Health Services Research Program at the Stanford Research Institute (now SRI International). A health economist and health services researcher, he received his doctorate in health services administration from UCLA and also holds master's degrees in public health and economics from UCLA and UC Davis, respectively. He has been principal investigator for more than 40 major research and demonstration projects. These include evaluation of the quality of care in Arizona's Medicaid managed care experiment (AHCCCS), the New Mexico project for the Community Intervention Trial for Smoking Cessation (COMMIT) community trial, and a national study of physician profiling. He recently completed a large Assistant Secretary of Preparedness and Response (ASPR)/Health Resources and Services Administration (HRSA) funded program to prepare Idaho's healthcare workforce for bioterrorism and disaster events through the application of innovative distance learning delivery systems. He has authored or coauthored more than 90 journal articles, four books, and numerous book chapters on healthcare delivery, health promotion, and healthcare financing.

Howard L. Smith, PhD, is professor in the Department of Management, former vice president (2007–2011) for University Advancement, and past dean (2006–2007) of the College of Business and Economics at Boise State University. He formerly served as dean (1994–2004) at the Anderson School of Management and School of Public Administration, University of New Mexico, Director of the Program for Creative Enterprise and the Creative Enterprise Endowed Chair (2004–2006). From 1990 to 1994 Dr. Smith served as associate dean at the Anderson Schools. He has published over 230 articles on health services, organization theory/behavior, and strategic management topics in journals such as the *Academy of Management Journal, Health Services Research, Health Care Management Review,* and *New England Journal of Medicine.* He has published six books on prospective payment, staff development, hospital competition, financial management, strategic nursing management, and reinventing medical practice, and published three books on nature literature: *In the Company of Wild Bears: A Celebration of Backcountry Grizzlies and Black Bears* (Lyons Press, 2006), *Mountain Harmonies: Walking the Western Wildernesses* (UNM Press, 2004), and *The Last Best Adventure* (CreateSpace, 2011). He also published *Taking Back the Tower: Simple Solutions for Saving Higher Education* with Greenwood Press/Praeger Publishers (2009).

Chapter 8

Steven Falcone, MD, MBA, is the chief operating officer, UHealth Faculty Practice, and associate vice president for medical affairs and associate executive dean for practice development, University of Miami Miller School of Medicine. He is also professor of radiology, neurological surgery, and ophthalmology, University of Miami Miller School of Medicine. Previously he served as the medical director of radiology services in the Department of Radiology and vice chair of the University of Miami Medical Group. Dr. Falcone is a delegate for the American Society of Neuroradiology to the House of Delegates of the American Medical Association. He obtained his MD and MBA degrees from the University of Miami and is board certified by the American Board of Radiology with added qualification in neuroradiology.

Michael J. Kelley, MBA, CMPE, is the vice chairman of the University of Miami Medical Group, the faculty practice plan of the University of Miami Miller School of Medicine, having previously acted as the director of satellite operations and ambulatory surgery for the Bascom Palmer Eye Institute. Mr. Kelley began his healthcare career in 1980 and has participated as a lecturer in numerous professional educational programs, with a focus on financial management. He has served on the executive committee as president of the Ophthalmology Assembly, Medical Group Management Association, and has chaired the American Academy of Ophthalmology's committee guiding the development of administrator skill levels. He received a BS in biology as a Faculty Scholar and an MBA with an emphasis in marketing and management at Florida Atlantic University. Mr. Kelley is active as a member of the Medical Reserve Corps, and has led first response teams for Hurricanes Katrina and Rita, as well

as acting as one of the chief administrative officers at the University of Miami Field Hospital in Haiti, following the earthquake of 2010.

Richard D. Norwood, CPA, FHMA, MBA, is the finance director of the Faculty Practice for the University of Miami Miller School of Medicine, where he developed and implemented several financial improvements such as incentive plans and revenue cycle improvement initiatives. Previously, he served as chief financial officer of clinics and hospitals at the University of Texas Medical Branch in Galveston, Texas, where he worked closely to align hospital and faculty interests in an academic setting. Mr. Norwood has acted as a consultant providing management and financial oversight at the Schools of Nursing, Allied Health Sciences, and Graduate School. His 35-year career in health began as a Medicare auditor and has included Catholic Health Care as the controller, as well as various financial leadership positions and consulting engagements in hospitals and HMOs providing interim management, implementation of hospital productivity management, and implementation of financial reporting for providers assuming risk.

Stephen G. Schwartz, MD, MBA, is associate professor of clinical ophthalmology at University of Miami Miller School of Medicine, and medical director of Bascom Palmer Eye Institute at Naples. He is the president of the Florida Society of Ophthalmology. Dr. Schwartz is board certified by the American Board of Ophthalmology and is a practicing vitreoretinal surgeon. He received a BS with honors in biological sciences at Cornell University, an MD at New York University School of Medicine, and an MBA at Northwestern University's Kellogg School of Management.

Chapter 9

Steven M. Andes, PhD, CPA, is a research assistant professor in the Division of Health Policy and Administration at the University of Illinois School of Public Health. He also teaches accounting, auditing, and healthcare policy analysis in the School of Continuing Studies at Northwestern University. He has also taught organizational design and behavior. Dr. Andes was the manager of the Policy Evaluation Group of the American Hospital Association and the manager of applied research of the American Osteopathic Association, in addition to his academic positions. He is a fellow of the Institute of Medicine of Chicago and is a member of the Illinois CPA Society, where he is a member of the Nonprofit Committee and chaired the Health Care Committee. His research, teaching, and consulting interests include practice efficiency, cost-benefit analysis, and the use of accounting information. He received his PhD from the University of Illinois at Urbana-Champaign.

Chapter 10

Lee Ann H. Webster, MA, CPA, FACMPE, has extensive experience with medical practices both as a practice administrator and as an independent accountant. Since 1997 she has served as practice administrator for Pathology Associates of Alabama, PC in Birmingham. She previously worked in national and local CPA firms, where she performed accounting, auditing, and tax services for clients in a variety of industries, including a significant amount of work for physicians and physician practices.

Lee Ann is a Fellow in the American College of Medical Practice Executives (ACMPE) and a certified public accountant in the State of Alabama. She is a past president of the Pathology Management Assembly of the Medical Group Management Association (MGMA) and a past chair of the ACMPE Professional Papers Committee. Lee Ann is a summa cum laude graduate of William Jewell College in Liberty, Missouri, and earned her Master of Arts in accounting from the University of Alabama.

Chapter 11

Elizabeth W. Woodcock, MBA, FACMPE, CPC, is a professional speaker, trainer, and author specializing in medical practice management. Elizabeth has focused on medical practice operations and revenue cycle management for 20 years. Combining innovation and analysis to teach practice operations, she has delivered presentations at regional and national conferences to more than 150,000 physicians and managers. In addition to her popular e-mail newsletters, she has authored seven best-selling practice management books and published dozens of articles in national healthcare management journals. Elizabeth is a Fellow in the American College of Medical Practice Executives and a Certified Professional Coder. In addition to a Bachelor of Arts degree from Duke University, Elizabeth completed a Master of Business Administration in healthcare management from The Wharton School of Business of the University of Pennsylvania.

Chapter 12

Margret Amatayakul, MBA, RHIA, CHPS, CPHIT, CPEHR, CPHIE, FHIMSS, is president, Margret\A Consulting, LLC, an independent consulting firm focusing on electronic health record (EHR) readiness, selection, implementation, adoption, and optimization strategies, as well as

HIPAA/HITECH privacy, security, and transactions and code sets assessment and compliance.

Margret's previous experience includes directing health information management services at the Illinois Eye and Ear Infirmary; associate professor, University of Illinois at the Medical Center; associate executive director, American Health Information Management Association; and executive director of the Computer-Based Patient Record Institute. In 1999, she formed her own consulting firm, providing health information technology (HIT) consulting services to hospitals, clinics, other providers, health plans, vendors, and federal policy advisory committees. She has helped hundreds of integrated delivery networks, hospitals, and clinics of all sizes select, implement, and optimize use of EHRs. She currently is also adjunct professor in health informatics at the College of St. Scholastica and a principal in Health IT Certification, LLC. She has written several books on EHR and HIPAA.

Chapter 13

Geraldine Amori, PhD, ARM, CPHRM, DFASHRM, is the vice president, Education Center for the Risk Management and Patient Safety Institute. In this role, she cultivates and coordinates professional development and education programs for insurers, brokers, and healthcare and consumer organizations nationally. In addition, she presents, teaches, coaches, and facilitates programs about risk management and patient safety issues.

Previously, Dr. Amori served as principal of Communicating HealthCare, which promoted the development of risk management skills and focused on communication issues in healthcare. She also served as risk manager for Fletcher Allen Health Care in Burlington, Vermont. Prior to that, she worked for nearly 10 years in mental health direct service and administration.

Dr. Amori is a nationally known speaker, facilitator, and consultant. She is a past president of ASHRM, as well as past president of the Northern New England Society for Healthcare Risk Management. In 2004, she received ASHRM's coveted Distinguished Service Award. She has a Master of Science degree in counseling and human systems from Florida State University and a PhD in counselor education from the University of Florida.

Dr. Amori is an advisor to Partnership for Patient Safety, a board member for the Northern New England Society for Health Care Risk Management, a member of the Council for the Madison-Deane Initiative for Palliative Care, and a lifetime member of the American Society for Healthcare Risk Management.

Chapter 14

Bruce A. Johnson, JD, MPA, brings both legal and management perspectives to healthcare-related legal issues. His more than 20 years of experience as a healthcare attorney and consultant with the Medical Group Management Association (MGMA) Health Care Consulting Group includes providing representation and services to medical groups, hospitals, academic practice plans, and other healthcare enterprises in a variety of operational, regulatory, and transactional matters.

Mr. Johnson has extensive experience in the application of the Stark self-referral prohibition, Medicare and Medicaid fraud and abuse, tax-exempt organizations, antitrust, and other legal issues to healthcare business transactions. He specializes in assisting clients in crafting effective relationships that promote business objectives in today's rapidly changing healthcare payment, delivery system, and compliance environments. He is a shareholder in the healthcare practice group of Polsinelli Shughart PC law firm, based in the firm's Denver office.

Mr. Johnson is a frequent speaker on various topics, including the application of the Stark law, physician compensation and compliance strategies, physician–hospital integration and alignment, and others. He is the author of numerous books and articles on healthcare-related topics, including serving as lead author of MGMA's *Physician Compensation Plans—State of the Art Strategies,* and was the originator of MGMA's StarkCompliance solutions web-based product.

Jennifer L. Weinfeld, JD, is counsel at Polsinelli Shughart PC. Her practice focuses on healthcare law and encompasses a variety of contract-related issues, regulatory counseling, and corporate transactions. Ms. Weinfeld's clients have included physicians, physician practices, physical therapists, hospitals, health systems, and professional corporations. She frequently assists clients in drafting and negotiating contracts including management services agreements, leased employee agreements, professional services and medical director agreements, and employment agreements for a variety of providers. She also advises healthcare providers on federal and state regulatory compliance issues including Stark, antikickback, and HIPAA.

Chapter 15

Peter D. Stergios, JD, focuses on labor and employment law. Mr. Stergios has authored articles, lectured, and appeared in print and television media on a variety of labor and employment subjects, including the effect of bankruptcy on labor relations, the scope of the federal laws against disability in professional sports, high-level executives as discrimination defendants, jury awards in discrimination cases, labor law developments, ethics for in-house counsel, alternative dispute resolution, and mandatory arbitration of discrimination claims.

His representation on behalf of employers includes labor contract negotiation; project labor agreements; interest and grievance arbitration; mediation; defending against strikes, boycotts, leafleting, and picketing; injunctions; advising employers in union organizing and corporate campaigns; whistleblower actions; defending against statutory discrimination claims before federal and local courts and agencies; designing of agreements mandating arbitration of statutory employment disputes and related advice; noncompete and confidentiality agreement litigation; counseling as to claims avoidance and statutory compliance; providing labor strategies in connection with mergers and acquisitions, and the conduct of related labor due diligence audits; and defending against court- and agency-based employment discrimination claims.

Mr. Stergios received his JD from Harvard Law School in 1972. He is rated a.v. (preeminent) by Martindale-Hubbell.

Jennifer Itzkoff, JD, is an associate at McCarter & English, LLP. She focuses her practice on labor and employment disputes. She has represented and advised a number of healthcare facilities on their employment practices, including internal policies in manuals and handbooks, hiring and firing decisions, wage and hour issues, employment discrimination claims, and whistleblower retaliation claims.

John M. McKelway, JD, is a partner in the McCarter & English LLP Labor and Employment Group. His primary area of practice is labor and employment law, including preventive counseling, employee relations, arbitration, litigation, and appeals before administrative agencies and state and federal courts.

Mr. McKelway counsels businesses and high-level executives on a variety of topics, including defense of sexual harassment, wrongful discharge, and whistleblowing claims; electronic monitoring and employee privacy issues; HIPAA and other concerns in the healthcare industry; sophisticated employment contracts and matters involving executive compensation; labor and employment issues in mergers and acquisitions; shareholder disputes in closely held corporations; state and federal wage/hour matters, including class and collection actions; union election campaigns and collective bargaining issues; pre-employment screening of job applicants; drug and alcohol testing; concerns involving AIDS and other disabilities in the workplace; and ERISA litigation. He has authored numerous articles and book chapters and speaks frequently on employment law subjects, including emerging privacy, security, and liability risks associated with the use of social media in the workplace.

Chapter 17

Michael R. Costa, JD, MPH, is a senior associate in the Health Business Practice Group of the 1,200-member international law firm of Greenberg Traurig, LLP, and focuses his practice on healthcare and nonprofit corporate matters. As part of his health law practice, Mr. Costa counsels various healthcare providers regarding contractual, business, and regulatory matters. He is a frequent lecturer before hospitals, medical practice groups, and legal associations on both regulatory and transactional healthcare issues and has published extensively in these areas.

Mr. Costa is a 1997 cum laude graduate of Suffolk University Law School where he served as technical editor on the *Transnational Law Review.* He is also a 2000 magna cum laude graduate of Boston University School of Public Health, where he was a dual concentrator in health law and health services management and administration. Mr. Costa serves as chair of the Massachusetts Bar Association Health Law Section Council and as a member of the communications subcommittee of the Boston Bar Association Health Law Section. He is also a member of the American Health Lawyers Association and American College of Healthcare Executives and is certified in Health Information Privacy and Security by the American Health Information Management Association.

Chapter 19

Richard A. Naegele, BA, MA, JD, has practiced law with the firm of Wickens, Herzer, Panza, Cook & Batista Co. in Avon, Ohio, for more than 30 years and oversees the firm's employee benefits practice area. He is a frequent lecturer on pension and employee benefits topics and has published numerous articles in tax and pension journals. He is a Fellow of the American College of Employee Benefits Counsel and member of the Board of Editorial Advisors of the *Journal of Pension Planning and Compliance.* Mr. Naegele received his BA and MA from Ohio University and his JD from Case Western Reserve University.

Kelly Ann VanDenHaute, BS, JD, is an attorney with the firm of Wickens, Herzer, Panza, Cook & Batista Co. in Avon, Ohio, in the firm's employee benefits practice area. Ms. VanDenHaute received her BS from Miami University and her JD from Cleveland-Marshall College of Law.

Chapter 20

Julie M. Brightwell, BSN, JD, CPHRM, earned her law degree from The Ohio State University College of Law. She also completed a Bachelor of Science degree in nursing and a certificate of nurse anesthesia.

Ms. Brightwell's experience includes surgical intensive care nursing, nurse anesthesia, and the practice of healthcare law. She has served as an adjunct faculty member on healthcare law issues for a college of nursing and a legal nurse consultant program. For the past 10 years she has been a faculty member of The Doctors Company Risk Management Certification Program, a 6-month distance learning program for healthcare risk managers. She has earned the Certified Professional in Healthcare Risk Management (CPHRM) designation. Her focus as director of patient safety programs is on developing patient safety educational programs for physicians, physician office staff, nurses, and risk managers.

Dan Bucsko, MBA, MHA, FACHE, CMPE, CPHRM, earned his MHA and MBA from the University of Pittsburgh and is certified as an Associate in Risk Management (ARM) and Associate in Claims (AIC). Additionally, he is board certified as both a Fellow of the American College of Healthcare Executives (ACHE), and as a Certified Medical Practice Executive (CMPE) with the American College of Medical Practice Executives (ACMPE), and is also a Certified Professional in Healthcare Risk Management (CPHRM).

Mr. Bucsko served in the U.S. Navy and Reserve and retired from the Air Force Reserve at the rank of Major after nearly 27 years of military service. He has over 10 years of underwriting and claims experience in addition to more than 14 years of healthcare administration experience, with many years in clinical settings.

Chris Morrison, Esq, is a health law attorney in Winter Park, Florida. He received his juris doctorate from the University of Florida College of Law in 1999. His legal experience includes medical malpractice and hospital liability defense, as well as a broad range of healthcare matters. He currently practices in-house for Adventist Health System/Sunbelt, Inc.

Darrell Ranum, JD, CPHRM, regional vice president of The Doctors Company, earned his juris doctor degree from Capital University in Columbus, Ohio, and graduated from Mid-America Nazarene University with a BS in biology. Mr. Ranum has served on many committees and boards, including the task force that created the Ohio Patient Safety Institute, the Ohio University Insurance Institute's Board of Advisors, and the Ohio Hospital Association's Risk and Insurance Management Committee. He also chaired the Hospital Insurance Forum's Education Committee, the board of an inner city charity health center, and the American Association for Accreditation of Ambulatory Surgery Facilities.

Mr. Ranum supervises a group of healthcare professionals who provide risk consulting services and education to hospitals, ambulatory care facilities, physician groups, and other organizations insured by The Doctors Company. He co-founded The Doctors Company/OHIC Insurance Risk Management Certification Program, a 6-month distance learning program cosponsored with Ohio University Without Boundaries. Mr. Ranum was recently named Risk Manager of the Year by the Ohio Society for Healthcare Risk Managers (OSHRM).

Susan Shephard, MSN, CPHRM, director, patient safety education, The Doctors Company, earned her master's degree in Nursing Administration from Medical Colleges of Virginia–Virginia Commonwealth University. She also received a Master of Arts in Management from Webster University and a Bachelor of Science in Nursing from St. Louis University. She holds the rank of Colonel (retired) in the U.S. Air Force, Nurse Corps. Ms. Shepard spent 7 years as a nurse and administrator surveyor for the Joint Commission on Accreditation for Healthcare Organizations (JCAHO) and was a highly acclaimed speaker for Shared Visions New Pathways, Ambulatory Care, and the AHA Continuous Readiness Program in Tennessee, Alabama, Mississippi, and Arkansas.

Ms. Shepard has over 30 years of leadership experience in acute care hospitals, ambulatory care systems, and health maintenance organizations, and in conducting comprehensive healthcare evaluations. She has expertise in change leadership, utilization management, complex organizations, managed care and wellness, staff development, strategic vision development and implementation, and multidisciplinary collaboration.

Chapter 21

Christian F. Bormann, AIA, NCARB, LEED AP, is an architect who has focused on the planning and design of healthcare facilities of all scales and complexities. He studied architecture at Princeton University, and afterwards was introduced to healthcare facility planning and design while an officer with the U.S. Army Health Facility Planning Agency. Chris managed the design of some of the Army's largest state-of-the-art teaching medical centers.

After the military, Chris obtained a master's degree in architecture from the Architecture and Health graduate program at Clemson University, which focuses specifically on healthcare facilities. At Clemson, Chris received an American Institute of Architects/American Hospital Association fellowship grant for graduate work. Since then, Chris has been planning, managing, and leading the development of complex healthcare facilities and was a Principal at Perkins+Will in New York City, where he managed the healthcare practice. Chris resides in Hunterdon County, New Jersey, with his wife, Holly, and their three children.

Sonya Dufner, FASID, has for the past 20 years focused on promoting fully integrated environments for the workplaces of both healthcare and corporate clients. As director of workplace in the New York office, Sonya works with global and national clients in rethinking processes and standards, bringing research, and benchmarking practical solutions into modern goals of improving productivity, collaboration, and attracting the best talent. Her background in interior design combined with her planning experience leads to an approach that synthesizes strategy and design. Her experience includes projects for clients such as ColumbiaDoctors, Massachusetts General Hospital, Mayo Clinic, United Nations, Thomson Reuters, Bank of America, and L'Oréal USA. Sonya holds a bachelor of arts degree in interior design from Michigan State University and is NCIDQ certified, a Fellow and national board member of the American Society of Interior Designers, on the advisory board of Design Ignites Change, a professional member of AREW and CoreNet Global, as well as a LEED Accredited Professional.

Jason Harper, AIA, LEED AP, is an associate principal and healthcare architect with Perkins+Will architects in New York City. Jason's expertise is as a designer and planner of healthcare facilities, where he has focused his career for over 20 years. Jason's experience includes project management, design, and planning efforts for many of the largest academic medical centers in New York and the Northeast region, including Maimonides Medical Center, Mount Sinai Medical Center, New York–Presbyterian, and Johns Hopkins Hospital. He has also served his clients by leading many healthcare design and construction projects, from large-scale new construction to small-scale renovations, at both inpatient and outpatient facilities. Jason attended Rensselaer Polytechnic Institute in Troy, New York, receiving both Bachelor of Science and Bachelor of Architecture degrees. Prior to joining Perkins+Will in 2007, Jason was a principal with Guenther 5 Architects in New York City.

John Rodenbeck, AIA, NCARB, LEED AP BD+C, is an architect who has focused on the programming, planning, and design of hospitals, clinics, and other healthcare facilities for over 20 years. He has written articles and spoken at healthcare events on various healthcare planning subjects. He has a Bachelor of Architecture from the University of Cincinnati and was a senior associate and medical planner at Perkins+Will in New York City.

Richard Sprow, AIA, is an architect who has specialized in the planning and design of healthcare and hospital facilities for 30 years. His experience includes more than 200 projects, ranging from small clinics and rural hospitals to major university teaching hospitals and medical schools. Mr. Sprow has written papers on healthcare planning topics and has led postgraduate seminars on planning issues at New York University and at Peking Union Medical College. He holds a Bachelor of Architecture degree from Pennsylvania State University and was a senior health planner with the New York office of Perkins+Will, where he directed programming, planning, and design projects for work in New York and China.

Practice Operations and Functions

CHAPTER

1

International Physician and Health System Practice: Can U.S. Reform Efforts Learn from Other Nations?

Grant T. Savage, PhD, MBA, BA
Mohamed Bouras, MS
Leo van der Reis, MD

The National Library of Medicine defines medical group practice[1] as: "Any group of three or more full-time physicians organized in a legally recognized entity for the provision of healthcare services, sharing space, equipment, personnel and records for both patient care and business management, and who have a predetermined arrangement for the distribution of income." Medical group practice—which also may refer to collaborative medical work by physicians—is grounded in the social and economic, as well as the preventive and curative practices of physicians. The physician's role as a healer has had many different facets since prehistory. From shaman to herbalist to surgeon to specialist, the role of the physician has been intertwined with social, economic, scientific, and technological change.

Throughout most of Western history—albeit, with some notable exceptions—physicians have had solo practices. However, beginning in the eighteenth century and accelerating rapidly in the nineteenth and twentieth centuries, several forces radically changed not only what physicians were capable of accomplishing, but also how and where their services could be accomplished in the United States and in Europe.

This chapter examines changes in the physician's role and traces the emergence of medical group practice in the United States and other industrialized nations. It is divided into three sections:

- Section one reviews the history of Western medicine, starting with Egypt; traces the origin of medical group practice up to the twentieth century; and concludes by noting the institutional forces influencing physician practices.
- Section two focuses on the modern development of medical group practice in the United States, notes the influence of healthcare financing on group practices, explores the impact of the Patient Protection and Affordable Care Act of 2010, and documents the benefits that medical group practices provide to physicians.
- Section three contrasts the financial access, cost, and quality of healthcare in the U.S. health system with those of 11 other countries, examines the growth of medical groups within these other countries, analyzes the systems of medical malpractice liability used by seven of these countries and the

United States, and concludes with a set of recommendations for improving health reforms in the United States.

■ Origins of Medical Group Practice

The Western notion of medical group practice has its origins in the ancient medical practices of the Egyptians (circa 2600–450 BC) and the Greeks and Romans (circa 600 BC–476 AD). Although the Egyptian and Greco-Roman frameworks for medical practice overlapped, separately these frameworks endured for 2,000 years each; together, they spanned nearly 3,500 years. The modern practice of medicine is the result of a paradigmatic shift in scientific thinking[2] that started with the Muslims (circa 750–1100 AD) and continued through the Industrial Revolution (circa 1760–1900 AD). Because ancient medicine is far removed from modern practice, the following sections delve into the Egyptian and Greco-Roman medical practices, and then briefly highlight the shifts in paradigmatic thinking about medicine that have implications for medical group practice from the fifth through the nineteenth centuries. Table 1-1 provides an overview.

Egyptian Medical Practices

Within the Western tradition, the earliest known physicians engaging in group practice served in the court and temples of the Egyptian pharaohs.[3] For the Egyptians, religious and medical practices were separate but intertwined, with three types of physicians: priests, magicians (*sau*), and professionals (*swnw*). As with the prehistoric practice of shamanism, religion and medicine were the purview of physician-priests.[4] Most notable among these physician-priests were those who worshiped the lion-goddess Sekhmet, the punisher of sinners; of slightly less note were those who worshiped Serqet, the goddess of breath who is identified with the scorpion.[5]

For illnesses without observable causes—such as infectious diseases—only magic, invoked through incantations or prayers by the priest- or magician-physicians (*sau*), could placate angry gods or confront and drive away demons and cure disease.[5-8] For these and other mystifying diseases, Egyptians believed that medicine used alone would only relieve suffering, but—when paired with magic—medicine allowed the patient to recover strength and vitality.[9]

Medical Practices, Physicians, and Specialization

Nonetheless, the medicine practiced during the 2,000 years of Egyptian reign included an impressive pharmacology, a rudimentary knowledge of human anatomy and the circulatory system, and a sophisticated approach to treating trauma-related injuries. Contributing to general health were beliefs and practices of personal hygiene and public cleanliness. The knowledge about medical practices was regarded as sacred and was codified in scrolls, which were available in scriptoriums called *Peri-Anhk* or Houses of Life. Religious beliefs that the body was the vessel for the afterlife prohibited physicians from dissecting and gaining a sophisticated understanding of human anatomy and physiology.[5-8]

Interestingly, the Egyptians employed physicians, at public expense, to care for the workers building the pyramids, as well as those working the mines and quarries. There also is some evidence to suggest that workers were allowed sick leave and were awarded pensions for physically incapacitating on-the-job injuries. Although evidence of medical practices in the military are scant, it is known that physicians accompanied and treated wounded soldiers and that standards of physical hygiene, including shaving facial hair and trimming hair, were enforced.[7]

Most medical doctors were the professional physicians (*swnw*), who could be either male or female. According to records from the Old Kingdom and First Intermediate Period (circa 2686–2040 BC), the professional physicians were organized hierarchically, with the *swnw* supervised by overseers of physicians (*imy-r swnw*).[5-8] Moreover, several authorities argue that the overseers reported to chief physicians, who were led by master physicians.[6-8] At the apex of the hierarchy were the inspectors of physicians who were subject to the Overseer of the Physicians of Upper and Lower Egypt.[5-8] Importantly, although some *swnws* were scribes—able to write and, thus, read medical texts—most were not. Given the extensive medical knowledge of the Egyptians, and the limited literacy of the physicians, this was probably a factor driving medical specialization.[5,6]

Implications for Medical Group Practice

The written and archeological evidence from the Old Kingdom (circa 2600 BC) through the Late Period (circa 600 BC) reveals that physicians became highly specialized. Physicians specialized in treating ailments of the eye, teeth, mouth, or stomach. They also specialized in women's health, including pregnancy testing, childbirth, and contraception.[5-8] With each physician specializing in the treatment of different body parts and illnesses, the physicians for the court of the pharaoh formed a *de facto* multispecialty group.[3] The major force that influenced physician practices during this period was the demand for organized labor for public projects like the pyramids.

Table 1-1 Historical Influences on the Formation of Medical Group Practice in Western Culture

Historical Period	Circa	Description	Physician Practice	Key Influences
Egyptian	2600–450 BC	The Egyptians were the first to organize medical groups, both to serve the courts of the pharaohs and to serve the general population. Medicine was specialized around illnesses and symptoms affecting each part of the body. Significantly, medical, religious, and magical practices were all drawn upon to treat illnesses. Multispecialist groups were formed because of medical specialization and the need to treat injured and sick workers for public projects, such as the pyramids, as well as to treat military-related traumas. Medical texts on scrolls were preserved in *Peri-Anhk* (Houses of Life) at Memphis and other cities. The Houses of Life served as scriptoriums, precursors to the libraries developed by the Greeks.	Multispecialty and solo practices	Organized labor for public projects; magical and sacred beliefs about disease
Greco-Roman	600 BC–476 AD (Western Roman Empire) 300–1000 AD (Eastern Empire)	The Greeks rationalized medicine, separating it from magical and religious practices. Their framework of the four humors allowed doctors and patients to have a shared understanding of why illnesses occurred and encouraged a systematic approach to treating illnesses. This framework encouraged physicians to be generalists and to work as solo practitioners. The Romans adopted and extended Greek medical practices. Roman innovations during its Imperial period included creating a medical staff and establishing hospitals for the military; providing public physicians for citizens in cities; and building public baths, aqueducts, and sewers. For both the Greeks and Romans, religious temples also were medical practice arenas and precursors of medical schools.	Mostly solo practices	Military hospitals and government policies establishing public health as a priority; humoral framework of disease
Islamic Empire	600–1100 AD	The followers of Mohammed not only created a new empire stretching from Spain to Northern Africa to Persia, but also helped develop the modern notion of the hospital as a place to operate on and treat the sick, regardless of class or wealth. Translating and drawing upon Greek and Roman books on medicine, Arab scientists and scholars advanced the knowledge of chemistry, as well as human anatomy and the circulation system. They also introduced the practice of inoculation to combat smallpox and other contagious diseases.	Mostly solo practices	Religious beliefs; scientific advancement and public hospitals; humoral framework of disease
Medieval and Renaissance (Western Europe)	500–1600 AD	With the support of the Roman Catholic Church, medical schools thrived during the late Middle Ages; the licensing of physicians was introduced, along with professional training and practice restrictions. During the Renaissance, Greco-Roman and Muslim medical practices were rediscovered and extended. The humoral theory of disease was challenged, as an accurate understanding of human anatomy and new understandings of circulation and chemistry were developed. Groups of physicians delivered healthcare for the military, taught and practiced in medical schools, and provided care in almshouses, dispensaries, and hospitals.	Mostly solo practices	Religious beliefs; schools of medicine and hospitals; humoral framework of disease
Enlightenment and Industrialization (Europe and North America)	1600–1900 AD	The germ theory of disease gradually became dominant, supplanting the humoral framework, as modern understandings of circulation and respiration were developed and infectious micro-organisms were discovered. New technologies (e.g., microscopes, vaccines, stethoscopes, antiseptics, radiology) added complexity to the practice of medicine. The new technologies stimulated specialization and the growth of multi- and single-specialty medical group practices, as well as hospitals.	Emergence of single- and multispecialty practices	Scientific and technological advancements; germ theory of disease

Greco-Roman Medical Practices

In contrast to the Egyptians, the Greeks emphasized the microcosm–macrocosm connection, the relationship between the healthy human body and the harmonies of nature. This philosophy can be traced to Empedocles (circa 450 BC), who

> . . . regarded the four elements, fire, air, earth and water, as "the roots of all things," and this became the corner stone in the humoral pathology of Hippocrates. As in the Macrocosm—the world at large[—]there were four elements, fire, air, earth, and water, so in the Microcosm—the world of man's body—there were four humours (elements), viz., blood, phlegm, yellow bile (or choler) and black bile (or melancholy), and they corresponded to the four qualities of matter, heat, cold, dryness and moisture. For more than two thousand years these views prevailed.[9]

Hippocratic Medicine

Egyptian medicine, as well as the philosophy of Ionia (western Asia Minor) and mainland Greece, influenced Hippocrates, who was born on the Greek island of Kos (circa 460 BC) into an aristocratic family, which was renowned for its medical knowledge. Hippocrates learned, practiced, and taught medicine in Kos, but he also traveled widely throughout northern Greece (Macedonia, Thrace) and died in Thessaly.[10] Hippocratic medicine is distinct from Egyptian and other ancient approaches to medicine because of its appeal to reason and observation, rather than to rituals and supernatural forces. For example, despite the basic stability of the four humors—the bodily fluids of blood, phlegm, yellow bile, and black bile—Hippocrates argued that people were affected by climatic and, especially, seasonal changes: "phlegm, cold and moist, prevails in winter; blood, warm and moist in spring; yellow bile, warm and dry in summer; and black bile, cold and dry, in autumn."[10] Hence, a person was healthy when the four humors were in equilibrium; illness caused the humors to become unbalanced, but climatic and seasonal changes also affected this balance. The role of the doctor was to apprehend both the type (diagnosis) and the probable outcome (prognosis) of the disease. Physicians should counter the imbalance in the humors of the ill person, allowing the power of nature to cure the disease.

Hippocratic medicine was also known for being patient-centered; the compendium of writings ascribed to Hippocrates and his disciples underscore the importance of careful observation, the writing of comprehensive medical histories, the provision of comfort to dying as well as recovering patients, and the injunction to do no harm to patients.[10,11] The significance of Hippocratic medicine is four-fold, in that it:

- Created a lofty role for the selfless physician—which has survived as a contemporary model for professional identity and behavior[12]
- Taught that the understanding of sickness was inseparable from the understanding of nature[13]
- Began the Greek tradition of teaching medical knowledge to nonfamily members, laying the foundation for modern medical schools[14]
- Enabled physicians to be trained in all aspects of medicine, reinforcing the notion of the solo, general practitioner

Alexandrian Medicine

Hippocratic medicine had its shortcomings because it lacked a clear understanding of the internal workings of the human body. The framework of the four humors was a speculative way to link external signs of health with the internal workings of the body. It would take numerous scientific contributions from Aristotle (circa 384–322 BC) to Galen (circa 129–216 AD), as well as major changes in ancient society, to arrive at a more developed understanding of human anatomy, pathology, and physiology.[13,14]

Importantly, many of the ancient advances in human anatomy and physiology are traced to the Greek studies of medicine in Alexandria, Egypt. The city was established by Alexander the Great in 332 BC, and was ruled by his foremost general, Ptolemy, and his descendants until the death of Cleopatra IV in 30 BC. Under both Ptolemaic and Roman rule, the library in Alexandria was the leading center for knowledge in the ancient world. About 300 BC, Ptolemy I established a university and school of medicine.[15] Studies of human anatomy and physiology briefly flourished in Alexandria as both dissection and vivisection of criminals was allowed.[13]

During this period (circa 300–250 BC), Herophilus and Erasistratus made notable discoveries and contributions to medical knowledge. An adherent to the humoral framework of Hippocrates, Herophilus studied the brain (which he regarded as the site of intelligence) and the spinal cord; both he and Erasistratus distinguished between motor and sensory nerves. Herophilus also investigated the eye, the alimentary canal (he is credited with naming the duodenum), the reproductive organs, and the arteries and veins. Erasistratus also contributed to the study of anatomy, accurately describing the four chambers of the heart and other aspects of the vascular and nervous system. Moreover, combining pneumatic theory with corpuscular theory, Erasistratus attempted to explain processes such as respiration, nutrition, digestion, and growth.[13,14]

Galenic Medicine

Galen, a central figure in medicine during the second century AD in the Roman Empire, would make the four humors the dominant framework for medicine until the Renaissance. Born in Pergamon (129 AD), a major Greek city in Asia Minor, Galen emerged as the leading medical authority in Rome during the reign of Marcus Aurelius (161–180 AD). Following his father's death and with his newly inherited wealth, Galen continued his medical education in Smyrna, Corinth, and Alexandria. He then spent several years (157–161 AD) in a prominent position as the chief physician for the gladiators in Pergamon before practicing his art in Rome (162–166 AD). His surgical, diagnostic, and therapeutic abilities were so extraordinary that when he briefly returned to his native Pergamon in 166 AD to avoid the plague, he was invited by the Emperor Marcus Aurelius to join him on his campaign against the Germanic tribes. Galen continued to practice in Rome until he died around 216 AD.[16]

Building on the work of Hippocrates, Plato, and Aristotle, as well as Herophilus and Erasistratus, Galen expanded the framework of the four humors, linking human temperament to the framework illustrated in Table 1-2.

Unlike Hippocrates, Galen argued that humoral imbalances can be located in specific organs (i.e., heart, gallbladder, liver, and head), as well as in the body as a whole.[16,17] Galen loosely linked these points of the body to Plato's notion of the tripartite soul: head (reason), heart (emotion or spiritedness), and liver and gallbladder (desire). As Boylan points out,

[T]he sort of just balance of the soul that Plato argues for in the *Republic* is also the ground of natural health. When one part of the soul/body is out of balance, then the individual becomes ill. The physician's job is to assist the patient in maintaining balance. If a person is too full of uncontrollable emotion or spiritedness, for example, then he is suffering from too much blood. The obvious answer is to engage in bloodletting (guaranteed to calm a person down).[16]

Moreover, drawing from Aristotle, Galen helped to systemize humoral theory further by linking the treatment of illnesses to the theory of contraries, categorizing various mixtures to account for the properties of drugs: "Drugs were supposed to counteract the disposition of the body. Thus, if a patient were suffering from cold and wet (upper respiratory infection), then the appropriate drug would be one that is hot and dry (such as certain molds and fungi—perhaps hinting at the potential of penicillin)."[16]

Galen not only excelled as a practitioner, but also as a critical empiricist and as a synthesizer of all existing medical knowledge. He experimented with live animals to study their nervous, circulatory, and muscular systems, and provided public demonstrations of his dissections of apes, goats, pigs, sheep, and other animals. Galen's body of writing included at least 300 titles, of which 150 survive on topics ranging from anatomy to physiology to surgery to philosophy.[17] Moreover, as a court physician (*archiatri sancti palatii*) for the Emperor Marcus Aurelius, Galen surmounted the stratification of society during Roman times, elevating the role of physician to what some consider its highest point.[18]

Physicians, Court and Public Practices, Military Medicine, and Public Health

Unlike the Greeks, the early Romans did not practice rational medicine, but relied on folk remedies passed down from father to son and, following Etruscan practices, on appeals to various deities. Like the Egyptians, the Romans believed that illnesses were caused by divine intervention. As the Greek city-states crumbled between 200 BC and 146 BC, the ruling Roman class began to

Table 1-2	Galen's Expanded Framework of the Four Humors[13,16]				
Elements	Seasons	Life Cycle	Humors	Quality	Temperament
Air	Spring	Childhood (morning)	Blood (heart)	Warm and moist	Sanguine (serene, unruffled)
Fire	Summer	Youth (noon)	Yellow bile (gallbladder)	Warm and dry	Choleric (bold, exuberant)
Earth	Autumn	Adulthood (afternoon)	Black bile (liver)	Cold and dry	Melancholic (stubborn, insolent)
Water	Winter	Old age (evening)	Phlegm (head)	Cold and moist	Phlegmatic (idle, foolish)

adopt many Greek practices, including the use of professional physicians. Some Greek physicians traveled to Rome to seek employment as free men; however, many physicians were purchased as slaves by wealthy Romans, who saved medical fees by having these slave doctors attend to the health of their families.[15,19]

Between the second and first century BC, the Roman Empire became a world power, encompassing numerous cultures and religions. Understandably, with the influx of foreigners in Rome—and because anyone could declare him- or herself a healer—the practice of medicine was in low repute and dominated by charlatans who claimed specialties in one or another disease. Roman decrees and laws would gradually change the status of physicians, starting with Julius Caesar's granting of citizenship to all professional physicians practicing in Rome, circa 50 BC,[20] and culminating in Hadrian's decree in 133 AD granting immunity from taxes and military service to public physicians.[19]

Beginning around 100 BC, the Romans established hospitals (*valetudinaria*) to treat their sick and injured soldiers, along with corps of field medics and hospital-based physicians. The care of soldiers was important because the power of Rome was based on the integrity of the legions. Both military and gladiator-based medical practices led to advanced surgical techniques, including the treatment of head fractures, limb amputations, suturing, ligatures, and cauterization. Diet and exercise also were emphasized, with soldiers undergoing intense training and receiving ample rations, including hardtack for sustained marches.[15,21]

Moreover, in matters of public health, the Romans surpassed both the Egyptians and the Greeks. For example, the city of Rome had an unrivaled fresh water supply, gymnasiums, public baths, domestic sanitation, and adequate disposal of sewage. The Romans placed cities and military fortifications carefully, avoiding or draining swampy areas while also assuring easy access to water.[15]

Implications for Medical Group Practice

On one hand, the widespread specialization found in Egyptian medicine diminished in Greco-Roman times as literacy, libraries, and a liberal education of physicians was supported. On the other hand, Greco-Roman medicine surpassed Egyptian medicine in its practices in surgery, pharmacology, ophthalmology, and internal medicine.[22,23] Following Hippocrates, Greco-Roman medicine focused on the patient's diet, exercise, and environment.

The most reputable physicians, such as Galen, were broadly educated and trained in all aspects of medicine.

As opposed to Egyptian practice, the sophisticated forms of Greco-Roman medicine encouraged physicians to enter solo practice to serve the wealthy ruling class and to aspire to serve the Emperor and his subordinates as *archiatri sancti palatii*. The imperial funding of public or municipal physicians (*archiatri populares*) recognized the need for greater access to medical care among the poor and working citizens of Rome and its provinces. Because these public practices were also a training ground for those studying medicine, a loose form of group practice was encouraged. Significantly, the empire also promoted a more structured group medical practice in military hospitals, along with the training of field medics and other mid-level providers.

From Islamic to Renaissance Medical Practices

The fall of the Western Roman Empire in 476 AD not only devastated Rome, but also shattered the institutions supporting public health and medicine throughout most of Western Europe. The immediate effect was the deterioration of medical knowledge and the corruption of practice, particularly in public health and the training of physicians; however, the long-term impact was mitigated by the libraries and institutions sustained by the Byzantine Empire and the Islamic Empire. Foremost among these was the library and university at Alexandria, which remained a storehouse and institution for medical knowledge and training. The growth of the Roman Catholic Church also contributed to the preservation of medical knowledge and its practical extension. The most remarkable attribute of this historical period was the seeds for a revolution in scientific and medical thinking that started with the Islamic Empire, grew during the late Middle Ages, and blossomed during the Renaissance.

Islamic Medical Practice

Fortunately for western medicine, the followers of Mohammed not only created a new empire stretching from Spain to North Africa to Persia, but also respected and embraced the study of medicine. Significantly, the Greco-Roman knowledge that was retained in the impressive libraries of the former Roman Empire, especially in Alexandria, came under the control of the caliphs of the newly founded Islamic Empire.

Through the process of translating into Arabic the Greek and Latin books on medicine and science, including Galen's extensive work, scholars and physicians advanced the knowledge of chemistry, as well as human anatomy, the circulation system, physiology, and biology. As their cultural and historical assumptions were questioned, these Islamic scholars and physicians responded by re-examining their own understandings of illness and health in light of the Greco-Roman theories and descriptions. Not surprisingly, this hermeneutic process often led to the discovery of errors and mistakes, as well as new insights into the causes, forms, and treatment of disease. Most significantly, Muslim and Christian scholars within the Islamic Empire contributed by systematically organizing, commenting upon, and extending the classical texts of Hippocrates, Aristotle, Galen, and others to create encyclopedias of medicine (e.g., Rhaze's *Liber Continens* and Avicenna's *Canon of Medicine*), as well as introductory texts and manuals on subjects ranging from ophthalmology to surgery to pharmacology. Moreover, Muslim and Christian religious and cultural beliefs developed the modern notion of the hospital as a place to operate on and treat the sick, regardless of class or wealth.[24,25]

Much of this remarkable scholarship and practice made its way into Western medicine through translations provided by Constantine the African, an eleventh-century Christian born in North Africa who immigrated to Italy, and by Gerard of Cremona, a Spaniard living in Toledo during the twelfth century who is credited with over 68 translated works. The Crusades and trade with the Islamic and Byzantine empires also disseminated medical knowledge and practice throughout Western Europe.[24,25]

Medieval Medical Practice

The practice of medicine in Western Europe during the Latin Middle Ages represented a fusion of classical, Christian, and folk or empiric medicine with the classical medicine becoming ascendant starting in the eleventh century. With the support of the Roman Catholic Church, medical schools thrived during the late Middle Ages; moreover, the licensing of physicians was introduced, along with professional training and practice restrictions.[26]

The Roman Catholic Church dominated many aspects of people's lives, dictating what to believe and how to live. Significantly, following Saint Augustine, the Church taught that disease was a punishment for sin, and that life was a burdened journey to be tolerated until death led to the bliss of an afterlife. These beliefs and Church dogma initially hindered medical research and development. However, the Church, through its religious orders, did preserve and translate into Latin the many extant medical works in Greek and Arabic; mandate charity care for the poor and sick, encouraging the development of hospices and hospitals; and, during the late Middle Ages, secularize medical studies and practice, separating them from religion.[25]

The institution that would most profoundly influence modern medical knowledge and training was the

university. The earliest and most prominent was the Salerno medical school in Italy (circa 1010). During that time, Constantine of Africa translated the major medical works of the Islamic Empire into Latin. These translations, as well as those of others, not only increased the number of people who read the works of Aristotle, Galen, and Avicenna, but also established Greco-Roman works as a canon of readings for medical students, the so-called "scholastic" medicine.[14] Many medical schools followed after Salerno: Montpellier and Paris in France and Bologna in Northern Italy. Many of the ideas that were generated at Montpellier are techniques that we still use today; in turn, clinical teaching and discussions were started at Bologna, as was the serious study of anatomy.[26]

Nonetheless, academic medicine was, as in Galen's day, not generally available to the lower classes and the poor. Academically qualified physicians often catered to the rich, and midwives, surgeons, barbers, and apothecaries provided their services to common folk.[26,27] Especially during the late Middle Ages, the Church assumed the task of caring for the sick and the dying, establishing hospices for the latter and hospitals for the treatment and recovery of the former. Particularly in urban settings, some of these hospitals were loosely affiliated with universities as a base for clinical training and staffed by salaried physicians and surgeons, a pattern that would accelerate during the Renaissance.[25,26]

Renaissance Medical Practices

The Renaissance, from the fourteenth through the sixteenth centuries, rekindled knowledge generation in Western Europe through the careful examination of Greek and Roman art, science, and philosophy. Technical advances helped to spread both ancient and new knowledge; for example, Gutenberg's printing press made books more quickly and cheaply and thus expanded their distribution among the population. Within medicine, both technical and scientific advances occurred as original Greek and Roman texts were re-examined. The humoral theory of disease was challenged as an accurate understanding of human anatomy, and new understandings of chemistry were developed, along with improved surgical techniques. At this same time, groups of physicians delivered healthcare for the military, taught and practiced in medical schools, and provided care in almshouses, dispensaries, and hospitals.

Both trade and craft guilds grew as the urban population increased in Western Europe during the Late Medieval period. The craft guilds for physicians, apothecaries, barbers, and surgeons, which were based on stabilizing the provision of crafts in towns and cities, helped to restrict entrance into a craft, institutionalized the master–apprentice relationship, and ensured both the quality of the services and the pricing for those services.[28] The transition from craft first occurred when English physicians successfully created a new form of protectionism by seeking and gaining professional licensure and self-regulation through the Royal College of Physicians in the early sixteenth century.[29] Licensure is now requisite for almost all healthcare professionals in Western nations, but this innovation marked an important step in creating the notion of a profession.

We would be remiss if we did not highlight the contribution of a number of key figures involved in medicine during the Renaissance. Among the most controversial of these pathfinders was Paracelsus (1493–1541), a Swiss-German physician, alchemist, philosopher, and astrologer. As a professor at the University of Basel, he publicly denounced Galen and Avicenna's ideas and burnt their works in 1528. Less than a year later, he was forced to flee for his life. Ironically, his background as a physician-surgeon treating soldiers during the many wars in Northern and Western Europe provided him with the same type of practical experience that Galen had treating gladiators in Pergamon. His textbook on surgery, *Dergrossen Wundartzney* (*Great Surgery Book*), published in 1536, brought him renewed fame and led to his treatment of the rich and powerful. However, his most remarkable contribution was to introduce, based on his medical practice and empirical observations, the scientific study of chemistry to the field of medicine.[30]

Another product of the Renaissance was the famous French surgeon Ambroise Paré (1510–1590), who rediscovered and further developed surgical techniques, while also establishing the professional role of the surgeon as an equal to academically trained physicians. Trained as a barber-surgeon at the Hôtel-Dieu (1533–1537) in Paris, where he learned anatomy and surgery, Paré was employed as an army surgeon in 1537. From this lowly regarded position, he became so well known for his skill and innovation that he became the royal surgeon for four successive French monarchs (Henry II, Francis II, Charles IX, and Henry III). A conservative physician who employed surgery as a last recourse, Paré was always in search of ways to humanely treat patients. For example, instead of dressing gunshot wounds with boiling hot oil—the standard practice—he found that a dressing of egg yolk, rose oil, and turpentine was more humane and effective. He is credited with reintroducing the use of ligatures, the tying of large arteries, thus replacing the standard procedure of cauterization. Paré also introduced the use of artificial teeth, eyes, and limbs, and developed

alternative surgical techniques for hernias that avoided the standard practice of castration.[31,32]

Andreas Vesalius of Brussels (1514–1564) produced Europe's most detailed and best-illustrated atlas of the human body at the age of 28 in 1543, with a revised edition in 1555. *On the Fabric of the Human Body* quickly became what the *Oxford Medical Companion* calls "probably the most influential of all medical works." His work undermined the reliance of anatomists on ancient books, especially the works of Galen, by showing that Galen based his human anatomy on animals such as the Barbary ape instead of human cadavers. For Vesalius and those who came after him, the human body, directly observed, was the only reliable source.[31] The work of Andreas Vesalius spurred others, and soon medical books were being published at a rapid pace. The French physician Jacques Dubois, better known as Jacobus Sylvius, named many blood vessels and muscles. He was the former instructor of Vesalius, but his work was not published until 1556.

While the science of medicine spread, the new understandings about the human body occurred because of changes in social mores. For example, in 1744, Albinus from Leyden, the most illustrious anatomist of his time, published, with ample comments, the long-lost anatomical *Tables of Eustachius*. Engraved on copper plates in 1552, these tables illustrated the results of the dissections of Eustachius. Albinus considered this work to be vastly superior to that of Vesalius. Significantly, the rivalry between the famous and flamboyant Vesalius and the almost unknown Eustachius marked the official acceptance of the dissection of the human body as a legitimate research and teaching method.[33]

Implications for Medical Group Practice

After the fall of the Roman Empire, scholars and physicians in the Islamic Empire continued to make scientific advances and established the hospital as a place to treat the sick regardless of social class. Throughout the Middle Ages, physicians continued solo practices as academically trained generalists connected to hospitals or universities affiliated with the Roman Catholic Church, although by the late Middle Ages, medicine became increasingly more secularized. While the Renaissance transformed medicine with the new discipline of therapeutic chemistry, revitalized the techniques for and outcomes from surgery, and elevated the study of anatomy, it also accelerated medical sociological trends already evident during the late medieval period. The most important of these trends for group medical care included the further development of schools of medicine and the use of teaching hospitals, as well as the waxing and waning of craft guilds for physicians, apothecaries, barbers, and surgeons. The major forces that influenced physician practices during this turbulent historical period were the developments of hospitals, medical schools, and universities. At the same time, the practice of medicine took on increased stature as an art and a profession.

Enlightenment and Industrialization

With the questioning of the humoral theory of Hippocrates and Galen, the Renaissance in Western Europe began a paradigm shift in medicine that reached fulfillment during the Industrial Revolution. The rapid pace of scientific discoveries during the next 300 years made the germ theory of disease dominant, supplanting the humoral framework, as modern understandings of circulation and respiration were developed and infectious microorganisms were discovered. New technologies (e.g., microscopes, vaccines, stethoscopes, anesthetics, antiseptics, and radiology) added complexity to the practice of medicine. Most importantly for our purposes, the new technologies stimulated specialization and the growth of multi- and single-specialty medical group practices, as well as hospitals.[15,34]

During the eighteenth and nineteenth centuries, medical care grew in sophistication, and specialization began to occur in many parts of Europe and North America, especially in major cities. However, most physicians remained generalists, practicing alone in small cities, towns, and hamlets. They faced competition from those practicing folk medicine, ranging from midwives to bone-setters to herbalists to apothecaries.[35,36] However, an important aspect of the profession for physicians was not only their academic training, but also their participation in experimental medicine and its discourse.[37] These distinctions would be used both in Europe and in the United States to further distinguish medical practice from its competitors, and further elevate the profession in terms of its legal and economic status.[29]

The industrialization of Western Europe and North America created major sociological changes that transformed the practice of medicine. The shift of populations from agrarian communities to urban centers created new markets and opportunities for physicians to specialize. At the same time, the concentration of people in cities spurred the growth of hospitals, dispensaries, and public health services.[34] These changes in health service organization were accompanied by major political and sociological changes: the elimination of slavery, the unionization of labor, and the voting rights of women and people of color.[38]

In the late nineteenth century, protection against the cost of sickness became a political issue in industrialized nations. Germany was the first country to establish a national system of compulsory sickness insurance that helped those who were wage earners in certain industries and trades. Besides medical attendance, it provided a cash benefit to make up wages while a worker was on sick leave. As an alternative approach to this issue, both in the United States and in Western Europe, health insurance companies were established in the nineteenth century, offering insurance against specific diseases and disabilities caused by sickness or accident. Both social and private health insurance encouraged the growth of medical groups.

Organized labor, advancements in science and technology, the emergence of qualified medical schools, and the dearth of hospitals in the late nineteenth century hastened the growth of medical group practice in rapidly industrializing nations. On one hand, advances in science and technology encouraged physicians to specialize and to work together in single-specialty clinics. On the other hand, the emergence of accredited medical schools, along with the requisite clinical training of interns and residents, produced *de facto* multispecialty medical practices. Medical schools such as Johns Hopkins University inspired the Mayo Clinic and other early multispecialty group practices. Moreover, these group practices filled a niche in small cities, towns, and rural areas of the nation that lacked the hospitals and solo practitioners of large urban areas.[34,39]

Conclusions about the Origins of Medical Group Practice

Figure 1-1 illustrates the variety of forces that influenced Western physician practices since around 2600 BC. Starting at six o'clock in Figure 1-1, these forces included

- *Hospitals* as workshops for physician practice and as curative places for the specialized treatments of diseases
- *Government policy* toward solo vs. group practice
- *Scientific and technological advancements* in medicine
- *Organized labor* and its medical needs
- *The military* and its medical needs
- *Medical paradigm* shifts
- *Schools of medicine*, which influenced professional standards
- *Managed care*, which influenced medical practice cost efficiency and quality

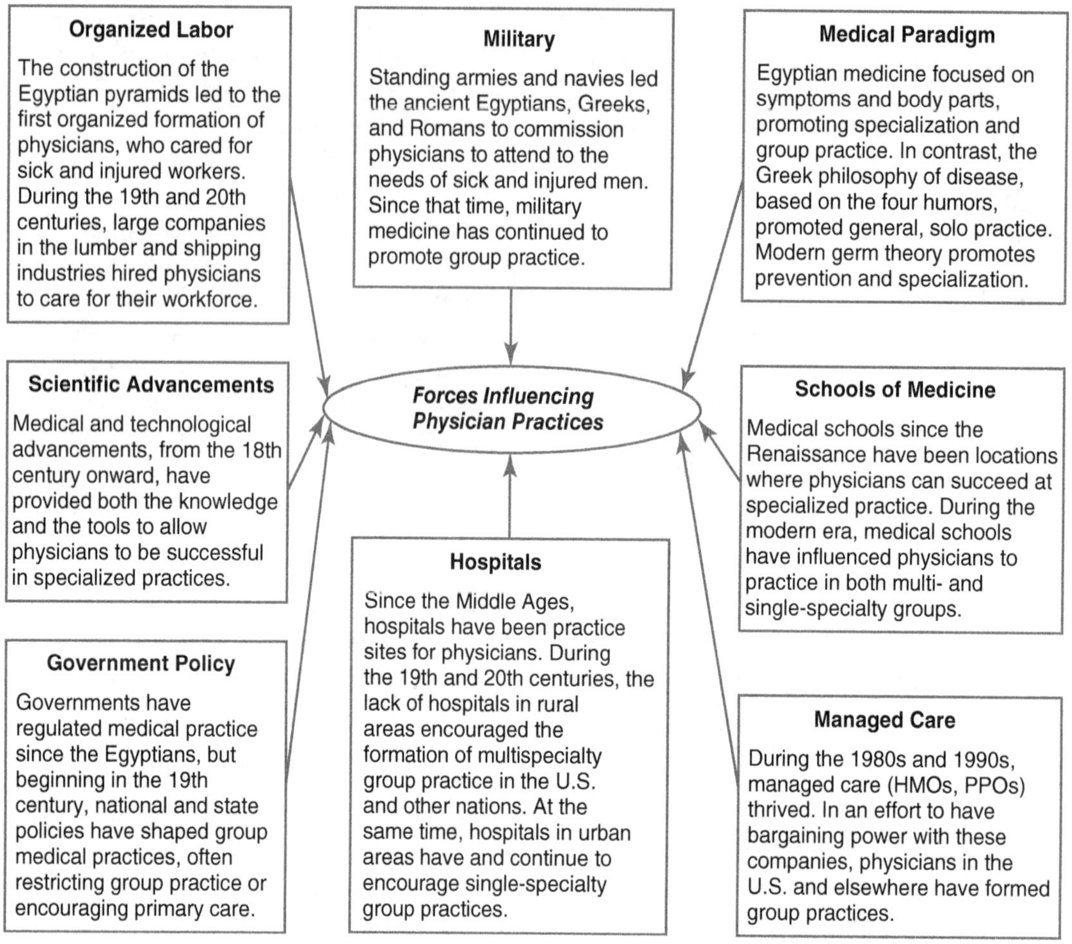

Figure 1-1 Institutional forces influencing physician practices.

In the next section, we will discuss medical group practice in the United States during the twentieth and twenty-first centuries.

Medical Group Practice in the United States

Our goal in this section is to analyze the contemporary conception of medical group practice in the United States. We begin with a historical account of groups of physicians practicing together. Next, we discuss how the financing of healthcare, whether market or government driven, has influenced groups of physicians to practice together in the United States. We then explore the potential impact of the Patient Protection and Affordable Care Act (PPACA) of 2010, and end this section by documenting the benefits that medical group practices provide to physicians.

The Development of Medical Group Practice in the United States

Despite the growth of single- and multispecialty group practices during the nineteenth century, most physicians in the United States were still engaged in competitive, solo practices as generalists. During the early twentieth century, a variety of forces influenced physicians to organize (see Figure 1-1), and group practice began to flourish in the United States under various forms. By 1932, the American Medical Association (AMA) recognized around 300 medical practice groups, with most groups averaging five to six physicians.[40] Four arenas for group practices took hold in the early twentieth century: the dispensary, the academic medical center, the industrial medical program, and the private medical clinic.[3] Each type of organization will be discussed briefly as it developed in the United States.

The Dispensary

The dispensary is the oldest of these four practice grounds for physician groups, with the first founded in Paris in

1630 by a wealthy Protestant physician and 20 of his colleagues—all of whom agreed to provide free services for poor, sick people. As originally conceived, the dispensary was a large, multispecialty group of healthcare practitioners, which, unlike hospitals, focused on ambulatory care. By 1900 there were around 100 dispensaries in large U.S. cities. Although U.S. dispensaries flourished until around 1920, they began to decline primarily because of the establishment of short-term, general hospitals (which increasingly functioned less as custodial homes and more as sites of medical treatment) and of public health clinics, with their focus on personal hygiene and health education.[3]

The concept of the dispensary has not died in the United States, however. The successors to these institutions are the federally qualified community health centers (CHCs) and rural health clinics that were established in the 1970s and 1980s as safety-net providers of primary care. Salaried physicians who focus on primary care (family practice, pediatrics, dentistry, and ophthalmology) typically staff these community health centers. Interdisciplinary teams of nurse practitioners, social workers, health educators, and others provide staffing to assist and extend physicians. As in the tradition of the dispensary, high quality care for the poor and needy is the focus.[41-44] The number of federally qualified CHCs increased from 750 centers in 2001 to 1,200 centers in 2007. In 2008, CHCs served a total of 17 million patients, 38.25% of whom were uninsured; this percentage represents approximately 14% of all uninsured Americans. In addition, another 5.3 million patients (or 35% of all the patients treated) were insured under Medicaid.[41] The 2009 American Recovery and Reinvestment Act (ARRA) committed $2 billion to federally qualified CHCs; the 2010 fiscal year federal budget was $2.19 billion. The 2011 fiscal year budget for federally qualified CHCs initially was to be the same as for 2010, but given the concerns over the federal budget deficit, the U.S. Congress funded the program at $600 million less than in 2010.

Academic Medical Centers

The first academic medical center in the United States was founded at Johns Hopkins University in Baltimore and spawned the establishment of similar practice groups around the country during the early twentieth century.[40,45,46] The spread of the Hopkins model of medical specialties (e.g., pediatrics, urology, etc.) solidified the notion of a multispecialty group practice.[47] Currently, more than 100 academic medical centers in the United States provide both medical school instruction and highly specialized care in ambulatory clinics and teaching hospitals.[52]

Reports predict that the United States will face a shortfall of between 20,000 and 46,000 doctors by 2025, renewing policy makers' interest both in the training of MDs and DOs and in changing medical school curricula, especially to increase the number of primary care physicians.[53]

Industrial Medical Programs

Industrial medical programs can trace their roots to the nineteenth-century lumber, mining, and railroad industries, all of which employed people in remote parts of North America. Both to create an incentive to work for these companies and to ensure that employees were productive workers, owners offered prepaid medical plans to prospective employees and hired physicians and other healthcare providers to deliver that care. Expanding this type of prepaid medicine to the public, however, was opposed by many local and state medical associations, in both urban and rural areas.[34]

Nonetheless, Donald E. Ross, MD, and H. Clifford Loos, MD, founded the first prepaid group practice in Los Angeles in 1929. The physician group existed for about 2 years, seeing municipal workers for a monthly price, before they were barred from the Los Angeles County Medical Society because of a strong resistance to prepaid medicine.[48] Also in 1929, Michael Shadid, MD, established a prepaid medical plan and a cooperative hospital for farmers in Elk City, Oklahoma (see http://www.gprmc-ok.com/about/index.html). Although many local citizens supported Shadid, the physician–hospital cooperative was not accepted by most of the medical community. Despite these early setbacks and limited acceptance by most physicians, prepaid medical group practices continued to grow in various parts of the United States. These and other prepaid medical plans from the first half of the twentieth century provided the impetus for health maintenance organizations (HMOs),[49] and most recently, accountable care organizations (ACOs). Both HMOs and ACOs will be discussed in more length in subsequent sections.

Private Medical Clinics

The first private medical clinic in the United States was established by Charles and William Mayo and had seven or eight staff members by 1900; it became a multispecialty practice early in its history with the addition of laboratory and x-ray specialists.[50,51] By 1929, the Mayo Clinic had grown to 895 staff members, 386 of whom were physicians.[40] Many of the physicians who trained at the Mayo Clinic used the same model to establish multispecialty group practices in other parts of the United States, and the number of private medical groups grew rapidly during the twentieth century, both in rural areas where there were few hospitals and in urban areas where specialty practices flourished.

Medical Group Growth in the United States: 1965–2009

There were 4,289 medical groups in the United States by 1965. Boosted by funding from the newly established Medicare and Medicaid programs, the number of both single and multispecialty medical group practices would increase at an almost constant rate during the next 15 years, to 10,762 in 1980. Between 1980 and 1984, moreover, medical groups grew to 15,485 (a growth rate of 43.8%).[52] This rapid growth in medical group practice formation was especially influenced by changes in the funding of Medicare, with its introduction of diagnostic-related groups (DRGs) and prospective payments for hospitals. Under this payment system, many hospitals suffered major reductions in Medicare payments, whereas ambulatory surgical centers and other ambulatory services provided by medical groups benefited.

By 1996, 70.9% of medical groups in the United States were single-specialty, 22.4% were multispecialty, and only 6.8% were family or general practice groups. Specialty medical practice encompassed medical (allergy, cardiovascular diseases, dermatology, gastroenterology, internal medicine, pediatrics, and pulmonary disease); surgical (general, neurological, obstetrics and gynecology, ophthalmology, orthopedics, otolaryngology, plastic, and urology); and other specialties (anesthesiology, diagnostic radiology, emergency medicine, neurology, pathology, psychiatry, and radiology). Depending on the type of group practice, the median size ranged from four to eight members, similar to the size of groups in the 1930s. Multispecialty groups with primary care physicians were generally the largest (mean of 27.2, median of 8 physicians).[52] These trends have continued into the twenty-first century, with the top five specialty practices in 2003 being internal medicine, pediatrics, family practice, general surgery, and obstetrics/gynecology.[53]

The Medical Group Management Association (MGMA) reported that in 1996 there were 19,820 groups (with about 32.2% of active physicians practicing in groups, based on AMA data). In 2003, the MGMA reported a slight decrease in the number of medical groups, 19,747, with about 30.2% of active physicians practicing in groups. However, by 2008, there were 39,944 groups, with about 75% of active physicians practicing in groups.[55,56] The latest available information from the AMA shows that in 2010, 77.4% of active physicians practiced in groups, with 45.7% in physician-owned medical groups, 26.2% in academic or hospital-owned medical groups, and 5.5% in urgent care centers, skilled nursing facilities, or ambulatory surgical centers.[54]

Interestingly, between 1996 and 2003, large groups with over 100 physicians increased their market presence, from 218 (1.1% of all medical groups) and 28.7% of the physicians practicing in 1996,[52] to 241 (1.2% of all medical groups) and 29.5% of the physicians practicing in 2003.[53] However, the most remarkable trend has been the rapid growth in the number of small to medium-sized group practices, from 19,506 in 2003 to 39,203 in 2008 (a growth rate of 200.9%).[53,55]

During the first decade of the twenty-first century, three interesting trends were evident. First, many medical groups purchased by financially stressed integrated health delivery systems during the early and mid-1990s were divested and transformed into smaller, stand-alone group and individual medical practices. Second, financially successful integrated delivery systems, including those directed by large medical groups—such as the Cleveland Clinic, Marshfield Clinic, and other large and dominant groups—actively purchased individual and small group practices, with this trend peaking around 2003. Third, physicians have been actively joining medical groups since 2003, typically as employees of either hospital-based health systems and networks, retail health clinics, or single-specialty groups.[54] Taken together, these three trends illustrate that there has been steady growth in exceptionally large medical groups in the United States from 1996 to 2003, with a tremendous surge in the overall number of medical group practices and the percentage of physicians practicing in them since 2003. The reasons for this remarkable growth in medical group practice in the United States are multiple and are intertwined with the influence of public and private funding.

In the following two parts of this section, we first explore how the financing of healthcare in the United States has influenced the growth of medical groups. We then examine the enactment of the 2010 Patient Protection and Affordable Care Act (PPACA) of 2010 and its current and potential impact on medical group practice.

The Influence of Financing on Medical Group Practice in the United States

To understand how the financing of healthcare services has affected medical group practice, we discuss the two major ways in which physicians are paid, note the perverse economic incentives associated with each, and point out the ways in which medical groups respond to each type of payment system. We then place these two models in historical perspective, tracing their growth patterns. Following this discussion, we point out how two initiatives associated with the PPACA of 2010 create a middle ground between fee-for-service and prepaid health plans.

Fee-for-Service Reimbursements

Most physicians in the United States receive fees for the health services they provide from Medicare (Part B, ambulatory services), Medicaid (the federal–state health insurance entitlement program), and employer-based health insurance plans. Currently, most employer-based health plans are set up as preferred provider organizations (PPOs), and physicians within these PPO networks discount their fees in exchange for a more certain volume of patients.

The economic incentives associated with fee-for-service payments are straightforward: Physicians receive more fees by providing more services of greater intensity to patients. Unfortunately, perverse incentives are associated with this production-based model for healthcare. Physicians may benefit, for example, by ordering unnecessary ancillary services or opting for surgical interventions (which garner higher fees) rather than other therapies that may be less risky but offer similar benefits. At best, patients who are subjected to additional ancillary services receive some marginal value of assurance regarding a correct diagnosis and/or course of treatment. At worst, patients who undergo surgery rather than alternative therapies potentially face the risks of complications or even death from surgery-related infections and medical errors. In other words, without quality controls in place, the production-based model encourages overutilization of services with marginal to negative benefit to the patient.

Under a fee-for-service model, medical groups in the United States benefit by owning and/or operating ancillary services and organizing around single-specialty services. Single-specialty groups are attractive because of their operational economies of scale and the market-based power (and pricing advantage) they often can generate relative to multispecialty groups and/or hospitals. This is especially true of surgical and other intensive specialties, which may also compete directly and/or partner with hospitals for patients.

Prepaid Health Plans

As an alternative, some employer-based health plans, as well as a subset of Medicare (Part C) and several state-administered Medicaid programs, operate on a prepaid basis. These health maintenance organizations (HMOs) pay physicians a per capita rate for the patients that

they agree to serve. A prepaid model also has perverse incentives associated with it for physicians, but they are the opposite of those associated with a fee-for-service model. Physicians potentially may benefit by delaying or forgoing patient visits and exams, not ordering some ancillary services to confirm diagnoses, or substituting low-cost drugs and other therapies in place of high-cost drugs and/or surgery. Again, without quality controls in place, the incentive to underutilize health services may harm patients by delaying needed therapies or surgery, increasing the likelihood of poorer patient outcomes, including death.

Under a prepaid model, medical groups benefit by organizing as multispecialties. Although ancillary services may be owned and operated by the prepaid medical group, these services become a cost, rather than revenue centers. Large multispecialty groups with a substantial number of primary physicians are favored under a capitated payment model because of their economies of scope, as well as scale. The primary care physicians within the group often act as gatekeepers to more expensive specialists, and the specialists receiving patient referrals from within the group are incentivized to minimize tests and services, including hospitalization. In addition, the larger the multispecialty medical group, the greater its market-based power and leverage to determine capitation rates.

The Historical Perspective

As previously highlighted, fee-for-service and prepaid models of payment have coexisted in the United States for decades. For most of the twentieth century, fee-for-service was the predominant U.S. payment model. With the growth in healthcare services spurred by Medicare from the mid-1960s through the 1970s, concerns about overutilization prompted both Medicare and insurance companies to introduce utilization review, preauthorization for services, and other measures to reduce costs. Although these forms of managed care are now standard features of most health plans, these controls did little to reduce the inflation in medical care costs. Employers, therefore, began seeking more aggressive efforts to control healthcare costs during the 1980s and 1990s. As a result, the prepaid model of HMOs became more favored by large employers during the 1980s; by the mid-1990s HMOs were also favored by most small and mid-sized firms.

The growth of HMOs was, in part, a market-based reaction to President Clinton's proposed healthcare reforms (1992–1993). Another reaction to those proposed reforms and to the prepaid model embodied in HMOs was the growth of integrated health delivery systems (IDSs), which were best able to provide all the health services needed for HMO beneficiaries. In turn, both HMOs and IDSs prompted the growth of large, multispecialty medical groups.

Although HMOs had initial success in reversing the growth in healthcare costs, much of this was due to a one-time reduction in the cost of physician and hospital services. At the same time as health costs began to inflate again in the late 1990s, there was a backlash from many employees who resented the delays and other limitations to health services that HMOs imposed. Employers, in response to their employees' complaints, settled on preferred provider organizations (PPOs) as a less constrained way to provide healthcare benefits. Thus, fee-for-service again became the more dominant payment model during the first decade of the twenty-first century, accelerating the growth of single-specialty medical groups, along with the proliferation of ancillary services within these and other medical groups.

Most recently, however, hospital-based and/or hospital-managed medical groups have seen explosive growth.[54] We believe this trend was triggered both by the policy discussions leading up to the PPACA of 2010 and its aftermath. Patient-centered medical homes (PCMHs) and accountable care organizations (ACOs) are two of the innovative initiatives authorized by the PPACA. On one hand, the Patient-Centered Medical Home initiative seeks to counter the fragmentation of care and overutilization of services under a fee-for-service model for Medicare patients suffering from high-cost, chronic illnesses. On the other hand, the Accountable Care Organization initiative seeks to create shared cost savings by encouraging greater integration of health services delivery among medical groups and hospitals, along with rehabilitative services, home healthcare, and nursing homes. Taken together, these two initiatives attempt to make the fee-for-service model under Medicare more quality-focused, constraining overutilization of services. The following discussion examines the current and potential impact of both ACOs and PCMHs.

Accountable Care Organizations and Patient-Centered Medical Homes

Although the primary purpose of the Patient Protection and Accountable Care Act of 2010 is to expand health insurance coverage, the PPACA also authorizes several experiments to curb healthcare cost increases by reforming healthcare delivery and insurance systems in the United States.[56] As stated in section 3022 of the PPACA, the transformation of the care delivery system is among the priorities of the healthcare reform.[57] To achieve this

transformation, the Centers for Medicare and Medicaid Services (CMS) are charged with implementing ACOs and PCMHs no later than January 1, 2012. Although the two models differ in their focus, they have the same common goal: to offer high quality healthcare for the American people at reduced cost.

The Accountable Care Organization

The term *accountable care organization* conveys the idea that healthcare professionals should coordinate (*organize*) their patient activities and be responsible (*accountable*) for both the appropriateness of their services and the outcomes they produce. The term was coined in 2006 during an exchange between Elliot Fisher (Dartmouth Institute for Health Policy and Clinical Practice) and Glenn Hackbarth (Chairman of the Medicare Payment Advisory Commission).[58] Since then, the notion of ACOs has captured the attention of healthcare practitioners, policy makers, and third-party payers.[59]

Many pilot programs in different states influenced the 2011 draft ruling on ACOs. For instance, in Vermont, various professional associations and state agencies (the state hospital association, the state medical society, the business community, the Vermont Department of Health, and the Vermont Department of Banking, Insurance, Securities, and Health Care Administration) assisted the legislature, three community hospitals and one tertiary hospital, and the state's three largest insurance companies in developing a pilot program in 2008. This pilot is intended to be among the first in the country to implement an ACO in 2011.

The results of this pilot program, according to a Commonwealth Fund report released in May 2010, show that ACOs require several factors for success. First, ACOs are not self-sufficient in that there is a need to strengthen the delivery of primary care at the community level to reduce their costs. Second, it is important to create voluntary connections among a network of primary providers with ACOs. Third, ACOs will not yield enough revenues to sustain their performance without a sufficient number of beneficiaries. At least 60% to 70% of the beneficiaries must be included in a shared savings strategy from all the third-party payers, both public and private. In a rural state, such as Vermont, with a small number of beneficiaries, a shared savings strategy will benefit primarily the consolidated third-party payers. Without strong coordination and governance, shared savings among the ACO partners will be minimal. Fourth, ACOs must have certain key resources, including the ability to manage the full care delivery continuum, robust health information technology for managing financial and clinical outcomes, and the leadership to implement the required changes within clinical and administrative processes to achieve high quality care within a reduced cost structure.[60]

The 429-page draft ruling for ACOs was released on March 31, 2011, by the CMS (for a summary, see http://www.commonwealthfund.org/Content/Publications/Other/2011/Proposed-Rules-for-ACOs.aspx). This ruling allows medical groups to participate as ACOs if they meet the following requirements as set forth in section 3022 of the PPACA[57]:

- They voluntarily accept to deliver the full continuum of care for at least 5,000 Medicare fee-for-service beneficiaries for a period of no less than 3 years. Note: Because these beneficiaries have the legal right to seek care from any Medicare-accepting provider, an ACO cannot restrict its assigned beneficiaries from seeking care from non-ACO member physicians and hospitals.
- They have a tax identification number and are legal entities under applicable state law, allowing them to receive and distribute shared savings; repay shared losses; and establish, report upon, and ensure compliance with requirements under the Shared Savings Program.
- They have a governing body with adequate authority to execute the ACO requirements; this body must be composed of at least 75% providers and include Medicare beneficiary and community stakeholder representation. Note: Nonproviders such as management companies and health plans, whose financial and managerial support might be critical for success, could be included.
- They have a leadership and management structure that includes:

  - An executive responsible for managing the ACO who is appointed by and accountable to the governing board
  - A senior-level medical director (board-certified physician) responsible for clinical management and oversight
  - Meaningful commitment by the ACO providers to clinical integration
  - A quality assurance and process improvement program with oversight from a physician-directed committee
  - An information technology infrastructure for collecting and evaluating clinical care services, including patient care experience and other quality and utilization measures

- They submit a plan for (1) promoting evidence-based medicine; (2) promoting patient engagement; (3) reporting internally on quality and cost metrics; and (4) coordinating care, especially for high-risk individuals.
- They submit a compliance plan showing how they will meet applicable legal requirements.

Lastly, the Center for Medicare and Medicaid Innovation (see http://www.innovations.cms.gov/initiatives), an agency that was established within the CMS in 2010, will evaluate the performance of ACOs in providing high quality care and reducing the cost of care.

Since the draft ruling was released, many commentators and critics have voiced their hopes and concerns about this new initiative.[61-64] Most critics of the ACO draft ruling have concerns about the short-term difficulties of both organizing physicians to share cost savings with hospitals and establishing shared governance structures with physicians. The other major concern is the level of financial risk that ACOs will have to assume if they expend more on care services than anticipated based on the proposed risk-adjusted, 3-year expenditure baseline for their assigned beneficiaries. Currently, ACOs would have to repay all reimbursed expenditures above 2% of the baseline, either from year one (track 2, with a 60% cost-sharing benefit and a 10% cap) or by year three (track 1, with a 50% maximum cost-sharing benefit and a 7.5% cap).

These are reasonable criticisms, especially if one considers which of the current types of healthcare organizations are prepared and eligible to become ACOs. The PPACA specifies that ACOs can be composed of (1) professionals in group practice arrangements, (2) networks of individual practices, (3) joint venture arrangements between hospitals and professionals, and (4) hospitals employing professionals. CMS proposes to expand ACO eligibility by including a subset of critical access hospitals. Drawing on these specifications, Shortell and his colleagues have speculated that ACOs could take the following organizational forms:

- Integrated health delivery systems (IDSs)
- Multispecialty group practices (MSGPs)
- Physician–hospital organizations (PHOs)
- Independent practice associations (IPAs)
- Virtual physician organizations (VPOs)

As detailed in the following sections, vertically integrated IDSs and MSGPs are the most viable forms for ACOs, with PHOs, IPAs, and VPOs as alternative organizational forms for ACOs, but with distinct shortcomings that will need to be overcome for them to succeed.[65,66]

Integrated health delivery systems (IDSs) take advantage of both vertical and horizontal integration to achieve efficient and high quality healthcare outcomes. Typically, IDSs have been formed through mergers of single- or multispecialty groups, and will include at least one hospital and possess their own health plan. IDSs may rely on physicians as employees and contract with other medical practice groups to deliver healthcare. Examples of medical group practices that are considered IDSs are the Dean Health System, the Geisinger Health System, and Marshfield Clinic. Most IDSs have the capacity to redesign their care processes, achieve economies of scale, implement electronic health records, incorporate knowledge management, develop strong teamwork, coordinate care among specialties, and be accountable for their performance. A key feature of IDSs is their flexibility to share and distribute cost-saving monies.[65,66] Based on this assessment, IDSs are most likely to qualify as ACOs, and most capable of assuming a high level of risk (i.e., track 2).

Multispecialty group practices (MSGPs) typically are less vertically integrated than IDSs, but they usually own or partner with a hospital in order to provide coordinated clinical care. Among the best examples of MSGPs are Mayo Clinic and the HealthCare Partners Medical Group. Unlike IDSs, which own their own health plan, MSGPs usually contract with health plans. Nonetheless, their governance structure enables them to share cost savings with physicians and hospitals.[65,66] Because MSGPs have developed strong leadership and coordinated mechanisms to provide care, they are well qualified to become ACOs and to assume a high level of risk (i.e., track 2).

Physician–hospital organizations (PHOs) strengthen the joint ownership and common interest of physicians and hospitals. Many PHOs were initially created in the late 1980s and early 1990s to leverage contract negotiations with health plans. To qualify to be ACOs, PHOs need to develop coordinated systems of clinical care among their members, ensure that common (or compatible) electronic health records are used, and have a platform and mechanism for sharing financial information. Without these additional steps, PHOs cannot achieve cost savings and meet ACO criteria.[65,66] Because of these shortcomings, PHOs and their associated medical group members may have difficulty qualifying as ACOs. Nonetheless, because of the resources of their hospital partners, PHOs probably have the capabilities to overcome such obstacles and to assume a low level of risk (i.e., track 1).

Independent practice associations (IPAs) originated as an organizational form and governance mechanism for independent medical groups and individual physicians to collectively contract with health plans. Some IPAs serve as quasi-multispecialty medical groups, implementing electronic health records and quality improvement and process redesign, while also partnering with hospitals. An outstanding example is Hill Physicians Medical Group. Medical group practice IPAs could qualify to be ACOs if they capitalize on their partnerships with hospitals, ensure the use of compatible electronic health records, and establish ways to share cost savings.[65,66] IPAs face many of the same shortcomings as PHOs and will have to negotiate agreements with their hospital partners in order to qualify as ACOs; like PHOs, IPAs could assume low levels of risk (i.e., track 1).

Virtual physician organizations (VPOs) typically are physician networks composed of small medical groups and individual physicians and are located mainly in rural areas.[65,66] They have the advantage of potentially partnering with rural health centers and/or federally qualified health centers under the proposed ruling for ACOs, making them eligible for a higher percentage of shared savings. As with IPAs, VPOs would need to capitalize on their partnerships with hospitals—especially critical access hospitals—to establish ways to share cost savings and to ensure the use of compatible electronic health records. Additionally, VPOs would probably need some financial subsidies from these and other partners to create and sustain the management and health information technology infrastructure for an ACO. Given these constraints, VPOs could, at best, assume low risk (i.e., track 1).

Under the proposed regulations, large, multispecialty medical groups and integrated delivery systems are most likely to qualify as ACOs, and to benefit from the Shared Savings Program. Single-specialty, nonprimary care medical groups often are members of either PHOs or, more likely, IPAs. As we have discussed, they face significant organizational and financial challenges to participate as a member of an ACO: They are less likely to become members of an ACO and typically will benefit less from such membership.

In contrast, primary care providers who are members of a single-specialty medical group will benefit from ACO membership. To manage the full continuum of healthcare costs effectively, ACOs require a strong network of primary care delivery.[67] Primary care physicians are in short supply,[68] and they are essential for generating cost savings through improving the care management of chronically ill Medicare recipients. Indeed, primary care physicians are essential for patient-centered medical homes, the other innovation in healthcare delivery mandated by the PPACA.

Patient-Centered Medical Homes

The Council on Pediatrics Practice introduced the term *medical home* in 1967 as a way to improve the delivery of care to children with special healthcare needs. The idea was that a medical home would be the place to centralize the medical records for these children.[69] This idea was debated, elaborated on, and expanded on during the next 40 years to include coordinating primary care, with a focus on the health of a local community. This expanded notion of a medical home was formally recognized in 2007, when four physicians associations—the American Academy of Family Physicians (AAFP), American College of Physicians (ACP), American Osteopathic Association (AOA), and American Academy of Pediatrics (AAP)—established seven Joint Principles of the Patient-Centered Medical Home. These principles are summarized as follows (see http://www.medicalhomeinfo.org/Joint%20 Statement.pdf):

1. Each patient has a *personal physician*, with a continuous relationship and focus on comprehensive care.
2. The medical practice is *physician-directed*, involving a team of care providers dedicated to the ongoing care of patients.
3. There is a *whole-person orientation* toward patients, taking into account their entire set of healthcare needs and arranging care with other health professionals.
4. *Care is coordinated and/or integrated* across the continuum of care and the patient's community via registries, information technology, health information exchanges, and the like.
5. *Quality and safety* are ensured through care planning processes, evidence-based medicine, performance measurement, mutual decision making, and the like.
6. *Enhanced access* to care is facilitated via open scheduling, expanded hours, and other forms of enhanced patient communication.
7. *Payment models* recognize the value added by a medical home.

The enabling of PCMHs is implied by the PPACA's requirements for ACOs, and is strengthened in the proposed regulations by the provisions for an increased cost-sharing percentage if ACOs partner with rural health centers and/or federally qualified health centers. Moreover, the Center for Medicare and Medicaid Innovation has launched a demonstration project focusing on medical homes within FQHCs (see http://innovations.cms.gov/ areas-of-focus/seamless-and-coordinated-care-models/ fqhc/) and is assisting states in developing Medicaid Health Home Plans, an option mandated by the PPACA.

Concluding Comments on Medical Group Practice in the United States

As noted earlier, large multispecialty medical groups potentially will benefit from ACOs, whereas non–primary care single-specialty groups will be much less likely to benefit. Hence, we believe further consolidation will take place among healthcare delivery organizations—including medical groups—as they seek to pool financial resources, take advantage of managerial and clinical expertise, and mitigate risks. Consolidation implies that multispecialty groups will continue to grow. We base this belief on research that demonstrates that physicians in medical groups vs. solo practice typically

- Increase their negotiating power with insurers[70]
- Improve the efficiency of their operations[71]
- Minimize the cost of their services[72]
- Improve their service quality[73]
- Increase their negotiating power with hospitals[74]
- Improve their quality of lifestyle[74]

Lastly, given the emphasis on primary care by the PPACA, single-specialty primary care groups should be sought-after partners for ACOs, and primary care physicians should see an increase in their current status and incomes. As the next section underscores, this emphasis on primary care providers to coordinate care is in line with the experiences of many other industrialized countries.

■ Medical Group Practice in 11 Other Nations

This section has four purposes: first, to contrast the financial access, cost, and quality of healthcare in the United States with that in 11 other countries; second, to examine the growth of medical groups in these other countries; third, to analyze how the United States and 7 of these countries deal with medical malpractice; and fourth, to provide recommendations for improving health reforms in the United States. We begin by comparing 12 national healthcare systems: Argentina, Brazil, Canada, Germany, Greece, Indonesia, Mexico, the Netherlands, Sweden, Turkey, the United Kingdom, and the United States. This is a diverse set of nations, representing a range of low-, middle-, and high-income nations, with gross national income per capita in 2010 ranging from

$4,200 (Indonesia) to $47,200 (United States) in U.S. dollars adjusted for purchasing parity (see https://www.cia.gov/library/publications/the-world-factbook/index.html). Whatever the level of per capita income, national healthcare systems can be characterized and evaluated in terms of who may be treated, for how much money, and with what expected outcome. Every healthcare system must deal with the tradeoff among issues of financial access, cost, and quality.

In the first part of this section, we focus on two factors that influence these issues: (1) financing, that is, how monies are mobilized and allocated for the provision of healthcare; and (2) how health services are organized, that is, who provides services and the relative weights placed on the provision of primary and tertiary care. We seek to answer the question, "How and to whom is healthcare provided, and with what effect?" The next part provides a brief review of the organization and financing within each national health system, focusing on three prototypes for achieving universal access. (For more detailed explanations of each country's health system, see Appendix A at the end of this chapter.) The final part provides a set of lessons learned from comparing these 12 national health systems, which will help inform the ongoing debate about the PPACA and possible paths for reforming healthcare in the United States.

The Financing, Organization of, and Outcomes from the Provision of Healthcare

Table 1-3 compares 12 national health systems on simple measures of financial access to, cost of, and quality of healthcare. The left-hand column lists each country according to its quality and cost performance. Within our 12-country comparison, Sweden anchors the high end, and Indonesia anchors the low end.

Financial Access to Healthcare

The access column in Table 1-3 incorporates information about how each nation organizes and finances its healthcare system. The assessments of access are based primarily on financial access because it is the most amenable to policy interventions and comparative data are most readily available on this aspect of access. National healthcare systems display three distinct configurations for ensuring universal access: (1) a government-owned, national health service (Sweden and the United Kingdom); (2) a national, compulsory social or private insurance (Canada); or (3) a mixture of compulsory social and private insurance (Germany and the Netherlands, respectively). Interestingly, both Greece and Turkey combine a national health service with a mixture of compulsory

social and private health insurance. Under the PPACA, the United States seeks near-universal financial access by (1) mandating private health insurance for those without employer-based coverage, and (2) expanding coverage under Medicaid to those with low incomes. The intent of the reforms is to gain near-universal coverage through a mixture of social insurance and compulsory private insurance, a combination of the approaches most similar to the recent health reforms implemented by the Netherlands and Germany.

Financing can be broken out into two aspects: the direct versus indirect provision of health services by various national governments.[75] Direct financing of health services occurs if the main health insurer or government—whether national, regional, or local—owns healthcare facilities and employs healthcare professionals, as in Greece, Sweden, and the United Kingdom. Indirect financing, in contrast, occurs if the main insurer or government contracts for the provision of various health services. For example, the provincial and regional governments in Canada, the sickness funds in Germany, and the insurance companies in the Netherlands contract with providers for health services. Indirect financing is also the primary mechanism used in the United States.

Costs of Healthcare

The percentage of gross domestic product (GDP) devoted to healthcare expenditures provides a convenient and meaningful ratio for comparing healthcare costs (see Table 1-3). Due, in part, to lower transaction costs,[76] the direct financing of healthcare in Sweden and the United Kingdom averages 9.6% of the GDP, and is less costly than the indirect financing in Canada, Germany, and the Netherlands, which averages 11% of the GDP. Figure 1-2 expands on this point and shows both the level of GDP and the international dollars (adjusted for purchasing power parity) per capita devoted to healthcare by each of the 12 nations in 2009. Taking into account the dollars per capita for healthcare is important, because less wealthy nations have to spend a greater percentage of their GDP in order to achieve comparable levels of funding. Nonetheless, the United States clearly spent much more on healthcare than any other country in 2009 (16.2% GDP; $7,410 per capita). Indeed, even when taking into account the influence of per capita GDP on health expenditures (i.e., wealthy nations typically spend more on health than poor nations), the United States spends far more than other nations of comparable wealth (i.e., Canada, Germany, the Netherlands, Sweden, and the United Kingdom). This holds true even when taking into account the increased demand for health services from

Table 1-3	Comparisons Among 12 Nations on the Financial Access, Cost, and Quality of Healthcare		
Country *Listed by Quality and Cost Results*	Financial Access *Degree and Form of Insurance Coverage*	Cost (2009) *Percentage of GDP for Healthcare*	Quality (2007) *Healthy Adjusted Life Expectancy (HALE) at Birth*
Sweden	Universal access via a devolved national health service with supplementary, private insurance	9.9% 0.5% Δ avg.	74 years 4.75 Δ avg.
Netherlands	Universal access within a compulsory system of private insurance with supplementary, private insurance and government subsidies	10.8% 1.4% Δ avg.	73 years 3.75 Δ avg.
Canada	Universal access within a devolved, single-payer system with supplementary, private insurance	10.9% 1.5% Δ avg.	73 years 3.75 Δ avg.
Germany	Universal access within a compulsory system of social insurance and substitutive, private insurance	11.3% 1.9% Δ avg.	73 years 3.75 Δ avg.
United Kingdom	Universal access via a devolved national health service with supplementary, private insurance	9.3% −0.1% Δ avg.	72 years 2.75 Δ avg.
Greece	Universal rights and variable access within a system of national health services (ESY), social insurance, and private insurance	10.6% 1.1% Δ avg.	72 years 2.75 Δ avg.
United States	Variable access within a system of employment-based voluntary insurance, social insurance, and public programs and services	16.2% 6.7% Δ avg.	70 years 0.75 Δ avg.
Mexico	Universal rights but variable access within a system of employment-based social insurance, public health services, and private insurance	6.5% −2.9% Δ avg.	67 years (2.25) Δ avg.
Argentina	Variable access within a multipayer system of employment-based social insurance, private insurance, and public health services	9.5% 0.1% Δ avg.	67 years (2.25) Δ avg.
Turkey	Universal access within a single-payer system that includes both publicly and privately owned health services	6.7% −2.7% Δ avg.	66 years (3.25) Δ avg.
Brazil	Universal rights but variable access within a system of national and contracted services, along with substitutive, private insurance	9.0% −0.4% Δ avg.	64 years (5.25) Δ avg.
Indonesia	Variable access within a system of employment-based social insurance and private insurance, with public health services	2.4% −7.0% Δ avg.	60 years (9.25) Δ avg.
12 Country Average		9.4% avg.	69.25 avg.

Source: World Health Organization. Global Health Observatory Data Repository. Accessed July 17, 2011, at http://apps.who.int/ghodata/#.

an aging population within the United States, and is due, in part, to the prices for services.[77]

Quality of Healthcare

Although the total cost of healthcare is a focus of many reform efforts in high-income countries, the current U.S. efforts to establish ACOs focuses on obtaining greater value for the money spent. Ideally one would like to compare national healthcare systems on the basis of clinical outcomes and quality of life. The right-hand column in Table 1-3 shows quality, based on a population measure of health-adjusted life expectancy (HALE); this is probably the single best proxy available for assessing health outcomes across the 12 countries in the comparisons.

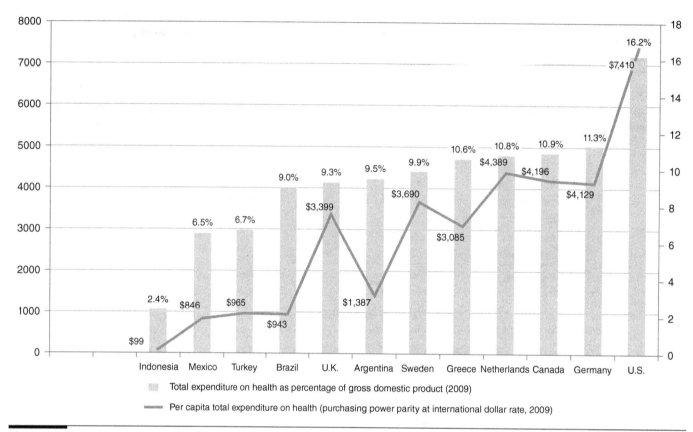

Figure 1-2 Comparisons among 12 nations on the percentage of gross domestic product and per capita spending on healthcare in 2009.
Source: Data from World Health Organization. Global Health Observatory Data Repository. Accessed July 17, 2011, at http://apps.who.int/ghodata/#.

HALE estimates the average number of years that a person can expect to live in "full health" by taking into account years lived in less than full health due to disease and/or injury. For example, the average HALE for the six high-income countries with universal financial access is 72.8 years; in contrast, the average HALE for both genders in the United States is 70 years, and the average HALE for the five middle- and low-income countries is 64.8 years.

Figure 1-3 shows how the United States fares in comparisons across the 12 countries on two measures of HALE when compared to two preventable healthcare outcomes—infant mortality and maternal mortality at birth. The health quality outcome index in Figure 1-3 subtracts the sum of the standardized scores for preventable deaths (infant and maternal) from the sum of the standardized scores for female HALE and male HALE. Although this is a crude measure of amenable healthcare quality, it does take into account both healthy life expectancy and the provision of maternal and infant care. Based on this outcome index, the United States is ranked seventh out of the 12 national health systems under comparison, the same point as the U.S. ranking in Table 1-3. All of the countries with higher rankings provide universal financial access to their citizens. Interestingly, the health

quality outcome index also suggests changes to the rankings listed in Table 1-3, with Germany and Greece moving up in the rankings by two and three places, respectively, and the United Kingdom, Canada, and the Netherlands falling in the rankings by one, two, and two places, respectively. These changes undoubtedly reflect the addition of infant and maternal mortality in the health outcome index. Taken together, infant and maternal mortality is an important proxy for health system quality because most birth-related deaths are preventable, assuming diet, living conditions, and healthcare provision are adequate. Significantly, that set of presumptions may be questionable not only in low- and middle-income countries with large inequities in family income such as Brazil (Gini Index: 56.7) and Mexico (Gini Index: 48.2), but also in the United States, which has had increasing inequities in family income distribution (Gini Index: 45.0).

A Framework for Understanding Health System Constraints

Under the PPACA of 2010, the United States is attempting to obtain better value for the amount of money it spends on healthcare. Given that countries such as Sweden, Germany, Greece, and the Netherlands obtain

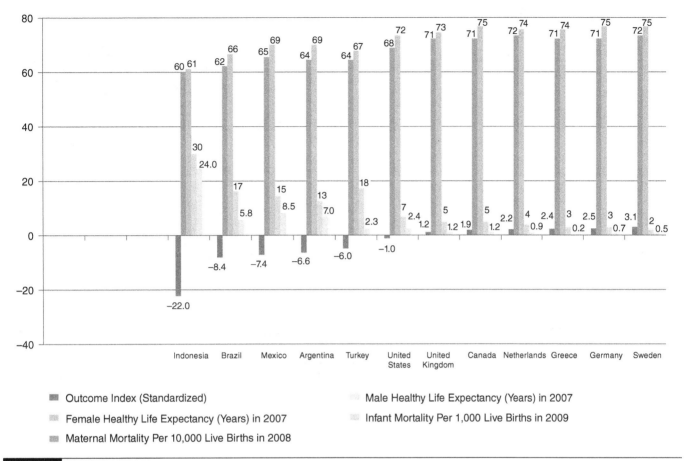

Figure 1-3 Comparisons among 12 nations on four healthcare outcome measures, ordered by standardized outcome index.
Source: Data from World Health Organization. Global Health Observatory Data Repository. Accessed July 17, 2011, at http://apps.who.int/ghodata/#.

better healthcare outcomes (see Figure 1-3) and spend less than the United States (see Figure 1-2), we should be able to learn some lessons by examining their healthcare systems, as well as the systems in Canada and the United Kingdom that obtain better cost–benefit ratios than the United States. At the same time, it would be wise to look at those middle- and low-income nations that also are addressing healthcare financial access, cost, and quality issues, particularly Indonesia, Mexico, and Turkey, which are all undergoing major healthcare reforms.

At the national level, both the allocation of healthcare resources and the funding sources for healthcare establish constraints on health system efficiency and effectiveness. Three health resource indicators, along with a health outcome indicator, help illuminate the diverse ways in which healthcare is organized. Figure 1-4 displays the density of hospital beds, nurses and midwifes, and physicians in each of the 12 countries, ordered by the total (combined) density of these three resources. The country with the highest combined density of these three resources is

Germany, whereas Indonesia has the lowest density. The outcome index reported in Figure 1-4 is the same standardized health outcome displayed in Figure 1-3. Typically, a country's health outcomes index improves with increases in the allocation of health resources. However, this relationship is not a one-to-one correlation. For example, the four countries with established, high-performing primary care networks—Canada, the Netherlands, Sweden, and the United Kingdom—display a greater reliance on nursing and midwifery in relationship to both physicians and hospitals than do most other countries. Usually, this configuration of resources is more efficient than other configurations, as illustrated by Figure 1-5, which orders the 12 countries by health resources efficiency. The health resources efficiency index divides the total health resource density (hospital beds, nursing and midwifery, and physicians) within a country by the GNP each country devotes to healthcare. It provides a way to compare the value—in health resources—that each country acquires given the monies each country deploys

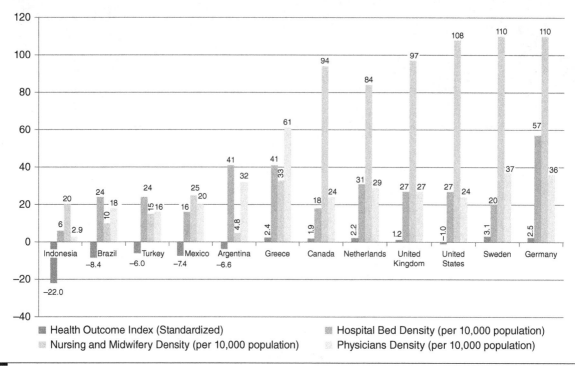

Figure 1-4 Comparisons among 12 nations on density of hospital beds, nursing and midwifery, and physicians, ordered by combined density.
Source: Data from Organisation for Economic Co-operation and Development. OECD Health Data 2011. Accessed July 17, 2011, at http://www.oecd.org/health/healthdata; and World Health Organization. Global Health Observatory Data Repository. Accessed July 17, 2011, at http://apps.who.int/ghodata/#

on healthcare. Based on this efficiency index, Germany, Sweden, and the United Kingdom obtain the most health resources for the monies they expend, followed by the Netherlands, Greece, Canada, and, remarkably, Indonesia. Brazil, in contrast, obtains the least amount of health resources for its monies. Interestingly, the United States' efficiency index is similar to that of Mexico, and

only slightly better than the health resources efficiencies achieved by Turkey and Argentina.

Although a country may expend its monies efficiently on healthcare resources, it may not garner much value from those resources. Figure 1-6 displays a healthcare effectiveness/health resources efficiency index, which divides the standardized health outcome index by

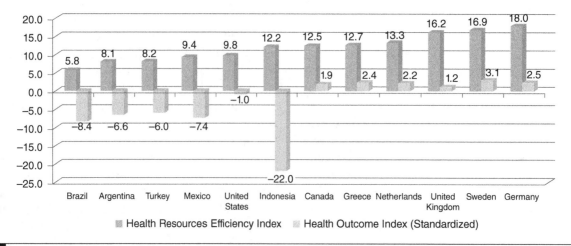

Figure 1-5 Comparisons among 12 nations on health resources efficiency and health outcomes, ordered by health resources efficiency index.
Source: Data from Organisation for Economic Co-operation and Development. OECD Health Data 2011. Accessed July 17, 2011. at http://www.oecd.org/health/healthdata; and World Health Organization. Global Health Observatory Data Repository. Accessed July 17, 2011, at http://apps.who.int/ghodata/#.

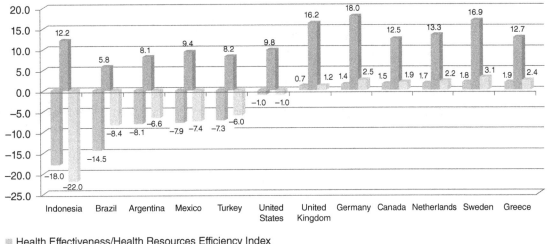

Figure 1-6 Comparisons among 12 nations on health resources efficiency and health outcomes, ordered by health effectiveness/health resources efficiency index.
Source: Data from Organisation for Economic Co-operation and Development. OECD Health Data 2011. Accessed July 17, 2011, at http://www.oecd.org/health/healthdata; and World Health Organization. Global Health Observatory Data Repository. Accessed July 17, 2011, at http://apps.who.int/ghodata/#.

the health resources efficiency index. The effectiveness/efficiency index provides a way to view how well each country achieves health outcomes relative to the health resources and monies it expends on healthcare. Based on this utilitarian viewpoint, Figure 1-6 shows that Greece, Sweden, and the Netherlands, respectively, achieve the best rankings, whereas Indonesia and Brazil achieve the lowest rankings. The United States' ranking (seventh) is the lowest among the high-income countries in this comparison, but is higher than any of the lower income countries.

Figure 1-7 compares the sources of revenue for health expenditures in each of the 12 national health systems. Taking into consideration the organization of these national health systems, these sources of revenue for health expenditures help explain both the flexibility and constraints facing each country. The three countries at the top (United Kingdom, Sweden, and Canada) and the two countries at the bottom (Germany and the Netherlands) of the figure offer universal financial access. The United Kingdom, Sweden, and Canada rely primarily on taxation; in contrast, Germany achieves universal financial access through compulsory social insurance and private insurance. The Netherlands achieves universal financial access via both compulsory private insurance and social health insurance. On one hand, financial access to healthcare within these national health systems does not come

without rationing and limiting access to secondary and, especially, tertiary healthcare.[78] On the other hand, mixing sources of funding and types of financing often leads not only to high costs, but also to limited financial access and poor quality outcomes.

Shared Concerns and Bases for Comparisons

The comparisons of the United States with these 11 countries raise a number of issues. Do these countries face the same social, economic, and demographic problems as the United States? On one hand, the industrialized countries we have examined to this point share many similarities with the United States; on the other hand, many of the middle- and low-income countries face greater social, economic, and demographic problems.

As Table 1-4 illustrates, one major demographic characteristic of the United States is its large population—ranging from 34.2 times the size of Sweden to 1.3 times the size of Indonesia. However, both Indonesia and Brazil have populations nearing the size of the United States. Another major characteristic of the United States is its per capita income; it is the highest in this comparison group, but is typically grouped with other high-income nations such as Canada, Germany, Greece, the Netherlands, Sweden, and the United Kingdom. Others in this comparison have moderate per capita incomes, except Indonesia. Both the United States and Canada

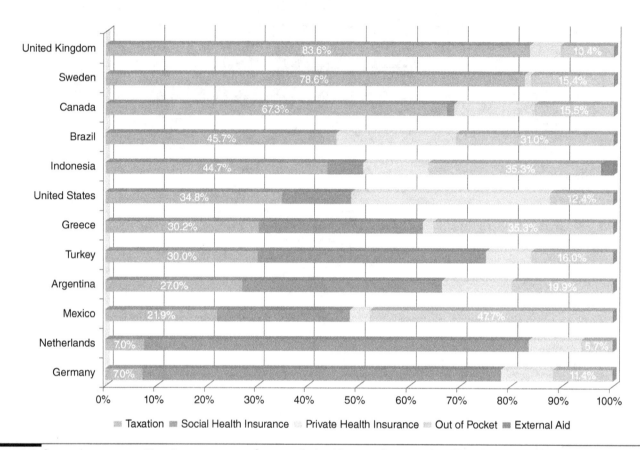

Figure 1-7 Comparisons among 12 nations on sources of revenue for health expenditures, ordered by reliance on taxation (2009).
Source: Data from World Health Organization. Global Health Observatory Data Repository. Accessed July 17, 2011, at http://apps.who.int/ghodata/#.

Table 1-4 Demographic, Economic, and Social Comparisons Among 12 Nations, Ordered by GDP Per Capita

	GDP Per Capita (Purchasing Power Parity U.S. dollars, 2010 est.)	Distribution of Family Income (Gini Index)	Land Area (square km)	Population (2011; in 1000s)	Population Density (square km)	Growth Rate (2011)	International Ranking by Population (2011)
Indonesia	$4,200	37.0	1,811,569	245,613	135.6	1.1	4
Brazil	$10,800	56.7	8,459,417	203,430	24.0	1.1	5
Turkey	$12,300	41.0	769,632	78,786	102.3	1.2	17
Mexico	$13,900	48.2	1,943,945	113,724	58.5	1.1	11
Argentina	$14,700	41.4	2,736,690	41,770	15.3	1.0	32
Greece	$29,600	33.0	130,647	10,760	82.3	0.1	76
United Kingdom	$34,800	34.0	241,930	62,698	259.2	0.6	22
Germany	$35,700	27.0	348,672	81,472	233.7	−0.2	16
Sweden	$39,100	23.0	410,335	9,089	22.1	0.2	90
Canada	$39,400	32.1	9,093,507	34,031	3.7	0.8	37
Netherlands	$40,300	30.9	33,893	16,654	491.4	0.5	60
United States	$47,200	45.0	9,161,966	311,051	34.0	0.9	3

Source: U.S. Bureau of the Census. 2011. International Data Base. Accessed July 17, 2011 at http://www.census.gov/population/international/data/idb/country.php; and Central Intelligence Agency. 2011. The World Factbook. Accessed July 17, 2011 at https://www.cia.gov/library/publications/the-world-factbook/index.html.

have moderate population growth rates, whereas all of the European countries have low growth rates, and the middle- and low-income countries high growth rates. Importantly, the high population growth rates in the middle- and low-income countries place special demands on their healthcare systems for prenatal, maternal, and childcare services, which are best met by primary care networks of providers. In addition, most of these countries have lower unemployment rates than the United States (9.7%), with only Greece (12%) and Turkey (12.4%) having higher rates in 2010 (see https://www.cia.gov/library/publications/the-world-factbook/index.html). Arguably, of the 11 other countries we have reviewed, the German and Dutch healthcare systems are the most comparable to the U.S. system. However, lessons can also be drawn from the United Kingdom's and Sweden's National Health Service and Canada's single-payer models, albeit with careful attention to the fundamental differences with the U.S. system.

Significantly, Canada, Germany, the Netherlands, Sweden, and the United Kingdom have been implementing various elements of managed competition in order to increase providers' efficiency when delivering healthcare, thus balancing the macro-management of financing healthcare practiced in each country with a quasi-market mechanism for micromanaging expenditures.[79] Healthcare systems like those in the United Kingdom and Sweden provide universal access to healthcare by relying primarily on taxes to fund the direct provision of care, but each country must ration health services in order to control costs. On one hand, the United Kingdom's network of primary care providers serve as gatekeepers, implicitly rationing by limiting access to specialists and hospitals, thus controlling costs. On the other hand, the already decentralized Swedish National Health Service uses explicit rationing, along with local control and coordination of services, to maintain high quality care, contain costs, and uphold universal access to basic health services. Rationing, of course, shifts the costs of elective health services to consumers, increasing out-of-pocket expenses.

An alternative to this prototype is Canada's tax-funded, indirect provision of care. The decentralized Canadian healthcare system achieves universal access, high quality, and moderate costs through implicit (e.g., primary care gatekeeping) and explicit (e.g., technology assessment) rationing of services. Like the Swedes, the Canadians have focused on coordinating care services, but also have been rationing by shifting elective service costs to consumers, increasing out-of-pocket and supplementary private insurance expenditures.

Both the German and Dutch models of compulsory health insurance provide universal access and achieve high quality, albeit through different combinations of public (social health insurance) and private insurance. Both have adopted certain U.S. managed care techniques and have introduced different forms of managed competition between insurers and providers to increase efficiency. Moreover, to counter the risk avoidance and resulting inequitable financial access inherent within any system relying on multiple social and private health insurance funds, both the Dutch and the Germans have introduced risk equalization schemes for insurers.

Implications for Medical Group Practice

In each of the high-income countries—indeed, in most developed countries—medical groups are becoming more common and, in many cases, larger.[80] This general trend seems to be accentuated in single-payer national health systems, which rely on primary care gatekeeping. For example, approximately 75% of the general practitioners (GPs) in Canada were in group practices in 2000,[81] as were 53% of the GPs in the United Kingdom during 2002.[82] Moreover, the trend of GPs being members of group practices is on the rise. In countries where the healthcare system is financed through taxation, the number of GPs who are members of a group practice is the highest, with 98% in Sweden and 92% in the United Kingdom. In Canada, the number of GPs who are members of medical groups also is high, with 90% in Quebec and 60% in Ontario. On the other hand, countries that have mixtures of compulsory social and private insurances, such as Germany, have the lowest rate of GPs as members of group practice, about 30%.[83]

Germany, the Netherlands, Sweden, and the United Kingdom are focused on becoming more coordinated healthcare systems, utilizing mechanisms similar to the U.S. notions of medical homes and accountable care organizations. These innovations have come about in part due to aging populations that experience more chronic illnesses, and in part to contain or reduce healthcare expenditures. For instance in Germany, a pilot program, *Gesundes Kinzigtal*, created a substantial efficiency gain through a shared savings contract with Gesundes Kinzigtal GmbH cooperating with a physician network and two healthcare insurers.[6] In 2007, similar programs were launched in Sweden to improve the coordination of care. As in the United States, coordinated care, health information technology, and patient-centeredness have been shown to achieve better health outcomes for treating patients within chronic care.

■ Lessons for the U.S. Healthcare System: Whither the PPACA of 2010?

The PPACA of 2010 is being challenged in U.S. courts, is the focus of congressional attempts to defund its provisions, and has been variously opposed and supported by numerous interest groups in the United States. Is it a reform that should be supported? If so, what provisions should be changed, if any, especially in light of the interests of single- and multispecialty interest groups in the United States?

Should We Allow Individual Health Insurance to Be Compulsory?

The U.S. healthcare system has been unique among high-income countries in relying on voluntary, employer-based health insurance for most of its population. The PPACA requires individuals to buy health insurance if they are not covered by employer-based health insurance and are not eligible for either Medicare or Medicaid. Opponents of this aspect of the legislation are currently challenging its legitimacy through the federal courts, claiming it violates the U.S. Constitution.

Regardless of the merits of such a challenge, mandating individual health insurance is a sound and pragmatic policy. On one hand, it reduces the burden placed on employers to provide health insurance as a benefit. Because this burden is voluntarily assumed, employers in the United States have been covering fewer employees and their dependents each year since 2007. On the other hand, such policies have been successfully enacted in both the Netherlands[84] (also see Appendix A) and Switzerland.[85] However, the PPACA penalizes employers, especially large employers, who withdraw health insurance coverage as an employee benefit. The rationale for this policy is to slow the exit from the employer-based health insurance coverage, making for a more orderly transition to individual-based health insurance. If the intention is to shift to individual insurance as the major means for financing health coverage, the United States should learn from the Dutch, who did not allow health insurance purchased through employers to continue, but required employers to pay to their employees a portion of that former benefit in salary.[86]

Indeed, if anything, the individual insurance mandate does not go far enough and should include long-term care coverage. Such is the case in Switzerland (mandated private insurance) and in Germany and the Netherlands (mandated social health insurance).[87] By mandating the purchase of long-term care insurance, both the federal and state governments would eliminate most of the public costs currently associated with Medicaid.[88] In turn, a long-term care insurance mandate would drastically lessen the fiscal burden of extending Medicaid coverage for all low-income, employable adults, making this aspect of the PPACA much more feasible in the United States.

In terms of mandating insurance coverage, the PPACA has at least two other deficiencies that should be addressed. A compulsory individual insurance model has several prerequisites, including (1) a basic set of services that every insurer must cover, (2) guaranteed issue to anyone seeking coverage from an insurer, (3) a fixed premium from the insurer for all those insured under the basic coverage, and (4) a post hoc risk equalization scheme. The PPACA allows a range of premiums (3 to 1 ratio based on age; 1.5 to 1 ratio based on other factors) for the same basic coverage and does not include a post hoc risk equalization scheme. This fourth element, especially, is necessary because it deters health insurers from making premiums unaffordable to high-risk individuals. On one hand, an insurer with sicker enrollees would have those costs offset by the risk equalization fund at the end of each year; on the other hand, an insurer with healthier enrollees would forgo a portion of the premium set aside in the risk equalization fund. The four elements, taken together, allow private insurance companies to offer basic insurance packages to anyone, without assuming untoward risk.

Should We Experiment with Patient-Centered Medical Homes?

Countries that have established integrated primary care services have had remarkable improvements in their population's health status. Brazil, Indonesia, and Turkey are exemplars of this trend in moderate- and low-income countries. Variations of this model are also deployed in Canada, Germany, the Netherlands, and the United Kingdom. Because the focus is on preventive and primary care services that enhance wellness within families and across generations, integrated primary care is more than a gatekeeping model for controlling access to high-cost, tertiary care. Within high-income countries with rapidly aging populations, various models of integrated primary care address the problems of chronic diseases and help to coordinate the continuum of care. The after-hours primary care collaboratives in the Netherlands, in conjunction with a national health information system, are one innovative way to address concerns about continuous, 24-hour access to care. The patient-centered medical home model in the United States provides a similar way to approach these concerns while reaping the benefits inherent in providing preventive and primary care to everyone.

To establish medical homes, the United States must address myriad shortcomings in its current system, including funding for such services, the maldistribution of primary care physicians relative to specialists, and the shortage of nurses. The PPACA provides some limited mechanisms for funding medical home services via ACOs, and does attempt to address the shortage of primary care providers. For example, the PPACA authorizes increases in both Medicaid and Medicare funding for primary care physicians, establishes the Community-based Collaborative Care Network Program for underserved and underinsured populations, expands the training and incentives for medical students choosing primary care as a specialty, and expands the training programs and funding for nurses. However, these provisions may be undermined easily if the U.S. Congress continues to underfund these initiatives, as it has the program for federally qualified community health centers.

We believe the United States needs to establish a special payment system within Medicare for patient-centered medical homes. Currently, physicians are not rewarded adequately for integrated preventative and primary care services that maintain the wellness, manage the chronic conditions, and coordinate the secondary and tertiary care of Medicare recipients. The United States could base such a payment system for primary care providers on the United Kingdom's system of GP payments, which uses a mix of capitation fees, fixed allowances for practice costs, bonus payments linked to quality processes and outcomes, and specific fees for enhanced services (such as coordination of care). Alternatively, the United States should look at the physician payment incentives that have been implemented in Ontario, Canada, for primary care physicians. Like those in the United States, Canadian physicians are paid primarily on a fee-for-service basis, so this initiative bears close examination.[89]

What About Accountable Care Organizations and Value-Based Purchasing?

Aligning the incentives for healthcare providers with the desired outcomes for patients, communities, and regional and national populations has been a major challenge for Canada, Germany, the Netherlands, Sweden, Turkey, and the United Kingdom. Each of these countries has and is experimenting with various forms of performance-based payment systems for hospitals and physicians, as well as other healthcare providers. For example, the United States should look carefully at the regional experiments in Germany to provide patient-centered, integrated care to improve the population health.[90]

As discussed previously, the PPACA authorizes CMS to establish ACOs, which can share cost savings with both the Medicare and Medicaid programs. The draft ruling clearly favors large multispecialty groups and, especially, integrated delivery systems that employ physicians. If implemented, such a policy will accelerate the growth of not only integrated health systems and large multispecialty groups, but also hospital-owned single-specialty groups. However, many medical associations oppose this corporatization of physician practice. They believe, moreover, that any long-term mechanism for sharing savings clearly will entail some sort of bundled payment for both hospital and physician services. Indeed, several of the commentators on the draft ruling urge CMS to propose an alternative to the fee-for-service model for physicians that would allow smaller medical groups to invest in cost-sharing mechanisms with hospitals, but without downside risks.[61,62] Currently, under Medicare's prospective payment system, hospitals are rewarded for being efficient; however, Medicare's fee-for-service system for physicians rewards them for providing services, not improving patient outcomes. The conundrum is to develop a system that will reward both efficiency and effectiveness. Given their experiments with bundled payments, CMS should look to the Germans[90] and the Dutch[91] for insights on how best to align incentives for physicians and hospitals.

Putting the Teeth Back into Evidence-Based, Comparative Health Assessments

Closely linked with the need to adopt an integrated preventative and primary care model is the need to improve healthcare by using evidence-based medicine and evidence-based management practices. Different countries are using various approaches, ranging from comparative effectiveness research for drugs (e.g., Germany and the United Kingdom) to establishing evidence-based guidelines for treating various diseases (e.g., the Netherlands and Canada) to safety registries for medical devices (e.g., Sweden).

Within the United States, evidence-based medicine is well recognized, and many guidelines have been developed by the Agency for Healthcare Research and Quality (AHRQ), but there remain significant delays in the adoption of best medical practices among physicians, hospitals, and other healthcare providers. The PPACA established the Patient-Centered Outcomes Research Institute (PCORI), but terminated the Federal Coordinating Council for Comparative Effectiveness Research (FCCCER). Although the PCORI is mandated to promote stakeholder engagement and to identify and conduct research that compares the clinical effectiveness of medical treatments, it lacks any authority to restrict the proliferation of healthcare technology, a major driver of costs in the United States. Although a comparative effectiveness (or health technology assessment) agency with such authority would certainly be controversial, it would be a proven way to limit the continuous health inflation that has plagued the United States.[92] Moreover, just as the FCCCER was terminated, part of PCORI's funding, along with its mandate, should be transferred to the AHRQ, because it is already engaged in conducting comparative effectiveness research.

Reducing Defensive Medicine by Reforming the Medical Liability System

A recent study by researchers from Harvard University estimates that the medical liability system cost the United States about $55.6 billion in 2008, with about $45.6 billion attributable to the costs of defensive medicine.[93] However, a major limitation of this study is the way it estimates indemnity and self-insured payments costs. Using a different methodology that does not rely on A.M. Best data, Towers Watson estimates that the tort system of medical malpractice liability cost the United States about $30 billion in payments (including administrative, indemnity insurance, and self-insured costs) and awards (including out-of-court settlements) in 2009. These expenses were increasing at an annual rate of 10% each year between 1975 and 2004, but have only increased by 0.5% per year since 2005.[94] Significantly, the Towers Watson figures do not include the costs attributable to defensive medicine, suggesting that the annual costs of the medical liability system in the United States may be closer to $75 billion.

The tort systems of medical liability in most other countries provide various ways to restrict the frivolous lawsuits that plague the United States. Tort systems are used for two reasons: (1) to compensate victims of medical errors, and (2) to deter the commission of such errors. However, most tort systems of medical liability are very expensive and time-consuming ways to compensate victims.[95] Tort systems also do little to deter medical errors, many of which are system-based rather than individual-generated.[96] Moreover, tort systems tend to encourage the practice of defensive medicine, even in countries such as the United Kingdom.[97] In contrast, a no-fault compensation system addresses the needs of victims in a cost-effective manner and eliminates the perverse incentives supporting defensive medicine. Allowing patients to pursue additional recourse for noneconomic and/or punitive damages provides a safeguard for the dereliction of provider duties to the welfare of the patient (see Appendix B later in this chapter).

Although most countries also use a tort system of medical liability to compensate patients and to deter malpractice by physicians and other healthcare professionals, a few countries have adopted no-fault compensation systems, and still others have hybrids of these two systems. The costs associated with tort systems of medical liability increased in all countries between 2001 and 2005, as medical malpractice insurance companies around the world faced large losses from claims. These losses led several insurers to withdraw from the market, making access to insurance more limited and making premiums more expensive for most providers. Nonetheless, these increases varied depending on the ways countries funded medical malpractice insurance and the policy limitations they placed on their tort systems. During this same time, no-fault compensation systems saw little increase in their overall costs.[97]

The costs associated with defensive medicine (i.e., the costs of additional medical services for patients ordered primarily for the purpose of minimizing physicians' liability risks) are driven by physician perceptions about risk.[93] Such perceptions are fueled by the U.S. tort system of medical liability, with all its uncertainties and inequities involving jury-based decisions regarding a plaintiff's economic and noneconomic compensation for alleged injuries. At the same time, the perceived risks of medical liability severely hamper the reporting of medical errors, undermining quality improvement efforts that would help mitigate medical liability.[98] Hence, we recommend that the United States look beyond caps on noneconomic compensation as a way to contain medical malpractice liability, and investigate hybrid systems of no-fault compensation that permit patients to sue for additional damages, as is done in the Swedish system. To reduce the lack of provider accountability inherent in the Swedish model, we also recommend making no-fault medical liability insurance compulsory for healthcare providers (both physicians and hospitals). Given the experience of countries such as Sweden and the Netherlands, we believe that such a change would significantly reduce the practice of defensive medicine and reduce liability-related costs, more so than simply reforming the existing tort system in the United States.[99]

In closing, the U.S. healthcare system can benefit from looking at the successes and failures in other systems. We believe that the polarizing discussions around the PPACA have been insular and caught up in ideology. For the most part, those within the debate have missed the opportunity to gain perspective and insight from other healthcare systems. We hope that policy makers and all healthcare stakeholders will begin to take a look around the world in order to improve the financing, organizing, and delivery of healthcare in the United States, and to take advantage of innovative medical group practices.

■ Appendix A: Financing and Organization of 12 Health Systems

We organize this appendix around three health system prototypes, based on their primary means of financing and organizing healthcare. The United Kingdom and Sweden exemplify the tax-funded, direct provision of health services prototype. Each of these countries has achieved universal access, relatively low costs, and moderate- to high-quality outcomes with their national health services. Canada's system of compulsory national insurance exemplifies a tax-funded prototype with indirect provision of health services. This system has achieved universal access, with moderate- to high-quality outcomes. The compulsory insurance prototype is exemplified by the German and Dutch systems, which indirectly provide health services funded by mandatory social and private insurance; these prototypes have achieved universal access and moderate to high quality, albeit with slightly higher costs. Lastly, we discuss those countries pursuing mixed models of these three prototypes, including Argentina, Brazil, Greece, Indonesia, Mexico, Turkey, and the United States.

■ Tax-Funded Models for Direct Provision of Health Services

Although both Sweden and the United Kingdom make use of National Health Services that provide universal access to healthcare to all of their citizens, they differ in the degree to which those services are decentralized and locally controlled. Nonetheless, each country recently has engaged in reforms to control expenses, reduce waiting times for specialized services, ensure the quality of care, and develop national health information networks.

The United Kingdom's National Health Service

All residents of the United Kingdom (England, Wales, Scotland, and Northern Ireland, as well as the island states of Guernsey, Isle of Man, and Jersey) are covered under the National Health Service, which is funded through national taxes. Within England, the Department of Health (DH) is in overall charge of the NHS, with a cabinet minister reporting as secretary of state for health to the prime minister. The department controls England's 10 Strategic Health Authorities (SHAs), which oversee all NHS activities in England. In turn, each SHA is responsible for the strategic supervision of all the NHS trusts in its area. The devolved NHS administrations of Northern Ireland (Health and Social Care [HSC][100]), Scotland (NHS Scotland[101]), and Wales (NHS Wales[102]) plan, organize, and manage their services separately.[103] In other words, as purchasers and providers of healthcare, the government entities for England, Northern Ireland, Scotland, and Wales retain the responsibility for health legislation and general policy. Healthcare expenditure planning takes place within each government's general public expenditure planning process. NHS funding for the following year is established during this process.

In 2009, taxes raised by the national government accounted for 83.6% of total expenditures on healthcare. Out-of-pocket payments included payment for nonprescription medications, ophthalmic and dental services, and private healthcare (although the latter may be covered through private health insurance). In 2009, out-of-pocket expenditures accounted for 10.4% of total healthcare expenditures. Both for-profit and nonprofit companies provide private health insurance, which accounted for about 6.0% of total health expenditures in 2009.[104]

Comprehensive health services are provided by the NHS, ranging from preventive to primary to acute to rehabilitative care. Within the NHS England, these services include inpatient and outpatient hospital care, physician services, inpatient and outpatient drugs, dental care, and mental healthcare. Citizens may choose a general practitioner within their locale, as well as have a choice for specialist care. All hospital and specialist services are supplied without charge to the patient; however, user charges occur for outpatient drugs, dentistry, and ophthalmology. These charges are regulated, depending on treatment, and may be waived (e.g., sight test) or subsidized based on income and other criteria.[105]

The following discussion of health system structuring, including hospitals and physicians, focuses only on the NHS in England, which provides services to the largest population segment in the United Kingdom. Secondary and tertiary care services are overseen by 175 acute trusts, which manage hospitals. There are also 60 mental health trusts and 12 ambulance trusts.[103] Primary care trusts (PCTs) not only organize and provide primary care services via general practitioners, dentists, opticians, and pharmacists, but also commission hospital and other specialist services for local populations. Currently, the 152 PCTs in England control about 80% of the total NHS budget.[103,106] Foundation trusts (FT) were first established in April 2004, and they have greater financial and operational oversight than do other acute trusts and mental health trusts within the NHS. The 117 FTs, including 33 mental health trusts, are subject to NHS performance inspection, but are independently regulated by Monitor (see http://www.monitor-nhsft.gov.uk/) rather than the by the SHAs.[107] Another recent innovation is care trusts, which provide both health and social services; there are currently eight pilot care trusts. Taken together, there are 235 acute trusts, specialist trusts, and foundation trusts.[103]

Hospitals

The 1,600 NHS hospitals and specialty centers are managed by the 235 NHS and foundation trusts noted earlier. Secondary and tertiary care services are provided in these locations; a subset of hospitals offer emergency care services, and specialty hospitals and centers offer mental health services.[103] In 2009, there were 2.7 acute care hospital beds per 1,000 people.[108]

Physicians

The British Medical Association negotiates with the Department of Health to determine the NHS payment systems for both general practitioners (GPs—primary care physicians) and consultants (physician specialists). The NHS has a well-developed primary care system made up of GPs, mid-level providers (e.g., midwives and practice nurses), and other healthcare professionals. This system will become more pronounced given the proposed reforms to the NHS if the Health and Social Care Bill 2011 is approved by Parliament. As currently proposed, the reforms will have GPs directing patients to specialist care and controlling most of the monies associated with those expenditures (see http://www.dh.gov.uk/en/Publicationsandstatistics/Legislation/Actsandbills/HealthandSocialCareBill2011/index.htm).

General practitioners may be independent contractors or salaried employees. However, most GPs are independent, self-employed professionals within partnership-based group medical practices. Whether as a member of a group medical practice, as a solo practitioner, or as a salaried employee, the GP provides preventive and primary care, acts as a gatekeeper to specialized care, and receives payments from a PCT. These payments include a mix of capitation fees, fixed allowances for practice costs, fees linked to quality processes and outcomes, and specific fees for enhanced services and the dispensing of drugs. Acute trusts and foundation trusts employ consultants on either a full-time (~40 hours) or part-time basis and pay them on a set salary scale based on seniority, with additional payments for extended services and clinical skills. As has been the tradition, both full-time and part-time consultants may supplement their salary by treating private patients.[109]

Sweden's National Health Service

The National Health Service covers all Swedish citizens, as well as immigrants and foreign residents. Although a basic package of care services is not set, the NHS typically provides preventive care, public healthcare, prescription drugs, inpatient and outpatient care, dental care, long-term care and rehabilitation, and mental healthcare services.[110] The NHS has three levels of organization: national (Ministry of Health and Social Affairs, National Board of Health and Welfare, as well as other regulatory agencies), regional (Swedish Association of Local Authorities and Regions), and local (20 county councils, the island of Gotland, and 200 municipalities). At the national level, the government sets forth principles and policies either through laws and regulation or through negotiation. The National Board of Health and Welfare typically represents the central government in negotiations with the Swedish Association of Local Authorities and Regions.[111] It also acts as the supervisory and advisory agency for health and social services, as well as the licensing agency for all healthcare personnel. On one hand, county councils have authority over primary and inpatient care, including public health and preventive care. On the other hand, the municipalities determine the housing, social support, and healthcare for the elderly and disabled.[110]

Patients are able to choose their principal healthcare provider. Choices may also be made concerning outpatient facilities and health centers in the county council. A referral may be necessary for care outside the individual's county council.[110] Income taxes are levied on residents with rates determined by county councils and municipalities. The average collective rate of taxation of local income is around 30%. Healthcare accounts for about 85% of total county expenditures.

In 2009, national, county, and municipal taxes accounted for 78.6% of total expenditures on healthcare. Out-of-pocket expenditures accounted for 15.4% of total healthcare expenditures. Dental and pharmaceutical copayments, as well as supplemental charges for private physicians, are the major costs associated with out-of-pocket expenses. Private health insurance accounted for about 1.2% of total health expenditures in 2009.[104]

Hospitals

Sweden has 73 hospitals. Specialty care is provided by 65 district/county hospitals; 60 of these hospitals provide 24-hour emergency care and are owned by county councils. Both secondary and tertiary care are provided by eight regional, academic medical hospitals.[111]

Physicians

Over 90% of physicians belong to the Swedish Medical Association (SMA), a union and professional organization for medical practitioners. The SMA negotiates general employment conditions (e.g., salaries, benefits, working hours) for its members through collective agreements, primarily with county councils.[112] In 2004, a total of 26,400 licensed physicians were employed in Sweden, with 21,900 employed within the NHS. Most physicians are specialists employed in hospitals (12,500, plus 5,000 licensed residents). The 4,400 general practitioners within the NHS serve as family doctors, but not as gatekeepers, and are employed by the county councils. Physicians employed within the NHS typically are paid a salary if they are specialists; general practitioners may be remunerated prospectively via capitation. Physicians in private practice (2000 in 2004) may set their own fee-for-service rates, but must adhere to county and national guidelines if they are to be reimbursed by the NHS and must have a contract with the county council. Otherwise these private practice physicians must use the regulated fee schedule or receive payment directly from the patient.[113,114] Basic care—preventive, primary, and public health—is provided at 1,000 public health centers. In addition to physicians, patients may receive care from district nurses and other mid-level providers.[111]

■ Tax-Funded Model for Indirect Provision of Health Services

Although Canada shares with Sweden and the United Kingdom a single-payer model of funding health services, it differs in that health providers are not employed by the state, and the federal or provincial governments typically do not own healthcare facilities. Ten provinces and three territories administer the Canadian system of Medicare, with the federal government recently instituting reforms to ensure equitable funding for, and access to, health services.

The Canadian Healthcare System

Canada indirectly provides health services through a tax-funded public system, which is accessible by all Canadians.[115] Citizens receive coverage for ambulatory services, inpatient services, prescription medications, physician services, community health services, disease prevention programs, and health protection programs. Home care is covered at varying levels.[116] Although the provincial and territorial governments oversee the provision of health services in their jurisdictions, the federal government is directly in charge of the healthcare services for the following groups: Royal Canadian Mounted Police, veterans, members of the armed forces, inmates in federal jails, Inuits, and status Indians (registered members of the First Nation).

Federal, territorial, provincial, and municipal governments share the costs of healthcare. In 2009, taxes accounted for 67.3% of total expenditures on healthcare. Supplementary private insurance accounted for 15.8% of total health expenditures, and out-of-pocket payments for 15.5%; these sources were used primarily for drugs and dental care. Social security accounted for the remaining 1.4% of public expenditures on health in 2009.[104]

Hospitals

Canadians were served by 535 general hospitals[117] (with about 1.8 acute care hospital beds per 1,000 people) in 2009.[108] Most hospitals are nonprofit, autonomous entities that provide inpatient and ambulatory services, diagnostic testing, and other services. Hospitals are staffed with physicians, registered nurses, licensed practical nurses, registered psychiatric nurses, aides, and various other healthcare professionals. In many hospitals, the staff works to provide patient care through a primary care team.

Physicians

In 2009, there were about 2.4 physicians per 1,000 people in Canada.[108] About half of all physicians are general practitioners, who act as gatekeepers for secondary and tertiary health services.[118,119] Most GPs and specialists are paid on a fee-for-service basis; their fee schedules vary based on provincial and territorial governments' negotiations with regional medical associations. Some GPs, such as community clinic physicians, and a few specialists, such as hospitalists, are salaried. Recently, some provinces have been shifting towards a mixed payment method for both GPs and specialists, combining fee-for-service with a salary or capitation component.[120]

For example, the provincial government of Ontario revised its physician services agreement with the Ontario Medical Association. This agreement not only increases base payments to physicians, but also incentivizes physicians to enroll unattached patients, to work collaboratively with other healthcare providers to coordinate patient care, to increase on-call coverage, to reduce avoidable emergency department admissions, to manage diabetic patient care, to increase psychiatric care services, and to enhance interdisciplinary care service for the frail elderly.[89]

■ Compulsory Insurance Model for Indirect Provision of Health Services

Both Germany and the Netherlands rely on compulsory health insurance that is used to purchase health services from various health providers. Recent legislation in both countries has reformed how and by whom health insurance is purchased. On one hand, the Dutch have implemented an individual mandate for private health insurance; on the other hand, the Germans have made access to health insurance both a right and a requirement within an employment-based insurance system. Significantly, as part of these reforms, both countries have also implemented risk equalization schemes to incentivize health insurers to compete on the basis of health quality and efficiency, while ensuring equitable and affordable access to a basic package of health services for all.

The German Healthcare System

Every German is eligible to participate in the statutory, social insurance system. Individuals above a determined income level have the right to obtain private health insurance. Because of the 2007 reforms, every individual must obtain either statutory or private health insurance.[121] In 2009, social health insurance accounted for 68.7% of health expenditures, and private health insurance accounted for 9.8%. Government taxes covered 7%, with out-of-pocket costs accounting for the remaining 11.4% of health expenditures.[104]

The chief system for financing healthcare is through contributions toward statutory, social health insurance funds (SHIs), which included about 220 funds in 2009.[122] The unemployed, the homeless, and immigrants are covered through a special sickness fund financed through general revenues. The benefits covered include health screening and prevention, nonphysician care, ambulatory medical services, inpatient care, home nursing care, dental care, and some types of rehabilitation. Copayments exist for pharmaceuticals, nonphysician care, dental treatments, ambulance transportation, and initial hospitalization or rehabilitation. Nonetheless, these charges are limited or exempted for those with low incomes or chronic illnesses, or who are under 18 years.[123]

The Federal Ministry for Health and the parliament are in charge of healthcare at the national level. Decision-making authority is shared between the federal government and the 16 *Lander* (states). One of their most significant roles is to oversee the sickness funds and voluntary insurance companies, assuring a level playing field for competition. Because sickness funds vary in their income and expenditures depending on their pools of insured

people, a compensation scheme operates to equalize these differences, requiring transfers of income from low cost sickness funds to sickness funds with high expenditures based on age, gender, and disability. Beginning in 2009, the risk equalization scheme also takes into account the morbidity of the insured population using 106 morbidity groups based on 80 diseases. The intent of this reform is to prevent risk selection by sickness funds, to improve care for patients with chronic or catastrophic illnesses, and to provide a level playing field in which sickness funds can compete based on quality and efficiency.[124]

Hospitals

In 2009, Germany had about 2,200 general hospitals[122] and about 5.7 acute care hospital beds per 1,000 people.[108] Private for-profit hospitals accounted for around 20% of the total, with nonprofit, private hospitals accounting for more than 40%.[125] However, all of these hospitals contract with the social insurance funds. Sources for hospital funding include operating costs from the sickness funds and investment costs from the *Lander*. The 1992 Health Care Structure Act and subsequent pieces of legislation introduced an inpatient prospective payment system. Representatives of the sickness funds negotiate with individual hospitals over prospective payment rates.

Physicians

In 2009, Germany had about 300,000 doctors[122] and about 3.6 physicians per 1,000 people.[108] Most GPs and specialists are self-employed and paid based on fee-for-service with budget ceilings. For services to patients covered by SHIs, the fee-for-service reimbursement is subject to some controls. SHIs and regional physicians' associations negotiate the total amount to be distributed to physicians under the fee-for-service payments. SHIs make the payment to regional physicians' associations for all their affiliate physicians, and physicians' associations distribute the payments among affiliated physicians based on the Uniform Value Scale and other additional rules. This fixed fee schedule includes performance bonuses for high quality care. For services to private patients, physicians are paid on a fee-for-service basis by private health insurance and receive out-of-pocket payments. Some GPs and specialists are salaried employees and work in hospitals. Both salaried GPs and specialists can also treat and bill private patients based on the fee schedule for privately insured patients.[120]

The Dutch Healthcare System

All citizens are covered under the *Algemene Wet Bijzondere Ziektekosten* (Exceptional Medical Expenses Act, or AWBZ), which provides funding for long-term, disability, and chronic psychiatric care. In 2006, the ZVW reforms were passed, which altered the structure of the sickness funds and private insurance for acute and primary care. Under the new financing scheme, individuals are no longer automatically enrolled in a health insurance plan. Rather, they are required by law to enroll in a plan of their choosing. This reform attempts to shift the Dutch system from supply- to demand-driven care. To attract members, insurance companies can offer competitive premiums for the basic benefits mandated by the government; many companies also offer extra, voluntary benefit packages for services not covered under the base package. Regulation of the system is provided for in the ZVW and is performed by two entities, the Health Care Insurance Board (CVZ) and the Health Insurance Monitoring Board (CTZ). When the Health Market Regulation Act was passed in July 2006, the CTZ merged with the Health Care Tariffs Board to form the Netherlands Health Care Authority (NZa).[126]

Hospitals

In 2009, there were 3.1 acute hospitals beds per 1,000 people.[108] For-profit and not-for-profit hospitals may be either privately or publicly owned. In 2006, the Dutch government passed legislation (*Wet Toelating Zorinstellingen* [WTZi]) that deregulates planning for hospitals and other providers, allowing them more autonomy for building and capacity decisions. However, the high-tech hospitals associated with academic medical centers remain centrally regulated.[86]

Physicians

In 2009, there were about 2.9 physicians per 1,000 people.[108] Less than a third of all physicians are general practitioners who provide preventive and primary care and serve as gatekeepers for secondary and tertiary care services. GPs may be paid via a combination of capitation and fee-for-service, with performance bonuses for preventive care services and managing chronic diseases. Most specialists are self-employed and paid on a fee-for-service basis. However, specialists working in university or municipality hospitals and physicians in training are paid salaries. They supplement their incomes by working at night or during the weekend.[120] With the reforms of the health insurance system, selective contracting with health providers has also started to occur, along with changes in the physician payment system.[127]

■ Mixed Models for Provision of Health Services

With the exception of Greece, all of the national health systems that follow mixed models for the funding and provision of health services have not yet achieved universal access to health insurance. Those nations include Argentina, Brazil, Indonesia, Mexico, Turkey, and the United States. Many of these countries have declared healthcare as a right, but rely on both public and private systems of care. The most common mix is one of social health insurance combined with tax-funded, direct and indirect provision of care. Regardless of the funding mix, all of these countries are attempting to reform healthcare to expand insurance coverage and access to care. We briefly review each national healthcare system, beginning with Argentina and ending with the United States.

The Argentine Healthcare System

The Argentine health system combines tax-funded, direct provision of health services through compulsory social and private health insurance with indirect provision of services. Around 10% of the population purchases private, substitutive health insurance. Treatment services, especially inpatient care, are emphasized. Other coverage available includes transplants, dental care, services for hemophiliacs, dialysis for chronic patients, and psychological care, but these are covered with variability among different social health insurance plans (*Obras Sociales*). Employees gained some freedom to choose among insurance plans in 1997. The reforms that have introduced managed care also have increased the burden of copayments (20–30%) by those covered by *Obras Sociales*.[128]

During 2009, private expenditures accounted for 33.6% of the total expenditure on health, of which 59.4% was out-of-pocket.[104] *Obras Sociales* accounted for 39.4% of health expenditures; taxation accounted for the remaining 27%.[129] Despite the creation of a National Health Services Superintendency under the Ministry of Health and Social Action,[130,131] the federal government does not play a central role in regulating healthcare. Rather, that regulation is the result of contracts among payers, intermediaries, and direct providers.[132]

Hospitals

In 2009, there were about 4.1 hospital beds per 1,000 people.[104] Beginning in the 1990s, attempts were made to decentralize public hospitals; 20 hospitals and some specialized centers or social programs became the responsibility of provinces. Several public hospitals were created as self-managed entities. Public hospitals receive funding from their jurisdiction and insurance like *Obras Sociales*, as well as from private insurance and out-of-pocket payments; however, they have suffered from poor reimbursements from these third-party payers.[132]

Physicians

In 2009, there were about 3.2 physicians per 1,000 people.[104] General practitioners in private practice work on a per-capita basis, and private specialists or physicians providing ambulatory services are paid on either a fee-for-service or per-capita basis. Public physicians are paid salaries.[133]

The Brazilian Healthcare System

Brazil relies on both a public and a private subsystem, and covers about 75% of the population through the public health sector. The public health system relies on taxes to provide or contract for health services. In 2009, about 23.3% of the population had private health insurance.[104]

The Ministry of Health is responsible for regulating standards of care. The public system provides most primary and secondary care, as well as emergency services. There are several types of private, supplementary health insurance with varying types of coverage. However, most affluent Brazilians opt for substitutive private health insurance, either provided through employment or directly purchased. Employer-managed health plans provide services for employees of large public or private organizations and offer a wide variety of services, including dental care. Both group medical companies and medical cooperatives cover substitutive services based on prepaid arrangements.[134]

Taxes at the federal, state, and municipal levels accounted for 45.7% of total health expenditures in 2009. Private expenditures on health accounted for 54.3% of total health expenditures in 2009, of which out-of-pocket expenditures accounted for 31% of all healthcare expenditures.

Hospitals

In 2009, there were 2.4 hospital beds per 1,000 Brazilians.[104] Inpatient care occurs mostly within private hospitals with reimbursement from public funds. In contrast, most outpatient care occurs in public institutions. In 2002, public hospitals accounted for only 31% of all hospital beds in Brazil. Most secondary and tertiary care is located in the most affluent and populated regions of Brazil. The federal government uses a prospective payment mechanism to reimburse both public and private hospitals. Each state receives funds based on quotas and is subject to financial caps.[135]

Physicians

In 2009, there were about 1.8 physicians per 1,000 people.[104] General practitioners do not play a gate-keeping role; specialist care is emphasized. Starting in 1998, financing of ambulatory services began to be distributed on a per-capita basis to municipalities. Health insurance companies incorporate both reimbursement and delivery of services within health provider networks, similar to preferred provider organizations in the United States. The number of doctors has increased dramatically over the past 30 years, with the number in private practice growing most rapidly.[136]

The Greek Healthcare System

The Greek healthcare system is a combination of tax-funded, direct provision (Εθνικό Σύστημα Υγείας [ESY], the national health service) and social insurance-funded, indirect provision of care. All citizens have access to physician services, outpatient and inpatient care, health promotion and disease prevention, prescription drugs, and dental care. However, variations in coverage still exist based on the social insurance fund. Most social insurance covers lost income due to illness or maternity; however, the largest four social insurers cover nearly every possible healthcare service or product, short of cosmetic surgery. Long-term care is covered almost exclusively by private funds and is relatively rare. Copayments for pharmaceuticals are 25%; out-of-pocket payments for private physicians, outpatient, and inpatient services vary.[137]

State and national taxes fund ESY. In 2009, taxation accounted for 30.2% of total health expenditures. National and employer-sponsored funds accounted for 32.4% of the health expenditures in 2009.[104] Private funding in the form of both insurance and out-of-pocket money funded the remaining 37.4% of the healthcare system in 2009, growing from 2.9% (GDP) in 1980 to 5% (GDP) in 2004.[138] As of 2009, out-of-pocket payments accounted for 35.3% of total health expenditures, and private insurance accounted for 2.1% of total expenditures.[104]

Hospitals

Private and public hospitals provide about 4.1 beds per 1,000 people.[108] Public hospitals are financed primarily by tax revenue, with the addition of social insurance funds and user fees. As of 2000, there were 139 public and 218 private facilities.[137]

Physicians

In 2009, there were about 6.1 physicians per 1,000 people.[108] General practitioners are supposed to serve a gatekeeping function by referring patients to specialized primary or other secondary care; however, that has not been the case. Relatively few physicians choose general practice.[139]

The Indonesian Healthcare System

The Republic of Indonesia's health system is a complex mix of private expenditures; tax-funded, direct provision of services; compulsory social insurance; and voluntary private insurance. In 2009, public expenditure on health accounted for 51.8% of total health expenditures, of which, 13.7% of expenditures were raised from social security payroll deductions and 1.8% from external sources. Out-of-pocket expenditures accounted for 5.3% of all health-care expenditures; private health insurance accounted for only 12.9% of total health expenditures.[104]

Government employees, the military, Indonesians employed in the formal sector, and the poor are covered under the Indonesian social insurance programs (*PT Askes, PT Jamsostek*). Private insurance covers a small percentage of the population. Public hospitals and out-patient facilities provide services for those without social or private insurance, estimated at 70% of the population. Both public and private facilities provide primary through tertiary services. Those covered by *PT Askes* receive services mainly in public facilities. Preventive and primary care are emphasized in public services. Patients pay user charges in public facilities.

Civil servants, civil service pensioners, the armed forces, and their families and survivors receive services from *PT Askes*, which is funded through payroll contributions of 2% and an additional 0.5% from the government. *PT Jamsostek* is a semicompulsory system for employees of firms with more than 10 employees and is also financed through payroll deductions of 3–6%, paid entirely by the employer. To address the substantial increase in the underserved and poor, the government instituted an additional program called the National Social Security System, or *Sistem Jaminan Sosial Nasional*. Launched in 2005, this program covers around 60 million people. It is administered following managed care principles, and receives a monetary contribution from the government.[140]

Hospitals
In 2005, Indonesia had 1,268 hospitals, 642 government and 626 nongovernmental. Of these hospitals, 995 were general hospitals and 273 were specialty hospitals.[141] In 2009, there were about 6 hospital beds per 10,000 people.[104] Policy analysts argue that the high level and unpredictability of user fees deters utilization of hospitals. Private hospitals (both for-profit and not-for-profit), which represent about half of all hospital facilities, are the dominant provider of inpatient care.[142]

Physicians
In 2006, there were 44,564 general practitioners and 12,374 physician specialists, supported by 308,306 nurses and 79,152 midwives. In 2009, there were 2.9 physicians per 1,000 people.[104] Because of the many rural villages throughout the nation's archipelago, Indonesia relies on 7,669 health centers to provide primary and

some secondary care. These include district health centers (2,077 with beds) that provide a wide range of medical, preventative, and obstetrical services. One or more physicians, with nurse support, staff these centers. Subdistrict health centers (5,592 without beds) provide limited medical services and are staffed by either a physician or a nurse. Transportation vehicles (all-terrain vehicles and/or motor boats) are available in most rural subcenters. Preventive and primary care is provided by integrated health centers; these are managed by the community, and provide maternal and child health, diarrheal control, family planning, nutritional development, and immunization services at the village level.[141,142]

The Mexican Healthcare System
Until recently, Mexico relied on a three-fold method of insuring and providing health services: (1) a national health subsystem (Ministry of Health and IMSS-Solidarity); (2) a set of compulsory employment-based social insurance subsystems (IMSS and ISSSTE), which covered approximately 50% of the population in 2000; and (3) a private health insurance market. Although about 50% of people were covered by social health insurance in 2000,[143] estimates of who had access to at least basic health services ranged between 70% and 90%.[144,145]

To address the needs of the uninsured, the Mexican health system recently underwent a massive reform, which allowed for the formation of the System of Social Protection in Health (SSPH). The reform focused on the 50 million uninsured Mexicans that had not been able to access healthcare services through the compulsory social health insurance programs that previously were in place. The SSPH program is funded largely by federal taxes, as well as contributions from municipal governments. Families also pay a small premium; however, the poorest 20% of families are exempt from the payment. The insurance component of the plan covers all individuals that are not covered by social security because they are self-employed, unemployed, or out of the workforce.[146,147] The System of Popular Social Security (SISSP), another form of social insurance, was implemented in 2006 to reduce the number of marginalized individuals in Mexico. In addition to providing housing and retirement benefits, the SISSP offers health services to the nation's poorest population.[148]

In 2009, out-of-pocket expenditures accounted for 47.7% and private insurance 4.0% of all healthcare expenditures. Taxes at the federal, provincial, and municipal levels accounted for 21.9% of healthcare expenditures. Depending on employment, social health insurance is financed through either bipartite employer and employee contributions or tripartite contributions that include federal funds; social health insurance accounted for 26.4% of total health expenditures in 2009.[104]

Hospitals

In 2009, there were 1.6 hospital beds per 1,000 people.[108] In 2006, Mexico had over 4,000 hospitals and 77,705 beds; however, only 1,047 hospitals were in the public sector. Nonetheless, the public sector accounts for most hospital beds. Also, whether privately or publicly owned, 86.8% are general hospitals, and most provide emergency and secondary care services.[148]

Physicians

Mexico had 2 physicians per 1,000 people in 2009, with most providing primary care.[108] In 2002, 45% of all physicians were specialists. Around 27% of physicians work only in private practice, where they are paid on a fee-for-service or per-capita basis; the remaining 73% are in public practice. Most physicians in public practice receive salaries, which they may supplement through private practice.[148]

The Turkish Healthcare System

Until recently, Turkey's health system was a combination of tax-funded, direct provision and social insurance–funded, indirect provision of care. This system provided financial coverage to about 85% of the population through some kind of public or private health insurance. In 2003, most people were covered through one of three forms of social health insurance: (1) the Social Insurance Organization (SSK; 46.3% of the population); (2) the Social Insurance Agency of Merchants, Artisans and Self-employed (Bag-Kur; 22.3% of the population); or (3) the Government Employees Retirement Fund (GERF; 15.4% of the population). Less than 1% of the population was covered by private insurance. Those without formal social or private health insurance were issued a Green Card, providing them with access to preventive, primary, and emergency care in the healthcare facilities managed by the Ministry of Health. However, as in Greece, informal, cash payments also existed, with most of it going toward physician services. Since 2003, Turkey has been implementing a Health Transformation Program (HTP) with the goal of establishing a national health service. The HTP objectives include improving governance, efficiency, user and provider satisfaction, and long-term fiscal sustainability.[149]

In 2005, all healthcare facilities that were part of the SSK were transferred to the Ministry of Health.[150] This change was one key element of the eight-fold plan underlying the HTP.[149] Other significant changes to the health system have included: (1) The integration of the social security and health insurance institutions (SSK,

Bag-Kur, and GERF) under one institution, the SSI; (2) unification of benefits and management systems (e.g., databases, claims, utilization review) across the different social health insurance plans; (3) movement away from fee-for-service and toward prospective-payment systems that include pay-for-performance incentives; (4) deployment of an integrated primary care system in about a third of the provinces; (5) increased hospital autonomy over resource allocations, coupled with greater accountability to the Ministry of Health; and (6) establishment of a single-payer system for all public patients via the 2008 Social Security and Universal Health Insurance Act.[149]

Taxes paid for 34.5% of total health expenditures in 2009. Out-of-pocket payments, including user charges, accounted for 20% of total health expenditures. Social insurance funded by employer and employee contributions accounted for about 37% of all healthcare expenditures. Private insurance accounted for 8.5% of all health expenditures in 2009.[104]

Hospitals

There were about 2.4 beds per 1,000 people in 2009.[108] The Ministry of Health owns and operates 850 hospitals, and 350 are privately owned. Certificate of need legislation restricts the growth of the private sector and reduces duplication of services with publicly owned hospitals. Payment mechanisms for both public and private hospitals are in flux; the Australian DRG prospective payment system has been piloted in 47 public hospitals. It is likely that a combination of prospective payments and global budgets will be used to control the costs of public hospitals.[149]

Physicians

Turkey had about 1.6 physicians per 1,000 people in 2009.[108] There are a relatively high proportion of specialists compared to general practitioners. Most physicians are paid salaries, and hospital-based specialists also are eligible for performance-based bonuses, which are adjusted to encourage full-time status. There is and has been concern about the current number of physicians being able to meet the demand in Turkey. To overcome this shortage, the Ministry of Health has opened new medical schools and implemented a family medicine–based integrated primary care initiative. Much of primary care has been the responsibility of midwives and nurses, but the integrated primary care initiative has increased the supply of family medicine physicians, both through rigorous training and an innovative payment system. Family physicians in the integrated primary care system initiative receive capitation payments, with incentive bonuses for preventive care services.[149]

The U.S. Healthcare System

The current U.S. health system comprises a voluntary, employer-based private insurance subsystem, social health insurance for the elderly, and tax-funded, direct and indirect provision of care. Health expenditures in 2009 were funded through a combination of taxation (34.8%), social health insurance (13.8%), private health insurance (39%), and out-of-pocket payments (12.4%).[104] Benefit packages vary with the type of insurance, but typically include inpatient and outpatient hospital care and physician services. Many private plans also include preventive services, dental care, and prescription drug coverage. User charges vary by type of insurance, but typically include outpatient and prescription drug copayments, as well as deductibles for hospitalization.

The federal government is the single largest healthcare insurer and purchaser. Medicare covers health services for the elderly, the disabled, and those with end-stage renal disease. Administered by the Centers for Medicare and Medicaid Services (CMS), Medicare covered 14.3% of the population in 2009. The program is financed through a combination of payroll taxes, general federal revenues, and premiums. Medicaid, a joint federal–state health benefit program, covers targeted groups of the poor (e.g., pregnant women, families with children, and the disabled). Medicaid is administered by the states, which operate within broad federal guidelines overseen by the CMS. It covered 14.1% of the population in 2009. The program is financed by federal tax revenues, which match tax revenues raised by each state. The ratio of matching federal funds varies for each state depending on its per capita income. The Children's Health Insurance Program (CHIP) is a state–federal health benefit program targeting poor children. CHIP is jointly financed by the CMS and the states and is administered by the states (see http://www.cms.gov/NationalCHIPPolicy/).

Private insurance is provided by not-for-profit and for-profit health insurance companies, and is regulated by state insurance commissioners. Individuals can purchase private health insurance, although most people receive employer-based insurance. Many large employers self-fund health benefits for their employees, using insurance companies as third-party administrators. Private insurance covered 66.7% of the total population, with 58.5% of the population receiving employment-based insurance in 2009. Private insurance, including that provided by employers, accounted for 39% of total health expenditures in 2009.[151]

Hospitals

In 2009, there were about 2.7 hospital beds per 1,000 people.[108] In 2007, the United States had 4897 community hospitals, of which 2,913 were not-for-profit, 873 were for-profit, and 1,111 were public (owned by state or local governments). In contrast, in 2007 the federal government operated only 213 hospitals (serving veterans, active members of the armed services, and native Americans). Hospitals typically are parts of organized delivery systems, with most U.S. community hospitals being a member of an integrated delivery system ($n = 2,730$) and/or a network ($n = 1,472$) in 2007.[152] For-profit, not-for-profit, and public hospitals are paid through a combination of methods: per diem charges, case rates, capitation, and prospective payments based on DRGs (diagnostic-related groups).

Physicians

In 2009, there were about 2.4 physicians per 1,000 people.[108] General practitioners usually have no formal gatekeeper function, except within some health maintenance organizations. Although the majority of physicians are in private practice, increasingly physicians are being employed by medical group practices, hospitals, health maintenance organizations, or organized delivery systems. They are paid through a combination of methods: charges, discounted fees paid by private health plans, capitation contracts with private plans or public programs, and direct patient fees.

■ Appendix B: Medical Malpractice Liability in Eight Health Systems

This appendix examines an important feature of health systems, how they handle the problems arising from medical malpractice. Medical liability systems differ in terms of the types of compensation they provide for the patients who are the victims of malpractice, as well as how such patients or their families may seek redress for damages. Such compensation may be economic (typically reimbursements for the costs of ongoing care, loss of wages, etc.), noneconomic (typically for pain and suffering), or punitive (typically to punish the provider and to deter others). Depending on the system of medical liability, patients who believe they are victims of medical malpractice may seek recourse through a tort entered into a court of law, through a no-fault compensation scheme, or some combination of these two systems. In the country vignettes that follow, we highlight the types of systems for medical liability, whether insurance is compulsory, the main features of the medical malpractice liability market, and any relevant government funding. Because our main source is a 2006 report from the Organisation for Economic Co-operation and Development on medical malpractice,[97] we cover a subset of the countries discussed in Appendix A: Canada, Germany, Greece, the Netherlands, Sweden, Turkey, the United Kingdom, and the United States.

Canada's Medical Liability System

Canada has a tort system that relies on proven error, and provides awards for economic and noneconomic damages. Liability is joint and several, with no caps. Punitive damages may be sought, but are seldom awarded. Insurance for physicians is compulsory in five provinces. In 2005, premiums of $310 million (Canadian) were collected by the Canadian Medical Protective Association (CMPA), which covers 95% of practicing physicians. Trends show claims declining on average. The CMPA fully funds the medical liability for physicians.

Germany's Medical Liability System

Like Canada, Germany also employs a tort system that relies on proven error, and provides awards for economic and noneconomic damages. Liability is joint and several, and insurance is compulsory for physicians, as well as for medical professionals in hospitals and other healthcare facilities. In 2002, there were 250 million Euros of claims, with large losses for certain specialties. Trends show claims are increasing for hospitals and other facilities. Fifty companies provide medical malpractice insurance.

Greece's Medical Liability System

Greece also has a tort system that relies on proven error, and it provides awards for not only economic and noneconomic damages, but also punitive damages. There are caps for GPs of $30,000 per claim and for hospitals of $90,000 per year. Insurance is voluntary. Trends show rapid increases in claims, and about 25% of providers cannot obtain coverage. Reinsurance is also difficult to obtain.

Netherland's Medical Liability System

As with the other countries discussed so far, the Netherlands employs a tort system that relies on proven error. It differs in that it has compulsory no-fault compensation for clinical trials; otherwise, insurance is voluntary. Both tort and no-fault systems provide awards for economic and noneconomic damages. The total premium (all providers) paid in 2005 was about 33 million Euros. Claims are capped for both physicians (1.25 million Euros/claim; 2.5 million Euros/year) and hospitals (2.5 million Euros/claim; 6 million Euros/year).

Sweden's Medical Liability System

Unlike the other countries discussed so far, Sweden employs a no-fault compensation system, with joint and several liabilities. Both economic and noneconomic damages are awarded, but there is low compensation for pain and suffering. Insurance is compulsory for all healthcare providers, and is available from several mutual companies. Patients have a right to sue for additional compensation based on the Patient Torts Act of 1997, which is capped at $730,000 per claim. There are about 10,000 claims per year, with approximately 35–40% compensated. Surgical and orthopedic specialists typically incur more claims than other specialties. There has been no increase in claims.

Turkey's Medical Liability System

Turkey employs a tort system that includes not only proven, but also presumed and no error. It awards both economic and noneconomic damages. Liability is joint and several. Compulsory insurance was introduced in July 2010 for all physicians. Prior to this requirement, four companies provided insurance. Leading up to the introduction of compulsory insurance, there was an increase in claims and in premiums.

The United Kingdom's Medical Liability System

The United Kingdom employs a tort system that requires breach of duty and causation to be established. It awards not only economic and noneconomic, but also punitive damages. Liability is determined on a case-by-case basis, and may be joint and several. Between 2001 and 2005, the awards for damages averaged about £500 million per year, with a 10% increase per year. The number of awards also increased by about 5% per year. Physicians employed by the NHS are covered by the state; three medical organizations provide insurance for non-NHS physicians.

◼ The United States' Medical Liability System

The United States employs a tort system that relies on proven and presumed error. It awards economic, non-economic, and punitive damages. Depending on state law, liability may be joint, or joint and several. Insurance is compulsory for physicians in most states. Some states have established Patient Compensation Funds, serving as an insurer of last resort. Virginia and Florida have no-fault compensation systems for birth-related neurological injuries.

References

1. Agency for Healthcare Research and Quality. 2010. Glossary. Accessed January 18, 2011, at http://www.qualitymeasures.ahrq.gov/about/glossary.aspx
2. Kuhn T. *The structure of scientific revolutions.* Chicago: University of Chicago Press; 1962.
3. Madison DL. Notes on the history of group practice: the tradition of the dispensary. *Medical Group Management Journal.* 1990;37:52–54, 56–60, 86–93.
4. Encyclopædia Britannica Premium Service. 2010. Shamanism. Accessed August 27, 2010, at http://www.britannica.com/eb/article?eu=117459
5. Nunn JF. *Ancient Egyptian medicine.* London: British Museum Press; 1996.
6. Centre for the History of Medicine, School of Medicine, The University of Birmingham. 2010. Medicine and surgery in ancient Egypt. Accessed August 27, 2010, at http://www.touregypt.net/featurestories/humansac.htm
7. Arab SM. 2010. Medicine in ancient Egypt: part 2 of 3. Arab World Books. Accessed August 27 2010, at http://www.arabworldbooks.com/articles8b.htm
8. Arab SM. 2010. Medicine in ancient Egypt: part 3 of 3. Arab World Books. Accessed August 27, 2010, at http://www.arabworldbooks.com/articles8c.htm
9. Osler W. *The evolution of modern medicine.* New Haven, CT: Yale University Press; 1921.
10. Vegetti M. Between knowledge and practice: Hellenistic medicine. In: Grmek MD, ed. *Western medical thought from antiquity to the Middle Ages.* Cambridge, MA: Harvard University Press; 1998:72–103.
11. Porter R. *The greatest benefit to mankind: a medical history of humanity from antiquity to the present.* London: HarperCollins; 1997.
12. Rosner L. The growth of medical education and the medical profession. In: Loudon I, ed. *Western medicine: an illustrated history.* New York: Oxford University Press; 1997:147–159.
13. Longrigg J. Medicine in the classical world. In: Loudon I, ed. *Western medicine: an illustrated history.* New York: Oxford University Press; 1997:25–39.
14. Jacquart D. Medical scholasticism. In: Grmek MD, ed. *Western medical thought from antiquity to the Middle Ages.* Cambridge, MA: Harvard University Press; 1998:197–240.
15. Encyclopædia Britannica Premium Service. 2010. History of medicine. Accessed August 27, 2010, at http://www.britannica.com/eb/article?eu=119072
16. The Internet Encyclopedia of Philosophy. 2010. Galen. Accessed August 27, 2010, at http://www.iep.utm.edu/g/galen.htm
17. Encyclopædia Britannica Premium Service. 2010. Galen of Pergamum. Accessed August 27, 2010, at http://www.britannica.com/eb/article?eu=36532
18. Greenhill WA. Archiater. In: Smith W, ed. *A dictionary of Greek and Roman antiquities.* London: John Murray; 1875:119–120.
19. Williams HS. 1999. Galen—the last great Alexandrian. The World Wide School. Accessed April 30, 2004, at http://www.worldwideschool.org/library/books/sci/history/AHistoryofScienceVolumeI/chap44.html
20. McCallum JE. *Military medicine: from ancient times to the 21st century.* Santa Barbara, CA:ABC-CLIO; 2008.
21. Encyclopædia Britannica Premium Service. 2010. Hospital. Accessed August 27, 2010, at http://www.britannica.com/eb/article?query=&ct=null&eu=119078&tocid=35526
22. Capasso L, Mariani CR. Ophthalmology in ancient Rome. *InterNet Journal of Ophthalmology.* 1997;2:1–8.
23. Encyclopædia Britannica Premium Service. 2010. Pedanius Dioscorides. Accessed August 27, 2010, at http://www.britannica.com/eb/article?eu=31063&hook=4323 - 4323.hook
24. Savage-Smith E. Europe and Islam. In: Loudon I, ed. *Western medicine: an illustrated history.* New York: Oxford University Press; 1997:40–53.
25. Agrimi J, Crisciani C. Charity and aid in Medieval Christian civilization. In: Grmek MD, ed. *Western medical thought from antiquity to the Middle Ages.* Cambridge, MA: Harvard University Press; 1998:170–196.
26. McVaugh MR. Medicine in the Latin middle ages. In: Loudon I, ed. *Western medicine: an illustrated history.* New York: Oxford University Press; 1997:54–66.
27. Rawcliffe C. *Medicine and society in later Medieval England.* Stroud, England: Alan Sutton Publisher; 1995.
28. Encyclopædia Britannica Premium Service. 2010. Guild. Accessed August 27, 2010, at http://www.britannica.com/eb/article?eu=39194&tocid=0&query=surgeon guild&ct=
29. Berlant JL. *Profession and monopoly: a study of medicine in the United States and Great Britain.* Berkeley: University of California Press; 1975.
30. Encyclopædia Britannica Premium Service. 2010. Paracelsus. Accessed August 27, 2010, at http://www.britannica.com/eb/article?query=paracelsus&ct=&eu=59828&tocid=0 - 0.toc
31. Rhodes P. *An outline history of medicine.* Boston: Butterworths; 1985.
32. Encyclopædia Britannica Premium Service. 2010. Ambroise Paré. Accessed August 27, 2010, at http://www.britannica.com/eb/article?eu=59902
33. Fahrer M. Bartholomeo Eustachio—the third man: Eustachius published by Albinus. *ANZ Journal of Surgery.* 2003;73:523–528.
34. Rosen G. *The structure of American medical practice 1875–1941.* Philadelphia: University of Pennsylvania Press; 1983.
35. Rosen R. Clinical governance in primary care: improving quality in the changing world of primary care. *British Medical Journal.* 2000;321:551–554.
36. Ramsey M. *Professional and popular medicine in France, 1770–1830.* New York: Cambridge University Press; 1988.
37. Estes JW. *Hall Jackson and the purple foxglove: medical practice and research in revolutionary America 1760–1820.* Hanover, NH: University Press of New England; 1979.
38. Link EP. *The social ideas of American physicians (1776–1976).* London: Associated University Presses; 1992.
39. Schneck LH. Health insurance for the "uninsurable." *Medical Group Management Journal.* 2000;47:48–52, 54, 56–57.
40. Schneck LH. Strength in numbers. Medical group practices fill vital niche in U.S. health care system. *MGMA Connexion.* 2004;4(1):34–43.

42 | Chapter 1: International Physician and Health System Practice

41. Shi L, Politzer RM, Regan J, Lewis-Idema D, Falik M. The impact of managed care on the mix of vulnerable populations served by community health centers. *Journal of Ambulatory Care Management,* 2001;24:51.

42. Carlson BL, Eden J, O'Connor D, Regan J. Primary care of patients without insurance by community health centers. *Journal of Ambulatory Care Management.* 2001;24:47–59.

43. Shi L, Starfield B, Xu J, Politzer R, Regan J. Primary care quality: community health center and health maintenance organization. *Southern Medical Journal.* 2003;96:787–795.

44. O'Malley AS, Mandelblatt J. Delivery of preventive services for low-income persons over age 50: a comparison of community health clinics to private doctors' offices. *Journal of Community Health.* 2003;28:185–197.

45. Fishbein RH. Origins of modern premedical education. *Academic Medicine.* 2001;76:425–429.

46. Harvey AM, Brieger GH, Abrams SL, McKusick VA. A model of its kind. A century of medicine at Johns Hopkins. *Journal of the American Medical Association.* 1989;261:3136–3142.

47. King LS. Medicine in the USA: historical vignettes. II. Medical education: the early phases. *Journal of the American Medical Association.* 1982;248:731–734.

48. Knight W. *Managed care: what it is and how it works.* 1st ed. Gaithersburg, MD: Aspen; 1998.

49. Kongstvedt PR. *Managed care: what is it and how it works.* 2nd ed. Gaithersburg, MD: Aspen; 2002.

50. Nelson CW. Origins of the private group practice of medicine. *Mayo Clinic Proceedings.* 1992;67:212.

51. Nelson CW. Origins of the name "Mayo Clinic." *Mayo Clinic Proceedings.* 1997;72:296.

52. Havlicek PL. *Medical group practices in the US: a survey of practice characteristics.* Chicago, IL: American Medical Association; 1999.

53. Smart DR. *Medical group practices in the US: 2004 edition.* Chicago: American Medical Association; 2004.

54. The state of the medical practice: Hospital ownership increases among MGMA practices. *MGMA Connexion.* 2011;1:32.

55. Gans ND. *Number of medical groups in the United States.* Englewood, CO: MGMA Center for Research; 2010.

56. Axelrod DA, Millman D, Abecassis MM. US health care reform and transplantation. Part I: overview and impact on access and reimbursement in the private sector. *American Journal of Transplant.* 2010;10(10):2197–2202.

57. U.S. Congress. *Compilation of Patient Protection and Affordable Care Act.* Washington, DC: 111th Congress; 2010.

58. Fisher ES, Staiger DO, Bynum JP, Gottlieb DJ. Creating accountable care organizations: the extended hospital medical staff. *Health Affairs.* 2007;26:w44–57.

59. Taylor M. The ABCs of ACOs. Accountable care organizations unite hospitals and other providers in caring for the community. *Trustee.* 2010;63:12–14, 24.

60. Hester J, Lewis J, McKethan A. *The Vermont Accountable Care Organization Pilot: A Community Health System to Control Total Medical Costs and Improve Population Health.* New York, NY:The Commonwealth Fund, May 2010. Accessed July 1, 2011, at http://www.commonwealthfund.org/Publications/Fund-Reports/2010/May/The-Vermont-Accountable-Care-Organization-Pilot-A-Community-Health-System-to-Control.aspx

61. Hatton D. 2011, June 2. Comment: Medicare Shared Savings Program: Accountable Care Organizations (CMS-1345-P). American College of Physicians. Accessed July 1, 2011, at http://www.acponline.org/running_practice/aco/acp_comments.pdf

62. Jessee WF. 2011, June 1. Comment: CMS-1345-P Medicare Shared Savings Program: Accountable Care Organizations. Medical Group Management Association. Accessed July 1, 2011, at http://www.mgma.com/WorkArea/DownloadAsset.aspx?id=1366447

63. Ginsburg PB. Spending to save: ACOs and the Medicare Shared Savings Program. *New England Journal of Medicine.* 2011;364:2085–2086.

64. Iglehart JK. The ACO regulations: some answers, more questions. *New England Journal of Medicine.* 2011;364:1–3.

65. Shortell SM, Casalino LP, Fisher ES. How the Center for Medicare and Medicaid Innovation should test accountable care organizations. *Health Affairs.* 2010;29:1293–1298.

66. Shortell SM, Casalino LP. Health care reform requires accountable care systems. *Journal of the American Medical Association.* 2008;300:95–97.

67. Rittenhouse DR, Shortell SM, Fisher ES. Primary care and accountable care—two essential elements of delivery-system reform. *New England Journal of Medicine.* 2009;361:2301–2303.

68. "Baby boom" contributes to bust: dealing with an increase in physician retirees and insured patients. *MGMA Connexion.* 2011;1:35.

69. Sia C, Tonniges TF, Osterhus E, Taba S. History of the medical home concept. *Pediatrics.* 2004;113:1473–1478.

70. Robinson JC, Casalino LP. The growth of medical groups paid through capitation in California. *New England Journal of Medicine.* 1995;333:1684–1687.

71. Lee PR, Grumbach K, Jameson WJ. Physician payment in the 1990s: factors that will shape the future. *Annual Review of Public Health.* 1990;11:297–318.

72. Kralewski JE, Wallace W, Wingert TD, Knutson DJ, Johnson CE. The effects of medical group practice organizational factors on physicians' use of resources. *Journal of Healthcare Management.* 1999;44:167–182; discussion 82–83.

73. Miller P. Summary report: 2002 medical group office management systems survey. *Journal of Medical Practice Management.* 2003;18:207–210.

74. Casalino LP, Devers KJ, Lake TK, Reed M, Stoddard JJ. Benefits of and barriers to large medical group practice in the United States. *Archives of Internal Medicine.* 2003;163:1958–1964.

75. Abel-Smith B. Cost containment and new priorities in the European Community. *Milbank Quarterly.* 1992;70:393–416.

76. Williamson OE. *Markets and hierarchies.* New York: Free Press; 1975.

77. Anderson GF, Reinhardt UE, Hussey PS, Petrosyan V. It's the prices, stupid: why the United States is so different from other countries. *Health Affairs.* 2003;22:89–105.

78. McKee M, Figueras J. For debate: setting priorities: can Britain learn from Sweden? *British Medical Journal.* 1996;312:691–694.

79. Reinhardt UE. Response: what can Americans learn from Europeans? In: Organisation for Economic Co-operation and Development, ed. *Health care systems in transition: the search for efficiency.* Paris: OECD; 1990:105–112.

80. Organisation for Economic Co-operation and Development. *Health at a glance: OECD indicators 2009.* Paris: OECD; 2009.

81. Canadian Institute for Health Information. *Canada's health care providers.* Ottawa: CIHI; 2002.

82. Royal College of General Practitioners. 2003. Profile of UK practices: RCGP Information Sheet No. 2. Accessed May 14, 2004, at http://www.rcgp.org.uk/information/publications/information/PDF/02_OCT_03.pdf

83. Bourgueil Y, Marke A, Mousques J. *Medical group practice in primary care in six European countries, and the Canadian provinces of Ontario and Quebec: what are the lessons for France?* Paris: Institute for Research and Information in Health Economics; 2007 November.

84. Maarse H. Health care reform—more evaluation results. *Health Policy Monitor.* 2009 April. Accessed December 5, 2011, at http://www.hpm.org/survey/nl/a13/1

85. The Henry J. Kaiser Family Foundation. 2011. International health systems: Switzerland. Accessed July 25, 2011, at http://www.kaiseredu.org/Issue-Modules/International-Health-Systems/Switzerland.aspx

86. Maarse H. Health insurance reform 2006. *Health Policy Monitor.* 2006 March. Accessed December 5, 2011, at http://www.hpm.org/survey/nl/a7/1

87. Organisation for Economic Co-operation and Development. *Help wanted? Providing and paying for long-term care.* Paris: OECD; 2011.

88. Census Bureau. *Medicaid—beneficiaries and payments.* Washington, DC: U.S. Census Bureau; 2011.

89. MacAdam M. Physician payment incentives. *Health Policy Monitor.* 2009 April. Accessed July 25, 2011 at http://www.hpm.org/survey/ca/b13/1

90. Hildebrandt H, Hermann C, Knittel R, Richter-Reichhelm M, Siegel A, Witzenrath W. Gesundes Kinzigtal integrated care: improving population health by a shared health gain approach and a shared savings contract. *International Journal of Integrated Care.* 2010; 10:e046.

91. Groenewegen PP. Towards patient oriented funding of chronic care. *Health Policy Monitor.* 2009 April.

92. Carey D, Herring B, Lenain P. *Health reform in the United States.* Paris: Organisation for Economic Co-operation and Development; 2009.

93. Mello MM, Chandra A, Gawande AA, Studdert DM. National costs of the medical liability system. *Health Affairs.* 2010;29:1569–1577.

94. Towers Watson. *2010 update on U.S. tort cost trends.* New York: Towers Watson; 2010.

95. Golann D. Dropped medical malpractice claims: their surprising frequency, apparent causes, and potential remedies. *Health Affairs.* 2011;30:1343–1350.

96. Waters TM, Budetti PP, Claxton G, Lundy JP. Impact of state tort reforms on physician malpractice payments. *Health Affairs.* 2007;26:500–509.

97. Organisation for Economic Co-operation and Development. *Medical malpractice: prevention, insurance and coverage options.* Paris: OECD; 2006.

98. Langel S. Averting medical malpractice lawsuits: effective medicine, or inadequate cure? *Health Affairs.* 2010;29:1565–1568.

99. Thomas JW, Ziller EC, Thayer DA. Low costs of defensive medicine, small savings from tort reform. *Health Affairs.* 2010;29:1578–1584.

100. Department of Health, Social Services and Public Safety. 2009. Health and social care in Northern Ireland. Accessed July 29, 2011, at http://www.n-i.nhs.uk/index.php

101. Scottish Government Health Directorate. 2009. About the NHS in Scotland. Accessed April 25, 2011, at http://www.show.scot.nhs.uk/introduction.aspx

102. Department of Health and Social Services. 2009. What is NHS Wales. Accessed April 25, 2011, at http://www.wales.nhs.uk/nhswalesaboutus

103. Department of Health. 2009. About the NHS. Accessed March 24, 2011, at http://www.nhs.uk/NHSEngland/aboutnhs/Pages/About.aspx

104. World Health Organization. 2011. Global Health Observatory data repository. Accessed July 17, 2011, at http://apps.who.int/ghodata/

105. Department of Health. 2009. NHS services. Accessed March 24, 2011, at http://www.nhs.uk/NHSEngland/AboutNHSservices/Pages/NHSServices.aspx

106. Healthcare Commission and Audit Commission. *Is the treatment working? Progress with the NHS system reform programme: health national report.* London: Audit Commission; 2008.

107. Monitor. 2009. Monitor: independent regulator of NHS foundation trusts. Accessed April 25, 2011, at http://www.monitor-nhsft.gov.uk

108. Organisation for Economic Co-operation and Development. 2011. OECD health data 2011. Accessed July 17, 2011, at http://www.oecd.org/health/healthdata

109. British Medical Association. 2009. British Medical Association: the professional association for doctors. Accessed April 25, 2011, at http://www.bma.org.uk

110. Glenngård AH, Hjalte F, Svensson M, Anell A, Bankauskaite V. *Health systems in transition: Sweden.* Copenhagen: WHO Regional Office for Europe on behalf of the European Observatory on Health Systems and Policies; 2005.

111. Swedish Institute. *Swedish health care. Fact sheet.* Stockholm: Swedish Institute; 2007.

112. Swedish Medical Association. 2009. Swedish Medical Association. Accessed April 25, 2011, at http://www.slf.se/templates/Page.aspx?id=2033

113. Swedish Medical Association. 2005. Physicians in Sweden 2005. Accessed January 27, 2006, at http://www.slf.se/upload/Lakarforbundet/Trycksaker/PDFer/In English/L%C3%A4karfakta_2005_eng_webb.pdf

114. Swedish Medical Association, National Board of Health and Welfare. *Working in Sweden: information for doctors from EU/EEA countries.* Stockholm: Swedish Medical Association; 2009.

115. Organisation for Economic Co-operation and Development. *OECD health at a glance—how Canada compares. Policy brief.* Paris: OECD; 2001 October.

116. Canadian Institute for Health Information. *Health care in Canada 2002.* Ottawa: CIHI; 2002.

117. Canadian Institute for Health Information. 2009. Number of hospitals and number of hospital beds, by province, territory and Canada, 1999-2000 to 2005-2006. Accessed August 23, 2009, at http://secure.cihi.ca/cihiweb/dispPage.jsp?cw_page=statistics_a_z_e - N

118. Canadian Institute for Health Information. *Canada's health care providers, 2007.* Ottawa: CIHI; 2007.

119. Pan American Health Organization. *Health in the Americas, 2007.* Washington, DC: PAHO; 2007.

120. Fujisawa R, Lafortune G. *The remuneration of general practitioners and specialists in 14 OECD countries: what are the factors influencing variations across countries? OECD Health Working Papers.* Paris: Organisation for Economic Co-operation and Development; 2008. Report No. 41.

121. van Ginneken E, Busse R. Mandatory health insurance enacted. *Health Policy Monitor.* 2009 May.

122. fur Gesundheit B. *Health care system and health care reform in Germany.* Accessed April 15, 2009, at http://www.bmg.bund.de/ministerium/english-version/healthreform.html

123. Busse R, Riesberg A. *Health care systems in transition: Germany.* Copenhagen: European Observatory on Health Systems and Policies; 2004.

124. Schang L. Morbidity-based risk structure compensation. *Health Policy Monitor.* 2009 April. Accessed July 25, 2011, at http://www.hpm.org/survey/de/b13/1

125. Busse R. Germany. In: Dixon A, Mossialos E, eds. *Health care systems in eight countries: trends and challenges.* Copenhagen: European Observatory on Health Care Systems; 2002:47–60.

126. Muiser J. *The new Dutch health insurance scheme: challenges and opportunities for better performance in health financing. Discussion paper.* Geneva: World Health Organization; 2007.

127. Van de Ven WPMM, Schut FT. Managed competition in the Netherlands: still work-in-progress. *Health Economics.* 2009;18:253–255.

128. Cavagnero E. Health sector reforms in Argentina and the performance of the health financing system. *Health Policy.* 2008;88:88–99.

129. World Health Organization, 2008. WHOSIS: WHO Statistical Information System. Accessed November 24, 2008, at http://www.who.int/whosis/en/

130. Pan American Health Organization. 2001. Regional Core Health Data System—country health profile 2001: Argentina. Accessed October 26, 2002, at http://www.paho.org/english/sha/prflarg.htm

131. Pan American Health Organization. Argentina. In: *Health in the Americas.* Washington, DC: PAHO; 1998:18–39.

132. Belmartino S. Reorganizing the health care system in Argentina. In: Fleury S, Belmartino S, Baris E, eds. *Reshaping health care in Latin America: a comparative analysis of health care reform in Argentina, Brazil, and Mexico.* Ottawa: International Development Research Centre; 2000:47–77.

133. Pan American Health Organization. Argentina. In: *Health in the Americas.* Washington, DC: PAHO; 2007:26–48.

134. Lobato L. Reorganizing the health care system in Brazil. In: Fleury S, Belmartino S, Baris E, eds. *Reshaping health care in Latin American: a comparative analysis of health care reform in Argentina, Brazil, and Mexico.* Ottawa: International Development Research Centre; 2000:103–131.

135. Pan American Health Organization. Brazil. In: *Health in the Americas.* Washington, DC: PAHO; 2007:130–153.

136. Almeida C, Travassos C, Porto S, Labra ME. Health sector reform in Brazil: a case study of inequity. *International Journal of Health Services.* 2000;30:129–162.

137. Tountas Y, Karnaki P, Pavi E. Reforming the reform: the Greek national health system in transition. *Health Policy.* 2002;62:15–29.

138. Petmesidou M, Guillen AM. "Southern-style" National Health Services? Recent reforms and trends in Spain and Greece. *Social Policy and Administration.* 2008;42:106–124.

139. Tragakes E, Polyzos N. *Health care systems in transition: Greece.* Copenhagen: World Health Organization; 1996.

140. Ramesh M, Wu X. Realigning public and private healthcare in southeast Asia. *Pacific Review.* 2008;21:171–187.

141. Indonesia Ministry of Health. *Indonesia country profile 2006: make people healthy.* Jakarta: Ministry of Health Republic of Indonesia; 2007 August.

142. Republic of Indonesia. 2002. Health care system. Accessed August 28, 2002, at http://www.depkes.go.id/ENGLISH/index.htm

143. Barraza-Llorens M, Bertozzi S, Gonzalez-Pier E, Gutierrez JP. Addressing inequity in health and health care in Mexico. *Health Affairs.* 2002;21:47–56.

144. International Clearinghouse of Health System Reform Initiatives. 2000. Prospects of the Mexican health care reform. Accessed October 26, 2002, at http://www.insp.mx/ichsri/country/reforma_mex.pdf

145. Gonzalez Block MA, Sandiford P, Ruiz JA, Rovira J. Beyond health gain: the range of health system benefits expressed by social groups in Mexico and Central America. *Social Science and Medicine.* 2001;52:1537–1550.

146. Frenk J. Bridging the divide: global lessons from evidence-based health policy in Mexico. *Lancet.* 2006;368:954–961.

147. Frenk J, Gonzalez-Pier E, Gomez-Dantes O, Lezana MA, Knaul FM. Comprehensive reform to improve health system performance in Mexico. *Lancet.* 2006;368:1524–1534.

148. Pan American Health Organization. Mexico. In: *Health in the Americas.* Washington, DC: PAHO; 2007:466–485.

149. Hurst J, Scherer P, Chakraborty S, Schieber G. *OECD reviews of health systems—Turkey.* Paris: OECD; 2008.

150. Tatar M, Ozgen H, Sahin B, Belli P, Berman P. Informal payments in the health sector: a case study from Turkey. *Health Affairs.* 2007;26:1029–1039.

151. U.S. Census Bureau. 2011. Health insurance. Accessed July 17, 2011, at http://www.census.gov/hhes/www/hlthins/hlthins.html

152. Health Forum. *Fast facts on US hospitals.* Chicago: American Hospital Association; 2008.

CHAPTER

2

Organization and Operations of Medical Group Practice

Stephen L. Wagner, PhD, FACMPE

Our Age of Anxiety is, in great part, the result of trying to do today's jobs with yesterday's tools.

—Marshall McLuhan

This chapter is divided into two parts. Part I covers the organization of medical group practice and deals with the various structures, characteristics, methods of governance, and other important issues related to the many forms of medical group practice. Part II discusses the operations of medical group practices and how these operations are organized into functional departments, or divisions in the case of large groups. The issue of quality and the management implications of quality are also addressed.

■ Part I: Organization

When Home State Mining Company opened the first medical practice in 1,870 to care for its growing workforce in the remote parts of the West, it could not have been predicted that medical groups would become such a significant modality for physician practice in the delivery of medical care in the United States. Although over 140 years have passed, consolidation of group practices

has been slow, and group practice size on average has remained small.[1]

The reason for this, very likely, lies in the nature of medical practice itself and the nature of technological uncertainty as described by James Thompson. Thompson classified technologies as being either long-linked, mediated, or intensive. Medical practice is an example of an intensive technology where a "customized response" to a given set of circumstances or contingencies is necessary,[2] as shown in Figure 2-1.

In addition, Robbins discusses the concept of decision maker divergence as a significant reason why organizations and decision makers' interests do not coincide. In this construct, the ability of an organization to grow and become

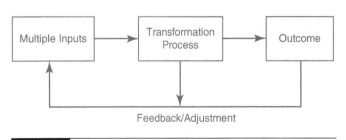

Figure 2-1 Thompson's intensive technology model.

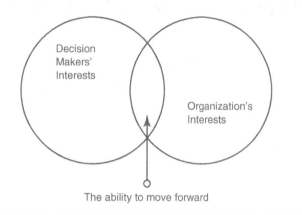

Figure 2-2 Aligned interest model.

efficient is directly related to the divergence of the interests of the decision makers,[3] as shown in Figure 2-2.

Regardless of the organizational challenges facing medical groups, many variant structures have been developed. In its simplest form, a medical practice can exist as a solo proprietorship with no formal organizational structure at all; a simple general partnership is the next step in the development of a group practice.

Taxonomy of Medical Groups

By definition, medical groups must contain at least three practitioners working within a common organizational structure. Groups share expenses and services and almost always bill under a single tax identification number. Special requirements for designation as a group practice are also defined by the U.S. Department of Health and Human Services Office of the Inspector General and will be discussed later in this chapter.[4] Furthermore, one can think of groups as being either confederate models, in which the practices tend to be loosely affiliated, or centralized models, in which the practices tend to be closely affiliated.

Figure 2-3 shows a taxonomy of medical groups and the relationship of the different forms. There are many variations in the structure of a group practice, but all typically fit into one of these categories.

Of course, this taxonomy is incomplete. Groups are also organized by single- or multispecialty status. Single-specialty

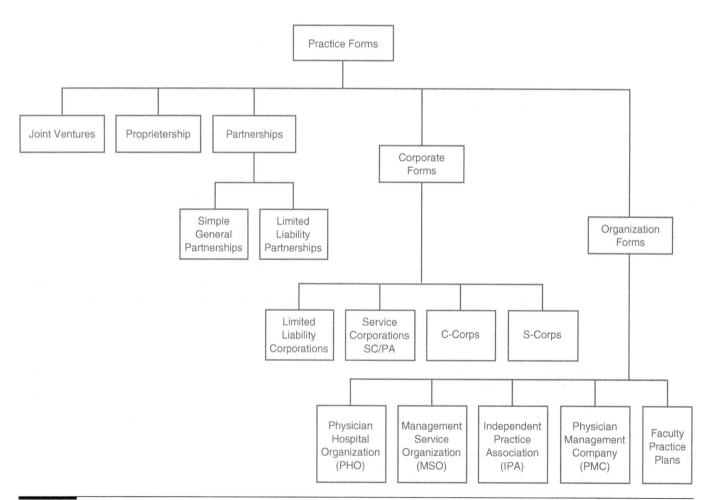

Figure 2-3 Taxonomy of medical groups.

groups are common in cardiology, surgical specialty, OB-GYN, pediatrics, orthopedics, behavioral medicine, rehabilitative specialties, internal medicine, neurology, and many others. The more divergent the specialties in terms of their economics and the nature of practice, the more difficult they can be to bring together under one structure.

The many organizational forms of medical groups have evolved in response to the needs and interests of medical practitioners as they have sought to adapt to a changing environment and to overcome the inherent nature of practices to stay small. In this sense, the medical group practice is a pragmatic entity. The definitions of each form are constantly varying and assuming characteristics of several forms.

One question needing to be answered when considering which group practice structure to use is: How will the structure influence the culture of the group and the governance system that the group envisions? As illustrated in Figure 2-4, the governance structure of a group affects the culture, which ultimately influences the operational nature of the group. For example, if there is not a centralized governance system and the culture of the group is biased toward significant physician autonomy, then operations will likely be variable with standardization lacking.

The degree of integration varies widely according to design and group type. Solo practices obviously have no integration with other practices, whereas in confederate models such as independent practice associations (IPAs) and management service organizations (MSOs), some

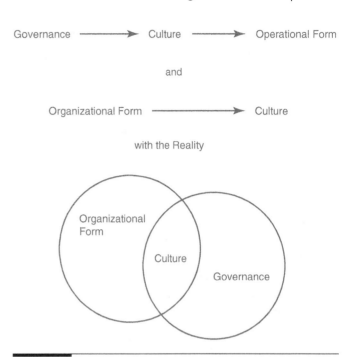

Figure 2-4 Governance.

services, identified in Figure 2-5 as "soft resources," are shared and integrated by the organization. In the fully integrated centralized group, all resources are shared.

Considerations for Structuring Practices

Choosing a practice form requires the consideration of a number of points. In general, organizational forms offer

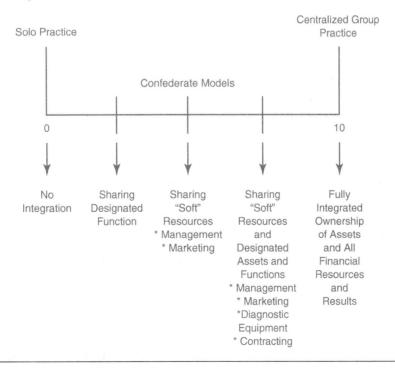

Figure 2-5 Integration spectrum.

different advantages and disadvantages to the physician and patients. They are generally related to:

- Liability of owners
- Control
- Continuity of the business entity
- Transferability of assets and ownership
- Capital formation
- Taxation
- Benefit plans

Virtually every state has adopted statutes that govern the formation and operation of corporations, partnerships, and other forms of commercial ventures. Since 1961, most states have special statutes specifically related to the organization of professional organizations. In some states, these are referred to as "service corporations," signified by the designation SC. In other states, the designation PA is used, which stands for "professional association." The principal feature distinguishing these organizations from other incorporated entities is that medical professionals are not protected by malpractice liabilities in an incorporated medical practice. A malpractice claim can and does pierce the corporate veil, and the physician is held liable individually for any acts of malpractice.

The other major difference in the treatment of PAs and SCs is in the area of taxation. These entities are essentially treated as individual taxpayers. They are taxed at the highest individual tax rates and are required to have a calendar year for their fiscal year for tax purposes. This was a response by the IRS to the use of the professional corporation by small practices to defer income between tax years.

In addition, centralized practice structures and confederate forms have different attributes that determine the level of satisfaction of the physician with the practice form. Figure 2-6 shows a list of several attributes that have been identified by physicians as being important to their satisfaction with practice. Centralized forms have a tendency toward certain attributes and confederate forms tend to move in the opposite direction.

Organizational Forms

A large number of practice structures and variations of those structures are possible for a medical practice. Although clear distinctions are sometimes made among these forms, they often have much in common and, in some cases, vary more by name than function.

General partnerships (see Figure 2-7) are the simplest form of group practice organization. Partnerships are created by a contract commonly referred to as a partnership agreement, which specifies the terms of the partnership.

	Group Practice Centralized	Confederation Models
Personal Physician Autonomy	↓	↑
Personal Flexibility	↓	↑
Services Offered	↑	↓
Capital Formation	↑	↓
Easy Patient Access	—	—
Quality	—	—
Efficiency/Standardization	↑	↓
Professional Interaction	↑	↓
Stability/Transferability	↑	↓
Shared Call	—	—
Operational Reporting	—	—
Decision-Making Process	—	—

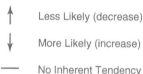

↑ Less Likely (decrease)

↓ More Likely (increase)

— No Inherent Tendency

Figure 2-6 Relative influence of practice structure on practice attributes.

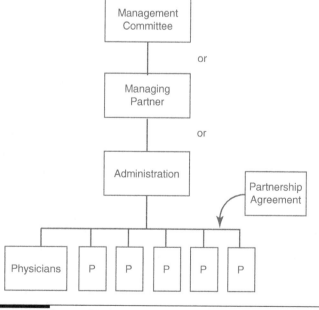

Figure 2-7 Partnership (straight partnership or limited liability partnership, LLP).

These entities are characterized by the following:

- There is an agreement on the nature of the enterprise. Two or more individuals (remember that a corporation is an artificial person in the eyes of the law, and therefore may form partnerships) agree to work together by contributing their assets, skills, and efforts in whole or part in the pursuit of the practice activity.
- Partnerships are pass-through entities for taxation. Profits or losses are divided in accordance with the partnership agreement, and the partners then declare those profits as income on their personal tax returns.
- General partners have unlimited liability for the debts and torts of the partnership and their partners.
- Upon the death of a general partner, the partnership ceases to exist.

The greatest advantage of a partnership is that it is easily formed. Partnerships are generally controlled by the owners, and decision making is usually by consensus.

Unlike a partnership, a corporation (see Figure 2-8) is an artificial person created by the law. However, state legislators have placed a number of limits on what a corporation can do and what its legal rights are. First,

Professional Associations (PAs)
Service Corporations (SCs)
C-Corp Section of Laws
S-Corp Section of Laws
Limited Liability Corporation (LLC)

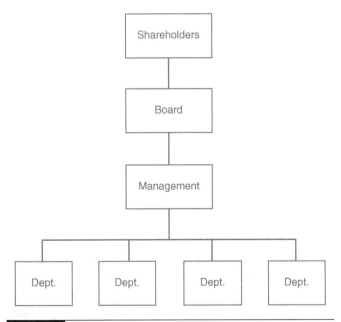

Figure 2-8 Corporate firms.

corporations have a right to buy and own assets, borrow money, enter into contracts, sell interests or shares in the ownership of the corporation, commit torts, may also commit crimes, and make income. They can be taxable or tax exempt, but are taxed under the corporate tax provision of the Internal Revenue Code. Ownership of the corporation is seen as having some level of independence from the corporation. Individuals that have an interest in the corporation are called shareholders. An important distinction between corporations and partnerships is that corporations and their shareholders can easily exchange their ownership interests without dissolution of the corporation. This allows a medical group practice to add shareholders and remove shareholders as needed while the integrity of the organization remains intact.

Although it is seen as a person under the law, a corporation does not have all the rights of a living person. A corporation may not vote and has no Fourteenth Amendment rights, so states may tax and impose fees on corporations for the privilege of doing business in a particular state.

Corporations are created by filing articles of incorporation in accordance with state law. A charter is then granted for the corporation to operate and engage in the lawful activities it was created to do. It is important to note that corporations may not practice medicine and may not be licensed to practice medicine. Furthermore, corporations, being constructs of legislation and having no free will, are required by law to operate according to their charter or bylaws. It is, therefore, essential that a group practice carefully consider the operating parameters established in its organizing documents.

Most large medical groups operate as corporations. Physicians typically join the practice under an employment agreement. Unlike publicly traded companies, becoming a shareholder in a group practice is usually not automatic and often requires more than a simple purchase of the stock. The incoming shareholder purchases the stock in the medical group in accordance with the stock purchase agreement. These agreements specify the terms for the purchase and sale of group stock and any restrictions related to its sale. One common restriction, for example, is that the stock must be sold back to the corporation upon death or departure from the practice for any reason. The use of a stock restriction agreement is extremely important, because, although states have statutes that require all members of a professional corporation to be licensed professionals, the state does not require that stock be sold to members of the existing corporation or to the corporation in the absence of a stock restriction agreement.[4]

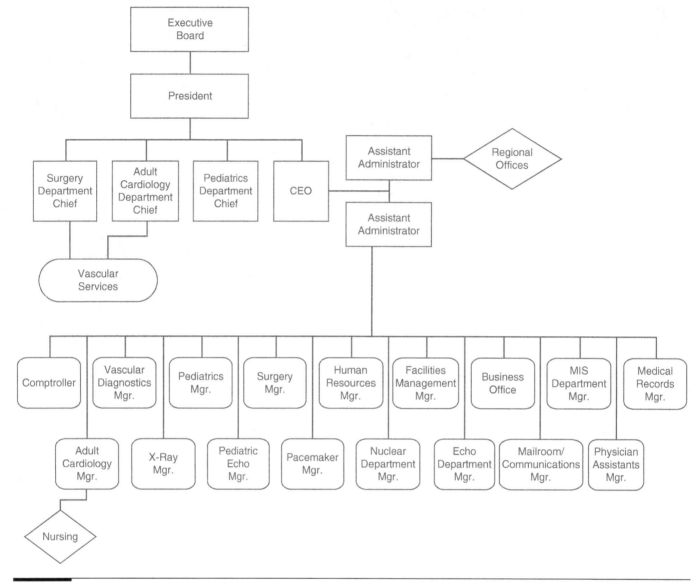

Figure 2-9 Group-practice organizational chart.

Figure 2-9 shows the organization of a typical group practice.

Hybrid Corporate and Partnership Forms

Although the corporate form is the dominant practice organizational form for medical groups today, they can vary in form.

The limited liability partnership (LLP) is a variation in the partnership form that has some characteristics of a corporation in the area of taxation and extends liability protection to its partners. Similarly, limited liability corporations (LLCs) and the S-Corp are variations of the corporate form and have some characteristics of the partnership. S-Corps, for example, are pass-through entities for taxation much like a partnership, but still have the corporate veil for protection from nonprofessional liability. A more detailed discussion of this can be found in J. Stuart Showalter's book, *Southwick's The Law of Health Care Administration*.[3(p251)]

Physician Hospital Organization (PHO)

One form of group practice that combines the hospital and the physician group or groups into a single organizational structure is the physician hospital organization (PHO; see Figure 2-10). This form usually occurs when a hospital or its parent company acquires a medical group through the purchase of the group practice's assets and the employment of the physicians directly by the hospital corporation or through a medical services agreement executed by the corporation.

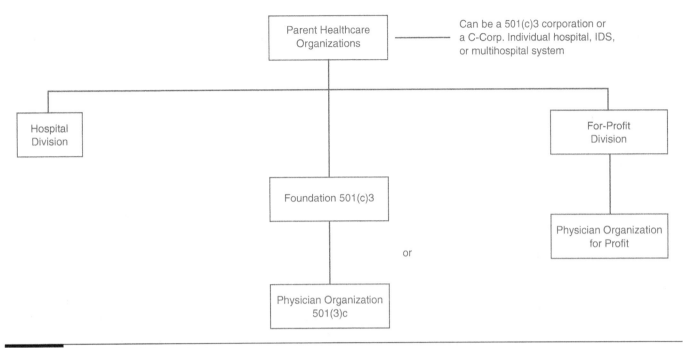

Figure 2-10 Physician hospital organization.

This form offers some clear potential advantages. Many arrangements that would be prohibited or very difficult and complex can be accomplished in the routine course of business for the PHO. This includes such things as joint marketing, contract negotiation for professional services contracts, managed-care contracts, purchasing, and the sharing of such assets as information technology. Another advantage is the access to capital for the purchase of increasingly expensive new technologies and practice development.

The major potential disadvantage is the loss of control over decision making and the potential inflexibility of a larger organization.

Management Service Organization (MSO)

Management service organizations (MSOs) are not actually medical groups at all; the MSO and the medical practice are usually two distinct organizations (see Figure 2-11). MSOs are entities that provide management service support to practices through a contract relationship. The MSO generally contracts with several practices to provide similar services. These contracts specify the nature of this relationship, which generally involves billing and collection of practice accounts receivable, personnel management contract administration, and most of the administrative functions of any medical practice. The advantage of this arrangement is the potential for having higher quality management and administrative service at a lower cost.

A large MSO has the ability to employ more highly skilled and, consequently, more expensive people in the organization and leverage more expensive technologies for more efficient operations because these costs can be spread over a larger number of physicians. In most cases, MSOs are capitalized by outside investors and are managed independently of the medical group.

The disadvantages are largely related to the difficulty of separating out these essential functions from the practice should the relationship with the MSO prove to be unsatisfactory. Once the arrangement is in place, it is extremely difficult to undo, rehire staff, and rebuild the necessary aspects of the practice operation. It is essential that practices contemplating such an arrangement do so with great care and due diligence. Performance

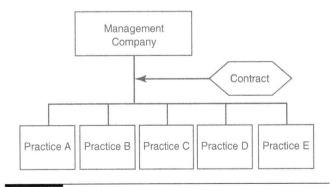

Figure 2-11 Management service organization (MSO).

benchmarks in the contract with procedures for resolving problems and potential compensation for fee relief for poor performance are advisable.

Practice Management Company (PMC)

Practice management companies (PMCs; see Figure 2-12) largely have fallen out of favor, with some notable exceptions. These entities essentially took the MSO concept a step further by serving as a vehicle to amalgamate practices under one corporation. Many of these organizations were able to tap large amounts of capital for acquisitions by becoming publicly traded companies. The advantage of this practice form is its ability to raise capital in the financial markets, but that has turned out to be as much a problem as an advantage.

The need to generate profits from aggregated businesses accustomed to distributing 100% of the income to the physicians as income seemed to be a clear problem with the model. PMCs simply could not live up to their promise of increasing income to physicians, improving group performance, and providing an acceptable return to public shareholders. PhyCor, one of the largest and oldest of the PMCs, was delisted by the National Association of Securities Dealers (NASD) in November 2000 after posting over a $400 million loss.[5]

In contrast, Pediatrix is a publicly traded medical group that has met with great success, even though its business model is similar to a PMC. The PMC is not a complete relic of the past, and as with many medical business models, it requires a careful examination of asset acquisition cost and operations to produce an optimal outcome.

Independent Practice Association (IPA)

An independent practice association (IPA) is a loosely affiliated entity that is not as widely employed today as in the recent past. Many IPAs formed when managed-care plans were seeking to contract with a smaller number of providers at discounted fees with the promise to direct larger numbers of patients to those providers. The IPAs often share risks with the managed-care plans and accept a defined number of patients while agreeing to provide care at a fixed price or capitated fee (see Figure 2-13).

IPAs are usually operated by a board or management committee derived from the practice participants and a professional staff.

The popularity of IPAs has waned as capitation and risk-sharing arrangements with physicians have declined. IPAs that experienced difficulties did so because it was often difficult to properly evaluate risk for the patient population being serviced. Managed-care organizations also had difficulty in providing enough patients to an IPA so that the risk associated with the contract was predictable in actuarial terms.

IPAs may also function similarly to MSOs by providing management services and a way for many practices to share resources. In the case of the IPA, however, such relationships tend to be partnerships between the practices, and the IPA agreement is actually a partnership agreement.

Typical Activities of Service Organizations (MSOs and IPAs) MSOs and IPAs serve a variety of functions for the practices they support, and in many respects can replace some or all of the administrative functions traditionally

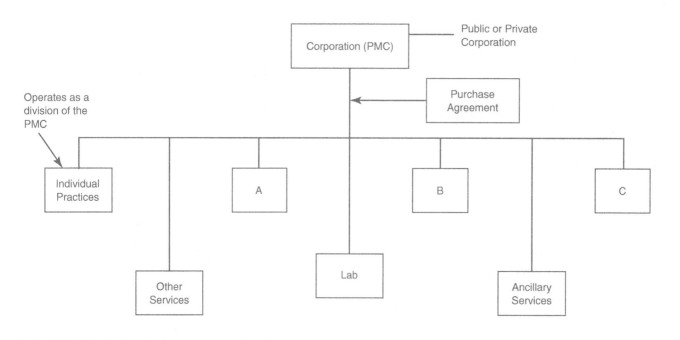

Figure 2-12 Practice management company (PMC).

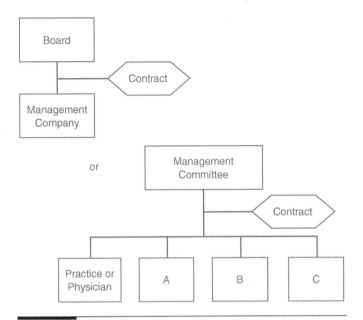

Figure 2-13 Independent practice association (IPA).

contained within the medical group. These services typically include:

- Assessing and developing local marketing plans
- Providing practice management support through the employment of professional managers
- Increasing coding expertise
- Developing a compliance plan
- Developing and complying with an Occupational Safety and Health Administration (OSHA) plan

MSOs and IPAs also offer:

- Practice assessment
- Billing assistance, or provide the billing function
- Wage and hour administration
- Practice positioning, by serving as a clearinghouse for managed-care contracts
- Telemedicine
- Promotion and other marketing activities
- Continuing medical education
- Quality initiatives
- Vendor leverage and other economies of scale
- Access to capital
- Data collection and management
- Contract administration

Faculty Practice Plans: Medical Foundation Model

Faculty practice plans are group practices within a university setting or integrated delivery system (IDS). They have sometimes been referred to as "clinics without walls." These organizations are mechanisms by which the medical school faculty or physicians servicing the IDS can

operate as a single large group practice (see Figure 2-14). These structures may be tax exempt under 501(c)3 of the Internal Revenue Code.

Faculty practice plans and medical foundation models offer several advantages to the physician practice.

- They allow several independent practices to come together and contract as a single entity, which may offer strength in numbers to the managed-care company.
- Because the organization is tax exempt in most cases, more flexibility is available to the physicians for certain employee benefits such as nonqualified deferred compensation plans.
- The legal barrier to joint activities with the parent organizations is greatly reduced because they are a single organization.
- In the case of a physician with a faculty appointment at a medical school, it simplifies the ability of the practice to provide teaching services and maintain a private practice at the same time, with less legal concerns and barriers, because these activities are coordinated by one administrative organization.

The greatest potential disadvantage concerns the complexity of the organization and some of the unique regulatory challenges of working within a tax-exempt environment. Many medical groups distribute all or most of the organization's income to the physician owners. IRS regulations have standards on reasonable compensation for employees of tax-exempt organizations, so care must

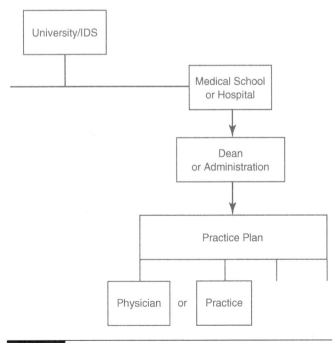

Figure 2-14 Faculty practice plan—foundation models.

be taken to properly implement compensation plans to avoid private inurnment.

Joint Venture (JV) Relationship

Joint ventures (JVs) are special partnerships. They are usually entered into for a specific project or service. They can be between medical groups, between hospitals and a medical group, or among other entities (see Figure 2-15). These entities are highly regulated by the Office of the Inspector General (OIG) of both the federal and state governments because of the potential for fraud and abuse. JVs are often permissible when there is a low potential for abuse or the potential for community good exceeds the potential for harm to the Medicare or Medicaid program.

Most JVs attempt to comply with the various regulatory requirements by fitting into one of a number of safe harbors:

- *Investments in group practices:* Physicians are protected when they invest in their own practice if the practice meets the physician self-referral (Stark) law definition of group practice. This does not apply to physician or group-practice investments in ancillary services joint ventures, but those ventures may qualify under other safe harbors.
- *Investments in ambulatory surgical centers (ASCs):* Certain investment interests in four categories of freestanding, Medicare-certified ASCs are protected: surgeon-owned, single-specialty, multispecialty, and hospital–physician owned. The ASC must be an extension of a physician's office practice for the physician to be protected as an investor.
- *Specialty referral arrangements:* A physician or entity is protected when referring a patient to another provider with the understanding that the patient will be referred back to that physician or

entity at a certain time or under certain circumstances. Referrals must be clinically appropriate.

- *Cooperative hospital services organizations (CHSOs):* CHSOs are relations between two or more tax-exempt hospitals to provide specific services, such as purchasing, billing, and clinical services, solely for the use of the patron hospitals. The CHSO can be supported through operational costs and payments from a CHSO to a patron hospital.
- *Joint ventures in underserved areas:* Raises the limit on investments in a venture in an underserved area by "tainted" investors—those who refer to or provide services to the entity—from 40–50% and allows unlimited revenues from referral source investors.
- *Practitioner recruitment in underserved areas:* Protects recruitment payments made by entities to attract needed physicians and other healthcare professionals to areas in need of health professionals. Places certain restrictions on patient percentages and payment time limits.
- *Sales of physician practices to hospitals in underserved areas:* Allows hospitals in underserved areas to buy practices of retiring physicians for the purpose of holding them until the hospital can find a new physician buyer. The sale must occur within 3 years.
- *Subsidies for obstetrical malpractice insurance in underserved areas:* Protects entities that pay malpractice insurance premiums for practitioners engaging in obstetrical services in areas in need of health professionals.[6]

In addition, there are five standards of the group practice safe harbor:

- Equity interests must be held by licensed professionals who practice in the group or by solo professional corporations owned by individuals who practice in the group.
- The equity interest must be in the group itself, not a subdivision of the group.
- The practice must meet the definition of a "bona fide group practice under the Stark law and implementing regulations."
- The practice must be a "unified business" with centralized decision making, pooling of expenses and revenues, and a compensation–profit distribution system that is not based on satellite offices operating as if they were separate enterprises or profit centers.
- Ancillary revenues must be derived from services that meet the Stark law and implement the regulations' definition of "in-office ancillary services."[7]

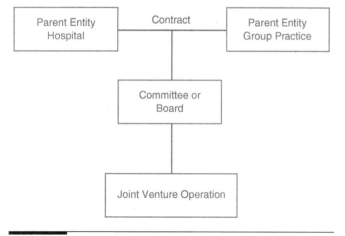

Figure 2-15 Joint venture (JV) relationship.

The complexity and extent of the various legal restrictions on JVs has made them less attractive as possible business models for group practice. The penalties can be so onerous that, frequently, JVs will not service patients with Medicare or Medicaid because the JV cannot qualify for harbor status. The most serious economic penalty for the medical group and its physicians is exclusion from the Medicare and Medicaid program.

Governance

One of the most significant issues for medical group practice today is the issue of governance. What makes a group practice a focused and effective organization has much more to do with how the governance structure is organized than the practice's legal structure. As Figures 2-16 and 2-17 illustrate, the effective interaction of governance and operational activities are essential for the execution of the group's mission. Such interaction also ensures that the organization's mission is advanced by monitoring operational and governing activities.

Medical groups are traditionally viewed as professional collegial organizations. They have many unique features, but some that affect governance include that the primary producers are all the owners (in many cases), the governed are also the governors (which leads to many

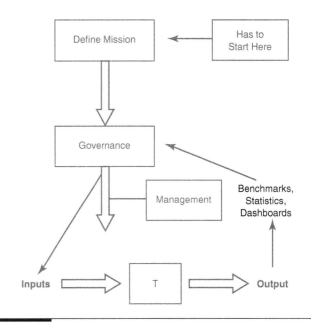

Figure 2-16 Group-practice governance.

policy quandaries), and the notion that "My view should be considered above all else."

This issue becomes more difficult, as well as more important, the larger and more diverse the group gets.

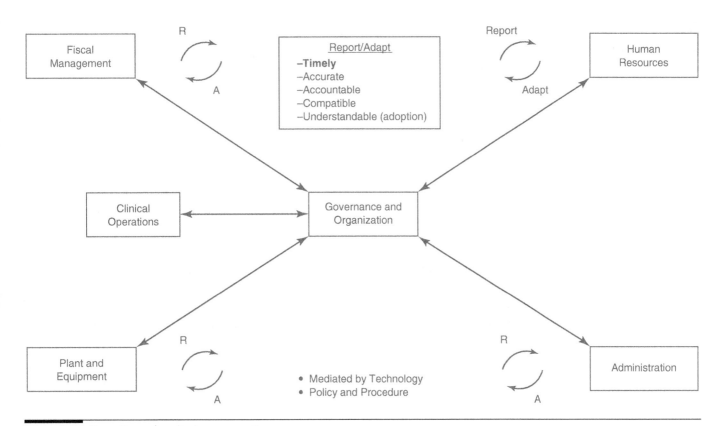

Figure 2-17 Operations of medical group practice.

As groups grow, the need for a more centralized form of governance becomes important for many reasons:

- It becomes more difficult for members of the group to find time and to get adequate numbers of the group together to make policies.
- Information disequilibrium increases. Some people are aware of and understand the issues, and some do not. This may be due to poor communication or the lack of time to understand the issue or to be informed.
- The geographic limitations of attendance at meetings, calls, and other necessary absences from meetings make it difficult to deal with important issues.
- There is a lack of interest in topics for discussion.
- There is a sense that members do not understand the issues or that their participation is not needed or welcomed.

The Role of the Governing Body

The governing body of the medical group must deal with a number of stakeholders in its quest to provide effective governance of the group, such as:

- Physicians in the practice
- Other physicians in the community
- Employees
- Patients and families
- Payers
- Federal, state, and local government
- Communities at large
- Hospitals

There is widespread agreement that the principle role of the board is to:

- Develop the organizational mission
- Provide institutional goals and target (and monitor them)
- Hire, evaluate, compensate, and interact with senior management (e.g., CEO)
- Be responsible for providing quality of care
- Deal with external constituents (media, community, and government)
- Monitor the organization
- Develop plans (financial and other)
- Evaluate its own performance as a body

In medical groups, most members of the board are physicians; although their duty is to the group as a whole, they may find it hard from time to time to let their own interests or the interests of their specialty take a back seat for the good of the whole. Much of this may be a matter of experience on a governing body, adequate structure in the group for operational concerns that address individual and specialty needs, and education. Members that value the group tend to have a much easier time serving in a nonparochial manner.

A Board Job Description

It is very important that every potential member of the board understand his or her role and the expectations of the job. As an example, the following is what a board prospect sheet might look like.

Member of the Board Job Description and Expectations

Purpose: To advise, govern, oversee policy and direction, and assist with the leadership and general promotion of the clinic so as to support the organization's mission and needs and to work closely with the administration of the clinic in order to achieve its goals.

Number of Members: Specify the number of members. The typical number is between 5 and 11, depending on the size of the group.

Major Responsibilities:

- Organizational leadership and advisement
- Organization of the executive committee officers and committees
- Formulation oversight of policy and procedures
- Financial management (to be defined)
- Reviewing and adopting a budget for the organization; reviewing quarterly financial reports, and assisting administration with budgetary issues as necessary
- Oversight of program planning and evaluation
- Hiring, evaluation, and compensation of senior administrative staff
- Review of organizational and programmatic reports
- Promotion of the organization
- Strategic planning and implementation

Length of Term: Specify length of term, which may be staggered.

Meetings and Time Commitment: Specify the time and location of meetings, such as, "The executive committee will meet every other Friday commencing at 7:30 a.m. and meetings will typically last one (1) hour (this may need to be revised)." An alternative is to have monthly meetings (2–3 hours) in the afternoon or evening (consider payment to participants).

Expectations of Board Members:

- Attend and participate in meetings on a regular basis and special events as possible.
- Participate in standing committees of the board and serve on ad hoc committees as necessary.
- Help communicate and promote mission and programs of the clinic.
- Become familiar with the finances and resources of the clinic as well as financial and resource needs.
- Understand the policies and procedures of the clinic.

Board and Committee Structure Establishing Committees: It shall be the responsibility of the executive committee to establish ad hoc and permanent standing committees as necessary to assist in the functioning of the clinic. Whenever possible, these committees should contain a representative of the executive committee to provide a proper liaison as well as an administrative staff person.

Typical Committees: Include finance, personnel, marketing, quality care, and technology. In an area where managed-care risk contracting is a significant part of the business environment, a utilization management committee is common to oversee the risk management of such contracts.

Board Selection

Board members are typically selected by election. Election rules are specified in the bylaws of the organization. It is extremely important that the bylaws be properly adopted and that the procedures adopted by the bylaws be adhered to carefully. Failure to follow an organizational process correctly could result in a challenge to the legitimacy of the process and invalidation under state law.

Board Retreats

An essential element of group planning and strategic activity is the board retreat. This event combines educational time, by internal and external speakers, with time to consider issues that are of strategic interest to the group. These issues are often related to:

- Growth
- Competition
- Change in or development of new services
- Examination of future scenarios and how they will play out: what their effect will or will not be on the organization
- A reexamination or development of a mission statement

Outside Board Members

Increasingly, groups are beginning to behave more like traditional business corporations. As part of this change, groups are adding outside persons to the board to improve the governance process and to bring new ideas and perspectives to the board. These individuals must be chosen carefully with consideration to a number of important criteria. An example of these selection criteria for a clinic's outside board member might be:

- Has a general understanding of the region, its business climate, political environment, and some of the key community drivers; has some perspective on healthcare and what is happening in the broad view
- A strategic thinker
- Willing and able to attend meetings
- Able to treat information discreetly
- Some experience as a member of a board
- No conflicts of interest or its appearance (not someone looking to do business with the clinic)
- General business acumen
- Someone who can contribute to but not dominate the board
- Someone who has a history of working well in a group setting—a good fit
- Willing to sign a confidentiality agreement
- Willing to accept fair compensation

The Process of Governance Change

Many groups have boards that consist of all of the physicians or all of the physicians that have reached full shareholder or partnership status. Although this method may address the perennial question of autonomy and control, it does little to improve decision making or the speed at which decisions are made. To improve the speed of decision making, many large boards elect an executive committee that has the ability to make certain decisions on behalf of the organization without the vote of the full board. For other decisions, typically those that are significant in magnitude, the executive committee develops preliminary information about a matter and makes recommendations to the board for voting.

Changing governance and modifying the manner in which the board operates is assessed through observations about the effectiveness of the board. Such assessments can be gained by using a survey instrument similar to the following:

Physician Survey

At the physician retreat, we agreed to examine the issue of group governance for the Good Clinic. This survey is intended to provide input to the committee to help guide the process.

Please rate the following statements based on how strongly you agree or disagree with each of these issues in your association with the Good Clinic.

| | Strongly Agree | | | | Strongly Disagree |

I. GOVERNANCE

1. The current governance practices of the clinic need to be changed. 5 4 3 2 1

2. I feel the executive committee could handle many issues without full board approval as long as I am kept informed of the process (e.g., last year's malpractice issue). 5 4 3 2 1

3. I feel the full board should meet less often. 5 4 3 2 1

4. I would be willing to allow a smaller group of physicians to make major clinical decisions so long as they are held accountable for their actions. 5 4 3 2 1

5. I would be willing to allow our clinic management greater autonomy in decision making for the clinic so long as they are held accountable for their actions. 5 4 3 2 1

6. We attend too many meetings on a regular basis. 5 4 3 2 1

7. There are too many physicians involved in the clinic decision-making processes. 5 4 3 2 1

8. The three divisions of the Good Clinic should be more coordinated in terms of their decision making, not less. 5 4 3 2 1

9. I would be willing to have less personal autonomy to expedite decision making in the group. 5 4 3 2 1

10. I would be willing to devote significant time to the governance of the clinic. 5 4 3 2 1

II. MISSION

1. The Good Clinic should offer comprehensive care to the region even if that occasionally means investing in technologies or staffing that may not be profitable. 5 4 3 2 1

2. I would be willing to make less money to preserve lifestyle issues such as time off. 5 4 3 2 1

3. In a few sentences, please describe your view on the mission of the Good Clinic.

Monitoring by the Board

It is important to develop a series of benchmarks that can be tracked by the board over time to monitor the progress and status of the group's performance. This includes quality indicators, such as results of quality initiatives, comparisons with peer databases, and financial indicators such as:

- Gross revenue per RVU
- Collections per RVU
- Profit/net income per RVU
- RVU per MD
- Operating cost per RVU
- Employee salary per RVU

Relative value units (RVUs) make excellent measurement tools because they have become a standard part of group-practice management and reimbursement systems.[8]

Benchmarks need to be understandable and communicate a clear message as to their meaning, be reproducible over time, and be timely (old news is no news, and it is not helpful for quickly reacting to changing situations). Benchmarks also need to measure a key competency or key success indicator for the practice.

Having discussed the structural aspects of group practice, Part II explores the functional and operational components found in most physician practices.

Mission

One of the most important, but often most neglected, aspects of a group practice organization is the lack of a clear mission statement that is consistent with the values of the organization's members. Here is an example of a mission statement:

The Good Clinic will provide care of the highest quality to our patients within an environment that is compassionate, ethical, and economically sound. We will accomplish this by:

1. Always putting patients first, maintaining clinical excellence, and seeking to improve care through research, system enhancement, innovation, and continuing education.

2. Being ethical in all of our dealings with patients, colleagues, employees, our hospitals, third-party payers, vendors, and our community.

3. Providing value to our patients, insurance carriers, and hospitals, and being seen as an asset to our community.

4. Having an effective organization that provides quality care, efficient service, effective communication, cost-effective treatment, and a competent and positive workforce.

5. Recognizing the value of the group—that we are greater than the sum of our parts.

6. Being focused on the creation of a positive environment that shows compassion and caring for our patients and our staff members.

7. Providing attractive salary and benefit packages that are competitive with all national standards, allowing the Good Clinic to attract and keep the most talented physicians and employees.

■ Part II: Operations

Administration

Nonphysician leadership and implementation of board policies is the principle role of medical group administration. This is accomplished by a coordination of the group's departmental functions to produce the desired outcome. One of the most critical activities is the translation of policy to procedure (see Figure 2-18).

Policies must be stated in terms of actionable steps and procedures that can be communicated to employees. Policies should be documented in a way that allows for consistent application of policy in a reproducible way.

The function of administration varies in groups depending on a number of issues:

■ Size matters. Larger groups often have more departments headed by professional managers that require less supervision and management by administration. In small groups, functions such as human resources (HR), marketing, and finance may be combined under the title of administration. In the context of this chapter, administration is synonymous with executive management.

■ How involved are the physicians in the management structure of the clinic? The physician administrator team has been recognized as an important success factor for groups.

■ The skill and education of the administrative group.

Administration generally falls into three board domains of group-practice administration:

1. The strategic, which can be either mission oriented or competitive in nature

2. The adaptive, reactive, or proactive

3. The operative, maintenance, or implementation

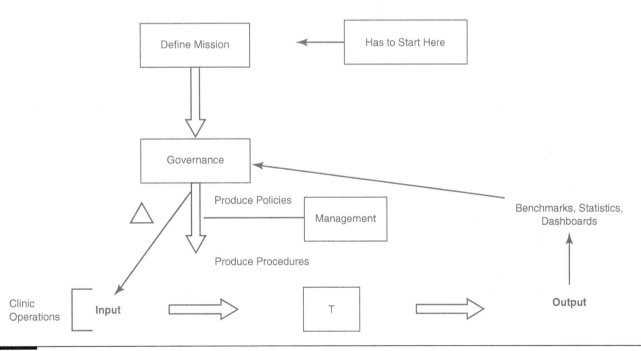

Figure 2-18 Policy and procedure development cycle.

Strategic planning and marketing are major functions found in the strategic domain. Michael E. Porter talks about three general aspects of strategy:

■ Cost leadership
■ Differentiation
■ Focus[9]

The medical reimbursement system does not provide a mechanism for strategies based on price. In the medical group system, pricing has very little to do with what is actually paid for a service, and price elasticity is not as relevant a concept as in most industries. Differentiation and focus have been the dominant strategies for medical groups. Group differentiators are becoming an increasingly important concern. Chief among these are quality and customer satisfaction. Focus is another widely used strategy. The single-specialty group and the specialty hospital are clear examples of focus strategies.

The American College of Medical Practice Executives (ACMPE) has developed an extensive document that seeks to define all of the critical areas of knowledge and skill necessary for an individual to be a successful administrator of a medical group practice. The ACMPE Body of Knowledge defines five general areas of competency for the group-practice administrator.[10]

1. *Professionalism:* Achieving and preserving professional standards
2. *Leadership:* Supporting the organization's strategic direction
3. *Communication skills:* Interacting and presenting information clearly and concisely
4. *Organizational and analytical skills:* Solving problems, making decisions, and developing systems
5. *Technical and professional knowledge and skills:* Developing the knowledge base and skill set necessary to perform activities unique to the job, role, or task within the eight performance domains or areas of responsibility:
   ■ Financial management
   ■ Human resource management
   ■ Planning and marketing
   ■ Information management
   ■ Risk management
   ■ Governance and organizational dynamics
   ■ Business and clinical operations
   ■ Professional responsibility

Best Practices

A significant body of research exists on medical group practices and the traits that distinguish better performing

organizations. According to data published by the Medical Group Management Association,[11] better-performing groups have the following characteristics:

■ Physician compensation usually rewards productivity.
■ There is excellent communication between physicians and administrative staff.
■ There is a productivity-oriented culture in the group.
■ An emphasis is placed on quality care, reputation, and patient satisfaction.
■ There is a physician administrative leadership team in place.
■ A good relationship exists with referral physicians.
■ Excellent control systems and budgets are used.
■ Cost structures are known and understood.
■ Central organization (delegation of decision making as opposed to consensus) is key.
■ The entire staff focuses on customer service.
■ New physicians are recruited to fit with the group and its culture.
■ Management is delegated to administration.
■ Administration is seen as professional colleagues and specialists in business.
■ A culture of respect is in place.

Risk Management

Another important function for medical group administration is in the area of risk management. The purpose of risk management is the mitigation of risk. Groups need an active risk management program. In very large groups, the function of risk management may be performed by an entire department within the organization or as a part of the legal department, but typically it is a part of administration. Risk management activities involve:

■ The purchase of insurance for physical assets and liability (fiduciary liability directors and officers, malpractice, and bonds); however, these activities are certainly not limited to those that can be insured against
■ Antitrust, fraud and abuse, criminal acts of all kinds, Health Insurance Portability and Accountability Act (HIPAA) violations, unfair trade practices, contract disputes, private inurnment issues, and Stark I and II, all issues that have the potential to cause considerable harm to the practice, even as much as malpractice suits can
■ The development of an effective quality assurance program, as described later in this chapter
■ Contract administration, which includes a number of documents common to all medical groups

Contracts and Other Legal Considerations

Healthcare, including the medical group practice, is one of the most highly regulated industries in the United States. It is essential that the well-managed medical group consider this and be familiar with this enormous body of law and how it applies to the practice. This information is also critical in the proper development of policies and procedures to ensure compliance and legal operation.

Although malpractice is the first subject to come to mind in a discussion of legal matters that affect medical group operations, it is by no means the only issue. These issues can be generally divided into the following categories:

Patient care issues: Standards of care, informed consent, medical records, advance directives, malpractice, and reporting requirements.

Business issues: Reimbursement, Medicare and Medicaid, Stark and antikickback rules, credit and collection, contracts with payers and vendors.

Employment contracts: A host of laws devoted to human resource issues.

Licensure issues: Physicians, physicians' assistants, nurses, nurse practitioners, and clinical laboratory, nuclear medicine, radiology, and cytology technicians are a key management concern for the medical group. Corporations and partnerships are also required to maintain business licenses, which requires filing with states in which the organization has been incorporated, and in which it operates.

Credentialing: Thousands of applications and renewals must be handled by this functional unit of the practice on an annual basis. Managed-care companies, hospitals, insurance companies, state regulators, and federal programs such as Medicare and Medicaid require an application for provider status and maintenance of pertinent records on a regular basis. Unfortunately, this activity varies dramatically from state to state and from company to company. A practice of 50 physicians could easily have over 2,000 pieces of credentialing that must be handled each year.

A medical license is required for each state in which the physician or other licensed professional practices. A practice also must maintain a Medicare provider number, a Medicaid provider number, and a provider number for managed-care organizations and insurance companies

such as Aetna, CIGNA, United Healthcare, and Blue Cross and Blue Shield (several across the country).

Contract negotiations: The complexity of contracts and the significant consequences of signing a "bad" contract make this a considerable duty for administration to either carry out this function or manage the process if it is delegated to a law firm or in-house counsel.

Patient Flow

Effective group-practice operations begin with a well-organized and -managed patient flow system. Front office activities include the scheduling of patients and preparation for their visit to the clinic, as shown in Figure 2-19. These systems are usually integrated with the information technology systems of the organization and may be divided into smaller department functions for:

- Registration
- Appointment scheduling
- Patient arrival and check-in
- Patient management during their visit
- Patient exit

The physical layout of the practice is also critical for efficient patient flow. The steps that patients need to follow in preparing for and receiving their services should be logical, communicated carefully to the patient (verbally and through well-written information), and prompted by well-done and informative signage, as well as the careful observation of a staff that is well trained in customer service and the hospitality arts. Employees for a well-managed medical group should always be selected for their ability to interact well with patients and visitors and not just for technical skill. It is often possible to teach technical information, but it is much more difficult to train for customer service attributes.

Because patient waiting is one of the most frequent sources of dissatisfaction, waiting areas should be comfortable, with plenty of reading material or other activities such as patient education, either in written form or as video material.

Billing, Credit and Collections, and Insurance

Managing the revenue cycle is an essential function for the successful medical group. This is a very dynamic process that is constantly changing because of revisions in billing requirements by payers and as information technology continues to improve. Most medical groups use medical-practice software packages that contain all of the subsystems necessary for the effective documentation of

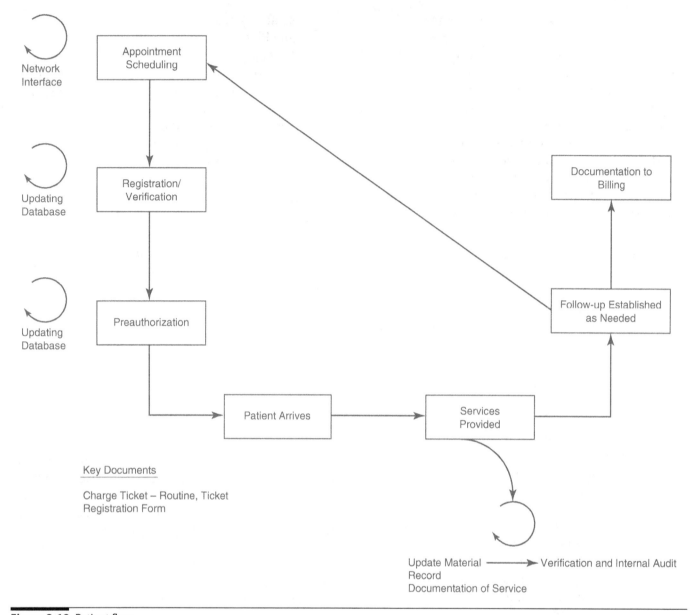

Figure 2-19 Patient flow.

service, entry of patient information, and service information. Almost all systems include:

- Scheduling and registration of patients and verification of services and payer information
- Patient information
- Billing functions, which include multiple fee schedules and billing requirements for each payer
- Managed-care requirements and procedures
- Reporting of billing and service information
- Multiple data entry options such as scanning, key entry, and downloading from wireless devices
- Accounts receivable and collections information and reporting

- Electronic claims submission and remittance of payments through electronic data interchanges (EDI)

These systems then provide for the creation of claims for reimbursement to Medicare, Medicaid, and all commercial insurance payers, as well as the creation of patient bills.

Although attempts have been made to standardize claims processing, almost no standardization of billing and payment processes exists among the more than 1,000 health insurers in the United States. (The Centers for Medicare and Medicaid Services [CMS] has created the standardized 1,500 claim form, however, and HIPAA has mandated some standardization of coding and submission of claims.) Among the areas of variability are:

- Patient eligibility verification procedures[12]
- Payer documentation requirements for certain procedures
- Bundling policies
- Modifiers and formats for explanations of benefits (EOBs)

The failure of our healthcare system to standardize the billing process has led to high error rates, denial of payments, and difficulty for everyone involved—the patient, the practice, and the payers.

The billing and collection process is covered by a significant number of rules and a large body of law. In addition, the billing process is very complex and varies greatly among payers. In an article published in the *New England Journal of Medicine*, authors Steffie Woolhandler et al. found that the cost of administration in the United States was $1,059 per person in 1999, compared to $307 in Canada. Although some are critical of the study and felt it overestimated the cost of the administrative burden of the U.S. health system (some $300 billion annually), no one doubts that the administration of our healthcare system is fragmented and cumbersome.[13]

Because these systems vary by their specific functionality, each system requires a significant amount of training by the medical group for all employees that will use the system. Many groups maintain training facilities for this purpose because the cost to the practice for having poorly trained employees can be substantial in terms of revenue loss and potential penalties by payers, not to mention the delay in receiving payment.

Figure 2-20 outlines the revenue cycle for most medical groups from the entry of patient service information until the claim is paid and the cycle is completed.

Medical Records

The maintenance and safekeeping of a patient's medical record is the principal function of the medical records unit. These records contain the proof of what was done, who did it, how it was done, why it was necessary to be

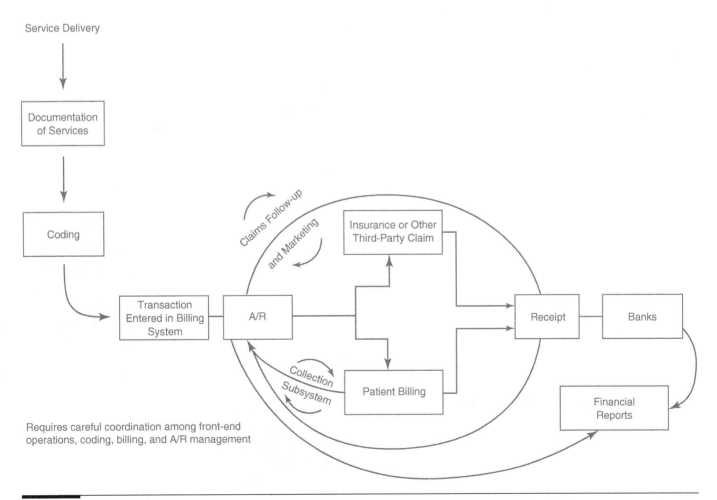

Figure 2-20 Revenue cycle.

done, and where it was done; in addition, it contains a plan for future care. One could argue with great success that this is the most valuable and important document within the medical practice.

Most group-practice records contain:

- Physician notes including a treatment plan and treatments provided
- Operative notes
- Laboratory test results and orders
- X-ray test results and orders
- All other ancillary services that may be applicable to the patient
- Communication from other providers in the form of letters or other forms of communication, such as copies of records
- Hospital records, such as discharge summaries, operative notes, and copies of test results from the hospital
- Consultative reports
- Treatment plan
- Demographic information about the patient
- Identification of the last organization to provide service to the patient
- Details of the admitting or receiving clerk
- Patient demographics
- Insurance or health plan information
- Relevant appointments
- Diagnoses
- Allergies
- Medication list
- Physician orders
- Anticipated goals (care plan), including rehabilitation plans
- Home health or hospice information
- Follow-up
- Nurse detail
- Self-care status
- Disabilities and impairments
- Equipment requirements
- Nutrition details
- Therapist details
- Social service detail

One of the great challenges of medical records management is completeness. Patient records come from so many sources, as shown in Figure 2-21.

HIPAA

The new emphasis on patient privacy has also led to new challenges. The Health Insurance Portability and Accountability Act of 1996 (HIPAA) is a very pervasive

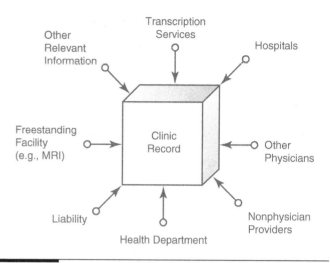

Figure 2-21 Sources of medical records information.

law that affects many aspects of group practice. The law deals with:

- Privacy of patient information
- Security of patient information
- Transaction and coding standards
- Patient identifiers[14]

It is essential that all employees are properly trained regarding HIPAA, and that all systems within the organization, including physical space, are vetted for HIPAA compliance.

Electronic Medical Records (EMRs)

One of the most dynamic areas of the medical group practice has been, and continues to be, the electronic patient record. After many years of development, however, electronic records are beginning to fulfill their promise of creating a reduced amount of paper records in the office. Although there have been electronic records systems for a number of years, and many of them have been capable systems, adaptations have been very slow, principally because innovation can be adopted only so quickly (see Figure 2-22). This fact can largely be attributed to the inherent difficulty of getting 100% adoption of the innovation, which is necessary to prevent the need to maintain multiple records systems.

Another problem is the multiple systems of medical records material; often there is a plethora of technological platforms and media formats. It is frequently impossible to find compatible ways to integrate the records, and these different medical records formats produce a regression to the lowest technological denominator. In many cases, it is paper. Scanning technology and the development of e-interfaces with computer systems, making them easier

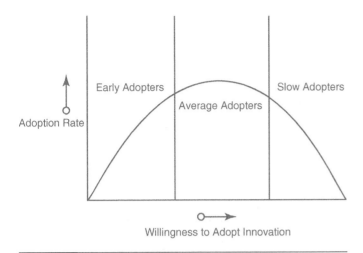

Figure 2-22 Adoptors.

to use, have overcome these issues. In addition, developers of systems are creating the ability to provide more linkages, either through using common computer code or by using common interface engines. Another positive development in the electronic records area is the precipitous drop in prices of storage media.

In spite of the inherent difficulties involved in the move to electronic medical records, this is a trend that will continue. In a survey of providers conducted by the

Medical Records Institute, the driving force for implementation continues to show an upward trend, as shown in Table 2-1.

Finance

The financial structure of medical groups is not substantially different, or at least should not be substantially different, from other organizations. One significant exception to this operation is the fact that most medical groups still maintain their financial records on a cash basis accounting system as contrasted to an accrual system. Cash basis systems recognize expenses when they are paid and income when it is received. Accrual systems recognize expenses when incurred and income when it is earned. Cash basis systems are analogous to the way our income tax system works and is undoubtedly a remnant of proprietorship, which must operate in this way. Another reason such a system has endured is at least in part the nature of medical receivables, which at times can be difficult to determine. In addition, the reversion to an accrual system once a cash system has been in place represents a formidable challenge because it requires the recognition of receivables as income. In addition, most medical groups are privately held, which means a strict adherence to generally accepted accounting principles (GAAP) is not required.

Table 2-1 Trends

	2002	2001	2000	1999
Improve the ability to share patient record information among health care practitioners and professionals within the enterprise	90%	83%	85%	73%
Improve quality of care	85	83	80	72
Improve clinical processes or work flow efficiency	83	83	81	67
Improve clinical data capture	82	78	68	61
Reduce medical errors (improve patient safety)	81	n/a	n/a	n/a
Provide access to patient records at remote locations	70	73	71	59
Facilitate clinical decision support	70	69	66	58
Improve employee/physician satisfaction	63	n/a	n/a	n/a
Improve patient satisfaction	60	59	54	40
Improve efficiency via previsit health assessments and postvisit patient education	40	38	36	n/a
Support and integrate patient health care information from Web-based personal health records	30	28	29	n/a
Retain health plan membership	9	9	7	n/a
Other	0	4	1	3
Responses to these questions	729	293	296	358

Financial systems typically maintained by a medical group are:

- Payroll
- Accounts receivable
- Billing
  - Insurance
  - Government third party
  - Self-pay
- Employee benefits
- Accounts payable
- Financial reporting
  - Balance sheet
  - Profit/loss statements (income statements)
  - Budgets
  - Variance analysis
  - Service and receipt (and its various forms)
- Financial control and audit functions
  - Internal
  - External

- Compliance
- Maintenance of fee schedules and charge masters
- Chart of accounts

Human Resources

The human resources department is responsible for the orderly management of the most important resource in the medical group practice, its people. As shown in Figure 2-23, this involves a large number of functions:

- Evaluation of positions needed by the organization
- Creation of position-control procedures
- Establishment and preparation of job descriptions
- Salary administration, which includes the establishment of pay ranges
- Recruiting, which includes seeking candidates, interviewing, and testing
- Credential evaluation and verification
- Selection of applicants

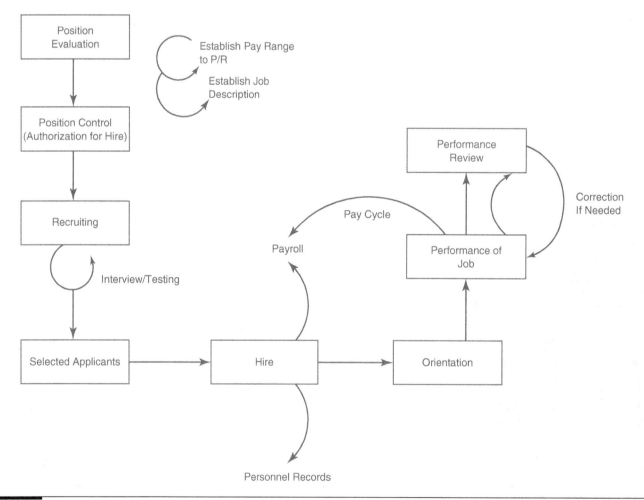

Figure 2-23 Human resources.

- Hiring and the required statutory and organizational documentation
- Orientation
- Evaluation of performance
- Documentation of work to payroll

In addition, administration of employee benefits is a vital function. Some benefit plans include the following:

- *Paid time off or PTO:* This is sick leave and vacation or personal time off.
- *Statutory benefits:* FICA, Medicare, FUTA, and state unemployment benefits.
- *Pensions:* Money purchase pensions, 401k and 457 (b) plans in the case of not for profits.
- *Insurance benefits:* Health, dental, life, and disability.
- *Section 125 plans:* These are special employee reimbursement plans that allow pretax reimbursement of certain expenses, such as noninsured medical expenses, copays, deductibles, and child care. They are so named because they are enabled by Section 125 of the Internal Revenue Code.

Another critical function of the human resources department is development and management of personnel policies, which cover a vast number and variety of issues beyond the scope of this book. However, a typical personnel manual, which contains an extensive list of issues that must be addressed by the human resources department, might look something like this:

Information Technology

Information technology (IT) is widely used for many of the functions found in medical group practices. Most larger medical group practices have now developed integrated networks to provide ready access to information and the ability to instantly update records and information related to various activities within the practice.

The IT department touches virtually every department in the clinic and provides the opportunity to share data and information and to easily access information for management and clinical use.

Often these networks include many subsystems that carry out a specific function, such as accounting, financial management, personnel and file maintenance, accounts receivable, accounts payable, billing, medical records, clinical reporting, quality assurance, and training. Figure 2-24

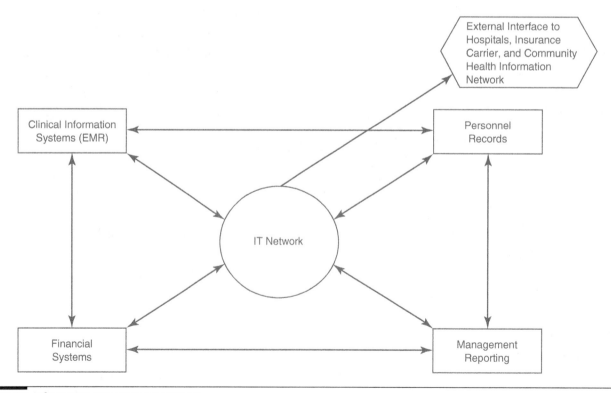

Figure 2-24 Information management systems.

shows a simplified schematic of a group-practice information system.

Increasingly, systems between organizations are being linked through network interfaces. In some cases, these networks become quite extensive and encompass many aspects of the medical community. Such systems are known as community health information networks (CHINs). A typical system includes:

- Patient portals
- Websites
- Clinical portals
- HIPAA compliance by monitoring and recording access to confidential patient information; unauthorized access can then be determined
- The ability to easily exchange information with authorized parties
- Links between different providers to share the patient's longitudinal care record

As the Internet has become faster and more available, especially high-speed access, the interaction of the medical group practice with all of its stakeholders has become increasingly possible.

The Internet has begun to significantly change how the group practice operates. Both clinical and business operations are involved in this revolution. The World Wide Web is cost-effective, makes possible ready access to information for review, and is a vehicle for updating records.

Web portals have become the key to an effective Internet strategy. The key element is the practice website. Frequently, a practice's website becomes the portal of entry to the practice, and not only serves as a vehicle for the prospective patient to obtain information about the practice, but also is increasingly becoming a method of two-way communication.

Websites should:

- Be easy to navigate
- Be updated frequently
- Contain accurate and relevant information, including such topics as services, directions, physician information, specialized care and services, policies, community activities, and research being conducted

Similar to the electronic availability of records, the notion that organizations can be connected to better service the patient is a concept that has been developing over the years. These CHINs will likely gain additional vigor as more emphasis is placed on patient-centered care.

The specialist referral process can create significant frustration for both referring physicians and patients which can be greatly reduced when the referring specialist is connected to the patient care network. In interviews with physicians, here are some of the most common statements and findings:

- Referral coordinators are often on the phone 20 to 30 minutes to get an appointment.
- Managed-care influences access and administrative burden.
- Appointments are difficult to get in a timely fashion.
- Despite the proliferation of information technology, the referral process continues to lack sophistication, clear customer interfaces, and information flow.
- Specialist feedback, when provided, is written and sent through the mail.
- Patient records are often misplaced.

Patient Communication and Access

Some 25% of patients use the Internet for health information.[15,16] The Internet is becoming the great "democratizer" of healthcare information. Patients, however, want that information to come from their physicians. In a recent survey of 400 patients with an average age of 59.1 years, 44.1% indicated they had access to e-mail; of those, 58.6% said they would like to communicate with their physician in this manner. Certainly, this finding supports the idea that healthcare is becoming a more collaborative venture between the physician and the patient.

Facilities Management

For smaller practices with a single location, facilities management may be a function within administration. The function of facilities management is to acquire and maintain the physical facilities of the organization. This involves:

- Leasing or purchase of the space
- Construction management of building or renovation projects
- Acquisition of fixtures, such as office furniture and equipment
- Maintaining the property and equipment to ensure that the clinic is able to function at all times

These activities may also be done through a series of outsourcing and maintenance arrangements, such as maintenance contracts, but the coordination and supervision of this function cannot be overlooked. Facilities that are in poor condition or not functioning not only are ineffective, but also can be a considerable liability to the practice.

Purchasing and Supply Management

The purchase of supplies and other necessary items for the practice requires special attention to the following concerns:

- Dependability
- Discounts for bulk orders
- Price and quality
- Relationship with current vendors
- Customization
- Market exclusivity
- Value
- Delivery schedules
- Guarantees
- Safety for the purchasing agent

The current state of the art in medical group management uses computerized systems to purchase supplies and equipment for the organization and to manage the supply chain for the practice. The characteristics of these systems are:

- A common catalogue (used to control items that are ordered). Many groups with automated systems have a difficult time controlling the number of sources and the scope of the items purchased. This is especially true in groups with a number of offices in different geographic areas.
- A rule-based established ordering program that requires authorization of purchases from the approved catalogue.
- A system to control and document receipt of goods and the accuracy of the ordered items, which provides an effective method to verify delivery of products and establish whether the order is correct in terms of quantity and price.

Important features included in many of the newer software products include:

- Online requisitioning (electronic catalogs incorporated)
- Transaction-based audit trails
- Online approvals and purchasing
- Automated faxing
- Internal messaging
- Request for quotation
- Electronic ordering capabilities
- Standing orders
- Freeform orders
- Rule builder
- Transaction-based reporting
- Predictive reporting

- Multiuser defined pick lists
- In/out status tracking
- Purchase order attachments
- Real-time status updates
- Purchase order consolidation

In addition to control, automated procurement provides the practice with better opportunities for inventory control and taking advantage of economies of scale when purchasing.

Clinical Activities and Departments

Medical group practice provides a large variety of patient services in addition to the physician visit. Physician services are often loosely divided into office-based services and hospital-based services, but the line is rapidly beginning to blur. Group clinic operations often include:

- Clinical laboratory services
- Radiology services
- Ultrasound
- Nuclear medicine
- Computerized axial tomography
- Nuclear magnetic resonance imaging
- Outpatient surgery, sometimes within the context of the ambulatory surgery center
- Dietary counseling services

Other clinical services such as preventive care are often organized into a unique department of the group practice.

The organization of each medical service department requires careful attention to a host of legal, licensing, and regulatory requirements. It also may be necessary in many states to obtain a Certificate of Need (CON) or other regulatory approval for certain services, depending on the cost of the service and the compliance of the service with community standards of care and state health plans.

Clinical services must be organized and managed by properly licensed and knowledgeable professionals. Such services also require adherence to standards that are established by various professional societies and credentialing bodies. Approval and certification of operations often are required by state departments of health and by major payers before payments are made on behalf of covered individuals.

Quality Assessment: An Important Focus

A major barrier to change and improvement activities in medical groups is the problem of variation. Variation equals cost. This variation, as noted earlier, is one inherent reason for the slow growth of group medical practice. In addition, the variability in the delivery of care has been associated with the fragmentation of quality and the inability to leverage economies of scale to any great degree in physician practice.

This has become one of the most important areas of concern for the medical group. The Institute of Medicine (IOM) released a report, "To Err Is Human,"[17] which has been a hotly debated topic, but nonetheless has strong support from the social science and economics disciplines. These are issues that everyone in group management needs to understand, and these issues should be the basis for quality assurance and risk management activities. Regardless of our feelings on the matter, there are many critics of the healthcare system and all of its components. These voices are increasingly being heard and simply cannot and should not be ignored. The medical group is a quasi-public organization, although most groups are privately owned. To illustrate this point, consider that 60% of all healthcare in the United States is paid for by government entities, and public scrutiny of healthcare and its regulations is increasing. Medical groups will continue to be a source of public interest and debate.

It is important to have some background on the nature of quality improvement and the critical need for it in the medical group. Unlike in most other industries, quality is difficult to define and measure for the typical consumer/patient. First, consider the asymmetric nature of healthcare, which is characterized by situations in which the parties on the opposite sides of a transaction have differing amounts of relevant information. Examples of asymmetric knowledge include:

- Vendors typically know more about the strengths and weaknesses of their products than do purchasers.
- Employees typically know more about their health problems than do human resource or health plan managers.
- Subordinates typically know more about the effort that they have put into assignments than do their superiors.
- Providers typically know more about the treatment options than do their patients.

Another widely discussed concern by critics of the medical industry is that physicians and other healthcare providers have the unique ability to create supplier-induced demand (SID). SID is characterized by a change in demand for medical care services associated with the discretionary influence of providers, especially physicians, over their patients. This is demand that provides for the self-interest of providers rather than solely for the patients' interests.

Critics of the healthcare system, and of physicians in general, have often pointed to small area variations (SAVs) as evidence of a physician's ability to increase the use of services. SAV was documented by John Wennberg,[18,19] and is defined as large variations in the per capita rates of utilization across small, homogenous areas for many medical and surgical procedures.

The Social Concerns for Healthcare Delivery

The detractors of our healthcare system do not stop with Wennberg and, in fact, go much further. In his book *Medical Nemesis*, Ivan Illich delivers a stinging indictment of the healthcare system. He says, "The major threat to health in the world is modern medicine. The medical community has actually become a great threat to people. Doctors and others (pharmaceutical industry) serve their own interests first. People become consumers and objects."[20] He identifies three levels of damage:

1. Clinical treatment actually often harms people. Patient safety has not been a high priority.

2. More and more problems are seen as amenable to medical intervention. Pharmaceutical companies develop expensive treatments for nondiseases.

3. Over 100,000 people a year die from adverse drug effects.

It is a new idea that everything, including labor and culture, can be assigned a market value. However, such a practice destroys traditional ways of dealing with death, pain, and sickness.

Thomas McKeown, a leading expert on social medicine and another prominent critic of our healthcare system, asserts in his book, *The Role of Medicine*, that the role of medicine and doctors in improving human health has been greatly overstated. Rather than through treatment of the disease state, disease is best addressed through prevention and only secondarily through treatment.

Longevity of life has increased through factors such as:

- Reduction in infectious diseases because of genetic reactions
- Better nutrition
- Elimination of infanticide

McKeown goes on to say medical research is of limited value and researchers too often focus on "basic research" at the expense of socially useful research.[21]

It is essential that we have programs to demonstrate quality care that is appropriate, cost-effective, and in the best interest of patients. We need to understand our outcomes and our process so we can better explain away the "black box" nature of the profession to our detractors.

Quality Improvement and the Effective Medical Group

The issue of the quality of the service provided by group practices is paramount to group-practice operations and the future of healthcare. In addition to the critics of healthcare services, paying for performance is becoming a reality. Being capable of responding to the changes in payment systems, such as pay or performance, starts with understanding what the medical group is really about. The first section of this chapter discusses the many structures and attributes of group practice. Organizing for delivery of quality has not been a central theme in group practices because many structural and operational considerations have been focused on issues other than the quality of care. The lack of standardization, the absence of any formal adherence to best practices, and the lack of formalized quality improvement for programs all contribute to a lack of progress in delivering quality service.

This is not to say that financial issues are not important. Medical group structures are not designed, or in some cases are antithetically designed, to invest in quality initiatives. The extreme short-term focus of financial performance is a chief culprit. Groups do not invest either financially or in the training needed to carry out large-scale improvement initiatives. Investment dollars can only come from the shareholders' pockets, a prospect that has long curtailed the development of modern medical groups.

In his book *Out of the Crisis*, W. Edwards Deming asks a question that should serve as the cornerstone of any group's quality initiative:

> What are you doing about the quality that you hope to provide to your customers four years from now?[22]

The issue of quality in the U.S. healthcare system is an increasingly important one as we begin to better understand what quality means. For most of history, quality has been virtually undefined. As Voltaire would have said, it is indeed "in the eye of the beholder." However, that is changing dramatically as the ability to measure quality evolves and expectations of the quality of health services become higher.

As mentioned earlier, variation, or put another way, lack of standardization, is a central theme throughout group practices. We know our healthcare system usually produces superior outcomes, so why the variations: different standing admission and discharge orders for patients, treatment protocols also vary for the same disease or condition, surgery vs. medical treatment, for example? There are many potential causes.

So what do we do about it? Quality must be a core value of medical group practice, and that value must be expressed by having a systematic way of monitoring and improving quality in the medical group practice.

Identifying Issues That Require Examination and Correction

There are many opportunities to evaluate the practice. Some of the most fruitful areas in which to find projects for quality improvement activities are:

- Patient satisfaction surveys
- Malpractice claims review
- Benchmarking clinical and nonclinical data
- Standards established by specialty societies
- Review and understanding of national data such as all of the departments of the National Institutes of Health (see http://www.nih.gov/icd) and the Agency for Healthcare Research and Quality (see http://www.ahrq.gov)

Initiatives on quality require a systematic approach to reduce the influence of bias and emotions on the process. Many techniques have been used, including:

- Total Quality Management (TQM)[23]
- Continuous Quality Improvement (CQI)[24]
- Six Sigma[25-27]

All of these processes use statistical measures to evaluate an identified process to determine the source of error and variation in outcome. There are many resources on the actual techniques, and the reader is referred to these sources for more complete information.

However, all of these techniques have the same fundamental premise. They all involve the following steps:

1. Plan and determine the process to be examined and a clear delineation of the process.
2. Measure the process activities.
3. Analyze using various statistical techniques. This can involve one or more of the tools shown in Table 2-2.

All of these techniques seek to identify the variation in outcomes and then assign the nature of the cause of variation or error. These are often referred to as special causes, such as human error, or common cause, which are the results of the process itself. An example of this might

Table 2-2	Methods for Measuring/Monitoring Quality
Technique	**Description**
Histogram	Shows the range and depth of variation in a group of continuous data
Frequency plot	Displays discrete "count" data (number of defects)
Process maps	Charts a series of tasks (rectangles) and decisions/reviews (diamonds), connected by arrows to show the flow of work
Pareto chart	Stratifies data into groups from largest to smallest
Time series plot or run chart	Chart show how things change from moment to moment, day to day, etc. (see Figure 2-25 as an example)
Scatter plot	Shows the correlation between two factors that vary by count or on a continuum

be billing error due to improper coding. Run charts are very commonly used to evaluate data for common and special causes, as shown in Figure 2-25.

Variation is depicted as upper- and lower-control limits once the data are plotted. The run chart then shows the natural variation in the system, or the areas between the upper- and lower-control limits. Special causes can then be said to be those that fall outside these limits.

These quality assurance (QA) processes depend heavily on virtually everyone involved in the activity being trained to use the measurement tools needed to evaluate the process. The time and expense involved in doing this is one of the major difficulties in having an effective process-improvement program.

One of the more popular systems being used in process improvement today is Six Sigma. It is interesting considering the level of performance that Six Sigma implies and what users of the system are able to achieve.[28] Six Sigma takes the absolute number of unacceptable outcomes as a

percentage of all outcomes to determine the sigma level, as shown in Table 2-3.

U.S. industry is seeking the Six Sigma level of performance as a quality standard. It is probably unrealistic to achieve this in group-practice activities. For example, can many medical groups produce an error rate less than 3.4 per million appointments, transaction postings, or filed claims? How about diagnostic or treatment errors? The usefulness of Six Sigma in the medical group practice remains to be seen; even if sigma level six is not achievable, improvement is certainly possible using tools such as Lean and other quality management concepts.

Another important issue is the concept of the Type I and Type II error. Type I errors in process improvement occur when the evaluator concludes incorrectly that the observed outcome is caused by the data point being considered. Figures 2-26, 2-27, and 2-28 show examples of a potential Type I error.[a]

It might be logical to conclude that group size would influence total medical revenue per FTE physician (as reviewed in Figure 2-26), but when regression analysis is carried out, R-squared is only 0.0001, meaning that this has almost no effect on the outcome. (R-squared is a measure of the percentage of cause that can be accounted for by the variable under analysis while holding all other variables consistent.) Figure 2-27 shows a similar analysis for cardiology groups who accept Medicare. Logic might say that groups with high percentages also have lower total incomes, but this is not true according to these data.

A final example of Type I error, as seen in Figure 2-28, shows the effect of commercial insurance on total income. The conclusion must mean that other factors are more

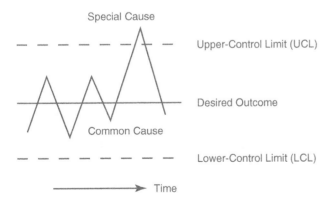

The greater the distance between UCL and LCL, the greater the variation due to systemic causes.

Figure 2-25 Chart control.

a. Charts in Figures 2-26, 2-27, and 2-28 were prepared with assistance from David N. Gans, MSHA, CMPE, MGMA Practice Management Resources Director, Denver, Colorado.

Table 2-3	Sigma Level Determination	
The absolute number of unacceptable outcomes per million observations	The percentage of unacceptable outcomes	The Six Sigma level
690,000	69.0000%	1.0
500,000	50.0000%	1.5
308,000	69.2000%	2.0
158,700	84.1300%	2.5
66,800	93.3000%	3.0
22,700	97.7300%	3.5
6,210	99.4000%	4.0
1,300	99.8700%	4.5
320	99.9800%	5.0
30	99.9970%	5.5
3.4	99.9997%	6.0

responsible for effects on total income than those examined. If action is taken to correct an erroneous cause of an effect, tampering occurs and then systems may actually become more variable.

Type II errors result from situations in which the cause is not recognized as being produced by the variable being analyzed. This is most likely caused by a failure in the process, improper data collection, or improper analysis. A type I error would conclude, for example, that drug A is better than the drug B, when in fact it is not. A type II error would conclude that drug A and B are equivalent when in fact the drug B is superior. In some cases the system may be so complex that it defies the use of these techniques. The results would be affected by the tendency

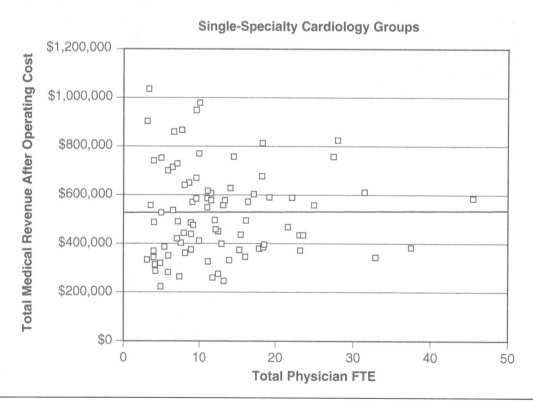

Figure 2-26 Revenue by number of FTE physicians.

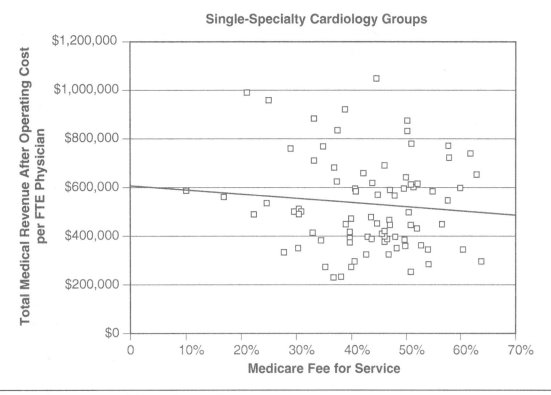

Figure 2-27 Revenue by percentage of charges from medicare.

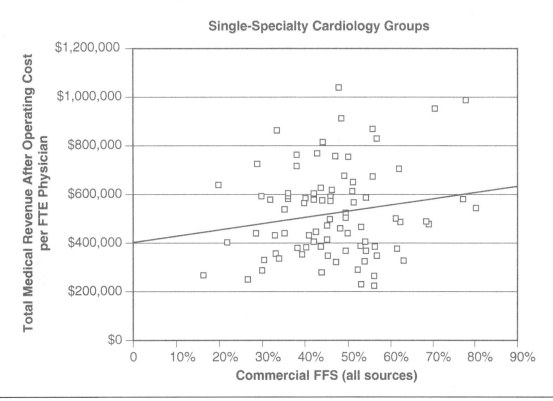

Figure 2-28 Revenue by percentage of charges from commercial insurance.

to undercontrol the process. This is the inherent nature of healthcare, and Type II errors are probable.

It is impossible to monitor all activities of the practice continuously in real time. Consider, for example, that in a large practice with 100 physicians, depending on the specialty, there can be as many as 1,000 visits a day, with other services adding thousands of additional transactions to the system, all of which have a "customized" feature. Control charts, the patient satisfaction survey, and the other techniques available to the practice are essential to help identify areas of the clinic that need to be examined in a systematic way.

Research

Many medical groups are engaged in significant research as part of the clinical activity of the group. This is almost always clinical research as opposed to basic research, and is usually divided into two general categories:

1. Premarket research
2. Postmarket research

This research is regulated by the Food and Drug Administration (FDA). As the name implies, premarket research is conducted prior to the FDA's approval to market the device or medication, and postmarket research is conducted to "monitor the ongoing safety of marketed products." This is accomplished by reassessing drug and device risks based on new data learned after the product is marketed, and recommending ways of trying to most appropriately manage that risk.[29]

The key players in the research department are:

- *The principle investigator (PI):* Usually this is a physician; the PI is responsible for conducting the clinical research.
- *The director:* Responsible for the administration of the project and often involved in the acquisition of projects.
- *Research nurses:* Conduct research, collect data, and manage the research information as well as reporting.
- *Support staff:* Assist the nurses and director in their duties by providing logistical support such as clerical work.
- *The institutional review board (IRB):* An independent body responsible for reviewing and approving proposed research involving human subjects. The role of the IRB is principally to help ensure that research is as safe as possible and that the potential benefits of the research outweigh any possible harm that could be caused to the experimental subjects.

A protocol is also needed. This is the written procedures and processes required by the project. It indicates which patients are eligible to participate in the research, what the endpoints of the research are to be, what measurements and data are needed, and what must be reported. Follow-up care of the subjects is also typically specified.

Figure 2-29 illustrates the process of medical research in the practice environment. As more new drugs and devices are discovered, research opportunities will continue to increase and become an increasingly important part of the medical group. Research also offers the advantage of intellectual challenge, and can be a source of great professional satisfaction.

Reform, New Forms, and Medical Practice Management

The U.S. healthcare system is caught up in a virtual whirlwind of information about the Patient Protection and Affordable Care Act of 2010 (PPACA),[30] and many people are trying to understand what reform means and how to respond to it. The overwhelming amount of information about this act puts healthcare practitioners in the position of trying to drink from a fire hose. Though little of the actual regulatory framework is completed, the bill is already enormous and it is likely that much of what is now known will change in some way. The wiser organizations are those focusing on the principles of the act, rather than the specific details. It is better to see the lake than just the ripple. With that said, this act will likely cause the most rapid transformation of an industry in U.S. history, so not to prepare and consider what is happening, to just wait and see, is probably a foolish approach.

Healthcare is discussed in the media or in political circles nearly every day. This discussion is often infused with a great deal of rancor and emotion. On the one hand, some believe very strongly that the plan goes too far. Indeed, there is a serious effort underway to repeal the reform bill, albeit few expect it to be successful; however, constitutional challenges are underway nonetheless. On the other hand, many believe the plan does not go far enough and does not focus enough on true reforms of the broken healthcare system. Regardless of providers' emotions and personal feelings on the issues of healthcare reform, they are involved in a trifecta of issues: access, cost, and quality. As illustrated in Figure 2-30, these issues are inextricably linked, and affecting the outcome of one issue will affect the others. Much of the debate and political activity has centered on how it is possible to obtain optimal outcomes for each of these important factors.

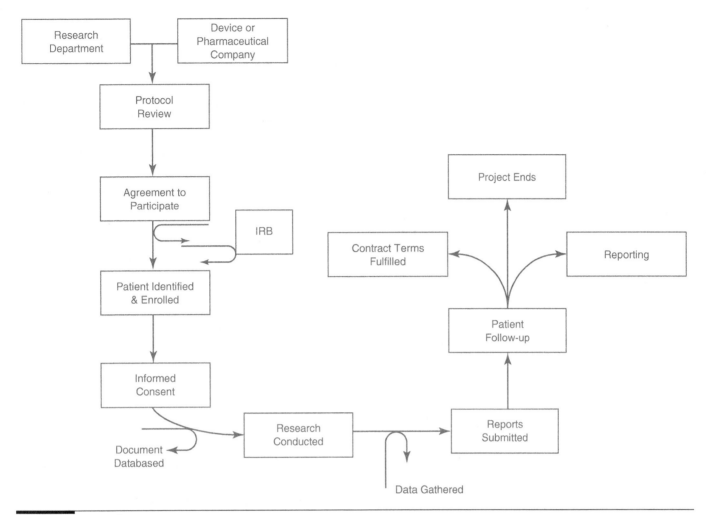

Figure 2-29 Research project.

The economic crisis makes healthcare reform an even more popular topic. In a recent article in *BusinessWeek* entitled, "USA, Inc.: Red, White, and Very Blue,"[31] Mary Meeker makes a compelling case that the nation is in a fiscal crisis: "By our rough estimate, USA Inc. has a net worth of negative $44 trillion. That comes to $143,000 per capita. Negative." She argues that this has much to do with our healthcare system and our Medicare and Medicaid programs. Indeed, the cost of healthcare is a major issue in U.S. society because it consumes almost 20% of gross domestic product. Because of this and many other reasons, it's clear that the time has come for change in the healthcare system. In her book, *Sudden Death*, Rita Brown wrote, "The true definition of insanity is doing the same thing over and over again and expecting a different result." In many ways this is what has occurred in healthcare. In spite of advancing knowledge and technology in medicine, the basic way care is delivered has changed very little. As was so eloquently stated by the Coen Brothers in the movie, *Oh Brother Where Art Thou*, we are still, "one-at-a timin'" it,[b] instead of taking a more population-based approach to health and healthcare delivery.

There is increasing recognition that the system has to change, and at the center of this change is the physician. The rules and administrative regulations such as

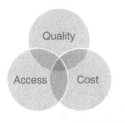

Figure 2-30 Healthcare issues.

b. *O Brother, Where Art Thou?* (2001). *Pappy O'Daniel*: I'll press your flesh, you dimwitted sumbitch! You don't tell your pappy how to court the electorate. We ain't one-at-a-timin' here. We're *mass* communicating!

precertification and complex policy restrictions will not improve consumer health and will only provide temporary relief from rising cost. Without improvement of health there is little chance of achieving the goal to reduce cost and improve access and quality.

The lack of collaborative approaches to care delivery has not served the goal of improving health very well. Unfortunately, healthcare has a tribal culture. Healthcare providers have lived in silos, independent and competing to provide increasing amounts of service to poorly informed patient populations. This has been driven by a payment system fraught with perverse incentives, regulation that often makes little sense, and so much focus on cost that the bigger picture of health and healthcare has been ignored. The complexity of the healthcare system is now beyond anyone's understanding. Karl Weick has aptly described this breakdown of understanding as a loss of "sensemaking."[32] (*Sensemaking* is the process by which people give meaning to experience.)

The healthcare profession must make an effort to return to sensemaking. One of the ways to do this is by understanding the most important pieces of the reform puzzle and how they affect the bigger picture of healthcare in the United States. Accountable care systems are one of these important pieces. The concept of an integrated delivery system (IDS) is not a new one by any means; however, the PPACA significantly increased the importance of this arena. The transition to more accountable care models and de-emphasis of activity-based reimbursement as a mechanism of payment has moved healthcare providers to consider new ways to organize and deliver care to large numbers of people and to consider care as a population management function rather than a series of care episodes.

Payment for outcomes, not just activities, also changes the strategic and operational focus. Value-based purchasing requires a major change in thinking about how to provide incentives to organizations and define success. The Public simply cannot pay for volume of service. We must pay for outcomes and quality.

The other major challenge will be the transition. Currently, physicians are largely paid based on production of services; few, if any, are prepared to make an abrupt switch to other reimbursement methodologies. Realistically, this transition is going to have to be an incremental process, but it will have to occur if the necessary fundamental change is to occur.

Basic Changes from PPACA

PPACA created a sea change in federal policy. In spite of the fact that the bill is thousands of pages long and will likely produced tens of thousands of pages of regulations, it has fundamentally created a three-legged policy stool for healthcare's future, focusing on the following:

- *Meaningful use:* The reform emphasizes the use of electronic connectivity to improve care for patients and the efficiency of that care. Figure 2-31 shows the three stages of meaningful use:
  - *MU Stage 1 (CMS Final Rule):* Provide patients with electronic copy of (and access to) their health information, discharge instructions, clinical summaries.
  - *MU Stage 2 (Concepts):* Offer secure patient-provider messaging and access to patient-specific educational resources; upload data from home monitoring devices.
  - MU Stage 3 (Concepts): Provide patients with access to self-management tools; capture accountable care organizations (ACO): electronic reporting on experience of care.
- *Value-based purchasing:* The value of service has to be seen as a function not only of the service, but also of the quality of that service. It is easy to measure dollars, but not so easy to measure the quality of care; however, electronic records and contemporaneous recording of care information will make this a feasible process and increase the accuracy and transparency of the data dramatically. These concepts can be expressed by the following equation: $Value = f \ cost \times quality$
- *Accountable care organizations (ACOs):* These organizations are a centerpiece of the legislation and represent a fundamental structure for the delivery of high quality lower cost care and population management. The ACOs may also include another innovative care model, the patient-centered

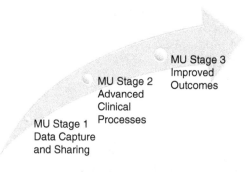

Figure 2-31 The stages of meaningful use building in their utility.
Sources: ONC HIT Policy Committee, 2010; MU Final Rule. 2010. Wagner SL and MR. Engaging patients in their health care using an interactive patient portal. Presented February 24, at the Healthcare IT Conference and Exhibition 11, Orlando, Florida.

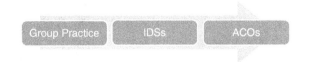

Figure 2-32 Group practices are one potential cornerstone for the ACO

medical home (PCMH). ACOs are a major focal point of reform, and physicians are an inherent part of ACOs because a physician organization must be the founding partner of an ACO (see Figure 2-32).

ACOs and PCMHs are receiving a lot of attention as potential solutions or responses to reform. Both seek to create structures that are more responsive to the issues raised by, and the goals of, reform. The PCMH actually fits nicely into the ACO model, which this chapter will touch on—at least as it has been conceived and piloted to date.

The ACO broadens the scope and depth of services offered by an organization and requires the full engagement of the medical practice. In fact, the medical practice is core to the ACO model. It requires a move from a silo mentality to a collaborative approach to care that will lead to meaningful clinical integration (see Figure 2-33).

PCMHs were more clearly defined and explored by in an article by Wagner entitled, "Chronic Disease Management: What Will It Take to Improve Care for Chronic Illness?"[35] The medical home has a number of definitions, but its essential elements are the provision of primary-based care and the coordination and management of other services through the primary care home.[36] The PCMH as proposed by Wagner is gaining a significant amount of attention and has now become a mainstream concept in accountable care. The National Committee for Quality Assurance (NCQA) now has guidance and certification guidelines for the PCMH.

Accountable Care and Accountable Care Organizations

The concepts of accountable care are not new. Many of the ideas embodied in the PPACA harken back to the days

when Paul Ellwood coined the term *health maintenance organization (HMO)*.[37,38] The key concepts are as follows:

- Collaborative business and care strategies
- Documentation
- Cost
- Connectedness

Health and Human Services Secretary Donald Berwick talks about accountability as the "triple aim" of reform:

- Population management
- Patient experience
- Per capita cost

At the heart of what organizations must do to create meaningful reform is this triple aim. Berwick's focus on these three fundamental issues is similar to what is being suggested by everyone, regardless of their political perspective.

The Accountable Care Continuum

Accountable care ranges along a continuum of care from solo practice to extensive employment of physicians in a large healthcare system (see Figure 2-34). The alignment of these physician practices allows a number of functions to be integrated and also allows for greater clinical integration and care delivery. This, at a minimum, includes having the following elements:

- Care standards
- Coordinated infrastructure
- Performance measurement and management
- Meaningful incentives for accountable care
- Joint contracting, bundled payments, and value-based payment models
- Virtual care networks based on specialties or service lines

As defined by the Centers for Medicare and Medicaid Services (CMS) in the March 31, 2011, publication,[39] there are a number of possible management and formal legal structures that would qualify as ACOs involving group medical practice:

- ACO professionals in group practice arrangements
- Networks of individual practices of ACO professionals

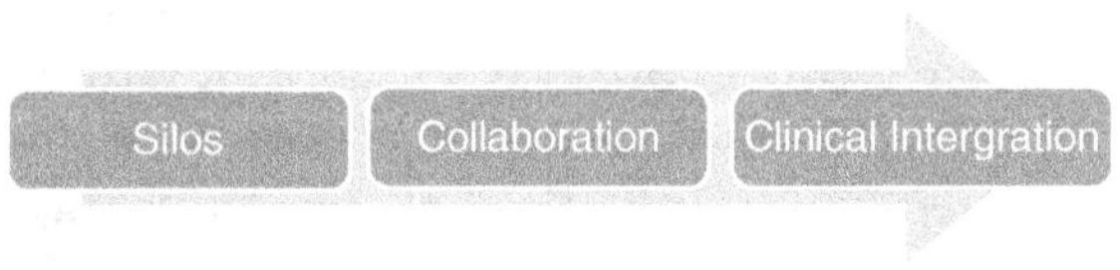

Figure 2-33 The integration of clinical services promises to improve quality by decreasing the fragmentation of care.

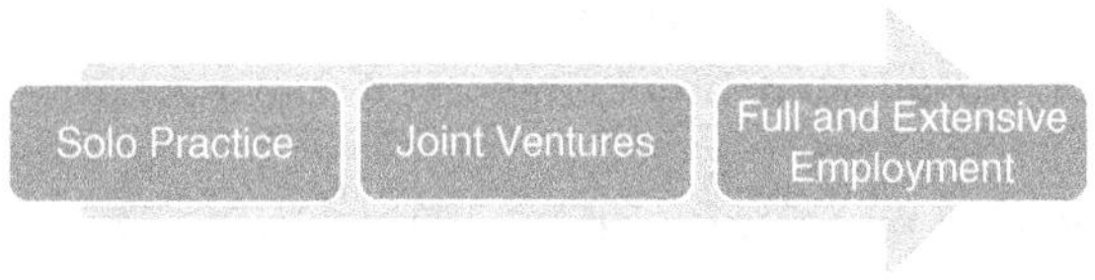

Figure 2-34 The integration of medical practice into IDS and ACO model.

- Partnerships or joint venture arrangements between hospitals and ACO professionals
- Hospitals employing ACO professionals
- Other groups of providers of services and suppliers deemed appropriate by the Secretary of the Department of Health and Human Services (DHHS)

Regulations have now been published by CMS that define specific requirements for the ACO.

- Each ACO will have shared governance and leadership that makes joint decisions in operations, and provide administrative and clinical systems.
- Each ACO must have an agreement with DHHS to participate in the ACO program for no less than a period of 3 years.
- A minimum of 5,000 Medicare beneficiaries are required.
- The ACO must both receive and administer payment of shared savings to participant organizations.
- The ACO must use patient and caregiver assessments or individualized care plans.
- The ACO coordinates care through the use of Telehealth, remote patient monitoring, and other enabling technologies.
- The ACO will promote evidence-based medicine and patient engagement.
- Each ACO must use specific quality measures identified by DHHS and also include care transitions across care settings. Additionally, this reporting will incorporate requirements of the physician quality reporting initiatives (PQRI).
- A benchmark must be established for each ACO's 3-year period with the most recent 3 years of "per-beneficiary expenditures" assigned to the ACO. When an ACO beats established benchmarks, a percentage of the difference may be paid to the ACO and the program will retain the remainder.[39]

One potential barrier to participation is the concern about taking financial risk for patients in the ACO. The current legislation provided substantial risk to providers and providers within the same ACO must determine how to share the risk of potential revenue shortfalls. The old method of payment reform—a method of financial engineering in which money is moved around the board and squabbled about, without any real change in what is done or how it is done—is no longer a viable reform methodology. That incessant need to shift risk will prevent true reform, which has to be born out of a collaborative model, not a competitive one.[40] Meaningful changes in the way care is delivered and in the way healthcare providers look

at performance are essential in the new era, regardless of what legal, regulatory, or healthcare market changes occur. The healthcare profession has kicked the can as far down the road as possible in dealing with fundamental system improvement.

In the end, accountable care has several imperatives: the first is to act. There must be uniform standards, open structures, and process that allow the "liquefaction" of information, allowing information to be easily shared and managed. These care models must have a code for prevention and managing care at their core, with local caregivers in a local environment connected to other networks and services either in a virtual way or in fact. These ideas will be expressed digitally and in a practice setting. In order to adopt truly accountable care, a team culture has to arise, one that is far beyond anything seen today. This team culture must pay serious attention to administrative capabilities and shared best practices.

The Effect of Scale on Reform Efforts

Scale is also significant, in two dimensions:

- *Size:* The practice must serve enough people to make economic and system scale a reality.
- *Depth of offerings:* One size does not fit all.

It may be a great irony that all the digital aspects and the size of developing organizations may actually allow healthcare providers to offer more personalized service. Banks can provide great service because customers provide services to themselves, on their terms, customized to meet their needs. The bank provides the platform, customers do the rest. Isn't more of this needed in healthcare? In a recent study presented to the Health Information and Management Systems Society 2011 Annual Conference (HIMSS11), Wagner and Solomon were able to show a significant effect on patient activation by using online self-management tools.[41] So patient engagement is a significant and currently missing ingredient in the U.S. healthcare system. Patients will need to be able to self-define what they need within the boundaries of sound medical practice. An example would be diabetes education. Currently many practices provide a single level of diabetic education. There is little reason this could not be interactive and self-managed, giving virtually an unlimited number of offerings unique to each patient's educational level, interest, and understanding. All of this allows healthcare providers to create incentives that further their cause, not distract and detract from it.

The rules and specifics of reform and these new structures will undoubtedly change, but in the end, future progress will depend on the answer an organization can give to these four questions:

1. *Are we prepared to govern in the new era of healthcare?* Developing leadership is imperative. Developing physician leadership will be essential and challenging.

2. *Do we have the management structure in place to deal with all of the tasks and requirements?* Developing new ways of collaboration and a culture of teamwork is imperative. Think about payments in a new way, not simply producing service.

3. *Do we have the infrastructure in place?* Developing infrastructure is imperative to being able to understand, manage, and account for care.

4. *Are we a patient-centered organization or can we be one?* Can this be done not just in name or by regulation, but in fact? Patient activation and engagement are imperative: we have to become a medical home in name and in spirit.

These are enormous cultural changes for many if not most healthcare organizations.[42] Are they up to the challenge? The reality is that they may have little choice. This may be the last opportunity to reform in a way that is transformational rather than draconian. Few, if anyone, really thinks the present situation is optimal or sustainable. Either healthcare leads change or change will drive healthcare: remember there is a choice.

Emergency Preparedness in Medical Groups

The assessment of risk and preparation for the unthinkable has significantly changed in recent years. Hurricane Katrina, September 11th, and the Fukushima Daiichi nuclear plant incident have caused people to think about these unexpected and often unpredictable events more carefully. What do these changes mean to medical group executives? Medical groups, especially those that are part of larger systems, may no longer simply be able to close their doors in emergency situations, but may need to become an integral part of the resilience of the community. If a large-scale disaster occurs, clinic offices and physician practices may need to serve as an important part of the emergency medical care delivery system. Certainly, the resources of the medical group could play a vital role, but it must be adequately prepared to be in a position to do so.[43]

Most medical groups have some sort of an emergency plan, but those plans deal largely with operations and business from an isolated and internal view. A plan of this nature only addresses the practice itself and frequently does not take into account how the practice fits into the context of the larger community. Medical practices need to consider their role in community preparedness and may seek to become a partner in the community emergency preparedness planning process. Every group will have to consider its own circumstances and how it might want to be involved or not, but this should be an active consideration rather than a decision made at a time of crisis.[44]

A large number of resources are available to medical groups trying to make decisions about emergency preparedness and their role in the context of the larger community. The Federal Emergency Management Agency (FEMA) has a large number of specific planning tools and other resources that are freely available and easily accessed from the Internet.

Your group might also want to consider being a part of the National Mutual Aid and Resource Management Initiative, which helps to provide medical personnel in emergency situations.[45]

Medical groups interested in emergency preparedness will need to focus on several important issues:

- Basic management of resources
- Organization
- Delegation of authority
- Coordination
- Communication
- Evaluation[46]

At a minimum, the organization needs to consider the following elements and what they mean to the group practice[46,47]:

- *Communication:* Communication strategies must be established to direct and communicate response information to staff, patients, families, and external agencies. There must be backup communication processes and technologies in place and a common terminology in use.
- *Resources and assets:* Resource and asset management strategies that continue to care for the group's staff and patients are essential for an emergency response. Plans must be developed to address inventories of resources as well as critical supply procurement, possibly from multiple vendors.
- *Safety and security:* During an emergency, it is crucial that the hospital control the movement of patients, staff, visitors, and volunteers within the hospital. Processes for hazardous material

management, decontamination, and control of access as well as egress must be developed, coordinated, and practiced with outside community partners.

- *Staff responsibilities:* Staff must be oriented and trained in their assigned responsibilities during an emergency based on a Hazard Vulnerability Analysis. The use of job action sheets and checklists to assist staff members could be instituted. Cross-training of personnel to perform other than normal duties during an emergency is an important consideration as well. An example of this would be training accounting staff to serve as patient transporters.

- *Utility management:* Hospitals must find alternative means to provide potable and nonpotable water, sanitation, fuel, and electricity. Memorandums of understanding and/or relationships with suppliers and emergency community managers can enhance implementation of this process in a time of crisis.

- *Patient and clinic support activities:* Fundamentally, protecting life and preventing disability are the goals of emergency management. A process for swift triage of those patients able to be discharged should be in place. Management of patient treatment should include attention to the special needs population as well as personal hygiene and sanitation. The ability to scale back noncritical operations or elective procedures to open up space and personnel for the emergency is also critical. Hospitals must be able to create a scalable response to meet the needs of the emergency.

Social Media for Medical Group Preparedness

Social media are becoming an increasingly important method of communications in today's society and may offer some especially attractive elements for emergency situations when more routine channels are down. The Centers for Disease Control and Prevention (CDC) provides information and resources for preparing for and responding to public health emergencies. The CDC has created four badges that healthcare organizations can copy and paste onto a website, social network profile, blog, or e-mail to provide people with access to information on how to prepare for emergencies like hurricanes or floods. Small computer applications are available, for example, CDC social media for badges, widgets, and content syndication and these may be useful in medical group emergency preparedness.[47]

References

1. Havlicek PL. *Medical group practices in the U.S.—a survey of practice characteristics.* Chicago: American Medical Association; 1999.
2. Thompson JD. *Organizations and action.* New York: McGraw-Hill; 1967.
3. Robbins SP. *Organizational theory: structure, design and applications,* 3rd ed. Upper Saddle River, NJ: Prentice Hall; 1990:191, 249.
4. Showalter JS. *Southwick's the law of health care administration,* 3rd ed. Chicago: Health Administration Press; 1999:81–89, 119, 251.
5. *Nashville Business Journal.* http://nashvillebizjurnals.com/nashville/stories/2000.
6. Redling R. New anti-kickback safe harbor rules or mixed bag for medical practices. *Medical Group Management Update.* 2000;39:5.
7. *Federal Registry.* Washington, DC: National Archives and Records Administration; 1999.
8. Glass K. *RVUs: applications for medical practice success.* Dubuque, IA: Medical Group Management Association, Kendall/Hunt; 2003.
9. Porter ME. *Competitive strategy: techniques for analyzing industries and competitors.* New York: Free Press; 1980.
10. American College of Medical Practice Executives. *Body of knowledge for medical practice management.* Denver, CO: ACMPE; 2001.
11. Medical Group Management Association. *Performance and practices of successful medical groups.* Denver, CO: MGMA; 2003.
12. U.S. Department of Health and Human Services. Health information privacy. Accessed April 25, 2011, at http://www.hhs.gov/ocr/hipaa
13. Woolhandler S, Campbell T, Himmelstein DU. Costs of health care administration in the United States and Canada. *New England Journal of Medicine.* 2003;349:768–775.
14. U.S. Department of Health and Human Services. Accessed April 25, 2011, at http://www.cms.hhs.gov/hipaa/hipaa2/default.asp
15. Health Information: Nursing Components and EHRs. Accessed December 2, 2011, at http://nursing-informatics.com/kwantlen/nrsg2220.html
16. *Patient satisfaction survey of 4000 patients at the Sanger Clinic, P.A.,* 2003. Accessed December 2, 2011, at http://nursing-informatics.com/kwantlen/nrsg2220.html
17. Kohn LT, Corrigan JM, Donaldson MS. *To err is human: building a safer health system.* Washington, DC: National Academies of Science, Institute of Medicine; 2000.
18. Wennberg J. Small area variations in health care delivery. *Science.* 1973;182:1102–1108.
19. Wennberg J. Dealing with medical practice variation: a proposal for action. *Health Affairs.* 1984;3:6–32.
20. Illich I. *Medical nemesis: the exploration of health.* New York: Random House; 1976.
21. McKeown T. *The role of medicine: dream, mirage or nemesis.* Princeton, NJ: Princeton University Press; 1980.
22. Deming WE. *Out of the crisis.* Cambridge, MA: Massachusetts Institute of Technology, Center for Advanced Engineering Studies; 1990:166.
23. Turzillo S. *Total quality management in the medical practice. The road seldom traveled.* Denver, CO: American College of Medical Practice Executives; 1992.
24. What is Six Sigma. Accessed December 2, 2011, at http://www.briefcasebooks.com/brue01.pdf
25. Pande P, Neuman R, Cavanagh R. *The Six Sigma way—how GE, Motorola and other top companies are honing their performance.* New York: McGraw-Hill; 2000:23–24.
26. Chowdhury W. *The power of Six Sigma.* Chicago: Dearborn Trade; 2000:29.

27. Six Sigma Systems. June 2001. What is six sigma and lean manufacturing. Accessed December 2, 2011, at http://www.sixsigmasystems.com/what_is_six_sigma.htm

28. Carey RG, Lloyd RC. *Measuring quality improvement in health care: a guide to statistical process control applications.* New York: Quality Resources; 1995.

29. *CFR - Code of Federal Regulations Title 21.* Accessed December 2, 2011, at http://www.accessdata.fda.gov/scripts/cdrh/cfdocs/cfcfr/CFRSearch.cfm?fr=56.102

30. 111th U.S. Congress. Public Law 111-148, The Patient Protection and Affordable Care Act. March 23, 2010.

31. Meeker M. USA, Inc. Red, white and very blue. *Bloomberg Business Week.* Accessed May 15, 2011, at http://www.businessweek.com/magazine/content/11_10/b4218000828880.htm

32. Weick K. The collapse of sensemaking in organizations: the Mann Gulch disaster. *Administrative Science Quarterly.* 1993;3:628-652.

33. ONC HIT Policy Committee, 2010; CMS MU Final Rule, 2010. Accessed December 2, 2011, at http://healthit.hhs.gov/portal/server.pt?open=512&objID=2996&mode=2

34. Wagner SL, Solomon MR. Engaging patients in their health care using an interactive patient portal. Presented February 24, 2011, at the Healthcare IT Conference and Exhibition 11, Orlando, Florida.

35. Wagner EH. Chronic disease management: what will it take to improve care for chronic illness? *Effective Clinical Practice.* 1998;1(1):2–4.

36. National Committee for Quality Assurance. Patient-centered medical home criteria. Accessed May 18, 2011, at http://www.ncqa.org/tabid/631/default.aspx

37. The Health Maintenance Organization Act of 1973 (Public Law 93-222).

38. Dorsey JL. The Health Maintenance Organization Act of 1973 (P.L. 93-222) and prepaid group practice plans. *Medical Care.* 1975;13(1):1–9.

39. Sec. 3022. Medicare Shared Savings Program. Accessed December 2, 2011, at www.healthreformwatch.com/wp-content/uploads/2010/03/senate_aco_language_sec-3022.pdf

40. McKethan A. Crossing borders: overcoming political barriers to technology-led economic development. In Kollmann T, Kuckertz A, Stöckmann C. (eds.). *E-entrepreneurship and ICT ventures: strategy, organization and technology.* Duisburg-Essen, Germany: IGI Global; February 2010. Accessed June 10, 2011.

41. Wagner SL and Solomon MR. Engaging patients in their health care using an interactive patient portal. Presented February 24, 2011, at the Healthcare IT Conference and Exhibition 11, Orlando, Florida.

42. American College of Medical Practice Executives. *Organizational governance and group dynamics.* Denver, CO: Medical Group Management Association; 2006.

43. Reilly M, Markenson D. *Healthcare emergency management: principles and practices.* Sudbury, MA: Jones and Bartlett; 2011.

44. Federal Emergency Management Association. *Make a plan.* Accessed June 10, 2011, at http://www.fema.gov/plan/prepare/plan.shtm

45. Federal Emergency Management Association. National Mutual Aid and Resource Management Initiative, glossary of terms and definitions. Accessed June 10, 2011, at http://www.fema.gov/txt/emergency/nims/507_Mutual_Aid_Glossary.txt

46. *Emergency management: what kinds of situations should be included in an organization's emergency management plans.* Accessed December 2, 2011, at http://www.jointcommission.org/standards_information/jcfaqdetails.aspx?StandardsFaqId=392&ProgramId=1

47. Federal Emergency Management Association. *Determine your risk.* Accessed December 2, 2011, at http://www.fema.gov/plan/determine.shtm

General References

Berglund RG. The world is working to improve health care. *Health Care Weekly Review, Special Reprint.* April 4, 2001.

Burney R. The JCAHO approach to medical errors. *American Society for Quality's 55th Annual Quality Conference Proceedings.* Milwaukee: ASQ; 2001:743.

Chaplin E. Comprehensive quality function deployment: beyond the seven basic quality tools. *American Society for Quality Health Care Division Newsletter.* 2001;1:5.

Eddy DM, Billings J. The quality of medical evidence: implications for quality of care. *Health Affairs.* 1998;7(1):19–32.

Galbraith J. *Designing organizations.* San Francisco: Jossey-Bass; 1995.

National Institutes of Health, National Library of Medicine. *HHS launches new efforts to promote paperless health care system.* Baltimore, MD: NIH; July 1, 2003.

Physicians practice compliance report. Denver, CO: MGMA; 2000;3(1).

Reinhardt U. The social perspective. In: Heithoff K (ed.). *Effectiveness and outcomes in health care.* Washington, DC: National Academies Press; 1990:Ch. 6.

Roper WL, Winkenwerder W, Hackbarth GM, et al. Effectiveness in health care. An initiative to evaluate and improve medical practice. *New England Journal of Medicine.* 1988;319(18):1197–1202.

Shewhart WA. *Statistical methods from the viewpoint of quality control.* New York: W. Edwards Deming, Dove; 1976.

U.S. Department of Health and Human Services. *NIH guide: transforming healthcare quality through information technology (THQIT)—planning grants.* Washington, DC: DHHS; November 20, 2003. RFA No: RFA-HS-04-010 (see NOT-HS-04-001).

Veney JE. *Statistics for health policy and administration using Microsoft Excel.* San Francisco: Jossey-Bass; 2003.

Wagner SF. *Introduction to statistics.* New York: Harper Perennial; 1991.

Participating Organizations

Agency for Healthcare Research and Quality (AHRQ): http://www.ahrq.gov

National Institutes of Health: http://www.nih.gov

Components of Participating Organizations

Clark F. Creating a community health care portal. *Advances for Health Information Executives.* August 2003:61–64.

Gans D. Following a road map to success. *MGMA Connections.* July 2003:26–27.

National Library of Medicine (NLM): http://www.nlm.nih.gov

Hannah K, Ball M (eds.). *Information networks for community health.* New York: Springer; 1997.

Powell JH. U.S. health administration costly. *Modern Healthcare.* August 21, 2003.

CHAPTER

3

Physician Leadership in Medical Group Practice

Gary S. Kaplan, MD, FACMPE, FACP

Although medical group practices have been in existence since the early 1900s, they have become much more prominent as a major mode of healthcare delivery over the past 50 years. Physicians increasingly choose to practice in a group practice for many diverse reasons. The implications of this emerging trend are significant.[1] Every year, more physicians just graduating from training programs choose to practice in a group practice setting, and established physicians are, increasingly, joining groups.[2] In fact, today the vast majority of newly graduating physicians are opting to join a group practice. There are many types of group practices within the United States, and each presents special issues, challenges, and opportunities.

Strong and committed leadership is increasingly recognized as a critical success factor. Those group practices and organizations having the most success in quality, safety, and economic performance are recognized as having superior leadership. New approaches to leadership are emerging, and increasing attention is being paid to partnering strong physician leadership with professionally trained administrators and managers. New organizational structures and the need for operational excellence necessitate the strongest possible leadership. Leadership for today and the future must possess change management

skills that will facilitate the changes and innovations essential to thriving in the years ahead.[3]

This chapter summarizes the foremost aspects of physician leadership and its implications for group practices of varying sizes and types. Physician leadership as a career pathway is also examined, along with current and future trends and opportunities.

■ The Evolution of Group Practice as a Preferred Model

Most graduates of residency training programs over the past decade have chosen to join group practices. This trend, noted for some time, is the result of the changing demographics of the physician workforce and healthcare economics. Multispecialty group practices continue to grow, and single-specialty groups of increasing size are prevalent in many communities. The solo practitioner is seldom found today in urban areas and is increasingly rare even in some of the most remote parts of the United States. The rationale for these trends is multifactored and includes clinical, business, and age-related determinants. With more and more clinical care delivered in ambulatory settings and increasing emphasis on quality, safety, and cost, the organizational structures in which this care is delivered take on great significance. Studies demonstrating enhancements in quality and safety correlated with structure are just beginning to emerge, and policy makers and industry leaders are paying a great deal of attention to structural models that could yield lower costs.[4-6] These structural phenomena go far beyond physician practices and include new partnerships among various provider sectors including hospitals, academic medical centers, health plans, pharmaceutical companies, home health agencies, and government.

In order to understand today's trends it is helpful to reflect on the history of ambulatory practice as it has evolved over the past century. Medicine has often been labeled a "cottage industry," and this was never more the case than at the beginning of the twentieth century. Ambulatory care was delivered by solo practitioners who were revered by their patients and were looked on as pillars of their communities. Following medical school they hung out the proverbial shingle and began practice. As the demands and complexity of primary care increased they began to form loose call-sharing arrangements, but preserved their strong focus on clinical autonomy and solo practice. This reinforced the role of the physician as primary caregiver and elevated the prestige of the general practitioner (GP), who many looked at as almost a member of the family.

The first real innovative structural breakthrough occurred when the Mayo brothers came together with a few peers and formed the first actual group practice in the United States in 1892, which became known as the Mayo Clinic around the turn of the century. The Mayo Clinic story is legendary; they demonstrated superior clinical results, breakthrough innovations, and the power of linking clinical care and academics. Their reputation developed rapidly, and patients and their families traveled long distances to get a definitive diagnosis and treatment at Mayo. Collaboration, collegiality, and partnership were beginning to be thought of as consistent with the very best healthcare delivery.

Within 10 years of its founding, the Mayo Clinic spawned the development of a small group of physician-led and physician-driven clinics across the United States. Several Mayo Clinic–trained physicians decided to set out on their own, and over the ensuing 10–15 years formed several group practices, now well known, around the country.[7] These included groups as prestigious as the Cleveland Clinic, Geisinger Clinic, Scott and White Clinic, Scripps Clinic, Marshfield Clinic, and Virginia Mason Clinic. All had in common Mayo Clinic roots, a commitment to excellence in patient care and academics, and strong physician leadership and influence. They were attractive to patients and to a segment of physicians with an affinity for teamwork and collaboration.

Over decades these clinics distinguished themselves for their quality and focus on coordinated care. Physicians joining these group practices knew they were joining a team of exemplary colleagues and were going to work in an environment of collegiality and intellectual stimulation. This did not always sit well with the local solo or small group physicians with whom these multispecialty groups were competing. Some of the multispecialty groups were labeled socialists and were feared as competitors. It became apparent that there was a certain type of individual who would thrive in a multispecialty group setting and others who were much more oriented to solo or small group practice.

Despite the attractions of the Mayo Clinic model, it was not a practice model that appealed to everyone. Many clinicians remained in solo practice; others began to see the benefits of group practice but wanted to form partnerships with only physicians in the same specialty. This was driven, in part, by primary motivating factors around call-sharing and ensuring a manageable workload, as well as economic and cultural factors. This was the beginning of the single-specialty group model; today we are seeing the full expression of this model in some massive single-specialty orthopedic, surgery, cardiology, and gastroenterology groups, among others. As the single-specialty group model has expanded and these groups grow, new business opportunities become apparent, including specialty hospitals, ambulatory surgery centers, and innovative partnerships.[8] Today these groups have great influence with insurance contracting and when negotiating leverage with hospitals and other stakeholders.

In the late 1930s and early 1940s, multispecialty groups coexisted with the still-dominant solo practitioners. As the labor movement emerged in the United States, new types of multispecialty group practices formed. These staff model health maintenance organizations (HMOs), most notably Kaiser Permanente in California and, several years later, Group Health Cooperative of Puget Sound, added another element to multispecialty group practices. These organizations focused on "health maintenance," and were reimbursed on a capitated or prepaid basis. The reimbursement approach was not fee-for-service and, thus, the incentives were heavily aligned with prevention. Some physicians were very attracted to this model of care and appreciated that there were no incentives to provide more services than what was actually needed. Interestingly, corporate practice of medicine laws in California necessitated that the physicians be in a separate organization from the health plan, and with both Kaiser and Group Health, physicians were inexorably intertwined with these organizations through long-term exclusive provider agreements.

Soon after their formation, these staff model HMOs drew criticism for having incentives that would potentially lead to the withholding of necessary or indicated diagnostic or therapeutic interventions. Though never clearly demonstrated, these anticipated consequences became the basis of a heavily financed and spirited campaign against health reform efforts in the 1990s. Because these HMOs were a hybrid of health plans and provider systems, other competing health plans were quick to criticize them as well.

Staff model HMOs have grown, and patients and physicians have seemed to stratify into those who love this care model and those who loathe it. Decades later, it appears that these HMOs were, in many ways, simply ahead of their time. Today, Kaiser has a dominant market position in California and selected other markets, and Group Health Cooperative is a strong force in the Puget Sound market. In recent years, other strong multispecialty group practices have chosen to form their own health plans and achieve more so-called vertical integration.

The late 1980s and early 1990s were interesting times for group practice structural evolution, because managed care was a hallmark of the Clinton healthcare reform efforts. Rapid cost escalations and increasing healthcare complexity were significant drivers in reform planning. Even before a robust national reform debate, several states passed reform legislation promoting managed care and increasing consolidation. There were predictions that there would be perhaps as few as three to six national healthcare systems. There was a major push towards growth, consolidation, and positioning to assume risk through capitation. The result was an interest in greater alignment of physicians and hospitals in order to assume risk and strengthen one's competitive position. The thought was that even if reform never happened, greater physician–hospital alignment would ensure filled hospital beds and secure referral revenue streams.

Hospitals began to acquire physician groups in almost all markets. Physicians were increasingly fearful of a future characterized by risk-bearing managed care, poor or no access to capital for growth and technology, an inability to fund their retirements, and little or no ability to grow and expand. Many physicians sold their practices to hospitals or hospital systems and became "employees" for the first time. These purchases were significant transactions, associated with the purchase of equipment,

medical records, and goodwill. Many of the physicians were given guaranteed long-term salaries without productivity requirements.

As it became apparent that managed care was not going to become predominant any time soon, and with the realization that hospitals were losing $50,000–$100,000 per primary care physician, the late 1990s were a time of considerable dissolution of many of these new employee relationships. Accordingly, many physicians returned to their previous practice structures or took early retirement.

The Institute of Medicine (IOM) report initially published in 2000, "To Err Is Human," dramatically changed the landscape for group practices and healthcare delivery across the United States.[9] This report clearly elucidated the distressing error rate and safety record within the healthcare industry. After a period of denial from the medical community, the report served as a major wake-up call, and radically revised the agenda for healthcare providers. Quality and safety became key issues and salient drivers of strategy as healthcare entered the twenty-first century. Focusing on improving safety and documenting quality, while moving from a culture of blame to one of improvement and accountability, represented a major change for the industry. Given this new quality imperative and the subsequent improvement roadmap outlined in a second IOM report, "Crossing the Quality Chasm," the priorities for physician and hospital leadership were fundamentally altered.[10]

By 2002 it became apparent that the "old economy" in healthcare had returned. Primary care practices had great difficulty remaining financially viable, and hospitals became increasingly aware of the poor economics associated with owning primary care practices. Medical school graduates began avoiding primary care specialties. Physicians that did surgery or procedures continued to command larger incomes and sought opportunities to expand their involvement in ancillary services as reimbursement for procedures declined. Some specialty physicians, for example, became involved in imaging centers, ambulatory surgical facilities, and so on. Hospitals and physicians became increasingly adversarial, with a breakdown in trust and increasing competition for the smaller, profitable portion of the healthcare dollar. Many hospitals began to disassemble their primary care practices, and managed care in most markets declined—precipitously.[11]

With the election of Barack Obama as President of the United States and with a Congress controlled by the Democratic party, momentum began to build again for healthcare reform. Reform had been a major campaign issue; Obama campaigned on a platform promoting comprehensive reform. Healthcare expenditures had climbed to over 17% of gross domestic product (GDP), and both the public and private sectors were facing double-digit annual increases in healthcare costs. It was obvious that the current trajectory of cost increases was unsustainable. Medicare and Medicaid represented the largest components of the federal and state budgets, respectively, and economic challenges resulting from the collapse of financial markets in 2008 created additional urgency. Large and small employers found that healthcare costs for their employees were a major factor in reducing competiveness in an increasingly global economy. Some were opting for defined contribution plans, or eliminating coverage altogether.

In addition to unsustainable cost escalation, the ranks of the uninsured and underinsured were swelling. Close to 50 million Americans were uninsured by early 2009, and the new President and Congress were determined to move towards universal coverage following the election of 2008. They envisioned a healthcare system that would, over time, provide coverage for all citizens, while improving quality, safety, and "bending the cost curve." This was a grand vision, but brought with it considerable controversy and difficulties. Following one of the most divisive congressional debates in decades, the Patient Protection and Accountable Care Act (PPACA) of 2010 was passed by a narrow margin. This represented a major step towards comprehensive reform and included insurance, payment, and delivery system reform.

The reforms clearly spelled out in the law, and changes implied or likely to result from the PPACA, represented significant strategic challenges and opportunities for group practices across the United States. Whether a small single-specialty group or a market-dominant integrated delivery system, change was coming, and new models of care and structures to succeed and thrive in this tumultuous environment were being proposed and implemented across the country. Some considered this overreaction, especially given political and judicial challenges to elements of the new law. Nevertheless, it was clear that many elements of reform were here to stay, and those organizations that were best prepared for the new environment were the most likely to succeed. Accordingly, the roles, responsibilities, and prominence of physician leaders in group practices were of more importance and a higher priority than ever before.

The PPACA focused on ensuring increased coverage in the early years of its implementation. Following implementation, provisions in the law called for significant delivery system and payment reforms. Beginning in the year 2012, the law called for incentives to create

accountable care organizations (ACOs), which would join together physicians and hospitals to create organizations able to share risk and provide enhanced coordinated care across the entire care continuum. For previously integrated multispecialty groups already affiliated with hospitals, this called for less change and disruption compared with single-specialty groups and multispecialty groups lacking hospital partners. This aspect of the law precipitated significant "deal-making," with many groups joining hospital systems, and an acceleration of the trend towards physician employment. Private practice groups began to explore new partnership opportunities as well. The question of whether hospitals, with their capital strength, or physicians would be in control of these new ACOs was hotly debated in numerous forums, spawning a new consulting industry to prepare physicians and hospitals for ACOs.

In addition to delivery system reforms, advocates of the PPACA hoped to stimulate new and innovative payment models. The fee for service (FFS) payment system that had been the predominant mode of reimbursement for most of the twentieth century needed to be modified. Numerous studies suggested that this volume-based reimbursement system was, in part, responsible for continuing cost escalation and that FFS incentives were misaligned with promoting the highest quality and safest care at the lowest possible cost.[12-16] Calls for value as the basis for payment, consistent with payment in most other industries, were widespread, and this was addressed in the PPACA.

Beginning in 2013, "bundled payment pilot projects" are to commence, and other value-based purchasing initiatives are either explicitly called for, or implied in, the new legislation. The ability to participate in these innovative payment demonstrations requires new approaches in group practice structure and care delivery.

Medical homes and similar innovative care models were piloted across the country, and hospitals sought to provide a "safe haven" for physicians concerned about decreasing reimbursement, the need for capital to finance growth and electronic health records, and overall security. It was obvious that reimbursement decreases were inevitable and independent physician practices would become increasingly vulnerable.

Going forward, strong physician leadership is undeniably a critical success factor; new ways of leading, collaborating, and aligning are imperative. The challenges and opportunities are both daunting and exciting. Group practices and hospitals have begun to seek out experienced physician leaders, and many physicians have begun to consider pursuing additional training to prepare for careers in leadership.

■ External Challenges

Physician practices face a multitude of external challenges, all of which need to be addressed in order to thrive in the future.

Reimbursement

Group practices continue to face increasing reimbursement pressures, a commonplace issue over the past several decades, but despite warnings and anxiety, the specter of profound reductions has not materialized as fact. A significant historical development was the Balanced Budget Act of 1997, which effectively reduced reimbursements to both physicians and hospitals for several ensuing years. This comprehensive bill created considerable concern and fear regarding inadequate reimbursement, and most of the provisions were attenuated as part of incremental congressional actions over the next several years. Reductions of selected physician payments have had substantial impact on group practices. This impact has been felt regardless of the predominant payment mechanisms for a particular group, and has seriously affected practices dependent on fee-for-service reimbursement as well as those in a primarily capitated environment.

Continuing declines in Medicare reimbursement rates relative to the costs of labor, supplies, and the like have been associated with relative declines in commercial payment rates as well. Although the overall cost of healthcare has been increasing far more than the rate of general inflation, relative payments to physicians and hospitals are being reduced. Absolute payment rates to physicians for certain services have also been cut, but nowhere near the amounts forecast to be associated with the Accountable Care Act of 2010.

Although at one time it appeared that the economics of healthcare would become a "zero sum game," and that enhanced payments in one area would adversely impact payments for other services, it is now apparent that both physician and hospital payments will decrease. Continued cost-shifting because of declines in payments from governmental payers will be limited in the future. Reimbursement challenges are drastically shaping the landscape, framing strategic options for group practices across the United States. Physician leaders find themselves challenged to lead and manage their group practices profitably in this hostile reimbursement environment.[17]

Payor and Purchaser Concerns

Much of the concern regarding reimbursement rates and the escalating cost of healthcare emanate from increasing employer–purchaser concerns. The employment-based commercial healthcare system continues to be under siege. Both large and small employers face significant economic challenges at a time requiring increased competition in a global economy. In all industries, the expense line item with the highest single rate of increase over the past decade has been that of employee and retiree healthcare benefits. Many industries continue to point to this as their greatest economic challenge and threat to their sustainability and competitiveness. After a period of low healthcare inflation in the mid-1990s, double-digit inflation rates, far exceeding increases in the consumer price index (CPI), have again become the norm. An example of this difficulty is the U.S. automobile industry, where, even several years ago, an individual vehicle price had embedded within it between $800 and $1,000 of cost to fund healthcare insurance for workers and their families—a burden not born by the Japanese and European automobile manufacturers.[18] The issue of retiree benefits is one of great concern as well.

The payer and purchaser communities are taking steps to mitigate this serious economic challenge. Employer coalitions such as Puget Sound Health Alliance, National Business Group on Health,[19] and Pacific Business Group on Health[20] have formed for a variety of purposes. Some are focused primarily on pooling resources to enhance purchasing power; others are interested in identifying characteristics of high-quality, efficient healthcare providers in order to channel employees selectively to these providers. Any perceived reduction in choice is met with some resistance from the workforce and unions; however, militancy on this issue has been tempered by overall economic concerns. Many employers are raising copayments and employee contributions to supplement the premium dollar provided by the employer. Each of these actions has an impact on the economics and strategies of group practices.

Competing in an individual, consumer-driven marketplace, where consumers actually have choice and incentive regarding provider selection, is already having substantial influence as leaders chart the course for group practices in the years ahead. In addition, the heightening emphasis on quality and the need to respond to purchaser coalitions such as the Leapfrog Group have already had significant impact.[21] Publicly reported metrics and calls for transparency on quality and cost are also having a considerable effect.

Governmental and Regulatory Issues

Group practices have struggled to cope with declining reimbursement, increasing purchaser pressure, and a constantly shifting environment, and governmental and regulatory factors have created further complexity over the past decade. The Medicare program and the Centers for Medicare and Medicaid Services (CMS) have undergone almost constant change, and their policies, procedures, and regulations are in flux. The problem of close to 50 million uninsured Americans continues to plague many communities and providers, and governmental programs, including Medicaid, are under tremendous pressure. The regulatory environment has become increasingly complex, and the passage of HIPAA (Health Insurance Portability and Accountability Act) had a dramatic impact. Even small group practices must put considerable resources into ensuring that they are fully compliant with all HIPAA regulations. The complexity of claims processing, billing, and coding have added further obstacles to care delivery.

Physician leaders must ensure their physicians and staff are fully engaged in learning and applying appropriate coding behavior, and recent actions by the Office of the Inspector General (OIG) suggest that stricter enforcement of rules and regulations is here to stay. Billing and coding practices, which previously were fairly routine, are now complex, and require significant attention within group practices. OIG investigations have led to both civil and criminal penalties, further accelerating the imperative that group practices approach this with appropriate diligence.[22] Some look to this regulatory environment as further evidence of a system run amok, whereas many in the public sector see this as protecting the public interest. Other regulatory issues gravely impacting group practices and on the agendas of many healthcare leaders are mandated benefits, including those for complementary and alternative medicine providers, as well as diverse legislative issues such as tort reform.

■ Internal Leadership Challenges

As the competitive environment evolves and external challenges mount, physician leaders increasingly focus inward to ensure that strategy and priorities are appropriate and that group practices are well positioned to survive and thrive in this chaotic environment. This often requires a shift in focus and significant change management challenges.

Recruitment and Retention

Perhaps the most pressing concern to physician leadership is the recruitment and retention of outstanding physicians. Although the issues differ between multispecialty and single-specialty groups, the need to ensure adequate numbers of quality physicians to meet patient demand and market

opportunities can be challenging. The recruiting process has become increasingly important in recent years, as physicians in several specialties are in seemingly short supply. New graduates, as well as those changing their practice venue, have greater choice and latitude. As noted, more are opting to join group practices and employment models. It is incumbent on physician leadership to design and implement recruiting approaches that are aligned with their individual group's mission and objectives. Academic credentials and experience remain important; however, there is increasing awareness of the need to identify individuals who will be a good fit within a particular group. What previously was a rather matter-of-fact, routine process now requires considerable rigor, planning, and follow-through.

Retention of quality physicians within group practices has emerged as a major challenge, particularly in today's competitive environment. This is as important as initial recruitment to physician leaders, because they have made considerable investments in their physicians over many years. Numerous issues affect recruitment and retention, requiring a thorough understanding and articulation of a group's "value proposition." This is more important than ever as options, particularly for highly paid doctors who conduct procedures and surgeries, as well as much sought-after primary care physicians, are numerous in a variety of private practice settings. As part of understanding the value proposition, one must understand the differential between income earning opportunities in different settings, as well as the rationale and foundational principles of internal group-practice compensation systems. These compensation formulas are undergoing extensive alteration as well, given the dynamic environment and continuing changes in specialty-specific reimbursement. We have come a long way from the "equal split" compensation methods present in the early multispecialty group practices.[23-25]

Among the many recruiting and retention challenges is an understanding of the tradeoffs that occur when one joins a group. As clinical care delivery and quality and safety imperatives have emerged, it has become increasingly apparent that complete independence and autonomy are no longer possible. An understanding of this as a physician enters group practice is critical, and the ability to articulate these factors is a core responsibility of group-practice leaders. Those who do it well, and fully understand the benefits of group practice, are most successful at recruiting and retaining physicians.

Cost Control and Efficiency

Many additional internal challenges face group-practice leadership. Declining reimbursement and rising costs of labor and technology have increased the focus on efficiency. Reducing expenses per dollar of revenue generated has, of necessity, become a priority for group-practice leadership, and this has definitely been accelerated by the PPACA. The previous approaches to reduced reimbursement focused on increasing volumes of visits and procedures. This resulted in less time available with individual patients and, predictably, serious decreases in both patient and physician satisfaction. Conventional approaches to cost cutting are limited in their effect; more aggressive approaches to re-engineering are required. This occurs most prominently in the larger, multispecialty groups; however, it is of increasing importance to smaller group practices as well.

The correlation between enhanced efficiency and improved quality and safety is also becoming more apparent.[26,27] Traditional quality improvement methods, although slow and cumbersome, have met with some success. More effective methodologies, borrowed from other industries, are being employed in innovative group practices at multiple locations across the country. Six Sigma methodologies promoted by consulting divisions of major U.S. manufacturers and vendors, such as General Electric, are being embraced by many physician leaders in group practices. Several organizations are embracing elements of the Toyota Production System and discovering many applications to healthcare.[28,29] Given the inadequate supply of healthcare workers in many disciplines, layoffs are no longer a first choice option as a strategy for cost control and efficiency. Although many of these factors have been most notable in hospitals, they also apply directly to most group practices across the United States.

Strategic Direction

As physician leaders and their administrative partners seek to meet the challenges of today's environment, a clear strategic direction is crucial. This represents another significant internal challenge, and it is often this planning process that facilitates necessary alignment within group practices. Issues requiring physician leadership include those related to growth strategies, as well as identification of areas for potential program contraction or elimination. Depending on the type of group-practice setting, it is necessary to focus on selective strategic growth, while recognizing, particularly in multispecialty group practices, that it is no longer possible to be all things to all people. Helping group practices become comfortable with simultaneous expansion and contraction requires strong, effective leadership. Identifying the optimal mix of service lines is not necessarily a simple task. Multiple

factors, including community need, profitability, presence of excellent clinicians, and payer mix, all enter into the strategic decision-making process. Payer mix modification and strategies to adjust a group's mix are also of growing importance as strategic direction is set.[30]

In recent years, there has been an increasing propensity to explore partnerships. These partnerships may take the form of specific specialty expansion, merger, and practice acquisitions with individuals or groups that complement a larger group's mission, as well as partnerships with community and academic hospitals and medical centers. As a result of the PPACA, market consolidation emerged as a significant trend in 2009–2010. Consolidation has occurred for many reasons, including establishing market dominance and pricing power as well as enhanced coordination of care and value creation. Motivation for consolidation varies considerably, and it is evident to many that strategies establishing market clout as a result of size may represent only short-lived gains. Strategic initiatives invariably require significant leadership attention and focus. At times, it is as important to understand what not to pursue as it is the actual pursuit of collaboration itself. In the final analysis, it is vital that physicians and staff participate in determining strategic direction and understand and support a group's mission, vision, and strategies. Alignment is critical to group-practice success, and physician leadership must prioritize and lead this work.

Credibility and Effectiveness

As the internal challenges facing group-practice leaders become increasingly complex, the leaders' credibility and effectiveness are of critical importance. Physician leaders traditionally have been selected because of seniority or perceived influence as well as clinical credentials. Today, new skills and approaches to leadership selection and ensuring leadership effectiveness are required. Establishing and maintaining credibility remains a prerequisite for success. In several large group-practice settings, chief medical officers and other physician leaders may now be full-time physician leaders. In many settings, and particularly smaller group practices, many physician leaders continue clinical practice. This certainly facilitates credibility and a connection to frontline patient care issues, and more importantly, distinguishes the physician leader from his or her professional management partner. It is the physician leader who often best articulates the group practice's values and ethics, and ensures that these are aligned within the professional staff. Many long-established group practices have deeply entrenched cultures, and some are presently undergoing cultural upheaval. In many ways, it is the leadership culture that becomes the organization or group culture, and the physician leader must approach these issues deliberately. The leader must maintain credibility while simultaneously promoting necessary group evolution and adjustment. Measures of effectiveness are changing as well, and include much more than average physician compensation in any given year. Credibility and effectiveness are a result of quality, safety, recruitment and retention, customer and staff satisfaction, and of course, economic performance.[31,32]

Pace of Change

Perhaps the greatest challenge facing group-practice leadership today is the unprecedented rate of change. The healthcare culture is quickly transforming, and consequently, the internal dynamics within group practices are constantly evolving as well. It is, of course, important to recognize that healthcare professionals, and physicians in particular, have historically been averse to change, and attempts at reform and redesign that proceed with excessive speed and without groundwork have frequently resulted in a short tenure for a given physician leader.

Helping physicians and members of the healthcare delivery team move out of their traditional comfort zones requires comprehensive change management skills. Applying basic principles of change management is critical to leading large scale change in the group practice environment.[33-35] Transformation is rapidly becoming a way of life in today's group practices, and requires considerable nontraditional thinking. Often this pro-change mentality must begin with physician leaders themselves, because leaders halfheartedly promoting reform are most often unsuccessful. Ron Heifetz, author of *Leadership on the Line*, suggests the need to help lead change by ensuring that teams stay in what he calls the "productive range of distress." [36] Effective leaders are able to modulate the "heat" so that teams feel discomfort with a dysfunctional status quo, while also recognizing that only so much change can be tolerated in any given period of time. The imperative that it is best to lead by example continues today. Physician leaders are faced with a variety of new dynamics, including generational differences within their groups, and this is reflected in a group's readiness to embrace and process rapid change and redesign of care delivery. Older physicians are even looking to early retirement as a preferred option when confronted with overwhelming metamorphoses in their daily work lives. Understanding the impact of specific changes on the individuals who work within group practices, and deliberately planning the best approaches to implement

and lead change, are important challenges for the physician leader.[37]

Stakeholder Management

A great challenge for physician leaders in today's healthcare environment is the application of new approaches to leadership and management of numerous diverse stakeholders. Modeling appropriate behavior is an important element of physician leadership, and as issues and requirements increase in complexity, new areas of focus are required. Whereas previously the emphasis was on facilitating outstanding individual performance, the new focus must be on encouraging and developing physicians as members of clinical teams. Physicians may actually serve as team leaders in various healthcare delivery venues, but are no longer able to focus solely on their work as individuals. With increasing complexity has come the necessity of optimizing team performance, and this requires physician leadership investment in staff satisfaction, overall quality metrics, and an understanding of complex systems. These new skills require new educational approaches and a willingness to revise one's leadership "mental model."

The physician leader as "coach" is a relatively new concept, and requires different skills than that of the physician leader as colleague, peer, or even boss.[38] Understanding the diverse stakeholders, and what their unique needs and requirements are, is crucial. Physicians, nurses, managers, and frontline staff all look to physician leaders in group practices for mentoring, setting of strategic direction, and ongoing coaching. The physician leader clearly sets the tone. Effective leadership requires an emphasis on collaboration and teamwork in both clinical and business endeavors. Although physicians have traditionally paid lip service to the concept of teamwork, one-on-one working relationships have predominated in both the ambulatory and inpatient settings. The single physician working with a single medical assistant or nurse is the long-standing, traditional office staffing model. Today, this may diminish efficiency and fail to bring all necessary skills and services to the patient.

The healthcare delivery team is increasingly subspecialized, and physicians must function in a much more collaborative mode. Physician leaders and their administrative colleagues can lead by example, forming strong leadership and management teams that achieve synergies that otherwise would not be possible. Finally, new opportunities for collaboration and teamwork exist within given communities between physician leaders and corporate and business community leaders, as well as suppliers and vendors. This collaboration and teamwork imperative demands new skills and approaches.[39,40]

The Disruptive Physician

Perhaps the greatest internal challenge to physician leaders remains that of the "problem physician." This has been a challenge in group practices since their creation, and it is unfortunate that only relatively recently has it been systematically addressed. Issues may range from quality-of-care concerns to behavioral issues that impact colleagues and staff. A great benefit of group practices for the patients they serve should be the ongoing peer review that exists within the group itself. This should lead to quality assurance approaches that ensure acceptable levels of care are being provided. The role of the physician leader in meticulously overseeing this quality assurance work is critical to identifying problems early during a physician's tenure within the group practice. No role is more important than that of quality oversight, and group-practice physician leaders must spend a significant portion of their time in this work.

Of comparable importance, however, is ensuring a safe, respectful work environment, which facilitates physicians and staff doing their very best work on behalf of their patients. We have all encountered difficult colleagues in our practice settings, and remember vividly the disproportionate amount of time and energy these individuals require from leadership and management. Many groups have experienced problems with individual physician behavior that can be extremely disruptive, disrespectful, and at times, abusive. The disruptive physician often insists on focusing on his or her individual needs at the expense of group goals and patient care. All too often meeting agendas are "hijacked," leading to dissipation of positive group energy.

This may be a function of individual personalities as well as of the hierarchical traditions within the profession. Historically, because of the high value placed on collegiality and conflict avoidance, leaders and physician colleagues have not directly addressed these behavioral concerns. The consequences have been considerable, and it is becoming increasingly clear that these behaviors are no longer acceptable. Confronting these issues is part of a new culture of accountability in healthcare.[41-45]

In addressing these issues, it is often helpful to be as data driven as possible. Several group practices have put a physician compact in place, resulting in clear expectations of group-practice physicians, as well as specifying what physicians have a right to expect from their group or organization.[46,47] These expectations form criteria upon which a physician leader can take action when behavioral or quality concerns emerge. Deliberate process should be followed exactly, and codifying this process prior to taking action and prior to actually having to deal with these difficult situations is helpful. Explicit, unambiguous written feedback and improvement plans should be an important component of every physician leader's work in today's environment. Sound human resource policies need to be understood and applied to physicians as well as staff. This clearly represents a new skill and role for physician leaders. It is one of the great burdens of leadership and of paramount importance to maintaining group integrity. Although individual physicians may choose to avoid expressing concerns regarding colleague behavior, one sees a great sense of relief and gratitude when these issues are addressed effectively by leadership.

◼ Clinical Care Delivery

Perhaps the most prominent changes in the role of physician leaders in group practice have been those required by transformations in clinical care delivery. The initial IOM report altered the landscape and brought into the public domain concerns regarding safety and quality.[9] Methods for addressing the unacceptable error rate leading to unnecessary morbidity and mortality have ensued. The healthcare profession has come to understand major areas in need of attention, including medication safety as well as handoffs between members of the healthcare delivery team and transitions in care.[10,48] These issues represent great challenges as well as opportunities for group practices. Although most of this increased awareness has centered on hospital-based care, similar issues exist in the ambulatory setting. What has been termed a "culture of blame" has contributed to a lack of awareness and the necessary subsequent action to improve patient safety.[49] Creating a culture of safety and focusing attention on these issues, utilizing best practices and deploying them consistently throughout group practices, is vital and requires strong physicianleadership.[50-55]

Embedded in many physician compacts is a commitment to identify and implement best practices. Guidelines and pathways to eliminate unnecessary variation that contributes to the high defect rate are necessary, and this requires mind-set changes on the part of individual clinicians. Without strong physician leadership, this does not occur. To many, being a physician and professional implies clinical autonomy, and in fact, many physicians fall back on their requirement to put the patient first as a rationale for autonomous decision making. Unfortunately, clinical autonomy is not always consistent with best practice, and an increasing awareness of the opportunities to create standard work, using evidence-based medicine guidelines, is beginning to become apparent in the highest-quality group practices. Group practices, like hospitals, are being challenged to move from a culture of blame to one of accountability and improvement. It falls upon physician leaders to lead the way.[55,56]

Physician leaders have a great opportunity to truly leverage the advantages of group practice. By virtue of being part of a group practice, physicians have the opportunity to pool their knowledge and experience to design effective approaches to patient care that can be standardized for the benefit of patients. The peer accountability that exists in the most highly evolved group practices can ensure that group practices and their healthcare teams deliver the very best care to their patients. Addressing challenging issues and always keeping the patient first is essential, and the physician leader is responsible for prioritizing this work. New tools such as electronic medical records and other information technologies can greatly facilitate this work, and understanding the importance of prioritizing precious capital dollars, as well as the intellectual capital and energy and commitment of member physicians, is an important task of leadership.

■ Evolution of the Physician Role

In order to understand physician leadership challenges and opportunities, it is helpful to review the evolution of the role of the practicing physician. This role has certainly changed, and commensurately, the needs and expectations of physicians have changed as well. Medicine has continued to evolve over the past two centuries. It was not until the mid-1800s that medicine began to emerge from its roots as a cottage industry.[57] Certifying bodies and formal school training were established during this period of time, and remnants of this cottage industry persist today. Inherent in the training experience is the process of acculturation that inculcates the traditions of medicine and establishes hierarchical perspectives among physicians.

Physicians are taught early in their training that they are at the top of the "food chain" in healthcare delivery. Unfortunately, a mind-set of omniscience and omnipotence often results. Despite an awareness of the dysfunction in present and traditional hierarchical models, only recently have medical schools begun to place emphasis on collaboration and teamwork.[58] The primary role of the clinician or caregiver remains the major component of the physician's identity. To a great extent, this is predicated on

independence and autonomy, and has led physicians into practice settings where the individual physician served as proprietor in a solo practice or owner in a small group practice. As groups grew in size, the role of partner and investor became important, and many physicians had to learn at least the rudimentary characteristics of small business proprietorship.

This dynamic has changed radically in recent years, with physicians becoming employees of group practices, hospitals, or other similar organizations. Many are joining group practices directly from training; others are choosing to become part of groups later in their careers, at times selling the assets of their practices. Some fit well into group practices; others have great difficulty. Group practices have spent considerable effort identifying the characteristics of physicians who can adapt seamlessly prior to hiring new physicians. The new role of employee presents unique challenges, and as noted, becoming a team member and potentially a team leader are new skills for physicians. The day-to-day practice experience has traditionally been built around intense one-on-one interactions, whether in the office, hospital, or operating room. Advocacy for patients is no longer predicated on these one-on-one interactions. The role and perception of physician as "hero" has dissipated somewhat with increasing consumerism.[59]

As the physician role has evolved from independent caregiver to effective team member and team leader, so have opportunities for physicians to develop new skills and interests. The role of the physician as teacher or mentor is evolving as well. Educational activities and mentoring of young physicians and colleagues, as well as nurses and other healthcare professionals, have focused in recent years on process improvement, team building, and leadership. The role of physician as teacher continues to be of great importance.

The role of physician as leader or manager is relatively new and of accelerating importance. Physicians' training has not adequately prepared them for this role and for many, their personality and experience seem poorly aligned for new leadership roles. Traditionally physicians often have relied on force of personality or their hierarchical "power position" as an owner or shareholder. They have counted on the deference of managers, nurses, and staff when conflict arises. Effectiveness in this pivotal new role requires new learning and developing new skills, particularly in areas of change management, care delivery redesign, strategic planning, and business principles and discipline. An understanding of these new requirements and the prior training and acculturation process leads to increasing recognition of the important role of the physician leader and manager and its criticality to the success of group practices today.

Spectrum of Group Practices and Implications for Leadership

There is a wide spectrum of group-practice types, and each has unique characteristics that require varying levels and models of physician leadership. Ensuring that physician leadership is appropriately matched with specific group-practice type, and exploring optimal models of leadership for specific types of group practices, is of considerable interest. Many different leadership models exist today, and each has strengths and weaknesses. Understanding these models and the role of the physician leader can facilitate group-practice success.

Small Single-Specialty Group

These groups typically have not placed a high priority on strong physician leadership. There is often a business manager or bookkeeper who has assumed the oversight of billing and collections, with little attention to staff development, enhancement of clinical care delivery, or teamwork. The physician leader is often the senior partner and may be called the managing partner. There is often no job description or salary designated for this role. These individuals may provide leadership by force of personality and seniority, and problem-solving is frequently ad hoc or reactive in nature. Maintaining the status quo and the physician income stream are key priorities. Only in recent years have challenges to this status quo precipitated more formal attention to leadership roles and responsibilities.

The need to become increasingly entrepreneurial has been an important factor in this recent role evolution, and many senior physician leaders in these types of groups are passing the baton to younger, more outwardly focused individuals. The leaders in these practice settings may only serve in their role for a brief period of time. In fact, leadership selection may often be on a rotational basis, leading to little continuity, a perpetual steep learning curve, and limited effectiveness.[60]

Small Multispecialty Group

This model presents considerable challenges beyond that of a single-specialty group. Understanding a group's mix of specialties and their important role in furthering the group's mission and strategies, as well as issues of growth and resource allocation, require considerable physician leadership. Recruitment and retention of physicians to multispecialty group practices present unique challenges as well. Some physicians are easily attracted to an environment where they work side-by-side with colleagues in multiple disciplines. Others feel it is critical that their primary allegiance be to their specialty, and have difficulty integrating into multispecialty practices.

A major flashpoint of conflict in these settings is physician compensation. Although design of compensation plans in these small, multispecialty groups may fall to the manager or administrator, implementation and support for these plans are essential to their success and highly dependent on physician leadership. Given what are likely time-limited opportunities for proceduralists to significantly enhance their income, the challenge to these multispecialty groups is to create and provide a value proposition that leads to recruitment and retention of highly paid specialists as well as primary care physicians. It is imperative that all physicians within these groups understand the significant role of each specialty and the need to provide market-competitive compensation. Failure to understand these important issues has led to fractionation and dissolution of many small multispecialty groups. Groups with effective physician leadership can find themselves able to survive and thrive in these turbulent times.

Large Multispecialty Group Practice

These groups, with over 100 physicians in multiple specialties, are present in most urban communities and selective rural settings across the country. They constitute many of the most prestigious group practices in the United States, and are often led by highly visible, prominent physician leaders. There are numerous historical examples of visionary founders providing strong, effective leadership during the development of these group practices. In recent years, many of the strong physician-dominated leadership structures have embraced team concepts in response to increasing complexity, economic challenge, and a realization that the model of strong physician-only leadership has many weaknesses and potential vulnerabilities.

Strong physician-centric leadership models most often have a physician leader noted for his or her clinical excellence and academic credentials. Stories abound of legendary physician leaders who ruled these groups with an iron hand. Administrators in these groups often were limited in their scope of work, and filled the role of accountant or business manager, with little involvement in strategy or quality improvement. Critics of this model have pointed out that many physician leaders only dabble in management, are often intolerant of detail, and do not appreciate the complexities required. Today, many of these large multispecialty group practices have embraced a true team model of leadership, with strong physician CEOs or medical directors working closely with professional administrators.

Economics and capital investment in information technology and facilities are among the primary issues facing these groups today. To move strategically an enterprise of significant size that is dominated by professionals, significant investment and business discipline are required. Physician leadership must be engaged in this work to effectively implement necessary change. Consultants often serve to augment leadership in these large groups and can contribute to effectiveness. At varying times, these groups require the full spectrum of physician leadership and management. They can be either nimble, change-oriented organizations or group practices deeply entrenched in maintaining the status quo. The vision and performance of physician leadership is often the determining factor.[58,59]

Academic Faculty Practice Plans

Academic faculty practice plans present unique challenges for physician leadership, and these challenges are often a function of established structures and hierarchies. These group practices have functioned for many years as independent departments, most often led by a strong department chair who has clear control of departmental budgets and resource allocation. These structures coexist within a loosely defined medical school framework, and there can be marked departmental rivalry. Their mission is not always clear, and tripartite objectives of patient care, research, and teaching can lead to serious conflict. The need to collaborate between departments often has not been established as a priority or an important success factor. The result is pronounced lack of alignment and much variation in terms of support of mission and strategies.

Care delivery and academic endeavors are most often individual based, with a mind-set of entitlement and autonomy among faculty. Leadership positions are most often attained as a result of successful academic careers, and many department chairs are those who have the longest curriculum vitae and most publications. Many of these organizations purport to have a team leadership model; however, interviews and discussion with executives in academic settings suggest that true partnership and collaboration may actually be the exception rather than the rule. Academic prestige for physician leaders is often coupled with a clear hierarchy and what seems to be subservience on the part of administrative colleagues.[58,59]

In recent years, academic medical centers have attempted to alter the dynamics of their faculty practice plans to compete with community-based practices and systems. The result has been a new awareness of the potential of strong physician leadership and willingness to tackle issues that previously were avoided. These issues include an unwieldy cost structure, a lack of horizontal collaboration between departments, and a lack of customer and marketplace orientation. The difficulties are numerous, and what some have termed "academic arrogance" further promotes aversion to change. The necessity for strong leadership in the establishment of business principles and discipline is made all the more urgent by actions by the Health and Human Services Inspector General and other regulatory bodies, and brought home dramatically by multimillion-dollar settlements following PATH (Physicians At Teaching Hospitals) audits.

Hospital-Based and Affiliated Practices

These practices are rapidly growing entities that emerged as a result of the specter of health system reform in the 1990s and have increased in size and influence in the past several years. Many hospitals and hospital systems chose to acquire and employ physicians and physician groups, partly in an attempt to hardwire market share for admissions and other hospital-based services. These initiatives seem logical, particularly in multihospital communities where hospitals were competing for admissions from community-based physicians. This acquisition frenzy is occurring even within communities with a single hospital and no competitors, as organizations focus on positioning to become ACOs.

A major challenge to physician leaders of practices linked to hospitals is an understanding of shared vision, mission, common goals, and strategies. Unlike many large multispecialty groups and integrated delivery systems, these organizations have their cultural roots and major focus within the hospital. These hospitals have functioned as workshops for physicians for many years, but have not engaged in the business and dynamics of physician group practices. At times, it may seem like different languages are spoken by group-practice leaders and hospital leaders. A lack of understanding of differing priorities often leads to conflict. A typical concern for hospital administrators and physician leaders is determining the appropriate setting for specific activities, such as common procedures or imaging studies, which can be done in either the ambulatory or hospital setting. Hospital-owned physician practices attempt to avoid these conflicts, but this is not always possible.[61]

Historically, physician leaders have served primarily as hospital chiefs of staff, with little or no authority. Recently, paid positions as hospital medical directors or affiliated practice medical directors have led to some authority and accountability. Physician leaders employed by the hospital have limited effectiveness if they are seen by their colleagues as serving solely as a "mouthpiece" for hospital administration. Hospital-based physician practices that are most successful are those rooted in strong community missions, coming together explicitly for the purpose of improving the health of their community. A common foundation and purpose, leading to common goals and strategies, is essential, and when this is in place, physician leaders have a chance to lead their organizations forward.

Organized Delivery Systems

These systems span the entire continuum of care, and may or may not be associated with a health plan or financing vehicle. They typically have a significant presence in both the ambulatory and inpatient arenas. Physician leadership of these entities requires sophisticated levels of expertise in a wide range of disciplines. By focusing on the entire continuum of care, these systems offer patients in communities optimally coordinated care for both routine primary care and the entire spectrum of complex specialty and critical care services. This model creates numerous synergies, while avoiding many of the traditional conflicts that occur between hospitals and physicians. Many of these delivery systems serve as so-called "academic halfway houses" and provide academic opportunities not found in most group practices. They do so without the structural encumbrances often present in academic settings.

These practices face significant capital challenges in order to fully capture the opportunities inherent in their model. Physician leadership is crucial to the success of these organizations, and many have a long tradition and history of strong physician leaders. Some of the most evolved team leadership models exist in these organizations because of their complexity and the vast array of skills required to provide effective leadership and management.[62]

■ Skills, Knowledge, and Competencies

Only in recent years has there been research leading to delineation of the leadership and management skills critical to success as a physician leader. Formalization of the physician leadership and management role in group practices is a relatively recent occurrence and has not been fertile ground for research or analysis. Much of what has been described is based on various authors' personal experience, as well as anecdotal observations. This field is rich for potential research and subsequent curriculum design based on research findings. This section explores some of the available data, and addresses leadership and management competencies, styles, and implications for developing future leaders.

American College of Medical Practice Executives Body of Knowledge

In 1996 and 1997, the American College of Medical Practice Executives (ACMPE), the professional development and credentialing organization affiliated with the Medical Group Management Association (MGMA), conducted a study designed to identify the roles and knowledge requirements essential to competent job performance of physician leaders and professional administrators. It also examined the relationships between them and the implications for organizational change. This study was commissioned, in part, because of the perception by ACMPE that physicians were taking on new and heightened leadership roles in group practices. The research inquiry was generated by the growing complexity of the healthcare delivery system and a need to better understand the competencies required to ensure that necessary leadership was in place.[63]

The initial study brought together a panel of experts in medical practice administration. These were predominantly administrators who came from a variety of practice settings, with different educational levels and years of experience. Specific performance domains, as well as the specific tasks involved in each area and the knowledge, skills, and abilities required to accomplish them, were examined. The second phase of the study involved questionnaires based on the identified domains and tasks. Analysis of the questionnaire results included a comparison of the responses of varying subgroups, including physicians and nonphysician respondents.

The study identified eight overall domains or areas of responsibility for group practice administrators. They were:

1. Financial management
2. Human resource management
3. Planning and marketing
4. Information management
5. Risk management

6. Governance and organizational dynamic
7. Business, including operations
8. Professional responsibilities

Specific skills or abilities making up each domain were then identified, resulting in a study that provided a helpful framework for examining roles and performance requirements of medical practice leaders.

Several key findings emerged, including a general agreement on the competencies required of medical practice administrators and physician leaders. Study participants agreed that their roles as physician and nonphysician leaders were very broad, but recognized the requirement for very specific skills and abilities in a number of key areas. Although each domain received high rankings in terms of importance from both administrators and physician leaders, specific activities within domains and the proportion of time allocated to these activities were not uniform, reflecting different prioritization. Subsequent focus groups were quite helpful in this regard, as noted below.

Domains that were felt to be of the most critical importance to both physician and nonphysician leaders were:

- Financial management, including budgeting, accounting systems, financial analysis, control systems, financial systems, cost statements, costs of operations, third-party contracts, retirement planning and investments, and the like
- Business operations, including operational planning, staffing schedules, ancillary support, facilities planning and maintenance, patient flow processes, accreditation, process improvement, and so on
- Human resources, including compliance with federal and state regulations, formulation of compensation and benefits programs, the creation and maintenance of job descriptions, employee appraisal systems, and the like

Survey respondents also noted that governance and organizational dynamics, which include change management, oversight of quality improvement efforts, governance systems, stakeholder relationships, and physician and staff teamwork, were areas that required disproportionate time and energy. One suspects that if the survey were done again today, these areas might become even more imperative.

Subsequent investigators conducted four focus groups of physician and nonphysician administrators to review this and other studies related to competencies. Interesting findings included a higher ranking by physician leaders of the tasks within the governance domain related to "ethical decision making and social responsibility." Similarly, administrators ranked "facilitating and managing change" within the governance domain much higher than did physicians. This higher ranking by nonphysician administrators was not surprising to the focus group participants. They saw leading change as a particularly difficult role for physicians and a fear by physician leaders of being labeled as "one of those administrators." It was also noted that "nothing can change without physician support." Other focus group participants stated that ethical and quality issues are often used by physicians as very powerful excuses for halting change efforts. Change management is an area where administrators can definitely help physician leaders to gain necessary skills and confidence, while supporting physician leaders to lead change efforts. This has significant implications for physician administrator team models of leadership.[58,59,62]

Physician Leader as Change Agent

An increasingly important role for physician leaders is as sponsors of major change efforts. It is no surprise that in an increasingly turbulent environment, considerable change is required. This is challenging even in stable environments, and during times of instability and upheaval, physicians and other professionals clearly tend to find ways to maintain the status quo. There are many compelling reasons for necessary change, including quality, safety, and cost imperatives. In addition, the economic adversity faced by most group practices necessitates decisive alterations in the way practices do their work and the processes involved in patient care delivery. Leading these initiatives is perhaps one of the most testing and uncomfortable roles for the physician leader.

There are numerous examples of successful change leadership in many industries, and these examples exist in healthcare and the group-practice setting as well. Likewise, there are numerous stories and vignettes of large-scale reformation that has not been successful, often because of failures of leadership. Physician leaders today must be students of change management and understand the complex organizational and individual issues that inherently promote resistance to change. Many of these issues are emotional in nature. Yet emotionally driven resistance to change can derail the most logical and fundamental reform efforts.

John Kotter's books, *Leading Change* and *The Heart of Change*, are increasingly popular, and the constructs he describes can be utilized in many industries, including healthcare.[33,34] The applicability and relevance are readily apparent. The eight stages of successful change described are:

1. Establishing a sense of urgency
2. Creating the guiding coalition
3. Developing a vision and strategy
4. Communicating the change vision
5. Empowering broad-based action
6. Generating short-term wins
7. Consolidating gains and producing more change
8. Anchoring new approaches in the culture

Looking at the eight-stage process of facilitating successful major change, it appears to be in many ways designed for the changes ongoing and required in healthcare.[3] We do indeed face a time of great urgency in many of our group practices. Marketplace realities, the regulatory environment, and concerns regarding safety and quality contribute to a sense of crisis. Guiding coalitions take many forms within our medical groups, and the challenge to leadership is to create a guiding coalition for positive change. Unfortunately, guiding coalitions to resist change can be prominent and assume disproportionate power all too often.

It is difficult to overemphasize the importance of a coherent vision and strategy. Physicians, like all staff, need to understand the strategic direction and their role in furthering strategic objectives. This is a critical role for physician leaders. Once that vision is understood, those leaders need to articulate that vision repeatedly, using all possible means. This requires a strong leadership team and often a network to "spread the word." Implementing change requires broad-based action, and physician leaders rarely, if ever, can accomplish this alone. Building broad-based support and then empowering others is essential. Piloting change initiatives in distinct areas of the group practice can generate short-term wins, which provide a foundation for further change and build momentum. Finally, as Kotter points out, changes must be anchored within an organizational or group-practice culture. This is often more difficult than it seems; the adage that "leadership culture becomes the organizational culture" is true in physician organizations as well. It is clear that the role of the physician leader in designing, managing, and implementing change is crucial to organizational success.[64]

Leadership Styles

Much has been written regarding leadership styles and their relative effectiveness. Most of the literature reflects observations and research in areas outside of healthcare; however, applications of findings and theories extend to the healthcare setting. There have been many classifications of leadership styles, coupled with theories as to when

to use each style and how to best assess and understand one's preferred style as a leader. Self-assessment programs, such as that developed by the ACMPE and the American College of Healthcare Executives (ACHE), are invaluable in identifying one's current skills and those needed for particular leadership roles.[65] Understanding one's leadership style is an important part of the self-assessment process. Self-reflection as to how one's style(s) meet the changing needs of the organization is important to developing the leadership approaches necessary for success.[66]

One effective classification of leadership styles is that brought forward by Goleman in 2000.[67] He describes six predominant leadership styles:

1. *Coercive:* Demands immediate compliance
2. *Authoritative:* Mobilizes people toward a vision
3. *Affiliative:* Creates harmony and emotional bonds
4. *Democratic:* Forges consensus through participation
5. *Pace setting:* Sets high standards for performance
6. *Coaching:* Develops people for the future

These styles actually are quite applicable to physician leaders in healthcare organizations and represent a continuum of approaches that are applied with varying effectiveness. Different styles may be required to meet specific issues and obstacles within an organization. These different styles may be optimally utilized by the same leader, and it may actually be the ability to ascertain the most appropriate and effective style for a given situation that can define the successful leader. Numerous examples of situations requiring specific styles are identifiable.

Coercive: This style certainly is required at times when dealing with the regulatory environment. Compliance with HIPAA rules is one example; so is appropriately following guidelines for billing and coding. It is incumbent upon leadership to be clear and to have a zero tolerance policy for deviation from what is required, which most often necessitates a coercive style.

Authoritative: This style can be used effectively when significant change is required and the physician leader plays a central role in defining and articulating a vision and rationale for change. Stating a compelling case for moving forward and mobilizing a guiding coalition may occur secondary to force of personality, as well as logical persuasion. An authoritative leadership style may be quite effective during these times.

Affiliative: The use of this leadership style recognizes that consensus is not always possible; however, decisions made by a leader or leadership team can be best implemented when there is broad-based support. A focus on harmony and relationship building often can serve as "glue" during difficult and challenging times.

Democratic: This style focuses on achieving consensus. It is a typical leadership style for physician leaders and has been particularly dominant in large, multispecialty group practices over the past 30 years. Many of these groups elected leaders and made consensus decisions regarding major strategic direction, large capital purchases, and the like. This style facilitates buy-in, and can be important for those decisions and initiatives that require vast majority support. However, it is, in many ways, responsible for the extremely slow rate of change historically present in many group practices.

Pace setting: This style functions in marked contrast to the more affiliative and democratic styles. High standards and targets for performance are set by leadership, and then well-aligned leadership structures are held accountable for striving to meet these standards. So-called stretch goals are often necessary to make even incremental progress, and knowing when to employ this style effectively is a useful skill for a physician leader.

Coaching: This is an important skill set for physician leaders to develop. Many leaders are increasingly recognizing their major responsibility for facilitating the career development of those with whom they work. This is an important component of talent development and succession planning, as well as skill-building for the future. This will be explored in more detail later in this chapter.

The most effective leaders are able to move from one style to another to meet specific needs. If an organization is in crisis, a leader may need to employ either a coercive or an authoritative style more frequently. Style changes can be confusing to the constituents within an organization, and it is critical for leaders to consider the impact of their behavior and style changes on their management team and others within the organization.[68]

There has been some early research on leadership styles and historical approaches to leadership in group practices. The role of the physician leader and physician manager has been slowly evolving, and most research indicated a predominance of the "middle of the road" style of leadership.[69] This style is often characterized by consensus and majority vote decision making, political maneuvering behind the scenes, and a minimal degree of collaboration. There is also a general reluctance to push too hard for task accomplishment along with fear of lowering morale. Although this has been a predominant mode of leadership in years past, this approach has not been universally effective in meeting current problems, and a blend of those styles noted in the previous list, with a marked reduction in consensus-type decision making, appears to be a necessary component of success.

Leadership vs. Management

Much has been written regarding leadership and management as separate but intertwined disciplines. Some have suggested that the skill sets required for effective management are quite different, and many times quite contrary, to those required for strong leadership. There has been little specific research on this within the healthcare sector; however, conclusions and concepts from work in other disciplines appear to be applicable to the group-practice setting. Clearly, there are distinct disciplines, and it is erroneous to use the terms "leadership" and "management" interchangeably.

One author and prominent leadership expert[70] looked at the discipline of management as creating order, setting impersonal goals, and requiring little emotional involvement.[67] He identified leadership as a discipline focused on changing the existing order of things, coupled with very personal goals and a high level of emotional involvement and intensity associated with the work. Another author[71] suggests that the manager's central function is to cope with complexity and develop methods for motivating others using organizational control systems and rewards.[66] This contrasts with the central function of leaders: to cope with change while inspiring and empowering followers to move forward towards a shared vision.

It would seem that both constructs have relevance to group-practice leadership and require, in part, different skills and training. These differences may resonate with some and be impetus to the physician leader–administrator team model of leadership, whereas to others this distinction may appear to be a false dichotomy. We have all encountered physicians who were very effective managers, with limited or no ability to inspire and lead change efforts. Conversely, strong leaders may have limited managerial competencies, and may be intolerant of the discipline required to be an effective manager.

Ideally, physician leaders can embody both leadership and management skills, and a skill assessment can lead to the development of a professional growth and improvement plan.[72] Practically speaking, it is the rare leader who is both an outstanding manager and inspiring leader; team structures can play a significant role in ensuring that the necessary skills are present. Emerging literature suggests that the presence of basic leadership and management practices within organizations are clearly correlated with the fundamental ability to achieve desired results. This has already been demonstrated by healthcare organizations that have chosen to pursue Baldridge Award designation and other recognition, and more evidence should be forthcoming.

Training, Education, and Experience

The recognition of physician leadership and management as a discipline that requires formal training and significant experience is relatively new. Most group practices have traditionally viewed physician leadership as something that is easy to do and made up of predominantly ad hoc activities requiring little time or investment. This continues to be the case in many smaller group practices. However, it is becoming increasingly apparent that approaching group-practice leadership as an important discipline with a specific body of knowledge, as noted earlier, is both advisable and necessary for organizational success.

There has also been much discussion of the question, "Are leaders born or made?" The answer to this question is by no means clear; certainly many skills must be acquired to perform effectively as a leader and manager. Certain personality characteristics appear to be more prevalent in strong leaders, and, of course, there are exceptions to every generalization. Some work suggests that certain medical specialties attract individuals with certain personality characteristics, and this would suggest possible research as to which specialists might make the most effective leaders, particularly in a multispecialty group setting.

A review of the literature reveals some interesting theories. Some relatively older studies looked at physician leadership styles, physician personality types, and other characteristics with implications for education and training. As a group, physicians in general were felt to have a low propensity for group behavior. Low-inclusion behavior, or a requirement for not feeling very much part of a group or team, seemed to be a skill that facilitated the often necessary need to function autonomously in the clinical realm.[69] It was also thought, however, that this relatively low need for inclusion resulted in less effectiveness as a physician leader or manager. The managerial role demands a high degree of interaction in an organizational setting.

Research indicates that physicians have a moderately high need to be in charge and attempt to get others to do what they want them to do. This fits with a high control orientation, which is reflected in traditional physician training. Physicians traditionally show a preference for remaining somewhat distant from others. This detachment may be reflective of the adaptive need to separate oneself from one's patients and their often life-threatening illnesses. These attributes are not necessarily helpful in developing leadership behavior.

These types of behavioral characteristics in early studies led to the recognition that there was a significant need for physician education in order to build effective leadership and management skills. Relatively few physicians have been formally trained in management and leadership, and those who abruptly find themselves in these positions often use styles and behaviors that have been only casually observed. This is not unlike the adoption of specific clinical approaches, where physicians may identify with a particular technique used by a more experienced colleague, and quickly adapt that to their own practice.[69]

An entire industry has emerged over the last 30 years to educate and train physician leaders. The American College of Physician Executives, the ACMPE, and other associations have created curriculum tracks for physician leaders. These organizations focus on the development of identified skills and competencies that can be of great benefit in preparing for management positions. Numerous academic institutions have created physician-specific certificate and degree programs in their schools of business, public health, and public policy. Several authors suggest that preparing for a management position is largely technical in nature and must be combined with adequate on-the-job experience.[73,74]

Although core management skills may be readily identified and subsequently taught, skills required for leadership roles might be quite different. Leadership roles are thought to require considerable self-awareness and character development, coupled with strong managerial skills.[75] Leadership, in many ways, is thought to be a "relational phenomenon." Leaders can exist in teams of varying sizes and within organizations at varying levels. In group practices, it is the leader who functions at the top of the organizational chart, who must articulate a vision and lead an organization to achieve its aspirations.

Competency in strategic leadership is critical for physician executives who must function in exceedingly complex environments. The ability to lead by the exercise of power and influence in a productive fashion is a challenging and important competency for the physician leader.

Much has been written about strategic leadership and the necessary abilities to perform strategic analysis and lead strategic change. These additional skills are imperative in group practices today. Much has also been said regarding leadership character. Character reflects personal values and integrity. Strong personal values and leaders who are recognized as having high integrity engender trust, and trust is a principal aspect of leading people toward the attainment of a common vision.

The question remains as to how to identify, train, and mentor physician leaders.[76] Many attributes of potential leaders are apparent as they perform their clinical tasks and join and participate in teams and organizational life. These personality attributes can lead to a readiness to acquire both leadership and managerial competencies via formal training and experience. One cannot overstate the benefit of on-the-job experience and strong mentoring. Physicians working with strong leaders and managers who take a genuine interest in their skill acquisition and professional development benefit greatly from this mentoring. Those lucky enough to have this experience are able to accelerate both formal and experiential training and build the skill sets necessary to succeed.

External Relationships

A major responsibility for the physician group-practice leader is to represent the group in a variety of settings and to be the public face of the group, its physicians, and staff. This requires a variety of skills and willingness to, at times, step out of the comfort zone within the walls of the practice itself. An understanding of the importance of many diverse external relationships is vital, and successful group practices support this leadership work.

Referral Relationships

Ensuring strong, collaborative referral relationships is one responsibility of leadership readily supported by group-practice physicians. It is easy to understand the necessity for channels of distribution that ensure a steady stream of patients into a group practice. Working with referring physicians to understand their needs and expectations is essential. Many specialty practices are highly effective in this work, but others seemingly miss an opportunity to solidify referral relationships by providing outstanding consultation and service. Physician leaders set the tone for others within their group, and must often lead by example in working with referring physicians. Identification of best practices within a group, using peer persuasion to ensure that referring physicians are treated with respect,

and providing a service orientation are all important. Communication is paramount and should be part of a distinct customer focus. Time spent working on referral relationships by physician leaders is generally highly valued by group members.

Hospital Relationships

Relationships with hospitals within a given community can take many forms and are a function of specific group-practice and hospital dynamics within a local community. These relationships may often take considerable amounts of time and energy, and there are many examples of collaboration and competition coexisting. Although both physician group-practice leaders and hospital executives often frame their conversations and public reporting of their interactions as striving for overall community benefit, their divergent goals and strategies historically have led to fragmentation, and impede care within the community. Major areas of friction revolve around the locale for provision of particular services. Hospitals have feared dissipation of profitable programs as they care for the severely ill, and competition from the many physician groups providing procedures and care previously performed in the hospital setting. From the physician perspective, declining reimbursements for professional services have been offset by expansion into traditional hospital domains. Physician-owned ambulatory surgery centers, imaging centers, and free-standing catheterization labs and lithotripters are examples of this phenomenon. Duplication of resources and overinvestment in technology beyond that supported by a given population has often been the result.[61]

With the emphasis on collaborative coordinated care, ACOs, bundle payments, and other aspects of the PPACA, hospitals and group practices are looking for ways to collaborate and be prepared for the emerging milieu.

Rarely have physician group-practice leaders and hospital executives worked together to thoughtfully plan and rationally approach resource utilization in order to serve the health and well-being of their community. Physician leaders must be engaged in working with their community hospitals; it is only through ongoing dialogue and improved understanding that competition can evolve into a collaboration that truly puts patients and the community first, and allows for optimizing quality and wise stewardship of community resources. This work is an important activity for physician leaders in group practices today.

Payers, Purchasers, and Employers

Physician leaders in group practices have traditionally deferred direct interaction with the payer and employer community to health plans, brokers, and consultants. This deference may actually be detrimental to the well-being of group practices, and in recent years direct communication between physician group-practice leaders and their purchaser community has led to fruitful collaboration. Credibility of physician leaders, in the minds of employers and businesspeople, is an important attribute upon which to capitalize. Despite concerns regarding escalating costs and the role of physicians and hospitals in driving these cost increases, mutual respect among business leaders and physician leaders of group practices still exists. Physician leaders are wise to seek input and ideas from colleagues in the business community. By building relationships and understanding, effective breakthroughs can occur.

There are many examples of purchaser coalitions and purchaser–provider relationships over the last several years that have led to pay-for-performance initiatives and new approaches to contracting. The Marketplace Collaborative Project at Virginia Mason Medical Center in Seattle, Washington, has resulted in dramatically lower employer costs in areas of their greatest expenditure, while improving quality and patient satisfaction.[77] These type of initiatives help group practices and their physicians move beyond the customary economic paradigms into approaches that can create win-win situations for all concerned.

Evaluators

Criteria to measure quality and outcomes have been sorely lacking in healthcare. In recent years a number of organizations have been created for the purposes of defining and measuring quality, and it is essential that physician leadership understand and engage in this important work. Those who are designing the metrics welcome physician leadership involvement, and it is only by participating that the leaders of group practice have their viewpoint recognized during the creation process. Organizations such as Leapfrog, HEDIS, and National Quality Forum, among others, are actively engaged in this work. Internet-based for-profit companies have established rating agencies using specific data sets. Metrics for performance measurement are changing as more is learned, and physician leaders should seek to build relationships both regionally and nationally in this domain. By having group-practice leaders involved, the mentality of "victim" so prominent in these chaotic times among physicians can be modified and channeled into participating in designing the solutions to our quality and safety dilemmas. Collaborating with and not resisting the evaluator is an important external relationship role for group-practice leaders.[78]

Social Responsibility and Public Policy

Although it is said all politics are local, it would appear that policy initiatives in the healthcare industry are being developed and implemented at the national, state, and local levels. The group-practice community and physician leaders have much to offer this public policy debate. One could argue that this involvement is necessary to ensure that the voice of the patients is truly heard. As group-practice leaders get involved in these discussions, it is critical that they be perceived as placing the overall community and patient care above their own selfish, economic interests. Unfortunately, all too often, physicians and hospitals are perceived as advocating only for their own individual interests, and the overall message is obscured. Physician leaders who engage in public health issues and recognize the plight of the underserved reflect very positively on their group practices in the eyes of others in the community.

It is particularly important that business executives as well as public officials understand group practices' commitment to community health. Involvement in issues not related to healthcare but critical to community well-being are also important, worthwhile endeavors. Volunteerism is necessary for any community to thrive, and encouraging a mind-set conducive to charitable purposes and volunteerism within the group-practice physicians and staff can be an important, visible, and rewarding role for physician leaders.

Professional Organizations and Associations

Today there is a myriad of professional organizations in which physician leaders participate. These organizations have many diverse purposes and varying effectiveness. Many physician leaders remain active in their specialty society, and despite considerable time in leadership and management, still identify predominantly with organizations such as the American College of Physicians, American College of Surgeons, and so on. These specialty societies, while representing physicians within a single specialty, have broadened their work to also include leadership, education, and training. Some physician leaders become quite active in group-practice associations and find this involvement quite rewarding.

It is often said that leadership is a lonely pursuit. Many associations serve the primary purpose of facilitating networking among leaders with much in common. The opportunity to share ideas and experiences, as well as the collegiality and support structures that ensue, are invaluable to the physician leader, particularly at times of change and challenge. Many have found that taking advantage of connections developed via participation in group-practice associations, such as the MGMA and the American Medical Group Association, enables one to quickly contact colleagues across the country to discuss challenging issues in real time. Many of these organizations have educational curricula, and organizations such as the ACMPE, the American College of Physician Executives, and the American College of Healthcare Executives have certification tracks as well.

Involvement in organized medicine is an endeavor that appeals to many group-practice leaders. The American Medical Association and state and county medical associations serve as political forces on behalf of their members. They have considerable influence in state capitals and Washington, D.C., as policy and legislation are brought forward. Although often the scene of interspecialty conflict and seemingly divergent purpose, many believe that participation and involvement are critical if a patient-focused agenda is to be brought forward. Given the prominence of healthcare as a high-priority public policy and political issue, the voice of physicians and physician leaders must continue to be heard; involvement in organized medicine may be more important than ever before.

Internal Relationships

Today's healthcare organizations are complex entities with many diverse, hierarchical, and matrix structures. Positive relationships between the physician leaders and physicians and staff within these organizations are critical to moving forward with common purpose and execution of strategic objectives. These constructive relationships do not just happen; they require deliberate, thoughtful approaches coupled with high levels of candor and trust.

Relationships with Staff and Faculty Physicians

Successful physician leaders are trusted and respected by the physicians within their group practice. They must build their credibility and trust over a period of time and often do so by building both personal and professional relationships. Leading by example is often an effective way to gain respect; however, one-on-one interaction, sharing experiences and challenging patient care dilemmas, and leading and participating in teams further the development of these very important relationships. Establishing relationships founded on trust leads to better execution and results. As part of this process, trust

facilitates a willingness to engage in productive conflict to circumvent the conflict avoidance that often allows situations to escalate out of control. This may have a detrimental impact on group cohesiveness and professional satisfaction. As Lencioni points out, trust facilitates productive conflict, which in and of itself leads to commitment and a willingness to be accountable within group practices.[79]

Important to building healthy relationships between the leader and staff and faculty physicians is the development of a culture of feedback. This, until recently, has been woefully lacking in healthcare, particularly among physician practices. Physicians historically have not been willing to give or receive feedback, and at times this has led to catastrophic consequences, both for group practices and the patients they serve. Many organizations are now actively promoting a culture of feedback, and some, such as Virginia Mason Medical Center in Seattle, Washington, require that every physician receive feedback via a 360-degree feedback instrument on an annual basis. Creating an environment where this occurs effectively falls to the physician leader, and this work succeeds to a large extent because of positive relationships that have been solidified over many years.

Relationships with Other Physician Leaders

Today, in many group practices of significant size, the physician leadership structure needs to go beyond the single physician CEO or medical director. It is critical that physician leaders work together as a team and align with the vision and strategic objectives of the organization.[80] Many physician leaders, including department chairs and others, have traditionally been chosen by their constituents. This electoral method of leader selection, although providing a semblance of physician control, inevitably leads to primarily politically driven decision making. This is most often not in the group practice's best interest. The relationship between physician leaders should be one that promotes peer accountability. Trust levels should be high and competition minimized such that leaders can truly hold each other accountable.

Physician leaders face difficult challenges; having leadership colleagues within a large group practice can provide crucial levels of support while reinforcing tough decision making. It is often necessary to change physician leaders to meet the needs of the current environment. Respected leaders must be respected clinicians, but being a respected clinician is not, in and of itself, a guarantee of strong leadership skills. Focusing on coaching and mentoring allows the growth of talent within the physician ranks to ensure a pool of individuals competent and interested in taking on leadership roles in the future. Depth of leadership within a group practice is an important success factor and critical to developing a cohesive physician organization.

Relationships with Nonphysician Leaders and Staff

Although it is true that physician leaders and staff physicians within a group practice clearly set the tone, it should not in any way be implied that only physicians are critical to the success of group practices. In fact, one can make the case that for many purposes the nonphysician staff and leadership are most important. It is being increasingly recognized that the importance of service as a component of overall quality, and many researchers indicate that service performance that builds customer loyalty can be of greater importance than perceptions of clinical quality in the minds of patients and potential customers.

Fostering collaboration with all members of the healthcare delivery team is crucial, and physician leaders play a very important and visible role in developing this collaboration. Traditional hierarchies must be overcome; the physician-centric mind-set can interfere with the development of effective collaboration. It is important to emphasize that physician leaders must nurture supportive relationships with administrators, managers, and all staff. By building these supportive relationships, leaders ensure that vision, mission, and strategy are effectively deployed throughout the organization. This alignment is critical to execution, but has not historically been a priority within group practices. Group practices that have achieved broad alignment throughout their organization are best able to cope with the rapidly changing environment and to execute new and innovative strategies designed to ensure that they thrive in the years ahead.

Physician Leader as Coach

The coaching style of leadership is becoming increasingly important within the group-practice setting. As noted, physicians and physician leaders have not traditionally been receptive to giving or receiving feedback, and coaching relies heavily on building a climate and culture of feedback.[68]

Research indicates that the coaching style works well, and is most effective when people on the receiving end are interested and receptive. This certainly is not always the case with physicians who have long prided themselves as having it all figured out. Managers today are being asked to help employees develop new skills and "be the best

that they can be," and those employees who understand their weaknesses and have the desire to cultivate new abilities can be most receptive to coaching. This cohort seems to be increasing among physicians, who recognize the need to adapt to a constantly shifting environment and work climate.[72]

Coaching leaders can help those they work with identify unique strengths and weaknesses and help them connect their personal and professional aspirations. An aspect of coaching that has been extremely helpful to many young physicians who hope to become leaders is the encouragement to establish long-term development goals and a work plan for achieving them. Leaders who excel at coaching are superb at delegating, and also recognize the necessity of occasionally tolerating short-term failures for the purpose of long-term performance enhancement. As healthcare organizations become increasingly complex, coaching styles need to be employed more frequently. Many leaders and managers are uncomfortable with coaching, and this often relates to the need to give ongoing performance feedback. Developing a style that facilitates delivering feedback in a constructive, open-ended fashion is a critical successful factor for physician leaders in the future.[81]

Physician Compensation Issues

One of the most challenging and historically important roles for physician leaders has been providing leadership for the design and implementation of physician compensation plans. These plans reveal the priorities, vision, and mission of individual groups, and have traditionally been of critical importance to sustaining the integrity of group practices. It is necessary for the physician leader to understand the subtle as well as overt messages that are transmitted to physicians, staff, and even patients as a result of a group's compensation plan. Physician compensation approaches have long been a source of conflict within many group practices and have evolved considerably over a period of years. Many early group practices were founded on a concept of total equality and "equal share." These plans provided little distinction among individual physicians and consequently few incentives for desired performance. As salaries increased and income opportunities developed among different specialties, it became clear that equal distribution of income would no longer work to sustain the all-important group-practice value proposition. To effectively compete, it became necessary, in multispecialty groups, to substantially differentiate the salaries for proceduralists from those of so-called cognitive physicians. Within single-specialty groups, it became clear that work effort was highly variable and that incentives needed to be aligned with desired performance.

In recent years, a wide range of plans has been used in group practices across the country. These plans seem to be constantly in flux; clearly, it is often necessary to change physician compensation plans for a variety of business and strategic purposes. Unfortunately, it is often a difficult and disruptive process, and therein lies the importance of physician leadership engagement.

It is clear in most industries that incentives should be carefully aligned with individual performance and organizational priorities. This has become the key foundational element in physician group-practice compensation plan design.[82] Even group practices embedded in traditional staff model HMOs, such as Kaiser-Permanente Medical Group and Group Health Cooperative of Puget Sound, have strayed from their standard step and range salary structure, which historically adjusts only by specialty and marketplace as contrasted with performance. It is becoming apparent that productivity incentives generate higher levels of productivity, and utilization of benchmark surveys from a variety of sources facilitates plan design and structure. Moving from a plan with little incentive for productivity to one that is predominantly productivity-driven has been shown to substantially improve organizational economics in the fee-for-service world still predominant in most communities.

Recently there has been considerable impetus to consider modifiers to productivity- driven compensation systems, as paying for value rather than volume becomes the focus. Measurable quality metrics and patient satisfaction are being used by some to balance predominantly productivity or salary compensation models. Productivity remains important, even in a value-driven reimbursement system, and should not be discouraged.

An important task for physician leadership is to ensure continuing balance between optimizing quality and service while also focusing on productivity and efficiency. Teaching and research may be added to the incentive system in some organizations that include these endeavors in their mission.

When it comes to physician compensation, individual physicians can often be singularly focused on the impact on them as individuals. The physician leader's responsibility is to keep the greater good of the group, as well as the mission and strategies of the group practice, clearly in focus.[83] At times this requires managing significant degrees of conflict and deploying one's personal power of persuasion and credibility. Many physician leaders have lost leadership opportunities because of their inability to effectively lead compensation change efforts. It is critical to always consider the impact of physician compensation plans on patient care processes and the delivery of a quality product. Unfortunately, the physician leader may discover this to be a lonely pursuit.

■ Collaboration and Teamwork

The ability to collaborate as team member and partner is a critical competency required in physician leaders who desire to take their organizations to the next level. It is such an essential competency that it warrants highlighting in this chapter. It is clear that a team leadership model can be extremely effective, bringing together diversity of skills and perspectives, having the ability to respond quickly to changing demands, and certainly reducing overdependency on single individuals. Team leadership models improve communication, enhance one's willingness to take risk, and are conducive to ongoing personal growth and development. These models have been increasingly recognized as having great value, and are being deployed to varying extents in group practices across the United States.[58,59]

The management literature in the late 1990s through today contains numerous articles and books on the value of teams used to accomplish the work within organizations. The literature indicates that "the team remains the most flexible and powerful unit of performance, learning, and change in any organization."[84] Despite promising results coming from Japan, U.S. industry has been slow to adopt the concept of multidisciplinary work teams, and healthcare certainly has lagged even further behind. The characteristics of teams that Katzenbach, Smith, and others believe lead to high performance include[84]:

- Bringing together complementary skills and experience, which create synergy beyond the individuals involved
- Providing a broader mix of skills and knowledge to respond to complex challenges
- Providing flexibility and responsiveness; as these demands change, the team can quickly change course

Labeling a group of people a team, however, certainly does not make them a team in function!

Throughout their medical education, physician leaders have been trained in the values of independence and autonomy. Developing leaders as part of a "learning team" requires new skills and organizational support. Research and experience suggest that there are definitely factors that facilitate the creation of a high-performance team, and they can be directly applied to that team created by the physician leader and the professional administrator partner. Suggested approaches include:

- Have clear, ambitious, and measurable team performance goals from the organization.
- Make a formal commitment to the team, educate yourself, and identify team role models.
- Develop a combined work agenda; identify and assign roles strategically. What are your goals for each item?
- Communicate via regular meetings; develop agenda items, but also keep time for unplanned conversation.
- Build trust, and agree to disagree if needed.
- Engage in self-evaluation and team evaluation.

Many have shared ideas on critical ingredients to building a learning team, one that is constantly growing, developing, and enhancing its performance. Suggestions include:

- Participate in formal leadership programs.
- Regularly complete 360-degree assessments of one's leadership skills and potentially share the results with your partner.
- Provide informal feedback and coaching for each other and debrief frequently.
- Share articles, books, and other instructive literature on leadership.
- Practice the art of giving and receiving feedback.
- Spend time together.
- Use conflict as a learning tool.
- Share self-assessment of strengths, weaknesses, and personality differences as a tool for building respect and trust.

Many pitfalls can occur in the process of striving to be part of an optimal team, and these are important for the physician leader to keep in mind. Some of the challenges to the team model of leadership include:

- A potential lack of accountability for performance and diffusion of responsibility
- A strong, charismatic physician leader who sees little value in teamwork
- Overuse of the team for all issues as opposed to selected deployment of team capabilities
- An overly high value placed on autonomy and individual recognition
- The personalities of team members

Some have written about pseudo-teams that in reality achieve little to no synergy from their work together.

However, the physician leader can derive great satisfaction from collaboration and teamwork, resulting in enhanced performance, stronger results, and high levels of professional satisfaction.[85]

Illustrative Leadership Vignettes

Some real-life situational vignettes serve as very effective illustrations of leadership challenges and optimal leadership behaviors. Following are brief synopses of events that have occurred in physician group practice and, furthermore, are commonplace occurrences in group practices today.

The Problem Physician

Dr. R. had been in practice for 7 years. He had distinguished himself as a superb medical subspecialist and was a much sought after consultant and educator. He enjoyed his consultative practice and built a loyal following of referring physicians, patients, and their families. He developed a reputation within the group practice as being always available, and never one to say no to a timely consultation. He chose to pursue numerous clinical interests, including diversifying into many areas related to his core specialty. His work volume continued to increase, and it became clear that he was not able to keep up with necessary documentation in a timely fashion. This became apparent when additional consultants would not find up-to-date chart notes and when routine compliance audits indicated lack of documentation for charges submitted.

His direct supervisor and physician leader was notified and confronted the issue. Dr. R. was very upset because he had never been criticized or given any feedback during his tenure within the group practice. Though initially denying that his workload was problematic, he agreed that he would quickly get up-to-date with his documentation and this would not occur again. There was little formal follow-up until it became necessary for physicians to move their offices. On the Friday of the weekend this was to occur, Dr. R. was on vacation, and his assistant willingly accepted the responsibility for facilitating his move. Early in the process she discovered over 150 charts and medical records contained within cabinets, drawers, under desks, and so on. She brought this to the attention of her supervisor, who brought it to the attention of the physician leader.

Another conversation occurred between the physician leader and Dr. R., and subsequently Dr. R. berated his assistant for lack of loyalty and "turning him in." Senior leadership within the group practice was notified and

Dr. R.'s behavior was found to be totally unacceptable. An immediate improvement plan was initiated, and clear consequences for lack of compliance with this plan were spelled out, up to and including termination from the group. The assistant was thanked by the organization's senior leaders for her courage and willingness to bring attention to issues that clearly were detrimental to patient care. Dr. R. subsequently complied with his improvement plan, and through additional counseling, feedback, and support, finally began to set limits, learned to say no, and began to thrive.

Several lessons emerge from this vignette that illustrate the importance of clear policies, procedures, and a willingness on the part of physician leaders to hold colleagues accountable. Clearly articulating the adverse impact of these and similar practices on patient care is important in providing context for behavioral change. Written documentation of problem behavior and agreed-upon improvement plans are critical and historically lacking within group practices. Follow-up and constancy are required in order to ensure that necessary performance improvements occur. Physician leadership has a key role in protecting the interests of patients, group-practice physicians, and staff, and in facilitating improvement work of all types.

Lack of Alignment

A large group practice in the early 1990s recognized the importance of developing clinical guidelines and pathways. It was clear that standardization and elimination of unnecessary variation were critical ingredients to ensuring quality, and a task force was appointed with clinical leaders who were passionate about quality initiatives. Over the next 2 years, several guidelines were developed using evidence-based medicine and consensus development with specialty physicians working collaboratively with primary physicians. There was considerable optimism that these guidelines would increasingly take hold within the organization and become the norm for clinical care delivery.

Unfortunately, adoption of the guidelines and compliance with recommendations coming from the guidelines task force were sporadic at best. Those who had invested significant time and energy in guideline development became frustrated, and it was clear that senior leadership had not prioritized this work in a way that would eventually facilitate its widespread implementation.

Simultaneously, the group practice was going through major changes in leadership, and subsequently, the organization CEO and senior physician leaders were elected by the physicians; much decision making was inherently political. Influencing or mandating practice pattern changes was impossible, given the political nature of leader selection and the desire of physician leaders to remain in their jobs. Despite a long history of collaboration within the group practice, it was clear that individual autonomy remained a very central value within the group.

With the election of a new CEO and senior physician leaders, it became apparent that the organization needed to change its decision-making process, as well as redefine the implied agreement or compact between the organization and its physicians. This occurred after considerable internal dialogue, and an appointment process to select physician leaders emerged. In addition, a group of frontline physicians was appointed to develop a physician compact that explicitly delineated the gives and gets between the organization and its physicians. Embedded in this compact was a commitment to follow established guidelines and pathways designed by the group practices' physicians and clinical leaders after review of all available evidence and experience. What was unique was codifying the responsibility for following agreed-upon best practices and committing to each and every patient that they would receive care in a manner that had been agreed upon as optimal.

The implications of the compact were widespread, and impacted physician behavior as well as clinical decision making. Recognition that once a best practice was identified it was incumbent upon every clinician to provide care utilizing this evidence was seemingly a breakthrough. Clarification regarding expectations of being a physician member of the group practice, and what every physician had a right to expect as benefits from this practice, helped to propel this organization forward, both clinically and economically.

Physician leadership with a willingness to challenge traditional approaches, in both governance and clinical care delivery, will increasingly be necessary in the years ahead.

Changing Leaders

A highly productive proceduralist specialty within a multispecialty group practice had recently been designated as a priority program. This suggested that the organization was interested in infusing significant resources to support growth, acquisition of technology, and positioning the clinical division as a premier program within the marketplace. This decision was predicated on outstanding outcomes, superb clinicians, and strong marketplace opportunity.

Although seemingly firing on all cylinders, it became clear that the clinical division was poorly prepared to take full advantage of its recent prioritization. Although it was composed of superb clinicians on an individual basis, they did not function as a team, and any suggestions of change were met with significant skepticism by the division leader. The division leader was a respected clinician, who had done a superb job of recruiting, and seemingly had prioritized maintenance of the status quo. He resisted any suggestions of change from senior leadership as potentially upsetting the apple cart, causing clinicians to leave the group to pursue other opportunities. Change was clearly necessary, and a cohesive strategic plan for the division needed to be crafted.

It became apparent to senior leadership that a division leadership change was necessary, and after much dialogue and one-on-one conversation, a change was made. An extremely intense, hard-working subspecialty clinician was appointed division head, to the surprise of most. He was believed to be the single individual who had the total respect of all clinicians, but most felt that he did not have an aptitude for, or interest in, leadership.

The results were astounding. The division moved aggressively forward with a collaborative team approach, and processes improved, leading to markedly enhanced efficiency. Strategic growth planning was initiated, and professional and staff satisfaction increased. Collaboration with other divisions in the group practice flourished.

This vignette illustrates the importance of aligning leadership with organizational objectives. At times it may be necessary to replace leaders who, under other circumstances, are excellent clinicians and more than adequate leaders. Leadership skills and approaches must be in sync with organizational and division needs. Difficult change may be a necessary prerequisite for progress, and at times it is necessary to help loyal and respected individuals return to full-time clinical practice. This is a difficult, but necessary, task of physician leadership.

■ Opportunities, Risks, and Vulnerabilities

The decision to seriously pursue a career focus as a physician leader should not be undertaken lightly. There are increasing opportunities, but each comes with risks and some may require giving up one's clinical practice. Being aware of the risks and one's own vulnerabilities is invaluable in making a wise career choice.

Physician Leadership: A Growth Industry

Recent years have seen the role of the physician leader emerge in a manner that suggests it is becoming a highly sought-after career pathway. This is, in part, a function of

supply and demand and the recognition of the criticality of physician leadership for group-practice success. This phenomenon has certainly increased in the past 20 years, and today various associations and certifying bodies are creating fellowships and masters programs designed specifically for physicians. Many major universities have identified executive MBA programs and certificates in medical management that have physician leaders and aspiring physician leaders as their major target market. There are many schools of thought regarding the necessary academic credentials for a physician leader in various settings. Experience continues to be an important attribute in the most highly sought-after candidates, and those with substantial long-term physician leadership experience are small in number.

The opportunities for physician leaders vary by organization type. Many hospitals and health plans are seeking physicians to fill full-time leadership positions, and many of these individuals come from group-practice positions. Likewise, group practices, which traditionally have looked within their own ranks for leaders to fill open positions, are now willing to work with recruitment firms to identify the best talent available from around the country.

Much can be said for developing talent within a given organization to facilitate succession planning. Knowledge of organizational culture, strategy, and personalities can be invaluable. At times, however, group practices have admitted that they suboptimize leadership selection because of an unwillingness to look outside their organizations. Numerous recruiting firms have begun to specialize in physician leadership recruitment, and all indicate this is a rapidly growing segment of their business.

For the individual physician leader, it is a rapidly changing environment. Many physician leaders assumed they would work in the same group practice for their entire careers, and now recognize that leadership opportunities may take them elsewhere. Willingness to relocate in order to take advantage of these opportunities is necessary. Many physician leaders now deliberately plan their career development pathways, and recognize the significant opportunities leadership provides. Many are looking to add diversity to their work life, moving beyond what some perceive to be the tedium of clinical practice, as well as income enhancement opportunities.

Measures of Success

As in most endeavors, medical group practices must have metrics of performance, and clear concepts as to what constitutes success. Medical practice leaders today are running complex businesses. Although the size and complexity of individual practices may vary, all are influenced by the diverse stakeholders that control the practice of medicine. These include physicians, partners or employees, third-party payers, regulators, and ultimately, the patient. Measures of success may vary depending on the stakeholder's perspective.

Historically, most measures of success for group practices have focused on financial indicators. Net revenue per physician, average physician income, and group-practice margin have been important metrics. Margin or profit available for retained earnings has gained importance, as the need to reinvest in facilities, technology, and human capital have become a priority. The annual MGMA report, "Performance and Practices of Successful Medical Groups,"[86] points out that success on financial performance indicators, such as profitability, cost management, productivity, capacity staffing, accounts receivable collection, and managed care operations, are critical ingredients to ensure that a group practice thrives and is able to continue to deliver care to its patients.

These metrics, however, have little to do with the metrics that are of primary importance to patients. Physician leadership in concert with professional administrator expertise is required to execute on these metrics as well as those that are not financial in nature. These metrics often tie to the patients' experience within the group practice, with quality outcomes and service being most prominent. Transparency of outcomes increasingly is becoming an issue, and the business community as well as government are working hard to distinguish characteristics of outstanding clinical care delivery. It is incumbent upon group-practice leadership to position its group effectively and to prioritize the generation and articulation of quality outcomes in order to succeed in the future. Other metrics, such as patient satisfaction, staff turnover and satisfaction, and appointment access, are critical indicators of leadership success.

The leadership team within the group practice is ultimately accountable for their results, and physician leaders should work closely with their boards, executive committees, and those in governance to clearly articulate the measures of success upon which performance is judged. Aligning priorities and leadership behavior with these measures of success is critical.

■ Barriers to Success

There are many potential impediments to the physician leader's success in the group-practice setting. Many are specific to the situation and relate to dynamics within an individual group as well as the personality and approaches of the physician leader. General themes emerge as one studies both successful and unsuccessful leadership across the United States. It is clear that serving as a physician leader is exciting, challenging, and in many ways a privilege. The opportunity to lead groups of professionals for the betterment of patient care and their communities can be an opportunity to fully use one's creativity, intellect, and passion, in very tangible ways.

Inadequate preparation and time commitment to this work is a primary barrier to success. Many physicians have thought that leadership and management were "no brainer" types of activities that presented little that could not be learned quickly and easily. The result has been many physician leaders who dabble in the realm of leadership, but have never seriously pursued advanced education or even networking opportunities to facilitate their learning or leadership development. This lack of appreciation of the complexity and the discipline required to be a strong physician leader can be a barrier to success.

An additional issue of significance to physician leaders is the conundrum of balancing clinical practice and leadership responsibilities. Approaches to this dilemma have taken many forms, depending on group culture and individual inclinations. Many group practices that choose their leaders from within expect their physician leaders to continue to practice. This is often preferred by physician leaders, because their roots and their core identity are more that of clinician than leader. This may also serve to enhance credibility, particularly when dealing with difficult change management around clinical care delivery issues. Other organizations feel they have evolved to the point that physician leaders are no longer expected to practice. This suggests recognition that physician leaders' identity must evolve from that of clinician to leader, and clinical practice becomes a distraction to one's core responsibilities. There is no one perfect model; however, lack of recognition of this dilemma, and efforts to excel in both clinical and leadership realms, often present a significant barrier to success. The result is an inability to focus in a way necessary to deal with today's issues.[87]

Among many additional barriers, it is important to highlight the necessary organizational attributes that must be present for leadership success. Group practices must value their physician leaders. This means supporting the leader in terms of time allocation, leadership development opportunities, and remuneration. It is critical that the leader be supported in a way that allows him or her to pursue activities in the best interest of patients and the group practice. This may at times represent a departure from the egalitarian and individual-centric nature of many group practices, and recognizes that a leader must have responsibility, accountability, and authority to do their best work. Alignment of organizational mission, vision, and strategies is critical, and lack of alignment and an unwillingness to support the leader may be insurmountable barriers.

In the final analysis, physician leaders must be capable of leading teams of people to their full potential. Recognition of the importance of teams and the importance of the physician leader, as well as leading teams and serving as team member and partner, are essential. Inability to do so represents a fundamental barrier to success that is difficult to overcome despite the presence of other strong leadership attributes. This is particularly true in today's complex healthcare environment, and it is clear that attributes that come with clinical training and are perceived as strengths in the clinical domain are no longer an asset, and can represent a significant barrier to group-practice leadership success.

■ The Future

The future is bright and with great potential for physician leadership in group practice. Continuous learning and focus as well as disciplined planning will be required. Bringing management principles and rigorous approaches to this work will be essential to success. This will include ongoing research, a willingness to learn from other industries, and a focus on developing talent and succession planning.

Succession Planning/Talent Development

Actively engaging in talent development and succession planning is a necessity for group practices to ensure that they do not suffer during leadership transition periods. Building a depth of leadership talent and prioritizing educational and development opportunities for young clinicians with leadership potential is very helpful. Formal mentoring programs are increasingly being developed by some of the larger group practices across the country. It is vital to actively engage in succession planning in a way that ensures an adequate pool of talent when leadership vacancies occur. Most large group practices and academic plans find they want to identify leaders from within their group practice as well as outside their organization so they will have the necessary leadership talent for their practice in the future.[88]

Research Opportunities

There are many further opportunities for research within the relatively new field of physician leadership. Further identification of specific competencies for physician leaders and those that might be applicable to specific group-practice types and cultures are of great interest and value. Leadership styles of physician leadership executives who have been identified with successful leadership contrasted with those who have been less successful are also of interest. Recent literature on emotional intelligence has generated much notice in academic and lay publications. The applicability of concepts of emotional intelligence to identifying those with significant leadership potential is of great interest. In addition, an understanding of which attributes of strong leadership can be taught and which seem to be much more inherent in one's character and personality are of great benefit to those organizations interested in creating a roadmap for effective physician leadership. Can all competencies be enhanced by formal training, or is formal training only effective in specific domains?

Finally, research opportunities on the role of physician leadership and organizational trust are of great importance to furthering the effectiveness of group-practice leaders. In times of change, trust is a precious commodity and lack of trust can be a major impediment to the kinds of breakthrough progress needed. There is considerable literature on issues of trust, and it is of great interest to study directly the roles of trust and organizational culture as they relate to the development of group-practice leadership cultures and their efficacy.

Lessons from Other Industries

Healthcare has traditionally been a very insular industry consumed by the belief that issues in healthcare are unique to healthcare. Healthcare has a quality and safety record that is not tolerated or acceptable in other industries. The "defect rate" in healthcare today was often attributed to medicine being an art, not a science. In reality, this defect rate is a function of processes that are inadequate, filled with unnecessary variation and waste. They are not always focused on the ultimate customer, the patient.

Over the last several years, there has been an increasing interest in lessons from other industries and the applicability of management lessons to healthcare. In reality, these so-called industrial approaches in manufacturing and other industries are directly applicable to healthcare, which is an aggregation of processes producing a product or service to benefit the patient. Six Sigma is one such approach, and new subsidiaries of organizations such as General Electric have begun to work with healthcare organizations to bring these innovative methodologies to healthcare. Lean manufacturing, as exemplified by the Toyota Production System, has also become an area of interest, and several organizations across the country have embarked on a journey to bring the principles of this system to healthcare. There is a myriad of lessons and principles from other industries that can and should be adapted to healthcare.[89] As healthcare has become more open to approaches beyond its historical care delivery and business boundaries, the beneficiaries are patients. Leadership within group practices as well as other healthcare settings needs to identify opportunities and be open to embracing any and all approaches that can improve the ability to deliver the safest, highest-quality care.

Leadership Lessons

There are many lessons that come from leadership experience. Drawing lessons from leaders who have been accountable for leading during times of revolutionary change has much relevance for today. There is much to learn, and successful leaders are lifelong students.

Some of the lessons learned include:

- Change sponsorship is a major role for today's leaders.
- An enterprising vision of success should be articulated and shared.
- Set ambitious goals for yourself and for teams.
- Tear down barriers to success.
- Embrace failure and learn from it.
- Celebrate achievements.
- Know your people and let your people know you.
- Go see for yourself what is really going on.
- Connect the dots constantly.
- It takes hearts and minds to succeed.
- Skeptics can become champions.
- Be accountable and hold others accountable.
- Leading change is hard work.
- Patients and staff depend on leaders being successful.

References

1. Garmendia J. More physicians choose to work in groups. *Jacksonville Business Journal.* October 20, 2003: A1.
2. Davis C. For group doctors, a winning model. *The New York Times.* February 1, 2004; 14WC:4.
3. Gabel S. Leaders key to success during organizational change. *American Medical News,* December 8, 2003; 46(46). Accessed December 7, 2011, at www.amednews.com/2003/bicc1208
4. Gillies R, Shortell S, Chenock K, et al. The impact of health plan delivery system organization on clinical quality and patient satisfaction. *Health System Research.* 2006;41(4).
5. Council of Accountable Physician Practices. *Employer and community partners with physician organizations.* Alexandria, VA: AMGA. Accessed August 27 2010, at www.amga-capp.org
6. Council of Accountable Physician Practices. *Delivery systems matter: shaping the future of health care.* Alexandria, VA: AMGA. Accessed August 27, 2010, at www.amga-capp.org
7. Ross A, Williams S, Pavlock E, eds. *Ambulatory care management.* Albany, NY: Dalmar, 1998.
8. Havlicek P. *Medical group practice in the US: a survey of practice characteristics.* Chicago: AMA Department of Data Survey and Planning; 1999.
9. Kohn LT, Corrigan JM, Donaldson MS, eds. *To err is human.* Institute of Medicine; Washington D.C.: National Academies Press; 2000.
10. Institute of Medicine. *Crossing the quality chasm.* Washington DC: National Academies Press; 2001.
11. Gerbarg Z. Physician leaders of medical groups facing increasing challenges. *Journal of Ambulatory Care Management.* 2002;25(4):1–6.
12. Congressional Budget Office. Rising health care costs: causes, implications, and strategies. Washington DC: CBO Publications; April 1991.
13. U.S. Federal Trade Commission, U.S. Department of Justice. *Improving health care: a dose of competition.* Washington DC: FTC; July 2004.
14. Bodenheimer T. High and rising health care costs, part 1: seeking an explanation. *Annals of Internal Medicine.* 2005;142:847–854.
15. Bodenheimer T. High and rising health care costs, part 2: technologic innovation. *Annals of Internal Medicine.* 2005;142:932–937.
16. PriceWaterhouseCoopers. *The factors fueling rising health care costs 2008.* Washington, DC:America's Health Insurance Plans; 2008.
17. Goldfeld N. An overview: physician payment reform. *Journal of Ambulatory Care Management.* 2000;23(1):39–44.
18. Hakim D. Their health costs soaring, automakers are to begin labor talks. *New York Times.* July 15, 2003: C1.
19. *A toolkit for action: the imperative for health reform: the position of the National Business Group on Health.* Washington, DC: National Business Group on Health, 2007. Accessed December 7, 2011, at www.businessgrouphealth.org/publications/
20. Baker L, Hopkins D. The contribution of health plans and provider organizations to variations in measured plan quality. *International Journal for Quality in Health Care.* 2010;22(3):210–308.
21. Leapfrog patient safety standards. February 2004. Washington, DC: Center for Studying Health System Change.
22. Miletich S. UW regents may be close to settlement. *Seattle Times.* January 26, 2004. Accessed December 7, 2011, at www.seattletimes.nwsource.com/
23. Berkowitz S. The development of a successful physician compensation plan. *Journal of Ambulatory Care Management.* 2002;25(4):10–25.
24. Stein JM. Successfully implementing a performance based compensation plan. *Medical Group Management Association Journal.* 2000 TZA1; 47(5):16–29.
25. Pierdon S, Eckrote B. Changing compensation plan: moving beyond last year's, this year's, and next year's. *Physician Executive.* 2004;30(1):26–29.
26. Dingley C, Daugherty K, Derieg MK, Persing R. *Improving patient safety through provider communication strategy enhancements.* Agency for Healthcare Research and Quality. Accessed December 7, 2011, at www.ahrq.gov/downloads/pub/advances2/vol3/Advances-Dingley_14.pdf
27. Rafferty AM, Ball J, Aiken LH. Are teamwork and professional autonomy compatible, and do they result in improved hospital care? *Quality in Health Care.* 2001;10(Suppl II):32–37.
28. Wysocki B. Industrial strength: to fix health care, hospitals take tips from factory floor. *Wall Street Journal.* April 9, 2004: A1.
29. Kenney C. *Transforming health care: Virginia Mason Medical Center's pursuit of the perfect patient experience.* New York: Taylor & Francis Group; 2011.
30. Kaplan G. Modifying your Service mix—a profitability strategy; *performance and practices of successful medical groups 2003 report*

based on 2002 data. Englewood, CO: Medical Group Management Association; 2003.

31. Bottles K. The good leader. *Physician Executive.* 2001; 27(2):74–76.

32. Lyons MF. Leadership and followership. *Physician Executive.* 2002;28(1):91–93.

33. Kotter JP. *Leading change.* Boston: Harvard Business School Press; 1996.

34. Kotter JP. *The heart of change.* Boston: Harvard Business School Press; 2002.

35. Kotter JP. *Force for change: how leadership differs from management.* Washington, DC: Free Press; 1990.

36. Heifetz R, Linsky M. *Leadership on the line: staying alive through the dangers of leading.* Boston: Harvard Business School Press; 2002.

37. Goodspeed RB, Gerbarg Z, Barrett DM. Physician Leadership: an interview with David M. Barrett, MD. *Journal of Ambulatory Care Management.* 2002;25(4):7–9.

38. Goleman D. *Working with emotional intelligence.* New York: Bantam; 1998.

39. Allred NJ, Wooten KG, Kong Y. The Association of Health Insurance and Continuous Primary Care in the Medical Home on vaccination coverage for 19- to 35-month-old children. *Pediatrics.* 2007;119(Suppl 1):S4–11.

40. Schoen C, Osborn R, Doty MM, Bishop M, Peugh J, Murukutla N. Toward higher-performance health systems: adults' health care experiences in seven countries, 2007. *Health Affairs.* 2007;26(6):w717–734.

41. Piper L. Addressing the phenomenon of disruptive physician behavior. *Health Care Manager.* 2003;22(4):335–339.

42. Peters JA. The devil in the doctor: how to cope with problem physicians. *MGMA Connexion.* 2003;3(2):50–53.

43. Kissoon N, Lapenta S, Armstrong G. Diagnosis and therapy for the disruptive physician. *Physician Executive.* 2002;28(1):54–58.

44. Hickson G. Deal with difficult doctors. . . . reduce claims payments. *Hardwired Results.* Accessed December 7, 2011, at http://www.studergroup.com/newsletter/Vol1_Issue11/index.html

45. Hickson G. *Discouraging disruptive behavior: it starts with a cup of coffee.* Nashville, TN: Vanderbilt University; 2009.

46. Silversin J, Kornacki MJ. *Leading physicians through change: how to achieve and sustain results,* American College of Physicians; Tampa, FL: Hillsboro Printing Company; 2000.

47. Silversin J, Kornacki MJ. Creating a physician compact that drives group success. *Medical Group Management Journal.* 2000;47(3):54–62.

48. Arora VM, Johnson JK, Meltzer DO, Humphrey HJ. A theoretical framework and competency-based approach to improving hand-offs. *Quality and Safety in Health Care.* 2008;17(1):11–14.

49. Nieva VF, Sorra J. Safety culture assessment: a tool for improving patient safety in healthcare organizations. *Quality and Safety in Health Care.* 2003;12(Suppl 2):ii17–23.

50. Cohen MM, Eustis MA, Gribbins RE. *Changing the culture of patient safety.* Oak Brook, IL: Joint Commission Journal of Quality and Safety; July 2003.

51. Brennan TA, Gawande A, Thomas E, Studdert D. Accidental deaths, saved lives, improved quality. *New England Journal of Medicine.* 2005;353(13):1405–1409.

52. Wachter RM, Pronovost PJ. Balancing "no blame" with accountability in patient safety. *New England Journal of Medicine.* 2009;361:1401–1406.

53. Pronovost PF, Goeschel CA, Marsteller JA, Sexton JB, Pham JC, Berenholtz SM. Framework for patient safety research and improvement. *Circulation.* 2009;119:330–337.

54. Wachter RM. *Understanding patient safety.* New York: McGraw-Hill Medical; 2008: 17–38.

55. Mohr JJ, Abelson HT, Barach P. Creating effective leadership for improving patient safety. *Quality Managed Health Care* 2002;11(1):69–78.

56. Marx D. *Patient safety and the "just culture": a primer for health care executives.* New York: Columbia University; April 17, 2001.

57. Lyons AS, Petrucelli RJ. *Medicine: an illustrated history.* New York: Harry N. Abrams; 1987.

58. Kaplan G, Patterson S. *The physician administrator team: an optimal model for leading medical practices.* Presented to the American College of Medical Practice Executives. Englewood, CO; 2001.

59. Kaplan G, Patterson S. *Effective balance with physician administrator teams.* Presented at the Medical Group Management Association Western Section; Colorado Springs, Co, 1997.

60. Stearns TH. How physician/administrator teams work in small groups: six steps to make it happen. *Medical Group Management Journal.* 1999;46(3):44–48.

61. Goldsmith J. Hospital/physician relationships: a constraint to health reform. *Health Affairs.* 1993;12(3):160–169.

62. Coddington DC, Moore KD, Fischer EA. *Making integrated healthcare work.* Englewood, CO: Medical Group Management Association; 1996.

63. American College of Medical Practice Executives. *Body of knowledge for medical practice, a note delineation study of medical practice executives.* American College of Medical Practice Executives. Englewood, CO: ACMPE; July 1999 and subsequent revisions.

64. Bujak JS. Culture in chaos: the need for leadership and followership in medicine. *Physician Executive.* 1999;25(3):17–22.

65. Guo K. An assessment tool for developing healthcare managerial skills and roles. *Journal of Healthcare Management.* 2003;48(6):367–376.

66. Goleman D. *Emotional intelligence: why it can matter more than IQ.* New York: Bantam; 1977.

67. Goleman D. Leadership that gets results. *Harvard Business Review.* 2000;78(2):78–90.

68. Ross A, Wenzel FJ, Mitlyng JW. *Leadership for the future.* Association of University Programs in Health Administration; Chicago, IL: Health Administration Press; 2002.

69. Schenke R. *The physician in management.* Falls Church, VA: American Academy of Medical Directors; 1980:34–43.

70. Zalezuick A. Managers and leaders, are they different? *Harvard Business Review.* 1977; 55(5):67–78.

71. Kotter J. What leaders really do. *Harvard Business Review.* 1990;68(3):103–111.

72. Stahl MJ, Dean PJ. *The physician's essential MBA: what every physician leader needs to know.* Sudbury, MA: Jones and Bartlett; 1999:191(2):208–213.

73. Keagy B, Thomas M. *Essentials of physician practice management.* New York: John Wiley and Sons; 2004.

74. Wenzel F, Wenzel J. *Fundamentals of physician practice management.* Chicago, IL: Health Administration Press; 2005.

75. Goleman, D. *Working with emotional intelligence.* New York: Bantam; 1998.

76. Ross A. *Cornerstones of leadership for health services executives.* Chicago: Health Administration Press; 1992:69–77.

77. Mecklenburg MD, Kaplan G, Story MD. *The marketplace collaborative project.* Center for Health Care Solutions at Virginia Mason Medical Center; Seattle, WA; 2007.

78. Epstein AM, Lee TH, Hamel MB. Paying physicians for high-quality care. *New England Journal of Medicine.* 2004;350(4):406–410.

79. Lencioni P. *The five dysfunctions of a team.* San Francisco, CA: Jossey-Bass; 2002.

80. Tichy NM. *Managing strategic change.* New York: Wiley; 1983:132–144.

81. Sperry L. *Becoming an effective health care manager: the essential skills of leadership.* Baltimore, MD: Health Professions Press; 2003.

82. Conrad DA, Sales A, Liang SY, et al. The impact of financial incentives on physician productivity in medical groups. *Health Service Research*. 2002; 37(4): 885–906.

83. Beck LC. Compensating group practice partners. *Physician Executive*. 2003; 29(2): 48–50.

84. Katzenbach JR, Smith DK. *The wisdom of teams*. Boston, MA: Harvard Business School Press; 1993.

85. Kaplan G, Patterson S. *Building team synergy*. Presented at Medical Group Management Association Executive Education Seminar; June 2005.

86. MGMA Best Practices Reports, 2000–2003.

87. Gill S, Lambert MJ. Life cycle of physician executives. *Healthcare Executive*. 2004;19(1):42–43.

88. Conger JA, Fulmer RM. Developing your leadership pipeline. *Harvard Business Review*. 2003;81(12):76–84.

89. Womack JP, Jones DT. *Lean thinking*. New York: Simon & Schuster; 1996.

Management of Nursing Services

Sheila Richmeier, MS, RN, FACMPE[a]

A revolution is occurring in medical practices across the nation—especially in primary care. Perhaps revolution is too strong of a word for some, but for those who are in the grips of those changes, revolution is the right word. This revolution has been coming for some time and the causes are many. Healthcare reform is here and evolving. Nursing services, therefore, are being affected by the changes, particularly those that involve a trend of physician practices integrating into large systems, improved health information technology, a shift to quality instead of quantity, and better care coordination and care management. The Institute of Medicine called for a transformation in the nursing profession in the following four areas:

1. Nurses should practice to the full extent of their education and training. The scope of practice rules vary across states and have varying effects on what activities a qualified nurse may perform.

2. Nurses should achieve higher levels of education through an improved education system to better manage more complicated patient needs and deliver high-quality care. Nurses are being called upon to fill expanding roles and need training in those competencies.

3. Nurses should be full partners with physicians and other healthcare professionals in redesigning healthcare in the United States, be accountable for their contributions to high-quality care, and work collaboratively with leaders from other health professions.

4. Effective workforce planning and policy require better data collection and improved information infrastructure.[1]

Change happens in healthcare on a regular basis. Why is this upcoming revolution different? In a recent study, healthcare executives cited several reasons why this one is for real:

- The fee-for-service model is of low value with high cost and variable outcomes.
- Shortfalls in healthcare funding in programs such as Medicare and Medicaid may lead to price controls.

a. Portions of this chapter reprinted with permission from the Medical Group Management Association, 104 Inverness Terrace East, Englewood, Colorado 80112. 877.ASK.MGMA. www.mgma.com. Copyright 2010.

- In the current economy of slow growth and high unemployment, the situation worsens.[2]

This chapter will explore the restructuring of medical practices related to nursing and how nursing is reacting to those changes. Nursing roles in a medical practice will be clarified along with different models of care being provided. How nursing fits into the overall workings of the medical practice will be reviewed. Finally, training and education needs will be discussed, with a look at management of nursing staff and how it may differ in the future.

Movement of Practices to Larger Systems

Because of many factors, medical practices are having to make difficult decisions regarding staying independent or joining larger practices or hospital systems. This section looks at that movement and the impact on nursing.

According to the Centers for Disease Control and Prevention (CDC), from 1997 to 2007 the total number of visits to physician offices increased from 787 million to 994.2 million, accounting for a slight increase in visits per person from 3 to 3.36.[3-5] Among other elements, volume (i.e., relative value units [RVUs]) is an important driver in the practice.

In addition to needing more volume to become financially sound, the practice also needs to look at minimizing expenses. The largest expense for any practice is staffing costs, which account for approximately 60% of total costs on average.[6] Nursing staff expense can be a significant portion, and will be higher if the practice has registered nurses. In the short term, replacing registered nurses with nonlicensed staff may reduce costs, and many practices have taken this action. In the future, as the role of the nurse changes, adding registered nurses may be more cost efficient and add more value to the practice. In addition to staffing, other expenses related to the clinical area that may need to be minimized are medical supplies, equipment, and non-revenue-generating service offerings.[6]

Independent physician groups may still demonstrate financial difficulties even though they increase the number or quantity of services provided or reduce expenses. Alignment with larger systems is another survival method. In 2008, research indicated that physicians were migrating to mid-sized practices in order to be better positioned.[7] According to the CDC statistics, the percentage of visits to independent solo physicians decreased 21% from 1997 to 2007, whereas larger physician groups (with 6–10

physicians) showed a 46% increase in visits. This would indicate the proportion of small practices (with one to five physicians) is dropping. Interestingly, ownership of medical practices by hospital systems showed a decrease from 15% to 10% from 1997 to 2007.[3-5]

Hospital ownership of medical practice is changing again. Many hospital executives are betting on physician integration, and when interviewed estimate that physician employment will increase from 10% today to 50% by 2015.[2] As part of the healthcare reform efforts since 2008, the creation of a new arrangement, accountable care organizations (ACOs), is driving medical practices to align with organized delivery systems. The ACO organized effort is focused on cost containment and quality accountability. Practices are seeking assistance due to capital constraints, reimbursement pressures, physician shortages, and the changing healthcare landscape.[8] The Medical Group Management Association (MGMA) cost survey of physician practices reflected this by reporting that hospital-owned practices increased from 25.6% to 49.5% from 2005 to 2008.[9] Practices are focusing on operational and financial aspects to ease growing reimbursement and cost pressures.

Advantages of larger systems include:

- Improved physician and hospital relationships leading to a more cohesive culture and greater buy-in for hospital strategies
- Care coordination among the hospital, specialists, and primary care, minimizing the risk of rehospitalizations
- Improving physician coverage and reducing the risk of physician shortages related to practice stabilization
- Optimal contract negotiations with managed care companies

Hospitals are trying new business models that allow the physicians to maintain operational control, reduce costs, increase efficiency, and provide for more adequate compensation plans. Providers are also able to better meet the growing payer demands for improved quality and bundled payment policies.[10]

Larger healthcare organizations will create challenges for the delivery of care. It may be complicated to create a unified culture with appropriate standardization while allowing for physician independence and operational control. Physician expectations and governance issues may create difficulties if not fully explored prior to the acquisition. Physicians are going from an independent culture to one of interdependence.[8] As hospitals acquire practices, the hospital system cannot impose its culture and operating procedures on the practice—they are different entities and need to be managed differently.[11] In addition, physician leadership as part of the larger organization will be a key element of success. New payment incentives will be tied to the ability to demonstrate high-quality clinical outcomes, coordinate care with multiple providers, and reduce the overall cost of care. The efficient combination of all these factors will create an effective ACO.[12]

Nurses are affected by the movement towards larger practices in the same ways as physicians are. Larger systems can be burdened with increased administrative procedures, operational controls, and standardization. For nurses who have practiced independence in a small group practice, interdependence within a large system may create additional burden. The benefits of a larger system are the available resources with technology, education, the ability to have adequate RN staffing, and others.

Movement to Health Information Technology

From 2001, the use of healthcare technology in physician offices has increased over 25%. Recently it was reported that physicians use technology for the following reasons: 61.8% were viewing lab and radiology results in the practice; 48% were accessing patient notes, medication lists, and problem lists; 32.2% were writing prescriptions; and 6.7% were communicating about clinical issues with patients by e-mail.[13] The CDC reported in a 2009 survey that 43.9% of doctors were using a full or partial electronic medical record system, which was a 14% increase between 2009 and 2001 (see **Figure 4-1**).[14]

The movement towards technology in a medical practice has been influenced by the belief that technology will reduce errors and automate existing processes. Health information technology should enable new capabilities that are difficult or impossible without it. Innovations can improve the following:

- Preventive care
- Chronic disease management
- Care coordination
- Non-visit-based care, or e-care
- Knowledge-based medication management[15]

Preventive care often is missed because of lack of payment for such services, or providers simply do not remember to ask the patient about age-appropriate screening. Having effective reminder systems at the point of care could improve care team education for patients to obtain key screenings and tests. Reporting can be done to manage preventive care across the entire population, and automated reminders can be sent to patients who fall outside the recommended guidelines. For example, a report on all women over the age of 40 who have not had their annual mammogram would generate a reminder to those patients. This system supplements the care provided in a simple, effective, and efficient manner.

Clinical decision support related to specific chronic diseases could be embedded in the electronic medical record (EMR) to allow the care team to quickly see how the care the patient has had compares to recommended evidence-based guidelines. The care team can immediately see the patient's condition and trends over time, and be alerted to any data outside of the guidelines. For instance,

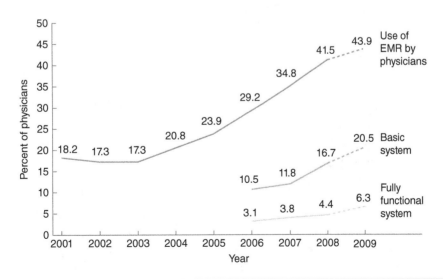

Figure 4-1 Percentage of office-based physicans with electronic medical records/electronic health records (EMRs/EHRs): United States, 2001–2008 and preliminary 2009.
Source: Woodwell, David, "National Ambulatory Medical Care Survey: 1997 Summary," Centers for Disease Control and Prevention, May 20, 1999.

the care team would be alerted to a diabetic patient who has not had a lipid panel in the past year. Real-time clinical decision making can occur in the exam room.

Proactive reporting could be done on the entire disease-specific population to send out automated reminders to provide better overall chronic disease management. For example, a report could be run on all diabetics for a particular physician, and those patients who have not received an HbA1c test (a specific blood test to manage diabetes) in the last year could be sent a reminder. In addition, a report could be run to determine all diabetics with an HbA1c greater than 13, indicating a need for more intensive care management by the care team. Health IT would allow the care team to get performance feedback on their management of chronic diseases. Sharing data often changes behavior.

EMR technology in integrated systems, if one system is integrated through all the practices, has allowed clinicians to coordinate and have connectivity among providers (i.e., hospital systems, specialist care, primary care, home health, etc.). The care team can easily look at the specialist role or the last hospital admission. This allows for better management of the patient's condition as well as transitions of care. Outside of integrated systems, disparate EMR systems create difficulty in sharing data.

A substantial amount of care is provided by the care team to patients before and after the office visit. With improved technology and payment incentives, this could increase significantly. E-visits could be performed instead of office visits for many minor acute care problems and more enhanced chronic care treatment. Monitoring a patient through a chronic disease portal or with tele-med technology could greatly improve the patient's engagement in his or her own care and provide convenience for the sickest patients.

E-prescribing helps prevent drug–drug interactions and inadvertent prescription of drugs the patient is allergic to, improves physician legibility, and helps automate managed care formularies. A knowledge-based medication management system allows for a seamless initial prescription and prescription renewal, as well as the application of comprehensive knowledge that supplements the providers' expertise.[15] The care team becomes more efficient with information at their fingertips and all in one place.

Meaningful regulations for electronic health records have required changes in medical practices across the nation, starting in 2010 through the Health Information Technology for Economic and Clinical Health Act (HITECH), which provides incentive payments to clinicians and hospitals. Requirements include using technology securely to achieve specific improvements in care delivery.[16]

Health information technology adoption reflects a tremendous change in the manner in which medical services are delivered. Improvement in data collection and the processing of that information affects the physician and nurse providing care. Technology can also address the ability to accommodate the need for medical knowledge in the patient exam room. Physicians can access medical information online at the point of care. In addition, the need for data to substantiate and improve quality in a physician's office is a strong driver for technology adoption.

Most nurses lack the necessary skills and abilities to use technology appropriately. Nursing IT competencies can be categorized as computer skills, informatics knowledge, and informatics skills. Computer skills include competency with basic software applications, administrative applications, electronic communications, data access and decision support, patient documentation and monitoring, education systems, research, and usability and ergonomics. Informatics skills include management; system requirements and selection, design, and development; fiscal management; implementation; analysis and evaluation; and system maintenance.[17-19] Resources, time, and training are needed to support nursing staff in recognizing gaps in their computer skills, obtaining education that shrinks those gaps, having greater access to high-quality information resources, committing to using information resources effectively to provide better patient care, and setting goals for improvement.[18]

The movement to health information technology affects nursing in a medical office in many ways. Better information at the point of care allows for better care. Information technology allows the nurse to make point-of-care judgments based on scientific knowledge and to rely on procedures and guidelines for standardized care processes. For nursing leaders, information technology helps to effectively manage resources, thanks to better reporting, which shows where care needs to be concentrated.

Movement to Quality

Another change is quality versus quantity. "Under the fee-for-service model, every patient touch produces revenue; under fee-for-value, every touch generates costs."[2] The change in focus is reflected in how physicians are reimbursed. From 2001 to 2005, physician compensation based in part on reporting of quality measures increased from 17% to 20% for physicians in group practice.[20] Financial incentives can create a nonvoluntary physician engagement strategy, and is currently being used to motivate physicians to make needed changes. Incentives that support the goals of the physicians will be most successful. Financial incentives should not create a conflict between the quality of care provided and the level of revenue.[21]

While physician offices are negotiating for their portion of healthcare reimbursement, other players in the healthcare system are also competing for a larger share. The United States spends more on healthcare than any other nation.[22] Spending in healthcare is escalating relentlessly with increasing evidence of waste. It is estimated that 30% of total healthcare dollars are spent wastefully in the following areas: (1) unexplained variation in the intensity of medical and surgical services, (2) misuse of drugs and treatments resulting in preventable adverse effects, (3) overuse of nonurgent emergency department care, (4) underuse of appropriate medications and nongeneric use, and (5) overuse of antibiotics for respiratory infections.[23]

Across the nation, in many different healthcare settings, there is a growing disparity among care provided and resources utilized to provide that care. Newspapers or journals print numerous accounts of variances in how treatment is provided for certain chronic conditions at different hospitals. Differences between regions of the country in dollars and utilization of services is common. Wide variations occur in hospital readmission rates, access, and prevention/treatment quality. For instance, in 2006–2007, the percentage of adult diabetics getting the recommended preventive care ranged from a low of 33% in Mississippi to a high of 67% in Minnesota. Hospital readmission rates among Medicare beneficiaries ranged from a high of 23% in Nevada to a low of 13% in Oregon.[24] Variances may represent inefficiencies in practice, and it is stated that fewer variations in practice would result in less unnecessary medicine and lower medical costs.[25,26] Other factors related to cost containment in a medical office are[24]:

- The lack of incentives in the current fee-for-service environment that rewards providers for providing more services regardless of quality
- Socioeconomic factors resulting in higher rates of disease and a higher number of uninsured patients among certain patient populations
- Inadequate state efforts to assist patients
- Lack of resources from the practice or patient
- Unhealthy lifestyles of patients
- Poorly coordinated care
- Inefficient use of resources

In the 1990s, patients, employers, and payers started expressing concerns about quality of care and started asking questions about what they were paying for. The 1999 Institute of Medicine (IOM) report, "To Err Is Human," brought quality in healthcare to the forefront; the subsequent release of "Crossing the Quality Chasm" by the IOM in 2001 focused on safety, effectiveness, patient-centeredness, timeliness, efficiency, and equity.[27,28] In 2007, the Institute of Healthcare Improvement (IHI) released the Triple AIM initiative, which further expanded the goals to improve the health of the population, enhance the patient experience, and reduce the cost of care.[28] Many efforts have been made to improve quality, such as clinical practice guidelines, electronic medical records, computerized provider order entry systems, multidisciplinary patient rounds, error reporting systems, and pay for performance, to name a few. Many of these have not been as successful as expected, and the assumption is that healthcare organizations have not implemented these changes effectively to realize real system change.[27]

Quality is assumed in a physician office, and the assumption that quality is high is most consistently measured with patient satisfaction scores. Patients value their physician, the staff, and the office setting itself. Patients perceive satisfaction/dissatisfaction upon assessing the value of the medical services provided and their individual cost, and the effort related to obtaining services.[29] However, questions have arisen about equating patient satisfaction with the quality of care provided. Patient satisfaction scores can be a partial measure of quality, if appropriately administered. Questions such as the ability to access the practice, the value of physician and nurse communication, and overall satisfaction with the care provided do measure certain quality aspects of the practice.[30] In addition, when these results are studied and areas of opportunity are corrected, quality of care can be improved in the practice.

Quality has several dimensions beyond patient satisfaction, however. Medical practices are shifting from a focus on medical care to a focus on healthcare. The practice wants not only satisfied patients, but also healthy patients. Instead of focusing solely on the sick, practices are starting to focus on keeping people healthy. As stated by the American Nurses Association, "Registered nurses are fundamental to the critical shift needed in health services delivery, with the goal of transforming the current 'sick care' system into a true 'health care' system."[31] Managing the patient's health instead of just his or her disease can lead to a reduction in overall future healthcare expenditures and a more satisfied patient, who will experience reduced hospitalizations, reduced disease, and prevention of illness. Quality in a medical practice is about the quality of care provided. This is where the change is occurring—quality instead of quantity.

Another measurement of quality of care is the use of evidence-based guidelines. Evidence-based medicine is defined as "the conscientious, explicit, and judicious use of current best evidence in making decisions about the care of individual patients."[32] The concept of the "art of medicine" indicates that physicians can synthesize all of the information about the patient, as well as all the patient's past experiences and knowledge, and then come up with the best solution for the patient's complaint. In the 1970s, it became increasingly evident that when faced with the same patient symptoms, two physicians could very well treat differently and often did. In the 1980s, studies concluded that physicians often were performing inappropriate procedures, and many treatments taken for granted by physicians were actually found to be ineffective when subjected to clinical trials. This led to a discussion regarding medical decision making and the ability of the physician to be solely responsible for individual patient care decisions without some outside assistance. The use of research evidence as the obvious new anchor for medical decisions was formed. The term "evidence-based" was first used by the *Journal of the American Medical Association* in 1990. Over the next 20 years, more and more organizations began to apply evidence-based guidelines. By the end of the 1990s, evidence-based guidelines were widely accepted.

Physicians are adopting this change. The proportion of primary care physicians reporting that evidence-based guidelines have had a very large or large effect on their practice has increased from 16.4% in 1997 to 38.7% in 2005. Specialists have shown an increase in the same time period from 18.9% to 28.2%.[20] These data are in tandem with the government's push for quality.

The Agency for Healthcare Research and Quality (AHRQ) and the Department of Health and Human Services (HHS) have reported progress and opportunities for improving healthcare quality. Efforts to improve quality include: (1) improving measurement, (2) removing barriers to quality care, (3) empowering providers with health information technology, and (4) establishing and sustaining partnerships to lead change.[26]

Often government initiatives spearhead change in the industry, especially in healthcare. The Centers for Medicare and Medicaid Services (CMS) started the quality initiative in home health with the Outcome and Assessment Information Set (OASIS) in early 2000; they then expanded it to hospitals and nursing homes with the Hospital Quality Initiative and the Nursing Home Quality Initiative. Quality reporting is now reaching medical offices with the Physician Quality and Reporting Initiative (PQRI).[33-36]

The use of quality initiatives also has quickly spread to the private insurance arena. Many insurance companies and government payers are now collecting and reporting clinical outcomes in the form of PQRI, Pay for Performance (P4P), Health Employer Data and Information Set (HEDIS) quality measures, utilization measures, and more. Most group leaders are reporting that they are measured for quality in at least one commercial health plan contract.[37]

Quantity is becoming less important and quality is becoming the key driver in care. Quality is the driver of many recent healthcare initiatives. Measures include coverage of preventive services and immunizations; PQRI incentive payments; establishment of the Center for Medicare and Medicaid Innovation to test innovative payment and service delivery models to reduce program expenditures; and creation of a nonprofit Patient-Centered Outcomes Research Institute to perform comparative effectiveness research to assist patients, physicians, purchasers, and policy makers in making informed healthcare decisions.[31,33]

Provider quality payments are now based on data collection and outcomes. Outside entities such as insurance companies can measure outcomes with data collected from claims, but the data are not always accurate due to the timeliness of claim processing. If providers want accurate data to be used to measure their outcomes, the practice must implement systems to collect and then manage the data.

The ultimate goal of managing clinical data is to have better overall healthcare outcomes for the healthcare system as a whole. Developing and implementing evidence-based guidelines has been a key method in addressing the variation in service utilization.[38] By managing diabetics better in the office setting, the physician can possibly prevent a hospitalization or an emergency room visit. By managing the preventive clinical outcomes, for instance, and ensuring influenza vaccinations are given to most patients, the care team may be able to prevent an outbreak of influenza in their community. By knowing what the childhood immunization rates are, the care team might be able to increase those numbers by having all team members encourage immunizations, thus preventing illness.

Nursing is affected in many ways by the increased movement towards quality; the role of the nurse in a medical office is undergoing radical changes in this realm. The increased use of protocols allows nurses to effectively manage patients as part of the team. The care team takes on the role of providing care. Each patient is treated with whole person care in the most appropriate manner. The mentality of "this is the way we always do things" has gone away, and evidence-based medicine now is used to standardize the treatment.[28]

Movement Towards Better Care Coordination and Care Management

Another movement is towards better care coordination and care management. One critical area of healthcare quality and cost is potentially preventable hospitalizations. These can be reduced if clinicians effectively diagnose, treat, and educate patients and if patients are engaged in their care. Preventable hospitalizations are a significant issue in regards to quality and cost. Many hospitalizations may have been prevented if individuals received high quality primary and preventive care. Hospitalizations may be prevented with timely diagnosis, treatment, and education for patients in the outpatient setting.[39]

Preventable rehospitalizations also are a significant cost to the healthcare system and often are avoidable. Causes for rehospitalizations are poor discharge procedures and inadequate follow-up care. A survey of rehospitalizations of Medicare beneficiaries completed in 2009 found that one of every five Medicare patients discharged from the hospital was readmitted within 30 days. Fifty percent of those patients readmitted were not seen within 30 days by a physician after discharge.[40] The elderly are often more prone to readmissions. The Medicare patient preventable readmission rate is 13.3%; the rate across all insured patients is 11%.[41] Persons with the highest rate of preventable admissions are patients:

- With heart failure, chronic obstructive pulmonary disease (COPD), psychoses, or intestinal problems and who have had various types of surgery (cardiac, joint replacement, or bariatric procedures)
- Who are taking six or more medications, who have depression and/or poor cognitive function, and/or who have been hospitalized in the previous 6 months
- Who are discharged on weekends or holidays[41]

Reasons cited for readmitting include limited or no access to posthospital care in the communities, inadequate information received about postdischarge care, poor coordination of care with primary care physicians or home health, or preventable errors and complications in the first hospital stay.[41]

Solutions for preventable hospitalizations and rehospitalizations are better management of the patients in the outpatient setting and better coordination with follow-up care.[41] Between 1994 and 2000, admission rates rose for COPD, hypertension, and pneumonia. However, hospital admission rates were reduced for treatment of angina, uncontrolled diabetes without complications, adult asthma, and pediatric gastroenteritis. The reductions are attributed to increased patient education, better environmental settings, enhanced awareness, and changes in medical technologies. The quality of primary and preventive care improved these conditions during this time period.[42]

The use of the emergency room (ER) for nonurgent care and for conditions that could have been treated in a primary care setting also is increasing the cost of care. It is estimated that 56% of ER visits are potentially avoidable. The average cost of an ER visit is over $500 more than the cost of an office visit.[43] Patients from all payer groups and ages use the ER for nonurgent care. Reasons cited include lack of timely appointments and after-hours care, poor care coordination, and often primary care offices send patients to the ER due to access issues. ER care is an enticing alternative because it provides an open door policy (patients can come at any time for anything), reassurance (patients will receive immediate feedback about their condition), and one-stop shopping (it offers a wide range of services).[43]

To change the quantity of use of the ER, primary care practices have to improve their access to care by providing weekend and evening hours, 24-hour telephone consultation services, and the ability for patients to receive care when needed from their physician.[43] Providing better access in the office setting may reduce the need to use the emergency room or urgent care centers. The patient who cannot get into the physician's office in a timely manner is more likely to use another method of care. Often, making it easier to see acute patients can provide continuity for the patient but also reduce the overall cost to the system. Patients who do not see their primary care provider with acute care needs often are told to follow up with them after the urgent care or emergency room visit, thus increasing overall healthcare costs.

Nursing in the medical office is becoming more intense. Patients can be managed more effectively in the outpatient setting; when they are admitted to the hospital, they are leaving sicker than ever before, therefore needing more intensive care in the medical office. Nurses' skill sets have to accommodate this change.

Nursing is affected by the movement to provide better quality because nurses are a key player in the care coordination and care management functions. Better coordination of care and management of patients with chronic illnesses in the medical office can reduce the number of hospitalizations, rehospitalizations, and ER visits. Care management processes allow for more optimal preventive and chronic disease management. Care coordination puts good systems in place to follow up on all those patients dismissed from the hospital, and allows the care team to better manage the patient posthospitalization with better medication management and assessment of patient status. Those patients will be better managed when they are dismissed from the hospital, thus reducing the need to return to the hospital setting.

Summary of the Revolution

There is an overwhelming need to transform the healthcare system, and nurses can play a fundamental role in the transformation of medical practices.[1,2] Physicians will not be able to make all the changes necessary in this revolution; nurses can provide the support and expertise needed.

Changes are occurring as the result of pilot projects across the country. Pilots look at different ways to reimburse medical practices and have been in progress since the early 2000s. These pilots may focus on care coordination, care management, health information technology, or access to drive down the costs of healthcare.

Payment reform accompanies these pilots—paying physicians to change their mindset of quantity being the driver. Most pilots have a quality reward that allows physicians to substantiate the need for improvement in quality or efficiency measures. The federal government, insurance companies, and large systems are providing funding for payment reform pilots.[44] The entire care team, including the nurse, contributes to the quality of care achieved in the office, and therefore should be included in the decisions and rewards. In one study from a hospital quality incentive program, it was noted ". . . that you cannot do anything in quality if you do not involve the nurses in a significant way." Nursing contributions include critical data gathering and analysis activities on which the incentive program and infrastructure exist. Nursing has a key role to play in improvement of quality.[45]

This quality initiative has forced practices to relook at the staffing and for nursing to start showing its value. Nursing in a medical office has changed from just rooming patients. It's about caring for those patients in the best manner possible to achieve the best outcome of health. Nursing has not done a good job at proving its worth in the practice with evidence of improved outcomes, critical thinking skills, or reduced adverse events. Nationwide, many practices have replaced RNs with nonlicensed staff because of the reduced cost and difficulty of determining the value of nursing.

The restructuring in the hospital setting in the 1990s led to replacing RNs with nonlicensed staff to reduce costs. The impact was studied by many, and nursing's value was determined as providing an improved quality of care—higher rates of RN staffing were associated with a 3% to 12% reduction in adverse outcomes. Patients in hospitals with high RN staffing were 4% to 12% less likely to develop UTIs, and surgical patients had an 11% lower rate of hospital-acquired pneumonia.[46]

The research in medical office nursing has not been as extensive, but the signs point to the need for rethinking the role of the RN. Physicians have been inundated with the tasks required to provide good quality care. In one study, family physicians are spending on average 45.8% of their time, or 3.7 hours per day, on acute care needs; 37.4%, or 3.0 hours, on chronic disease; and 16.8%, 1.3 hours per day, on preventive medicine. If they were to meet the current clinical guideline requirement, the same physician would have to work a total of 21.7 hours per day.[47] In other words, physicians alone cannot provide quality care. There is a growing need for the nurse to return and have an active role on the care team in the medical office.

New competencies will be needed in physicians' offices in a quality/value-based marketplace. These include:

- Clinical risk management
- Care model management for episodes, diseases, and populations
- Population management
- Predictive modeling
- The use of integrated multidisciplinary teams for complex patient care and patient engagement[2]

Nursing is well positioned to play a leading role in all of these competencies.

In the next section, nursing roles, nursing models, and new care models will be explored.

■ Nursing Roles

Prior to delineating the roles of each staff member, the following sections provide an explanation of the two distinct types of clinical staff—licensed and nonlicensed. Tasks that can be performed will often be determined by this distinction.[48]

Licensed Staff

Licensed staff are regulated by a state agency, sometimes called the board of nursing, which defines nursing practice through a nurse practice act. This practice act defines how the nursing board regulates the practice of nursing and nursing education. Most importantly, the board of nursing defines nursing for that state. It is important to know the regulations as they relate to the practice of nursing in the state. These can be obtained by searching for "board of nursing" and the state of practice in any search engine. If a nurse will practice in two states concurrently, both states' regulations should be reviewed. Although all states regulate nursing in their own unique way, there are similarities among them. Most state practice acts include reference to the following:

- Protection of the public
- Licensure requirements for competence in nursing practice
- Accountability for conduct
- Educational requirements of nursing schools

Protection of the Public

The ability to use the term "nurse" is limited for the protection of the public. It is against the law to identify someone as a nurse if they are not licensed as a nurse. It misrepresents the educational background and experience to patients who think they are speaking with a nurse when in actuality they may be speaking with a medical assistant. Nursing and office staff must be careful to clarify this with the public.

Registered nurses or practical nurses are licensed through the board of nursing. The nurse practice act defines licensure requirements, including payment of fees, qualifications of applicants, examinations required, refresher courses, and titles.

In general, nursing offers several entry levels to practice, from a 1-year technical degree to a 4-year bachelor's degree and beyond (see also **Table 4-1**).

- *Licensed practical nurse (LPN)/licensed vocational nurse (LVN):* LPNs and LVNs are trained in the technical side of nursing—administering medications, performing treatments, and assisting in caring for the patient. They require a 1- or 2-year program that enables the individual to sit for the practical or vocational nurse licensure exam after completion.
- *Associate degree registered nurse (ADN):* An ADN is able to provide and manage patient care in the hospital, home, or clinic setting. After completing a 2-year program, students are given a degree and are able to sit for the registered nurse licensure exam.
- *Diploma-prepared registered nurse:* Although this was a very popular way to train RNs many years ago, only one or two programs are still available. This individual is employed by the hospital while the hospital prepares him or her to become a nurse. The focus is on patient care. Graduates are given a diploma upon completion, which allows them to sit for the registered nurse licensure exam.
- *Bachelor's degree with a major in nursing (BSN):* This RN has been trained in nursing, but also has a more rounded general education. There is an emphasis on critical thinking, theory, and management of patients and other staff. The graduate has an opportunity to sit for the registered nurse licensure exam.
- *Master's degree/doctoral degree:* Advanced education in nursing is available in fields such as education, administration, and clinical applications. Advanced registered nurses are all trained for independent and collaborative practice. Licensure is usually obtained prior to entering into these degree programs.

After an individual has completed a course of education, he or she must write to the board of nursing requesting permission to sit for a board exam. Each state regulates nursing education and requirements to sit for boards. The board also regulates the retaking of the exam if an individual does not pass the first or subsequent attempts. Nurses who are waiting to take boards may work as a graduate practice nurse (for an LPN/LVN) or a graduate nurse (for an RN). If supervised, they

Table 4-1	Roles of Different Types of Nurses in a Medical Office		
	Education Requirements	Roles	Other
LPN/LVN	1- to 2-year vocational degree	Patient care—technical component Administer medications, perform treatments, assist in care of patient	Requires supervision by RN
RN: ADN	2-year associate degree	Provide and manage patient care including IV therapy	
RN: Diploma	3-year diploma	Provide and manage patient care including IV therapy	Education provided by hospital program
RN: BSN	4-year bachelor's degree	Critical thinking, theory, and management of patients and staff	
RN: MS or MSN	6-year master's degree	Advanced degrees may be given for nursing administration, nurse practitioner, nurse anesthetist, or nurse clinician	

may perform all the functions of an LPN/LVN or RN, respectively. When they pass boards, they are then called LPN/LVN or RN. If they fail boards, they can no longer work in the capacity of a nurse. They can be employed as nursing assistants until they pass the exam. Each state regulates how many times an individual may sit for boards before he or she must complete additional requirements to be able to retake the exam.

Nurses have to be licensed in the state for which they will practice; they can hold licenses from several states as long as they maintain the requirements of licensure from each state. A temporary license is issued while the state verifies the licensure of that individual.

Licensure requires payment of fees every 1 to 2 years to the state board of nursing. Some states require continuing education hours to maintain licensure; others do not. This is stated in the nurse practice act of each state.

Accountability for Conduct

The nurse practice act defines standards of practice for nursing and unlawful acts, and outlines unprofessional conduct. This usually includes handling of complaints, disciplinary procedures, and licensure restrictions.

Licensure verification can be done through most boards of nursing for a fee. If you cannot verify licensure with past employment, licensure verification is a good measure. Each month, a board of nursing also will report numerous disciplinary actions and/or suspensions of nursing licenses on its website or through a monthly publication.

The board of nursing for each state regulates nursing. Any scope of practice or disciplinary incident should be reported to the board of nursing for the state where the act occurred. Examples of this are a nurse self-prescribing narcotic medication, helping him- or herself to narcotics, or willfully harming a patient. The board then sets up a hearing in which the nurse is given parameters to keep or lose his or her license. Licensure is a very serious matter, and rightfully so. It should never be taken lightly because it does take considerable work to obtain a nursing license.

Educational Requirements of Nursing Schools

Nurse practice acts define the approval process for nursing schools, including the requirements of the curriculum, facilities, and faculty. Surveys are conducted to ensure requirements have been met. Most nursing boards also define position statements in relation to nursing practice. Position statements further define nursing from the board of nursing's point of view. They usually are developed around controversial or hot topic issues. One position statement noted among most nursing boards is delegation of unlicensed nursing personnel.

Unlicensed Staff

Unlicensed staff are used in a medical practice to provide patient care. This is a broad category with many different titles. In the nursing industry, unlicensed staff are grouped under the name unlicensed assistive personnel (UAP). These positions range from someone who works in a practice who has completed no formal education program to those who have completed a formal program and gained certification. Generally nursing staff are either medical assistants (MA) or nursing assistants (NA).

Generally, nursing assistants have completed an 8- to 12-week course that allows them to complete a nursing assistant exam and become a certified nursing assistant. They should have a diploma to verify their training. The training reviews patient care (e.g., how to give a bath, position a patient, assist a patient to move, and take vital signs). However, many people call themselves nursing assistants although they have completed no training.

Medical assistants undergo formal training, which may be a 1- to 2-year program. It is much more extensive than a nursing assistant course, and usually includes technical components such as giving injections and drawing blood. Medical assistants are usually trained in office functions such as medical records and front desk duties. They will have either an associate degree or a diploma from a medical assistant school. Some become certified after training.

Various certification programs exist for different specialties. Each specialty has different initials and certifications. After NAs and MAs receive certification, a C is placed before their initials—CNA or CMA. Specialty certification exists for areas such as general surgery; surgical technologists complete a 1- to 2-year course on surgery.

The specific training and expertise of unlicensed assistive personnel can be confusing because there are many credentials available. Asking for a certificate or diploma can add clarity. There may be incongruence between the initials given and the actual training received. Due diligence in asking questions and doing research prior to hiring may prevent problems in the future.

When delegating tasks, the RN must know the role, skills, and competencies of the person to whom they are delegating the tasks. A job description is a good place to start in understanding their role. To delegate a task, the RN should spend sufficient time explaining and reviewing the task. Having the task demonstrated back to the RN helps to ensure the task has been fully understood. If the task is new to the unlicensed staff, documentation of the delegated task should be completed and perhaps included in their personnel file for future reference. An open line of communication and adequate follow-up after the task has been delegated can reveal any issues with completion of the delegated task. If the task is a lengthy one, the progress should be evaluated on a regular basis until completion of the goal. Coaching may be needed to correct or encourage completion of a task that was delegated.

Each state has differing views on delegation and who is ultimately responsible for the delegated task. Some states have determined that nursing is responsible for all delegated nursing tasks whereas others deem the delegated staff member to be responsible. Researching a particular state's rules will help the RN and physician understand their responsibilities.

Experience as a Factor

Experience is a key determinant as to whether the staff will be able to perform the job tasks. It would be difficult for a new graduate nurse to provide phone triage in a family practice without experience in a hospital setting. Experience can have many benefits for unlicensed staff also. If a physician has invested time educating a medical assistant over the course of several years, that MA will know which questions they can answer and which require the physician's attention. An experienced surgical tech will be able to answer certain questions more appropriately regarding pain after surgery if they have assisted with positioning the patient during surgery and understand the surgical procedure. Often when UAPs first start in the practice, they will be unable to give that information to patients without adequate training and experience.

Physician and practice liability is greatly reduced by the experience of the nursing staff, especially with phone triage. A less experienced nurse may give advice to the patient that is detrimental to his or her well-being and consequently results in legal action in the future.

Determining the RN Role in the Office

It is sometimes difficult to determine the need for and benefit of having an RN in the medical office. Often, administration and physicians look at profit margin and determine they cannot afford a registered nurse, and thus make the decision to hire a nonlicensed nursing staff to carry out nursing tasks. Although an RN may not be needed to escort a patient from the waiting room to the exam room (rooming) or to stock rooms, the RN may add value to the practice, allowing the physician to see more patients, spend more time with patients, and provide the care that justifies the medical degree he or she spent many years obtaining.

As healthcare reform becomes a reality, the need for RNs has become amplified. There are many benefits of having an RN in the practice; often these benefits are intangible such as increased patient understanding of the treatment protocol or disease process, reduced risk of patient hospitalizations or rehospitalizations, improved reputation of the physician and office, reduced malpractice claims, reduced compliance and training costs, increased professionalism of the office, and improved work environment for the physician. Tangible benefits may be an increased ability for the physician to perform those functions and use the skills that they were educated to perform, instead of handling administrative and clinical oversight of nonprofessional staff. Another benefit is the ability of the office to have a true team caring for the patients, with each member supporting patient care and not always depending on the physician to provide all the care.

The RN role in the medical office should be thought of in the same manner as the physician's role in delegating tasks. If the RN is freed up to perform those tasks she or he went to nursing school to perform—critical thinking, advocacy, patient education, care coordination—the team functions at the highest level possible.

Nursing functions can be divided into the following categories:

- *Facilitation of operations:* Ordering supplies, rooming patients
- *Nursing procedures:* Medication administration, vital signs, diagnostic testing
- *Nursing process:* Determining how best to assist patients through diseases, problem-solving concerns
- *Telephone communication and triage:* Determining patient needs and prioritizing those needs
- *Advocacy:* Working with patients to obtain better care
- *Patient education:* Teaching patients about their disease and health
- *Assisting with high tech procedures:* Assisting and preparing patients for procedures, monitoring patients, post-op care, and follow-up
- *Care coordination:* Coordinating care across many spectrums
- *Quality improvement:* Care management of patient clinical outcomes

When nursing tasks are analyzed, some activities can easily be delegated if taught and supervised appropriately. The following list of nursing tasks could be performed by nonlicensed staff:

- Rooming patients, including chart prep, vital signs, and history taking
- Assisting the physician with simple procedures

- Diagnostic testing procedures including EKG, spirometry, waived lab testing (simple lab and other tests that the physician practice is able to conduct in the office, as determined by the Clinical Laboratory Improvement Act [CLIA])
- Review of medication lists
- Acquiring samples
- Stocking rooms
- Supply management
- Insurance precertification and follow-up
- Referrals to specialists
- Communicating with community resources
- Simple nursing procedures, such as removing sutures and dressing changes

More specialized and complicated tasks also can be delegated with intense training and competency validation. A nonlicensed staff person could perform the following:

- Injections, including allergy, subcutaneous, and intramuscular (requires extensive teaching)
- TB testing
- Vaccinations
- Wound care
- Medication refills
- Answering the phones and taking messages
- Simple patient education

Because of the need for critical thinking skills and expertise in the following activities, a licensed nurse would be better suited for the following:

- Phone triage in which the nurse gives the patient advice or nursing care over the phone, reviews symptoms, or provides teaching
- Administration of chemotherapy, IV medications, or complex injections
- Care management and care coordination for complex patients
- More extensive patient education, patient engagement, and self-care education

When making the decision on how to staff a physician's office, three factors should be considered:

1. How does the cost differ between the two options?
   - *Direct costs:* Salary, benefits
   - *Indirect costs:* Supervision costs—will extra staff or physician time be needed to supplement or supervise?
2. What are the required tasks of the position, and what activities can the staff member perform independently without supervision?

3. What are the outcomes desired by physicians, administration, and other nursing staff?
   - Supplement physician tasks
   - Add clinical capabilities
   - Physician, staff, or patient satisfaction
   - Clinical outcomes management

There have been few studies as to whether substitution of lower-paid staff for RNs always translates into lower cost per visit. Having an RN in the practice will enhance clinical performance. Nurses' training on the nursing process is an ideal fit for implementing chronic care management protocols. RNs can add value to the team in the form of better outcomes for the physician and the practice. Although there may be better outcomes, hiring an RN does increase the cost to the practice; however, that cost can be mitigated by allowing the physician to perform other functions that might generate revenue to offset the cost difference. An example of this is a physician who typically spends 1 hour per day answering phone messages created by the front office. In addition, she spends 30 minutes approving refills for patients. After an RN is hired and takes on these two responsibilities, the physician can see four more patients in that same time period, thereby generating revenue that offsets the cost of the RN.

Evolving Nursing Roles

There are an increasing number of roles for nurses in a medical practice and ambulatory care. Nurses are needed to provide patient education and to work with patients with chronic disease to manage their illnesses more effectively. Roles in quality improvement and outcome measurement should follow the increased focus in this area. Care management and care coordination roles will be more prevalent as outcome measurement and chronic illness care develops. The care manager typically seen only at insurance companies will be either in the medical office or an independent case management or care management agency. They assess the patient; develop the plan of care for the complex, high utilization patients; and work with team members to enhance quality of care and reduce cost across a variety of settings.

Nurses also will be asked to take a greater role in technology as healthcare becomes more technologically advanced. Nurses can play a key role in development, customization, and support for health information technology due to their knowledge of the clinical aspects of care. Telenursing, including remote monitoring, is just emerging as an area that could be further developed and specialized. Virtual care is just now being realized. Online clinics may be in the future, and phone advice nurses will play a larger role.

The 15-minute visit can no longer accommodate the increasing acuity of patients in a medical office. Recent research studies found the following:

- Fifty percent of patients leave the office without understanding the advice they received.
- In 25% of visits, patients were unable to express their concerns at all.
- Fifty-two percent of primary care physicians report not having enough time to spend with their patients.

Physicians need assistance in providing better care to their patients.[49-51] The complexity of tasks the provider is responsible for leads physicians to embrace assistance with the care they provide in the form of mid-level clinicians and nurses.

Nursing can take a leading role in the transformation of the healthcare system. As stated at the beginning of this chapter, a revolution is happening in medical offices, and nursing will be a key player. New roles and opportunities for nurses are expanding, and each of the following will be looked at in depth in the following sections:

- Care management and care coordination roles
- Nursing leadership roles
- Nursing informatics roles
- Nurse practitioner or advance practice nursing roles
- Professional nursing education roles

Care Management and Care Coordination

A wide range of knowledge is required to manage more complex chronically ill patients. A team including nurses, pharmacists, social workers, physicians, nurse practitioners, and other providers will need to work together to find and carry out solutions for the patient to remain in the outpatient setting. Collaboration among specialists, hospitals, and disciplines will have to be the norm instead of the exception to coordinate the patient and population's care needs.

Care management is a broad term used to describe the process of managing the entire patient population assigned to one physician or care team. Most often it is found in primary care offices; however, in some specialty offices such as oncology, care management is also a key role of the nursing staff. Care management includes managing chronic illnesses and preventive care by engaging patients further in their healthcare.

The entire care team is involved in care management by determining the needs of individual patients as well as the entire population. Preplanning for the visit determines the previsit needs, and nursing staff can better prepare the patient for the one-on-one with the provider. For example, protocols can be used by nonlicensed staff to provide testing (HbA1c, lipid panel) or procedures (foot exam, weight) prior to a 3-month return visit for diabetes or heart disease.

Providers using clinical decision support at the point of care have information that enables them, in collaboration with their patients, to make good decisions based on specific circumstances. The patient's information is compared electronically to evidence-based clinical guidelines, and the provider is reminded to perform recommended immunizations, chronic disease care, and preventive care. Clinical decision support is most useful when it fits with the existing workflow of the practice and becomes seamless for the entire care team, providing reminders throughout the visit without having to stop and remember protocols.[52,53]

Technology such as registries can assist the nurse care team to compile data, analyze the data, and find care opportunities; patients can then be notified and engaged to obtain further care. In some cases, insurance carriers provide outcome data to providers in order to assist them in providing quality care. Because it is based on claims data, however, accuracy is a problem. It is better for the data to be generated and processed within the practice. A registry tool gathers data from disparate sources (pharmacy data, claims data, lab data, EMR data, practice management data), combines it, and creates reports that allow the nurse to determine opportunities in care. For instance, for preventive care, a report run on women who have not received recommended yearly cervical cancer screening could provide a patient list for needed appointments. In addition, the registry can provide lists of patients needing mammograms or other preventive health measures. Registry tools also can be used for chronic disease measures and can stratify the patient population of a specific disease. For instance, diabetics with HbA1c results of greater than 13 may need more intensive care management by the care manager with frequent visits to the provider. Those patients with HbA1c results in the range of 9–12 may need to visit a diabetic nurse educator and receive more frequent e-mails or provider visits. Those patients with a result of less than 9 may just need to be managed by the assigned primary care team. Registry tools are outside the EMR in most cases, but there is a move for EMR vendors to embed the registry tool within the EMR for ease of use.[54]

Work is being done throughout the country in defining the roles of care management. One example, the Center for Health Care Strategies, a national non-profit organization dedicated to improving the quality of publicly financed care, came to a consensus definition of care management and developed the Care Management Framework to be used by Medicaid programs nationwide. The following components were used: identification, stratification, prioritization, intervention, evaluation, and payment/financing. Tools and strategies were defined, including health risk assessments, predictive models, surveys, evidence-based practices, medical home (a new model of primary care), physical/behavioral health integration, quality outcome measurement, and pay for performance.[55]

A component of managing the patient's care is coordinating all the care across many different healthcare providers. Care coordination is defined as "a function that helps ensure that the patient's needs and preferences for health services and information sharing across people, functions, and sites are met over time."[56] For instance, when a patient enters the hospital, the nurse coordinates that hospital admission by sending orders, a medication listing, and progress notes to the hospital so treatment can be coordinated more completely. When the patient is dismissed, the nurse obtains reports about the hospital stay including history and physical, medication list, and discharge summary so the patient can be treated appropriately.

Likewise, when a patient is sent to a specialist, the nurse will need to gather information (e.g., medications, progress, and reason for referral) to send to the specialist. After the visit, the consult report is obtained so care can be coordinated with specialist care. On the other hand, a nurse in the specialist office may have to coordinate care by obtaining information from the referral physician, hospitals, or diagnostic testing facilities prior to the physician visit. After the specialist visit, the nurse coordinates surgery, treatment, or further diagnostic treatments, and assists in sending information back to the referring physician. Often care coordination functions can be performed by different members of the care team in unison.

Care coordination is a cornerstone of quality health-care. "Health care cannot be of high quality without being delivered in a coordinated, efficient manner."[56] Care coordination is important for patients with chronic diseases because they usually receive care in several locations and from several providers. As these patients move through the complex healthcare environment, they have difficulty managing their own care. Care coordination involves managing more intensely those patients who are heavy users of the system, such as those who have multiple chronic conditions. Essential elements of good care coordination are a written care plan and communication following the visit. This may be facilitated by the EMR, which prints a summary of the visit, orders and self-care activities, medications, and a problem list for the patient to take home. Communication allows the care team, the patient, and his or her family to share progress and decision making.[56]

Self-management support education is a nursing action that enables patients to care for themselves by encouraging daily decisions to improve health-related behaviors. Patients become more informed about their conditions and take an active role in their treatment. Strategies that can be used are collaborative decision making, establishing an agenda, information giving, assessing readiness to change, and goal setting. When patients take a more active role in their care, clinical outcomes improve and the collaborative relationship between physician/nurse and patient allow for better overall health. Nurses are taking a larger role in providing self-management support and are supplementing the patient education activities of the provider.[57]

Patients need to become engaged and have a continuous relationship with their physician, both primary and specialty care. Care management/care coordination has become more difficult in today's world because patients often determine their own need for specialist or hospital care. Engaging the patient to inform the practice about their "other" healthcare activities is very important to managing the patient's care. The appropriate use of specialty care to supplement primary care services can lessen the complexity of the system for the patient. Often patients need assistance in determining when to use a specialist. Patients who are included as part of the team can be more informed and make better healthcare decisions.

New roles such as nurse care managers or care coordinators are emerging for nurses who have training in the clinical and behavioral treatment of chronic disease. These nurses may be nurse practitioners, advance practice nurses with additional degrees, or RNs with additional training and experience. The nurse care manager works with the sickest patients, developing a relationship to better assist the patient to manage their disease more effectively. The use of protocols, managing transitions between inpatient and outpatient settings, acute assessment and listening skills, and a greater attention to the intensity of care make these nurses successful. Often care managers are shared among several practices. The minimum qualification of nurse care managers is the RN level.[58]

Another form of care management/care coordination is the health coach. One practice created three levels of health coach—one for medical assistants and two for RNs (RNI, RNII). The RNII position migrating to full care management responsibilities is tasked with:

- Oversight of the disease registry database
- Conducting a previsit chart review
- Working with patients and families on self-management support
- Coordination of care across the care continuum
- Involvement in quality improvement activities

Initial results demonstrated positive clinical outcomes and improved job satisfaction among the staff and physicians.[59]

Diabetic nurse educators are emerging as specialized care managers focusing on the person with prediabetes or diabetes and their caregivers. The diabetic nurse educator facilitates the patient's self-care knowledge and ability. Using evidence-based standards, the diabetic nurse educator engages the patient to improve his or her clinical outcomes and health status.[60]

Nursing Leadership

One role that is becoming more important is nursing leadership. Moving into uncharted territories and the development of new roles will require nurses to lead to a greater extent. From the nurse who cares for the patient on the phone to the nurse manager or administrator who oversees clinical operations, there is a need for more sophisticated nursing managers and leaders in the medical office setting. Medical office nursing requires clinical experience and strong communication skills. Knowledge of financial and reimbursement systems, as well as business expertise, is needed to effectively and efficiently manage care.

Nurse leader competencies include the ability to enhance technology skills that facilitate mobility and portability of nursing staff. Technology needs and expertise of the nursing staff will be on the forefront as healthcare changes. Expert decision-making skills give the leader the ability to react to a rapidly changing healthcare environment. The ability to create a quality culture with the use of research findings to provide better patient care and a patient safety culture will allow for a safer and more effective care system. Collaborative and team-building skills will allow the nursing leader to engage nursing and other members of the healthcare team such as pharmacy, physicians, social work, administration, and others. A good nursing leader can engage others to assist in transitioning nursing into new roles. Finally, the ability to envision a

professional nursing role in the medical office setting and striving to improve the overall abilities and competencies of the nursing staff will lead to more recognition of this important role.

Nursing Informatics

Electronic technology can and will change the healthcare delivery system. The improvement in quality and often cost allow for better care. Physician offices have been slow to adopt the technology because of several factors. In particular, many systems have not grasped the true essence of care and the eloquence of the physician–patient relationship. Nursing informatics with a focus on the clinical side is emerging as a bridge to better understand the complexities of patient care and the ability to improve efficiency.

During EMR transition, physicians often are given tasks that normally would be handled by other team members. Many technology companies fail to understand that having the physician do more does not maximize his or her care delivery. The physician's workload often doubles if the EMR implementation is not well thought out.

Nursing can have an impact on streamlining only those items that require the physician's knowledge and skill and directing them to him or her. Thinking about those processes and how or if the EMR will change them is very important in planning for an EMR. If an EMR is in place, looking at all the responsibilities of the physician and determining those tasks that need his or her expertise and delegating to others on the team are vital in making technology work efficiently for the practice.

New technology is emerging regularly for both the clinical and administrative portions of a practice. New EMRs, registries, patient portals, chronic disease portals, and endless other tracking and clinical documentation advances are being tested. The design of the exam room and how technology can be incorporated to improve efficiency are also being tested. New surgical and specialty offerings occur on a regular basis. Interfacing between tools in the office and the EMR has already been initiated at many levels. Much progress can be expected as medical office leadership realize the potential of automation and point of care technology.

New technology also is emerging in other areas of nursing practice. The ability to complete referrals or preauthorizations online, or by using Wi-Fi instead of having a paper form to fill out is the start of automating insurance connections. Ordering tests through a portal instead of having a lab requisition and having tests return to the office without having to touch paper are some of the technological advances. Others will continue to emerge.

Technology is probably the biggest and greatest improvement that will be seen over the next decade as medical practices try to catch up with the technology revolution. The development of better user interfaces, transfer technology, and telecommunications technology are just a few of the areas we might see vast improvements in. The accessibility of the data will be a key driver to improve outcomes and reduce cost.

A nursing informatics specialist combines clinical knowledge with the efficient use of technology. This will be a powerful combination in the future of medical office nursing.

Increasing Roles for Nurse Practitioners and Physician Assistants

Nurse practitioners and physician assistants are playing an expanded role in medical offices. Some of the reasons include:

- The U.S. population is projected to increase by 18% between 2005 and 2025.
- The senior population is increasing. By 2030, one-fifth of Americans will be over the age of 65.
- There has been an increase in patients with chronic disease. Conservative estimates indicate 45% of Americans have a chronic disease; 83% of Medicare beneficiaries have one or more chronic illnesses.
- There has been a decrease in graduating medical students, especially those specializing in primary care.
- There has been an increase in women primary care physicians, who typically work fewer hours.[61,62]

One reason to add mid-level providers is to conserve more expensive physician labor. If tasks can be performed using a lower level of professional training, then higher-level, more intense services can be reserved for physicians who are uniquely equipped to handle them. Teams that make a greater use of nurse practitioners or physician assistants may see lower labor costs per visit. Nurse practitioners have been trained to have superior patient education and communication skills.

Nurse practitioners can play active roles in managing their own patient panel or supplementing the care provided to a physician's panel of patients. There are not enough physicians to provide the care that will be needed in the future, especially in primary care. There will be an increasingly bigger role for nurse practitioners to provide more care.

Nursing Educators

An educational support system that teaches and develops leaders in medical office nursing will help the medical office nurse to have a positive impact on efficiency. Nurses who understand the changing role of the medical office nurse are needed as educators who can provide teaching that augments the knowledge base of the leader and the staff nurse.

Standard nursing education today spends very little time on specific needs of the medical office nurse. Most programs have a community care nursing curriculum that includes education and experience in community health centers, home health, hospice, public health, schools, universities, occupational health, and other ambulatory care settings. There is very little focus on the medical office and the needs of a nurse who wants to specialize in that area. However, a good office nurse will have a background in nursing in hospitals and other community settings that will assist her in managing patients in the medical office setting. In addition to adding more content and educators to formalized nursing programs, there is a need for better processes and leadership in the medical office setting in regards to orientation, competency, and ongoing training.

Medical offices' administrative practices can often hinder education, because new staff are usually needed, and the newly oriented are often put on the job with minimal training. Whether the nurse has to formalize orientation or it is provided, it is important for reasonable amounts of time to be taken initially to understand the office in areas of policies and procedures, the functioning of various departments (scheduling, billing, front office), patient education resources, technology applications, reimbursement, and external regulations.

As the nurse becomes better acquainted with his or her responsibilities, the office in general, and the various processes, he or she can then define how to fit into the practice. There may not be a set role for the RN; the RN may find that the role requires re-engineering. This may take time, especially if the role is new to the practice. Even if the role is not new, there may be some preconceived ideas regarding what a nurse should do, and the nurse will have to clarify and re-educate those around them.

Understanding the roles of all team members is the first step in identifying the nurse's role as a medical office nurse. If there is a job description, it might give the nurse some insight into what is possible. There are numerous resources and organizations that may also provide guidance. Talking to other nurses in other medical offices can help to clarify the nurse's role—especially if they have experiences that match your goals. Having frequent discussions with the physician(s) will help clarify matters for all. Together, a clear role can be defined.

Each employee needs training throughout his or her career with the practice and must stay updated on procedures, practices, and products. Ongoing training can be as simple as having a 10-minute training session at every nursing meeting on various subjects, or having bimonthly training sessions in various topics. This is extremely helpful for unlicensed assistive personnel because it is a good way for them to gain more knowledge.

Other Nursing Roles in the Practice

Nursing can function in other areas of the practice such as radiology, nuclear medicine, lab, therapy services, pain management, cosmetic treatments, billing, or retail that require the skills of a nurse. For instance, an RN can be an integral part of the radiology team. In addition, the nurse can help monitor patients, give medications, provide venous access, and inject IV medications or dyes. Often the RN is borrowed from another department if there is not a full-time need in the department. These roles may expand as this revolution takes on momentum.

■ Nursing Models

There are numerous ways to utilize nursing staff in a medical office. This section provides a look at the most common nursing models used in physician offices.[48] There may be variations in how each of these models is used, and hybrids can be used to serve the variances from one practice to another.

To illustrate how a nursing model may work for an office, a family practice of five physicians and two midlevel providers will be used in the following examples.

Primary Nursing

Primary nursing is one RN to one physician or provider; tasks include overall management of the patient panel with the provider—rooming patients, assistance with

procedures, phone care or triage, follow-up, care coordination, and all other duties related to taking care of patients in a medical office. Primary nursing is seldom used with RNs in a medical office due to cost; variations are often used with the one-on-one team—one nursing staff is assigned to one provider (see **Figure 4-2**). Primary nursing for the medical office has the following characteristics:

- Nursing staff can be medical assistant, LPN, or RN.
- Each nursing staff has the full responsibility for patient care.
- If nurses are used, they have a high level of autonomy and responsibility.
- The patient is provided a continuous relationship with one nursing staff for all of his or her needs.
- An integral role of primary nursing staff is to establish communication between physician and patient and other team members.
- A primary role is to assist the provider in taking care of his or her entire panel—phone management, rooming patients, follow-up, care coordination, and so on.
- Advantages include the one-on-one relationship the nursing staff establishes with the patient, and the efficiency of the one-on-one relationship between the physician and the nursing member.
- Disadvantages include a large workload for one nursing staff member.

Often there is a combination of RN, LPN, and MA staff that work one on one with providers in any given practice. The determination of whom to hire may depend on availability, physician desire, and/or other factors. Sometimes roles are different for the RN, LPN, or MA but often they assume the same role throughout the practice, regardless

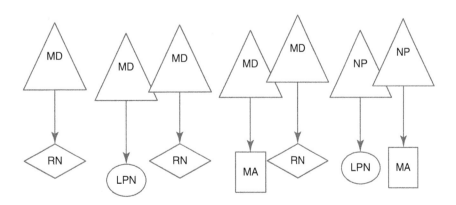

Figure 4-2 Primary nursing.

of level of education or expertise. Many practices could not afford a one-on-one RN–physician staffing model as reimbursement issues became prevalent. They chose to replace RNs with MAs or LPNs as positions opened.

A wide range of activities exists depending on the skill set of the particular primary nursing staff. Physicians delegate tasks according to skill set, licensure, and often experience. This can create scope of practice issues and, depending on the ability or inability of the provider to delegate, a higher workload for the physician/provider.

Team Nursing

Team nursing looks at utilizing the skills and expertise of the RN for those tasks that require her or his expertise and license, and delegating supporting tasks to other members of the team. An example of a team nursing setup is shown in **Figure 4-3**. The Internet defines a team as a group of people with a full set of complementary skills required to complete a task, job, or project. Team members (1) operate with a high degree of interdependence, (2) share authority and responsibility for self-management, (3) are accountable for the collective performance, and (4) work toward a common goal and shared reward(s). A team becomes more than just a collection of people when a strong sense of mutual commitment creates synergy, thus generating performance greater than the sum of the performance of its individual members. Better performing teams have good leadership, a clear division of labor, training of team members, and team-supporting policies. A highly functioning team can increase efficiency and productivity as a whole.

The following are some characteristics of team nursing:

- Personnel work together to provide care for a group of patients under the direction of the RN and/or physician.

- It requires extensive team communications to ensure consistent patient care.
- Small teams take care of the entire patient panel.
- It involves autonomy and shared responsibility and accountability.
- More staff are available to provide more care.
- Advantages include shared workload and responsibility.
- Disadvantages include increased organizational complexity, insufficient time for team planning and communication, and decreased job satisfaction in delegating tasks.

In a medical office, team nursing can be very useful and cost effective. The RN could be used for phone triage and teaching. The MA could be used to room patients, stock rooms, and assist the RN as needed. However, the communication needs to be consistent and well thought out. Communication could be from physician to RN and then to MA or it might be from physician to RN and MA and then between RN and MA.

Learning how to work together as a team can create efficiencies throughout the organization. A new concept, team-based care means that every team member, including providers, has knowledge of their role and is maximizing their knowledge and training. Tasks that do not require the expertise of a team member can be delegated to those members providing support. For instance, rooming patients does not require the expertise of the physician or RN, so that task can be delegated to nonlicensed staff. Another example would be phone triage. Physician expertise is not usually required to triage patient concerns; an RN can triage those calls and ask for physician expertise when needed. Tasks such as rooming patients, stocking rooms, and assisting with simple procedures could be delegated to the medical assistant, whose training and knowledge can be maximized to provide good

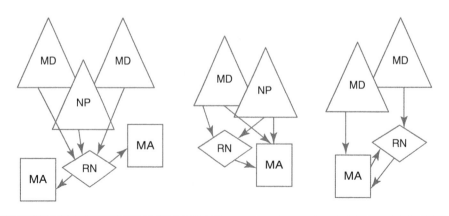

Figure 4-3 Team nursing.

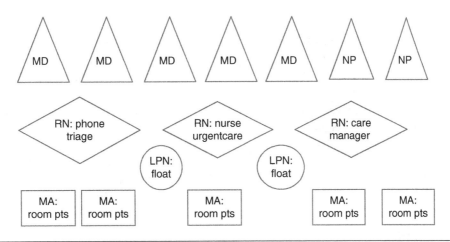

Figure 4-4 Functional nursing.

care. To maximize the use of the team, each task should be analyzed for the complexity and abilities of those completing the task. Each team member's abilities should be examined and understood by all. Matching abilities to tasks creates a high functioning team.

All members of the team need to communicate on a regular basis to ensure everyone is functioning with the same set of information. Sometimes daily huddles or quick meetings can facilitate an update to maximize the team's use. Regular department and staff meetings also support the team concept. Physicians can teach staff to better manage patients with regular communication, whereas nurses can facilitate more integrated care by communicating regularly with nonlicensed or administrative staff.

The right size and composition of the team are driven by the needs of the patient population, the complement of skills and capacity of team members, the quality of the organizational support, the ability of the needs of the patients to be served by external resources, and the degree to which leadership values the team concept.

Functional Nursing

Functional nursing is similar to team nursing in that each member of the team has responsibilities. However, instead of a team, each member works at his or her job function for the team as a whole. For maximum efficiency, nursing staff are given certain tasks to perform for a group of patients (see **Figure 4-4**). Characteristics of this approach are:

- Specific tasks are assigned to certain individuals.
- Repetitive motion increases efficiency.
- There is a wider variation in team members—RN, LPN, or MA—assigned to specific tasks.

- Training on simple task performance provides efficiency and competency (e.g., checking blood pressure, bathing, stocking supplies).
- Advantages include efficiency.
- Disadvantages include fragmented care, the possibility of overlooking patient needs, and low job satisfaction. Also, physicians/providers may struggle with whom to ask to do what.

This model works well in medical practices if it is combined with the team concept. All team members know their roles and they work to the top of their abilities and licensure. Each team member is responsible for certain functions and is held accountable.

In summary, it is possible to create many different structures of nursing care dependent upon the practice and nursing actions needed. Each medical office needs to look at what tasks are needed to be performed and then determine, from these tasks, how nursing actions affect each team member and the structure of the practice. The ultimate goal is to provide the best care for the patient in a cost-effective, quality manner.

■ The Future Medical Office

Many new care models are being piloted to improve efficiency and change outcomes in medical offices. An Internet search found new care models such as the Clinical Caring Model, Patient-Centered Care, Relationship-Based Care, patient-centered medical homes, Chronic Care Model, Evercare Care Model, Living Independently for Elders, Comprehensive Rural Care Collaborative, and Values Driven System.

Primary care has been striving to improve the work and satisfaction of physicians for several years, and some new and exciting models are emerging. Technology has taken on a life of its own in the medical office and it will impact future care in many different ways. Managing the entire patient population and providing care in new care management models are showing promising rewards right now.

A few promising models that have been used more commonly in primary care—patient-centered medical homes and the Chronic Care Model—are explained in the following sections.

Patient-Centered Medical Homes

In early 2000, the leading physician organizations for family medicine, internal medicine, and pediatrics created a list of principles to be implemented if primary care was to survive in the future. The number of primary care physicians is declining, as is the number of residents who are interested in primary care. Many potential primary care physicians are choosing specialty care instead of primary care to seek higher wages and better working hours.

The joint principles that were created and agreed upon led to more interest in taking care of the entire patient through a continuous relationship with a primary care physician, providing more access, managing patients across a continuum, and using technology effectively. The name for all of this was the patient-centered medical home. The Patient-Centered Primary Care Collaborative lists the following joint principles[63]:

- *Personal physician:* Each patient has an ongoing relationship with a personal physician trained to provide first contact, continuous, and comprehensive care.
- *Physician-directed medical practice:* The personal physician leads a team of individuals at the practice level who collectively take responsibility for the ongoing care of patients.
- *Whole-person orientation:* The personal physician is responsible for providing for all the patient's healthcare needs or taking responsibility for appropriately arranging care with other qualified professionals. This includes care for all stages of life, acute care, chronic care, preventive services, and end-of-life care.
- *Integrated care:* Care is coordinated and/or integrated across all elements of the complex healthcare system (e.g., subspecialty care, hospitals, home health agencies, nursing homes) and the patient's community (e.g., family, public and private community-based services). Care is facilitated

by registries, information technology, health information exchange, and other means to assure that patients get the indicated care when and where they need and want it in a culturally and linguistically appropriate manner.

- *Quality and safety:* These are hallmarks of the medical home:
  - Practices advocate for their patients to support the attainment of optimal, patient-centered outcomes that are defined by a care-planning process driven by a compassionate, robust partnership among physicians, patients, and the patient's family.
  - Evidence-based medicine and clinical decision-support tools guide decision making.
  - Physicians in the practice accept accountability for continuous quality improvement through voluntary engagement in performance measurement and improvement.
  - Patients actively participate in decision making, and feedback is sought to ensure patients' expectations are being met.
  - Information technology is utilized appropriately to support optimal patient care, performance measurement, patient education, and enhanced communication.
  - Practices go through a voluntary recognition process by an appropriate nongovernmental entity to demonstrate that they have the capabilities to provide patient-centered services consistent with the medical home model.
  - Patients and families participate in quality improvement activities at the practice level.
- *Access to care:* Enhanced access to care is available through systems such as open scheduling, expanded hours, and new options for communication between patients, their personal physician, and practice staff.
- *Payment for services:* Payment appropriately recognizes the added value provided to patients who have a patient-centered medical home. The payment structure should be based on the following framework:
  - It should reflect the value of physician and nonphysician staff patient-centered care management work that falls outside of the face-to-face visit.
  - It should pay for services associated with coordination of care both within a given practice and between consultants, ancillary providers, and community resources.

- It should support adoption and use of health information technology for quality improvement.
- It should support provision of enhanced communication access such as secure e-mail and telephone consultation.
- It should recognize the value of physician work associated with remote monitoring of clinical data using technology.
- It should allow for separate fee-for-service payments for face-to-face visits. (Payments for care management services that fall outside of the face-to-face visit, as described above, should not result in a reduction in the payments for face-to-face visits.)
- It should recognize case mix differences in the patient population being treated within the practice.
- It should allow physicians to share in savings from reduced hospitalizations associated with physician-guided care management in the office setting.
- It should allow for additional payments for achieving measurable and continuous quality improvements.

What has evolved out of the principles is the patient-centered medical home. The medical home concept was created in the pediatrics community 40 years ago to help take care of chronically ill pediatric patients in a more comprehensive manner. This same concept is now being applied in various forms in many primary care specialties.

Pilot programs led by insurance companies and big integrated delivery systems have given funding to primary care practices to test this new model of care. It is starting to catch on and create excitement in the primary care community. Reimbursement is being tested with these pilot programs to pay for quality and care management/care coordination in addition to paying per visit as the current system allows.

The patient-centered medical home creates a medical office environment that is patient centered with a continuous relationship with a primary care provider. It focuses on patient access to that provider through appointments, e-mail, or phone for acute, preventive, and chronic needs. The primary care provider provides care management and care coordination for his or her panel of patients to better manage their conditions across the continuum. Evidence-based medicine is stressed and incorporated in the day-to-day operations so that care is delivered consistently and effectively. The use of technology helps to improve the

efficiency of the practice. The healthcare team provides a collaborative relationship with the patient to engage him or her in management of healthcare needs. Managing the practice more efficiently and effectively leads to better quality care and outcomes—financial, clinical, and the satisfaction of providers, staff, and patients.

The patient-centered medical home concept can be expanded to other healthcare providers such as hospitals, specialists, and community agencies, who can collaborate to coordinate the care of the patient. The patient remains at the center of care and all efforts are tailored to facilitate better health. This concept stresses the importance of relationship building. The patient builds a relationship with the primary care physician, who collaborates with referring providers and other agencies including hospitals to take care of the patient in a comprehensive manner.

Although the name is somewhat limiting, the concept of providing more efficient, cost-effective care is here to stay. Focusing on evidence-based medicine in addition to experience-based medicine can lower healthcare costs and provide better outcomes. The RN's role in the medical home is evolving, with particular attention focusing on care management and care coordination.

Chronic Care Model

Another model used frequently in primary care is the Chronic Care Model, developed by Ed Wagner, MD, MPH, in the 1990s. It is a widely adopted approach to managing chronic care in a medical practice. Healthcare delivery is changed using interrelated system changes, making the practice more patient-centered and providing evidence-based care. A proactive approach requires physicians to develop systems that include the following elements:

- Proactive interactions between physicians and patients
- Self-management support empowering patients to take greater responsibility for their care
- Decision support tools that assist the care team to provide recommended care
- Clinical information systems that track the care of individuals and populations[58]

The Chronic Care Model utilizes the entire team to identify patients and seize opportunities to provide comprehensive chronic disease care. RNs can have a significant impact in chronic care. Outcomes include improved clinical measures, physician satisfaction, patient satisfaction, and financial outcomes.[65]

In summary, nursing's role in the medical office is undergoing a significant change. There are many changes occurring, and the future will be very exciting.

References

1. Institute of Medicine. *The future of nursing, leading change, advancing health.* October 2010, Washington DC.

2. Main T, Weil R. The view from healthcare's front lines: an Oliver Wyman CEO survey. Oliver Wyman Health and Life Sciences. Accessed February 25, 2011, at http://www.oliverwyman.com/ow/pdf_files/The_View_from_Healthcares_Front_Lines_An_Oliver_Wyman_CEO_Survey.pdf

3. Woodwell D. National ambulatory medical care survey: 1997 summary. Advance data from vital and health statistics; no 305. Hyattsville, MD; National Center for Health Statistics; 1999.

4. Hsiao CJ, Cherry DK, Beatty PC, Rechtsteiner EA. National Ambulatory Medical Care Survey; 2007 summary. National health statistics reports; no 27. Hyattsville, MD; National Center for Health Statistics, 2010.

5. Centers for Disease Control and Prevention. Latest data on ambulatory medical care in America, 1999 fact sheet. Accessed January 27, 2011, at http://www.cdc.gov/nchs/pressroom/99facts/97namcs.htm

6. Gans D. Managing costs. *MGMA Connexion.* February 2007:16–18.

7. Shih A, Davis K, Schoenbaum S, Gauthier A, Nuzum R, McCarthy D. *Organizing the U.S. health care delivery system for high performance.* Washington, DC: Commonwealth Fund; August 2008.

8. Strode R, Beith C. Something old is something new again, structuring physician practice acquisitions. *Healthcare Financial Management.* July 2009:78–82.

9. Wong J. Hospitals are buying private medical practices. *Richmond Times Dispatch.* January 9, 2011.

10. Chew K. Integration opportunities: hospitals and doctors reconsider alignment. *MGMA Buyer's Guide 2010.* 2010:10–11.

11. Boggs S. Physician practice and hospital revenue cycle drivers, what's the difference? *Healthcare Financial Management.* September 2010:40–44.

12. Fink J, Hartzell S. From acquisition to integration, transforming a hospital into an ACO. *Healthcare Financial Management.* October 2010:90–98.

13. Boukus E, Grossman J, O'Malley A. Physicians slow to e-mail routinely with patients. Center for Studying Health System Change. Issue brief no. 134. October 2010. Accessed February 10, 2011, at http://www.hschange.com/CONTENT/1156/

14. Hsiao CJ, Beatty P, Hing E, Woodwell D, Rechtsteiner E, Sisk J. Electronic medical record/electronic health record use by office-based physicians: United States, 2008 and preliminary 2009. Centers for Disease Control and Prevention. December 2009. Accessed February 10, 2011, at http://www.cdc.gov/nchs/data/hestat/emr_ehr/emr_ehr.htm

15. Park T, Basch P. *A historic opportunity: wedding health information technology to care delivery innovation and provider payment reform.* Center for American Progress. http://www.americanprogress.org; Washington, DC: May 2009.

16. Blumental D, Tavenner M. The "meaningful use" regulation for electronic health record. *New England Journal of Medicine.* 2010;1–4.

17. Westra B, Delaney C. Informatics competencies for nursing and healthcare leaders. American Medical Informatics Association. Accessed February 26, 2011, at http://www.ncbi.nlm.nih.gov/pmc/articles/PMC2655955/

18. Pravikkoff D. Readiness of US nurses for evidence based practice: many don't understand or value research and have had little or no training to help them find evidence on which to base their practice. *American Journal of Nursing.* 2005;105(9):40–51.

19. Moran M. Prediction: in seven years electronic records the norm. *Psychiatric News.* 2007;42(1):5. Accessed February 26, 2011, at http://pn.psychiatryonline.org/content/42/1/5.1.full

20. O'Malley A, Pham H, Reschovsky J. Predictors of the growing influence of clinical practice guidelines. *Journal of General Internal Medicine.* 2007;22:742–748.

21. Chaixl-Couturier C, Durand-Zaleski I, Jolly D, Durieux P. Effects of financial incentives on medical practice: results from a systematic review of the literature and methodological issues. *International Journal for Quality in Health Care.* 2000;12(2):139–142.

22. Agency for Healthcare Research and Quality. Key themes and highlights from the National Healthcare Quality Report. *National Healthcare Quality Report.* 2009.

23. New England Healthcare Institute. *Waste in health care.* 2008, Cambridge, MA.

24. Scorecard reveals wide variances in health care access, quality, and cost from state to state. *Managed Care Outlook.* December 1, 2009:1–6.

25. Institute of Medicine. *Crossing the quality chasm: a new health system for the 21st century.* March 2001, Washington, DC.

26. Agency for Healthcare Research and Quality; National Healthcare Quality Report, 2009 Fact sheet, health care costs; Rockville, MD.

27. Nembhard I, Alexandar J, Hoff T, Ramanujam R. Why does the quality of healthcare continue to lag? *Academy of Management Perspectives.* February 2010;24–42.

28. Rutledge V, Huber D, Mathews J. Progression of strategies used by a healthcare system preparing for healthcare reform: past and present. *American College of Healthcare Executives.* 2010;27(1):13–27.

29. Kim YK, Cho CH, Ahu SK, Goh IH, Kim HJ. A study of medical services quality and its influence upon value of care and patient satisfaction—focusing upon outpatients in a large-sized hospital. *Total Quality Management.* 2008;19(11):1155–1171.

30. Bleich S, Ozaltin E, Murray C. How does satisfaction with the health-care system relate to patient experience? *Bulletin of the World Health Organization.* 2009;87:271–278.

31. American Nurses Association. *Health care reform: key provisions related to nursing.* 2010, Silver Spring, MD.

32. Eddy D. Evidence-based medicine: a unified approach. *Health Affairs.* 2005;24(1):9–17.

33. Medical Group Management Association Government Affairs Department. How healthcare reform provisions affect your practice. May/June 2010:18–21, Englewood CO.

34. Centers for Medicare and Medicaid Services. Home health quality initiatives overview. Accessed February 11, 2011, at https://www.cms.gov/HomeHealthQualityInits/01_Overview.asp

35. Centers for Medicare and Medicaid Services. Hospital quality initiatives overview. Accessed February 11, 2011, at http://www.cms.gov/HospitalQualityInits/01_Overview.asp

36. Centers for Medicare and Medicaid Services. Physician Quality Reporting System overview. Accessed February 11, 2011, at http://www.cms.gov/PQRI/01_Overview.asp

37. Mehrotra A, Pearson S, Coltin K, Kleinman K, Singer J, Robson B, Schneider E. The response of physician groups to P4P incentives. *American Journal of Managed Care.* 2007;13(5):249–255.

38. Baker N, Whittington J, Resar R, Griffin F, Nolan K, Institute for Healthcare Improvement. *Reducing costs through the appropriate use of specialty services.* Innovation Series. 2010, Cambridge, MA.

39. Agency for Healthcare Research and Quality. Preventable hospitalizations: a window into primary and preventive care. 2000. Accessed January 27, 2011, at http://archive.ahrq.gov/data/hcup/factbk5/

40. Jencks S, Williams M, Coleman E. Rehospitalizations among patients in the Medicare fee-for-service program. *New England Journal of Medicine.* 2009;360:1418.

41. National Priorities Partnership, National Quality Forum. *Preventing hospital readmissions: a $25 billion opportunity.* November 2010, Cambridge, MA.

42. Agency for Healthcare Research and Quality. Preventable hospital-izations, executive summary. Accessed January 27, 2011, at http://www.ahrq.gov/data/hcup/factbk5/factbk5a.htm

43. National Priorities Partnership, National Quality Forum. *Reducing emergency department overuse: a $38 billion opportunity.* November 2010, Cambridge, MA.

44. Patient-Centered Primary Care Collaborative (PCPCC). Pilots and demonstrations. Accessed February 10, 2011, at http://www.pcpcc.net/pcpcc-pilot-projects

45. Kurtzman E, O'Leary D, Sheingold B, Devers K, Dawson E, Johnson J. Performance-based payment incentives increase burden and blame for hospital nurses. *Health Affairs.* 2011;30(2):211–218.

46. Agency for Healthcare Research and Quality. *Hospital nurse staffing and quality of care.* March 2004:1–7, Rockville, MD.

47. Yarnall K, Ostbye T, Krause K, Pollak K, Gradison M, Mechener L. Family physicians as team leaders: "time" to share the care. *Preventing Chronic Disease—Public Health Research, Practice, and Policy.* 2009;6:A59. Centers for Disease Control and Prevention. Accessed February 10, 2011, at http://www.cdc.gov/pcd/issues/2009/apr/08_0023.htm

48. Richmeier S. *Leading your clinical team: a comprehensive guide to op-timizing productivity and quality.* Denver, CO: MGMA Publications; 2009:67–69.

49. Roter D, Hail J. Studies of doctor-patient interaction. *Annual Review of Public Health.* 1989;10:163–180. Accessed February 26, 2011, at http://www.annualreviews.org/doi/abs/10.1146/annurev.pu.10.050189.001115

50. Center for Studying Health System Change. Health Tracking Physician Survey Methodology Report. September 2009. Accessed February 26, 2011, at http://hschange.org/CONTENT/1085/

51. Marvel M, Epstein R, Flowers K, Beckman H. Soliciting the pa-tient's agenda, have we improved? *Journal of the American Medical Association.* 1999;281(3):283–287. Accessed February 26, 2011, at http://jama.ama-assn.org/content/281/3/283.full.pdf

52. Patient-Centered Primary Care Collaborative. Clinical decision support in the medical home, an overview. Accessed February 11, 2011, at http://www.pcpcc.net/guide/clinical-decision-support

53. Agency for Healthcare Research and Quality. *Adult preventive care timeline.* April 2006; Rockville, MD.

54. Metzger J. Using computerized registry tools in chronic dis-ease care. California Healthcare Foundation. February 2004. Accessed February 11, 2011, at http://www.chcf.org/~/media/MEDIA%20LIBRARY%20Files/PDF/C/PDF%20ComputerizedRegistriesInChronicDisease.pdf

55. Center for Health Care Strategies. Care management definition and framework. 2007. Accessed February 11, 2011, at http://www.chcs.org/usr_doc/Care_Management_Framework.pdf

56. National Quality Forum. Care coordination. October 2010:1–12.

57. Bodenheimer T, MacGregor K, Sharifi C. Helping patients manage their chronic conditions. California Healthcare Foundation. June 2005:4–55. Accessed February 11, 2011, at http://www.familydocs.org/files/HelpingPatientsManageTheirChronicConditions.pdf

58. Wagner E. The role of patient care teams in chronic disease man-agement. *British Medical Journal.* 2000;320:569–572.

59. Sweskowski D. Office-based health coaches: creating healthier communities. *Group Practice Journal.* February 2008;41–45.

60. Burke S, Cornell S, Crawley C, Kadohiro J, Kanzer-Lewis G, Schreiner B. Competencies for diabetic educators: a companion document to the guidelines for the practice of diabetic educa-tion. American Association of Diabetes Educators. Accessed March 3, 2011, at http://www.diabeteseducator.org/export/sites/aade/_resources/pdf/competencies.pdf

61. Zerechi M. *How is a shortage of primary care physicians affecting the quality and cost of medical care?* Philadelphia, PA: American College of Physicians, 2008:3–5.

62. Bodenheimer T, Chan E, Bennett H. Confronting the growing bur-den of chronic disease: can the US health care workforce do the job? *Health Affairs.* 2009;28(1):64–74.

63. Patient-Centered Primary Care Collaborative. Joint principles of the patient centered medical home. Accessed February 11, 2011, at http://www.pcpcc.net/joint-principles

64. Coleman K, Austin B, Brach C, Wagner E. Evidence on the Chronic Care Model in the new millennium. *Health Affairs.* 2009;28(1):75–85.

Recommended Resources

Gauthier S. *Governmental accounting, auditing, and financial reporting.* Chicago: Government Finance Officers Association; 2011.

Governmental Accounting Standards Board. http://www.gasb.org

Governmental Accounting Standards Board. *Codification of governmental accounting standards, 2011–2012.* Norwalk, CT: Financial Accounting Foundation; 2011.

Mead DM. *An analyst's guide to state and local government financial state-ments.* 2nd ed. Norwalk, CT: Financial Accounting Foundation; 2011.

Human Resources Management in Group Practice

Michael A. O'Connell, MHA, FACHE, FACMPE

Over the next 5 years, with the advent of significant healthcare reform in the United States, our healthcare systems, processes, and organization will dramatically change unlike any other time in history. Although legislation has been passed, the policies and procedures to implement its intent are still being written, and the policies continue to evolve throughout the individual 50 United States and within the federal government. With this reform will come cascading changes in the way healthcare is delivered and tremendous challenges for the medical practice leader, the physicians in the medical group, and their employees. These challenges will revolve around the ability to perform more effort with fewer resources and to streamline operations around patient safety, quality, and measurable outcomes. Thus, human resources management in group practice will need to change to meet the dynamic and evolving changes of healthcare.

The field of human resources management has evolved over time from a function primarily involving hiring and terminating employees to a recognized profession. As organizations experience change, human resources professionals provide the change management support necessary not only to change in reaction to external forces, but also to implement internal change effectively and efficiently.

The options for organizational investment in human resources management have never been greater. With the advent of computer technology, the Internet and intranets, and e-mail as tools for data management and transfer, the field of human resources management has changed dramatically. Human resources management computer systems and software are available for all sizes and types of organizations. Utilization of intranet, Internet, and e-mail capabilities allows for the dissemination of information to more employees at a significantly greater speed than previously experienced. As a result, there has been a proliferation of companies that provide a range of human resources management products and support.

The legal and labor law environment that influences human resources management has grown exponentially complex with the continual enactment and revision of laws and accompanying regulations. A significant portion of the legislation to which organizations are subject falls to human resources professionals to interpret and implement.

The demographics of the population in the United States have changed, causing a dramatic shift in the labor market. Many older employees are continuing to work longer than in previous generations. There is a shrinking availability of well-qualified replacements for those employees who do retire. The change in the immigrant population is having an impact as many employers find that they must deal with employees who are not proficient in the English language. The recruitment of the right employee for the right job at the right time has become more of a challenge, not only from the perspective of the availability of candidates, but also from the perspective of the need for compliance with the new and changing laws and regulations that apply to employment.

All of these factors point to the necessity for group practices, particularly larger ones, to make appropriate investments in human resources management. Human resources professionals must be well-educated, have highly developed communication skills, be technologically skilled, and be able to manage change.

◼ Organizational Investment in Human Resources Management

Any organization with employees knows it is necessary to invest in human resources management. At each stage in an organization's development, the type of human resources management support that is needed evolves. A start-up organization needs recruitment and hiring of the key employees to begin the business. The focus is on the development of employment contracts and competitive salary and benefits packages. Organizational policies and procedures are written. Employee orientation and training programs are developed. The human resources manager for a small organization is typically a generalist with the appropriate education and experience necessary to provide all of the human resources support the organization needs. In addition, the smaller group practice may contract with third parties to provide some of the human resources support, such as payroll or benefits administration.

For smaller organizations, an option for providing human resources management is to use a professional employer organization (PEO). A PEO becomes the employer of record for the organization's employees. The PEO shares the responsibility and liability for the employees. It manages the compliance with labor laws, maintains the employee files, processes the payroll, administers the benefits, and files the payroll taxes and reports. The work done by the employees is managed by the large group practice. Both the PEO and the group practice have responsibility for the hiring and terminations. The advantage of a PEO for an employer is the reduction in risk to the group

practice, the ability to focus resources on the business of the practice, and the group purchasing power that the PEO has for contracting for benefits for the employees. By having the employees employed by a PEO, a smaller organization can provide its employees with benefits that normally can only be provided by much larger organizations. A PEO also reduces or eliminates the need for an organization to invest in human resources management staff and systems.

As the group practice matures, the human resources function continues to support employment of the appropriate type and number of employees as well as working with the organization to retain the well-qualified, experienced employees that it already has in place. A well-developed compensation and benefits program must be in place to ensure the organization is providing competitive pay and benefits to employees compared to the market, and that pay equity within the organization is maintained.

In larger groups the focus also shifts to the training and education of employees, in particular the training of supervisors. Well-trained supervisors are the key to employee retention. More often than not, employees leave an organization because of a poor supervisor. In addition, training is provided to ensure that key competencies are in place and up-to-date for all employees. Succession planning includes the training of employees in preparation for their moving into other roles within the organization.

A formal performance management program is necessary to ensure that employees receive regular feedback on their job performance and to provide a method to address any performance issues that might exist.

Human resources management is also a key function to have involved in any organizational change. Human resources professionals work with the organization in evaluating the impact that any change might have on the workforce, to develop the communication about the change, and to work with the supervisors in managing the employee reaction to organizational change.

As organizations grow and change, the human resources management area evolves as well. The human resources professional's responsibilities change, and many may be specialists in their particular area. For example, the large group practice may have a vice president of human resources and human resources directors reporting to the vice president. Each director is responsible for a particular area of human resources such as employment, employee/labor relations, compensation and benefits, and human resources information systems (HRIS).

Human Resources and Technology

Human resources management requires data management. The more information can be stored electronically, the easier it is to access the data and use them for organizational needs. The tracking of information includes:

- Employee data for payroll processing, benefits administration, legally required reporting, and to track licensure and certification expiration information
- Position information to manage the positions held by employees, to develop organizational charts, and to develop and maintain the compensation structure for the organization
- Transaction tracking to measure the human resources activity from the perspective of volume and effectiveness. Examples of transaction tracking and the resulting reporting include:
    - Tracking hires and terminations and developing staffing metrics such as the rate of employee turnover, cost of turnover, cost per hire, time to fill, and time to start, for each part of the organization, as well as for the organization as a whole
    - Compensation changes to manage, to budget, and to enforce equity in compensation among employees in similar positions

As a result of technological advances, organizations have more choice in purchasing the appropriate HRIS support. The market for HRIS provides comprehensive systems for all sizes and types of organizations. A large group practice can purchase the software and hardware to own and run HRIS in-house; however, it is not necessary for an organization to invest a significant amount of capital in order to access the HRIS necessary to run the business. There are HRIS suppliers that act as service bureaus selling access to their system without requiring the client to invest in the hardware and software.

These arrangements with service bureaus range from basic access to the HRIS to a full-blown outsourcing of the human resources function. Many of these companies have a range of options from which organizations can choose for human resources support. The Internet has made it possible for human resources service bureaus to provide access to their systems from any location worldwide.

In addition, the Internet has changed the way information is provided to employees. Organizations are using the Internet, an intranet, or both to establish employee self-service, allowing employees to access policies and procedures, organizational news, job postings of open positions, payroll and benefits information, hours worked, work schedules, and vacation information. These systems can be programmed to allow employees not only to view their personalized information, but also to make changes. For example, employees can be given access to change their address or tax exemptions, apply for vacation time off, and request schedule changes.

This technology revolutionizes the type of work on which the human resources investment is spent. The more mundane clerical tasks can be automated, the more time the human resources professional can spend on higher-level work supporting the organizational strategy.

Another alternative, as an organization grows, is to invest in hiring human resources staff and contracting with a third-party administrator for transaction processing of benefits and payroll. The human resources function can also be supplemented with consultants specializing in various areas of human resources management including employment, employee and labor relations, and compensation management.

The staffing of the human resources function for organizations is determined based on the size and complexity of the organization, the amount of control the organization prefers to have over all of its operations, and where the organization is in its development. A BNA survey done in collaboration with the Society for Human Resource Management (SHRM) found that for 2003 "the median ratio of human resources staff to total headcount is 1.0 HR staff for every 100 employees served by the HR department."[1]

Evaluation of Positions Needed by the Organization and Preparation of Job Descriptions

Small medical groups have staff that may assume a variety of diverse tasks and duties, but as a medical group grows in size, staff become more specialized in a certain area or function. For example, a human resources (HR) specialist in a small medical group may handle all aspects of recruitment, training and development, benefit administration, and workers' compensation claims, yet in a large medical group, an HR specialist may handle just one aspect of benefit administration such as tuition reimbursement. The evaluation of a new position needed by a large medical group requires involvement from the manager, the HR department, and a medical group committee. These three groups help lead the organization to plan and implement the new position. The manager is best suited to identify what is needed within the department. The HR department is able to help facilitate the process for getting the position description established. The medical group committee has the diversity and breadth of membership to evaluate the position and determine if it is approved and how it fits within the organizational structure.

A sample position description for the position of coding and education specialist, or the CES position, demonstrates the range of responsibilities inherent in the job. The medical group has decided that it needs a person to help the organization code its medical services and provide coding education for its physicians and staff. The proposed position accomplishes two key functions: financial improvement and compliance. The position is being created to help improve physician documentation, coding of services from that documentation, and better financial reimbursement brought on by improved documentation. The position should also help the medical group address compliance with managed-care plan requirements and demonstrate a commitment to compliance through ongoing education and audits.

Determining Job Scope

Preparing for a new position requires collection of information, verification of the information for accuracy, creation of the position description, and determination of position requirements. The collection of information may involve talking with other organizations that have comparable positions, seeking sample position descriptions from other organizations, and reading professional literature. In addition, professional associations provide useful resources for the medical group to consider.

With the CES position, because the medical group didn't previously have this position in its organization, it investigated other entities through personal interviews to see what they had in place. It also collected sample position descriptions and read literature from professional magazines on coding. This information served as a baseline for determining what specific information was needed for the CES position in the medical group.

Verifying Information for Accuracy

After the job scope information is collected, it needs to be verified for accuracy. The information may be dated or not relevant to the medical group. Certain tasks or duties may not apply based on how the medical group is organized. For example, the CES may physically review encounter forms and enter charges into the computer system, whereas another organization may have charge entry handled by another person. Other organizations

might assume specific responsibilities and not be needed in the new position description whereas other functions need to be added because they are not addressed in other positions. These aspects must be considered when reviewing the information.

Creating a Position Description

The writing of the position description needs to follow the medical group's format. Many organizations have a planning sheet that helps the author of the position description determine its components.

The new position description helps determine the type of employee to recruit and clarifies how the position fits within the organization. It helps the committee determine how this position benchmarks with other comparable positions within the organization. The position's authority and responsibility establish how it fits within the medical group. The position structure determines the acceptable pay range and leads the manager to recruit the appropriate person.

Position Description

Components of the position description include:

- *Title:* The title reflects the nature or function of the position. For example, a biller handles multiple billing functions, whereas a payment poster handles only posting of monies.
- *Statement of duties:* "Other duties as assigned" is usually the last item listed on the position description; the primary duties of the position are listed based on order of significance or frequency of use.
- Full-time or part-time
- *Reporting relationship:* Determining the reporting relationship helps to define the level of authority the position has within the medical group. Reporting to a manager, supervisor, or team leader is different than reporting to the medical group CEO.
- Key responsibilities or essential functions
- *Educational and experience requirements:* The educational level helps define what external requirements are needed to fulfill the position. If a clinical position requires the person to be an RN, it eliminates an LPN, medical assistant, or dietician from applying for the position.
- *Special skills or abilities:* Stating that a person needs special skills helps to screen out those people that lack those skills. For example, if prior experience with certain computer software is required, then people without that skill are not eligible for the position. Or if a physician needs board certification in a specialty and lacks that certification, then that physician won't be considered.

Job Analysis Interviews

Sometimes a position needs to be evaluated or reevaluated through a series of steps. Whether the group chooses to use a consultant or handle the work internally, it is important to reevaluate all positions within the organization periodically through the steps of job analysis interviews, observation of work flow, and completion of forms. The job analysis interviews involve meeting one on one with the person who holds the job along with people who work with that person performing the job. These observations allow the functions of the position to be committed to writing. The second step is to observe the person performing the job functions and determine if there is a gap between perceived and actual functions. The final phase is completion of forms by both the internal reviewer and the employee in the position. Through this exercise, they determine if their forms match in job analysis. Many times, the position description does not accurately reflect the full nature of the position and needs to be revised.

Committee Review

Although a committee could be seen as a bureaucratic mechanism for creating and evaluating position descriptions, a well-functioning committee can be an invaluable asset for the medical group. The committee is meant to be an interconnection to other components of the organization and benchmark comparable positions to where the position fits within the organization through assignment of a pay grade, pay range, or employment status (exempt or nonexempt) to determine whether the position qualifies for overtime and what the appropriate salary range should be.

The multidisciplinary committee can review the proposed position, place it into an appropriate pay grade, and determine any factors or issues prior to the position being approved and posted for consideration. The committee helps facilitate communications and determines any political or controversial issues that need to be addressed. It also determines the appropriate grade that the position falls into so that the manager knows what the range of wages will be. **Table 5-1** describes a sample pay grade table into which a position would fit. For example, if a position fit within pay grade C, the position could be brought in anywhere in that range depending on the person's experience, qualifications, and competition in the marketplace. Because of the shortage of medical coders nationally, a medical group may want to bring a person into the range at a higher level than an entry level. This strategy can be achieved by either moving the position into a higher-level range or moving the staff to a higher level within the current range.

Table 5-1	ABC Medical Group Salary Ranges		
Salary Grade	**Minimum**	**Midpoint**	**Maximum**
A	$10,816	$13,900	$17,056
	$5.20	$6.68	$8.20
B	$11,232	$14,539	$17,900
	$5.40	$6.99	$8.60
C	$11,575	$15,200	$18,720
	$5.65	$7.30	$9.00
D	$12,188	$15,900	$19,552
	$5.86	$7.64	$9.40
E	$12,818	$16,700	$20,500
	$6.16	$8.02	$9.85
F	$13,520	$17,576	$21,600
	$6.50	$8.45	$10.38
G	$14,248	$18,512	$22,776
	$6.85	$8.90	$10.95
H	$14,976	$19,448	$23,816
	$7.20	$9.35	$11.45
I	$15,704	$20,400	$25,168
	$7.55	$9.80	$12.10
J	$16,536	$21,424	$26,416
	$7.95	$10.30	$12.70
K	$17,368	$22,500	$27,700
	$8.35	$10.81	$13.31
L	$18,304	$23,700	$29,120
	$8.80	$11.39	$14.00
M	$19,240	$24,900	$30,700
	$9.25	$11.97	$14.75

Job Evaluation

Positions in the group practice must be evaluated to determine the worth of each position to the organization and in relationship to other positions in the practice. There are established job evaluation methods from which an organization can choose or the evaluation method may be internally developed so it is tailored to the unique needs of the group. In either case, a systematic method must be chosen in order to maintain consistency of job evaluation across the organization.

Some examples of job evaluation include:

- *Job ranking:* Establishes a hierarchy of positions based on the relative importance of each position to the organization.
- *Job classification:* Positions are grouped into salary grades. Each salary grade has a job group or class description that is used to determine the positions that fit into that grade.

■ *Point-factor method:* Assigning points based on the compensable factors of positions. Compensable factors are the position responsibilities that add value to the group. Compensable factors may include the level of responsibility the job holds, the skill required for the position, the amount of effort to perform the job, whether the position supervises other employees, and what the working conditions are for the position. There may be multiple levels with associated point values for each compensable factor established. The total point value for the evaluated position determines into which salary grade a position falls in relationship to all other positions within the organization.

■ *Factor comparison method:* Complex method that ranks jobs on established compensable factors and values based on dollars and a weighting strategy. This method is not frequently used because it tends to be relevant only for organizations in very stable markets not impacted by inflation.

■ *Market comparison method:* Evaluates positions based on their worth to the organization from a determination of the market value of each position.

In addition, a determination must be made of the status of each job under the Fair Labor Standards Act (FLSA) for designating whether the job is eligible for overtime pay (nonexempt) or can be exempted from the act and not paid overtime (exempt). The FLSA provides guidelines to aid organizations in making the appropriate determination. However, this must be done carefully and the regulations must be adhered to or the penalties to the organization can be costly in the form of payment of past overtime and fines as well as loss of reputation.

Regardless of the job evaluation method chosen, the organization must be able to demonstrate that positions have been established and are evaluated based on the work that is actually being done, have written job descriptions, are reviewed on a regular basis (optimally annually), and are of value to the organization in fulfilling the mission and strategy.

■ Recruitment and Hiring

Recruiting in a large medical group can be a challenge because of the conflicting nature of seeking a large pool of candidates to consider versus the cost required to process the candidates. As with most positions, the manager wants the position to be filled "yesterday" and struggles with the gap left from the vacant position. If a person gives at least a 2-week notice prior to leaving the position, the organization should have just enough time to approve filling the soon-to-be-vacant position and advertise its opening. Recruiting puts strain and stress on the medical group because the opening places stress on the people that need to either fill the vacancy through overtime or train an agency person to learn the functions in a short period of time.

However, if the position is a new one to the organization, the organization has some additional time to recruit. Once a position description is written and approved, the manager completes a job bid form that initiates the recruiting process. The form has information on it to help the recruiter know what is needed. The form includes the title of the position, and refers to the appropriate position description, pay range, and special qualifications or needs. Some forms have an indication of the position's productivity score. This information may delay position recruitment if productivity isn't at 100% or above. This productivity figure assists in the control of departmental budgets and avoids filling positions that may not need to be filled if department volume has declined or flattened.

The Philosophy of Recruitment

Having an internal posting period to allow internal candidates to apply for the position opening sets a strong message to the employees that the organization promotes from within the organization. However, this approach loses its impact if the medical group doesn't work diligently to ensure hiring talented people for the long term.

For example, filling a vacancy with an internal candidate that is not qualified for the position and lacks the experience and training necessary to do the job well can lead to a higher employee turnover. If the medical group is committed to hiring people from within the organization, it also needs to be committed to employee education and training to solidify a successful employee fit with a position.

Position Posting

The posting of a vacant position allows employees to know of vacancies. This posting is in writing through some kind of job board and provides a brief overview of the position and requirements and the name of the person handling the recruitment. The internal posting also includes a time frame of how long it will be posted internally (e.g., 3–5 days) prior to an external job posting. In this way, employees must respond promptly to an internal posting and bid for that position.

In today's tight job market where there are many vacancies due to shortages of certain types of personnel, such as nursing, professional coders, and diagnostic technologists, the internal bidding process becomes less of an issue because the group lacks the talent needed for the position. In these situations, while an internal bid is placed, an external process is set in motion to look for a job candidate within the area or even establish a state, regional, or national search.

Use of External Recruiters

As medical groups grow, the internal recruiter may not be able to spend the time, effort, and energy needed to recruit for positions new to the medical group. For example, if a new service is being added to the group, the initial process to obtain qualified people may be outsourced to an external agency. Many times a high-level position is outsourced to an external recruiting firm because of the complexity of the search, resources needed to complete the search, and political implications of the position. An external search firm can handle difficult searches, especially one that is confidential and requires no advertising.

Recruitment Methods

One of the most common ways to recruit for a position is to place an advertisement in the newspaper. It reaches a broad audience and usually solicits responses. The advertisement in the regional Sunday newspaper reaches the largest audience, and local newspapers reach a much smaller audience. In healthcare, although newspaper advertisements work well for general jobs, such as nurse, receptionist, and clerk, more specific or specialized media should be used for highly technical and specialized positions. A physician opening is usually not listed in the local newspaper, but in professional publications and professional society newsletters.

Television and cable television have become used to pursuing innovative recruiting methods, with some companies creating a bundled package of cable TV and newspaper ads. These methods are pursued especially in difficult-to-place areas.

Professional journals and magazines reach a larger, national audience and require greater resources for recruitment including monies to pay interview candidates for travel, lodging, meals, and mileage. Such periodicals are more commonly used to recruit physicians, high-level health executives, technical directors, and difficult-to-recruit positions (such as professional coders and nurses).

An employer website makes it easier for people to know of openings in the organization without having to read the newspaper or going into the HR office. It also allows candidates to submit a resume online and thus simplifies the recruitment process. In a difficult recruiting market, an organization that provides a website shows an orientation and commitment to the use of technology in its daily workings.

Temporary agencies are used to cover staff vacancies until a position is filled and sometimes leads to the temporary worker becoming the permanent worker. In this situation, the medical group pays a placement fee to the agency for recruitment of the temporary person. Although many temporary workers don't want to work permanently and wouldn't consider a permanent placement, some workers use the temporary agency as an opportunity to pursue varied jobs and locations to test the organization's culture and work environment.

It is important to note that for higher-level positions, executive search firms often are used because in many cases the best candidates are not really looking for a job change and are unlikely to respond to ads. In these circumstances, the search firm, in addition to using more traditional techniques such as those just described, use networking with the intent of identifying qualified candidates who may not be looking for another job.

Acceptance of Job Inquiries

Smaller medical groups may pursue candidates without ever having the applicant complete a job application, but it is highly unlikely for a large medical group to have this kind of arrangement. Regardless of size, all employers should have an established application process used consistently for all jobs. This goes a long way in reducing exposure of the organization to Equal Employment Opportunity (EEO) discrimination claims.

A job inquiry requires completion of a job application to ensure waiver of liability, to follow federal requirements, and to collect consistent information on each candidate. Although a cover letter of inquiry and resume may be attached to the application, all potential candidates must complete an application. An accurate and complete job application helps the organization pursue truthful candidates. As information is verified on the application, it allows the organization to screen out certain people who falsify answers to questions or include data that are not correct.

The type of information requested on the application should include:

- Basic demographic information
- Education
- Work history and references, including a release allowing contact with former employers to perform reference checks

- Criminal record (Disclosure of a criminal record may not automatically disqualify an applicant from a job. Each situation must be judged on its own merits as it relates to the job responsibilities.)
- Waivers, including employment-at-will, if applicable
- Authorization and release by the applicant to allow verification of all information
- Statement to the effect that the information provided is truthful
- Applicant signature

As part of the development of the application form, a legal review of the form should be performed to ensure that there is no negative EEO impact.

Completed applications should be reviewed for any information that may not be complete or clear, and follow-up calls made to applicants to obtain the missing, incomplete, or unclear information. Information on the application that may lead to additional discussion with the applicant, and could be areas for concern, include significant gaps in employment, changing positions on a frequent basis (if that is unusual for the type of position and the industry), and reduction in levels of responsibility.

Selection Process

Organizations have selection processes in place to ensure that legal guidelines are followed and that the most qualified person is hired for the open position. Timely processing of applications and communication with applicants is critical from the perspective of filling open positions as expeditiously as possible and in preserving the reputation of the organization for investing in positive employee relations.

The completed application forms are reviewed to filter out those applicants who do not meet the minimum qualifications for the position as defined in the job description. Those who do not meet the minimum qualifications for the job are notified that they will not be considered for the position. For internal candidates who do not meet the minimum qualifications for the job, this is an opportunity for a developmental discussion with the employee to let them know what they need to do to qualify for a similar position in the future.

Qualified candidates should be scheduled for interviews as soon as possible to reduce the potential for the candidate to be hired by another organization and to help the candidate build a positive image of the group practice.

Verification must be made of information critical to the successful performance of the job. The candidate is asked to provide copies of certificates, licenses, and diplomas. Educational institutions are contacted to verify education. Professional or state agencies are contacted to verify certifications and licensure. Former employers are contacted to verify employment.

The Interview

HR may be involved in the interview process to perform an initial screening of what appear to be qualified candidates based on the information provided on the applications. The supervisor of the position is the critical person in the interviewing process and performs the more in-depth interviews. The supervisor should, at a minimum, interview the final candidates for the position. This requires the training of supervisors in interviewing skills and techniques. The interviewing process, once established by the organization, should be consistently applied to all candidates for all positions.

There are many types of in-depth interviews. A structured interview is one in which the same questions are asked of all of the candidates. The targeted or patterned interview covers questions about the same knowledge or skills area, but the questions are not necessarily the same from one candidate to the next. An interviewer in a stress interview uses an aggressive approach to test the reactions of the candidates to a stressful situation. A directive interview is where the interviewer asks very specific questions and maintains firm control of the interview. When an interviewer asks open questions, providing general guidance to the candidate, the nondirective interview is being used. In this type of interview, the response to the last question sets the direction for the next question asked of the candidate. A behavioral interview in which the interviewer asks questions about past experiences the candidate has had and how the candidate handled the situations results in more objective information than the other types of interviews.

Panel interviews are sometimes used when there are multiple interviewers for a position and there is pressure due to time and expense. Panel interviews can be more stressful for the candidates. The panelists should have assigned roles and questions to cover during the interview. To make the environment less threatening for the candidate, seating arranged in a circle or more casual arrangement is recommended.

Interviewing skills that are important to obtain the best results include establishing a good, open communication with the candidate; carefully listening to what the candidate has to say; paying attention to the candidate's nonverbal behavior (however, this is subjective and should not weigh heavily in the decision regarding selection); asking questions relevant to the job; providing good information to the candidate about the job;

and taking notes that can be used later when evaluating candidates.

The questions that are asked by an interviewer should be specifically related to the job for which the candidate is interviewing. Questions other than those to evaluate the candidate's qualifications for the job should be avoided in order to comply with civil rights laws and the federal Equal Employment Opportunity Commission (EEOC).

Some organizations use tests to help screen candidates for positions. Tests should be used only if they are job related and have been proven to be valid and reliable in predicting success on the job.

Pre-employment substance abuse screenings are commonly used, in particular by employers that have established themselves as a drug-free workplace under the federal Drug-Free Workplace Act. Usually the substance abuse screening is done only on the candidate to whom the position has been offered on the condition of successfully passing the screening. In addition to substance abuse screenings, group practices screen for tuberculosis.

Many organizations also perform background checks. Checks for criminal activity may be required based on the type of care being provided by the group practice and the patients the practice serves. As mentioned earlier, the discovery of criminal convictions does not necessarily exclude a candidate from consideration for a position. Each situation must be reviewed independently based on the requirements of the job.

Background checks of credit reports are regulated by the Fair Credit Reporting Act (FCRA) and by the Fair and Accurate Credit Transaction Act (FACTA). The employer must advise the candidate or employee that a background check is going to be done and must obtain the employee's written authorization to obtain a credit check. Before any adverse action is taken as a result of the background check, such as withdrawing an offer of employment, the individual must be given a copy of the report and a copy of "A Summary of Your Rights Under the FCRA," which can be obtained through the Federal Trade Commission (FTC).

■ Orientation

Orientation of employees has become more complex for medical groups as federal, state, and regulatory agencies and accrediting bodies place greater demands on the healthcare institution. A medical group provides a general employee orientation program for all new employees hired within the organization. The programs vary, but usually provide basic information about the practice, its vision, mission, goals, and objectives. The orientation should include information about the group's procedures and policies, benefits, and safety issues, such as fire safety, infection control, and risk management.

The following are some of the areas that a medical group may cover in an employee orientation:

- *Tour of facility:* The tour allows the group to showcase its facility and allow people to see certain parts of the facility that the employee may not normally see. For example, a medical records clerk may not have the opportunity to visit the ambulatory surgery center, even though she may pull records for it daily. Seeing parts of the organization helps the employee to be connected to how her job connects to other groups.
- *Introduction to the president of the medical group:* A senior leader can help set the tone and focus of the medical group. Employees may not get to meet or interact with senior leaders on a daily basis, and this leadership can share the vision, philosophy, mission, and goals of the medical group.
- *Review of employee expectations:* Every employee has probably worked at another organization that has different expectations and rules. Many times employees make mistakes based on misunderstandings of what is expected of them. For example, an employee that came from a flextime environment may come into work tardy thinking incorrectly that the new environment provides flextime when it does not. Articulating expectations helps establish a core foundation of understanding.
- *Review and signing of position description:* A written position description is critical to all medical group employees. Whether it is done at a group orientation or department level, the reviewing and signing of the position description gives each employee a signed document showing what is expected. This process helps avoid unnecessary problems in the future.
- *Review of employee handbook:* The employee handbook should be designed to help the employee better understand the organization and the employee's role in it. The handbook is meant to guide the employee through various policies, procedures, and expectations and to be used as a reference and resource for the employee. Usually the handbook has a disclaimer that it is not meant to cover all of the organization's procedures and policies in detail, and that it should be used as a guideline.

- *Review of benefits and completion of paperwork:* Numerous forms need to be completed for the proper processing of benefit information. Primary source information needs to be verified and documented (e.g., place of birth, photo identification), data must be collected for an employee to be signed up for benefits, and an employee needs to choose benefits options from various choices provided by the employer.
- Review of policies:
  - *Time and attendance:* Reviews time record process, overtime, payday, and distribution of checks; explains policies regarding excessive tardiness and absenteeism and required process for notification of absence
  - *Personal appearance and uniform requirements:* Defines what kind of dress is acceptable in the work environment
  - Rest periods/breaks
  - Eating and smoking areas
  - Use of employee identification badges
  - Fair treatment
  - Sexual harassment
  - On-the-job injuries
  - Acceptance of gifts
  - Parking
  - Safety/security
  - Family Medical Leave Act
  - Office of the Inspector General (OIG)/corporate compliance/Health Insurance Portability and Accountability Act (HIPAA)
  - Occupational Safety and Health Administration (OSHA) training
  - Infection control training
  - Safety training (fire, electrical, disaster, emergency)

The individual department also provides an orientation that is more specific to the duties and tasks required of the employee. This orientation serves to reinforce the general orientation.

In addition to the general orientation, an ongoing orientation sheet may be used to help guide the supervisor or manager on a self-orientation. This tool lets the manager know what is expected and how to learn expected competencies. It also allows each person to manage the information individually and customize learning based on personal needs.

For certain staff members, a checklist may be used along with listed competencies to demonstrate that a person can't perform a certain function until those skills are mastered.

For example, a nurse needs to demonstrate that he is able to perform a urine dip test correctly and able to interpret the results correctly. Until this task is mastered successfully, the nurse cannot perform this task without supervision.

■ Employee Education and Training

The Malcolm Baldrige National Quality Award program was developed in 1987 and has served as an impetus for many companies and medical groups to pursue a stronger orientation to improving its customer focus and satisfaction. Statements such as service excellence, continuous quality improvement, quality improvement, and total quality management are commonplace in many medical groups today. Each of these efforts focuses on improving clinical and service outcomes through a team approach.

To ensure that the focus is maintained, medical groups, particularly large ones, have committed to a significant amount of employee training and education. It is believed that through focused education and training of employees to prioritize the right things, the medical group can improve its productivity, service, growth, satisfaction, and, ultimately, its financial performance.

As with any medical group, the organization must commit to providing the resources necessary to train its workforce. Whether the resources are put into individual departments or allocated through a centralized training function, providing resources for training and development are critical for the organization's future success. Because adult learning requires a diverse approach, a medical group should offer many modes of training: one-on-one tutor/student style, interacting with others, or self-directed modules.

Classroom Style vs. Group Simulation

The classroom style is the more traditional approach. Held in an auditorium, conference room, or training room, it offers an opportunity for the trainer to provide a review of the material to be learned. With the advances in technology, some medical groups are using computers, audiovisual equipment, video cameras, and computer software to enhance learning. Simulations of clinical care allow staff to respond to real-life situations and learn how to handle a problem by interacting with others.

Use of Computer-Directed Programs

A variety of training formats allows the adult learner to customize learning to fit his or her individual needs. Recently, computer-directed programs have helped some medical groups achieve staff knowledge of the new HIPAA regulations and requirements by having each person take a self-directed computer study. The training software not only allows the medical group to track who has completed the program, but also monitors that every person achieves a minimum score on the program.

Internal vs. External Function

Some medical groups have outsourced part of their training function. For example, in-house training may be done for nursing education, but all computer education may be handled by an external company that has a computer training room with experts who exclusively train on certain computer software. This approach changes as the organization changes. A medical group may contract out for computer training, but eventually bring it in-house by hiring a person to handle that function based on ongoing needs. As technology needs change, so does the training function.

Train the Trainer

Every new function or task in an organization challenges it to consider how the training will occur. Training is an expensive function, and it is hard to measure the immediate effects and impact of its success. When a major change occurs in a medical group, such as implementing an electronic medical record, the group needs to determine not only how training will occur, but also who will provide that training. "Train the trainer" is the practice of hiring an external consultant to train key staff in the medical group. The employees, in turn, are expected to train all staff on the function. It becomes a logistical challenge of time and project management, but one that works well if the trainers have the skills and expertise to handle the project.

Other Training Approaches

If a medical group values training, it provides extensive internal in-service education opportunities to help its staff. These programs help the manager and supervisor focus on individual management skills needing development. Also, employee in-services provide consistent, reliable learning and create a tracking mechanism to ensure that everyone has learned the information.

Training approaches that provide monies for external workshops and seminars are limited to fewer people because the organization usually cannot afford to send an entire team for training. Instead, a smaller group is often sent to be trained as "trainers" so that they can then return to the medical group to train the rest of the staff. Tuition reimbursement for college and university coursework is another resource to support training for the organization. Such resources also support a professional development plan for succession planning within the medical group.

■ Evaluation of Performance

The evaluation of performance is critical for every employee, and the approach is as varied as the methods of evaluation. Because the position description serves as the baseline for the evaluation, the key responsibilities and position responsibilities serve as the foundation for the evaluation. Ideally, supervisors provide feedback to employees on a continuous basis. The feedback should be provided at the time the behavior is observed, and it should be in line with the accomplishment. The feedback for positive performance should be done publicly, if possible. A powerful way to show appreciation to an employee who has gone well beyond expectations is to send a thank you note to the employee's home. Showing your appreciation to the employee at the employee's home where the employee's family will see it sends a strong, positive message about the organization to the employee and the family.

30- and 90-Day Review

Employee retention is fundamental to the success of any organization. The cost of turnover to an organization is significant. It includes not only the recruitment costs to fill a vacant position, but also the cost of lost productivity and the impact on employee morale when the organization is understaffed. Costs to consider include:

- *Separation costs:* Unemployment compensation, administration of COBRA benefits, time spent on exit interviews
- *Replacement costs:* Time spent on recruiting, advertising costs, time to screen and interview candidates, pre-employment testing costs, the cost of orientation materials and time
- *Training costs:* Time of the trainers, supervisor, and coworkers to train the new employee
- *Productivity costs:* Lost productivity while position is vacant and during the time the new employee is orienting to the job

To retain employees, asking for employee feedback is necessary, and no time is more critical than an employee's first 90 days on the job. Every employee benefits from a formal review of his or her performance after 30 days and after 90 days on the job. A 30- and 90-day review allows a formal opportunity for the manager and employee to review job expectations, accomplishment of goals and objectives, and focus on areas that need improvement. From this evaluation comes a work plan or assessment of additional support that the employee needs to exceed expectations of the job.

Quint Studer, in *Hardwiring Excellence*,[2] recommends that at 30 days the supervisor ask the employee four key questions. The first question is to find out from the employee how what they have experienced on the job compares to what they were told when they were interviewing. The second question is to ask the employee what is being done well. Third is to find out from the employee what was being done at their last place of employment that worked well and that the group practice should consider implementing. The fourth question is to ask if there is anything with which the employee is uncomfortable or that would make the employee want to leave. These questions and the employee's responses set up perfectly for the 90-day review. The information gleaned from the 30-day review must be used to clarify misunderstandings, provide appropriate support, and benefit the employee in their orientation period. If possible, any recommendations they make should be implemented or an explanation provided as to why implementation cannot be accomplished.

Annual Evaluation

A particular component of a medical group's long-term success is its ability to measure its employees' performance and apply that knowledge to ways for the employee to improve performance incrementally and over time. It is a difficult process requiring solid, objective judgment and clear expectations.

The formal, structured annual performance review is used by large organizations and guides the supervisor to assess the employee's performance through an official form. This form reflects the philosophy of the organization and reflects which components are measured and emphasized and which components are not acknowledged. Generally, employees are rewarded for behaviors the organization values. If the organization has a strong organizational priority on customer service, then the evaluation form should have an evaluation of an employee's customer service orientation and behaviors. Or if the organization has a strong financial accountability orientation, then the form requires measurement and accomplishments on cost control, productivity, and revenue enhancement strategies. An annual performance review helps the organization to measure whether the employee is aligned with its priorities and is a way to identify poor performance and inconsistent behaviors. On the other hand, an evaluation form that doesn't link its organizational priorities with employee behavior may find that its outcomes are inconsistent with what it measures. This kind of problem happens in an organization that has an old evaluation form that has not been updated to reflect new organizational priorities.

Performance management needs to evolve and change as the organization changes. For example, when a medical group chooses to pursue a new organizational approach and commitment, such as service excellence and teamwork, it needs to change its evaluation process including the form and how the evaluation is conducted. Defining and measuring performance along with providing appropriate feedback are key elements in any evaluation process. As medical groups begin to pursue new organizational priorities, it has been found that new venues for evaluation arise. The following evaluation tools are four examples of how organizations have further developed their evaluation process.

Annual Self-Evaluation and/or Assessment

As part of the performance evaluation process, a self-evaluation helps both the employee and supervisor to assess progress made during the last year and incorporate goals into future plans. Giving the employee the opportunity to provide a self-evaluation may initially be met with employee resistance. Employees may not feel comfortable doing a self-evaluation because it forces the employee to be part of the evaluation process instead of the evaluation process being one sided. The supervisor can help the employee with a self-evaluation by providing a form to complete or a format to follow. The submitted information guides the supervisor in potential conflicts that may exist between the supervisor and employer. For example, an employee could give him- or herself high marks for teamwork, whereas the supervisor evaluates the employee as below average. This disparity helps the two to discuss expectations and differences of opinion and resolve possible conflicts. In another example, a supervisor may rate an employee as exceeding expectations whereas the employee rates him- or herself as meeting expectations. In this scenario, the employee thinks he or she can perform better but the supervisor believes the employee is a high performer. Both parties can discuss the differences and clarify the perspectives.

The self-evaluation includes not only a past performance section, but also a developmental plan for the future. This written format gives the employer and employee a forum to dialogue on the employee's future goals and objectives. The self-evaluation is an invaluable tool to set both short- and long-term goals and potential training and development needs.

360-Degree Evaluation

Instead of performing an annual evaluation or self-evaluation, some organizations provide a 360-degree evaluation for its management staff. The 360-degree tool has the manager identify two to three people who report to him or her, two to three peers, and his or her supervisor.

These people complete an evaluation form on the manager along with the manager's self-evaluation and submit it to an independent company that compiles the information into a format. The manager and his or her supervisor receive the compiled report, which serves as a vehicle to determine how the employee perceives him- or herself compared to the opinions of others. This developmental tool may be completed once every 3 to 5 years and serves to help focus development on certain areas.

Physician, Patient, and Staff Review of Employee

In organizations that value teamwork and cooperation, evaluations from physicians and staff along with any patient satisfaction surveys that identify the employee are used along with feedback from the supervisor. This assessment allows a more balanced assessment of the employee's feedback. **Exhibit 5-1** contains a sample form that can be used to help seek feedback from physicians and employees. For example, a supervisor was going to provide a poor evaluation on an employee; however, he sought evaluations from physicians, staff, and patients. Their evaluations came back very positive. A conflict existed in that the supervisor saw poor performance, but the physicians and staff saw exceptional performance. The supervisor needs to sort out whether the evaluations are accurate and sincere, or whether they reflect popularity or a resistance to documenting poor performance. Written evaluations by this group may also require a one-on-one verbal review to determine whether the evaluator doesn't feel comfortable writing things down, but is willing to verbally discuss problems, issues, and concerns.

Performance Appraisals

The annual performance appraisal is an important opportunity for the manager (and others) along with the employee to address past performance, current issues, and future activities, efforts, and goals. It must be positive, constructive, and address specific areas of job performance. Concrete examples must be given for both exceptional and poor performance so that the employee understands what behaviors are considered exceptional or poor by the organization. The evaluation is an opportunity for the two parties to participate in measuring past performance and establishing future performance expectations. **Exhibit 5-2** shows a sample evaluation form that measures an employee's performance in the areas of technical excellence, customer service, adaptability, efficiency and effectiveness, and managerial responsibility (if applicable). This form allows the supervisor to weigh each category in terms of importance and provide feedback to the employee based on a range of performance expectations. This form acknowledges that an employee receives a rating based

on annual performance. This rating is converted into a merit increase for employees with better ratings receiving a higher performance rating. In this example, an overall rating of "Exceeds Expectations" can bring a 4% merit increase for the employee whereas a "Meets Expectations" can bring a 2% merit increase, and an "Unsatisfactory Expectation" warrants no merit increase and development of a performance improvement plan.

Discipline. What does discipline mean to an organization? Corrective action is intended to provide feedback to an employee to correct a behavior. Progressive discipline sets parameters on what behaviors are unacceptable and how those negative behaviors will be communicated to the employee when change is necessary. Large medical groups usually have a progressive discipline process that clearly establishes expectations as well as consequences if the expectations are not met. The discipline process may be different for the staff and physicians. The purpose of having a constructive discipline process is: (1) to establish guidelines to ensure that the environment is efficient, productive, and orderly; and (2) to provide standards and rules governing performance and a procedure for consistent, nondiscriminatory application of the rules with the intent of providing quality patient care.

When it becomes necessary to correct the actions of an employee for poor performance or for acts contrary to established policies and procedures, or to ensure that the medical group's best interests are being served, reference may be made to pre-identified categories. These categories relate the severity of the offense to the corrective action. The categories are not all-inclusive, and employees may be corrected for action not specifically designated. Certain situations may require deviation from the guidelines outlined. The policy does not apply to employees who are in their new hire period or per diem or temporary employees. The policy applies to part-time and full-time regular status employees.

Recorded Conference. For rule infractions considered less serious, a recorded conference may be the first step in the corrective action process. It consists of a conference between the supervisor and employee that should be documented in writing and placed in the employee's personnel file. Examples of behavior for which a recorded conference may be initiated as the first step of the corrective action process include:

- Work area absence without permission (e.g., leaving work without clocking out)
- Extended lunch time or breaks without permission (e.g., taking a 30-minute break instead of a 15-minute break)

Exhibit 5-1 **Peer Evaluation**

In order to evaluate each employee's performance more accurately and with greater objectivity, employees, coworkers, and/or physicians are asked to share in the evaluation process. Please rate the following categories accordingly:

1: Needs Improvement   2: Below Average   3: Average   4: Above Average   5: Excellent

Any ratings of a 1 or 5 must be explained in the comments section.

I. Professional Skills

A. Job Knowledge   1 2 3 4 5
   (Working knowledge of job)
B. Quality   1 2 3 4 5
   (Accurate, thorough, neat)
C. Creativity   1 2 3 4 5
   (Proposal of new ideas, better ways of doing tasks)
D. Judgment   1 2 3 4 5
   (Making decisions)
E. Productivity   1 2 3 4 5
   (Significant volume of work efficiently in specified time)
F. Initiative   1 2 3 4 5
   (Seeks out new assignments and additional tasks)
G. Adherence to Policy   1 2 3 4 5
   (Safety, conduct, office policy)

II. Other Skills

A. Interpersonal Relationships   1 2 3 4 5
   (Cooperate with and communicate appropriately)
B. Reliability   1 2 3 4 5
   (Relied upon to complete tasks)
C. Availability   1 2 3 4 5
   (Attendance record)
D. Independence   1 2 3 4 5
   (Extent performs work with little or no supervision)
E. Seeks Resources to Maintain Knowledge and Skill   1 2 3 4 5
F. Demonstrates Ability and Willingness to Be Flexible with Assignments to
   Meet the the Needs of the Office   1 2 3 4 5
G. Ability to Establish Priorities in Meeting Office Needs   1 2 3 4 5
H. Responds Appropriately in Crisis   1 2 3 4 5
I. Maintains Confidentiality   1 2 3 4 5
J. Shares Knowledge and Expertise with Others   1 2 3 4 5
   (Is a team player)
K. Works Towards Office Goals   1 2 3 4 5

Comments: _____

- Loitering during scheduled work time or during off-duty hours (e.g., staying in work area after shift and creating disturbances with employees)
- Smoking or eating in unauthorized areas (e.g., eating in surgical area that should have no food in it due to the sterile environment)
- Conducting personal business on work premises (e.g., selling products during work time)
- Violation of parking rules (e.g., parking in a no parking zone for the work shift)
- Improper attire or appearance (e.g., wearing jeans or denim when not part of the dress code)

Exhibit 5-2 Cleveland Health Network Annual Performance Management Evaluation Form

CLEVELAND HEALTH NETWORK
Annual Performance Management Evaluation Form

DATE: _____

NAME: _____

SUPERVISOR: _____

EMPLOYEE NO.: _____

DEPARTMENT: _____

LOCATION: _____

General Instructions:

The performance appraisal process must be job specific. Assess the employee's actual job performance during the appropriate appraisal period and reference the key job responsibilities as identified in the formal job description. Check the corresponding box that best describes the actual level of performance for each of the performance dimensions included in the appraisal. Specific examples and comments to substantiate the ratings are encouraged.

Overall Rating Definitions:

Too New to Rate

The employee has been on the job for less than 3 months, and there has not been sufficient opportunity to evaluate performance.

Unsatisfactory*

The employee's overall performance on the job meets few or none of the established goals/standards. The employee should not expect to continue employment unless overall performance significantly improves within a specified period.

Needs Improvement

The employee's overall performance on the job is inconsistent with job requirements and does not meet one or more established goals/standards. The employee's performance in identified areas must improve.

Achieves Expectations

The employee's overall performance on the job is consistent with job requirements. The employee successfully meets established goals/standards.

Exceeds Expectations

The employee's overall performance consistently surpasses job requirements and the established goals/standards. The employee demonstrates a superior level of work and an exceptionally high level of proficiency throughout the rating period.

*Requires establishment of Performance Improvement Plan for the employee.

(continues)

Exhibit 5-2 **Cleveland Health Network Annual Performance Management Evaluation Form (continued)**

Technical Excellence: Includes the technical skills and expertise that enable an employee to make sound technical judgments, to provide or support quality care, and to otherwise successfully perform in the position.

☐	☐	☐	☐
Unsatisfactory	**Needs Improvement**	**Achieves Expectations**	**Exceeds Expectations**
Demonstrated job knowledge and understanding is not sufficient to meet the quality, safety, and technical goals and standards established for the position. Decisions are rarely sound or practical.	Demonstrated job knowledge and understanding is not consistently sufficient to meet the quality, safety, and technical goals and standards established for the position. Decisions are not consistently sound or practical.	Demonstrated job knowledge and understanding is sufficient to meet the quality, safety, and technical goals and standards established for the position. Employee's decisions are consistently sound and practical.	Demonstrated job knowledge and understanding is exceptional. Employee's decisions are consistently sound, practical, and based on thorough analyses.

Specific Examples and/or Comments:

_____
_____
_____
_____
_____
_____

Customer Service Orientation: Includes teamwork, attitude, behavior, interpersonal skills. and problem-solving skills that enable an employee to respond to internal and external customer needs and expectations in a positive manner.

☐	☐	☐	☐
Unsatisfactory	**Needs Improvement**	**Achieves Expectations**	**Exceeds Expectations**
Poor service orientation. Does little to contribute to the satisfaction, productivity, and development of others, including new employees and/or students. Unresponsive to employee or supervisor suggestions for service improvement.	Positive, but inconsistent service orientation. Occasionally contributes to the satisfaction, productivity, and development of others, including new employees and/or students. Not consistently responsive to employee or supervisor suggestions for service improvement.	Positive service orientation. Readily contributes to the satisfaction, productivity, and development of others, including new employees and/or students. Responsive to employee and supervisor suggestions for service improvement.	Exceptional service orientation. Makes extraordinary effort to contribute to the satisfaction, productivity, and development of others, including new employees and/or students. Initiates and implements suggestions for service improvement.

Specific Examples and/or Comments:

_____
_____
_____
_____
_____
_____

Adaptability: Includes initiative and flexibility to accept and master changes in function, equipment, technology, and/or departmental needs, and the dependability to adhere to attendance and other CHN policies.

☐	☐	☐	☐
Unsatisfactory	**Needs Improvement**	**Achieves Expectations**	**Exceeds Expectations**
Demonstrates very little independent thinking in addressing problem. Resists accepting new tasks and reacts negatively to change. Rarely contributes to departmental needs. May require corrective action.	Demonstrates some independence in addressing problems, accepting new tasks, and adjusting to changing work conditions—but is inconsistent. Occasionally initiates opportunities to contribute to departmental needs. May require corrective action.	Consistently demonstrates independence in addressing problems, accepting new tasks, and adjusting to changing work conditions. Consistently initiates opportunities to contribute to departmental needs.	Consistently demonstrates initiative and independence in addressing problems. Assumes formal/informal leadership role in adapting to new tasks or changing work conditions. Demonstrates exceptional initiative in seeking opportunities to contribute to departmental needs.

Specific Examples and/or Comments:

_____
_____
_____
_____
_____
_____

(continues)

Exhibit 5-2 **Cleveland Health Network Annual Performance Management Evaluation Form (continued)**

Effectiveness and Efficiency: Includes the quantity and quality of desired work, as well as the organizational skills necessary to perform successfully.

☐	☐	☐	☐
Unsatisfactory	**Needs Improvement**	**Achieves Expectations**	**Exceeds Expectations**
Quality and/or quantity of work is insufficient. Work is frequently sloppy and incomplete, with unacceptable number of errors. Requires constant direction, close supervision, and/or corrective action.	Quality and quantity of work is not consistent. Work is occasionally sloppy and incomplete, with occasional errors. Requires direction in specific areas and regular supervision.	Quality and quantity of work is consistent. Work is neat and complete with few errors. Meets established departmental standards and requires infrequent direction or supervision.	Quality and quantity of work is exceptional. Work is neat and complete. Errors are rare. Requires minimal or no direction.

Specific Examples and/or Comments:

_____
_____
_____
_____
_____
_____

Managerial Responsibility (if applicable): Includes overall accountability for assigned work group relative to operational goals, personnel requirements, and budgetary constraints.

☐	☐	☐	☐
Unsatisfactory	**Needs Improvement**	**Achieves Expectations**	**Exceeds Expectations**
Specific and predetermined performance goals are not attained. Ineffective and inefficient management of budget and personnel issues (i.e., staffing, FTE compliance, performance management, EEO/Affirmative Action and corrective action).	Specific and predetermined performance goals are not consistently attained. Management of budget and personnel issues (i.e., staffing, FTE compliance, performance management, EEO/Affirmative Action and corrective action) is not consistently effective or efficient.	Specific and predetermined performance goals are consistently attained. Management of budget and personnel issues (i.e., staffing, FTE compliance, performance management, EEO/Affirmative Action and corrective action) is consistently effective and efficient.	Specific and predetermined performance goals are surpassed. Management of budget and personnel issues (i.e., staffing, FTE compliance, performance management, EEO/Affirmative Action and corrective action) is consistently effective and efficient, and demonstrates exceptional leadership, administration, and initiative.

Specific Examples and/or Comments:

_____
_____
_____
_____
_____
_____

OTHER (if applicable): _____

Unsatisfactory Work	**Needs Improvement**	**Achieves Expectations**	**Exceeds Expectations**
_____	_____	_____	_____
_____	_____	_____	_____
_____	_____	_____	_____
_____	_____	_____	_____

(Note: Criteria must be identified for each performance rating in this performance dimension.)

Specific Examples and/or Comments:

_____
_____
_____
_____
_____
_____

(continues)

Exhibit 5-2 **Cleveland Health Network Annual Performance Management Evaluation Form (continued)**

Developmental Plan/Goals, Objectives, and Target Dates:

_____
_____
_____
_____
_____
_____

Employee Comments: (Employees are encouraged to add job-specific comments that are appropriate to the evaluation and future performance.)

_____
_____
_____
_____
_____
_____

Overall Rating:

An employee's overall performance summary should be determined as follows:

The performance rating for each performance dimension should be identified in the column labeled "Performance Rating."

The weight for each performance dimension should be identified in the column labeled "Weighting." The weights should be established in multiples of 5%, with the total equaling 100%.

The performance rating multiplier corresponding to the assigned performance rating should be identified in the column labeled "Multiplier."

The point value is determined for each dimension by multiplying the assigned weight by the performance rating multiplier and should be identified in the column labeled "Point Value."

The point values for each dimension should be added with the total points being used to classify the employee's overall performance summary.

Performance Dimension	Performance Rating	Weighting	Multiplier	Point Value
Technical Excellence	_____	_____ x	_____ =	_____
Customer Service Orientation	_____	_____ x	_____ =	_____
Adaptability	_____	_____ x	_____ =	_____
Effectiveness/Efficiency	_____	_____	_____ =	_____
Managerial Resp. (if applicable)	_____	_____ x	_____ =	_____
Other (if applicable)	_____	_____ x	_____ =	_____
		100%	Total Points	_____

Overall Performance Summary:

☐ Too New to Rate

☐ Unsatisfactory* (below 76)   ☐ Achieves Expectations (88–95)

☐ Needs Improvement (76–87)   ☐ Exceeds Expectations (96–100)

*Requires establishment of Performance Improvement Plan for the employee.

PERFORMANCE RATING MULTIPLIER	
Exceeds Expectations	—1.00
Achieves Expectations	—0.90
Needs Improvement	—0.80
Unsatisfactory	—0.70

The employee's signature does not necessarily infer agreement or disagreement with one's performance assessment. The signature merely signifies that the employee was given the opportunity to discuss his/her past performance and future potential with his/her immediate supervisor.

In addition, the employee's signature does reaffirm his/her understanding as to the importance of confidentiality of information, specifically, the acquisition release. Discussion or other use of confidential information for purposes other than to conduct normal authorized business activities is strictly prohibited.

Employee's Signature: _____ Date: _____

Supervisor's Signature: _____ Date: _____

Administrative Approval: _____ Date: _____

- Inefficiency, incompetence in work duties performed (e.g., failing to perform job duty during work shift)
- Unauthorized telephone use (e.g., making long-distance personal calls without permission)
- Attendance (e.g., showing up late for work without prior permission)

Written Corrective Action. The written corrective action is a document summarizing the performance problem or incident detrimental to the customer, inability to follow established policy, or the failure to respond to supervision. A written corrective action serves as notice that continued infractions will not be tolerated and that performance must improve to meet expectations. Examples of behavior for which a written corrective action may be initiated as the first step of the corrective active process include:

- Inappropriate treatment or behavior toward a customer
- Conduct prejudicial to the best interest of the medical group
- Careless, indifferent, or negligent job performance including unsafe or unsanitary practices
- Careless neglect or unauthorized, improper use of company property or equipment
- Collecting money or accepting gratuities for personal use
- Failure of good behavior or neglect of duty
- Repeated or chronic infractions with no evident improvement in performance or conduct

Suspension or Final Written Corrective Action. An unpaid suspension or final written corrective action in lieu of suspension may occur when performance continues to be detrimental to customer or patient satisfaction or when a serious performance problem exists. Depending on the seriousness of the incident or behavior, the employee may receive a suspension or final written corrective action as the first step of the corrective action process. Suspensions should be scheduled so that patient care and consistency of service do not suffer, but as close to the infraction as possible. Examples of behavior for which a suspension may be initiated as the first step of the corrective action process include:

- Possession, use, or sale of alcohol, narcotics, or controlled substances on the medical group premises or reporting to work under the influence of alcohol or narcotics as evidenced by:
  - Inability to perform assigned work
  - Presentation of undesirable attributes (e.g., breath, attitude, uncooperativeness)

- Insubordination or refusal to perform a reasonable assignment after having been instructed to do so
- Sleeping on the job
- Disorderly conduct
- Failure to conform to professional standards
- Any other critical failure of good behavior or serious neglect of duty

Termination. Termination may occur as the final step in the corrective action process. Termination may occur for serious offenses or for continued performance problems impacting the customer or patient. Examples of behavior for which immediate termination may be initiated as the first step of corrective action include:

- Threat of or actual physical or verbal abuse of patients, visitors, or employees; inappropriate treatment of any patient for any reason
- Falsification of any official medical group records (e.g., medical records)
- Illegal or dishonest act
- Damage or theft of property
- Absence from work without justifiable reason or without reporting for two consecutive working days
- Unauthorized possession, use, copying, or revealing of confidential information regarding patients, employees, or medical group activity
- Unwelcome sexual advances, requests for sexual favors, or other verbal or physical conduct of a sexual nature with an employee, visitor, or patient
- Harassment in any form, including harassment based on race, gender, religion, and national origin such as offensive jokes, ridicule, and racial, religious, sexual, or ethnic slurs
- Improper use of leave of absence
- Conviction of a felony relevant to the employee's position
- Solicitation and distribution of literature
- Any other gross neglect of good behavior or gross neglect of duty

Policy Interpretation

For all disciplinary action, policy interpretation is the responsibility of the HR department. The disciplinary action or progressive discipline process is meant to give appropriate feedback to the employee in a formal way. This constructive feedback for desired results is meant to provide the employee with measurable accomplishments, instill individual accountability and responsibility, and facilitate the desired behavior. The supervisor can serve as a mentor, coach, and facilitator of the process and help the employee understand the desired results.

If the communication requires multiple areas of behavior change, the supervisor may choose to use a performance improvement plan (PIP) for the employee. This tool focuses on below-average or substandard performance and provides an action plan for needed change. The plan is time-specific and allows the employee to receive periodic feedback. For example, an employee may receive a PIP for inappropriate interactions with patients. The PIP would provide the employee with customer service training and weekly feedback sessions between the supervisor and employee on improvement in the desired results. Failure to achieve desired results can lead to additional disciplinary action up to and including termination. The

PIP's intent is to help the employee be successful and shepherd the process along the way.

Exit Interviews

When an employee submits a resignation to the medical group, it is important for the HR department to meet with the employee prior to his or her leaving. **Table 5-2** is a form that can be used by the department to determine the reason or reasons that the employee is leaving the organization. It is critical that the employee be met with in person to determine the reason(s) for the departure. Many times what is said to coworkers versus what is said to an HR person behind closed doors is different. The

Table 5-2	**ABC Medical Group Exit Questionnaire**

1. What was the most important factor influencing your decision to come to ABC Medical Group?

Reputation of ABC Medical Group	Educational Opportunities
Career Advancement	Employee Referral
Salary/Benefits	Practice Specialty
Other:	

2. What most influenced your decision to leave ABC Medical Group? (Please check one.)

Other Employment	**Personal Reasons**	**Job Dissatisfaction**
Closer to home	Relocation	Supervisor
Return to prior job	Family responsibility	Type of work
Better shift/hours	Child care	Shift/hours
Better position	Marriage	Staffing
Better wages	Health/illness	Other
Return to school	Retirement	
Military service	Other:	

3. Please check a rating for each category that best represents your opinion:

	No Opinion 0	Poor 1	2	Average 3	4	Excellent 5
Your Salary						
Your Benefits						
Educational Opportunities						
Promotional Opportunities						
Communication of Policies						
New Hire Orientation						
Departmental Orientation						
Work Environment/ Equipment						
Job Satisfaction						
Cooperation Within Your Department						
Morale in Your Department						

Comments on any of the above: _____

feedback can be helpful to determine if there are any opportunities to create improvements in the organization, whether it is better benefits, work schedule, supervision, or education and training.

Labor Relations

Organizations that:

- Invest appropriately in the compensation, benefits, training, education, and development of employees
- Hire and train supervisors to manage employees well
- Establish fair and reasonable policies and procedures that are consistently applied
- Communicate and listen effectively and openly
- Treat employees as a team member of the organization

may never need to deal with a union.

Employees decide to join a union:

- If they do not believe that their basic needs are being met by the employer
- If the employer is arbitrary in its dealings with employees
- If there is little or no job security
- If employees are not made to feel a part of the organization
- If they are not treated with respect
- If there is little or no opportunity for advancement or leadership within the organization.[3(pp4-6)]

Union activity is governed by the National Labor Relations Act (NLRA), which is enforced by the National Labor Relations Board (NLRB).

An initial contact with a union may occur through an employee or employees contacting the union or by a union organizer contacting employees. The union may organize employees from inside the group practice. Employer recourse is limited other than by adopting a no-solicitation policy, which prohibits union, or any, solicitation of employees during work hours. A union may pay people to be hired by the target employer. This is known as salting.[3(p116)] Unions also distribute leaflets, hold off-site meetings, visit the homes of employees, make telephone calls, use the Internet, try to gain media attention, and picket the employer.

The employer does have rights in a union organizing campaign. Management can communicate with their employees reasons for the employees to keep the group practice free from unions. Management can discuss with employees the potential for, and impact of, union strikes, but cannot try to coerce employees by making promises if the employees vote against the union. Management can use supervisor meetings as a vehicle for communicating with employees about the union, discuss the costs versus the benefits of the union, use an outside consulting firm to support the group-practice effort to defeat the union, and explain that improvements the employees are looking for can be accomplished without a union.

Unions use authorization cards to determine if employees want union representation. The NLRB does not order a union election unless at least 30% of the eligible employees sign authorization cards.[3(p119)]

Recognition of a bargaining unit may occur if the employer grants recognition or witnesses the majority status of the union (by, for instance, counting the authorization cards), or if the NLRB orders the company to recognize the union because of the company having committed unfair labor practices, or by an NLRB election.

Unfair labor practices on the part of the employer include using threats, interrogating employees, promising employees anything in exchange for not voting for the union, and spying on union activities.[3(p136)] Supervisors can use the acronym *TIPS* to remember these unfair labor practices. Employers cannot use interference, discrimination, or retaliation against employees who support the union. It is an unfair labor practice for an employer to try to dominate or support a union unlawfully. Another unfair labor practice is refusal by the employer to bargain with a certified union. Remedies by the NLRB for employer unfair labor practices can include sanctions against the employer in the form of cease-and-desist orders or an order to bargain with the union.[3(p143)]

Unfair labor practices may be filed against the union with the NLRB. Examples of union unfair labor practices are when unions threaten or use physical violence against employees, threaten economic sanctions, strike against or boycott a third-party employer, require the employer to hire more employees than is necessary for operations, or refuse to bargain in good faith over wages, hours, and conditions of work. Unions must fairly represent their members, cannot induce the employer to unfairly discriminate against an employee (by, for example, threatening to strike if the employee is not fired), and cannot charge unfair union dues.[3(pp144-146)]

The NLRB investigates claims of unfair labor practices, files a charge if sufficient evidence is discovered, and determines a settlement. If the settlement is not accepted, a hearing is conducted by an administrative law judge (ALJ). The ALJ issues the "decision and order" at the close of the hearing. If the decision of the ALJ is not followed, the NLRB can file in the U.S. Court of Appeals to seek enforcement.[3(p149)]

Once a union is recognized, a collective bargaining agreement is negotiated between the union and the employer. The collective bargaining agreement covers employment conditions such as wages, benefits, and working conditions. In addition, the collective bargaining agreement usually includes a formal grievance procedure to be used to address disagreements between employees and the employer. Normally the first step in the grievance process is to file the grievance with the immediate supervisor. If the grievance cannot be resolved by the employee's union representative and the supervisor, the grievance proceeds to the next level of management and union representation. If the grievance is not successfully resolved, it goes to the highest level of management for the employer and to a member of the union grievance committee or a higher-level union representative. The final level of the grievance process is for the grievance to go before a third-party arbitrator. Usually the representatives at the arbitration hearing include the highest level of management for the employer or legal counsel, the union president, a national union representative, or legal counsel of the union. The decision of the arbitrator is final and binding.

Employees may come to believe that a union is not properly representing them. The employees' recourse is to file a petition with the NLRB to have the union decertified.[3(p129)] An agent of the NLRB then performs an investigation. If the investigation finds that the petition has appropriately raised the question of the union properly representing the employees, a secret-ballot election can be held. The employer is constrained from activity during the decertification process, similar to the constraints in place during a union election. If the employees vote as a majority to decertify the union, the union can no longer represent the employees.

Total Compensation Administration

It is critical for the large group practice to have a well-defined total compensation philosophy and strategy that matches the organizational mission and strategy. The goal is to ensure that the practice retains employees that it needs by remaining competitive with the market and by maintaining internal equity among employees with similar positions within the practice.

The organizational culture also drives the compensation strategy. The organization with a primary focus on the profit of the organization as a whole and no focus on individual achievement structures a more paternalistic compensation strategy. In an organization with a culture emphasizing individual accomplishment, more focus is on incentive and performance-based types of pay. Organizations such as large group practices may do best to establish a compensation strategy with a balanced mix of focus on profit and encouragement of individual achievement, because the two are not necessarily mutually exclusive.

In analyzing the market for competitive position as it relates to total compensation, the large group practice needs to determine whether its compensation strategy matches the market, leads the market, or lags behind the market. Depending on the financial resources of the practice and the positions in question, the compensation strategy can involve a combination of all three approaches to the market.

Salary surveys are used to determine whether the organization is competitive with the market. If the organization has the available resources, salary surveys may be done internally. Many organizations opt to use external salary surveys, which can be obtained through an outside consulting firm. There are professional or industry organizations that perform regularly scheduled salary surveys. Organizations that participate in the salary surveys usually receive the survey results at a discounted fee or at no cost.

Salary survey data, along with the structure of the jobs in the organization, are used to develop the pay grades and ranges for all of the positions in the group practice. Pay or job grades are used to group jobs with the same value to the organization so that they are paid within the same pay range or at the same pay rate. The number of pay grades is determined to meet the needs of the organization based on the size and complexity of the group practice, the number of clearly differentiated jobs, and the pay practices of the organization.

Pay ranges are established as the minimum, midpoint, and maximum of each pay grade. Pay ranges vary based on the types of jobs within the range. Properly structured pay ranges should overlap to allow for the differentiation between experience levels of employees in different ranges. For example, a highly experienced employee in a lower pay range job could earn more than a less-experienced person in a job in the next higher pay range.

Large, complex organizations may, over time, develop too many pay grades and the differentiation between pay grades is lost and the effectiveness of the pay grade structure degrades. These organizations may elect to use broadbanding,[4(p54)] which is the combination of pay grades resulting in fewer, broader pay grades. Organizations may choose this strategy to simplify the pay grade structure, allow for flattening of a highly hierarchical organization, and better enable employee job mobility. However, for some organizations with a compensation philosophy of many levels and a defined "career ladder," broadbanding is not optimal. Broadbanding also allows for salary expenses to more easily expand because of the wider ranges and the ability of employees to achieve higher pay in the same range. Internal pay equity is more difficult to maintain because of the larger difference between the minimum and the maximum of the ranges, and employees have less opportunity for promotion. An organization that adopts broadbanding as a strategy should also develop a well-structured succession plan for positions that includes lateral job moves as an objective. The appropriate communication of this strategy and the eventual rewards for employees who take advantage of lateral opportunities helps to alleviate some of the issues posed by broadbanding.

Assuming that the group practice has established a set of competitive pay ranges, human resources is able to determine whether the group practice is paying an individual competitively compared to the market by calculating the compa-ratio[4(p53)] for the employee's pay. The compa-ratio is determined by dividing the individual employee's pay rate by the midpoint of the pay range. The midpoint is considered to be the market rate for the job. For example:

$$\text{Compa-ratio} = \text{Pay Rate} \div \text{Midpoint}$$

Employee earns \$8 per hour. The midpoint is \$9 per hour.

$$\$8.00 \div \$9.00 = 0.89 \text{ or } 89\%$$

Employees with a compa-ratio below 1.0 are being paid below the pay range midpoint, or market rate, and those with a compa-ratio above 1.0 are being paid above the midpoint of the range.[4(p53)] An analysis is next done to determine whether it is reasonable for an employee to be paid above or below the midpoint of the range. It may be reasonable based on the employee's experience and performance or if the organization has adopted a market lead or lag pay strategy.

Total compensation includes direct and indirect compensation. Direct compensation is the pay and cash awards provided to employees. Indirect compensation is the benefits that organizations make available to employees.

Direct Compensation

There are a range of direct compensation methods, as described in the following sections.

Base Pay

Base pay is the base amount the employee is paid per hour or on a fixed salary. Base pay systems include the following:

- Single- or flat-rate systems pay each employee in the same job the same pay rate.
- Time-based step-rate systems base the pay rate on how long the employee is in the job. There is a set schedule for pay increases.
- A step-rate with variability-based performance factors allows the size and/or timing of the pay increases to vary based on performance that is significantly above or below what is considered the norm.
- A combination step-rate and performance pay structure uses a strict step-rate structure up to the job rate. Pay increases above the job rate can be achieved only by superior performance.
- Performance-based or merit pay systems base increases on individual performance. Performance-based systems are challenging to administer. What the organization considers as high performance must be well defined and measurable. It is necessary to train supervisors to provide defendable performance appraisals. A comprehensive communication strategy should be used to roll the program out to the organization so that employees understand and buy into the process. In addition, the merit increase budget must be large enough to effectively differentiate among levels of performance.
- Productivity-based systems determine pay based on employee output. Piece-rate systems are an example of productivity-based systems.
- Knowledge-based systems base pay on the level of knowledge the employee has in the field represented by the position.
- Skill-based systems base pay on the number of job skills the employee has. Employees increase their pay by increasing their number of skills.
- Competency-based systems are based on the level of performance of competencies or job skills the employee can perform.

Differential Pay

Differential pay may include payment to:

- Provide incentive to employees to work specific shifts
- Attract employees to work in less desirable locations
- Compensate for the labor market in a particular part of the country
- Pay for an employee being on call or available to be called in to work
- Pay for call-back time when an employee is called in to work

■ Pay for business travel
■ Pay when there is no work available for the employee

Incentive Pay

Incentive pay programs are for motivating employees for high levels of performance. These programs work best when a high proportion of the employees' pay is incentive, or at-risk, pay. Incentive pay must be tied to specific measures such as organizational profits, patient satisfaction, productivity, or other established organizational metrics. Incentive programs may be at the individual, group, or organizational level. Some examples of incentive programs for the individual are sales commissions, productivity or piece-rates, cash bonuses, and recognition programs (i.e., length-of-service awards, extraordinary contribution). Group incentive plans can take the form of gain-sharing plans or performance incentive programs. Gain sharing is when the group shares in the organizational gains for superior performance. Group performance incentives are based on measurable goals the group must achieve. Organization-wide incentive plans include profit-sharing plans, deferred profit-sharing plans, performance-sharing plans, and stock ownership plans.

Select Pay Programs

There may also be pay plans for select or critical employees within the large group practice or for individuals who are outside of the organization and play a major role for the group practice. This may include executives, sales personnel, physicians and other professionals, and outside directors of the organization. Some of the plans for which these individuals may qualify, in addition to base salary, include annual incentives, perquisites (or "perks"), parachute clauses for loss of job or change of control of the organization, long-term incentives, commissions, bonuses, dual-ladder career progression for nonmanagement key employees, and maturity curves for time spent in a professional field. Outside directors' incentives may include base pay or a retainer, incentives for attending meetings, some benefits provided by the organization, perquisites, stock options, and some form of retirement accounts.

Internal Pay Equity

An important part of the management of compensation within an organization is to maintain pay equity among employees in jobs with the same value. Human resources will, on a regular basis, study employees' pay rates in relationship to each other to find any inequities that may have developed over time. An example of how pay inequities are established is when, due to market pressures, new employees with less experience are hired at pay rates at or above the pay existing employees are receiving. This leads to pay compression where less- and more-experienced employees are being paid very similar rates. In order to avoid pay compression, organizations need to continuously keep up with market changes or inflation by adjusting pay ranges. To alleviate or avoid compression, all employees should be paid to match the market; to do this, the more experienced employees can be provided with bonuses or other benefits can be provided.

Circumstances can arise in which employees are paid outside of the pay range for their job. An employee's pay rate might be highlighted because it is above the pay range. This can occur as a result of the reduction of the maximum of the pay range for the employee's job, or an employee at the maximum of a pay range receives an increase that puts his or her pay over the top of the range. An alternative is to provide an employee at the top of the pay range with a lump sum increase rather than an increase to their base rate. This keeps the employee's pay rate within the range, but can result in reduced employee morale. If there are a number of employees with highlighted pay rates, it may be a signal for the organization to examine their pay ranges against the market to determine if the ranges should be adjusted and to evaluate if the jobs affected should remain in that pay range.

When pay ranges are adjusted up to match the market or as a result of inflation, there may be employees whose pay rate may be identified as a variance because it falls below the pay range. Employees in this situation should be given a pay raise to bring them to at least the new minimum of the pay range.

Indirect Compensation

Indirect compensation is the benefits that an organization is either legally required to provide or, to remain competitive, must voluntarily provide its employees. In analyzing the organizational strategy for employee benefits, the HR professional reviews the organizational mission and strategy, the characteristics of the employee population, any benefits that are currently provided, the benefits provided by similar size organizations in the market, and the benefits commonly provided by similar organizations in the same industry. In many markets, the large group practice is competing for employees with other group practices and with healthcare organizations such as hospitals or integrated delivery systems.

According to the SHRM/SHRM Foundation 2003 Benefits Survey, for the health industry, the cost of mandatory benefits, including FICA and unemployment, is equivalent to 21% of salary. Voluntary benefits, other than leave benefits, were 19% of salary.[5]

Government-mandated benefits include Social Security, Medicare, unemployment insurance, workers' compensation, COBRA, and the Family and Medical Leave Act (FMLA).

The list of voluntary benefits frequently offered by employers in the health industry, according to the SHRM/SHRM Foundation 2003 Benefits Survey, is shown in **Table 5-3**.

The group practice must determine the level of investment in employee benefits that fits into the financial strategy of the organization. The level of employer and employee contributions to the cost of each of the benefits can then be established. The employee contribution to benefits may be before tax or after tax. The establishment of a cafeteria plan or Internal Revenue Code (IRC) Section 125 plan, allowing for the pretax deduction of certain benefits costs, can be an additional benefit for employees by reducing their taxable income.

Once the benefit program for the group practice is established, communication of the program is key to

Table 5-3	**Benefits Frequently Offered by Employers in the Health Industry**
Family-friendly benefits	Dependent-care flexible spending account
	Flextime
	Family leave above required federal FMLA leave
	Telecommuting on a part-time basis
	Compressed work week
Housing and relocation benefits	Temporary relocation benefits
Healthcare benefits	Prescription drug program coverage
	Life insurance
	Dental insurance
	PPO (preferred provider organization)
	Mail-order prescription program
	Mental health insurance
	Contraceptive coverage
	Vision insurance
	Medical flexible spending account (IRC Section 125 for all expenses)
	Employee assistance program
	Vaccinations on-site (example: flu shots)
	Chiropractic insurance
	Wellness program, resources, and information
	CPR training (first aid)
	HMO (health maintenance organization)
	Healthcare premium flexible spending account (IRC Section 125 cafeteria plan allowing for premium conversions)
	Supplemental health accident insurance
	Long-term care insurance
	Well-baby program
	Health screening programs (high blood pressure, cholesterol, etc.)
	Intensive care insurance
	Critical illness insurance
	Work-life newsletter or column
	Accelerated death benefits (for terminal illnesses)
	Smoking cessation program
	Cancer insurance
	On-site medical care
	(continues)

Table 5-3	Benefits Frequently Offered by Employers in the Health Industry (continued)
Personal services benefits	Professional development opportunities (seminars, conferences, courses, etc.)
	Professional memberships
	Casual dress day (one per week)
	Free/discounted uniforms
	Food services/subsidized cafeteria
Financial and compensation benefits	Payroll deductions (e.g., flexible spending account, 401(k))
	Direct deposit
	On-site parking
	Defined contribution retirement plan
	Undergraduate educational assistance
	Graduate educational assistance
	Incentive bonus plan (executive)
	Credit union
	Automobile allowance/expenses
	New-hire referral bonus
	Shift premium
	Employee discount on company services
	Incentive bonus plan (nonexecutive)
	Laptop for travel or personal use
	Shift premium
	Individual investment advice
	Loan to employees or emergency assistance
	Sign-on bonus (nonexecutive)
Business travel benefits	Employee keeps frequent flyer miles
	Paid long-distance calls to home while on travel
	Per diem for meals
Leave benefits	Paid holidays
	Paid bereavement leave
	Paid jury duty
	Long-term disability
	Paid vacation
	Short-term disability
	Paid sick leave
	Paid time-off plan (sick, vacation, personal days, all-in-one plan)
	Floating holidays (other than personal days)
	Paid personal days (aside from sick, vacation, and floating days)
	Time bank of vacation leave (donate vacation leave to other employees)
Other benefits	Holiday parties
	Summer picnic
	Ice cream socials
	Halloween parties

Source: Excerpted from SHRM/SHRM Foundation. 2003. SHRM/SHRM Foundation 2003 Benefits Survey.

employee understanding and appreciation of their benefits. A comprehensive communication strategy includes, for example, employee meetings at which benefits are explained; written materials supplied including summary plan descriptions, and contact names and numbers for the employees to use if they have questions; and websites on the Internet or group-practice intranet that the employees can access for information.

Employee Engagement

With the advent of healthcare reform come new expectations for healthcare leaders. A new set of skills is needed as cuts in reimbursement and new methods of payment challenge medical groups to improve operations beyond traditional past efforts. The changes are unprecedented, and require a complete refocus on ways that physicians, hospitals, medical groups, patients, medical practice administrators, and the community interact with each other. The new leadership skill sets need to better prepare the medical practice leader to lead effective change for the medical group to succeed. Leading change needs to translate to leading the workforce to change as well. Leaders can't effect change without eliciting teams of employees to embrace that change and make it happen. The ability of leaders to engage employees to embrace the new changes required under healthcare reform is key. Medical practice leaders and employees will need to be ready to implement numerous actions to improve clinical and operational efficiencies, increase patient satisfaction, enhance quality and patient safety, support clinical integration, and use the tools and data from the electronic medical record and information technology to effect change. Employees need to develop their own set of skills to better prepare them for the changes in healthcare. That transformation revolves around employee engagement.

Employee engagement is not just employee satisfaction. "An engaged employee is involved in, enthusiastic about, and committed to his or her work."[6] "Engagement relates to satisfaction and loyalty, but also explains unique information related to how individuals perceive their daily work life within their workgroups."[7] So why is it important to have highly engaged employees? "People who are satisfied with their companies are proud, are more likely to stay, and are advocates both of their companies as places to work and of their products and services."[7] Engaged employees are key to the future success of medical groups of physicians and leaders to achieve the many opportunities and challenges of healthcare reform. And with that knowledge, medical practice leaders need to understand the importance of employee engagement in achieving positive outcomes.

This employee engagement section is not meant to be all-inclusive and comprehensive, but to serve as a primer to help the medical practice leader better understand areas to focus on when working with employees. Employee engagement references are listed at the end of the chapter. The following areas of focus with employees will help the medical practice leader to be successful:

- *Medical practice engagement:* If an employee sees the medical group working to improve its relationship with employees by trying to understand employee concerns and acting on its behalf to incorporate them, employees are more likely to be engaged in the medical group.
- *Job importance:* Every job is important because if it wasn't, it wouldn't exist in the medical group. However, the way employees interact with each other places a different value on each job and results in employees either not seeing the full value of their job or not putting themselves fully into accomplishing the job. The medical group needs to work on ways to help each employee better understand the importance of his or her job. Doing so will result in employees providing better service to each other and the patients.
- *Job expectations:* It is not uncommon in a medical practice for the "other duties as assigned" in the job description to become primary parts of the job responsibilities. The employee then can become frustrated and angry because he or she does not have the resources or training necessary to do the job. The expectations of the job do not match the daily responsibilities of the job. As a result, the employee is more focused on struggling to make the job work than on helping the medical group to achieve successful outcomes.
- *Career and improvement opportunities:* Most employees want opportunities to improve themselves, their skills, and their abilities, and to advance within the organization. The medical practice leader needs to work with each employee to understand his or her talents and skills and help him or her focus on strengths. Each employee has a skill set that needs to be developed, and the manager can help facilitate opportunities to help the employee improve.
- *Feedback:* Constructive feedback is usually welcome, but inconsistently given to employees because it takes time, may involve a crucial

conversation, can be uncomfortable, and requires an artful way to communicate without offending an employee. Feedback of any kind involves a dialogue between the manager and employee that helps align the employee's performance with the manager's expectations. Feedback can be as simple as a comment and as complex as a formal written performance appraisal. Regardless of the feedback method provided, it is important that feedback be timely and consistent.

- *Working relationships:* Employees need to have positive working relationships with team members and manager to achieve high engagement. Many times an employee leaves an organization due to poor working relationships. The employee does not feel heard or does not feel that others recognize his or her value to the organization. An employee can see coworkers as a second family, and wants to have someone who cares about him or her. A caring environment allows the employee to try new things in a safe environment, dialogue with others without judgment, and know that there is always someone who supports him or her when help is needed.

- *Values, mission, greater purpose:* Every organization has a set of formal and/or informal values that shape how it operates. The values may be broad qualities expected to be provided in every transaction, such as service or quality, or may be specific behaviors expected, such as respect, professionalism, or tolerance. Sometimes they are hard to define, but we know they exist when we experience them. Engaged employees need to know how their job fits into the overall scheme of the organization. Finding a higher purpose, understanding the company's mission, and living the values energizes employees to achieve greater outcomes of quality and safe patient care.

- *Communication:* If communication is so widely understood as a key component to achieving effective outcomes, why is it so poorly done? Effective communication allows the employee to better understand what is going on in the medical group. It allows him or her to see how something needs to be done, how a function needs to change, or what impact an event will have on daily work. Effective handoff communication reinforces the importance of teams communicating with each other to accomplish a task. A medical receptionist who doesn't know that the computer system is going down can't prepare to care for patients with manual systems. Employees want to be involved and know what is

happening in the medical group. Without appropriate communications, the impact can be devastating.

- *Reward and recognition:* All employees want some kind of recognition, but the type of recognition varies for each employee. For example, a manager decided to recognize an employee's excellent work in a public form. Although the manager was pleased with how he gave recognition, the employee was embarrassed and didn't want that kind of recognition. As a result, the employee stopped trying to provide excellent service in fear of getting publically recognized again. That's why it is important to find out from each person how he or she wants recognition. Usually, a simple "thank you" is all that is needed. Other ways are a thank you note, an announcement in a newsletter or memo, or an acknowledgment before a group of people. There are numerous ways to recognize employees. The important approach is to find out the kinds of things that an employee values in terms of rewards and work to provide those incentives.

■ Physician Recruitment, Retention, and Resource Enhancement

It is both simple and complex to understand the importance of integrating physicians into the culture of the organization. The medical group leaders need to come together to define what kind of medical practice they are and what kind of medical practice they are not. This strategic visioning provides focus for the vision, mission, and values of the medical group and provides clarity to their purpose. Physicians want to believe in what their medical practice does. Excellent performance happens when physicians are strongly attached to having a purpose in life. Physicians want to make a difference, and knowing how the difference will be accomplished in a medical group appeals to the physician's sense of purpose and mission. Following are medical practice areas that need to be determined to help communicate to physicians the parts of the practice that make up the whole:

- *Clinical practice:* What kind of clinical practice is offered? Is there an opportunity to teach medical students, residents, and/or fellows? To do clinical research or national studies? To do community outreach, lectures, or charity work at an indigent clinic? Can a new clinical program be trialed? Is there openness to being on the forefront and piloting a new theory (the medical home) or implementing a new technology (e-prescribing)? Can a specialized population of the community be targeted (e.g., diabetics, the elderly, the underserved, those with a chronic disease)?

- *Compensation:* What kind of compensation is offered? Is it based on fair market value? Is it based on productivity or incentives? Is the compensation fixed, salary based, or variable salary based on collections? Are there payments for achieving quality, patient safety, and patient satisfaction measures? Is there recognition for attendance at meetings and committees, and for providing a leadership role? Is citizenship recognized?

- *Benefits:* What kind of benefits are provided and how do they complement the medical group's vision? Do benefits includes the following: paid time off; health, dental, and/or vision insurance; short- and long-term disability insurance; pension plans; malpractice insurance with tail coverage; tuition reimbursement; continuing education allowance for keeping current in the marketplace; car and travel allowances; provision of cell phone or laptop computer; or relocation assistance?

- *Work hours and call coverage:* What kind of work hours are expected during the week? Does the medical group provide any call coverage? Is the physician expected to be on call every evening and weekend? Can the physician spend time with family without interruption?

- *Location, location, location:* A physician has many factors to consider when deciding whether to work for a medical group, including location. For example, some medical groups provide services throughout the world, throughout the United States, or in a region, state, county, or city. Those offerings may be a factor for a physician who wants to stay with a health system with the opportunity to relocate throughout her or his professional career. Or it may be a factor for a physician to decide to work with a smaller group that won't expect relocation in the future. Also, the location of the practice in an urban versus rural setting, by the mountains or by water, by major metropolitan or resort areas, are all factors for a physician to decide the type of practice he or she can work in.

- *Medical practice resources:* If a physician has been trained in an electronic medical record (EMR) environment in a residency program, it is unlikely that she or he will go into a setting without an EMR in the future. There are too many efficiencies learned to give up in future settings. Also, physicians value

anything that makes their job easier to see patients, so any resource that supports that effort is valued. Some of those resources may include number of ancillary support staff provided, provision of mid-level providers, answering service, billing support, professional coders, number of exam rooms provided, and type of equipment and supplies provided.

- *Physician contract:* A contract is a communication between the medical group and the physician that outlines the mutual agreement shared between them. What it says and doesn't say speaks to the culture of the group, its values, and the services it provides. Important factors to consider in a contract are:
  - Is there is an income guarantee for practice start-up?
  - What is the risk of losing the job? Is a 1-year or multi-year contract provided?
  - Is there a noncompete clause if the physician leaves the group?
  - Who are the decision makers that could end the contract?
  - What kind of timeline is given to end an agreement?
  - Does the medical group provide malpractice tail coverage when the agreement ends?

- *Practice flexibility:* The practice structure helps define how the physician's values align with the practice's needs. For example, if the position requires the physician to work early mornings to handle hospital rounds and the physician has young children that need to get off to school and doesn't have alternate arrangements, can the medical group rotate the physician's responsibilities to another function to allow the physician to meet personal needs? Or is the medical group so small (e.g., two other partners) that this kind of arrangement would be unacceptable without creating strife and difficulty with the other partners who are already covering other morning responsibilities? Newly graduating residents and fellows have different personal priorities than physicians who graduated in earlier decades. More professional options are being sought including part-time versus full-time positions, positions that can flex up and down in hours based on the care of children and aging parents, and positions that allow the physician to pursue additional pursuits. The variety of personal options considered include everything from the ability to take time off to volunteer at an indigent mission in another county to taking time off to write a book, travel around the world, or take 3-day hiking trips.

- *Medical practice promotion opportunities:* When a physician begins working in a new setting, he or she wants to know how the new practice will be promoted. Is it as simple as "If we build it, the patients will come," due to strong pent-up demand, or will it take time and numerous communication mechanisms to market the start-up? Will the group support a variety of communication methods including direct mailings, newspaper advertisements, open houses, speaking engagements to community groups, Yellow Page advertising, and social media blogs?

- *Citizenship:* Physicians are part of the community. They are leaders who are expected to be good citizens and participate in various business and social events. The medical group needs to define the focus of physician involvement in the community including participation on community boards, attending social events, mentoring and coaching others, serving on hospital medical staff committees, and performing internal administrative duties (e.g., board meeting attendance, interviewing other physicians and staff, reviewing policies and procedures).

The Human Resources of Physicians

The landscape of healthcare is changing due to healthcare reform. In this new environment, leaders can't continue to use the same tools and skills sets and still be successful. The bar is being raised to higher expectations. This is especially telling in developing a culture where physicians want to work. The balance of supply and demand has changed, and it is becoming increasingly difficult to recruit a physician. The number of physicians is decreasing and the demand for physicians is increasing. This dynamic presents new challenges for the organization recruiting a physician. Gone are the days when a casual conversation between two physicians at a medical convention leads to a physician joining a group with little structure and a "handshake" agreement. In today's competitive marketplace, a physician candidate has numerous choices and is "shopping" for the arrangement that best meets both professional and personal goals.

Clinical Practice

Clinical practice encompasses what clinical duties the physician is expected to perform. Clearly defining those expectations will avoid wasting valuable time for both the physician and organization. For example, if a group wants to recruit a family medicine physician who will provide both inpatient and outpatient services, it is worth clarifying the need with a physician who is currently only providing outpatient services. Also, if a physician plans to change clinical focus (e.g., hospitalist to outpatient services), the group needs to assess the physician's previously learned skills and their transferability to a new setting. Whether through physician proctoring or physician peer review, the group needs to assess whether the physician has the clinical skills necessary to meet the job's needs. The level of structure, problem solving, and proactive listening done in aligning the practice's needs with the physician's needs will determine the future success of physicians staying in the practice. Otherwise, a physician will leave the medical practice due to poor mentoring and orientation processes.

Compensation

If a physician in a private practice joins a hospital-based practice where compensation transitions from a productivity model to a fixed salary without any incentives, the organization needs to determine consequences when physician volume drops without a change in pay. Due to healthcare reform changes, future compensation models will need to include new metrics including:

- Expense reduction in use of products, services, and work flow redesign
- Reductions in hospital length of stay
- Reductions in cost per adjusted hospital discharge
- Achievement of Medicare Hospital Core Measures
- Appropriate documentation in the electronic medical record
- Keeping patients out of the hospital and managing chronic disease in an outpatient setting
- Reducing hospital readmission rates
- Achieving appropriate *Hospital Consumer Assessment of Healthcare Providers and Systems* (HCAHPS) scores
- Reduction in hospital-acquired infections

These measures, along with many others, are dynamic and are not vetted among physicians and hospitals. The physician compensation model will continue to change as the healthcare reform model evolves.

Lifestyle

Recently, a family physician in his seventies retired from a busy practice. He worked every day of the week including Saturdays and Sundays; worked 3 nights a week; saw patients in the office, hospital, and nursing home; and served as medical director of a home care agency. All his patients loved him and he was the epitome of compassion and service. But he was also someone that was difficult to replace because his work ethic did not match that of physicians starting a practice. It is important for a medical group to be open about changing practice lifestyles and work ethic priorities. In the above-mentioned scenario, it took recruitment of 2.5 physicians to replace the work previously performed by this physician. The medical group determined that it was not realistic to find only one physician to recruit into the retired physician's practice. It took a blended model to accomplish the same tasks.

More often than not, physicians want to know what is expected of them. They want to understand the call coverage responsibilities, the volume of telephone calls expected, and the frequency of those calls. The more that a medical group can provide clarity and structure and address varied lifestyle requests, the more likely the physician will not only come into the job with realistic expectations, but also stay with the practice for the long term.

Benefit Options
Baseline physician benefits are expected in today's healthcare market. What differentiates a medical practice are the benefits that allow a physician to pursue his or her personal interests. Those nontraditional benefits may include:

- Getting time off to provide missionary work for 1–3 weeks
- Receiving a laptop computer or other personal device to keep in touch with others through social media
- Receiving credit for providing free services at an indigent clinic
- Provision of on-site daycare services for the physician so that he or she can visit with the child during the day
- Flextime for care of aging parents or a child with special needs
- Extra pay for conducting research, publishing in a professional journal, presentations at national associations, or extra patient work

Being prepared and addressing these types of benefits up front helps the medical group to better define its culture and how benefits support those efforts.

Location
The practice setting helps define how the physician will practice medicine. It is important to determine where the physician will practice including exam rooms, office space, and equipment used.

Practice Promotion
How the medical group communicates the services provided is important for the practice. It's about developing the relationships needed to get the job done. How the medical group promotes the services to the physician makes all the difference in the success of the physician. It's more than just sending out a brochure or putting an advertisement in the newspaper. It's about getting the word out and building rapport with other physicians, patients, staff, and the community to accomplish the goals of the practice. The collegiality and collaboration experience becomes a core value of the practice.

Citizenship
A successful physician must be a strong leader in the community and in the medical group. The new physician needs to be appropriately on-boarded to what is expected throughout the year. What kind of social functions will the physician be expected to participate in? What meetings does the physician need to attend in the medical group? At the hospital? These types of questions will help both the group and physician be in sync in expectations.

Leadership
The physician of the future needs to be a leader in his or her specialty, a patient advocate, and a teacher to others. Healthcare reform will require physician leaders to embrace new sets of skills to navigate through very difficult and challenging times.

■ Conclusion

The beginning of the twenty-first century has pushed healthcare leaders to focus on creating a culture of service. The physician, employee, medical practice leader, and patient create a team working towards health. The traditional lines of employer–employee are broken down as everyone works to exceed the patient's expectations. With the human resources function, medical groups are moving human resources from traditional models to becoming a strategic partner. Restructuring continues to incorporate principles of collaboration, partnership, service, the value proposition of cost and quality, and development.

Quality and safety have become the cornerstones of the medical group, and those medical groups that are able to provide quality at a competitive cost will have long-term success. This focus on quality and safety will help create successful job models with an eye toward improved performance, working toward excellent results, and focusing behavior changes that lead to strong patient satisfaction and highly engaged employees. Those medical groups able to create influence and positive change in a high-quality and cost-effective manner will be the future healthcare leaders.

The human resources function serves as the corporate steward of its resources—its people—and directs the physicians and staff along with salaries and wages, benefits, reward and recognition, performance, training, and employee engagement to fit within the medical group's culture and its vision, mission, and values.

References

1. BNA. *HR department benchmarks and analysis 2003*. Arlington, VA: The Bureau of National Affairs: 2004:4.
2. Studer Q. *Hardwiring excellence*. Gulf Breeze, FL: Fire Starter; 2003:174–176.
3. Society for Human Resource Management. The SHRM learning system: module five, employee and labor relations. Alexandria, VA: SHRM; 2002.
4. Society for Human Resource Management. The SHRM learning system: module four, compensation and benefits. Alexandria, VA: SHRM; 2002.
5. Society for Human Resource Management/SHRM Foundation. 2003 benefits survey. Table I–2. Accessed May 15, 2004, at http://www.shrm.org
6. Gallup. Employee engagement impact 1, Cleveland Clinic manager training. Cleveland, OH: 2008:7.
7. Gallup Consulting. Overall satisfaction: what is it worth? Position Paper. Gallup Consulting: Gallup, Inc.; 2008:1.

Resources

American College of Medical Practice Executives. *Defining the profession: a guide to the body of knowledge for medical practice management*. Denver, CO: ACMPE; 2001.

Beeson SC. *Practicing excellence: a physician's manual to exceptional health care*. Gulf Breeze, FL: Fire Starter, 2006.

BNA. *HR department benchmarks and analysis 2003*. 2004.

Chapman E. *Supervisors survival kit*. New York: Macmillan; 1990.

Cleveland Health Network Management Services Organization. *Employee materials*. Independence, OH: Author; 2004.

Colan L. *Engaging the hearts and minds of all your employees*. New York: McGraw-Hill; 2009.

Cook S. *The essential guide to employee engagement: better business performance through staff satisfaction*. Philadelphia: Kogan Page; 2008.

Federal Trade Commission. A summary of your rights under the Fair Credit Reporting Act. Accessed May 16, 2004, at http://www.ftc.gov

Harris J. *Getting employees to fall in love with your company*. New York: AMACOM; 1996.

Jennings K, Stahl-Wert J. *The serving leader*. San Francisco, CA: Berrett-Koehler; 2004.

Macey W, Schneider B, Barbera K, Young S. *Employee engagement: tools for analysis, practice, and competitive advantage*. Malden, MA: Valtera; 2009.

Medical Group Management Association. *RX for business success: joining a medical practice for physicians*. Denver, CO: MGMA; 2005.

National Association of Professional Employer Organizations. PEO industry information. Accessed May 16, 2004, at http://www.napeo.org

Pollard JW. *The physician manager in group practice*. Englewood, CO: Center for Research in Ambulatory Health Care Administration; 1995.

Pritchett P. *The employee handbook of new work habits for the next millennium: 10 new ground rules for job success*. Rummler-Brache; 1999.

Pritchett P. *The employee handbook of new work habits for a radically changing world: 13 ground rules for job success in the information age*. Pritchett and Associates; 1994.

Ross A, Williams S, Schafer E. *Ambulatory care management*. Delmar; 1991.

Society for Human Resource Management. The SHRM Learning System. 2002.

Society for Human Resource Management. SHRM research. 2002 staffing metrics survey. Accessed May 16, 2004, at http://www.shrm.org

Society for Human Resource Management/SHRM Foundation. SHRM/SHRM Foundation 2003 benefits survey. Accessed May 15, 2004, at http://www.shrm.org

Studer Q. *Hardwiring excellence*. Gulf Breeze, FL: Fire Starter; 2003.

Townsend PL, Gebhardt JE. *The executive guide to understanding and implementing employee engagement programs*. Milwaukee, WI: ASQ Quality Press; 2007.

CHAPTER 6

Marketing Healthcare Services

Roberta N. Clarke, MBA, DBA

The role of marketing in any medical practice or healthcare organization should be a reflection of the milieu in which it operates, the competition it faces, the markets it serves, and the regulatory, technological, political, and clinical environment within which it must function. When one or more of these change, marketing strategy must change as well. There is little doubt that much is changing in the health sector, largely driven by the unanimous agreement by those in health policy and management that healthcare costs must be driven down. The result is a changing set of demands placed upon the marketing function in healthcare organizations and medical practices now and in the coming years.

Although highly variable across the healthcare field, the level of marketing sophistication has increased in many larger healthcare organizations. However, physician practices generally still lag in their understanding of marketing as a strategic and tactical tool rather than merely being a quick fix, a magic bullet to attract more patients, more referrals, and more business of any kind. Some continue erroneously to view marketing as public relations, an undervalued function itself, but not in any way the equivalent of marketing. Others, particularly health insurance and managed-care organizations, historically defined marketing largely in terms of sales and

promotional activities. Far too often, healthcare organizations have created their own definitions of healthcare marketing without taking into account the data collection and analytical components of marketing. As a result, they either have developed marketing strategy in a vacuum or, possibly worse, have failed to develop a cohesive and comprehensive marketing strategy at all.

To use marketing appropriately, it is first necessary to have a clear understanding of what it is. Leaders in the field of marketing cite the American Marketing Association's definition: "Marketing is the activity, set of institutions, and processes for creating, communicating, delivering, and exchanging offerings that have value for customers, clients, partners, and society at large."[1] They further define marketing management as "the art and science of choosing target markets and getting, keeping, and growing customers through creating, delivering, and communicating superior value."[2]

In order to carry out this process, marketers rely on tools called the marketing mix, often referred to as the 4 P's: product and/or service, price, promotion, and place (also thought of as distribution, channels, and access). Often, the promotional component of marketing, which includes (but is not limited to) advertising, sales promotion, collateral materials, direct mail, telemarketing,

171

web-based promotion, social networking capabilities, events, selling, and price promotion, has been mistaken for the equivalent of marketing. Although an important part of marketing, promotion and communication are only one aspect of marketing. All the tools in the marketing mix must be considered together in developing a marketing strategy because they are closely interrelated. To rely on one or two marketing tools to the exclusion of the others is to invite disaster. The marketing mix can be viewed as a jigsaw puzzle; unless all the pieces of the puzzle are in place, the puzzle is not complete. It takes only one tool in the marketing mix, one piece of the puzzle, to be out of place for the marketing strategy to fail.

As marketing sophistication in healthcare has increased, resulting in greater recognition of the analytical component of the marketing function, the use of marketing intelligence, databases, and market research has become more common. Healthcare organizations can, as a result, better understand their market, their competition, the operational performance of their own organization and the impact of that performance on their customers, and the regulatory, technological, legal, and healthcare environments within which they must function. Furthermore, their increasing use of marketing performance benchmarks allows them to evaluate the effectiveness of their marketing efforts. The use of dashboard technologies and tools, which measure the achievement of operational goals, has provided another set of metrics that allows the organization to assess how it is performing on key performance indicators (KPIs); many of these KPIs are tied to marketing strategy targets.

Marketing is a process that involves the collection of market-related, competitive, and other relevant intelligence; performance of market research; assessment of internal performance; an environmental market scan; careful analysis of all available data, coupled with consideration of the organization's strategic plan; and finally, the development of marketing strategy and tactical marketing plans. Ultimately, there must be an evaluation of the results of marketing efforts in order to improve future investment in the marketing function. There is a tendency to confuse marketing with strategic planning. A strategic plan relies heavily on market planning, which may explain the confusion. Strategic planning is the effort to align the organization's mission, resources, and capabilities with its external environment, its current and potential markets, and its competition. It not only must extend beyond marketing planning to include financial, human resource, technological, regulatory, operational, and information system considerations, but also must build on the values and mission of the organization.

There is consensus among marketers that data collection and analysis should precede marketing strategy, which should then be followed by marketing plan development, implementation, and control. Healthcare marketers are not in agreement, however, about whether marketing should have a heavy consumer focus or instead emphasize business-to-business marketing. Nor do they agree on the value of, and relationship between, customer satisfaction and customer loyalty, nor on the appropriate allocation of resources between customer attraction and customer retention. These are key issues for any organization. If the mission statement and strategic plan of the healthcare organization do not address these considerations—and many of them do not—then the marketing efforts may be focused on goals that do not reflect the values of the organization.

Marketing Mission and Objectives

The function of healthcare marketing is difficult to define; changing incentives in the healthcare system can turn what had been the traditional mission and objectives for marketing upside down. Healthcare marketing efforts historically attempted to increase the volume and usage of hospitals, medical practices, nursing homes, and other medical care providers. The introduction of managed care and capitation modified the objectives of most healthcare providers to aim to minimize volume or use and, as a result, cost. When this first happened in the 1980s, success no longer was defined in terms of high occupancy rates and a high volume of patients or procedures, but in terms of the ability to keep the cost of "covered lives" low. As managed-care organizations and employers continued to transfer the capitated risk for patients onto the providers with whom they contracted, these providers found themselves forced to assume a "womb to tomb" approach to caring for patients. Some responded by then applying marketing to a variety of tasks, from promoting patient compliance (i.e., encouraging patients to follow through with all their physicians' instructions with regard to medications, exercise, lifestyle, and so on) to educating patients about the appropriate time to see the physician.

Part of the premise of managed care and capitation was a limitation in consumers' choice of medical provider, whether physician, hospital, diagnostic provider, or allied health provider. Massive resistance by consumers to these limitations caused insurers to lessen these restrictions. Business and industry responded by attempting to measure and ensure medical care quality; to decrease medical errors, which carry both a human and a financial cost; and to reintroduce greater consumer choice, requiring these entities to yet again reform their mission and objectives. However, once again, payment for volume of services delivered became a more dominant incentive and objective for healthcare marketers. Managed-care organizations sought to increase the size of their memberships; holding the top or second place market share in a local and regional market became a compelling aspect of brand strength for these organizations. Hospitals, after downsizing, attempted to maintain a high occupancy level in order to cover their fixed costs. Similarly, providers sought to attract a sufficient quantity of patients to maintain an acceptable level of income and of quality in performing certain surgical and other procedures.

The newest, and possibly soon to be revoked, healthcare legislation now being discussed embrace both old and new incentives, once again causing the marketing mission and objectives to be redefined. Accountable care organizations (ACOs), whose structure is still open-ended (and may ultimately take a number of different forms), are expected to rely on a number of incentives: pay-for-performance, bundled payments and shared savings, adherence to evidence-based medicine, better teamwork, and systemically built communications networks between physicians, hospitals, and other clinically trained providers, all tied in some form to a medical home, also as yet undefined but likely to be defined in terms of primary care providers (PCPs). Once again, the proposed ACO approach to healthcare reimbursement and delivery asks for providers to take a womb-to-tomb approach; some have referred to this as "managed care in drag." Medicare has proposed assigning patients to a particular ACO and PCP based on which providers they visited the most in the previous year (determined by billed charges). The currently proposed ACOs will not, as did earlier managed care forms, necessarily restrict patient choice with limited networks or gatekeeping, even while holding the ACO providers responsible for patient charges and outcomes contributed to by providers that are not a part of the ACO.

One likely marketing objective, then, for primary care providers is to be designated as the medical home for a high volume of patients. Specialists and hospitals will have the marketing objective of wanting to be part of the ACOs of many busy primary care providers so they can receive a high volume of referrals from these PCPs. Volume therefore will continue to be a marketing objective. A second marketing objective would seem to follow from the proposal that providers can earn bonuses if they meet certain quality and cost goals (quality/up and

costs/down); in addition to being able to earn bonuses, providers will also assume financial risk so that if costs are higher than the spending targets, providers stand to lose 5–10% of any spending over the targeted spending goals. So the second marketing objective would be keeping the patient within one's own ACO so that spending can be controlled and quality measures, determined either by the government or by insurers, are attended to as part of the patient's care. This second marketing objective will require far greater understanding and use of social marketing and customer service, if the ACO is to achieve success.

Anyone who defines the marketing objectives of a healthcare organization as simply seeking to increase volume has underestimated the complexity of the new healthcare marketplace. The necessity of conceptualizing organizations as parts of larger systems—currently as part of one or more ACOs—requires a recognition of multiple and sometimes conflicting marketing objectives.

One of the tasks, then, of the marketing function is to define carefully the full range of the organization's objectives. An accountable care organization must simultaneously seek a high volume of assigned patients and foster either a low volume of usage or at least less costly usage. Even this is simplistic, however. It is necessary to encourage certain types of visits, for example, for preventive care and early diagnosis of disease, but to discourage visits for certain nonacute symptoms, such as sore throats that are likely to disappear by themselves with no treatment within a week. Each of these objectives, even if directed at the same market or individual customer, may require a different marketing strategy.

The Competition Defined

The same complexity in the healthcare environment that leads to multiple marketing missions and objectives also requires a more systematic and skilled approach to defining the competition. A competitor often is defined as any organization that lessens the likelihood of another organization achieving its desired marketing exchange. In the not-so-distant past, one looked only at organizations that carried the same category title as competitors; hospitals competed only with other hospitals, and nursing homes competed with other nursing homes, for example. Even so, there was some overlap between types of providers. An inpatient psychiatric unit of an acute care hospital might have competed with a freestanding psychiatric hospital; physical therapists, chiropractors, and orthopedic surgeons might all have competed for the same patient with chronic acute low back pain. With greater demand being placed upon the healthcare system to address unmet needs, we now see greater intercategory competition. Given the impending shortage of primary care physicians that was forecast and affecting patients well before the Affordable Care Act was on anyone's radar screen, we now can expect to see increasing use of nurse practitioners and physician assistants as substitutes for and competing for the patients of primary care physicians. We can further expect the expansion of MinuteClinics, walk-in medical clinics in CVS stores that employ nurse practitioners and physician assistants to carry out the routine tasks of a primary care physician. The competition for a primary care physician practice may now no longer be a primary care physician nor delivered in a traditional practice setting. The same principles may be found across the field of healthcare delivery.

The formation of systems, including ACOs and hospital systems, expands the definition of competitors. The uncertainty of future membership in these healthcare delivery systems makes it unclear who may be a competitor today and yet be a collaborator in the future. Among hospitals that had combined to create one unified health system, some later broke apart, their partnerships disbanded, and the previous partner hospitals were soon vying to take away each other's business. This uncertainty as to who is or will be friend or foe makes it more difficult to invest in competitive positioning strategies or to develop strengths and competencies based on a competitor's strengths and weaknesses.

The Changing Environment

The current healthcare environment promises confusion in identifying the competition. Organizations not only have to ask themselves, "What business are we in?" but also have to ask about the competition, "What businesses are they in? What businesses will they be adding tomorrow? Which providers and organizations that contract with us now will choose to contract with our competitors tomorrow?" This difficulty in defining long-term competitors arises even when ACOs and managed care do not play a significant role in the competitive environment. As physician practices have become increasingly able to acquire and operate diagnostic capabilities that once resided only inside of hospitals, and as they found that they could perform certain types of surgeries that required neither a full-fledged operating room nor the backup of wide-ranging hospital services, these practices have become competition to the hospitals on whose staffs they serve. As stated by Berenson et al.:

Because many services performed in hospitals can safely and conveniently be performed in ambulatory settings physicians have become owners of entities directly competing with hospitals for patients in a new medical arms race. Hospitals and medical staff physicians face growing tensions.... Although there are increasing expectations that health systems challenges will lead hospitals and physicians to collaborate, in many markets the willingness and ability for hospitals and physicians to work together is actually eroding.[3]

Peaceful coexistence between healthcare entities can rapidly change when new competitive activities of one entity threaten to erode the revenues or market share of the other. The vertical integration of a variety of healthcare organizations into systems can make competition out of customers. For example, one can envision that an ACO, with which one physician specialty group contracts to provide care to the ACO's patients, may now instead choose to contract in the same service area with a competing physician specialty group, making competitors of the two former collegial practice groups. Yet, it may not be wise for the rejected physician specialty group to launch a marketing offensive against that ACO, because it might once again contract with the ACO in the future. Few healthcare vertical integration relationships specify exclusivity; the relationship of the ACO with the competing specialty practice does not prevent it from once again developing a relationship with the first practice as well.

Alternatively, organizations that were once ardent competitors may become part of the same system. Sometimes they continue to offer the same services they provided before becoming part of a system; other times, the system expects them to complement each other rather than compete. The former instance is an example of a federation, the latter of a partnership. An even more extreme competitive change is the merger of two or more former competitors. Such mergers abounded in the late 1990s as healthcare providers and managed-care organizations concluded, at least at that time, that the greater size, geographic coverage, and service coverage produced by a merger made them more marketable. Some merged entities appear to demonstrate that this is true. In California, seven entities, formed from combining a number of smaller healthcare provider organizations, control more than one-third of all California hospitals and licensed beds. The ability to compete in the California market depends in part on whether one is part of one of these large entities. On the other hand, some well-known mergers are not doing well at all. Many well-known in addition to lesser-known mergers formed from the mid-1990s through the mid-2000s have since either fallen apart or are performing badly from a financial perspective. The Allegheny Health, Education, and Research Foundation in Pittsburgh, a well-publicized $1.3 billion entity encompassing teaching hospitals, community hospitals, and a medical school, went bankrupt in July 1998. CareGroup, a combined group of Harvard teaching hospitals and smaller community hospitals in Massachusetts, showed deficits for a number of years, and has to divest itself of some of its constituent parts in order to stay afloat financially. In Rhode Island, the state's two biggest hospital systems, after trying twice a decade apart to merge, finally declared it a failure in 2010. Gabel noted that the mergers and acquisitions in managed care, the shift from vertically integrated staff models to virtually integrated network models, and the increased patient cost sharing (including capitating primary care physicians) have not improved patient satisfaction or quality of care.[4]

In the long term, the widely held belief that the larger merged entities function more effectively and are more marketable may or may not hold true, particularly if several network members suffer from poor quality service and poor management and, thus, potential customers elect to use other networks. Some networks may be trading away long-term marketability for short-term assumed economies of scale and presumed competitive advantage. The economies of scale that a number of merged healthcare organizations have expected have not always materialized in the basic services that they provide. This could be seen in the attempts of a large floundering hospital in lower Manhattan (N.Y.), St. Vincent's Hospital, to merge or form a network with other nearby hospitals. Having attempted and failed to merge with two significant teaching hospitals in Manhattan, N.Y.U. Medical Center in 2009 and Mt. Sinai Medical Center in 2010, St. Vincent's then sought to create a network with other hospitals like itself, believing that there would be strength in size. However, this proved not to be the case, as described in a local newspaper:

> The hospital seemed doomed to failure for many years, going back to the 1990s, when the decision was made to form a network with other New York City Catholic hospitals. . . . "It was probably the biggest mistake that St. Vincent's ever did," Webb [the COO of St. Vincent's] said. A number of the other hospitals were already in terrible shape when they teamed up with St. Vincent's and it wasn't long before they were going out of business.[5]

Smaller merged entities may not offer marketing advantages either. The heavy cross-functional dependence of many medical specialties and services, for example, prevented two hospitals that had formally merged from eliminating certain specialties from one hospital and placing them solely in the other, originally a goal of the merger in order to cut costs. Both hospitals needed infectious disease, cardiology, nephrology, endocrinology, psychiatry, otolaryngology, and other diagnostic and treatment capabilities in-house for their inpatients. The inconvenience, cost, and possible clinical repercussions of having to move a patient from one hospital to the other because the necessary diagnostic equipment was not available in the first prevented the hospitals from eliminating the services as they had initially planned. This scenario has been repeated around the United States.

The more common result of hospital mergers essentially has been to eliminate one of the hospitals as an acute care hospital. The eliminated hospital may become a substance abuse center, rehabilitation provider, walk-in facility, chronic care center, congregate living quarters for the elderly, or a housing center for needy women and infants, for example. These are valuable services for which there may be more demand than for the acute care services that the hospital facility used to provide. This process is not one of merging with the competition, however, as much as it is a process of eliminating the competition. The weakest hospitals begin to provide nonacute care services, whereas the stronger hospitals with which they merged remain in the acute care business. The merger of hospitals with more equal status is less likely to result in the closure of one of them, but it is not yet proved that there are significant economies of scale to be achieved when these hospitals both continue to operate as acute-care facilities.

There is an argument to be made that healthcare entities that do not truly merge, but that sit down together at the negotiating table, may gain market power. Massachusetts General Hospital (MGH) and Brigham & Women's Hospital formed a corporate entity, Partners HealthCare. The two hospitals did not merge their services, however. To the contrary, once Partners was created, MGH added a maternity unit to its long list of service units, in spite of the fact that the Brigham & Women's Hospital already had the largest maternity service in New England. The true advantage of creating Partners was not to prevent the two hospitals from competing with each other, but rather to give the two hospitals more negotiating power when they met with insurers and managed-care organizations to agree upon reimbursement rates and terms. Similar advantages may accrue to ACOs and insurers that, in merging, grow in size and in the geographic area they cover; this allows them to offer employers greater coverage for their employees through contracting with a single insurer or ACO rather than forcing the employers to have to sign contracts with a number of insurers or ACOs to cover their employees. That benefit provides the larger ACO or insurer greater negotiating power.

However, it also brings with it the troubling possibility that very large ACOs may bring about the opposite effect on costs sought by the creators of the ACO concept. The previously noted Partners HealthCare was the subject of investigation by the Massachusetts State Attorney General in 2010 because the rates at which it was being paid were much higher than the rates at other hospitals; at the same time, there appeared to be no quality justification for these higher charges:

Now that the nation has embarked on a course toward universal health care, it is more important than ever that the government go after cost drivers in the system. In Massachusetts, that means addressing the power some hospitals have to demand rates much higher than others get for identical procedures. So it is encouraging that the US Department of Justice is investigating possible antitrust violations by Partners HealthCare, the parent of Massachusetts General Hospital and Brigham and Women's Hospital.

The market clout of Partners—and that of hospitals with geographic monopolies, like Berkshire Medical Center in Pittsfield—pushes rates up and contributes to annual increases in insurance premiums that greatly exceed the cost-of-living index. That was one conclusion of a report earlier this year by Massachusetts Attorney General Martha Coakley. Coakley's report found that higher hospital rates did not reflect greater quality of care or complexity of cases. Yet costs to the system rose as consumers flocked to high-prestige settings with higher costs but not necessarily higher quality.

That makes the need for government action all the more crucial. The playing field for providers, insurers, and consumers must be level and transparent. There are other areas of the country where dominant hospitals have much the same pricing power as Partners does.[6]

Many dominant hospital systems are also already well ahead in the development of ACOs and are recruiting primary care and specialist physician practices into their ACO network. Sutter Health, one of California's largest health systems with 24 acute-care hospitals and large numbers of physicians who have already signed exclusivity contracts with the system, has some of the highest hospital prices in the state. In geographic areas where it is dominant, health insurers will be unable to offer policies to employers unless Sutter's ACO offerings are included. This removes pricing power from the insurers. Sutter's market share in these geographies will allow it to command significantly higher prices. It may also allow it to be less accountable for the ACO-promised better quality as, again, insurers in these geographic regions will continue to make Sutter ACO offerings available. This concern was raised in a *New York Times* article:

Consumer advocates fear that the health care law could worsen some of the very problems it was meant to solve—by reducing competition, driving up costs and creating incentives for doctors and hospitals to stint on care, in order to retain their cost-savings bonuses. "The new law is already encouraging a wave of mergers, joint ventures and alliance in the health care industry," said Prof. Thomas L. Greaney, an expert of health and antitrust law at St. Louis University. "The risk that dominant providers and dominant insurers may exercise their market power, individually or jointly, has never been greater."[7]

Mergers outside the healthcare industry may provide a glimpse of the future. The period of high-flying mergers and acquisitions in the general commercial sector subsequently led to a less than exciting and sometimes traumatic period of divestitures and fraudulent conveyances. Businesses that had merged later discovered that the gains expected from the mergers were not to be found. Idiosyncratically, parts of the healthcare industry have exhibited the same cycle of merger followed by divestiture. Until provider networks become more stable, the naming of competitors may be possible only on a short-term basis.

Analysis of Competitive Position

The development of a good marketing strategy requires an analysis of the organization's competitive position. Customer-oriented analysis is one possibility; this approach involves determining who the customers are, what benefits and values they seek, and how well the organization is providing those benefits and values to the customers compared to how well the competition is doing so. Then, if one or more of the competitors are doing a better job of delivering the desired benefits to the customer, the organization investigates further to determine which of the competitors' activities it needs to emulate or, if possible, surpass in order to equal or exceed the competition.

Competitor-oriented analysis, a second form of competitive analysis, involves benchmarking. With this technique, the organization regularly compares its performance on key performance attributes and benefits desired by the customer against the "best in class." Benchmarking allows the organization to get a sense of context; it provides the organization with answers to questions such as: Where do we stand in the marketplace? How far behind the strongest or best competitors are we? What will it take for us to draw ourselves up to an equal level of performance with our best competitors?

Another useful tool is a perceptual map. An organization positions itself and its competitors along a two-axis grid according to the variables that the two axes represent (see **Figure 6-1**). For example, consumers often compare hospitals on the basis of whether they are teaching hospitals (or whether they provide tertiary care) or community hospitals (which provide nontertiary basic acute care). They also often compare hospitals on the basis of their nursing and support staff care being friendly, warm, and responsive, and on the nurse-to-patient ratio. Through the use of market research, a hospital can ask a sample of consumers in its service area to rate it and its competing hospitals on these two attributes. Then, using these research findings, the hospital can position all the hospitals that the consumers rated along these two axes (see Figure 6-1). In addition, the hospital can, with further research, determine where the consumer segments in the market are positioned. For example, the people inside the oval marked <1> care primarily about being in a tertiary

care or teaching hospital, even if that means not receiving the friendliest or warmest care. For them, a community hospital, such as hospitals E, F, or G, would not be satisfactory. Those who fall inside the oval marked <3> prefer to go to the local community hospital. They obviously trust the community hospital to provide adequate acute care, and they want the friendliness and warmth that they feel a community hospital is more likely to provide. Clearly, this would be the segment to which hospital E would appeal. Those in the oval marked <2> are not willing to sacrifice friendly, warm care, nor do they want to forgo the capacity for tertiary care. Hospital B best meets their needs, followed by hospital D. In comparing the position of the consumer segments with the position of the various hospitals on the perceptual map, it becomes apparent that hospitals C, F, and G may want to modify their positioning in the marketplace to attract a larger portion of the existing market segments.

Innovative Sources of Competition

Competition sometimes comes from unexpected places. Disruptive innovations, often dismissed in their earliest stages because they represent something other than "business as usual," have the potential to change the market landscape and the market's behavior. One example of this is MinuteClinic and similar retail health clinics. MinuteClinic, a subsidiary of CVS Caremark Corporation, is the largest of the retail health clinic chains. The clinics are staffed by nurse practitioners (NPs) and physician assistants (PAs), follow rigid evidence-based medical protocols, and limit what they treat to the most common acute medical problems that NPs and PAs are able to treat. MinuteClinic visits are very affordable relative

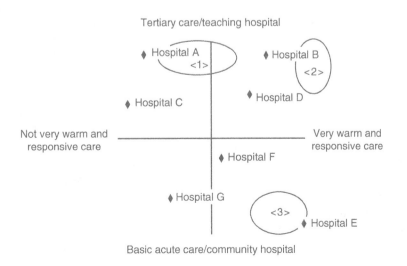

Figure 6-1 Medical practices: two-axis grid.

to the cost of a visit to a physician's office, and especially in contrast to an emergency room visit. MinuteClinics are also very accessible; located in CVS pharmacies, they require no appointments, taking patients on a first-come, first-served basis, and are open 7 days a week, into the early evening on weekdays, as well as weekends during the day. They combine aspects of the accessibility of a hospital emergency room with an even lower price than a visit to the physician's office.

Originally dismissed as "mall medicine," these retail-based health services are now being recognized for their innovative approach to dealing with high healthcare costs coupled with a growing shortage of primary care physicians. Many young physicians are choosing to work fewer hours than their predecessors,[8] meaning less time available to see patients. Added to this, the Patient Protection and Affordable Care Act (PPACA) promises to add 16 million people to the Medicaid rolls by 2014, yet many PCPs have already indicated an unwillingness to bring new Medicaid patients into their practices due to low Medicaid reimbursement.[9] The increase in previously uninsured people who will be covered by health insurance under the new law is expected to dramatically exacerbate the physician shortage that had already been predicted years before, during the Bush administration.

In light of this shortage, MinuteClinic's innovative approach seems to target the problem directly by bringing down costs and increasing access. Insurers have begun to integrate MinuteClinics and similar services into larger healthcare networks (with many of these networks soon to become ACOs) where the clinics will become part of the local healthcare system. MinuteClinic will also be well able to address one of the pillars of the ACO concept, that of medical homes, because more than half of all MinuteClinic patients are medically homeless. Moreover, as pointed out in a presentation by Dr. Andrew Sussman, the president and COO of MinuteClinic, along with Dr. Joe Jabre, the founder of TeleEMG.com, another innovative medical solution, it makes little sense for physicians, after 12 years in school, 4 years in college, 4 years in medical school, and another 3–8 years in internship and residency, to spend their time doing throat cultures and similarly less demanding tasks when these can easily be performed by NPs and PAs. As both innovators pointed out, "we cannot afford the current system."[10]

Many innovations in the healthcare sector are technological in nature. Some compete with current service providers; others complement them. There are, for example, a mind-boggling number of apps (software applications) that provide medical information or address ways of keeping healthy. There are drug reference apps like Epocrates, a popular resource that contains information on both prescription and over-the-counter drugs, and general reference apps like the Merck Manual, which contains information on thousands of medical issues. There are also websites to which patients may turn to learn more about their disease as well as to network with each other. One example is the website, PatientsLikeMe.com. Because patients input data on the website on the efficacy and side effects of their medications and on the outcomes of their treatments, they may know more than do their physicians about the newest ways to deal with their disease, a situation considered by some physicians to be a bit unsettling. Still, in 2007, the company (PatientsLikeMe.com) won recognition as one of the "15 Companies that Will Change the World" from CNN Money.[11]

Many innovations address problems that the healthcare world had yet to successfully solve. Project RED, the shortened name for the Project Re-Engineered Hospital Discharge, targets preventable hospital readmissions. The Agency for Healthcare Research and Quality (AHRQ) cites 4.4 million hospital stays as resulting from preventable causes. The physician behind the innovation, Brian Jack, stated: "There are loose ends, there are communication problems, there is poor quality information, there is poor preparation, there is fragmentation of care, and there is great variability. . . . It is no surprise that there are many adverse events post discharge."[12] At the heart of many preventable readmissions lie poorly coordinated care, including unreconciled medications; still-pending test results and still-needed tests; poorly communicated discharge instructions; and rushed staff who don't have adequate time to spend with patients who are leaving the hospital. His innovative solution to this problem was to create a virtual discharge assistant named Louise, a software program that, relying on the input of information from a discharge advocate, generates a thorough posthospital care plan that includes information about medications (how much, how often, what the pills look like), follow-up appointments, and other instructions relative to caring for oneself after leaving the hospital. Although a discharge advocate, who may be one of the always extremely busy nurses, spends some amount of time with the patient discussing the discharge plan, Louise, presented on-screen as an animated face with a pleasant voice, can "talk" with patients, answering questions that are routinely asked by patients leaving the hospital, can show emotion, and can ask each patient questions that require the patient to respond to be certain that he or she is paying attention and that the patient actually understands the information presented. This frees up the nurses to carry out their other duties for which there is no substitute innovative solution.

Could one say that Project RED competes with nurses, in that it replaces the nurse for part of the discharge process? The answer is yes, but with hospitals keeping their nursing staff numbers low in order to control costs, this type of competition, which lessens the burden on hospital nurses, is a welcome form of competition. The AHRQ reported that the use of Project RED's virtual discharge assistant prevented one emergency room readmission for every 7.3 discharge patients, resulting in significant cost savings.[12]

Innovations in healthcare may evoke fear and concern in some due to their direct competitive nature, or they may bring about relief because they successfully tackle problems that have not previously been solved. Either way, the flow of healthcare innovations will continue.

■ Business-to-Business Marketing

The need to market to businesses and organizations, referred to as industrial, business-to-business, or organizational marketing, remains as strong as ever. Whether the target market consists of employers, the government, insurers, physician groups, healthcare oversight groups like the Leapfrog Group, or managed-care and accountable-care organizations, the nature of business-to-business marketing remains the same: Marketers must be skilled in organizational analysis in order to understand to whom to sell and what to sell. Failure to identify the decision-making unit or buying center, as it is called in a business-to-business marketing setting, is likely to result in unsuccessful marketing efforts. Thus, marketers must know who within the organization plays the roles of initiator, influencer, decider, purchaser, gatekeeper, and user.

Historically, for example, pharmaceutical companies hired salespeople to sell existing and new drugs to physicians, who then prescribed or recommended them to their patients. In this scenario, the physician was the decider, and the patient was the user (and often the purchaser as well). Increasingly, however, organizational healthcare providers such as hospitals and health insurers are examining the cost and efficacy of the various drugs available and using their findings to create formularies that specify the drugs that their physicians may prescribe. The individuals who select drugs for the formularies (e.g., infectious disease physicians, pharmacists, quality assurance nurses) are now the initial deciders. The practicing physician can decide on a drug only within the limited set of formulary drugs (unless the patient alerts the physician of his or her willingness to pay out of pocket for a specific medication). A pharmaceutical company that continued to sell its drugs only to physicians and did not attempt to address the formularies might unnecessarily lose significant business. Pharmacy benefit managers, who are often employed by pharmaceutical companies to contain pharmaceutical costs for employers or insurance entities, continue to sell to physicians; in recognition of the influence and decision-making power of hospital and insurer organizations in the purchase of pharmaceuticals, their marketing efforts remain within the limits of the drugs approved for the formulary.

A buyflow map permits a more systematic analysis of a buying center. It traces the buying process through the customer's recognition of need that presumably must be met through the purchase of a good or service, specification of a technical product or service, potential supplier identification, solicitation of proposals, selection of a supplier, negotiation of the final contract, and performance evaluation. The map identifies who, within the customer's organization, participates in each step of the process, in what order each person affects the process, and where the process slows and may need the further attention of the supplier (marketer).

Organizational buyers are fewer in number than are consumers (individual buyers), but they represent larger overall volumes of purchases. For example, a physician can "sell" more streptococcus test services to a preferred provider organization (PPO) than to an individual consumer or family within 1 year. Because of the smaller number of business buyers, the investment in analyzing their buying center behavior may be less, even though the potential purchase volumes are greater.

The analysis of an organization's buying centers may take at least two forms. Snowball research within the target organization entails asking the individuals within the organization thought to be involved in the purchase to identify all others within the organization who might also influence the particular purchase. The analysis proceeds by determining the role that each named individual plays, soliciting from those individuals more names, identifying the roles of those newly named, and continuing until no new names are given. The sum of this type of information usually allows the marketer to detect who plays what role in the decision-making unit/buying center.

Focus group research is the other most common source of information in organizational analysis. This approach generally involves a number of similar organizations rather than just one. For example, a medical device and equipment company had traditionally sold to hospitals, as part of its wide product line, clinical networks on which hospitals could run their clinical devices such as telemetry and patient monitoring. The company was now planning to enter the LAN (local area network) data network arena, hoping that it could persuade hospitals of the value of combining the company's clinical and medical device wireless networks with the hospital infrastructure wireless networks. The clinical network sales process usually relied heavily on clinician input to the decision-making unit; in fact, clinicians were usually the ultimate decider in the purchase process. However, the company was uncertain who should be the target of its promotion and personal selling for the product solution that combined the clinical and data networks. They specifically needed to identify the influencers and deciders within the hospital IT departments who would drive the hospital to pursue the company's proposed single network strategy. Therefore, the company held six focus groups with a variety of people in both the related clinical departments and the IT departments in order to assess who would be the likeliest deciders and influencers in the purchase of this new product.

The expansion of the marketing of certain healthcare products and services is going beyond traditional organizational buyers to include consumers. The reclassification of certain previously ethical drugs (those that consumers could buy only with a prescription from a physician) to over-the-counter (OTC) drugs, and the decreasing influence of physicians over which drugs may be prescribed for a patient (because of pharmacy benefits managers, and insurer and hospital formularies) have resulted in a dramatic explosion in pharmaceutical advertising directed to consumers. This direct-to-consumer advertising boom for prescription as well as over-the-counter pharmaceutical products has caused such pressures on physicians to prescribe according to the patient's wishes that many physicians have become incensed at their loss of power; some health insurers are supporting political efforts to limit the extent of this advertising, given that the most heavily advertised products are also often among the most expensive in their product categories, although not necessarily the most efficacious.

Patients are playing a more active role in determining their own treatment, sometimes appropriately so, sometimes not. In recognition that some products and services should remain in the business-to-business marketing domain, the Food and Drug Administration (FDA) has stepped in, determining on a case-by-case basis whether certain genetic tests sold directly to consumers should instead be supplied only through physicians or if at least the results should be delivered only through physicians. These include tests for inherited disorders such as cystic fibrosis, breast and ovarian cancer, and Alzheimer's disease, as well as tests that purport to

predict how a patient will respond to a particular drug. The accuracy and reliability of the tests is not yet well determined, because the field is new, emanating from the U.S. Human Genome Project, which began in 1990. Of equal concern is the potential for misuse of the tests, mistakes in the testing process, and misunderstanding of the test results.[13]

This movement of greater influence and decision-making power being placed in the hands of consumers, called participatory medicine, is clearly unstoppable. The rise of social networks like Facebook and PatientsLikeMe.com allows patients to find each other and discuss the progression of their diseases and treatment efficacy. Type in the name of almost any disease in the "Search" box of Facebook and you will find one or more disease-specific discussion groups, fundraising groups, groups that converge to underwrite drug research and development and help direct research priorities, and other forms of disease-related online communities. The decision-making unit in business-to-business settings is now increasingly likely to have consumers actively participating in one or more decision-making roles. Marketers whose expertise had in the past been limited only to organizational selling must also learn how to market directly to consumers.

■ Derived Demand

Some marketers believe that consumer marketing should not require as much attention as does business-to-business marketing in the healthcare marketplace. They rationalize that employers make the first choice of health plans, before the individual employees are given any purchase choices, and that health plan members sometimes must choose their physicians or hospitals from panels approved by their health plan. Therefore, they conclude that the individual plays a less significant role in healthcare purchase decisions.

This set of beliefs does not take into account derived demand. For example, a hospital is trying to convince the management of a new health insurer to the area that it should be the insurer's primary hospital. Although factors such as the hospital's willingness to negotiate on price and the extent to which it can provide the full range of medical care will influence the insurer, the desirability of the hospital to the insurer's potential members is a key consideration. If the insurer's potential members consider the hospital unacceptable as the insurer's primary hospital, then the insurer itself will be a less attractive health plan and will have difficulty enrolling members. The insurer derives its demand in part from the attractiveness of the hospital(s) to which it sends patients, as well as from the physicians who are on its panel.

In essence, derived demand requires a two-stage marketing process. The marketer must develop a set of products and services to appeal not only to the immediate customer, but also to the customer of the immediate customer. In the near future, a large medical group practice could choose to make itself attractive to an ACO by agreeing to significant discounts. To reduce costs sufficiently to permit these discounts, however, the medical group may understaff and, as a result, deny quick or easy access for patient/physician visits to all but the sickest patients. Although the discounts initially may be appealing to the ACO, the lack of access would soon become apparent to the patients, would make the medical practice unattractive to them, and would cause them to steer away from this practice in future enrollment periods. Thus, the ACO would derive little long-term demand from consumers through contracting with this practice. Ultimately, with little derived demand, this practice would become unattractive to the ACO. Medical groups that denied non-life-threatening but needed care to patients in the hope of cutting costs enough to earn the promised ACO bonuses would also suffer from a decline in derived demand, once the patients had accumulated enough experience with the practice to recognize that the practice was placing its financial concerns above patients' concerns.

With the right information available, derived demand offers marketers an opportunity to influence business-to-business buyer behavior. Any healthcare provider (of significant size) that can produce credible market research to establish consumer preference for its services within its target market area is in a good position to negotiate with insurers, employers, ACOs, other organizational buyers, and potential contract partners; the stated consumer preference indicates that the provider can bring to the organization derived demand for its services. Similarly, these other entities do their own consumer preference research to identify the providers that are so attractive to consumers that their presence on the healthcare provider list overwhelms the need for a significant discount from them.

The key to using derived demand is information—market research data on consumer preferences and on consumers' intended use or purchase behavior. Customer repeat purchase and retention data are also useful information here. The relatively unsophisticated research that continues to characterize many healthcare marketing efforts does not uncover derived demand very well. Asking consumers if they prefer hospital A to hospital B may establish a preference for one over the other, but it does not assess any tradeoff that consumers may be willing to make, such as accepting the less-preferred provider for a specified lower premium or more convenient location. To capture this level of information, it is probably necessary to do a trade-off analysis, commonly called conjoint measurement. This market research methodology requires the identification of those variables that appear most likely to affect a buyer's purchase decision (in a specific, not generic, type of purchase situation). These variables include those that make it possible to measure the attractiveness to the consumer at different levels, such as a $5 vs. $10 vs. $20 copay per visit. Each of the variables, at different levels, is combined with other variables and presented as a package to the consumer interviewee, who is asked to assess the attractiveness of the overall package. For example, a shortened version of two packages for a PPO might be

Option A

- $5 copay
- Primary care visits with nurse practitioner
- Acute illness appointments available within 48 hours
- Admits to most preferred hospital in the area

Option B

- $20 copay
- Primary care visits with a physician
- Acute illness appointments available within 24 hours
- Admits to moderately preferred hospital in the area

The consumer is asked to rate the preferability of several of these packages. Using an algorithm, conjoint analysis can determine which variables at which levels prove to be most attractive to the consumer, and when to trade off one variable for another. Most healthcare organizations do not have the capability to carry out this type of market research and analysis in-house, but market research firms should be qualified to do so. Over time, healthcare marketers may add this type of research to their expected set of skills. Other research approaches, recommended by Berry and Parasuraman, include transactional surveys, which focus on customers' most recent service experiences with the organization rather than the totality of their experiences; mystery shopping in both one's own and competing services to evaluate the quality of services delivered; focus group interviews; service reviews (a formal process of periodic visits with customers to discuss the service relationship); customer complaint and inquiry systems; employee field reporting and surveys; and a system to track and analyze operating data, such as service response times and waiting times.[15]

Some network managers have failed to take derived demand into account. For some, the natural tendency has been to put together the lowest-cost hospitals and practices. As a result, their provider list may not have tertiary care facilities, the local women's health center, or a specialty children's hospital, for example. The network managers' assumption underlying this choice of providers is that low cost will outweigh all other considerations. This is the philosophy being espoused by the Steward Health Care System, the new name given by the private equity purchaser, Cerberus Capital Management, to the former financially ailing Caritas Christi health system, which was composed largely of Catholic hospitals in the eastern part of Massachusetts. All the Caritas Christi hospitals were suffering from poor financial performance, with only 40 days of cash available in the whole system in March 2009. Since the subsequent purchase of Caritas Christi, Steward has purchased a number of other small hospitals, most also in poor financial shape. The marketing strategy underlying the purchase of Caritas Christi, as well as of the small hospitals purchased since the name change, was spelled out in an article in the local newspaper. The article, referring to the Steward CEO, was subtitled "He stunned the medical world by getting a private equity giant to buy a group of debt-drowning community hospitals."[16] Speaking of the CEO of Steward, it said:

> As he sees it, through investment in information technology and bricks-and-mortar hospitals, he will be able to offer a highly integrated "accountable care organization" that gives patients quality care, close to home, thereby keeping costs down. The key is insisting that patients get all but the most complex care from their community hospital, rather than seeking treatment for pneumonia or a broken arm at a big shop like Mass. General.[16]

The challenge that Steward now faces is that of both consumer demand and derived demand. Consumers were not visiting these hospitals in sufficient numbers to keep them financially solvent before the Cerberus purchase. The private equity firm's investment in IT and bricks-and-mortar might bring small changes in consumer preference, but not enough to keep patients away from the more expensive teaching hospitals when they feel that they need to receive their medical care there. Although ACOs will be responsible for holding healthcare costs down and will therefore find value in lower-cost hospitals, the better run ACOs will understand derived demand and will recognize that Steward's marketing strategy is unlikely

to work. This is especially true because ACOs cannot, as the Steward CEO suggested above, "insist that patients get all but the most complex care from their community hospital."[16] The public acceptance of the ACO model is predicated upon consumer choice. Consumers in the United States have been raised in a healthcare environment where they have chosen their medical providers based on perceived healthcare quality first, particularly when it comes to acute and inpatient care. For many patients, cost is secondary to access to preferred high-quality providers. Moreover, if those for whom cost is the primary concern find, once in the network, that they are unhappy with the quality of the services, they are likely at the next purchase decision-making point or enrollment period to search out another network or ACO, even at a slightly greater cost. Failure to consider derived demand may be effective in the short run, but it is likely to create a higher turnover of customers in the long run.

◼ Consumer Behavior: Availability of Information

The overwhelming availability of healthcare information has changed the way consumers make their healthcare choices. This flow of information began as a small stream two decades ago and has now hit flood stage. In the early 1990s, employers were beginning to collect information that they could share with their employees. For example, three large employers (GTE, the former Digital Equipment, and Xerox) surveyed a sizable sample of their employees regarding their satisfaction with their healthcare providers, including managed-care organizations, and reported the results to all geographically relevant employees.[17] This "report card" on healthcare providers and managed-care organizations presumably allowed employees to compare these organizations intelligently and make informed choices. The National Committee on Quality Assurance (NCQA) has been producing report cards on health plans since the mid-1990s; report cards of various types, mainly local and regional, began to appear with greater frequency in the late 1990s and early 2000s. By the late 2000s, NCQA health plan ratings represented a combination of Healthcare Effectiveness Data and Information Set (HEDIS) ratings, Consumer Assessment of Healthcare Providers and Systems (CAHPS) scores, and NCQA accreditation scores. The Patient Protection and Affordable Care Act of 2010 (PPACA) links health plan reimbursement rates for Medicare Advantage to these report cards, based on ratings of how well the plans manage chronic disease conditions, keep their members well through the use of preventive screenings and use of vaccines, show responsiveness to their members, respond to complaints and customer problems, and deliver supportive telephone customer service. Further ratings appear in the form of the Physician Quality Reporting Initiative, which was expanded in 2010 as part of the PPACA. It reports on 131 clinical quality measures as part of a physician quality reporting system. The Centers for Medicare and Medicaid Services has now posted these data on a "Physician Compare" website.

In theory, consumers should be able to make well-informed choices because so much information about health plan performance is provided. The website ConsumerHealthRatings.com provides health insurance plan ratings from the perspective of consumers, hospitals, and physician groups. On the site, consumers can find multiple sources of health plan ratings, including from J.D. Power, The Street.com, *U.S. News & World Report*, and *Consumer Reports*. The ratings movement has now spread with increasing velocity beyond hospitals and health insurers to physician practices. As a *New York Times* article reported: "Medical groups that perform heart bypass surgery are now being rated alongside cars and toaster ovens in *Consumer Reports*."[18] Local magazines all over the country provide an annual list of the best regional physicians and hospitals. The Massachusetts Department of Public Health offers ratings of all the state's skilled nursing facilities on its website, and updates them every 6 months, based on semiannual surveys of the facilities. HealthGrades (www.healthgrades.com) allows users to search for ratings on over 5,000 hospitals and more than 15,000 nursing homes for a small (less than $10) fee. Further, HealthGrades provides wide-ranging physician-specific information including languages spoken, insurance accepted, awards won, and ratings by other patients in response to questions like "Would you recommend your physician to family/friends?" and "Do you trust your physician to make decisions/recommendations that are in your best interests?"

Many other sources have added or are adding themselves to the list of healthcare information providers who provide comparative information on healthcare providers and insurers. Angie's List, which originally focused on home improvement services, now also rates clinicians. Some state websites also list malpractice litigation decisions and state oversight findings. Even Yelp, a city-by-city website started in 2004 to allow people to rate local businesses (and which reported that more than 45 million people had visited a Yelp website in the month of January 2011 alone) carries consumer ratings (1–5 stars), comments, and complaints on all types of health and medical services.

From a marketing and consumer behavior perspective, the implications are enormous. Historically, the dissonance reduction model of consumer behavior, under which consumers make a high involvement (i.e., very important) decision with very little information, has characterized most annual healthcare enrollment or purchase behavior. To assure themselves that they are not making the wrong decision, consumers often choose what they perceive to be the safe choice: the most well-known organization, the organization recommended by the benefits clerk (the most immediately available expert to someone who is enrolling in a healthcare plan at work), or the organization in which they already have been enrolled, where the feeling of safety is based on personal experience. Rarely, in the recent past, have consumers incorporated valid, objective, and comprehensive provider and insurance carrier information into their decision-making process,[19] in no small part because the information had not been available.

Consumer Behavior: Information Search and Use

The growing availability of new information on healthcare providers and carriers suggests that a far larger portion of the population will behave, or at least try to behave, according to the complex buying behavior model. The basic assumption of the complex buying behavior model is that all purchase behavior is information based; consumers compare and contrast purchase alternatives, form intelligent opinions regarding the alternatives, and purchase based on these informed opinions. For those able to analyze the somewhat complex information related to healthcare plans, hospitals, and physician practices, the option to behave according to the complex buying behavior model may now be available. Many health plans and some physician practices now list the physicians online, noting those who are willing to take more patients, sometimes indicating languages spoken in the practice, and occasionally the office hours. Along with online information from sites like the NCQA, this information should allow consumers to do research and obtain information about their healthcare choices. Marketers should be sensitive to consumers' desire for data and should constantly be attuned to what the data say about the quality of the organization's healthcare services. For the marketer, this database should be a welcome addition (if it does not already exist) to the tools used for continuous quality improvement.

Unfortunately, it is clear that consumers are not receiving all the information that they want. Moreover, some of the attributes important to the consumer, such as the denial of access to a specialist when it is necessary, are difficult to measure. Consumer self-reports of needing to see a specialist may be inflated; patients may think they need a specialist when, in fact, they do not. The reporting organization, on the other hand, has an incentive to downplay the number of reports of denied access to specialists. Because the task of measuring a void, of measuring what did not happen, is usually more difficult than measuring what did happen, this information is generally not reported, yet it is exactly this type of information that will be particularly important if and when ACOs become a major structure of delivery in the healthcare landscape. Because primary care physicians will once again, as they did under managed care, be expected to be the gatekeepers (i.e., to steer patients to acceptable but cost-effective options for their care) of care, there are already reports of concern that they—and the rest of the ACO—will have incentives to curb spending and as a result also curb the use of specialists and other more expensive options for care in order to earn the bonuses promised for keeping costs down.

Other types of consumer-desired data not only are not measured, but also represent the type of data that the provider may not wish to have measured. Most people, for example, before selecting a health plan or PCP would want to know the average amount of time one must wait to make a nonurgent appointment with the PCP. Many components of service quality, such as waiting time, physician's acceptance and knowledge of alternative medicine, and willingness to take on top-down medical protocols when he or she does not think that the protocol is in the best interest of the patient, are difficult to measure, sensitive in an organizational political sense, and therefore not reported.

More significantly, research has shown that consumers are not using much of the data provided to them. In their study, Tumlinson and associates provided a wide range of information to consumers.[20] These researchers found that, although consumers consider specific plan benefits, premium costs, and out-of-pocket costs essential information when choosing a healthcare plan, they seldom use such information as the ratings of plans by independent experts, the percentage of members who are satisfied with the overall plan, and comparisons in the convenience of the administrative paperwork. Other research has shown that consumers do not use much of the information provided, particularly if it cannot be easily and readily understood.[21,22] Scanlon et al. found that, when presented with seven health plan report cards, only 34% of consumers used them at all

in making their health plan selection.[23] The elderly, in particular, have difficulty in utilizing the information presented to them in health plan report cards.[24] Hibbard and associates discovered that even employers (that is, the managers within companies who were responsible for selecting healthcare plans for the company's employees and who should have been knowledgeable about healthcare plan data), did not use much of the information made available to them, nor did they seek out other information that could have allowed for a more informed purchase choice.[25] Therefore, it appears that, even if far more data were available, many healthcare purchasers may continue to act according to the dissonance reduction model.

One reason for the failure to use available information is lack of medical literacy, a subject that has received significant attention recently. The same skills that would allow someone to analyze the complex information now available to make informed healthcare purchase choices are also the skills that would allow someone to be medically literate. It has been estimated that roughly 80 million adults, that is, 36% of the adults in the United States, suffer from limited health literacy.[26] The AHRQ reported, not surprisingly, that the elderly, those with less education, minorities, and the poor were more likely to demonstrate limited medical literacy. They were also more likely to suffer from a greater number of hospitalizations, greater use of emergency rooms, lower vaccination rates, and poorer medical outcomes, suggesting that their care is more costly. The AHRQ studies examined not only print literacy, but also numeracy (the ability to use and understand numbers) and reported that the two are highly correlated. Because many of the online health provider and insurer ratings as well as health report card ratings are numerical, for those 80 million adults with health literacy difficulties, these information offerings are of little help if they cannot be understood.[27] The care of those with medical literacy challenges tends to be more costly, so all providers in one or more ACOs would be wise to recognize the need to address the medical literacy challenges faced by those patients for whom they will be held financially accountable. Recognizing the importance of this issue, in April 2011, the Centers for Disease Control and Prevention set up a website, www.cdc.gov/healthliteracy, entitled "Health Literacy: Accurate, Accessible and Actionable Health Information for All," to provide guidance to those in the healthcare system who recognize the need to address failure to comprehend needed health-related information. Available information is not truly available if it is not intellectually accessible.

Consumer Behavior: Integrity and Validity of Information

Much depends not only on the availability of the data, but also on the integrity and validity of the information. For example, there is a great deal of generic healthcare and medical data on the Internet. Between 60% and 80% of consumers in the United States have sought health information on the Internet and, as reported in early 2008, consumers were as likely to get their health information from the Internet as they were to get it from their physicians.[28] It can empower patients and give them a great deal of information about their diagnoses and potential treatments, but it can also mislead them. No one is charged with reviewing studies or data cited on the Internet, in contrast with refereed medical journals; yet, one of the two most common reasons for logging on to the Internet is to obtain health information. Currently, there is no way to judge how much of this information is correct and how much may do harm. The PPACA does include plans for a healthcare.gov website, which will provide healthcare information as well as information on insurance coverage. Although the information on this site will be well vetted and will therefore likely be valid, this will not stop consumers from seeking information on other sites as well.

Another problem arises if the aggregation of healthcare data changes its meaning. For example, the healthcare services within healthcare organizations are of variable quality. An aggregation, averaging, or collapsing of the data makes them easier for everyone to use; some of the consumers report excellent experiences, whereas others report terrible experiences, which could average out simply to mediocre experiences. Failure to note the extremes could easily mislead those who wish to use and are capable of using the full range of data. A healthcare organization with a bimodal distribution of satisfaction ratings could hide the high level of dissatisfaction on the low end by reporting only means or medians. Moreover, Nuovo et al. reported that medical researchers generally report their findings in a way that makes the results seem better than they are.[29] Of 359 studies in leading medical journals, only 18 reported absolute risk reduction; the rest reported only relative risk reduction, which artificially magnifies the reduction of risk and the benefit provided from the intervention or treatment.

It may be difficult to promulgate objective information. One method of reporting aggregated information that can help to overcome this problem is to provide not only the means and medians, but also more complete information on the unaggregated data: How many answer categories were there? What percentage of the respondents fell into the lowest category? What percentage fell into the highest category? (If the audience were sufficiently sophisticated, one would report in terms of standard deviations.) A survey of customer satisfaction ratings with answers ranging from 1 to 5 (where 1 is extremely satisfied and 5 is extremely dissatisfied) may show a mean rating of 3 for both HMO A and HMO B. This may suggest that the HMOs are performing similarly in terms of satisfying the customer. However, if only 2% of those rating HMO A responded by rating it a 5, but 14% of those rating HMO B gave it a rating of 5 (which HMO B offset with a high number of 1 ratings), the potential customer may be far more likely to experience extreme dissatisfaction in HMO B than in HMO A.

Some marketers may find themselves under pressure to use the data to portray their healthcare organization in the best possible light, even if that portrayal is misleading or incomplete. In this scenario, a marketer takes the single best rating or set of ratings and positions the organization on that one rating or set while ignoring the other ratings. For example, a hospital may receive very high ratings on nursing care while receiving average or below-average ratings on maintaining its physical plant, having up-to-date diagnostic equipment, having a wide array of specialists, and providing coordinated care. The hospital management, in the interests of best representing the hospital, may then advertise that the hospital provides some of the best nursing care in the area.

From a policy perspective, the danger is that many consumers will rely on the advertisements, which may represent predigested information, rather than on the full body of information available. Few advertisements are likely to provide information that portrays the organization negatively, after all; the job of advertising is generally to sell the organization, not to de-market it. (De-marketing is the act of making a product, service, or organization less marketable.) The subjugation of available and/or required data from informing the consumer to selling the consumer has been a common practice in other industries and can be expected in the healthcare industry as the government, employers, or other outside bodies require the collection of outcome, medical error, and satisfaction databases. Although the consumer and employer may wish, if they could, to use the collected data and act by the complex buying behavior model, the act of analyzing large amounts of data is foreign to most people.[30] The natural tendency, then, is to substitute the predigested data, as presented in an advertising form or in a format that is oversimplified by the data collectors.

It is not yet reasonable to assume that the relevant data will be available. One problem in reporting customer quality perceptions and satisfaction data is the failure of senior management in many healthcare organizations to budget for the measurement of the data.[31] New requirements by the government, by accrediting organizations, or by employers force healthcare organizations to budget for the collection of such data, but because this is still relatively new for most healthcare organizations, the data measures continue not to be standardized from organization to organization. What one hospital or ACO labels as a condition leading to high consumer satisfaction (e.g., a 30-minute wait for urgent care) may be labeled as unacceptable by another hospital or ACO. These differences make it even more difficult for consumers to compare and contrast healthcare organizations intelligently.

As a result, the dissonance reduction model is likely to remain the predominant model of consumer behavior in the healthcare field, as it is in many other industries. Most people do not have the capacity or the desire to wade through the data and turn them into usable information, or they do not trust the integrity of the data. The healthcare industry does not yet have an independent, unbiased agency that can collect all the data that the consumer or employer would want, that could obtain an agreement among all the players in the healthcare industry regarding what information is the most relevant, that could objectively analyze it, and then present it in a trustworthy predigested format.

■ Consumer Behavior: The Role of Digital Communication

Electronic communication media have empowered patients as nothing else has ever done. They provide 24/7 access to health information that was heretofore not available to consumers unless they were willing to put in hours of library research. Because of the speed at which information is made available and updated electronically, digital media also sometimes allow the patient who is diligent in seeking the newest medical news to know of the latest medical research even before the patient's physician knows. This is a particularly likely scenario for patients with a chronic disease; over time dealing with their medical problem, they may become experts in their own disease, identifying and sometimes contributing to the most relevant and useful websites with regard to their specific disease and stage of disease. This last aspect, that of the patient contributing to the knowledge base about a disease, represents a paradigm shift in the creation and sharing of medical knowledge.

PatientsLikeMe (www.patientslikeme.com) is a social networking site in which patients dealing with the same disease talk to one another, identifying for each other successful and less successful treatments, discussing what to expect at various stages of the disease, and offering advice and comfort to each other. Because the patients report in real time how they are responding to specific treatments, with these responses often charted so that the website visitors can immediately learn, for example, if some new medication is causing unusual side effects or is performing better than the standard of care medication, not only patients visit these sites, but so do the pharmaceutical companies whose drugs might be used by the patients reporting on the site. Physicians, to serve their patients, and researchers also make use of this very current information.

Although PatientsLikeMe is the best known website of this type, it is certainly not the only one, and its colleague sites are fast expanding. ViroPharma launched a website to serve patients with the rare disease hereditary angioedema; previously, patients with orphan diseases (that is, rare diseases affecting small numbers of people) could seldom locate others with the same disease, making it nearly impossible for them to share their symptoms and disease-specific knowledge with others like them. Similarly, Genzyme, with the only drug available to treat Pompe disease, had multiple websites for patients with this disease; the websites not only allowed the patients to connect with each other, but also made it possible for Genzyme to monitor and immediately address any issues that patients raised about the usage of its drug.

This ability to connect and share information with other patients with the same medical issues was captured in a recent online article title "Patients Take On Expanded Role":

> "The patients are becoming much more involved in their own treatment. . . ." Among the factors empowering patients are the move towards personalized medicine, customizing health care based on genetic variability; a growing emphasis on "wellness" in an aging population through disease prevention; and the rise of social media enabling patients and doctors to form online communities. . . .
>
> . . .the drug Tysabri, made by Weston-based Biogen Idec Inc., is a popular topic among multiple sclerosis patients who register to take part in discussions on the Cambridge-based website Patients Like Me. While it is one of the most effective treatments for reducing MS relapse rates, it

can cause a rare brain infection known as PML, or progressive multifocal leukoencephalopathy, in about 1 of 1,000 patients.

Noting that Biogen Idec has developed a test to screen for the infection, Benjamin Heywood, president of Patients Like Me, said, "Patients are definitely talking about the risk-reward equation." . . . patients suffering from a variety of diseases and chronic conditions are overcoming what formerly was a stigma of discussing with others the progression of their illnesses and how they respond to different treatments. "People are realizing more and more the incredible value of sharing medical information."[14]

The popularity of digital media applications to maintain and improve one's health as well as to provide symptom and disease information continues to grow. The *Wall Street Journal* relates that, in the field of just diet and exercise, more than 400,000 apps (an application for a smartphone or other digital media) exist that can be accessed on mobile devices such as iPhones, iPads, Androids, and Blackberries. These include software applications such as Eat This, Not That; Fooducate; Nike+ GPS; and Hundred PushUps.[32] EverydayHealth.com, one of the fastest growing consumer health websites, not only provides an enormous breadth and depth of information on diseases, drugs, symptoms, food, fitness, health metrics, blogs, and a social network, all accessible from one's computer, it also has 23 health-related apps for mobile devices. One app involves a trainer from *The Biggest Loser*, another has a calorie counter. There are apps for physicians as well, such as the one featuring well-known physician Dr. Kevin Pho, who writes the blog KevinMD. Health information also can be found on Twitter, and one can click to have specific health tweets delivered automatically to one's smartphone.

The effect of the combination of immediate and easy access to the newest, most up-to-date content can result in a dramatic change in the patient's power within the decision-making unit. Whereas historically, it was the physician telling the uninformed patient what illness the patient suffered from and what the right course of action to take was, it may now be the patient who comes to the physician with an informed guess about the diagnosis (although it is also quite common that these informed guesses are wrong) and about the proper treatment plan. The patient may also know in advance of the physician that some new research has appeared that may affect the current decision regarding treatment efficacy. The empowerment of the patient has been viewed by many

as a significant paradigm shift, and indeed it is. However, it would be wise to keep in mind that there are still many patients who have little interest or, in some cases, little capability to trudge through the mountain of health and medical information now available. These patients will continue in many cases to turn to their physician for traditional guidance and decision making.

■ Consumer Behavior: Adoption of Innovation

In a world that is increasingly fast paced in terms of technological as well as other types of change, marketing must address not only selective demand marketing (i.e., "choose our brand over other brands"), but also the marketing of innovative offerings where the challenge is creating primary demand for a new product or service the market has not yet bought. An innovation also may represent significant change in behavior for the customer; any time a marketer has to change customer behavior, the marketing challenge can be daunting. The reasons for this were recognized back in the 1960s by Everett Rogers's definitive study on the adoption of innovation. He identified five segments, each operating somewhat differently in its willingness to and speed with which they would adopt new products or services, regardless of the type of industry being discussed. The segments varied in their speed to adopt from the fastest, the innovators, who represented 2.5% of the market, to the early adopters (13.5%), to the early majority (34%), the later majority (34%), and finally the laggards (16%). The adoption of innovation curve could be characterized as a bell-shaped curve, with the height of the curve at the line between the early and later majority. What is most notable is that it is very difficult to move the height of the curve to the left (that is, to get adoption to happen faster), closer to the innovators who are always the first to adopt.[33]

The innovators are two standard deviations to the left of the height of the curve, meaning that they are quite different from the majority (who fall within one standard deviation of the average adoption rate) in their willingness to adopt. Innovators tend to be risk takers; they also are often the best informed, most knowledgeable people in the product or service field. Because of this, they usually serve as key opinion leaders in their professional or work communities. The pharmaceutical and medical device industries have incorporated this knowledge into their marketing strategies, relying heavily on innovative physicians and researchers not only to carry out research on new drugs and medical devices, but also to speak at national conferences, to write in medical journals, and to become spokespeople for innovative products and services.

The pharmaceutical and medical device industries often find it easier to gain adoption of new products and services because, even though they may be innovative, they often do not require much if any behavior change from the market. A new cholesterol pill requires virtually no change in behavior at all from the physician, save for the writing of a different drug name on the prescription pad. (There should, of course, be after-the-fact monitoring of the patient for signs of side effects and ascertainment of efficacy, but these often don't play a role in the adoption of low-risk medications.) Many new medical devices do require the physician (often a surgeon) to retrain in order to learn the new system, hardware requirements, and so on related to a new medical device. This makes the adoption of more innovative products somewhat more difficult in this part of the health sector.

Equally difficult challenges are found in the service sector of the healthcare industry because most innovations in the provision of health services are disruptive. A prime example facing many medical practices today is the adoption of electronic medical records (EMR). The American Recovery and Reinvestment Act of 2009 provides physicians with incentives to adopt and meaningfully use electronic medical records. Further, because ACOs will require the clinical integration of hospitals and physician practices, this can really only be done through the use of EMR. Although incentives should certainly help motivate adoption of EMR, the challenges posed by the need to train physicians and other clinical staff in terms of order entry for medications and recording patients' medical histories on the computer will be costly and time consuming, requiring significant changes in work habits. This explains why 79% of surveyed hospital administrators were concerned that they would face resistance as they attempt to gain adoption of EMR by both physicians and other staff.[34] Clearly, adoption is easier to gain among those whose behaviors are not as ingrained. Younger staff have already shown a greater propensity to rely on iPads, given that they have grown up more tech-savvy. Some medical schools are requiring their medical students to use iPhones and/or iPod touch units, because of the immediate availability of medical references and medical images, and the ability to perform remotely such tasks as reviewing x-ray images. For medical students who are already conversant with technology lingo and applications, the use of EMR will come readily; they will fall into the early adopter or early majority category, depending upon the timing. Still, there will be

many physicians who will drag their feet, if only because the demands on their time are so great that they will engage in the necessary training in the use of EMR only when there is no other option. These are the late adopters or possibly laggards, some of whom may find ways to avoid EMR adoption altogether.

The lesson that marketers must understand is that, in order to market an innovation, one must first identify and solicit the active involvement of the key opinion leaders. In the health sector, these people can often be found in the academic positions in leading medical and other medically related professional schools. Because they usually carry out research, they are familiar with other key opinion leaders' research, and are aware of the newest practices, drugs, medical devices, and so on. They also are the professionals who often carry out the research that can bring about innovation. The respect held for them as innovators (the 2.5% who create the innovations or are the very earliest adopters) then leads the early adopters to feel safe in taking the risk of adopting a new relatively unknown technology, service, drug, or medical device. The late adopters come into play when the innovation has been used by enough of the market that the risk in use of the innovation has largely disappeared. The late majority will adopt later due to peer pressure, regulations, or heightened incentives; these individuals would possibly otherwise never adopt the innovation, a behavior that often characterizes the laggards. The marketing task to move an innovation through the adoption of innovation curve changes as one moves through the curve.

■ Differentiation: Quality

Marketers look to three variables that matter to consumers and, therefore, could act as differentiators: quality, cost, and access. The NCQA provides the Healthcare Effectiveness Data and Information Set (HEDIS) for quality management purposes; it is used by the vast majority of health plans in the United States to measure healthcare quality and healthcare services performance. Definitions of quality are anything but consistent across healthcare studies and healthcare consumers. The way in which the NCQA measures quality includes a number of early disease detection tests that many consumers perceive as largely irrelevant, for example. The measures of service quality that are now standard in the service marketing literature do not apply particularly well to healthcare settings. The focus on medical errors as a significant indicator of quality resulted in two reports from the Institute of Medicine, the more recent of which, "Crossing the

Quality Chasm," cites six dimensions of quality: timeliness, safety, effectiveness, efficiency, equity, and patient-centeredness, although one of the authors of the report, diverging somewhat from the report itself, states that "patients' experiences should be the fundamental source of the definition of quality."[35]

One of the most significant questions now being asked about healthcare quality as it concerns choices made by physicians in their care of patients is overtreatment. A *New England Journal of Medicine* article suggested that "unnecessary or inappropriate tests and procedures account for as much as 20% of health care expenditures" and noted these are wasted healthcare dollars that will be penalized under the ACO bundled payment system.[36] The concept of overtreatment is not new, however, having first been introduced by the work of John Wennberg, the pioneer in the research on regional variations in medical care. His research found that physician practice patterns varied dramatically based not on patient need, but on the way in which communities of physicians were trained to practice or chose to practice and on a number of non-patient-related factors. Using Medicare data, Wennberg introduced the Dartmouth Atlas of Health Care over a decade ago, visually demonstrating in multicolored maps of the United States the enormous variations in the use of medical resources and in the choices made by physicians in treating their patients. As noted in a summary of a *Journal of the American Medical Association* article, "Whether Chronic Diseases Are Diagnosed May Depend on Where You Live,"[37] on regional variations in medical practice and outcome:

> The likelihood of Medicare patients being diagnosed with a chronic disease may depend on where they live, a disparity that makes it more difficult to assess the quality of care patients receive, a new study finds. Certain groups of Medicare patients in regions with the most diagnoses also had a lower case-fatality rate for chronic conditions such as coronary artery disease and kidney failure, but the reasons for that are unclear, the researchers reported.
>
> It would stand to reason that whether a person is diagnosed with a chronic disease has to do with how ill they are, the researchers said. But instead, the findings suggest that chronic disease diagnosis is influenced by the "intensity of health care" in a particular region, which includes how many doctors and specialists are operating in a particular region, access to those doctors and the likelihood of doctors to send you to a specialist or to order lab and imaging tests.

> "The study suggests disease diagnosis is not only a property of the patient, but associated with the intensity with which health care is delivered in a region," said senior study author Dr. John Wennberg.[38]

Agreement as to what constitutes "quality medicine" is not close at hand. The debate continues to rage as to whether patients over the age of 50 should receive a colonoscopy vs. a sigmoidoscopy, whether bariatric surgery on obese teenagers constitutes good-quality medicine or is merely an undeclared clinical trial on an intervention whose long-term outcomes are unknown, and whether back pain should be treated by surgical intervention vs. other nonsurgical interventions. On this last point, a rheumatologist authored a book whose title testifies to too aggressive treatment: "Stabbed in the Back: Confronting Back Pain in an Overtreated Society."[39] Similarly, overtreatment across the health services, medical device, and pharmaceutical sectors of the health industry were documented in another well-received book, "Overtreated," by a former *Newsweek* writer.[40] Differentiation based on quality may very well focus in the future not merely on the traditional view of safety, but also on what diagnostics are used and what treatments are delivered that offer no value to the patient (and could possibly harm them).

■ Differentiation: Access

Healthcare plans also compete on the basis of location and other distribution/access issues. Location is the most obvious issue; physician practices, hospitals, outpatient facilities, and other healthcare providers make choices relative to the areas in which the served market works and lives. Acquisition of other providers and plans has become a fast-growing mode of expanding geographically within the healthcare market. Convenience of location clearly is one of the key decision factors people use in selecting their healthcare providers and in deciding to stay with those providers.

Even the definition of access may mean different things to different people. One person may speak of access as the ability to get an appointment with the physician on the same day; someone else may mean the ability to see a specialist at will; and a third may define access as the ability to find a physician who is willing to take new patients and whose office is closer than 30 minutes away.

The addition of roughly 32 million more consumers to the ranks of the insured is likely to exacerbate medical access issues, particularly access to primary care because there is already a shortage of primary care physicians. Reports of having to wait months to get an initial appointment with a new primary care physician are not uncommon. Given the ACO premise that every patient ought to have a medical home and that the medical home should usually be a primary care provider, the current and growing shortage of primary care physicians threatens the underlying proposed (although not currently clearly defined) structure of ACO delivery. The insufficient capacity in the U.S. medical system to make primary care easily accessible explains why corporations like CVS are building MinuteClinics inside their pharmacies as speedily as they can, while maintaining stringent training standards. They are doing so because they recognize an unmet need for access to primary care and, as a good marketing organization, they are trying to address that need. Other ways of expanding access are being considered in the form of redesigned care delivery models such as group visits, extended hours, electronic visits (e-visits), telemedicine, and e-mail and web portal access to one's healthcare provider.

Clearly, these and other factors can differentiate one provider or insurer from another. For a healthcare plan, the composition of benefit packages is one source of differentiation. Does it include drug coverage? Is there a large deductible? Does it allow self-referral to an obstetrician/gynecologist? To what hospitals can plan members be admitted? Many of these provisions can allow for differentiation between plans and can give the consumer (and employer) a real choice. In geographic areas where the benefit packages of the different healthcare plans are quite similar and the panel of physicians and hospitals offered are nearly the same, consumers seeking points of differentiation between plans will have to rely more heavily on satisfaction and service attributes, on location of physicians and facilities, and on other factors that the plan chooses to use for differentiation purposes, such as free membership in a health club. The implication for marketers is that they must attend to those areas where they can effectively differentiate themselves.

■ Differentiation: Price

One of the easiest areas of differentiation conceptually involves pricing. It does not require extensive advertising, promotion, and education to demonstrate a lower price. The ability to maintain a competitively low price is dependent on having a low cost structure, however. If a low cost structure does not result from significant reengineering of the service process so as to continue to deliver a consumer-perceived high quality of service,

but rather results from limited coverage, denial of access to services, long waits, and so on, differentiation on the basis of pricing will be advantageous only in the short run. Members dissatisfied with the level and quality of service will opt to join competing plans (even though they may be higher priced) in the next reenrollment period. From a marketing standpoint, the ability to differentiate on price means that price-sensitive consumers are given the choice of buying less service or lower quality (at least lower perceived quality) for less money; conversely, price-insensitive consumers are given the choice of buying more and paying more for the choice. Also, true innovation, which may entail vastly different prices (both higher and lower) is possible. The result should heighten the ability of organizations to differentiate themselves and should enhance consumer choice. This characterizes consumer-directed health plans, which have high deductibles, low premiums, and use of a portion of one's income on a tax-free basis when applied to qualified medical expenses. Whether some consumers interpret consumer-directed health plans as being less expensive, given the lower premiums—and whether in the long run they actually cost the consumer less—is as yet unclear.

A differentiated approach supports the concept of customer-responsive marketing. It allows the organization to segment the market; develop a product, package, or set of services that meets particularly well the needs and wants of that specific segment; and to differentiate itself from its competitors. Unfortunately, the marketplace has not yet focused on quality or access as much as it has focused on price (although access is playing a greater role in consumer choice, particularly when the consumer defected from a previous provider or insurer due to access). Therefore, price competition has been fierce, and differentiation on the basis of factors other than price has been limited.

In reality, pricing decisions are not nearly as straightforward in the healthcare industry as in most other industries. Regulations often dictate prices for healthcare services, for example, and retroactive denials of payment after the delivery of services are common. Normally, organizations set a price floor (below which the price does not fall) at the cost of producing the service. As in most service environments, fixed costs are high for healthcare, whereas variable costs are low. Determining the full cost of a service can be quite difficult, because it involves a somewhat arbitrary distribution of fixed costs among the various services that share the fixed costs of overhead. Because each organization can allocate overhead in a different way and competitors have different overhead structures, different providers of service have different costs for any specific service. Healthcare providers face fierce price competition in many parts of the United States and often feel compelled to try to match the low price of their competitors. If they are unsure of the full cost of the service in question, they may price the service below its true fixed cost in order to match competing prices. Furthermore, if regulated prices are based on the market's low prices, which arose from a mix of fierce price competition and uncertainty about services' full costs, then these low prices can be regulated into long-term existence. The decreasing amount of cross-subsidization in the healthcare market exacerbates the problem. Historically, those who had "good" insurance (usually fee-for-service or, until diagnosis-related groups [DRGs], Medicare) cross-subsidized those with "poor" insurance (e.g., Medicaid) and those without insurance. Those with "good" insurance paid a higher price for the same procedure, room, or diagnostic test, thus compensating for those with "poor" insurance. This cross-subsidization was viewed as serving the public good, ensuring that all who needed healthcare would receive it. As more healthcare providers came to see themselves as businesses and as price competition intensified, healthcare organizations sought increasingly to price their services as low as possible in order to make themselves as marketable as possible. This left little room for cross-subsidization.

Yet another way in which pricing decisions are not straightforward in healthcare is evident in the way in which healthcare organizations try to raise their prices by segmenting patients according to their insurance coverage. For example, Wildwood Health Care Center, an Indianapolis nursing home owned by Vencor, Inc., the fourth largest nursing home in the United States, had a significant number of nursing home patients who were covered by Medicaid. Wildwood indicated that it was losing money on these patients, however, because Medicaid was willing to pay only $82 per day. Because Wildwood could not persuade Medicaid to raise the reimbursement to be closer to the $125 per day that private-pay patients paid, Wildwood sought to raise the aggregate price mix of its patients by forcing out its Medicaid residents. It then planned to admit only private-pay patients in the future so that all its patients would then be paying $125 per day.[41] Their inability to change regulated prices may cause healthcare organizations to aim their marketing strategies at those segments of the market whose prices or reimbursement rates are already the most favorable. In this way, some healthcare providers differentiate themselves on price indirectly by directly targeting well-reimbursed market segments.

The emergence of concierge medicine, where physicians narrow their practice size to include only those who are willing to pay a fee ranging often into the thousands of dollars, demonstrates another evolving form of differentiation in medical care. Initially written off as being the domain of a few greedy physicians, concierge medicine is now recognized as being fueled by physicians who want to spend more time with their patients than they are able to under the constraints of many organizational productivity requirements, by patients who want more time with their physicians and are willing to pay for it, and by both wanting what they view as better-quality medicine.

■ Other Sources of Differentiation

Implicitly, many healthcare plans now are differentiating themselves by serving certain market segments particularly well. Disease management programs single out those with a specific condition (e.g., asthma or diabetes) and provide specialized services related to that condition. This is an application of one-to-one marketing and is dependent on information systems that can collect member information to identify those in need of specific services. For example, a program that focused on asthmatic patients would keep track of such occurrences as how many times an asthmatic patient needed to go to hospital emergency departments within a 6-month period and how many times the patient had filled a daily medication (to help determine if the patient was using the medication as often as prescribed) and tailor its services to that patient. Someone who had paid multiple visits to emergency departments in a short period of time probably would need more training in how to use the small diagnostic peak flow meter instrument that allows the patient to assess his or her air intake and how to use the inhaler medications that can arrest the development of the asthma incident before it requires an emergency department visit.

Healthcare providers who contract with managed-care plans seek to differentiate themselves to employers, to managed-care plans, and to consumers. The ways in which they differentiate their services should vary according to the audience. Although a hospital's ability to capture data on resources used in serving its employees may impress an employer, the employees may see little value in these data and want information instead on the post-surgical therapies offered by the hospital. Again, using the power of technology, a hospital can engage in one-to-one segmentation to differentiate itself. It can, for example, identify all patients coming for breast cancer surgery and arrange for all those patients to talk to a volunteer from Reach for Recovery, to receive literature on breast reconstruction if they have had a mastectomy, and to consult a representative from the local store that specializes in clothing for patients who have undergone breast surgery. Hospitals also are differentiated in some cases on the basis of characteristics inherent in their incorporation, such as Catholic, Jewish, Adventist, public city, private psychiatric, or specialty children's hospitals.

■ Customer Retention

Many consumers have felt that they must remain with their current health insurance or health plan in the belief that a preexisting condition precludes them from switching to a different provider organization. The promise of the Health Insurance Portability and Accountability Act (HIPAA), a law that was intended to guarantee consumers continued healthcare insurance when they changed jobs, has not been fulfilled because the premiums have been exorbitant and some insurance companies have discouraged their agents from writing these policies. As a result, many consumers who appear to be highly loyal to a healthcare provider or plan may simply fear losing their coverage. If the healthcare system ever develops in a way that allows these captive consumers to switch from one plan to another without penalty, healthcare plans would have a greater incentive to keep their members satisfied and their marketers would have to work harder at maintaining a high enrollment level. (In reality, everyone in the health plan, not just the marketers, would have to work toward this end, because anyone who comes into contact with or potentially has an impact on a member could enhance or lessen member retention.)

The belief that consumers have few options because many employers have in the past limited the number of options available to their employees is not fully correct. According to *Business & Health*, "Managed care has not put an end to choice. . . . Nationwide, nearly two out of three workers whose employers provide health coverage had a choice of plans. Even many employees whose firms offered only one health plan had options. According to the AAHP [American Association of Health Plans], 90 percent had coverage with a non-network component."[41] Consumers who have more choices switch plans more often. Because the choice of healthcare plan is a high-involvement decision, however, consumers must be convinced through advertising, personal selling, word of mouth, or some other form of promotion that their new choice of healthcare plan is a safe choice. Alternatively, if their satisfaction with their current choice is so low as to be untenable, consumers may switch to a new insurer

or physician, in the hope of avoiding replication of the problems that are causing them to defect.

Historically, the marketing efforts of healthcare providers and health insurers have appeared to focus more intently on attracting patients, customers, and members than on retaining them. Hospitals and medical group practices that have formally engaged in marketing have relied heavily on tactics such as promotion and advertising to the detriment of the more strategic functions of marketing. Insurers and health plans have done the same, with an additionally heavy use of sales personnel to market the product. Managed-care or capitated penetration has now reached such a high level, however, that it no longer draws its new members from the indemnity sector, but rather draws them from other managed-care or capitated plans during reenrollment periods. The net result is that one managed-care plan steals market share from a second plan while the second plan attempts to steal market share from the first. Taken together, these events challenge healthcare organizations to find new ways to retain patients and members. No amount of advertising, promotion, and selling can retain a customer who is unhappy with a service, unless that customer has no choice; promoting great nursing care or short waits will not counteract a patient's own experience of nonempathic and abrupt delivery of care. The focus of marketing efforts, if retention is the goal, shifts away from advertising, promotion, and selling to the provision of visibly good service quality.

Service marketers and academics in the last 15 years have been trying to measure and quantify service quality. Parasuraman and associates devised a now well-accepted model of service quality that has been applied to healthcare settings with mixed results.[42-44] Although this model, called the SERVQUAL instrument, may not apply fully to healthcare settings as it was developed, it is likely to fit healthcare consumer behavior better with modification over time. It measures constructs such as reliability, responsibility, tangibles, assurance, and empathy. Once its measures are better related to healthcare consumers' satisfaction, marketers will be able to rely on it and other validated measures of customer-defined quality in their search for ways to retain customers.

Those in healthcare marketing often fail to examine the consumer decision to stay with a provider. Even though it costs five times as much to capture a new customer as to keep an existing one),[45] most healthcare organizations continue to define marketing as encouraging trial (capturing new patients or members) rather than retaining members. This is not a wise choice fiscally, given the higher cost of attracting new customers. Greater effort should be directed toward retaining existing customers.

One reason for the failure of healthcare organizations to address customer retention is that most do not have information systems designed to identify retention variables.[46] It is the rare hospital, group medical practice, or outpatient rehabilitation facility, for example, that can easily produce a list of patients who have been using its services for more than 2 years and those who have used them for less than 1 year. Even more difficult is the task of identifying patient or member defectors. Few physician practices are aware of when patients leave their practices. Those patients who request their medical records are only a small subset (estimated to be approximately 13%) of the total number who defect.[47] The number of defectors from health plans is estimated to be 20%, meaning that the average health plan would have to replace the equivalent of its whole membership every 5 years.

Further, physician practices do not collect or input their patient data in a way that would allow them to retrieve information on lost patients. The most likely method that could be used to identify defected patients would be through the billing records; however, the billing system was developed to capture dollars, not patient defection information. As a result, most systems cannot pull up this information when asked to do so.[48] Even managed-care plans, which have annual enrollment periods that make it easier to distinguish years of use, cannot generally identify those who have voluntarily disenrolled. If an organization cannot identify those who have chosen to go elsewhere (presumably to a competitor), then the organization cannot learn from them what it can do better in the future so as to keep its members (or patients).

Customer service and a variety of service marketing issues, such as managing the service process experience so that the customer can project a positive outcome based on a positive process experience, have become a major focus of continuous quality-improvement efforts. Most larger healthcare organizations have instituted total quality management, continuous quality improvement, or some other form of patient/member-based reengineering process management that is designed to deliver a seamless service and, if introduced to the organization correctly, to build long-term relationships with its customers rather than a series of one-time transactions. Very often, only those with authority over the operations of the organization can solve what marketing research identifies as dissatisfaction caused by poor service. If patients are kept waiting for an average of 2 hours to get a laboratory test, the marketing resolution of the dissatisfaction requires modifying the operational component by expanding the capacity of the laboratory (e.g., adding technicians, space, equipment, information systems, or some combination of these).

The area of distribution and access is only one of the battlefields where the fight to retain customers will be fought. The concept of access always has been a sensitive one to consumers of healthcare. Time access is a constant and consistent source of irritation, if not anger, in healthcare market research; waiting for an appointment, waiting for a procedure or test, and waiting for the results of tests all have caused great customer dissatisfaction and have conveyed a sense of poor service.

The continuing movement of most of the marketplace into cost-saving–oriented health plans, where one of the primary cost-saving measures is based on denial of access (presumably in the positive sense of forgoing unnecessary care or substituting equally adequate, but less expensive care), expands the sensitivity of the issue of threatened access. Denial of access is most often seen as negative, such as denial of access to choice of provider, denial of access to any specialist without the gatekeeper's approval, or denial of tests deemed to be too expensive for 98% of cases. Healthcare organizations have seen and can expect to see much higher levels of dissatisfaction stemming from perceived (or real) access problems. Some health plans already have noted this and have removed the barriers that prevent members from seeking medical specialist care on their own, without having first to seek the permission and referral of their primary care physicians.

Physicians, too, have become highly sensitive and vocal about denial of access. In great numbers in the past, they have described to their patients and the press the barriers presented by the managed-care gatekeepers whose job it was to assess the need for tests, procedures, and care, supposedly in the interests of the patients. The physicians often viewed the gatekeepers as those who deny patients needed care in the fiscal interests of the organization. In fact, the denial of access may be based on a legitimate recognition that unnecessary tests and care are driving up healthcare costs. Anecdotally, consumer dissatisfaction stems from real fears of improper denial of access. In market research, consumers say things such as "What if an x-ray can't show the problem, and I really do need an MRI?" "What if my physician is right, and I really do need this surgery?" "What if my physician gives up too easily, and doesn't fight for the surgery I need?" When gatekeepers were young, inexperienced, or possibly not well trained in specialty areas, as happened in the managed-care plans of the past, denial of access became not only a marketing and retention problem, but also an ethical and clinical problem that cut to the very heart of the healthcare business and the practice of good medicine. The same issue promises to arise under the ACO vision of healthcare, only it appears that the primary gatekeeper once again will be the primary care physician. If a patient seeks alternative opinions from physicians not in the patient's ACO and those non-ACO physicians disagree with the initial conclusions of the patient's ACO physician, the result may be conflict and potential liability. Some primary care physicians have addressed this in part by setting up concierge or boutique medical practices where the dramatically decreased size of their practice allows them greater knowledge of and discussion with the patient in exchange for a significant fee for increased service, which can be categorized largely as increased access to the physician.[49]

One marketing task, then, in addressing retention is to explain denials of access to consumers and physicians in such a way that they can appreciate and agree with the decision, assuming that the rationale to deny is wise. Alternatively, the task is to examine the denial process to ascertain that denials are not, in fact, inappropriate. Unless this is done, dissatisfaction may be manifested not only through increasing retention problems, but also through medical malpractice suits and angry verbal assaults in the press. Either way, the healthcare organization places itself in long-term fiscal jeopardy if its retention rates drop dramatically. But there are other reasons for customer defection beyond denial of access.

Customer Satisfaction

Many of the regional and national healthcare accrediting organizations require the healthcare organizations that they accredit to collect and share customer satisfaction information. The obvious assumption is that organizations want to satisfy their customers and should do so. It is not yet clear, however, whether customer satisfaction correlates with customer retention; that is, are satisfied customers loyal customers? There is anecdotal information to suggest that the correlation might not be as high as one would expect.

Service Recovery

Dissatisfied customers have the potential not only to go to a competitor, but also to spread negative word of mouth about the organization's services. Instead of being a missionary (one who speaks enthusiastically in favor of the organization and recommends it to others), a dissatisfied customer is more likely to be a market terrorist (one who says negative things about the organization and tries to dissuade people from using its services). The cost of counteracting the efforts of a market terrorist can be quite high. The advertising and promotion undertaken by the organization do not have nearly the credibility of a former or current customer who can cite specific instances of bad service. The ability of patients to go online to websites such as Angie's List and Yelp, where they can post complaints about specific named providers, gives them the potential to broadcast their dissatisfaction to hundreds or thousands of people. Therefore, it is in the organization's best interests to keep its customers happy.

Keeping customers happy is not merely a matter of providing the routinely good service that customers expect. The real test of a service organization's ability to satisfy its customers is its ability to solve problems. No organization is perfect; all organizations sooner or later make a mistake or inadvertently provide poor service. The true test of an organization's service competence is its ability to recover after a service problem occurs.[50]

It is essential to anticipate service problems rather than simply to respond to them. Management must decide in advance the amount of flexibility that employees should have to solve customer problems on the spot and the amount of resources that should be available to employees for the purposes of service recovery.

Some organizations do not believe that their employees are capable of responding to service problems appropriately. In these organizations, a customer who feels that a service has been of poor quality must tell not only the front-line employee of the problem, but also the employee's immediate superior and anyone else in the chain of command who must be part of the problem resolution effort. This repeated explanation of the source of dissatisfaction, often two or more times, runs contrary to good problem resolution or service recovery, which dictates that the customer should have the problem resolved as quickly as possible. Each time the customer has to "tell the story" about the problem without obtaining resolution of the problem, the customer becomes increasingly uncertain that the problem will be resolved; customers frequently will resort to magnifying the problem in telling it to the next level in the organization in the hope that maybe this time it will be resolved. Any person who has suffered through this process is ripe to become a market terrorist in communicating about this organization.

In contrast, good service recovery organizations provide both flexibility and resources at the front line so that problems can be solved or addressed in a fashion that satisfies the customer immediately. In order for this approach to work effectively, the organization must inculcate its employees with an understanding that an important part of their job is to recognize and solve customer problems—whatever it takes. Educating employees to the concept of the lifetime value of a customer supports this outlook. If a physician practice patient stays with that practice for an average of 10 years, bringing in an average of $1,200 a year, then the lifetime value of the patient is $12,000. If a patient of the practice becomes upset because she spent $15 ($30 round trip) for taxi fare to be on time for her doctor's appointment, only to find that the physician was not in that day and no one thought to call her, it makes sense, given her long-term value to the practice of $12,000, to reimburse her for the $30 taxi fare. The tradeoff of $30 in order not to risk $12,000 seems more than reasonable for the service recovery.

Measurement of Customer Satisfaction

Ways of measuring customer satisfaction vary, as do the reasons for measuring satisfaction. First, many healthcare providers have been trying to measure customer satisfaction more aggressively in the past decade because of the requirements of accrediting organizations and employers. Often, these accrediting organizations require the use of standardized measures to allow comparisons across healthcare facilities. Although this requirement has obvious value, it also has drawbacks. Standardized measures usually are generic in nature, so they apply equally well to all the healthcare organizations using them; however, generic measures are generally so broad and nonspecific that they do not give the healthcare organization enough information to identify and correct problems revealed in the customer satisfaction research. For example, a poor rating on a patient survey for the Joint Commission (JCAHO) may alert a hospital to the fact that there is a problem, but may not indicate what the specific problem is, thereby limiting the hospital's ability to correct the problem. Thus, although standardized customer satisfaction studies are valuable for the purpose of providing industry report cards with needed information, they are not generally managerially useful.

Second, satisfaction is known to be in part a function of the amount of choice the customer had in the purchase decision.[51] Thus, satisfaction ratings are likely to be lower among healthcare plan members whose employers gave them no choice of healthcare plan than among members who had at least some choice of plan, even if only one other choice. This then raises the question, exactly what is being measured in customer satisfaction research? Choice at the time of purchase becomes one of the key items reflected in customer satisfaction studies rather than customer satisfaction with the organization's performance after purchase.

Third, the interpretation of customer satisfaction research often focuses on the nature of the customers. Medicare managed-care plans, for example, have recently been prone to explaining their low patient satisfaction ratings as a function of the age of the people who are the subjects of the research. Their assumption is that older people are, by definition, more dissatisfied. Studies have shown, however, that patient or member characteristics account for only 9% of the variation in customer service research; the rest is due to the performance characteristics of the organization itself.[52]

Fourth, some satisfaction studies in the healthcare industry have biased the response categories by loading them too heavily in the positive direction. For questions such as "How satisfied are you with your care?," for example, they have provided the answer categories highly satisfied, somewhat satisfied, satisfied, not satisfied. Because the respondent has three positive (satisfied) categories from which to choose and only one negative category, there is a bias toward a positive response. The willingness of many in the industry to interpret any of the top three categories as satisfied exacerbates the problem. The public has become cynical about the multitude of managed-care plan advertisements claiming 94%, 95%, 98% (and so on) customer satisfaction levels. In reality, only those who answer in the most positive response category are truly satisfied and likely to return to the organization for services. More than half of those in the second highest category can be expected to defect to a competitor. Obviously, customer satisfaction studies are neither simple to devise nor simple to interpret; when performed correctly with the appropriate expertise, however, they can be quite valuable.

■ Data-Driven Marketing

The most sophisticated user of customer and marketing data in the health sector is the pharmaceutical sector. As noted in a complaint filed with the Federal Trade Commission (FTC) in November 2010:

> As consumers increasingly go online seeking advice and information about possible forms of treatment for a variety of health and medical issues, they face an array of sophisticated and non-transparent interactive marketing applications. A far-reaching complex of health marketers has unleashed an arsenal of techniques to track and profile consumers, including so-called medical "condition targeting," to eavesdrop on their online discussions via social media data mining; to collect data on their actions through behavioral targeting; to use viral and so-called "word-of-mouth" techniques online to drive interest in prescriptions, over-the-counter drugs, and health remedies; and to influence their subconscious

perceptions via pharma-focused "neuromarketing." . . . Digital marketing raises many distinct consumer protection and privacy issues, including an overall lack of transparency, accountability and personal control, which consumers should have over data collection and the various interactive applications used to track, target, and influence them online (including on mobile devices).[53]

The filing contains concerns about the collection and use of market and consumer data. Cited, for example, is online data collection that can "identify, track, profile, and target an individual consumer based on information seeking behaviors related to illnesses or symptoms."[53] The complaint also notes eavesdropping on people on social networking sites and applying sophisticated analytical tools to predict future disease-specific behavior.

This type of data collection and analysis need not be performed in stealth mode, nor need it be viewed as deceptive or detrimental to the patient. It should, however, be transparent enough for the individual to object to its collection and use if they wish to do so. The contrast to this type of behavior is to be found on the service side (as opposed to the pharmaceutical side) of the health sector; hospitals and physician practices capture precious little information on their customers, in part because of the late adoption of digital media, coupled with HIPAA, which seems to suggest that no data should be collected in the interest of protecting patient privacy. In fact, HIPAA does not prevent the collection and use of patient data; it does, however, protect patient privacy. The two are highly distinguishable.

Correctly and ethically performed marketing always has been data driven. A marketing function that is fully supported will be given the tools with which to do its job. Insufficient data support, whether for internal data capture and analysis; market research; or market, competitive, and other external data analysis, cuts at the very heart of the marketing function. Healthcare organizations that hope to thrive in the future must expect to position marketing not only as a creative function, but also as a data-driven, analytical, and strategic function.

References

1. The American marketing association releases new definition for marketing. American Marketing Association Press Release, Chicago, IL, January 14, 2008.
2. Kotler P, Keller KL. *A framework for marketing management* (4th ed.). Upper Saddle River, NJ: Pearson Prentice Hall; 2009:3.
3. Berenson RA, Ginsburg PB, May JH. Hospital-physicians relations: cooperation, competition, or separation? *Health Affairs.* 2007;26(1):w31–w43.
4. Gabel J. Ten ways HMOs have changed during the 1990s. *Health Affairs.* 1997;16(3):134–145.
5. Anderson L. "St. Vincent's postmortem: why Village hospital died. *Downtown Express.* June 15, 2010;23(7). Accessed April 10, 2011, at http://www.downtownexpress.com/de_374/stvincents.html
6. Boston Globe Editorial. *Boston Globe.* April 30, 2010: A18.
7. Pear R. Consumer risks feared as health law spurs mergers. *New York Times.* November 20, 2010:A1.
8. Harris G. More physicians say no to endless workdays. *New York Times.* April 1, 2011:A1.
9. Cunningham P. State variation in primary care physician supply: implications for health reform Medicaid expansions. Research Brief, Center for Studying Health System Change. March 2011. Accessed April 10, 2011, at http://www.hschange.com/CONTENT/1192/
10. Sussman A. Disruption innovation panel, Boston University health sector management program event. Boston, MA, March 22, 2010.
11. PatientsLikeMe. Business 2.0 and CNN Money recognize PatientsLikeMe as one of its "next disruptors: 15 companies that will change the world." Accessed April 10, 2011, at http://www.patientslikeme.com/press/20070826/7-business-20-and-cnn-money-recognize-patientslikeme-as-one-of-its-next-disruptors-15-companies-that-will-change-the-world
12. Agency for Healthcare Research and Quality, U.S. Department of Health and Human Services. Re-engineered discharge project dramatically reduces return trips to the hospital. *Research Activities Online Newsletter.* March 2011; No. 367.
13. Bloss CS, Schork NJ, Topol EJ. Effect of direct-to-consumer genomewide profiling to assess disease risk. *New England Journal of Medicine.* 2011;364:524–534.
14. Weisman R. Patients take on expanded role. *Boston Globe.* March 22, 2011. Accessed April 11, 2011, at http://articles.boston.com/2011-03-22/business/29352119_1_patient-advocacy-health-care-diagnoses-and-treatments
15. Berry L, Parasuraman A. Listening to the customer—the concept of a service-quality information system. *Sloan Management Review.* Spring 1997:65–76.
16. Swidey N. The health care doctor. *Boston Globe.* February 6, 2011. Accessed March 11, 2011, at http://www.boston.com/lifestyle/health/articles/2011/02/06/how_caritas_christi_ceo_ralph_de_la_torres_wall_street_gamble_will_rock_main_street_health_care/?page=1
17. Winslow R. Three big firms survey workers to evaluate, improve health care. *Wall Street Journal.* October 8, 1993:B3.
18. Grady D. *Consumer Reports* is rating surgical groups. *New York Times.* September 8, 2010:A18.
19. Smith H, Rogers R. Factors influencing consumers' selection of health insurance carriers. *Journal of Health Care Marketing.* December 1986:86–98.
20. Tumlinson A, Bottigheimer H, Mahoney P, Stone E, and Hendricks A. Choosing a health plan: what information will consumers use? *Health Affairs.* May/June 1997;16(3)229–238.
21. Hibbard J, Jewett J. What type of quality information do consumers want in a health care report card? *Medical Care Research and Review.* 1996;53(1):28–47.
22. Hibbard J, Jewett J. Will quality report cards help consumers? *Health Affairs.* May/June 1997:218–228.
23. Scanlon D, Chernew M, Sheffler S, Fendrick AM. Health plan report cards: exploring differences in plan ratings. *Journal on Quality Improvement.* January 1998:5–20.
24. Hibbard J, Slovic P, Peters E, Finucane M, Tusler M. Is the informed-choice policy approach appropriate for Medicare beneficiaries? *Health Affairs.* May/June 2001:199–203.

25. Hibbard J, Jewett J, Legnini M, and Tusler M. Choosing a health plan: do large employers use the data? *Health Affairs*. December 1997:47–63.

26. Fox M. Low health literacy equals poor results. *National Journal*. March 28, 2011. Accessed April 4, 2011, at http://www.nationaljournal.com/healthcare/low-health-literacy-equals-poor-results-study-finds-20110328

27. Berkman ND, Sheridan SL, Donahue KE, et al. *Health literacy interventions and outcomes: an updated systematic review*. Evidence Report/Technology Assessment No. 199, AHRQ Pub. No. 11-E006. Rockville, MD: Agency for Healthcare Research and Quality; March 2011.

28. Sarasohn-Kahn J. The wisdom of patients: health care meets online social media. April 2008:18. Accessed June 16, 2010, at http://www.chcf.org/publications/2008/04/the-wisdom-of-patients-health-care-meets-online-social-media

29. Nuovo J, Melnikow J, Chang D. Reporting number needed to treat and absolute risk reduction in randomized clinical trials. *Journal of the American Medical Association*. June 5, 2002, 287(21):2813–2814.

30. Hibbard J, Harris-Kojetin L, Mullin P, Lubalin J, Garfinkel S. Increasing the impact of health plan report cards by addressing consumers' concerns. *Health Affairs*. October 2000, 19(5):138–143.

31. Baker M. Software for shaping up. *Wall Street Journal*. March 21, 2011:R2.

32. Rogers, EM. *Diffusion of innovations*. New York: Free Press; 1962:247.

33. Hobson K. Will there be enough primary-care physicians to treat new Medicare patients? http://blogs.wsj.com/health/2011/03/18/will-there-be-enough-primary-care-physicians-to-treat-new-medicaid-patients, March 18, 2011.

34. Berwick D. A user's manual for the IOM's "quality chasm" report. *Health Affairs*. May/June 2002, 21(3):80–90.

35. Griner PF. Payment reform and the mission of academic medical centers. *New England Journal of Medicine*. 2010;363:1784–1786.

36. Welch HG, Sharp S, Gottlieb DJ, Skinner JS, Wennberg JE. Geographic variation in diagnosis frequency and risk of death among Medicare beneficiaries. *Journal of the American Medical Association*. 2011;305(11):1113–1118.

37. Woodside A. What is quality and how much does it really matter? *Journal of Health Care Marketing*. 1991;11(4):61–67.

38. Medline Plus. Whether chronic diseases are diagnosed may depend on where you live. Accessed March 29, 2011, at http://www.nlm.nih.gov/medlineplus/news/fullstory_109871.html

39. Hadler NM. *Stabbed in the back: confronting back pain in an overtreated society*. Chapel Hill, NC: University of North Carolina Press; 2009.

40. Brownlee S. Overtreated: why too much medicine is making us sicker and poorer. New York: Bloomsbury USA; 2007.

41. Data watch—employee choice: alive and well. *Business & Health*. February 1998:58.

42. Moss M, Adams C. Evictees relish nursing homes' reversal. *Wall Street Journal*. February 11 1998:Bl–B12.

43. Parasuraman A, Zeithaml V, and Berry L. A conceptual model of service quality and its implications for future research. *Journal of Marketing*. 1985;49(2):41–50.

44. Shewchuk R, O'Connor S, and White J. In search of service quality measures: some questions regarding psychometric properties. *Health Services Management Research*. 1991;4(1):65–75.

45. Headley D, Miller S. Measuring service quality and its relationship to future consumer behavior. *Journal of Health Care Marketing*. 1993;13(4):32–41.

46. Heskett JL, Sasser WE, Wheeler J. *The ownership quotient: putting the service profit chain to work for unbeatable competitive advantage*. Harvard Business Press; Boston, MA2008.

47. Clarke R. The first step in addressing voluntary disenrollment. *Health Care Strategist*. December 1997:7–9.

48. Clarke R. Costs and prevention of patient defection. *Journal of Medical Practice Management*. July/August 2001:11–14.

49. Clarke R. Measuring patient loss. *Journal of Medical Practice Management*. January/February 2002:2–5.

50. Brennan TA. Luxury primary care—market innovation or threat to access? *New England Journal of Medicine*. April 11, 2002: 1165–1168.

51. Spreng R, Harrell G, and Mackoy R, et al. Service recovery: impact on satisfaction and intentions. *Journal of Services Marketing*. Spring 1995:49–58.

52. Ullman R, Hill J, Scheye E, and Spoeri R, et al. Satisfaction and choice: a view from the plans. *Health Affairs*. May/June 1997:209–217.

53. Clarke R. Measuring consumer satisfaction. Paper presented at the Health Care Policy and Regulation Workshop, Rutgers University, New Brunswick, NJ, December 9, 1994.

54. Chester J, Mierzwinski E, Simpson JM, Dixon P. *Before the Federal Trade Commission: in the matter of online health and pharmaceutical marketing that threatens consumer privacy and engages in unfair and deceptive practices*. Washington, DC; 2010, Accessed at www.ftc.gov/os/2010/11/101123publiccmptdigitaldemocracy.pdf

CHAPTER 7

Public Health and Private Physician Medical Practice Preparedness: Can We Be Medically Prepared for the Next Disaster?

Denise O'Farrell, MPH
Howard L. Smith, PhD
Keri D. Black, PhD, CFNP
Annette Phillipp, PhD, MPH
Lawrence F. Wolper, MBA, FACMPE
David N. Gans, MSHA, FACMPE
Neill F. Piland, PhD

It has become increasingly obvious to many people around the world that large-scale natural and man-made disasters are occurring with regular frequency. When considering recent massive earthquakes, tsunamis, tornadoes, droughts, floods, hurricanes, fires, nuclear reactor meltdowns, terrorism, civil wars, and associated maladies, it is clear that a disaster could be visiting our neighborhoods, cities, states, or nations sometime very soon. Although governmental and nongovernmental organizations are primarily responsible for planning responses that adequately address these massive disruptions, there remain many questions about the integrity of those plans and society's ability to galvanize resources that mount a corresponding effort to minimize adverse impacts associated with any disaster.[1]

Serious concerns have been expressed about public health and medical preparedness.[2] Numerous authorities argue that the National Disaster Medical System (NDMS) is not prepared to handle pandemic outbreaks.[3-5] Furthermore, after examining national survey data from medical practice administrators collected by the Medical Group Management Association (MGMA), Phillipp and colleagues concluded that private physicians are not being integrated into disaster preparedness, despite recognition by physicians responding to the MGMA survey that a threat of disaster is very probable for their community.[6] If frontline medical and healthcare personnel are not prepared to respond to large-scale disasters, the implications for morbidity and mortality are daunting.

The purpose of this chapter is to better understand the state of public health and medical practice disaster preparedness. First, the traditional, historical relationship of public health agencies to private sector medical care delivery is reviewed vis-à-vis all-hazard preparedness. Second, the interaction, communication, cooperation, and training that exist between the public health sector and private medical practice are critically analyzed. Third, the primary care setting is examined as a key player in disaster preparedness and response. Fourth, the preparedness of private medical practices to coordinate with public health entities during times of planning and crisis is assessed. Fifth, an agenda is outlined for where improvements can be made and the necessary requirements essential to implementation. Finally, the implications for healthcare practice and research are considered.

Historical Relationships Between Public Health and Medicine Related to Emergency Preparedness

As one of the first places people will go to seek treatment, private medical practices are essential to emergency response planning. It is a fact that physicians have not been extensively involved in disaster preparedness, a situation that should, and can, be resolved. It is important to understand, from a historical viewpoint, how medicine and public health were traditionally brought into the preparedness field.

The American Medical Association (AMA) and the American Public Health Association (APHA) have been in existence for 164 and 139 years, respectively. According to Brandt and Gardner, in 1872, when APHA was founded, 80% of the membership was made up of physicians.[7] Significant differences have existed between the fields of medicine and public health. Public health has largely been focused on disease prevention with a populations-based approach, whereas the medical field has been committed to curing sick individuals. Brandt and Gardner interpreted the antagonistic relationship that arose between public health and medicine as follows: ". . . the medical professional became more homogenous and powerful, medicine increasingly viewed public health interventions as a potential infringement on the doctor-patient relationship."[7(p709)]

Foundation of Preparedness

Public health and private medical physicians were partnering on health preparedness as early as 1940. An article in *American Public Health*, "Health Preparedness," described the formation of federal committees related to health preparedness for men preparing to go to war.[8] With registration for the Selective Service looming, and the possibility of a draft, it stated, "the shadow of war—even total war—is over us for the first time in our history."[8(p1466)] Manpower was acknowledged as being the greatest single resource in the United States. It was believed the Selective Training and Service Act would garner nearly 16.5 million men, with 2 to 4 million of them requiring comprehensive physical exams.

In September 1940, President Franklin D. Roosevelt signed an order to establish a Council on National Defense, as well as a National Health and Medical Committee. The National Health and Medical Committee consisted of Surgeons General from the Army, Navy, and Public Health Service, and the Division of Medical Sciences of the National Research Council. The committee was authorized to use the medical equipment and services of the these organizations. The concluding sentence of the "Health Preparedness" article is interesting on two accounts. First, it is written as if women did not work in the field at the time, and second, it indicates that physicians and public health workers will work together for the sake of an emergency. It states: "Physicians and public health men have always shown such a spirit and no doubt will respond in the present emergency."[8(p1468)]

Nearly 10 years later, another major shift in preparedness activities began to form. In 1949, the Civil Defense era began. The overarching goal during this time was to protect civilian health in the event of an attack. In the spring of 1950, and with the permission of the U.S. Atomic Energy Commission, 148 physicians from 38 states received training related to medical concerns following a chemical attack.[9]

In June 1950, the Resources Board recommended to governors to arrange for their state health commissioners to become the state civil health services directors and for local health commissioners to become the local civilian defense health services directors. This recommendation was considered to be considerably important by members of the APHA. Keifer said, "Civil Defense Health Services include first aid and ambulance services, emergency hospital systems, casualty services, health supply systems (including provision of blood and blood derivatives), laboratory, sanitation, nutrition, veterinary, mortuary, and similar services."[9(p1487)] Mutual aid agreements (i.e., sharing of medical supplies and personnel) were encouraged between cities up to 20 miles away from one another, for outside support.

The article "Civil Disturbance and the Health Department," by John Hanlon in the *American Journal of Public Health*, discussed the decline in civil defense activities within health departments after World War II. However, events associated with the Vietnam War and societal change witnessed an increase in rioting as a trend within U.S. cities. Subsequently, civil defense programs returned. On June 23, 1967, riots in Detroit, Michigan, created a surge of patients flowing into the healthcare system for treatment. Because public health activities were curtailed during the riots, many public health nurses served as sanitarians and hospital nurses, as well as taking on other roles and responsibilities. Other healthcare professionals also volunteered their expertise during this time. A total of 43 people were killed and 467 people were injured during the Detroit rioting.[10]

Following several major natural disasters, the Disaster Relief Act was passed in 1974, followed by President James

Earl Carter's Executive Order 12127, which merged over 100 federal agencies with disaster and emergency response roles and responsibilities into the Federal Emergency Management Agency (FEMA). The end of the Cold War allowed Director James Witt to redirect more of FEMA's limited resources from civil defense into disaster relief, recovery, and mitigation programs. When state and local emergency response agencies become overwhelmed, they can request assistance from FEMA through the governor of their state.[11]

In 1984, thousands of people died as a result of a toxic chemical release by Union Carbide, in Bhopal, India. As a result of this disaster, in 1986, Congress passed the Emergency Planning and Community Right-to-Know Act, commonly referred to as SARA Title III. The congressional act required the formation of local emergency planning committees (LEPCs) to address hazardous chemical releases. LEPCs include elected officials, emergency medical personnel, hospital personnel, fire departments, law enforcement, community groups, environmental groups, media, and owners and operators of covered facilities.[12]

This historical foundation of disaster preparedness allows us to observe similar parallel efforts that were launched as a result of one of the boldest acts of terrorism on the United States on September 11, 2001.

Strengthening Emergency Responses After September 11, 2001

Public health was once again brought into the fold of emergency health response as a result of the events surrounding September 11, 2001. Four planes were hijacked by al-Qaeda and crashed in suicide missions. American Airlines flight 11 crashed into the World Trade Center North Tower and United flight 175 crashed into the South Tower. American Airlines flight 77 crashed into the Pentagon, and United flight 93 crashed into a field in Shanksville, Pennsylvania.[13] The final death toll cannot yet be ascertained. It is estimated that nearly 3000 people died on that tragic day, but emergency first responders continue to die as a result of exposure to toxic chemicals and substances while sifting through debris during response and recovery operations. It was a devastating time for the United States and dozens of other countries who had citizens aboard the four flights. Again, war loomed around the corner.

Less than 2 weeks later, letters were sent through the U.S. Postal Service to media and government facilities containing *Bacillus anthracis*. The highly aerosolized letters caused a total of 22 suspected or confirmed cases of inhalational or cutaneous *B. anthracis*. Five confirmed inhalational cases resulted in death. The Centers for Disease Control and Prevention (CDC) provided recommendations for antimicrobial postexposure prophylaxis to prevent inhalational anthrax. Ciprofloxacin and doxycycline were the front-line antibiotics used for prophylaxis. There were 10,300 people meeting the specific criteria for treatment; however, 32,000 people initiated the 60-day course of treatment. People exposed to high levels of the aerosolized *B. anthracis* were also given the option of receiving the anthrax vaccine and additional antibiotics.[14]

Creation of the Public Health Emergency Preparedness Program

In 2002, Congress authorized, and the CDC signed, cooperative agreements with U.S. states and territories to establish the Public Health Emergency Preparedness program. In turn, state health departments contracted with local public health departments to accomplish preparedness and response activities related to bioterrorism, infectious disease outbreaks, and other public health threats and emergencies. Local health departments were to enhance the ability to respond to terrorism, infectious disease outbreaks, and natural disasters.[15] Initially, the program required Public Health Emergency Preparedness personnel to work on the following topics:

- Assessment/planning
- Surveillance/epidemiology
- Laboratory capacity: biologic agents
- Health Alert Network
- Communications/information dissemination
- Education and training

Hazard vulnerability assessments were performed for assessment and planning benchmarks. To increase disease surveillance, additional epidemiologists were hired at the state and local levels. Although laboratory capacity was likely bolstered in large municipalities, rural areas condensed laboratory capacity to state-level testing for biologic agents. Public information officers were hired at local health departments with the mandate to disseminate information and perform risk communication during large-scale real-world events.

Communication was significantly hindered during the September 11th response because first-responder agencies such as law enforcement and fire departments could not communicate with one another, because their communications equipment was not compatible.[16] Thus, compatible system-based communications became a high priority for all emergency response agencies, including public health agencies. Because of the significant financial commitment needed to buy interoperable communications equipment, and the complexities related to a system in which all response agencies can communicate with one another, it continues to remain one of the main priorities and activities of all agencies participating in emergency response.

One critically important method of communication between public health and providers is by means of the national, state, or local health department Health Alert Network (HAN) system. At the national level, the CDC's HAN system sends time-sensitive information impacting the public's health via e-mail messaging on a 24/7 basis, 365 days of the year.[17] State and local health departments have HAN systems in place to transmit health alerts, advisories, and updates via e-mail and fax (see **Table 7-1**). At the federal, state, and local levels, HAN messages are sent not only to physician offices, laboratories, and clinicians, but also to police and fire departments, county commissioners, and essentially any personnel who work to protect the public's health during emergencies, natural disasters, and infectious disease outbreaks.

Education and training programs related to biologic agents were developed for public health personnel and emergency first responders. According to the CDC, the U.S. public health system and primary healthcare providers must be prepared to address various biological agents, including pathogens that are rarely seen in the United States. High-priority agents include organisms that pose a risk to national security because they[18]:

- Can be easily disseminated or transmitted from person to person
- Result in high mortality rates and have the potential for major public health impact
- Might cause public panic and social disruption
- Require special action for public health preparedness

Table 7-1	Categories of Health Alert Messages
Health Alert	Conveys the highest level of importance; warrants immediate action or attention
Health Advisory	Provides important information for a specific incident or situation; may not require immediate action
Health Update	Provides updated information regarding an incident or situation; unlikely to require immediate action
Info Service	Provides general information that is not necessarily considered to be of an emergent nature

Creation of the National Bioterrorism Hospital Preparedness Program

In 2002, the National Bioterrorism Hospital Preparedness Program (NBHPP) was established. Administered through the Health Resources and Services Administration, within the U.S. Department of Health and Human Services, its main focus is to enhance the ability of hospitals to respond to biologic attacks and terrorism.[19] Similar to the Public Health Emergency Preparedness program, this program is typically housed within local health departments.

Program coordinators for the NBHPP were tasked with forming a planning group, or coalition, of the following groups:

- Hospitals
- Emergency medical services regional consultant
- Local transport and nontransport EMS agencies
- Local emergency planning committees
- Outpatient facilities
- Community and migrant health centers
- Rural health clinics
- American Indian/Alaskan Native healthcare facilities
- Other healthcare entities that serve as vital points of entry into the healthcare system

Getting participation from members of these groups was not without challenges. In rural areas, in particular, it was exceedingly difficult to get emergency medical services (EMS) agencies involved, because 75% of their crews are volunteers with full-time jobs. In addition, in many areas, hospitals are in competition with one another, and forming a regional healthcare system requires collaboration. Hazard vulnerability assessments and the likelihood of a large-scale disaster greatly impacting patient care during a surge event created a "for the good of the community" mentality among members.

In the timeline of events, the next guidance released to emergency response planners was when the U.S. Department of Homeland Security released its National Response Plan. It shifted away from a bioterrorism focus to an "all-hazards approach" and aligned with the Homeland Security Presidential Directive-5, which incorporated information on domestic emergencies and the utilization of the National Incident Management System (NIMS).

In anticipation of a long-overdue influenza pandemic, President George W. Bush signed into law the Pandemic and All-Hazards Preparedness Act (PAHPA), Public Law

No. 109-417, on December 19, 2006. The purpose of PAHPA was "to improve the Nation's public health and medical preparedness and response capabilities for emergencies, whether deliberate, accidental, or natural."[20] PAHPA had broad implications for the field of emergency preparedness and response activities. It amended the Public Health Service Act to establish the Assistant Secretary for Preparedness and Response; provided new authorities for a number of programs, including the advanced development and acquisitions of medical countermeasures; called for the establishment of a National Health Security Strategy; and restructured the National Bioterrorism Hospital Preparedness Program to what is now known as the Hospital Preparedness Program.

After Hurricane Katrina occurred in the Gulf region of the United States in 2005, new guidance on processes and a multijurisdictional coordinated response necessitated updates to *Medical Surge Capacity and Capability*, and a second edition was released in 2007.[21] The initial *Medical Surge Capacity and Capability* was created in 2004 by the CBA corporation as a methodology for managing medical

and health responses to major emergencies and disasters. A well-known phrase in the emergency response field is that "all disasters are local." Thus, the program was developed with local healthcare organizations being the first point of entry for a medical surge (Tier 1), and as a situation escalates, other tiers are brought in to respond, until federal support is requested in Tier 6. See **Figure 7-1** for a visual representation of the *Medical Surge Capacity and Capability* management and organization strategy.

As per NBHPP program and grant guidance, members of the regional planning groups, which could be considered a coalition of sorts, were given a set of benchmarks to enhance their ability to respond to a biological attack. Grant funding allowed hospitals to purchase equipment, supplies, and training in order to strengthen their emergency response capabilities. Since the program began, the focus areas have included:

- Hospital bed capacity
- Isolation capacity
- Laboratory capacity

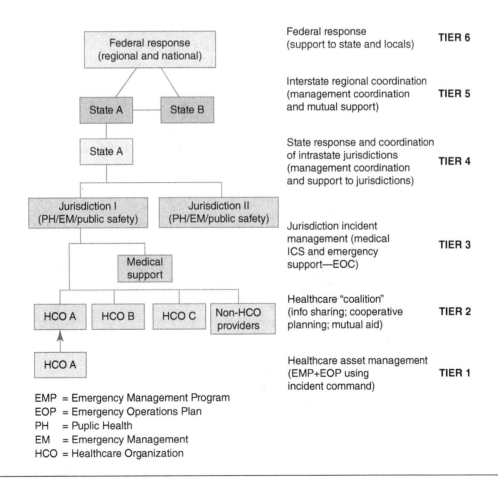

EMP = Emergency Management Program
EOP = Emergency Operations Plan
PH = Puplic Health
EM = Emergency Management
HCO = Healthcare Organization

Figure 7-1 Medical surge capacity and capability management organization strategy.

Source: Barbera JA, Macintyre AG, Knebel A, Trabert E. (Eds.). *Medical surge capacity and capability: a management system for integrating medical and health resources during large-scale emergencies* (rev. ed.). CNA Corporation; 2004.

- Healthcare personnel deployment
- Personal protective equipment
- Decontamination
- EMS mutual aid plan
- Surveillance and tracking
- Education/training
- Bioterrorism disaster exercise
- At-risk population planning
- Hospital evacuation
- Alternate care site planning
- Mass fatality planning
- Interoperable communications
- Mutual aid agreements
- Mobile medical assets

Nationwide, billions of dollars have been spent on equipment and supplies, and subsequently, training on how to use these supplies. Equipment and supplies purchased with grant funds have included portable negative pressure isolation units and decontamination units; mass casualty response trailers; personal protective equipment such as gowns, gloves, and N95 masks and respirators; cots; body bags; laboratory equipment; IV poles; evacuation stair chairs; and interoperable radio equipment to communicate with prehospital emergency responders as well as responders such as law enforcement and public health.

Success stories associated with the purchase of equipment and supplies shows a significant return on investment. Some items are dual purpose and can be utilized on a day-to-day basis while other supplies and equipment are stored for a surge capacity event. Rural hospitals, often without a respiratory therapist on staff and without ventilators for their patients, purchased a portable autoventilator to transport patients to a larger hospital with the goal of saving the patient's life.

One challenge faced by NBHPP groups is the mandate to develop plans to establish and operate an alternate care site. There are two scenarios in which this might be needed. One is an infectious disease outbreak or a mass casualty scenario in which the hospital is faced with an uncontrollable surge of patients, affecting its ability to adequately treat patients; the other scenario is one in which a portion or all of the hospital must be evacuated because its safety has been compromised. Supplies and equipment have been purchased for this possibility. If the second scenario occurs, hospital personnel accompany patients to the alternate care site.

This second scenario became a reality on May 22, 2011, when a Level 5 tornado hit the hospital in Joplin, Missouri. Hospital personnel and community-based responders were forced to evacuate the hospital and treat hundreds of patients in alternate care sites and triage locations throughout the community. However, if it is a surge capacity situation, the hospital staff will most certainly be working overtime shifts and be unable to go to an alternate location to care for patients at an overflow site. Specifics would need to be addressed, but it is hoped some practices close in order to manage patient care at an alternate care site.

The education and training benchmark of the grant requires NBHPP participants to learn about the National Incident Management System (NIMS) and the Incident Command System (ICS). The NIMS is an approach to incident management that is applicable to all jurisdictional levels and across functional disciplines. It is vitally important that all responders understand how a multijurisdictional response will take place when it includes fire, law enforcement, public health, public works, and so forth. They must form a unified command response operation to achieve the goals set forth in the incident action plan and work as partners on all aspects of emergency response operations.

The Incident Command System (ICS), developed and used by fire agencies in California since the 1980s, contains common terminology, a manageable span of control, and position-based job assignments.[22] See **Figure 7-2** for an example of the upper section of the Incident Command System structure.

Drills, tabletop exercises, and functional and full-scale exercises to evaluate emergency response plans also are

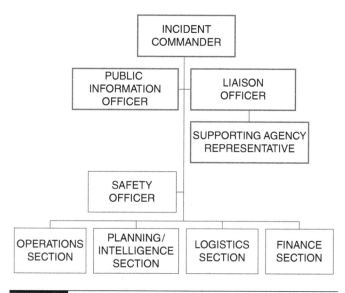

Figure 7-2 Incident command system organization chart for command staff and general staff.
Source: Department of Homeland Security. National Incident Management System. 2004. Accessed at http://www.dhs.gov

required by the NBHPP grant. They are regularly executed at the local, state, federal, and tribal levels. When completed, participants meet to debrief and discuss what aspects of the exercise went according to plan and make suggestions to improve identified gaps and weaknesses in their emergency response plans. Scenarios normally reflect probable emergencies specific to the area and available resources. These can include tornados, hurricanes, floods, chemical spills and exposures, and other likely scenarios.

As a result of issues experienced during the Hurricane Katrina response, new focus areas were added to the NBHPP, including planning for mass evacuation and mass fatalities. At-risk populations had long been a focus area, but Hurricane Katrina brought renewed concentration to the topic as a result of the suffering of the at-risk populations in New Orleans and other affected areas. Many groups fall within the category of at-risk or special needs populations. These terms have been used interchangeably for the past several years. The NBHPP requires continuous focus for at-risk planning, specifically for children, pregnant women, and the elderly. Planners also work with agencies who regularly work with mobility, transportation, independence, and communications needs as well.

Finally, in order to solidify the work being done by NBHPP groups, the program coordinators are required to establish a Health and Medical Surge Capacity Annex and distribute it to members of the regional healthcare system planning group as well as county emergency managers. It contains information on each of the focus areas listed earlier.

Emergency Preparedness for Private Practices

According to the article "Emergency Preparedness: Planning for the Worst, How to Establish a Plan that Will Keep Your Practice Running Should Disaster Strike," when prioritizing between disasters and coding errors or audits, disaster response planning may fall to the end of the priority list.[23] For example, that was to the detriment of one family physician who lost his entire practice due to a fire in his community. He had invested more time and effort in the reimbursement aspect of his practice's operations than in planning for a disaster. Fortunately, he received support from neighbors, friends, the community, and patients to rebuild. He now understands the importance of a disaster response plan. Similarly, Hurricane Katrina impacted thousands of physicians and many were unable to re-establish their practices.

Physicians are encouraged by oversight agencies to ensure compliance for their practice related to emergency planning. The Centers for Medicare and Medicaid Services (CMS) and the Occupational Safety and Health

Administration (OSHA) have specific requirements pertaining to emergency response plans and activities for healthcare practices. However, according to one source, OSHA does not send government officials to practices to ensure disaster plans are in place.

Various resources are available to assist physicians and their practices with all aspects of emergency preparedness. The CMS website contains healthcare provider guidance titled "Emergency Preparedness for Every Emergency." It states, "health care providers should make every effort to include any potential hazards that could affect the facility directly and indirectly for the particular area it is located. Indirect hazards could affect the community but not the providers, and as a result interrupt necessary utilities, supplies, or staffing."[24] It emphasizes that practices will be able to continue to provide care to their patients if they have a disaster response plan in place when a disaster occurs and essential services are disrupted. The site provides links to tools for emergency checklists and effective healthcare planning.

In order to ensure safety for employees, OSHA requires workplaces to determine hazards that may affect the safety of its employees. Its manual, *2011 OSHA Manual for Physicians*, assists physicians, dentists, and veterinarians in ensuring employee safety. It contains information about Emergency Action Plan (1910.38), OSHA's Emergency Preparedness and Response Guidance for Pandemic Influenza, as well as other hazards found in offices such as exposure to bloodborne pathogens and mercury, emergency evacuation, and so on.[25]

Additional resources are available for physicians' practices through various medical professional associations. One of the more proactive associations, the AMA provides the tools needed for education, training, and disaster plan development. An online web-based system called Management of Public Health Emergencies: A Resource Guide for Physicians and Other Community Responders contains sections on weather-related and other natural disasters, and meeting the mental health needs of victims, families, and responders. It also provides information on biologic, radiation, and chemical emergencies, as well as mass trauma, explosive events, and terrorism.[26]

The AMA also worked with subject matter experts and published *What to Do Before, During, and After an Emergency or Disaster: A Preparedness Toolkit for Office-Based Health Care Providers*. This checklist contains information on how to develop emergency response plans, defines roles and responsibilities regarding communication, and provides responses to challenges the individual practice encounters during a disaster. This is often referred to as continuity of operations planning (i.e., developing plans for alternate locations if the physician's office is destroyed by a disaster and how to begin providing services again within a 12-hour time period).[27]

The American Academy of Pediatrics (http://www.aap.org/) and the American College of Emergency Physicians (http://www.acep.org/) developed forms dedicated to emergency preparedness for children with special needs. These forms provide templates for physicians and parents to complete an emergency information form to give to providers during a disaster. On the website, an open letter to healthcare professionals working with pediatric patients states,

> This important document represents the culmination of years of work on the part of both organizations to create a tool that will assure prompt and appropriate care for Children with Special Health Care Needs. Now, when these patients present to emergency departments or health care professionals with an acute illness or injury, physicians, parents, EMS professionals, and nurses will be able to use the Emergency Information Form as a tool to transfer critical information.[28]

■ The Level of Interaction, Communication, Cooperation, and Training that Currently Exist Between Public Health and Medical Private Practice

Recruitment of Medical and Non-Medical Professionals into the Medical Reserve Corps

Following the events of September 11, 2001, many public health and medical professionals sought ways to offer their services. Although heroic and admirable, when spontaneous volunteers arrive at a disaster site it can be to the detriment of emergency operations. In the 2002 State of the Union Address, President George W. Bush encouraged Americans to volunteer in support of their country and announced the creation of the USA Freedom Corps. As a result, the Office of the Civilian Medical Reserve Corps was created within the U.S. Surgeon General's Office. The Medical Reserve Corps' mission is "to engage volunteers to strengthen public health, emergency response and community resiliency." The Medical Reserve Corps (MRC) program is administered at the national, state, and local level. Local Medical Reserve Corps units are largely housed within public health departments.[30]

The Medical Reserve Corps reports show 973 Medical Reserve Corps units in 50 states, the District of Colombia, Guam, the U.S. Virgin Islands, Palau, American Samoa, and Puerto Rico, with 203,815 volunteers enrolled in the program. See **Figure 7-3** for a representation of where Medical Reserve Corps units are located throughout the United States.[30]

According to the Department of Health and Human Service's Frequently Asked Questions related to ESAR-VHP (Emergency System for the Advance Registration of Volunteer Health Professionals), the critical/priority medical professionals being sought include the following:

- Clinical social workers
- Mental health workers
- Pharmacists
- Physicians (allopathic and osteopathic)
- Physician assistants
- Psychologists
- Registered nurses
- Respiratory therapists

Although it is known as the "Medical" Reserve Corps, nonmedical volunteers, including ham radio operators, information technology support personnel, data entry technicians, and clerical support personnel, also are being recruited by many units throughout the United States.

See **Figure 7-4** for a graph showing the number of registered MRC volunteers by type.[30] These data were collated from information provided by unit leaders on the national MRC website.

The Office of Civilian Medical Reserve Corps has provided core competencies for each MRC volunteer to achieve. Training can be accomplished through independent online training with FEMA, can take place on other emergency preparedness sites, or can be provided in the classroom by unit leaders. At a minimum, training should include orientation to local and regional emergency response plans, an introduction to NIMS and ICS, and information on the specific job responsibilities volunteers may have during an emergency response based on their skill sets and expertise.

Throughout the country, MRC volunteers have been participating in drills and exercises. They were activated in large-scale real-world events such as response efforts for Hurricane Katrina and H1N1 mass vaccination clinics, as well as disasters at the local level.

MRC volunteers also are encouraged to assist with public health initiatives, to develop and advocate for individual or family emergency kits, and to keep contact information up-to-date in case emergency activation is needed.

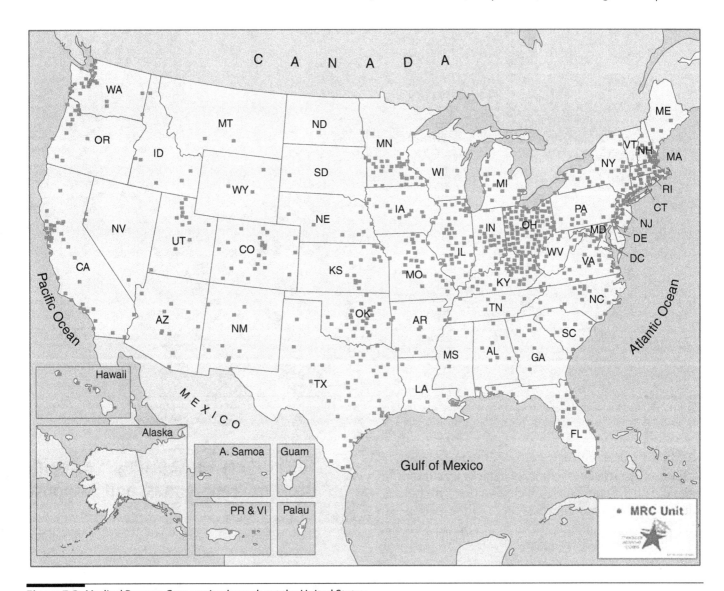

Figure 7-3 Medical Reserve Corps units throughout the United States.
Source: Office of the Civilian Volunteer Medical Reserve Corps, Office of the Surgeon General. *FY 2011 quarterly progress report*. Washington, DC; 2011.

Emergency System for Advance Registration of Volunteer Health Professionals

The Department of Health and Human Services (HHS) has implemented a national volunteer registration program: the Emergency System for the Advance Registration of Volunteer Health Professionals (ESAR-VHP). The system was designed to be a web-based, secure system for MRC volunteers to register and provide contact information *before* an emergency occurs.[31] Prior to this, emergency advance registration systems were developed and typically managed at the state level. After volunteers provide contact information, areas of expertise, and credentials on the ESAR-VHP, local MRC unit leaders are given access to this information and can validate the credentials.

Emergency planners have been making sincere efforts to inform the public that spontaneous volunteers can disrupt response operations. Nonetheless, concerned citizens will continue to step forward to help their community in a time of need and will report to the disaster site before being formally activated. If they are not MRC volunteers, the ESAR-VHP system can enroll spontaneous unaffiliated volunteers as both a tracking and accountability mechanism.

National Disaster Medical System

A federally coordinated system, the National Disaster Medical System (NDMS), exists under the tutelage of DHHS. As with the Hospital Preparedness Program,

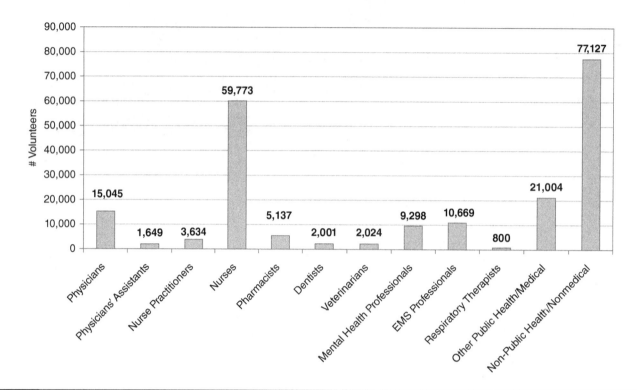

Figure 7-4 Number of medical reserve corps volunteers by type.

Source: Office of the Civilian Volunteer Medical Reserve Corps. Overview of the MRC. Accessed at http://www.medicalreservecorps.gov/QuestionsAnswers/Overview

NDMS is housed within the Office of Preparedness and Response. Its mission is to provide temporary support for federal, tribal, state, and local capabilities with personnel, supplies, and equipment. People with experience in emergency management and forensic science are being recruited, as are medical and public health professionals with specific areas of expertise and specialties. Teams within the system are:

- National Disaster Medical Assistance Team (DMAT)
- National Disaster Mortuary Team (DMORT)
- International Medical Surgical Response Team (IMSRT)
- National Veterinary Response Team (NVRT)

Deployed members of the teams are compensated as federal intermittent employees and protected under the Federal Tort Claims Act if a medical malpractice claim is filed. Response components include[33]:

- \Medical response to a disaster area in the form of personnel, teams and individuals, supplies, and equipment
- Patient movement from a disaster site to unaffected areas of the nation
- Definitive medical care at participating hospitals in unaffected areas[32]

■ The Primary Care Setting as a Key in Disaster Preparedness and Response

In a local disaster, primary care providers (PCPs) should expect that established patients and their families along with new patients will turn to them for treatment, education, and advice.[33–35] It seems fitting that when patients are experiencing a loss of normality, the familiarity of the primary care clinic and staff would provide comfort and reassurance. It is therefore essential, according to the Agency for Healthcare Research and Quality,[36] that each primary care office has prepared an emergency response plan that is coordinated with a regional systems approach.

PCPs should encourage both established and new patients to seek their care for several prudent reasons. First, much of the array of acute and chronic physical and mental health issues that commonly occur after a disaster are within the scope of practice for PCPs. Providing in-clinic care to patients with acute injuries would also defer them from an overcrowded emergency department (ED). The patient volume in an ED during and after a disaster can quickly surpass surge capacity. Crowding not only is problematic, but also has been found to reduce the quality of care, which subsequently worsens outcomes.[37] Furthermore, exposing vulnerable populations, such as children, to the immediate aftermath of other ED victims expressing physical and mental anguish may be psychologically traumatizing.

Additionally, healthcare is most efficient and comprehensive when made available from a provider who knows the patient and has ready access to healthcare records. In contrast, the ED staff is likely unfamiliar with the patient's healthcare history. Patient familiarity is particularly relevant for medically complex patients with underlying chronic health conditions. Finally, patients have been found to comply more willingly with their PCP's advice than that of an unfamiliar provider, particularly when there is an established relationship of trust.[38] PCP directives toward treatment, precautions, and follow-up instructions would be better adhered to, resulting in improved health.

Altered Primary Care Standards During a Disaster

In anticipation of a disaster with mass casualties, the provider focus shifts from individual care to maximizing the total number of lives saved. Decisions about who will receive care and how care is delivered often entail altering normal standards of care. Altered standards of care are standards that are legally acceptable when adequate resources are not available to meet the usual standard of care.[39] Complex care decisions regarding care allocation and decisions for the good of the greatest number are protected from liability under altered standards of care if they are provided in good faith and lack gross misconduct.

Shifting from normal standards to alternative standards of care in a disaster may be decided on a state, local, or clinical level. Who assumes responsibility for adopting alternative standards of care should be decided in predisaster planning by clinicians, local and state officials, lawyers, ethicists, and community stakeholders. Alternative care standards include, but are not limited to, the following areas as outlined by AHRQ[40]:

- *Liability of providers and institutions for care provided under stress with less than a full complement of resources:* The plan may have to provide for "hold harmless" agreements or grant immunity from civil or criminal liability under certain conditions.
- *Certification and licensing:* Although it is important to ensure that providers are qualified, it is also important to have flexibility in granting temporary certification or licenses for physicians, nurses, and others who are inactive, retired, or certified or licensed in other states.
- *Scope of practice:* It may be necessary to grant permission to certain professionals on a temporary

and emergency basis to function outside their legal scope of practice or above their level of training. For instance, physicians may be asked to practice outside their specialty. Nurses may be required to perform physician duties.

- *Institutional autonomy:* If organizations and institutions cede their authority in order to participate in a unified incident management system in a crisis, the plan may have to address the legal implications for those organizations.
- *Facility standards:* Standards of care that pertain to space, equipment, and physical facilities may have to be altered in both traditional medical care facilities and alternate care sites that are created in response to the event.
- *Patient privacy and confidentiality:* Provisions of the Health Insurance Portability and Accountability Act (HIPAA) and other laws and regulations that require signed releases and other measures to ensure privacy and confidentiality of a patient's medical information may have to be altered.
- *Documentation of care:* Minimally accepted levels of documentation of care provided to an individual may have to be established, both for purposes of patient care quality and as the basis for reimbursement from third-party payers. It is prudent to pre-prepare a checklist-type documentation to include necessary information, yet allow for a quicker turnaround of patients.
- *Property seizures:* Provisions may have to be made to take over property, including facilities, supplies, and equipment, for the delivery of care or to destroy property deemed unsafe.
- *Provisions for quarantine or mass immunization:* In anticipation of a biological event, the plan will have to address the establishment and enforcement of isolation, quarantine, and mass immunization and provisions for release or exception.

In comparison to the legal protection offered for licensed practitioners through the altered standards of care, volunteers and those who do not have a professional duty to respond are relieved of medical liability for acts performed in good faith under the Good Samaritan provision.

Types of Patients Anticipated During a Disaster

There will be an initial thrust of patients when a disaster occurs. Patients also may seek primary care appointments in situations where a threat is imminent, but not yet locally actualized. When first hearing about a hazard or pandemic occurring elsewhere, patients in another community may seek palliative care to address various fears and pseudosymptoms. Under this scenario, patient volume may gradually slow down as the pandemic moderates in that other community only to resurge if the threat actualizes within their area. Otherwise healthy individuals may present themselves as new patients following a disaster if they are referred by family members or are in the proximity of the clinic.

Initial triage for the volume of patients presenting in a disaster situation may be the most important role for a primary healthcare provider. Priorities change from providing the best care to every patient to maximizing the number of survivors. The influx of patients could be appropriately triaged through the skills of a nurse specifically trained in disaster response.

A staggering influx of patients is expected following a disaster. Some hazards, such as biological or chemical toxicity, may take weeks or months for symptoms to manifest. In addition to the potential chronic sequelae directly caused by the disaster, patients with underlying chronic conditions may present with disease exacerbation. For example, respiratory disorders such as chronic obstructive pulmonary disease (COPD) or asthma may be aggravated by environmental toxins as well as psychological stress. Essential medications and services, such as oxygen and dialysis, may not be readily available, which would further intensify chronic health conditions. Finally, studies have consistently shown increased healthcare demand secondary to the development of posttraumatic stress disorder (PTSD) and other psychological stress as people recover from the disaster.

Primary Care Communications

Because communications in a disaster area are often significantly compromised, it is important to convey preparatory education to patients and staff predisaster. Prior to the event, communication goals should be to educate the public about safety within the home and family, precautions, appropriate self-care, when to use healthcare, and what can be expected of the primary care office in the event of a disaster. Unfortunately, only 17% of primary care physicians have been found to discuss family emergency response plans and community evacuation with patients.[41]

During a disaster, it is imperative that all staff communicate a unified message to their patients to avoid confusion or distrust. Of course, daily directives and information from local, state, and federal health agencies may change frequently, so up-to-date postings may be required daily. Making provisions for communication in languages other than English may be necessary. To reach patients, a clinic website could be developed announcing the current status of the disaster, hours the clinic will be open, and what services will be available. Other communication avenues may include patient e-mails, posters or signs outside and inside the office, and radio announcements.

Staff Considerations in the Primary Care Setting

Staff education should include, at a minimum, the proper usages of emergency medications and equipment, current life-support certification in both adult and pediatric populations, and written emergency protocol.[42] Human resources issues, such as protection, overtime pay if available, and anticipated expectations for the immediate time of and after the acute incident, are important to address with staff as well. Cross-training staff for essential tasks is vital prior to the disaster in the likely event of inadequate resource distribution. For example, perhaps receptionists can learn the basics of billing and housekeeping. Laboratory workers may be trained in taking vital signs or how to order supplies.

Staff members face a complex decision as to whether to report to work during a disaster. Based on research reviews, Chaffee found that the most common reasons for healthcare workers opting not to report to duty include concern for family and loved ones (including pets), personal health threat, the perceived individual value and importance in contributing to the response effort, and availability of personal protective equipment needs.[43] Staff needs, and subsequent disaster work participation, should be met with available family care, clear work objectives, and fair compensation. Protective equipment and training on disaster-specific precautions must be available to ensure that staff members do not become secondary victims.

Primary Care and Rural Health

Rural areas face unique and multifaceted challenges when natural or man-made disasters occur. Specific problems related to rural preparedness include a paucity or lack of local health departments to coordinate emergency responses, surge capacity, resources, and surveillance. In addition to a shortage of hospitals and specialty care, rural areas are often served by volunteer EMS. A lack of funding for EMS translates into inadequate disaster relief training and equipment, and uncertainty in response availability.[43–45]

Geographically, rural areas may be particular vulnerable to natural or man-made biochemical and nuclear disasters because many nuclear power facilities, uranium and plutonium storage facilities, and missile launch facilities are located within rural areas.[46] What constitutes a mass casualty event in a rural area may be on a different scale than in an urban area. For example, 10 victims from a manufacturing accident may exceed rural health surge capacity whereas 100 victims might be accommodated within a metropolitan hospital.

After a terrorist event in an urban area, it is anticipated that many will flee to rural areas that are perceived as "safer." The potential evacuee population surge from neighboring urban areas could increase the population of a rural area by 50% to 150%. This overwhelming population increase could disrupt or even cripple rescue and response efforts. Another concern of mass fleeing from urban areas is the large number who may evacuate through these areas, consuming fuel, food, water, and sanitation resources as they travel to their destinations.

Multidisciplinary teams of support workers will be needed to seek out and transport and treat affected individuals and families. Such outreach teams should include a medical provider, basic supplies, and transportation to safe areas and medical facilities. Alternatively, staffed mobile clinics ("clinics on wheels") could be an ideal way to reach and immediately treat those in isolated areas. Utilization of a mobile unit would also defer ED use during a disaster.

Coordinating with other organizations and clinics providing trauma and disaster relief could increase resources that would translate into more patients being seen. Perhaps two or more rural-based clinics could temporarily pool their resources within a locally centered clinic or to accommodate a larger volume of patients. Another rural strategy may include an alert system that is able to reach geographically remote families whether they are outside in the fields or in the home.

Many of the challenges of providing pre- and post-disaster care will be tackled by primary care providers. Working collaboratively with relief organizations, PCPs provide education and guidance to patients and staff as well as accommodating an increased volume of patients in the acute and chronic stages of disasters. Healthcare switches from an emphasis on the individual to population care delivery that is made more efficient and legally protected through alternative standards of care. Despite the sequelae of a natural or man-made disaster being unforeseen, foresight and preparation, regardless of the location or size of the primary care clinic, are vital for community health. Core competency in disaster care and a well-organized plan to provide care to the staff, patients, and community in a time of crisis is one of the many and diverse services from the primary care clinic.

■ Level of Success in Medical Practices' Preparedness to Interact with Public Health and Perform During Times of Planning and Crisis

Disasters and emerging infectious diseases seemingly are becoming commonplace, and interaction between public health and medical practices is essential. This is especially the case for emerging infectious diseases, as was seen during the severe acute respiratory syndrome (SARS) outbreak in 2003 and the novel 2009 H1N1 influenza A outbreak in 2009–2010, which had a major impact around the world.

Severe Acute Respiratory Syndrome, 2003

In 2003, severe acute respiratory syndrome (SARS) emerged as a new coronavirus and spread to 27 countries. In total, there were 8096 cases and 774 deaths. Of the 8096 cases, 1074 were healthcare workers. Quarantine of healthcare workers and other people exposed to the virus was one means of preventing the spread of disease. In the United States, public health officials must occasionally order isolation for confirmed tuberculosis cases, but it is done as a last resort when the patient will not self-isolate. Physicians are encouraged to be mindful of this possibility and the impact another SARS-like illness may have on personnel.[47]

2009–2010 H1N1 Response

Five years after SARS, scientists and public health professionals were predicting that the next pandemic would emerge at any time. It was largely believed the major threat was avian H5N1, which could become easily transmissible and lead to the next pandemic. It was also believed the pandemic would originate in a foreign country, and the United States would have ample time to prepare its borders and ramp up response efforts. That was not to be the case.

In March–April 2009, two children in southern California and one child in Mexico sought and received medical care for respiratory infections, and later recovered. A sample from one of the patients being tested by a scientist from the CDC found it to be an unsubtypable influenza A virus that had never been seen before.[48] After additional testing, it was determined to be a triple-reassortant virus, and was quickly termed "swine flu," although it also contained human and avian strains.

Additional cases began to be seen in Texas and New York. By May 2009, all 50 states in the United States had confirmed cases, as did 43 countries around the world. The World Health Organization officially declared a pandemic in June 2009. It appeared as though this was the pandemic that had long been predicted.

Appropriately named "2009 novel H1N1 influenza A," or simplified to H1N1, the pandemic required an increased amount of interaction among public health, medical practitioners, community health centers, schools, pharmacies, media, and the general public. The CDC's Advisory Committee on Immunization Practices recommended the following:

> People at highest risk for complications from this virus, or those caring for high risk individuals who cannot receive vaccination, receive the vaccine first. These target groups included pregnant women, people who live with or care for children younger than 6 months of age, health care and emergency medical services personnel, anyone 6 months through 24 years of age, and people 25 through 64 years of age at higher risk for 2009 H1N1 influenza because of certain chronic health conditions or compromised immune systems.[49]

While a monovalent H1N1 vaccine was being developed, health education messaging to mitigate the spread of influenza was disseminated through public health, medical providers, schools, businesses, media, and social networking sites. The educational campaigns emphasized covering coughs and sneezes, frequent hand washing, and staying home when sick. Information was also provided in an attempt to deter the "worried well" from inundating healthcare and hospitals and to seek care only when certain signs and symptoms were present.

MRC volunteers assisted with H1N1 response, including answering H1N1 hotlines and working at mass vaccination clinics as registrars, health educators, vaccinators, and data entry technicians. Although there was great variation in how volunteers were used during the H1N1 response throughout the country, in many instances their presence allowed local health department personnel to continue day-to-day functions with little interruption to essential public health services.

When the monovalent vaccine became available, it was shipped to each state and then on to local health departments for mass vaccination clinics at schools, churches, and other public venues. Although largely a public health effort, the vaccine was distributed to pediatrician and obstetric practitioner offices as well as pharmacies to immunize the at-risk population. Antiviral medications also were released from the Strategic National Stockpile as a means to assist in medical countermeasures.

The CDC later concluded that the primary care provider's role is substantial in addressing widespread epidemics of this nature. This view was captured in a document titled *Abbreviated Pandemic Influenza Plan Template for Primary Care Provider Offices: Guidance from Stakeholders*. The introductory paragraph said,

> With the emergence of the 2009 pandemic H1N1 influenza, the importance of primary care provider's (PCP) role in the community healthcare system has become increasingly evident. Often serving as the entrance into the healthcare system, PHP offices are likely to play a large role in alleviating surge on the hospital emergency department. As such, PCP offices should integrate their pandemic influenza plans into their community's plan. However, anecdotal evidence has shown that many PCP offices lack these plans.[50]

There are countless opinions on H1N1 response efforts from the local, state, federal, and tribal levels. Some express that the situation was overblown. If asked, many public health professionals and scientists would likely say H1N1 was a preview to a much more virulent strain of influenza—something akin to the 1918 influenza pandemic with greater morbidity and mortality rates, estimated to have killed 50 million people. The lessons learned from H1N1 are still being evaluated, and emergency response planners are adjusting their plans in order to prepare for the next pandemic.

■ Improvements that Should Be Made in Emergency Preparedness and Requirements Essential to Implementation

Strategies listed within the National Health Security Strategy point to inclusion of health professionals such as physicians and nurses:

> Develop and maintain a workforce for public health (including epidemiologists, lab scientists, and other experts), health care (physicians, nurses, dentists, pharmacists, and other health care professionals), and emergency management, all with the knowledge and skills to respond to an incident; provide opportunities for continuing education, training and exercising; create workforce policies (e.g., identification and management, licensing and credentialing, liability protections, and competencies and standards) that will facilitate an effective response.[51]

In March 2011, the CDC's Office of Public Health Preparedness and Response released *Public Health Preparedness Capabilities: National Standards for State and Local Planning.*[52] It builds on the preparedness and response foundation found in the Pandemic and All-Hazards Preparedness Act; U.S. Department of Homeland Security Directives 5, 8, and 21; and the National Health Security Strategy. Fifteen public health capabilities were framed by stakeholders. Numbered and listed alphabetically they are as follows:

1. Community preparedness
2. Community recovery
3. Emergency operations coordination
4. Emergency public information and warning
5. Fatality management
6. Information sharing
7. Mass care
8. Medical countermeasure dispensing
9. Medical material management and distribution
10. Medical surge
11. Nonpharmaceutical intervention
12. Public health laboratory testing
13. Public health surveillance and epidemiological investigation
14. Responder safety and health
15. Volunteer management

Of these 15 capabilities, physicians have a clear responsibility over mass care, medical countermeasure dispensing, medical surge, and nonpharmaceutical interventions. In fact, they should be involved in every capability listed.

On March, 30, 2011, U.S. President Barack Obama replaced Homeland Security Directive 8, which addresses national preparedness and planning, with Presidential Policy Directive/PPD-8. The directive lists goals, systems, building and sustaining preparedness, reports, and roles and responsibilities. It introduces new terminology, indicating the President wants to see an "all-of-nation" approach to preparedness. It states:

> This directive is aimed at strengthening the security and resilience of the United States through systematic preparation for the threats that post the greatest risk to the scrutiny of the Nation, including acts of terrorism, cyber attacks, pandemics, and catastrophic natural disasters. Our national preparedness is the shared responsibility of all levels of government, the private and nonprofit sectors, and individual citizens. Everyone can contribute to safeguarding the Nation from harm. As such, while this directive is intended to galvanize action by the Federal Government, it is also aimed at facilitating an integrated, all-of-Nation, capabilities-based approach to preparedness.[53]

As public health delves into the National Health Security Strategy, the 15 public health capabilities, and the all-nation approach to preparedness as set forth in PPD-8, it will work to incorporate private practices on a broader basis. Physicians can take the initiative and contact their local health department about becoming more active in emergency planning and response in their community, and by joining their local Medical Reserve Corps unit.

■ Implications for Healthcare Practice and Research

The preceding background is essential for understanding how and why medical practices and their physicians could do more in preparing for large-scale catastrophic events. The implications of this historical perspective and review of current methods for addressing disasters provide insights on where improvements can be made through practice, theory, and research in order to achieve enhanced preparation and service delivery in times of inordinate crisis.

Medical Practice

Although considerable federal and state funding has been allocated to disaster preparedness planning, the fact remains that medical providers—particularly physicians—remain disengaged from the planning process and respectfully disconnected from meaningful integration into a viable system of disaster response. Admittedly, gains have been made in recent years (from large federal investments) in involving doctors from the private practice sector in the disaster response infrastructure. However, the most extensive progress involving physicians has been made in larger institutional settings such as hospitals (National Bioterrorism Hospital Preparedness Program) and specialty or multispecialty group practices. More limited progress is evident for physicians associated with smaller private practices, especially those that do not have an expansive administrative infrastructure that can manage preparedness relationships on behalf of clinical staff members.

A central factor in the failure to integrate private physicians in a viable manner ultimately relates to incentives.

Public health authorities have not created a set of incentives with sufficient value that encourages physicians to become more involved with disaster preparedness. To be certain, a relatively small percentage of physicians have volunteered for participation in the National Disaster Medical System, and signing up to participate does not necessarily imply active involvement in either associated planning or service delivery when a disaster does occur. Like most busy professionals, physicians have a very full agenda, and usually more demands for their time than time available.

A viable set of incentives must not only entice physicians to be integrally involved in more mundane efforts to establish disaster response structures and processes prior to a disaster occurring, but also to be deeply active if and when a disaster does occur. As experts on disaster management have observed, a sudden onslaught of energetic volunteers who are not conversant with proper disaster response procedures and protocols can rapidly exacerbate an already catastrophic situation. Perhaps many physicians avoid the predisaster planning stage because they are so inundated by demands from their existing practice. They reason that when a disaster occurs they can simply step up and volunteer their services. This naiveté not only undermines the formulation of efficient service coordination practices, but also contributes further to a crisis in progress.

In many respects this disconnect argues persuasively for a common set of protocols that all medical practices and their clinicians follow under catastrophic circumstances. Unfortunately, public health policy has yet to devise a functional system of remuneration to pay for these services that would help build a better relationship between physicians and emergency response. Without clear guidelines there can be great uncertainty about whether physicians are delivering care pro bono as volunteers or as paid members of a well-orchestrated medical system. An enlightened society desires the latter, but that implies allocating health and medical care resources that are already quite scarce.

In addition to analytically focusing on the precise level of patient care reimbursement that physicians may obtain for participation in service delivery during disasters, attention should be directed to the issue of patient referral. Physicians and medical practices that lend their much-needed skills to the care delivery system during catastrophes ultimately stand to gain patient referrals that can translate into a long-run patient load advantage as a disaster is ameliorated. In effect, disaster service delivery enables a physician or medical group to showcase skills in particular areas of medical care. Patients receive services under very trying circumstances, which can heighten the clinician–patient bond and may pay off in effective word-of-mouth advertising. This can not only create a short-run economic advantage, but also establish a channel for attracting new patients.

This potential to attract new patients to a practice should be closely examined by physicians and their medical groups. Because probabilities favor the occurrence of more disasters in the future, it makes sense that physicians would want to be part of an encompassing solution at the same time that they contribute to a disaster's resolution. It is prudent for physicians to want to be at the forefront of efforts that make a demonstrable contribution to disaster remediation. It is not only consistent with professional mores, but also part and parcel of community building.

Finally, physician integration with community- and region-wide disaster preparedness is consistent with best practices in medicine. An evolving professional medical ethic accentuates participation in community and regional endeavors rather than isolation and opting out. Given the continuing technological complexity associated with medical care delivery, all physicians are dependent on other institutional providers as well as colleagues within their fields. Thus, active engagement in disaster planning and service delivery should be a generally accepted concept of best practice across general practitioners, specialists, and subspecialists.

Research

Disaster planning and preparedness fall within many of the widely supported conceptual frameworks underlying the disciplines of medicine, public health, and healthcare management. Failure to broadly inculcate physicians in disaster preparedness has more to do with the implementation of a concept rather than controversy about whether disaster response is a worthwhile societal goal. In this sense, the theoretical underpinnings of medical practice and health system efforts to respond to large-scale catastrophes are for the most part stable. The integrity of the concepts is not necessarily in question, whether approaching disaster preparedness from prevailing models from systems design, organizational theory, public policy administration, operations management, emergency medical care delivery, or hundreds of other disciplinary concepts. In this respect, fruitful research should focus on the implementation of disaster response concepts as opposed to the underlying conceptual frameworks.

A very promising area for future research in disaster planning vis-à-vis medical practices and physicians is that of strategic advantage. It should be clear to physicians that their engagement in disaster planning serves as a prelude to channeling more attention, and hence patient referrals, to their practices. A disaster does not have to occur for there to be added value in participating in the design of response systems. More exposure to health and medical system authorities with the potential to direct patients to specific practices offers a distinct return on invested time in connecting with the disaster response community.

Based on the literature and judging from reports about physician practice behaviors, medical groups and physicians do not perceive the strategic advantage(s) of becoming active members in disaster preparedness planning and they may not recognize the long-term benefits from affiliations with response systems whether or not a catastrophic event occurs. Research should be directed at uncovering the causal factors for physician resistance to participation. Studies could clarify whether the problem relates to overwhelming time constraints associated with busy practices. If this is verified, additional research can ascertain which methodologies are most promising for informing physicians about the value-added propositions associated with disaster planning, and which tactics to present. If the problem involves other factors associated with daily medical care delivery, these causal factors can also be identified and appropriate strategies designed to minimize their adverse impact.

A rich area of research can be found in the area of incentives; that is, what types of incentive plans can be devised to encourage medical practice and physician interest in disaster preparedness. Public policy research might explore the alternative remuneration strategies and tactics for engaging physicians. Attention should focus on determining a viable system of incentives for engagement for both predisaster planning and service delivery during a catastrophe. Perhaps reimbursement differentials can be devised that support higher payment rates during a catastrophe for those who were engaged at a predetermined threshold in the planning process. Alternatively, a reimbursement scheme might more effectively address the planning phase with the implied benefit being a distinct pipeline to patients during the crisis. Under this model, payments to physicians and medical groups could be benchmarked against criteria essential to receiving payment.

Research can probe the amount of incentive necessary to elicit a positive engagement by physicians and medical practices. In many cases, medical professionals want to see at least some modest revenue stream from doing the right thing; that is, participating in planning and systems design before a catastrophe occurs. They understand the value of their time while simultaneously preferring to be connected with important projects that shape their communities and practices. Often a relatively modest honorarium/reimbursement is sufficient for physicians to justify (to themselves) why they should be engaged in disaster preparation as opposed to the plethora of other opportunities—personal and professional—that implore them to invest time.

Healthcare policy research should delve into the issue of forming a common protocol for all medical service providers during catastrophic disasters. As it currently exists, physicians have no formal expectation that they will participate in either the planning or actual delivery of services in the event of disasters. Although the medical field continues to carry on a discourse about expectations for physicians in times of crisis, it is also essential to begin articulating models for what minimum engagement looks like, including a range of options for providers to consider that best meets their abilities, resources, and experiences.

Healthcare policy research could make fruitful inroads to determining a short-run agenda of engagement while in-depth research examines more complex incentive, remuneration, and best practice models. Given the considerable resources that have already been invested in medical preparedness, there may be opportunities to identify innovative short-run solutions that bridge gaps, thus substantially improving the prospects for a more immediate and robust quasisystem of medical response to crises.

Getting physicians involved has been and remains a difficult problem. Given a total of 900,000 physicians who are licensed to practice medical care and an estimated 100,000 physicians who are linked to disaster response, there are opportunities for researching a variety of methodologies to achieve higher participation. This is one challenge for which we cannot turn to medical schools for a solution. The expectation that physicians will cooperate in planning for disasters and in actually delivering services is a laudable goal for the healthcare system. On the other hand, focused research studies and wide-scale demonstration projects could provide short-term improvement, even if such tactics have fundamental shortcomings that can be remediated over the long run.

Another area for research should target those physicians who are actively participating in medical disaster planning and preparedness. What are the characteristics of these physicians? What motivated them to become involved? Answers to these questions may shed light on how to engage nonparticipants. In the same vein, research should assess outcomes. Of those physicians involved in disaster medicine, do they tend to be more fiscally savvy practitioners? How does financial success correlate with engagement? By the same token, research should delve into outcomes. Do physicians who commit to disaster planning and preparedness deliver a higher quality of care? Are physicians more likely to engage in preparedness planning after a disaster has affected their community or practice? Are quality outcomes more aligned with actively participating physicians who maintain a vibrant practice with a clear consciousness for assisting their community and region when disasters occur? Alternatively, research can validate whether physicians without sufficient fiscal and quality care abilities are those that gravitate to disaster medicine.

■ Toward Enlightened Medical Care in Time of Disaster

Ten years ago, Alexander and Wynia conducted a study of 1000 randomly selected physicians from the Masterfile of the American Medical Association to study their sense of preparedness following the attacks of September 11, 2001.[54] After removing those who were not reachable by mail or who were ineligible, 56% responded. Most respondents (80%) indicated that they would care for victims of bioterrorism even though they did not perceive a professional compulsion to do so. Some 55% indicated that they should treat victims even if it endangered their (the physicians') health. In contrast, only 21% expressed that they were well prepared to play a role in clinically managing a bioterrorist event.

It is not clear whether any progress has been made in increasing physician willingness to assist in disasters or bioterrorist events during the intervening decade since the Alexander and Wynia study was completed. Over the past 10 years, the government has launched many programs designed to address disasters and terrorist activities. Several of these initiatives have promoted disaster preparedness to ensure public health safety; others have attempted to integrate physicians in networks as a critical response. Nonetheless, it is not clear whether physicians are prepared to play the considerable roles that may surface with widespread tragedy.

In many respects, programmatic initiatives to ensure disaster preparedness have been unable to make progress as far as physicians are concerned. Root causes for this disconnect are related to professional remuneration, risk, and opportunity costs. More attention and discourse could be focused on the economics of physician roles in disaster response. Although the public may naively assume that physicians and medical practices will step up after a catastrophe like a bioterrorist attack, providers themselves are less certain. In part this is due to unanswered questions about what they will receive in return for their professional services and from whom; what litigation risks they expose themselves to when they are called on to treat patients for conditions with which physicians perhaps have minimal familiarity; and what other personal and professional activities they might pursue instead of disaster response.

As this chapter has demonstrated, there is a lengthy history surrounding medical preparedness that is founded on governmental intervention for the public's welfare. Thus it is not surprising that many physicians, who are accustomed to interfacing with governmental entities relative to reimbursement for their services, now seem somewhat reticent to volunteer for duty. At the heart of more effective disaster preparedness and response in medical care are many unanswered questions, not the least of which includes payment for services rendered as well as reimbursement for valuable time spent in planning initiatives.

This disconnection between providers and the disaster preparedness system offers a rich environment for applied research. Despite this overwhelming need, a fully robust research agenda into disaster preparedness in health and medicine has not been formulated or funded, owing largely to budget shortfalls and an apparent belief that it is first necessary to fund response systems even if the proper design variables and their relationships are not entirely understood. Until fundamental questions surrounding incentives, risk, and opportunity costs are addressed, it is probable that physicians and medical practices will continue to occupy the fringe in disaster preparedness. This is a lamentable situation that will be much more discouraging should large-scale catastrophes continue to occur as has been predicted.

References

1. Wise R, James J, Dauner D, Dwyer M. Looking at health system disaster preparedness. Straighttalk. Special advertising supplement and educational section provided by PricewaterhouseCoopers. *Modern Healthcare.* September 2008.

2. Delaney JB. The National Disaster Medical System's reliance on civilian-based medical response teams in a pandemic is unsound. *Homeland Security Affairs.* 2007;3(2):1–9.

3. O'Toole T. *Fighting pandemic flu from the front lines.* House Committee on Homeland Security Subcommittee on Emergency Preparedness, Science and Technology. 109th Congress. February 8, 2006.

4. Qureshi K, Gershon RR, Sherman MF, et al. Health care workers' ability and willingness to report to duty during catastrophic disasters. *Journal of Urban Health: Bulletin of the New York Academy of Medicine.* 2005;82(3):386.

5. Balicer RD, Omer SB, Barnett DJ, et al. Local public health workers' perceptions toward responding to an influenza pandemic. *BioMed Central Public Health.* 2006;6:99–115.

6. Phillipp A, Stokes CD, Tivis R, et al. Are medical offices prepared for the next disaster? *Journal of Medical Practice Management.* 2009;25(2):97–99.

7. Brandt A, Gardner M. Antagonism and accommodation: interpreting the relationship between public health and medicine in the United States during the 20th century. *American Journal of Public Health.* 2000;90(5):707–715.

8. Atwater R, Hiscock I, Maxcy K, et al. Health preparedness. *American Journal of Public Health.* 1940;30(12):1466–1468.

9. Kiefer N. Role of health services in civil defense. *American Journal of Public Health.* 1950;40(12):1486–1490.

10. Hanlon JJ. Civil disturbance and the health department. *American Journal of Public Health.* 1970;60(3)470–474.

11. Federal Emergency Management Agency. FEMA history. August 11, 2010. Accessed February 2, 2012, at http://www.fema.gov/about/history.shtm

12. Idaho Bureau of Homeland Security, State of Idaho. *Local emergency planning committee handbook.* 2009. Accessed December 19, 2011, at http://www.bhs.idaho.gov

13. National Commission on Terrorist Attacks Upon the United States. The 9/11 Commission report. 2004. Accessed December 19, 2011, at http://www.gpoaccess.gov/911/pdf/fullreport.pdf

14. Jernigan DB, Raghunathan PL, Bell BP, et al. Investigation of bioterrorism-related anthrax, United States, 2001: epidemiologic findings. *Emerging Infectious Diseases.* 2002;8(10):1019–1028.

15. Centers for Disease Control and Prevention, Office of Public Health Preparedness and Response. Funding guidance and technical assistance to states, localities, and territories. Accessed at http://www.cdc.gov/phpr/coopagreement.htm

16. Brandt A, Gardner M. Antagonism and accommodation: interpreting the relationship between public health and medicine in the United States during the 20th century. *American Journal of Public Health.* 2000;90(5):707–715.

17. Centers for Disease Control and Prevention. Health alert network. 2011. Accessed at http://www2a.cdc.gov/HAN/Index.asp

18. Centers for Disease Control and Prevention. Emergency preparedness and response. Bioterrorism agents/diseases. Accessed at http://emergency.cdc.gov/agent/agentlist-category.asp

19. U.S. Department of Health and Human Services. Hospital preparedness program overview. FY02 to present and beyond. Accessed December 19, 2011, at http://www.phe.gov/Preparedness/planning/hpp/Pages/overview.aspx

20. Public Law 109-417. Pandemic and All-Hazards Preparedness Act. December 19, 2006. Accessed December 19, 2012, at http://frwebgate.access.gpo.gov/cgi-bin/getdoc.cgi?dbname=109_cong_public_laws&docid=f:publ417.109.pdf

21. Barbera JA, Macintyre AG, Knebel A, Trabert E. (Eds.). *Medical surge capacity and capability: a management system for integrating medical and health resources during large-scale emergencies* (rev. ed.). CNA Corporation: Alexandria, VA, 2004.

22. U.S. Department of Homeland Security. National Incident Management System. 2004. Accessed December 19, 2011, at http://www.dhs.gov/xlibrary/assets/foia/mgmt_directive_9500_national_incident_management_system_integration_center.pdf

23. Defino T. Emergency preparedness: planning for the worst. How to establish a plan that will keep your practice running should tragedy strike. *Physicians Practice.* 2006;16(13). Accessed December 19, 2011, at http://physicianspractice.com/display/article/1462168/1589690

24. Centers for Medicare and Medicaid Services. Health care provider guidance. Emergency preparedness for every emergency. 2011. Accessed December 19, 2011, at http://www.cms.gov/SurveyCertEmergPrep/03_HealthCareProviderGuidance.asp

25. Occupational Safety and Health Administration. Physician OSHA manuals. The 2011 OSHA manual for physicians. Accessed December 19, 2011, at http://www.oshamanual.com/medical_OSHA.html

26. American Medical Association. Management of public health emergencies. A resource guide for physicians and other community responders. Accessed December 19, 2011, at http://www.ama-assn.org/ama/pub/physician-resources/public-health/center-public-health-preparedness-disaster-response/management-public-health.page

27. Gebbie KM, James JJ, Subbarao I. *What to do before, during, and after an emergency or disaster: a preparedness toolkit for office-based health care practices.* American Medical Association: Chicago, 2009.

28. American Academy of Pediatrics. Emergency preparedness for children with special health care needs. Accessed at http://www.aap.org/advocacy/emergprep.htm

29. Division of the Civilian Volunteer Medical Reserve Corps. Overview of the MRC. Accessed at http://www.medicalreservecorps.gov/pageView?path=About

30. Division of the Civilian Volunteer Medical Reserve Corps, Office of the Surgeon General. Accessed December 19, 2011, at http://medicalreservecorps.gov/HomePage

31. U.S. Department of Health and Human Services. Frequently asked questions about ESAR-VHP. Accessed December 19, 2011, at http://www.phe.gov/esarvhp/Pages/default.aspx

32. U.S. Department of Health and Human Services. Public health emergency. National Disaster Medical System (NDMS) response teams. 2011. Accessed December 19, 2011, at http://www.phe.gov/Preparedness/responders/ndms/teams/Pages/default.aspx

33. Freedy JR, Simpson WM. Disaster-related physical and mental health: a role for the family physician. *American Family Physician.* 2007;75(6):841–846.

34. Soeteman RJ, Yzermans CJ, Spreeuwenberg P, Lagro-Janssen TA, Van den Bosch W, Van der Zee J. Changes in the pattern of service utilisation and health problems of women, men and various age groups following a destructive disaster: a matched cohort study with a pre-disaster assessment. *BMC Family Practice.* 2008;9(1). Accessed December 19, 2011, at http://www.medscape.com/viewarticle/586216

35. Toback SL. Medical emergency preparedness in office practice. *American Family Physician.* 2007;75(11):1679–1684.

36. Agency for Healthcare Research and Quality. *Altered standards of care in mass casualty events: bioterrorism and other public health emergencies.* AHRQ Pub. No. 05-0043. Rockville, MD: AHRQ; 2005.

37. Bernstein SL, Aronsky D, Duseja R, et al. The effect of emergency department crowding on clinically oriented outcomes. *Academic Emergency Medicine.* 2009;16(1):1–10.

38. Cheraghi-Sohi S, Risa-Hole A, Mead N, et al. What patients want from primary care consultations: a discrete choice experiment to identify patients' priorities. *Annals of Family Medicine.* 2008;6(2):107–115.

39. Agency for Healthcare Research and Quality. *Altered standards of care in mass casualty events: bioterrorism and other public health emergencies.* AHRQ Pub. No. 05-0043. Rockville, MD: AHRQ; 2005.

40. Olympia RP, Rivera R, Heverley S, Anyanwu U, Gregorits M. Natural disasters and mass-casualty events affecting children and families: a description of emergency preparedness and the role of the primary care physician. *Clinical Pediatrics.* 2010;49(7):686–698.

41. Toback SL. Medical emergency preparedness in office practice. *American Family Physician.* 2007;75(11):1679–1684.

42. Chaffee M. Willingness of health care personnel to work in a disaster: an integrative review of the literature. *Disaster Medicine and Public Health Preparedness.* 2009;3(1):42–56

43. Health Resources and Services Administration. Rural communities and emergency preparedness. April 2002. Accessed December 19, 2011, at ftp://ftp.hrsa.gov/ruralhealth/ruralpreparedness.pdf

44. Hsu CE, Mas FS, Jacobson HE, Harris AM, Hunt VI, Nkhoma ET. Public health preparedness of health providers: meeting the needs of diverse, rural communities. *Journal of the National Medical Association*. 2006;98(11):1784–1791.

45. Meit M, Redlener I, Briggs TW, Kwanisai M, Culp D, Abramson DM. Rural and suburban population surge following detonation of an improvised nuclear device: a new model to estimate impact. *Disaster Medicine and Public Health Preparedness*. 2011;5(Suppl1, ePub):S143–S150.

46. World Health Organization. Global alert and response. Summary of probable SARS cases with onset of illness from 1 November 2002 to 31 July 2003. Accessed December 19, 2011, at http://www.who.int/csr/sars/country/table2004_04_21/en/index.html

47. U.S. Department of Health and Human Services. H1N1 timeline: meeting the challenge. Accessed December 19, 2011, at http://www.flu.gov/news/blogs/timeline.html

48. Centers for Disease Control and Prevention. Questions and answers. Vaccine against 2009 H1N1 influenza virus. Accessed December 19, 2011, at http://www.cdc.gov/h1n1flu/vaccination/public/vaccination_qa_pub.htm

49. Centers for Disease Control and Prevention. Abbreviated pandemic influenza plan template for primary care provider offices: guidance from stakeholders. Accessed December 19, 2011, at http://www.cdc.gov/h1n1flu/guidance/pdf/abb_pandemic_influenza_plan.pdf

50. U.S. Department of Health and Human Services. National health security strategy of the United States of America. December 2009. Accessed December 19, 2011, at http://www.phe.gov/preparedness/planning/authority/nhss/strategy/documents/nhss-final.pdf

51. Centers for Disease Control and Prevention, Office of Public Health Preparedness and Response. Public health preparedness capabilities: national standards for state and local planning. March 2011. Accessed December 19, 2011, at http://www.cdc.gov/phpr/capabilities/Capabilities_March_2011.pdf

52. Obama B. *Presidential policy directive/PPD-8*. Washington, DC: The White House; 2011. Accessed December 19, 2011, at http://www.fas.org/irp/offdocs/ppd/ppd-8.pdf

53. Alexander GC, Wynia MK. Ready and willing? Physicians' sense of preparedness for bioterrorism. *Health Affairs*. 2003;22(5):189–197.

Monitoring and Controlling Physician Organizations

Physician Practice: Organization, Management, and Operation

Michael J. Kelley, MBA, CMPE
Steven Falcone, MD, MBA
Stephen G. Schwartz, MD, MBA
Richard D. Norwood, CPA, FHMA, MBA

Total U.S. healthcare expenditures totaled almost $2.5 trillion during 2009, representing almost 18% of the U.S. gross domestic product and over $8000 per person. Almost $506 billion was spent on direct physician and clinical services. Although substantially less than the expenditures for hospital care ($759 billion), the impact of physician practices on the healthcare industry is greater than the raw numbers would suggest.[1] It is estimated that 50% to 60% of healthcare costs are directed by physicians.[2] Physicians not only personally perform medical services, but also admit patients to the hospital, order hospital- and nonhospital-based services, prescribe drugs and therapeutic treatments, and order disposable and durable medical equipment and various ancillary and home healthcare services.

The physician and physician group sectors of the industry traditionally have been highly fragmented and vertically isolated. More recently, the physician sector has had to respond to radical changes in the medical environment, undergoing change consistent with, and often in conflict with, other sectors of the industry.

■ Forms of Physician Practice

There are four major forms of physician practice: individual or solo physician practice, single-specialty group practice consisting of two or more physicians, multispecialty group practice, and physician practice management companies (PPMCs). Two other forms are physician staffing services and hospital-employed physicians. Any of these forms may be either hospital-based or independent. The proportion of hospital-based medical practices appears to be increasing. A survey performed by the Medical Group Management Association (MGMA) reported that hospital-owned practices accounted for 55% of all respondents, an increase from 50% in 2008 and about 30% in 2003.[3]

Solo Practice

Solo practice is the choice of only a very few individuals currently embarking on a medical career. Only 5.5% of physicians under the age of 35 years are reported to be in solo or two-physician practices. Physicians in solo practices often cite the freedom and self-determination made possible by independence as major benefits. With no other physicians involved in the practice, a solo practitioner can make business decisions and develop a practice style and work ethic without the need to consult associates. The practice is able to directly meet the personal needs of the practitioner in terms of balancing income, scheduling, and professional interests.

The autonomy and flexibility of solo practice is not without costs—financial, professional, and personal. Solo practitioners frequently have lower average earnings than members of a group practice. It also can be difficult for a solo practitioner to develop areas of special interest or competence within the field of medicine due to the time constraints of constantly being available to patients and referring physicians. The lower total revenue stream makes it difficult, if not impossible, to hire professional managers to run the practice, and those employed, including the physician-owner, must often perform multiple roles within the business. It is also fair to speculate that the lack of collegial exchange of opinion and information can hinder professional growth, at least to some extent.

Of increasing importance, solo practitioners, particularly those who do not have a highly specialized area of practice, may have difficulty obtaining and retaining managed-care contracts. This lack of individual negotiating power tends to lead to lower contract rates for the physician, unless he or she becomes affiliated with an external contracting organization such as an independent practice association (IPA) or preferred provider organization (PPO).

The autonomy of solo practice also creates a corresponding responsibility for all aspects of the practice. Delegation of areas of responsibility among other physicians is not possible; in most cases, specialized administrative business personnel are financially unaffordable; and decisions need to be made without the benefit of alternative opinions and group decision making. The time spent managing the necessary business activities detracts from the time available for patient care activities.

A solo practitioner may function as a self-employed individual or as an employee of the corporation that the physician wholly owns, whether a subchapter S or subchapter C corporation. Selection of the specific form of practice is determined in conjunction with legal and financial planning experts. Each form has its own specific tax planning issues, including the deductibility of certain expenses, retirement plan options, and taxation of fringe benefits. In addition, there are legal consequences including, among other things, the degree to which the practitioner's estate is protected from ordinary business liabilities and uninsured professional liabilities.

Single-Specialty Group Practice

Single-specialty group practices are a common form of practice. In a single-specialty group practice, all the physicians practice within the same field of medicine. This does not mean, however, that the practices need to be identical. For example, an ophthalmic single-specialty group might incorporate subspecialties of the eye, such as retina, cornea, oculoplastics, and glaucoma.

Physicians in group practice may enjoy a number of benefits. Historically, compensation for group practicing physicians, whether single- or multispecialty, is frequently higher than for solo practitioners. Although often cited as a reason for group success, there is little evidence that economies of scale are created in a group. In fact, group physicians frequently have a higher expense ratio than do non–group-affiliated physicians. Group practices, however, often are able to make larger capital investments.

Two factors lead to this increase in capital investment. First, group practices tend to have substantially larger financial resources and cash flow. There is a general tendency toward greater predictability of financial performance due to diversification of both providers and services, and a lessened reliance on the performance of any one individual physician. As an example, cross-coverage during times of vacation, illness, and disability do not shut down the income stream; frequently, another physician in the group has some excess capacity that will generate revenues from the absent physician's existing patient population.

Second, there may be additional favorable capital investment opportunities. New equipment often can be profitably utilized in a group setting because higher aggregate numbers of patients are available to amortize the capital equipment cost. A new laser, for example, might not be a cost-effective investment for a solo practitioner because the physician's patient population does not generate enough utilization. When that same investment analysis occurs in a four-member group, the utilization theoretically increases an additional 300%, making resultant positive cash flow and profitability more likely.

Additionally, these practices often are able to employ more highly trained support staffs that are not required to multitask. Group practices often have specialized personnel devoted to diagnostic procedures requiring little direct physician involvement. The physician gains productivity by, essentially, outsourcing the technical component of the service and concentrating on the provision of professional services. In other words, those tasks that require skill, but do not require professional decision making (the art of medicine) can be performed by nonphysician employees who are compensated at a lower rate. A solo physician, by way of contrast, typically must personally perform most or all aspects of the service.

Group practice makes more affordable specialized staff members who are able to concentrate their efforts and learned expertise on billing, insurance, finance, and operational matters. These nonphysician operational specialists are able to manage the increasingly complicated insurance-imposed precertification processes and utilization limits, and the group can more successfully and profitably contract with managed-care organizations. Solo physicians are often unable to support the costs associated with management of the administrative processes and must either outsource these services with the associated loss of control or perform these services personally and often less effectively and efficiently than those with specific expertise.

The experience level and training of the nonphysician leadership in group practice settings is also different from the management found in solo practices. In solo and small groups, the office manager frequently will not have earned a college degree, but will have many years of on-the-job experience in clinical or financial positions performing multiple functions within the practice. Group practices, by contrast, have increasingly sought professional managers with formal education, frequently requiring a master's degree or CPA certification. Many of these managers also will have achieved certification through professional associations, such as the MGMA's Certified Medical Practice Executive (CMPE) program, or as a Fellow in the American College of Medical Practice Executive (FACMPE) programs.

This may help explain both the higher expense ratios and the higher incomes of physicians in group practice, a setting in which physicians generally see more patients per week while working a comparable number of hours.[7] The physician in a group practice also can achieve lifestyle benefits from delegating responsibilities, reduced call schedules, and cross-coverage during times of vacation, illness, or disability.

Casalino et al. investigated physicians practicing in groups of greater than 20 members. The most highly cited benefits were leverage with health plans (80%), economies of scale (46%), and profit from ancillary services (26%). Improved quality was cited by only 15% of respondents. Physician desire for autonomy and difficulty in intraphysician communication were cited by 49% as a barrier to large group formation. Lack of capital, IT, and investment was the second most-cited barrier (30%), closely followed by the cost of regulatory mandates for capitated patients (26%) and a perceived lack of physician leadership (24%).[4]

Offsetting the advantages of group practice is the need to develop consensus among physicians regarding practice philosophies and administrative policies. The difficulty of this task, combined with the inherent interpersonal relationships, causes a large number of group practices to end either in dissolution or with the departure of individual physician members, reported at a rate of 6.1% annually.[5]

This often can be traced to failures in the physician recruiting process. During the recruiting process, physicians often spend insufficient time gaining an understanding of each other as individuals, and determining the compatibility of personality traits, leadership styles, and expectations. More often, an inordinate amount of time is focused on the medical experiences and scholastic achievements of the candidate. The individual physicians who are part of the same group should ideally have the same vision, goals, and objectives. The costs, both personal and financial, associated with disassociation can be extremely high.

Multispecialty Group Practice

A multispecialty group practice shares many of the characteristics of a single-specialty group practice, but will include a range of specialties. Such groups might include primary, secondary, and tertiary care. Often these types of groups exist in a managed-care or academic organization. Many advantages can be cited for this model of practice. Multispecialty group practices tend to be, by their nature, larger than single-specialty groups. Many patients will have more than one significant medical problem, thereby creating opportunities for cross-referral to physicians within the group practice. A diabetic patient, for example, may require an endocrinologist to assist in the management of blood sugar levels, an ophthalmologist to treat diabetic retinopathy, a neurologist to treat diabetic neuropathy, and a wound specialist to care for diabetic foot ulcers. The size of the enterprise can produce opportunities whereby each practitioner can benefit from the professionally developed corporate administrative systems and cross-marketing plans. Multispecialty group practices often can position themselves as regional centers, drawing both self- and physician-referred patients from a larger geographic area than they would otherwise enjoy.

Offsetting these cited advantages are a number of problems associated with operating a large enterprise. The number of physicians in a multispecialty group can make governance a difficult issue. In the typical single-specialty group practice, each physician may play a role in the governance of the enterprise. In the typical multispecialty environment, governance is accomplished through an executive committee with a chief medical and administrative officer. Income and resource allocation may become rancorous subjects. Primary care and surgical specialties are often at odds because of financial and professional conflicts. Primary care physicians frequently seek to be subsidized by the higher revenue–producing specialists and subspecialists for whom primary care generates referrals, patient volume, and surgical cases.

Notwithstanding the negative issues associated with group practice, many physicians believe the support services generated by the group and the presence of ancillary services, as well as the freedom from administrative and managerial tasks, can offset the disadvantages. Group practice, whether single-specialty or multispecialty, is a growing force in the healthcare industry. Mergers and affiliations are becoming more common given the changes in the healthcare marketplace. Many healthcare experts predict the trend toward group practice medicine will accelerate and become an increasingly attractive choice for physicians beginning medical careers, as well as an alternative to be considered by solo and small group members. The trend toward consolidation often is viewed as a natural economic result of increased competition within the larger healthcare market.

Group practices, both single-specialty or multispecialty, may be formed under different legal entities. A partnership is an unincorporated form of practice that can be established as a vehicle for group practice. Group members own and distribute practice income based on their partnership agreement. There are clear disadvantages to partnerships with regard to liability issues. Each partner may be held individually responsible for the acts of any other partner related to the operation of the partnership. In some states, limited liability partnerships (LLPs) afford some protection from creditors that is unavailable to general partnerships.

Group practices are more often incorporated as either subchapter S or C corporations. The group physicians act as employees of the corporation. The governance of the group is carried out under the articles of incorporation and bylaws of the corporation. Not all group physicians need to be shareholders and officers of the corporation. Indeed, it is common for physicians new to the group to work for some period of time before they are offered the opportunity to purchase stock in the corporation.

Increasingly, physicians are not being offered ownership in the group. Rather, they are compensated through incentives that recognize the role they play as individuals in the achievement of the corporate mission. This can include phantom stock plans, bonuses based on productivity, incentives for proper utilization, retention bonuses, and other rewards for tangible and intangible achievements. The lack of partnership or ownership opportunity, however, may be a factor that limits the group's ability to recruit if other practices in the same market space offer this opportunity.

Factors for Physician Recruits and Employers to Consider

When investigating group practice opportunities, physicians should not overlook the personal and business relationships that are characteristic of group practice. Group practices are, in a social and economic sense, group partnerships. Individuals need to reconcile expectations about standards of care, professional competency, financial matters, social and personal behaviors, personality, and ethics. This is particularly true, and may be difficult to reconcile, when more experienced and seasoned physicians are hiring younger, less experienced physicians of a different generation. Generational differences can result in a completely different concept of how many hours constitute a workweek, and the younger and older physicians may be at odds. To some older physicians, limits on residency program training time (such as the 80-hour workweek maximum) may be seen as a lack of commitment and a loss of work ethic in the new generation of doctors.

The recruitment or affiliation process should start with the basic requirements, including licensure and clinical competence acceptable to all parties. Thereafter, the process should be driven by the factors that will influence professional and group success. How will the candidate "fit in" in terms of life goals? Is there a compatibility of styles, approaches, and decision making? Are the expectations of the senior members achievable? Will the junior associate essentially act as an overflow for the other group members, or be expected to develop an individual practice through practice-building activities, such as seminars, physician entertainment, and civic involvement? The goal of all parties should be to achieve a viable, pleasant, and profitable long-term relationship, and the decision process needs to be handled with this in mind. The importance of taking a more behaviorally based approach to joining a group practice cannot be overstated.

Physician Staffing Companies

Physician staffing companies, which directly employ providers and contract service to hospitals, is another physician practice model. Firms such as Mednax, Sheridan Health Services, and Cogent-HMG are exhibiting growth as they staff specialists, such as pediatrics, anesthesia, and hospitalist services, as subcontracted providers of essential hospital services. These firms frequently provide services regionally or nationally, focused on hospital-based specialty and subspecialty care.

Hospital-Employed Physicians

Recognizing that physicians drive hospital admissions and services, there has been renewed attention to recruitment and direct employment of providers since 2000. Hospitals are employing physicians both to defend existing service lines from erosion and as a growth strategy to expand service volumes. In general, employed physicians direct admissions and outpatient services to their hospital. Changes in provider reimbursements are reducing incomes of specialists, and the acquiring hospital will face the need to subsidize physician employment costs as a result.

Cited advantages that positively impact physician employment by hospitals include[6]:

- Improvements in negotiated fee schedules with health plans
- Reduction in costs through group purchases
- Access to healthcare engineering and IT infrastructure and expertise
- Access to hospital capital for clinical service line introductions
- The ability for physicians to balance professional and personal time through the elimination of managerial oversight roles required in running a physician practice

Physician Practice Management Companies (PPMCs)

PPMCs are organizations that exist primarily to perform nonclinical services that support the delivery of healthcare services. Several factors have led to their existence. Entrepreneurs, including hospital organizations, healthcare professionals, venture capitalists, and Wall Street, realized that healthcare represents an important segment of the economy. Physicians were increasingly aware of both their role in the delivery system and the threat posed by the evolution taking place in the nonphysician segments of the industry. The consolidation of hospital systems; the emergence of large, powerful, and restrictive health plans; and the diminishing role of indemnity insurance gave rise to new concerns, business imperatives, and strategic choices. Some large multispecialty groups are now positioned to negotiate for exclusive contracting

relationships with large insurers. These new arrangements have the potential to affect revenue, not only to the physicians, but also to a web of interdependent organizations (**Figure 8-1**).

Another driving force that led to the PPMC industry was the exponential growth in the complexity associated with operating the nonclinical activities of the physician practice. Authorization processing, contracting with managed-care organizations (MCOs), and compliance with federal guidelines all created new administrative burdens that some physician practices were ill-prepared to perform. Theoretically, business practices used in other industries, such as consolidation and specialization of activities, could improve both the effectiveness and efficiency of the operation, leading to increased revenues and profits. Also significant is the need for capital to invest in data processing, to implement capitation systems, and to build new cost-effective business and administrative systems.

PPMC Structure

There are a variety of PPMC structures. Equity model PPMCs purchase the assets of the physician practice and manage, through supervisory oversight, the nonclinical activities of the practice, including employment of all nonphysician personnel, supplies contracting, and centralized accounts receivable and payable management. At the time the PPMC purchases the physician practice, an exchange of cash, notes, and equity in the PPMC occurs at a negotiated value. This value is derived from an estimate of the value of the cash flow that the PPMC will derive through a contract that entitles it to a percentage of profits, frequently between 10% and 30%.

Service model PPMCs also emerged to provide management services to physicians without acquiring the practice. These often take the form of management service organizations (MSOs). MSOs provide, on a fee basis, selected management services, which can include managing contracting activity for the practice or a group of practices that are affiliated with an independent practice association (IPA) or other network. MSOs may provide centralized billing and collection activity, centralized group purchasing systems, and discounted consulting services. Frequently, these organizations are capitalized by the physicians themselves as a way to build aggregate negotiating power. The difference between the models is that the practice remains in the ownership of the physicians. Some industry leaders foresee expanded growth of the MSO industry, due to the increasingly complex IT infrastructure needed to teach quality, compliance, and coordinated care.

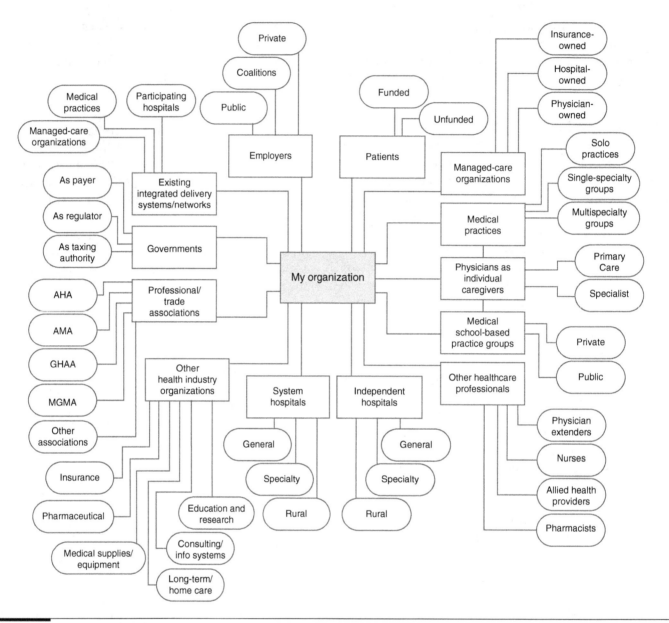

Figure 8-1 Healthcare stakeholders.

Source: Reprinted with permission from the MGMA Center for Research, 104 Inverness Terrace East, Englewood, Colorado 80112-5306; 303-799-1111. www.mgma.com. Copyright 1995.

■ Healthcare Funding Plan Evolution

Faced with the high cost of, or the inability to obtain, traditional medical insurance, organizations began to experiment with alternative delivery systems and insurance mechanisms in the 1920s and 1930s.[7,8] In 1965, a survey conducted by the U.S. Department of Health, Education, and Welfare identified 582 prepaid medical plans.[7(p13)] For the overwhelming majority of Americans, traditional fee-for-service medicine was the only available option. It wasn't until the 1970s and 1980s that managed-care plans showed significant growth. Nearly half of all employees covered by employer-sponsored group health plans were enrolled in managed-care plans by 1991. The report noted that 25% were enrolled in health maintenance organizations (HMOs), 22% were in preferred provider organizations (PPOs), and 5% were in point-of-service (POS) plans.[8] Managed care continued to expand its penetration as healthcare expenditures grew. By 2002, 26% of employees were enrolled in HMOs, 52% in PPOs, and 18% in POS plans.[9]

Since the year 2000, the percentage of employees choosing HMO coverage has shrunk from 30% to 19%, while high-deductible health plans with a savings option (HDHP/SO) have grown to approximately 13% of the covered employee market. Similarly, PPO growth has continued, while POS has declined and traditional indemnity plans have virtually disappeared from the marketplace.[10]

Although many physicians decry the complexity, utilization rules, and preapproval process that complicate managed-care participation, net incomes of physicians that participate in managed care average more than $28,000 more than those who do not participate. Those physicians with managed care representing 25% to 50% of practice revenues had incomes more than $44,000 higher than nonparticipants (**Figure 8-2**).[11]

"Managed care" is a widely used phrase, but one that is not necessarily easily defined. Strictly speaking, managed care could be defined as medical care being directed and paid for by a third party, generally an insurance company. Under strict interpretation, this would define virtually any insurance policy or government program as a managed-care program. Few policies or programs contain no restrictions on the services an insured party can obtain. Virtually all have limits on overall

spending, types of services covered, and frequency of services provided. Managed-care plans can be sponsored by a profit or nonprofit organization and may reimburse physicians on a capitated or discounted fee-for-service basis. Services can be provided by salaried healthcare providers or by contract with independent physicians. They may have large open or closed panels of providers. They can function by directly providing medical services or through the indemnification or reimbursement of incurred costs. On the basis of just these five characteristics, 32 permutations are theoretically possible. On a more general basis, though, managed care is defined as care that offers comprehensive benefits delivered by selected providers and that provides financial incentives for members to use providers who are members of the plan.

Health Maintenance Organizations (HMOs)

HMOs are medical care organizations that are responsible "for the provision and delivery of a predetermined set of comprehensive health maintenance and treatment services to a voluntarily enrolled group for pre-negotiated

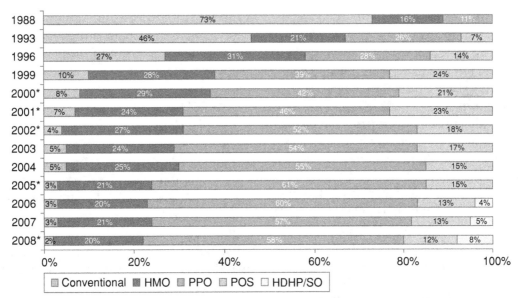

* Distribution is statistically different from the previous year shown (*p* < .05). No statistical tests were conducted for years prior to 1999. No statistical tests are conducted between 2005 and 2006 due to the addition of HDHP/SO as a new plan type in 2006.

Note: Information was not obtained for POS plans in 1988. A portion of the change in plan type enrollment for 2005 is likely attributable to incorporating more recent Census Bureau estimates of the number of state and local government workers and removing federal workers from the weights. See the Survey Design and Methods section from the 2005 Kaiser/HRET Survey of Employer-Sponsored Health Benefits for additional information.

Figure 8-2 Distribution of health plan enrollment for covered workers, by plan type, 1988–2008.
Source: Henry J. Kaiser Family Foundation. Distribution of health plan enrollment for covered workers, by plan type, 1988–2009. Kaiser Fast Facts. September 2009.

and fixed periodic capitation payment."[12] Cowan defines five common characteristics shared by such plans[13]:

1. A defined population of enrolled members
2. Payment by the members determined in advance for a specific period of time and made periodically
3. Medical services provided on a direct service basis rather than on an indemnity basis
4. Services provided to patients by HMO physicians for essentially all medical needs with referrals to outside physicians being controlled by HMO physicians
5. Voluntary enrollment by each family or member

In an HMO, a primary care provider (PCP) typically is responsible for determining what services are necessary and who will provide the services for enrolled patients. The PCP becomes the "gatekeeper" for the patient's access to services. In the event the patient seeks care on a nonemergent basis from any healthcare provider not authorized by the PCP, payment is typically denied for the services. The effect of this healthcare delivery model is that it limits the services received by the patient to those deemed medically necessary by the primary care provider and attempts to eliminate duplicative or unnecessary costs. A frequently cited problem of traditional fee-for-service medicine is that the provider receives a direct financial benefit from ordering additional tests and procedures. Under the HMO model, the provider receives no financial benefit from the tests and referrals initiated. In fact, in the event that utilization targets are exceeded, the PCP may be penalized for excessive healthcare costs incurred by the patients for whom he or she has accepted medical and financial responsibility.

Patients have the least amount of choice about the medical care and provider selection in an HMO plan. Because all care is directed by the "gatekeeper," the gatekeeper may view the need for care as less urgent, or unnecessary, than the patient does. Further, patients may desire to obtain specialty care from well-known physicians and academic medical centers that are not part of the HMO's panel. Should they, nonetheless, want to obtain the care from non-HMO physicians, they will have to pay the cost of the care completely out of pocket, with no benefits coverage.

There are three models for organizing physicians in an HMO: the staff model, the group model, and the IPA model.

Staff Model HMO

In the staff model HMO, physicians are salaried employees of the HMO. They furnish care exclusively to members of the HMO, with the HMO responsible for all nonclinical management. In some cases, these physicians are given incentives to control costs through bonus mechanisms that reward the physician for controlling costs and lower utilization.

Group Model HMO

In a group model HMO, the physicians are organized as a multispecialty group. These groups often have their own separate legal entity and contract with the HMO to provide services to its members. The group receives a direct capitation payment from the HMO, which has been predetermined by negotiation, and may be entitled to supplemental payments based on the profitability of the HMO. The group then compensates individual physicians based on either a salary, productivity, or utilization basis, or a combination of all three methods.

The group model HMO can result in significant risk shifting to the group practice. Inasmuch as the physicians often are the owners of the group practice, their net income can be directly affected by services provided to HMO members. Incentives to hold down overall healthcare costs can take two forms. First, there may be prenegotiated accruals, or withholds, payable in the event costs are under budget. Second, higher profits can be generated internally within the group through the lower costs associated with the provision of fewer services.

The physician group often provides services to patients who are not members of the HMO, as well, and may operate that component of the group practice on a traditional fee-for-service basis.

IPA Model HMO

An IPA (independent practice association) is a legal entity composed of physicians and physician groups, each of which functions as a separate and independent practice. Under an IPA model HMO, large panels of physicians contract with the HMO to provide health services within a defined geographic area. Traditionally, physicians have been paid on a fee-for-service basis, but at a rate that discounts their customary charges. In many cases, the fee schedule is set by a discount to or a multiple of the Medicare fee schedule. A portion of the discounts, referred to as withholds, may be paid to physicians if a surplus exists after payment of hospital, external, and administrative costs.

Faced with the desire of insurers to decrease their claims cost risk, some IPAs are developing capitated payment agreements. Under such an agreement, the IPA contracts to provide specified services at a fixed cost per beneficiary per month. The IPA then controls utilization issues within its organization and compensates individual practitioners for care on either a discounted fee-for-service or capitated basis. IPA physicians often derive a large percentage of their practice income from traditional fee-for-service patients. One of the cost control weaknesses of this model is that the overwhelming majority of the physician's income is still generated on a fee-for-service basis with the smaller remainder being dependent on the IPA's cost behavior. Physicians continue to receive the bulk of their income from the number of examinations, procedures, and tests they perform.

Preferred Provider Organizations

PPOs (preferred provider organizations) are similar to IPAs in that physicians function on a fee-for-service basis. Unlike the HMO model, in which there usually is a primary-care gatekeeper who controls the services provided to enrollees, PPO-enrolled patients are free to make their own choice of member providers. PPO physicians enter into an arrangement with the sponsoring organization, often an insurance company or hospital-affiliated organization, and agree to a discounted fee for service. By offering the discount and thereby maintaining access to patients converting from traditional indemnity plans, the physicians hope to stabilize or increase the size of the patient population they service.

Subscribers typically are free to seek the care of physicians outside of the PPO panel, but are penalized by receiving a lower rate of reimbursement, resulting in a higher out-of-pocket cost to the beneficiary. PPOs often incorporate low copayments and limited or nonexistent in-network deductibles in order to create an incentive for patients to obtain discounted care and remain within the PPO panel. The patients may opt out of the panel and seek care elsewhere if they feel value is generated equal to the higher cost associated with out-of-network services. Unlike HMO patients who have no coverage outside of the plan, PPO subscribers receive partial reimbursement of their out-of-network medical services, subject to copays and deductibles. PPO physicians typically do not share in any withhold pool and receive no direct incentive to hold costs down. The physician practices medicine on a discounted fee-for-service basis; income is directly related to the value and volume of services rendered.

High Deductible Health Plans

Recently, employees have had the option of enrolling in high-deductible health plans with a savings option (HDHP/SO). HDHP/SOs are defined as (1) health plans with a deductible of at least $1000 for single coverage and $2000 for family coverage offered with a health reimbursement account (referred to as HDHP/HRAs) or (2) high-deductible health plans that meet the federal legal requirements to permit an enrollee to establish and contribute to a health savings account (referred to as HSA-qualified HDHPs).

A health reimbursement arrangement (HRA) is a tax-qualified plan offered in conjunction with a high-deductible health plan, and is funded by the employer for each participating employee. It pays for eligible healthcare expenses typically covered under the medical plan. Employer-contributed funds that were not used to pay claims can be carried over to the next year to cover future healthcare expenses, an incentive to employees to use their personal HRA wisely. If funds are exhausted, the employee is responsible for satisfying the remaining deductible before the plan begins to pay. If the employee changes jobs, the money stays with the employer.

A health savings account (HSA) is a tax-advantaged medical savings account available to employees enrolled in an HDHP. The funds are a pretax employee contribution to their account and are not subject to federal income tax at the time of deposit. HSAs are owned by the individual, which differentiates them from the company-retained funds in an HRA. HSA funds may be used to pay for qualified medical expenses at any time without federal tax liability. Withdrawals for nonmedical expenses are treated very similarly to those in an IRA in that they may provide tax advantages if taken after retirement age, and they incur penalties if taken earlier.

Rand Corporation studied first-year results for enrollers in HDHPs and found an average 14% decrease in health spending compared to a lower deductible plan, and that savings were greatest among those with deductibles over $1000. Of concern was the finding that childhood vaccination rates, mammography, and cervical and colorectal cancer screening rates all fell, even when the deductible was waived.[14]

Accountable Care Organizations

One of the newest models of healthcare delivery is the accountable care organization (ACO). The ACO model is based on three principles[15]:

1. It is an organization composed of providers collectively responsible for the entire continuum of patient care.
2. The ACO distributes payments to providers in a way that slows spending growth.
3. It invests in infrastructure and care redesign processes to promote effective and efficient patient care.

The emphasis is on the medical providers as the parties collectively responsible for the cost of care, rather than through the types of cost control models in place at a HMO, where utilization is controlled through specific service approval or direct capitation. Objective and subjective indicators, including patient satisfaction scores, well-defined quality measures devised from evidence-based medicine, and coordination of care are important components of the organization's revenue and cost distribution model.

Examples of the metrics used to evaluate quality and effective care include:

- Rate of adverse events following an intervention
- The control of blood glucose levels in diabetic patients
- Rate of central line injections
- Rate of communication between specialists and primary care providers
- Rate of emergency room (ER) visits and associated admissions
- Risk-adjusted cost of care

Organizational Structures of ACOs

Review of the literature, as well as the proposed structures of Medicare pilot projects, outline the variety of approaches that can be taken to create an ACO. Clearly, many existing large health conglomerates such as academic medical centers and integrated health systems already possess a breadth of providers and facilities that can support the formation of an ACO. Additionally, they also have a governance structure and payment distribution process that can overcome one of the initial barriers to formation.

Additionally, existing well-organized multispecialty groups, physician hospital organizations (PHOs), and IPAs aggregate the breadth of providers needed to serve the patient care continuum, but in varied degrees of integration. One would expect that higher degrees of integration at academic and integrated health systems and PHOs could ease the ability to undertake ACO formation, whereas the absence of hospital involvement in an IPA would raise the difficulty of successfully forming an ACO.

Deloitte proposes seven core competencies and associated critical success factors needed to operationalize an ACO. These are shown in **Table 8-1**.

Opinions vary on whether this approach can successfully achieve the goal of improved care and outcomes and reduced costs. The transition from a largely fee-for-service–based physician compensation model to a system that rewards teamwork, cost control, and evidence-based medicine is not easily achieved. Likewise, institutions such as academic and integrated health systems present an outward appearance of integration that masks internal dynamic tensions among individuals, physicians, hospitals, and management over the allocation of a diminished or slowed revenue model, an implicit measure of ACO success. Structuring aligned incentives is difficult, at best.

ACOs also require new infrastructure creation to support coordination, cost control, and the capture of the metrics of performance that demonstrate the improvement in the effectiveness of care. Although there are limited existing measures of quality of care, such as the Physician Quality Reporting System (PQRS) used by Medicare, the very limited number of quality metrics would be insufficient to measure the care of many conditions, as well as coordination of patient care and effectiveness. The concept of the ACO model represents a theoretical transformative step in the evaluation of healthcare, but whether it can achieve the organizational support, technological backbone, provider integration, and patient support needed is largely unproven at this point.

System Comparison

All of these care models share a common goal: the reduction of healthcare costs. They vary substantially in the method and degree of control they exert on the individual practitioners. Not surprisingly, the lowest physician costs are typically found where control of physician activity is highest (**Table 8-2**). Indemnity insurance, the traditional insurance program in which patients are free to choose any physician for any healthcare problem, has the highest costs. PPOs, which are the least restrictive of the managed-care models regarding physician selection, are also the most expensive managed-care product. HMOs, with the highest levels of physician control, are generally the lowest-cost model.

Accessing Analytical Capabilities to Manage Physician Organizations

A common theme among all of the strategies needed for a physician to enjoy business success in the future is the need to manage the increasingly complex and capital-intensive resources needed to effectively collect, analyze, and process data. The capital needs are not just financial in nature, but increasingly include the human capital that can create efficient workflows and processes to drive down costs and increase effectiveness. Processes such as advanced revenue cycle management and clinical flow improvements from Six-Sigma and Lean Management approaches require skill sets that are not widely available

Table 8-1	Accountable Care Organizations: A New Model for Sustainable Innovation

Core Competency	Critical Success Factors
Leadership	Ability to: Develop strong teams and shared culture Mediate stakeholder priorities Clearly, regularly, and consistently communicate vision, strategy, and direction to internal and external stakeholders Change direction when necessary Innovate
Governance	Design and execute strategy and management performance goals Leverage cultural strengths and neutralize cultural challenges Access and deploy capital efficiently to implement strategy Recruit and retain competent leadership Use fact-based planning to engage trustees Leverage profit with purpose
Operational management	Incorporate clinical performance measurements (safety, efficacy, effectiveness, costs, outcomes, satisfaction, productivity, efficiency) to optimize accountability and gainsharing Contract effectively with health plans and employers to leverage capabilities and performance Align supply chain vendors in collective gainsharing and achieve optimal purchasing efficiency. Manage regulatory compliance
Clinical management	Manage clinical pathway adherence by care teams Redesign and align population-based health management processes with evidence-based guidelines Coordinate care across patient conditions, services, and settings over time Manage patient behavior and implement patient outreach, adherence, and self-care
Infrastructure and IT	Build and make effective use of information technologies for healthcare delivery and administration at provider, patient, and system level Integrate systems and aggregate data across multiple sites of care Synthesize data into dashboards for management decision making Leverage IT infrastructure to reduce paperwork and workflow inefficiency
Risk assessment	Identify and mitigate the impact of at-risk populations of patients Identify and interdict operational problems that pose risk
Workforce	Effectively design and allocate a healthcare workforce Optimize workforce productivity in a team-based incentive structure Control fixed and variable costs for workforce through innovation in HR design Manage outsourced relationships and strategic partnerships to cost-effectively enhance core competencies

Source: © 2010 Deloitte Development LLC. All rights reserved. *Accountable Care Organizations: A New Model for Sustainable Innovation*. Produced by the Deloitte Center for Health Solutions.

Table 8-2	Relative Costs of Managed-Care Models	
Model	**Control on Physician Activity**	**Costs**
Indemnity insurance	Low	High
Preferred provider organization (PPO)	Moderate	Moderate
Health maintenance organization (HMO)	High	Low

in the healthcare field, and may be prohibitive in cost for the small to medium-sized physician practice.

Part of the pressure for physicians to go to work for hospitals and health systems is related to this growing need for intellectual and financial capital. Many large systems have the required infrastructure to acquire and provide the resources for the employed physicians.

Management service organizations (MSOs) offer an alternative option to obtaining the needed skill sets without becoming a direct employee of a hospital (although some hospitals use MSOs to service their employed physicians). Serving more than 5600 physician clients,

MedSynergies president, J.R. Thomas, speaking during a personal conversation, defines the role of the MSO as "packaging information for physician leadership, leading to the development of processes that enable physicians to better treat patients."

Operational Aspects of Physician Practice

The operations of a traditional physician practice can be divided into a few key functional areas.

Resource Management

Operations management in a physician setting is similar to that of any other organization. The goal is to maximize long-term net revenue through the efficient utilization of resources. Resources include plant and equipment, physicians, ancillary staff, and time. A number of resource costs are fixed, including rent and many other occupancy expenses. Other expenses, such as supplies, are variable in that they rise and fall in direct relation to the volume of production. Some expenses, such as staffing costs, are semivariable in that they can be changed only in an incremental fashion, with a minimum level of cost that is essentially fixed within a specific range of activity. For example, a receptionist is necessary whether the physician sees one or six patients per hour. Hence, the cost is fixed if volumes stay in the range of one to six patients per hour, in this example. Once the capacity of the receptionist to adequately perform the duties is exceeded, even if by only one patient per hour, another receptionist needs to be hired to prevent downstream service impacts.

Operations management seeks to provide sufficient services at the lowest possible cost. For most medical practices, the highest-cost resource is the physician staff. Effective utilization of this resource requires that the physician's activity be concentrated in areas where he or she is uniquely qualified: the practice of medicine.

Principles of Staffing

Physician efficiency may be improved by delegating some aspects of patient care to lower-cost nonphysician staff. For example, many scientific measurement aspects of medicine, such as vital signs, weight, and height, can generally be performed by clinical assistants or physician extenders. Measurement activities take time, and time is the limiting resource for many physicians. When an activity is performed by physician extenders, the physician may increase the number of patients served as a result of the time savings. The art of medicine, a function that

can be performed only by a qualified provider, includes the cognitive function, the evaluation of quantitative and subjective data, followed by the definition of a disease management plan. Practices that utilize staff for measurement activities and physicians for the cognitive functions tend to have higher revenues than models utilizing fewer physician extenders.

Appointment Scheduling

The appointment scheduling process is one of the key variables in physician productivity. The goal of the process is to have the physician render medical care as continuously as possible during scheduled hours, while minimizing patient waiting times and staff overtime costs.

There are four basic types of appointment scheduling: standard segment, wave, resource-based, and open-access scheduling.

Under a standard segment system, the number of patients the physician sees per hour is divided into 60 minutes and scheduled in equal segments. If a physician sees six patients per hour on average, an appointment is scheduled every 10 minutes. Unfortunately, this system can be inefficient. If an individual patient requires less than the allotted 10 minutes, the physician may experience wasted time during which no patient is available. Alternatively, if an individual patient requires more than the allotted 10 minutes, the schedule will be disrupted and the physician becomes a bottleneck. The physician, therefore, essentially has three choices: work through a scheduled break (such as a lunch break), if one is available; try to catch up by spending less than 10 minutes with the next patient(s), which may lead to dissatisfaction; or run the rest of the day behind schedule.

Standard segment scheduling becomes even more problematic if multiple sequential steps are required for each patient. Many practices require each patient to be "worked up" by a physician extender prior to the physician encounter. For example, most pediatricians' offices have a technician or nurse measure the child's height and weight. If an individual patient requires additional time during this preliminary step, then the technician or nurse becomes a bottleneck. The physician's schedule becomes disrupted even if the physician is running on time.

In one high-volume ophthalmology practice the flow for most new patients is as follows[16]:

- Registration (5 minutes)
- Technician work-up (10 minutes)
- Optometrist evaluation (15 minutes)
- Ophthalmologist evaluation (15 minutes)
- Surgical coordinator (20 minutes)

Analysis of this patient flow helps to answer the common question: Why does my doctor always seem to run late? In general, physicians and medical administrators do not appreciate having their practices compared to assembly lines, but many of the fundamental operational principles are comparable. The short answer to this question is that, typically, doctors' schedules become delayed due to queues, or groups of patients waiting to be processed at one or more steps in the patient flow. In a multistep process, queues tend to form in the presence of statistical variability and dependent events.[17]

There is statistical variability because these times represent average times: at any given step, some patients will require less time, but some patients will require more time. In the ophthalmology practice studied, the "average" patient completes all 5 steps in 65 minutes. However, if a patient requires an extra 5 minutes to register, and this time is not "made up" by completing one or more subsequent steps in less time, then the patient completes the total encounter in 70 minutes.

The statistical variability is compounded by the presence of dependent events; that is, each step can commence only after the previous step has been completed. Therefore, if a patient takes 10 minutes to register (5 minutes longer than expected), he or she cannot progress to the next step, technician workup. If the technician cannot work up an alternate patient (if, for example, no other patient has progressed through registration at this time), then these 5 minutes are "lost" and all subsequent patients are delayed by 5 minutes, unless the time can be recovered some other way. In this manner, short individual delays become magnified as the day progresses. Two general strategies may be employed to reduce queues. If queues form in the presence of statistical variability and dependent events, then it stands to reason that reducing variability and allowing events to proceed out of sequence would be beneficial. For example, variability may be reduced by standardizing procedures to the extent possible (standard examination forms, etc.). Additionally, when possible, processes should allow for alterations in the sequence of events. For example, if there is a backup of patients (bottleneck) at registration, perhaps some patients may be diverted to the technician workup stage and returned to registration afterwards. Alternatively, staff may be cross-trained so that individual employees may "float" to the area of greatest demand.

Wave scheduling attempts to offset statistical variability by intentionally establishing a queue of patients. Under the same assumptions as for standard segment scheduling, a wave schedule would have three patients scheduled at the top of the hour and three scheduled at the bottom of the hour. Thus, if the first patient takes 5 minutes to be seen, the physician can move on to the next patient, who is already available to be seen. The second and third patients, however, may experience substantial wait times under this system.

A hybrid solution, called the modified wave, combines aspects of segment and wave scheduling. If a physician sees, on average, six patients per hour and the minimum visit is 5 minutes, appointments would be scheduled from the top of the hour in six 5-minute intervals until half past the hour. (That is, patients may be scheduled at 9:00, 9:05, 9:10, 9:15, 9:20, 9:25, and 9:30.) This ensures that the physician is always busy, but the fourth, fifth, and sixth patients may experience substantial wait times.

Another alternative scheduling method is based on time units. Typically, the 5-minute exam has characteristics that are distinct from the 15-minute exam. The 5-minute exam might be a routine postoperative exam and represent one unit of time, whereas the 15-minute exam would be an initial new patient visit using three units of time. By determining the type of exam, the number of units of time it will take can be determined. This can help to reduce patient wait times, which are stressful on both physician and patient, while reducing or eliminating periods of physician inactivity.

One of the most complex yet most effective scheduling methods looks at resource allocation. Each component activity of the medical service is analyzed and identified with a corresponding resource requirement. These resource components include technicians and nurses, physicians, diagnostic and surgical equipment, exam rooms, and waiting areas. Resource allocation looks at the availability of each of the resource components, seeking to maximize utilization while minimizing costs and reducing patient waiting times. Additionally, resource allocation requires that you forecast demand; planning includes making decisions about the demand for each type of appointment, whether it is for new patients, follow-up appointments, or surgical cases. Although complex, this sophisticated tool creates the most efficient and cost-effective schedules.

Open-access scheduling is an emerging method that seeks to have patients come to the office on the day of their call. By matching provider supply and patient demand, the method, used primarily by larger primary care providers, is designed to expeditiously meet patient needs, resulting in fewer no-shows and higher revenues. Open access has the advantage of providing services to the patient based on the patient's needs and wants, a powerful driver of patient satisfaction in today's competitive healthcare environment. This model presumes, however, that no insurance authorization or precertification is required prior to the patient's visit. Hence, open access is most prevalent in primary care practices, for which authorization of visits is frequently unnecessary.

Physician Billing

In the U.S., physician billing practices are unlike any other professional billing practices. This is due to many reasons, including the use of a third-party payor system. In addition, many physicians are uncomfortable discussing billing with their patients and prefer to delegate this to non-physician staff members.

CPT Coding

In order for both physicians and their patients to be properly reimbursed for services by insurers, the procedure or procedures performed must be identified. Medicare, Medicaid, and most other third-party payors utilize the American Medical Association's Physicians' Current Procedural Terminology (CPT)[18] to describe the services provided to the patient. This process of reviewing the service and categorizing it is referred to as coding. The CPT book (updated every year) contains some basic coding information, as well as thousands of defined services or procedures. Each of the described procedures is defined by a specific five-digit code.

Under some circumstances, a code must be reported with one or more additional two-digit modifiers that identify relevant additional information needed to determine the amount or type of service performed. There are 25 surgical modifiers commonly used for surgical procedures and an additional 6 that refer to the evaluation and management sections of the CPT code. For example, modifier -50 identifies that a bilateral procedure was performed during the same operative session; modifier -54 identifies that the surgical care was provided by the billing physician and that another physician provided the preoperative and postoperative components of the surgical procedure.

Some physician activities require the use of Centers for Medicare and Medicaid Services (CMS) Healthcare Common Procedural Coding System (HCPCS, pronounced "hicpics") descriptors. Level II codes are a series of national codes that describe supplies, injectable drugs, and physician and other healthcare provider services not described in the CPT (HCPCS Level I), as well as dental services.[15] A third level of descriptors, HCPCS Level III, includes local codes used by the Medicare carrier to describe services and activities for which national coverage has not been determined. The number of local codes is decreasing as Medicare and other private and governmental insurers move toward a uniform national payment policy.

Care must be taken when coding, for many reasons. It is important to accurately reflect what services were provided, and miscoding may result in civil and criminal investigations. Accurate coding is important not only to ensure that the service was provided as described, but also to avoid the unbundling of charges. Unbundling occurs when a procedure is broken down into discrete components rather than being identified by the procedure code that defines the entire service. The reason that unbundling represents an incorrect coding method relates to the way in which the value of procedures is determined. The value of the work performed by improperly componentizing the procedure would be significantly greater than the work value that would derive from the global or bundled procedure. In other words, the sum is greater than the whole.

As an example, during the repair of a retinal detachment by scleral buckling, a physician may inject air or gas, use cryopexy to seal the tear, and drain subretinal fluid. Each of those three procedures has its own discrete CPT code. When taken as a whole, they are regarded as components of CPT code 67105; repair of retinal detachment (**Exhibit 8-1**). The amount paid if the procedure were broken down by components would be significantly greater than that billed under the "global" code.

Evaluation and Management Coding

CPT coding also includes physician evaluation and management (E&M) services. "Evaluation and management services" is the term applied to what most people would consider "a visit with the doctor." This can take place in a variety of settings, such as the physician's office, a hospital room, a nursing home, or the patient's home. The level of intensity of the visits also can vary from a blood pressure check by a nurse to a comprehensive examination for a life-threatening disease.

CMS works in conjunction with the AMA and other industry groups, expending significant effort in an evolving process to measure the complexity and intensity of these widely variable activities. Major revisions to the process occur every several years; the trend is to make the evaluation and management coding system less subjective and easier to interpret and audit.

The purpose of the coding structure is to accurately evaluate the relative value units (RVUs) associated with the activity. The site of service (e.g., hospital or office) has an impact on costs associated with the provision of service. For instance, when a physician provides services within the hospital, the cost of delivery for the services borne by the physician is lowered by the fact that the physician has not borne the cost of supplies and staff.

Exhibit 8-1 Example of Bundled Codes

Billed Code

67105—Repair of retinal detachment, one or more sessions; photocoagulation (laser or xenon arc) with or without drainage of subretinal fluid

Bundled Codes

67015—Aspiration or release of vitreous, subretinal, or choroidal fluid, pars plana approach (posterior sclerotomy)

67101—Repair of retinal detachment, one or more sessions; cryotherapy or diathermy, drainage of subretinal fluid

67141—Prophylaxis of retinal detachment with or without (e.g., retinal break) drainage, one or more sessions; cryotherapy, diathermy

67145—Prophylaxis of retinal detachment (e.g., lattice degeneration) with or without drainage, one or more sessions; photocoagulation

67208—Destruction of localized lesion of retina, one or more sessions; cryotherapy, diathermy (e.g., small tumors)

67210—Destruction of localized lesion of retina; photocoagulation (laser or xenon arc)

67227—Destruction of extensive or progressive retinopathy, one or more sessions, cryotherapy, diathermy (e.g., diabetic retinopathy)

67228—Destruction of extensive or progressive retinopathy, one or more sessions; photo coagulation

67500—Retrobulbar injection; medication (separate procedure—does not include supply of medication)

92504—Binocular microscopy (separate diagnostic procedure)

Source: CPT codes only © 2002 American Medical Association. All rights reserved.

Hence, the compensation of the physician for the service episode is lower than when the same service is provided in the physician office, where the physician bears the cost of supplies and staffing.

Documentation Guidelines for Evaluation and Management Services Seven components are recognized in defining the level of E&M services. These are:

- History
- Examination
- Medical decision making
- Counseling
- Coordination of care
- Nature of the presenting problem
- Time

History, examination, and medical decision making are the key differentiating components in the overwhelming majority of evaluation and management services. The other components are important only when the majority of the time is spent counseling and coordinating care. Four types of patient history can be selected for proper coding: problem-focused, expanded problem-focused, detailed, and comprehensive. Each type, at varying levels of detail, encompasses the following categories:

- *Chief complaint:* A concise statement that describes the primary reason the patient presented to the physician, including symptoms, problems, conditions, diagnoses, and physician recommendations for return visit.

- *History of present illness:* A chronologic description of the development of the patient's current illness from the first sign or symptom (or from the last visit) through the present time. This description should include the location, quality, severity, duration, timing, context, modifying factors, and associated signs and symptoms of the illness.

- *Review of symptoms:* An inventory of body systems obtained through questions intended to identify the patient's current or previous signs or symptoms. The recognized systems are constitutional symptoms, eyes, ears, nose, mouth, throat, cardiovascular, respiratory, gastrointestinal, genitourinary, musculoskeletal, integumentary, neurologic, psychiatric, endocrine, hematologic/lymphatic, and allergic/immunologic.

- *Past medical and surgical history:* The patient's previous experiences with illnesses, operations, injuries, and treatments.

- *Past family and social history:* A review of pertinent medical events in the patient's family, including hereditary diseases and risk factors; and a review of previous and current social activities, including marital status, occupational status, and exposure to alcohol, tobacco, and recreational drugs.

Diagnosis Coding

The *International Classification of Disease (ICD)*, published by the World Health Organization, is used to code a diagnosis or diagnoses applicable to the service rendered. The

U.S. Public Health Service and CMS mandate the use of the ICD manual for their programs. Approximately 1300 pages in length, the manual lists thousands of diagnoses. Each diagnosis is given a unique three-digit code, which can be further subclassified with an additional two digits, if necessary. The ICD coding of disorders resulting from impaired renal function, 588, is shown in **Exhibit 8-2**.

ICD-10 is scheduled to be operationally required by CMS on October 1, 2013. Its impact on physician practice will be disruptive because of the increase in the number of diagnostic codes from 14,432 to 69,368; changes in the structure, detail, and rules; as well as substantial impacts on the cost of training coders, coder productivity implementation of software systems, and the need for better primary documentation by the physician in order to avoid coders needing clarification from the physician before claims may be submitted or resubmitted.[19]

ICD-10 does, however, better support the ability to identify risk, severity, and complications of care, a critical need in the functions associated with ACOs. The higher level of specialty associated with ICD-10 will facilitate care pathways that differentiate between low-risk, low-acuity presentations of disease states and more complex presentations with associated comorbidities and needs for additional levels of medical intervention.

Exhibit 8-2   ICD-9 Codes for Disorders Resulting from Impaired Renal Function

588   Disorders resulting from impaired renal function
  588.0 Renal osteodystrophy
      Azotemic osteodystrophy
      Phosphate-losing tubular disorders
      Renal:
          dwarfism
          infantilism
          rickets
  588.1 Nephrogenic diabetes insipidus
  Excludes: diabetes insipidus NOS (253.5)
  588.8 Other specified disorders resulting from impaired renal function
      Hypokalemic nephropathy
      Secondary hyperparathyroidism (or renal origin)
  Excludes: secondary hypertension (405.0–405.9)
  588.9 Unspecified disorder resulting from impaired renal function

Source: Reprinted with permission from ICD-9-CM, Practice Management Information Corporation.

Methods of Physician Reimbursement

In some medical specialties, such as cosmetic surgery, prices are simply set by individual surgeons, similar to non-medical professions such as accounting or law. For most physicians, however, prices are determined largely by third-party payors.

Usual, Customary, and Reasonable

Many indemnity insurers use (or used to use) what is referred to as the usual, customary, and reasonable (UCR) methodology, or a close variant thereof. Under this method, the insurer collects a database of charges for each service submitted by all similar physicians in a geographic area. The insurer then sorts these from the lowest charge to the highest and limits payment to a determined percentile. Some commercial carriers will pay at the fiftieth percentile of the charge array, whereas some others may pay as much as the ninetieth percentile charge. This is referred to as the "customary charge." The fee that the individual physician normally charges for the procedure is the "usual charge." The third fee that the insurer considers is a "reasonable fee." This fee allowance can vary based on documented special circumstances of the case, but generally is considered to be the average of all physician charges for the same service, in the same geographic area. The insurer will pay the lower of the usual or customary charge, unless a reasonable-fee adjustment is warranted. An example of a UCR system is shown in **Exhibit 8-3**.

Exhibit 8-3   Determination of Allowable Fee Under UCR Method

Table of Historical Charge Data

Physician	$		
Dr. Smith	75		
Dr. Gomez	60	..	90th Percentile
Dr. Casper	55		
Dr. Felix	50		
Dr. Felix	50	..	50th Percentile
Dr. Singer	47		
Dr. Alex	45		
Dr. Alex	45		
Dr. Jones	40		

Examples—Insurer pays 90th percentile

I   Dr. Smith submits charge for $75. Insurer allows $60. Charge exceeds 90th percentile UCR.

I   Dr. Felix submits charge for $50. Insurer allows $50, the usual fee for Dr. Felix.

I   Dr. Alex submits charge for $75. Insurer allows $45 based on his historical charges.

Relative Value Systems and Resource-Based Relative Value Systems

As early as the mid-1950s, payers began investigating a method of physician payment based on relative values. Under relative value payment methodologies, the economic cost of providing a service is the basis under which it is reimbursed. Physician time and training, the intensity of the service, and practice and malpractice expense components are factors that comprise the economic costs of providing a service. Rather than a reimbursement system based on historic charges, a relative value system quantifies the resources necessary to perform a service.

Relative value systems, when properly constructed, also have important utility as a management tool. They offer the opportunity for an organization to measure the resources necessary to deliver services and to compare them to an independently derived value. An organizational efficiency measurement can then be derived. Services can be measured in terms of both cost and revenue on an individual basis.

Relative value systems also provide organizations with a method to quantify the number of units of service provided. This method provides a productivity benchmark that is unaffected by changing case mix and fee schedules. Many practices track, as part of their financial management systems, the number of patient encounters. Relative value system–based management recognizes that some encounters and services are worth more than others. For example, the AMA has established that a comprehensive consultation with a physician expends 4.86 units of resources, whereas a comprehensive established patient visit expends 2.37 units.

Relative value systems also are useful in the measurement of the costs involved in providing care under capitated systems. The organization can track the number of units of service it provides and the capitated payment to compute the reimbursement per unit of service. By comparing the payer's reimbursement per unit of service to the organization's cost to provide a unit of service, management can make informed decisions about the profitability of managed-care contracts.

The most significant relative value system in terms of impact on the industry was adopted in 1992 by Medicare. The resource-based relative value scales (RBRVS) system came into effect because of the belief that the historical Medicare payment structure favored subspecialty and surgical procedures rather than primary care. Many feel that there is a serious inequity when primary care physicians, such as family practitioners, are earning significantly less than subspecialty surgeons.

Determination of Relative Values. The principal researchers that developed the relative value system used by Medicare and most other payers were a team of Harvard researchers commonly referred to as the Hsiao Team, named after its principal researcher. They surveyed a cross-section of physicians in multiple specialties to determine the amount of physician work involved in a number of described encounters/services. Physician work took into account the amount of time, intensity of effort, and technical skill required to provide the service. The physicians evaluated the work components relative to other defined encounters, indicating their perception of the amount of work involved in the task. These work values were then cross-linked against all of the procedures surveyed. The intent of the study was to have a uniform scale under which all physician activities could be evaluated. The Health Care Financing Administration (HCFA) then adapted and expanded on the work done by Hsiao to develop a schedule of work values for all covered Medicare procedures. Beginning January 1, 1992, the Medicare-approved fee for any service could be defined by calculating the following formula:

$$\text{Payment} = (\text{Work} + \text{Practice Expense} + \text{Malpractice}) \times \text{CF}$$
$$[(\text{RVUws} \times \text{GPCIwa}) + (\text{RVUpes} \times \text{GPCIpea}) + (\text{RVUms} \times \text{GPCIma})] \times \text{CF}$$

Where:

RVUws = Physician work relative value units for the service

RVUpes = Practice expense relative value units for the service

RVUms = Malpractice expense relative value units for the service

GPCIwa = Geographic practice cost indices (GPCI) value reflecting one-fourth of geographic variation in physician work applicable in the fee schedule area

GPCIpea = GPCI value for practice expense applicable in the fee schedule area

GPCIma = GPCI value for malpractice expense applicable in the fee schedule area

CF = Conversion factor (dollar denominated)

After the work components had been valued, two additional values had to be determined: practice expense and malpractice expense. The practice expense component reflects the overhead costs associated with providing the service. Practice expense and malpractice expense components were calculated by reviewing their historical costs, which were based on specialty-specific overhead ratios. The practice and malpractice expense ratios for a particular service were calculated to reflect a weighted average based on all the specialties performing the services.

During the consideration on the OBRA-89 legislation, debate arose over the need for adjustments to the fee schedule to account for variations and geographic costs. Geographic practice cost indices (GPCIs; pronounced "gypsies") were developed to make geographic adjustments against each of the fee schedule components. The practice expense GPCI was intended to account for geographic variations of office rents, employee wages, and other operating expenses. The malpractice GPCI was used to adjust the malpractice component of the cost in order to reflect the varying costs of malpractice liability insurance in different localities. The third factor, the physician work component GPCI, was the most controversial. Rural physicians complained that it was unfair to reward urban physicians with higher incomes simply because they practiced in areas with higher costs. They persuasively argued that physician cost of living was directly linked to the attractiveness of the location. Compromise was reached where only one-quarter of the geographic variations of physician GPCI would be used to adjust the payments.

After the work, practice expense, and malpractice components are determined and geographic costs are adjusted, the sum is multiplied by the conversion factor. The conversion factor is a monetary multiplier and is used nationally to compute the reimbursement level. The conversion factors can be adjusted annually to meet Congress's budgetary goals. For example, Medicare created a Sustainable Growth Rate (SGR) mechanism to control expenditures for physicians' services. The SGR formula has consistently created a situation where the computed value would create very large and cumulative cuts to the conversion factor, with resultant large cuts to the physician payments. Negative updates have been expected every year since 2002, although, as of this writing, Congressional action has averted payment reductions since 2003. In order to avoid these reductions, Congress and the administration have historically funded the Medicare program at a level that results in small positive changes to the overall level of payments to physicians.

The Billing and Collection Process

After the task of defining the service and linking it to its appropriate diagnosis is completed, the billing and collection phase of the physician reimbursement process begins. Each physician or group needs to create a billing and collection policy, a written set of procedures under which patients are expected to pay for the services they receive. A number of factors need to be considered when determining the payment policy. Does the group expect payment at the time of service (PATOS)? The advantages of this payment system, one of which is a rapid payment cycle with a low level of accounts receivable outstanding at any point in time, have to be weighed against the potential loss of patients who resent the unwillingness of the provider to bill the insurance companies for their appropriate balances. Patients may choose to obtain their services from competitors who offer more liberal collection policies.

The group or physician also needs to decide whether it will become a Medicare participating provider. Under this reimbursement option, the physician agrees to undertake the responsibility of collecting 80% of the approved charge directly from the Medicare carrier, making the patient responsible for only the 20% copayment and deductibles. Again, the socioeconomic characteristics of the target market need to be considered.

Insurance Submission. After the CPT and ICD codes have been selected for the encounter, claims are submitted to insurance companies for payment. Claims can be submitted on paper, often on universal billing forms, or electronically, if the practice is automated. Each year, greater numbers of practices use electronic billing, because payment often is made more quickly, important management information can be produced, and submission costs can be reduced. The payer applies its own rules when processing the claim. It may reject a charge based on inappropriate use, such as billing a follow-up visit as a new patient encounter. The insurer also may apply a fee screen (an automated edit of information). The fee screen will approve payment only for charges with specific diagnoses related to the services rendered. The rationale behind these fee screens is that tests and procedures are valid only for a limited range of diagnoses and appropriate patient types. For example, Medicare will not pay for a fundus photograph (a photograph of the retina) when the diagnosis is cataract (cloudiness of the lens).

Insurance companies often will reject unbundled codes, which represent multiple components of a global service. The insurance companies often adopt their own internally developed fee screens. These screens also may incorporate frequency-of-use limitations. This trend has continued to accelerate in both the private and governmental insurer fields as software is developed to enforce compliance with the insurers' disease management criteria.

The Accounting Process. In order to evaluate the efficiency of the billing process, the physician should establish an accounting system that collects all the pertinent information. One of the commonly used systems is the chart of accounts developed by the Center for Research in

Ambulatory Health Care Administration (CRAHCA).[21]

Gross charges are defined as the full value of medical services provided before any adjustment. Gross charges are then reduced by the following items:

- Charity adjustments
- Contractually agreed-upon reimbursement discounts (i.e., the difference between the charge and what the insurer allows on an assigned claim)
- Courtesy adjustments (such as for clergy or volunteers)
- Employee discounts

The result is the adjusted (net) gross charges or the maximum amount of payment that could be collected if all payers (insurers and patients paying co-insurance and deductibles) met their obligations. Net gross charges then become the collection goal of a physician practice.

The next step in the collection process is to record all cash payments collected from patients or the amount paid on their behalf by insurance companies and other payers. Noncash adjustments are referred to as payment allowances. These noncash adjustments are composed of bankruptcies, settlements, and provision for bad debts. Any remaining balance after the deduction of these items would represent a change in the accounts receivable.

The importance of timely and careful evaluation of the collection process cannot be overemphasized. Disruptions of cash flow can have major negative impacts. First, if fees are not collected in an efficient manner, the practice could suffer a liquidity crisis and be unable to meet its ongoing obligations. Second, and perhaps more important, the older a receivable is, the less likely it is to be collected. As the time period between the rendering of the service and demand for payment increases, patients will rationalize reasons why the fee was too high or they didn't receive what was expected. There is a greater perceived value to the service at the time the service is rendered.

Financial analysis and operational measurement generate numeric ratios and values that can be used to benchmark the organization's collection activity. These tools are utilized by well-run organizations, irrespective of the size of the organization.

Billing and Collection Systems

A physician practice has a number of options, manual and computerized, under which it can manage the billing and collection process. There are effective manual accounting systems, adequate for smaller practices that operate under a payment-at-time-of-service collection policy. The two common manual accounting systems used are the double entry system and the pegboard system.

A double entry system uses a charge and payment journal and individual records for each patient that list the individual's charges and payments, referred to as a ledger card. When a charge is incurred, it is entered into the charge and payment journal, as well as the ledger card. Thus, there is a double entry for each account activity.

The pegboard system improves on the double entry system by relying on a single-entry system. The ledger card is aligned in such a way that activity recorded in it also is recorded on a day sheet (listing all the day's transactions) by the use of carbon or duplicating paper. The entry also simultaneously creates the bill. Such systems, however, rely heavily on manual clerical functions for repetitive billing and aging of receivables. Both of these approaches are rudimentary and create only limited management information, and would likely only be found as legacy systems.

The overwhelming majority of practices operate computerized systems for a number of reasons. Most computerized collection systems are able to generate standard health claim insurance forms efficiently, a process that is very inefficient for manual systems, requiring work that duplicates efforts performed in the charge-posting activities. The overwhelming majority are capable of electronically transmitting these claims to Medicare carriers and other insurance companies. Many systems are capable of posting remittances electronically, as well. The net result is faster and more accurate turnaround of claims payments. Computer systems also can be programmed to generate bills to patients without interrupting normal office procedures. Outsourcing solutions that print, fold, and mail statements and collection letters without using the practice's clerical staff also can be used. In addition, most of these systems include computerized patient scheduling capability.

More sophisticated computer systems are able to pre-edit insurance submissions as well. By applying diagnosis and procedure linkages, submission errors due to miscoding or inappropriate unbundled charges can be prevented or corrected prior to submission. This helps to control the costs associated with the processing of denials, manual resubmission of claims, and telephone hearings with the insurer. It also flags inappropriate practice patterns, reduces the inflation of gross charges that can occur through inappropriate and uncollectible charge entry, and speeds the collection of patient copayments, as well as payments made by insurers.

Of particular importance is the ability to generate an aged accounts receivable and other analyses. These reports categorize the age of a receivable, which is calculated as the number of days since the service was rendered. This is an extremely important benchmark to monitor because of the previously described loss of collectability over time. Such a system also can be set up to force manual review, followed by the write-off or placement with collection agencies of uncollected debts.

Computerized collection systems also help reduce labor costs associated with manual systems. Submission of insurance claims on behalf of Medicare patients, now required by law, requires the repetitive entry of demographic and policy information. Many individuals will expect the practice to generate commercial insurance claim forms as well. This activity helps to expedite the payment of physician services to the patient. Basic computer and software packages capable of handling small practices are available for less than $5000, although systems for large groups can exceed $250,000. When such systems are bundled with an integrated electronic health record and interfaces for laboratory and other ancillary services and pharmacy, such systems can require multimillion-dollar, long-term commitments for integrated health systems.

The need for information about the practice also makes computerization valuable, particularly in a managed-care environment. The data entered in the course of recording account activity can give important insights into the demographics, case mix, and referral patterns in the practice. The ability to identify changes and extrapolate trends allows the physicians and management to react proactively. Increasingly, practices use the demographic and diagnosis information contained in the computer's database to interact with patients through targeted newsletters and other communications calculated to aid patient retention and service utilization of discretionary healthcare purchases, such as cosmetic surgery and aesthetic services and supplies.

Computerized billing and collections systems need not be owned by the practice. The practice can contract with an independent billing organization referred to as a service bureau. A service bureau functions solely to collect payments owed to physicians and other healthcare providers. By providing a collection function for a number of physicians, economies of scale and attention to the collection process can be achieved that may not occur within the physician's practice, with its focus on patient care. Service bureaus typically are paid on a percentage-of-collection basis, and this motivates them to collect efficiently and promptly.

This is not to disparage in any way the ability of a physician's own employees to effectively collect patient accounts; many can and do achieve results comparable to or better than those provided by service bureaus.

Management oversight, training, and system design always are the keys to a successful collection procedure, whether the activity takes place within the physician's office or through a service bureau. The efficiency of the collection function can be compared to collection data compiled by independent sources. A number of organizations, such as the MGMA, collect benchmarking data indicating gross and adjusted collection rates, as well as accounts receivable aging data.

■ Evaluation of Managed Care

Few physician practices can afford to ignore opportunities presented by managed-care contracting. Some specialties, such as cosmetic plastic surgery, are unaffected by insurance requirements because there is generally no coverage. However, nonparticipation in insurance plans limit these specialties' access to patients seeking insured reconstructive surgery following trauma or removal of cancerous lesions. Physician groups that enjoy a monopoly in their marketplace also can remain relatively resistant to the fee controls that can be a part of managed-care contracting, but may suffer a diminishment in patient demand due to higher out-of-pocket costs.

Contracts and Opportunities

The majority of managed-care contracting continues to take the form of negotiated discounts. These may be a percentage reduction in the charge. Most frequently, prices are set at a premium or discount to the Medicare fee schedule or other relative value system. Patients pay a copayment amount, which may be fixed or a percentage of the amount allowed for the services.

It is important to understand the current or projected market share of the prospective MCOs. The reimbursement that a physician accepts under the contract is often heavily dependent on the projected volume of services that the practice will gain, retain, or forfeit through nonparticipation. Careful intelligence and networking, along with requests for information from the MCO, should include:

- A general plan description
- The number of covered lives in the marketplace
- Affiliated insurance companies
- Sample provider contract
- Financial status of the plan
- Payment terms and copayments
- Withhold amounts
- Authorization processes and guidelines

Inasmuch as any arrangement with an MCO requires substantial administrative time and expense, the practice should focus its MCO contracting efforts on those plans that offer the best reimbursement terms and meaningful populations of patients.

Management of the patient mix among private pay, discounted, and capitated patient populations is essential. A useful analogy is often made between a physician practice and an airplane. Each day planes/physicians roll out to start a schedule. To be maximally efficient, the plane/schedule has to be full. To maximize revenue, the plane/physician wants to provide as many first-class seats/full-fee patients as possible, followed by business class seats/discounted PPO patients, filling the remainder of the plane/schedule with discounted advanced booking/capitation seats. If the plane/physician books too many advance-booking seats/capitation patients, revenue suffers because first-class seats/full-fee patients and business class seats/discounted PPO patients cannot be accommodated. The mix of filled seats/office appointments is critical to maximize profit. Yield management models can be used to adjust this mix.

Authorization Process

Many managed-care contracts require some level of authorization before providing services to the insured. These may be quite limited, as in general indemnity policies where authorization may be necessary only prior to a nonemergency hospital admission. Other tightly controlled plans, such as HMOs, may require preauthorization for any visit to a physician other than a primary care physician, have restrictions on approved hospitals and home health services, and require authorization for diagnostic testing and office-based surgical treatments. It is important for the physician services organization to set up a system that provides the pertinent information to the appropriate personnel in a timely fashion; that is, before the services are rendered. A practice can incur significant losses through poor authorization control, and every member of the staff needs to be attuned to strong authorization compliances.

Capitation is another method by which MCOs contract with physicians for services. Under capitation, physicians agree to provide a designated list of services to patients for a fixed payment, per member per month (PMPM). Risks are thereby transferred from the insurer to the physician to control costs associated with the listed procedures. In essence, the physician becomes the insurance company for risk associated with the amount and level of care provided.

In order to set capitation rates, the physician practice, utilizing the data derived from actuaries, attempts to project the amount and cost of service the population

will require to be served adequately. The age, sex, and employment status of the population can have important cost implications. The cost of providing eye care escalates dramatically in senior populations, whereas the cost of obstetric care is very low in patient populations that are skewed to middle-aged and older individuals. Specialty-specific analysis is necessary to understand fully the population of patients that is the subject of the bid. Frequently, stop-loss provisions are included to protect the physician from extraordinary costs, such as those associated with organ transplants or complications that can require extremely intensive therapies.

■ Financial Benchmarking

Financial benchmarking, often referred to as ratio analysis, is an important management tool necessary for sound practice management. Benchmarks are numerical indexes, used regularly and systematically, measuring overall performance or the performance of a specific target process (see **Exhibit 8-4**). Although it is a numeric index, the data reviewed may consist of either quantitative or qualitative measures.

Two levels of benchmark comparison are possible. First, the organization compares its performance against past or projected performance in order to evaluate trends. Second, the organization may compare and contrast its performance with external data compiled by organizations such as the MGMA, covering larger populations of self-reporting organizations. Benchmarks are useful in that they:

- Summarize complex information
- Allow early detection of financial problems
- Help in the management of payables and receivables
- Provide a framework for revenue and expense budgeting
- Allow the monitoring of re-engineered processes
- Provide a method to measure the performance of objectives identified during the practice's periodic goal-setting exercises

For analysis to be appropriate and sensitive, the design of the benchmarking system needs to consider the comparability, consistency, predictability, and relevance of the measure. When comparing ratios, particularly to externally derived benchmarks, it is important to understand the characteristics of the external measure. Is the group in the same specialty? Are there geographic or demographic biases? Is the data set composed of high-performing practices rather than "average" organizations?

Exhibit 8-4 **Examples of Ratio Types**

Liquidity Ratios

$$\text{Common Ratio} = \frac{\text{Current Assets}}{\text{Current Liabilities}}$$

$$\text{Quick Ratio} = \frac{\text{Cash} + \text{Marketable Securities} + \text{Accounts Receivable}}{\text{Current Liabilities}}$$

$$\text{Receivable Days} = \frac{\text{Accounts Receivable}}{\text{Net Collections}/365}$$

Profitability Ratios

$$\text{Write-Off Ratio} = \frac{\text{Charge Adjustments and Allowances}}{\text{Gross Charges}}$$

$$\text{Adjusted Collection Percentage} = \frac{\text{Gross Charges} - \text{Allowances and Adjustments}}{\text{Net Collections}}$$

Capitalization Ratios

$$\text{Fixed Asset Ratio} = \frac{\text{Total Operating Revenue}}{\text{Fixed Assets}}$$

Activity Ratios

$$\text{Surgery Yield (Specific type of) or Laser Yield} = \frac{\text{Total Patient Visits}}{\text{Surgeries (or Lasers)}}$$

$$\text{New Patient Ratio} = \frac{\text{Total Patients}}{\text{New Patients}}$$

Consistency refers to measurement of the item being reported. Are expenses carefully and uniformly classified by the reporting sites? Do all the reporting practices recognize a given expense within the same general ledger account? Predictability is another important feature of good indexing. Does the measure offer insight into future organizational or financial performance? And is that insight relevant or meaningful?

There are four types of practice ratios:

1. *Liquidity ratios:* The ability of the practice to meet payment obligations
2. *Profitability ratios:* The difference between the organization's expenses and revenues
3. *Capitalization ratios:* The relationships between debt and equity
4. *Activity ratios:* The relationships between input and output

The most commonly used liquidity ratios are the common ratio (current assets divided by current liabilities) and the quick ratio, expressed as the sum of cash, marketable securities, and accounts receivable divided by current liabilities. When the ratio falls below 1 in either case, the practice will likely experience a cash shortfall in meeting its current expenses, necessitating the use of additional liability financing. When using the quick ratio, care must be taken to value properly the accounts receivable. An unrealistic valuation—that is, one that does not properly quantify the bad debt and contractual allowances—will result in a quick ratio that misstates the ability to meet short-term obligations.

Although not strictly a measure of liquidity, receivable days and payable days measure the effectiveness of the collection process and the time lag in paying expenses. Receivable days are expressed as accounts receivable divided by annual net collections divided by 365 days. The measure determines the velocity at which services are converted into revenue. Gross or adjusted receivables can be used for the calculation, with adjusted receivables providing the best measure of velocity. Receivable days can be impacted by rapid insurance processing and submission, PATOS, and timely bad debt adjustments, all of which will reduce the number of days. Prepaid revenue, such as capitated payments received in advance of rendered services, will also cause a reduction in this important ratio. Rapid growth, whether cyclical or sustained, will, conversely, extend the number of days.

Payable days (current liabilities divided by annual operating expenses less depreciation divided by 365 days) measures the velocity at which expenses are being paid. This ratio is affected by periods of growth as well, because expenses during these periods often exceed the norm.

Cash management requires attention to both numbers; a growing number of days in either measure can signal a coming liquidity crisis.

As with many accounting ratios, the best numbers to work with are based on accrual rather than cash accounting. Accrual-based accounting minimizes the effects of seasonality and timing, prepaid revenues and expenses, and other distortions caused by the failure to recognize payables, such as the need to fund retirement plan contributions. The careful tracking of profitability ratios has become increasingly important. The write-off ratio—the difference between gross charges and recognized revenue—has increased dramatically with the growth of managed care–associated discounts, as well as Medicare fee schedules. If professional fees are set at a high level to maximize indemnity payments, the write-off ratio will be greater than for a practice with lower fees and equivalent collection efforts.

It is also increasingly important to perform analysis on a by-payer basis. A careful review will allow the determination of the actual percentage of total claims paid by the payer. This not only indicates the extent to which the payer is adhering to the negotiated fee schedule, but also allows the observation of the impact of disallowances, bundling, and noncovered services.

It is important that physicians and managers understand the differences between allowances and adjustments. Adjustments reduce the gross charge to the amount that can be theoretically collected. For example, if a procedure is charged at $125, and the associated Medicare allowed amount is $100, the account is credited with a $25 adjustment. The maximum amount legally collected on the patient's account is $100. In the event the patient failed to make the 20% copay, the account would be credited with a $20 allowance for bad debt (**Table 8-3**).

Allowances are the differences between gross charges and net revenues, and include such items as bad debts, settlements, and hardship adjustments extended by the physician after services are rendered. Bearing these issues in mind, the adjusted collection ratio (gross charges less adjustments divided by net collections) is the best measure of collection effectiveness.

Accounts receivable aging ratios also allow the measurement of collection velocity. Aging analysis tracks the proportion of total accounts receivable that fall within 30-, 60-, 90-, and 120-day-old periods since the charge was incurred. Several important factors must be considered. For example, consider similar periods. If the practice experiences seasonality, such as tourism inflows, these ratios will fluctuate a great deal. As the practice experiences an upswing in charges, the percentage of accounts in the older "buckets" will diminish. Likewise, at the end of the cycle, the older buckets will increase in percentage because of the wave effect. Why is it important to track receivables carefully? As stated earlier, consumer payment habits have shown that the longer a bill is deferred, the less likely it is to be paid. Excessive percentages of accounts more than 120 days old may indicate a suboptimal collection effort or a lack of discipline in the review of accounts for write-off or referral to a collection agency.

There are also important operational (or activity) ratios that can be either financial or nonfinancial measures. Examples of financial activity ratios are the percentage of nonphysician (staff) payroll expenses expressed as a percentage of revenue. Likewise, many practices track the percentage of revenues paid in the form of payroll and nonpayroll discretionary expenses distributed to the physicians and physician–owners. Other financial ratios include revenue per physician day worked, percentage of revenue generated through surgical codes, and average charges per patient.

Nonfinancial activity ratios are also important. The new patient ratio (new patients divided by total patients) is an often-tracked ratio in surgically based practices. Most surgically based practices experience the highest charges at the initial time period shortly following the new patient registration. Following surgery, there is often a period during which the surgeon provides follow-up care at no charge, or provides low-revenue office visits. The new patient ratio acts as a leading indicator of practice charges and is also sensitive to changes in referral patterns, advertising effectiveness, and patient-to-patient referral.

There are important caveats associated with all ratio analyses. Ratios provide measurement, not answers. There is no "correct" answer, and no single ratio can provide a good measure of practice "health." Some ratios may actually be counterintuitive on face value. For example, it is commonly believed that a low overhead ratio is an indication of a well-run practice. Yet, there is evidence

Table 8-3	Allowances Versus Adjustments
Physician fee	$125
Medicare allowed amount	$100
Adjustment	$25
Amount paid by Medicare	$80
Patient co-pay*	$20

* If the patient fails to make this 20% co-pay, the $20 would be considered allowance for bad debt.

that group practices with higher overhead ratios generate higher incomes to the physicians and physician–owners, because of higher levels of capital investment and wider service offerings. The physicians are taking home a small portion of a larger pie—but the slice is bigger than the larger slice of a small pie.

Other important factors also impact the ratios. Environmental differences, such as inner city locations and poor local economies, negatively impact collection ratios, as does high managed-care penetration. Differences from the norm can be part of a strategic plan. Practices that take aggressive marketing positions, such as high advertising levels, to stimulate the demand for services will have higher expense ratios than the norm. Practices also may offer low margin services in order to provide comprehensive care.

Practice philosophy and strategy also can have important impacts on the numbers. The physicians may have a heavily referral-based practice that has adopted the position that no one is turned away on the basis of ability to pay. Or, the physician may enjoy a more casual, less hurried approach to practice. Conversely, staffing costs might be increased through scribing and dictation costs in order to maximize physician productivity.

Ratio analysis needs to be undertaken carefully with an understanding of the practice, its goals, and the environment in which it practices. It is most valuable as a comparative measure within the practice, an indicator of change in relative performance over a comparable pertinent prior period measure. It becomes relatively less valuable as the measure is applied in comparison to other practices in the same specialty, and increasingly less relevant when compared to practices in dissimilar specialties and markets.

Notwithstanding these weaknesses, it is important to benchmark in order to carefully measure the impact of internal change, as well as performance, against the peer group. Benchmarking and ratio analysis are powerful tools that turn raw data into more meaningful information.

Benchmarking tools are available through professional organizations such as the MGMA. Annually, the MGMA produces the Physician Compensation and Production Survey in addition to other annual resources that are published by the MGMA.

A significant question for any practice is the physician direct cost and how that cost relates to market competitiveness. Also relevant is determining how physician compensation correlates with physician productivity. MGMA benchmarking surveys offer several choices of ratios useful for comparative purposes: collections by physician, gross charges by physician, and work RVUs per physician.

The analyst should consider issues of data availability, reliability, and consistency as part of the review process. Unfortunately, it is not unusual for a practice to not have RVU data available. In other instances, quality of RVU data may be impacted by the use of pseudo-codes (codes created for procedures not in the CPT code book), proper uses of modifiers, and coding accuracy within the practice.

The MGMA surveys, as well as surveys created by specialty societies and other industry groups, utilize other ratios for benchmarking physician compensation as it relates to productivity. Physician compensation by physician gross charges is another ratio example. Gross charges can be impacted by the pricing methodology existing at the practice. Some providers will set pricing based on a reference point, such as a markup on the Medicare Charge Allowable. Other pricing decisions may reflect prices generally found in the marketplace, and still other pricing decisions may reflect the desire to stimulate demand for strategic initiatives or capitalize on brand strength. These are all pricing strategies that have an impact on gross charges, and it would not be unusual for a large organization's price schedule to reflect the impact of several of these pricing strategies.

One of the weaknesses of this ratio is that prices do not always bear a direct relationship to more objective measures of productivity. The schedule of procedure and service prices will lead to the perception that the physician is generating a level of productivity that is misleading.

The MGMA's Physician Compensation and Production Survey includes other valuable information that adds to a deeper understanding of the relationship between productivity and compensation. Physician compensation per work RVU is an available metric that removes the impact of the pricing strategies outlined previously; payor factors, such as highly discounted fee schedules common in clinics serving the underinsured; as well as the effectiveness of the collection and billing process.

Physician compensation as a percentage of collections is another commonly used benchmark that has the advantage of adding revenue as a measure of productivity; ultimately, it is revenues that provide the cash flow to support the clinical operation. The drawback is that the measure lacks the objectivity of standardized work units that RVU-based measures provide.

All of the measures can be benchmarked within several dimensions such as geographic region, physician specialty, gender, and length of physician employment. Surveys provide information that will allow the comparison of the provider measure against the data continuum, such as the twenty-fifth percentile, fiftieth percentile, or seventy-fifth percentile. The use of these ratios can aid in the operation of physician compensation or incentive plans or in understanding practice financial performance or individual physician contribution to the practice. In practice, the analyst will often need to reconcile the different results provided by the various measures, because they will frequently produce dissimilar results. Practitioner subspecialty distinction may result in a survey group too small to be statistically meaningful; practitioners may provide services in several different provider classifications; and the provider compensation may be based on other, nonfinancial dimensions, such as professional prominence, research strengths, or the need to enhance a service line to offer comprehensive services. These are just a few examples of confounding real world examples that make what one might think would be a simple process more complex than suspected.

A strong knowledge of the practice financial data, the marketplace, and the mission of the organization is needed to provide the organization's management team with the contextual framework to create well-conceived, well-aligned, and financially viable compensation methodologies.

References

1. Centers for Medicare and Medicaid Services. National health expenditures 2009 highlights. Accessed March 24, 2011, at http://www.cms.gov/NationalHealthExpendData/downloads/highlights.pdf
2. Coddington DC, Keen DJ, Moore KD, and Clarke RL. *The crisis in healthcare: Costs, Choices, and Strategies.* San Francisco, CA: Jossey-Bass; 1990:38.
3. Matthews AW. When the doctor has a boss. *Wall Street Journal.* Accessed December 11, 2011, at http://online.wsj.com/article/SB10001424052748703856504575600412716683130.html
4. Casalino LP, Devers KJ, Lake TK, Reed M, Stoddard, JJ. Benefits of and barriers to large medical group practice in the United States. *Archives of Internal Medicine.* 2003;163:1958–1964.
5. The Economy Plus Flexibility Keep Physicians in Practice. *Newswise.* Accessed December 12, 2011, at http://www.newswise.com/articles/view/549601/
6. Larson JG. *Defense vs. offense: hospital employment of physicians.* Health Leaders Media. Accessed December 11, 2011, at http://www.healthleadersmedia.com/content/LED-210946/Defense-vs-Offense-Hospital-Employment-of-Physicians##
7. Hyman H. *Health planning: a systematic approach.* Gaithersburg, MD: Aspen; 1975:10–13.
8. Health Insurance Association of America. *Source book of health insurance data.* Washington, DC: HIAA; 1992:116–117.
9. American Medical Association. *Physician socioeconomic statistics* (2000–2002 ed.). Chicago, IL: AMA; 2002:8.
10. Employer Health Benefits 2011 Annual Survey. Accessed December 11, 2011, at http://ehbs.kff.org/?page=charts&id=1&sn=5&ch=564
11. Havlicek P, Eiler M (Eds.). *Physicians in medical groups: a comparative analysis.* Chicago, IL: American Medical Association; 1993:7
12. Shouldice R, Shouldice K. *Medical group practice and health maintenance organizations.* Washington, DC: Information Resources Press; 1978:10.
13. Cowan D. *Preferred provider organizations: planning, structure and operation.* Gaithersburg, MD: Aspen; 1984:5.
14. Tocknell, MD. *HDHPs associated with 14% decline in health spending.* Health Leaders Media; Accessed December 11, 2011, at http://www.healthleadersmedia.com/page-1/HEP-264431/HDHPs-Associated-With-14-Decline-in-Health-Spending##
15. Fisher ES, McClellan MB, Bertko J, et al. Fostering accountable healthcare: moving forward in Medicare. *Health Affairs.* 2009;28(2):w219–w231. Accessed December 11, 2011, at http://content.healthaffairs.org/content/28/2/w219.abstract
16. Miguel MF, Bowen HK. *Ophthalmic consultants of Boston and Dr. Bradford J Shingleton. Harvard Business School case 9-697-080.* Cambridge, MA: Harvard Business School; 1997.
17. Goldratt EM, Cox J. *The goal: a process of ongoing improvement* (3rd ed.). Great Barrington, MA: North River Press; 2004.
18. American Medical Association. *Physicians' current procedural terminology.* Chicago, IL: AMA; 1993.
19. Nichols JP. *ICD-10 physician impacts. Advisory board research report.* Washington, DC: Advisory Board; 2010:3–10.
20. Practice Management Information Corporation. *ICD.9.CM.* Los Angeles, CA: PMIC; 1993:270.
21. Schafer E, et al. (Eds.). *Management accounting for fee-for-service/prepaid medical groups.* Englewood, CO: Center for Research in Ambulatory Health Care Administration; 1989.

CHAPTER

9

Accounting and Budgeting for Medical Practice Managers

Steven M. Andes, PhD, CPA
David N. Gans, MSHA, FACMPE

Accounting and budgeting are central to business decisions. Accounting is the language of business. Businesses use accounting to record, monitor, and report their financial condition. Businesses use budgets to translate their goals and objectives into what they expect to spend and earn. Budgets are the accounts in the accounting system "dressed up" and arranged to support a business decision. For example, a practice decides to buy an electronic billing system using both cash and borrowing. The accounting system contains the accounts for the billing system, the cash, and the borrowing. The budget uses the information in the accounting system to translate that decision into capital assets, cash, and debt. This chapter focuses on what practice managers need to know about both accounting and budgeting, and how one supports the other.

■ The Major Types of Accounting

There are three major types of accounting: financial, tax, and managerial. Financial accounting is used primarily for creditors, lenders, and governmental bodies.

It describes the practice's financial position and helps investors and creditors determine the relative risk for investing or lending to the practice. Financial statements are important outcomes of financial accounting. Financial accounting has standard rules, terms, and procedures, which are called generally accepted accounting principles (GAAP). A nongovernmental agency, the Financial Accounting Standards Board, used to be the ultimate authority for GAAP; however, since the Sarbanes-Oxley Law of 2002 (Public Company Accounting and Investor Protection Act, PL 107-204, 116 Stat 745), the Public Company Accounting Oversight Board (PCAOB, www.pcaobus.org) is now the final authority for GAAP for publicly traded corporations. Although the PCAOB is technically not a government agency, the Securities and Exchange Commission, which is a governmental agency, appoints the chair and the members, and approves its rules, standards, and budget. The FASB however remains the authority for GAAP as it relate to other businesses and organizations.

The purpose of tax accounting is to determine a practice's tax liability, rather than its risk to lenders. Tax accounting, therefore, does not follow the same rules as financial accounting. Congress and state legislatures, not the financial accounting community, formulate and interpret the principles of tax accounting.

Managerial accounting is used primarily for members of the practice. It focuses on business decisions. It helps identify what services are profitable. It also feeds more directly into the budget and into performance assessment than does financial accounting. Managerial accounting has no official set of rules; rather, it offers a set of tools that managers can use to make their practices more efficient and effective. For a comparison of financial and managerial accounting, see **Table 9-1**.

The Institute of Management Accountants (IMA, www.imanet.org) is an important organization that promotes managerial accounting and develops new managerial techniques. However, it is not the final authority for managerial accounting, as the PCAOB and the FASB are for financial accounting.

The Practice Manager's Responsibility for Accounting and Budgeting

The practice manager is responsible for both accounting and budgeting. Practice managers are the liaison between the medical staff, who have the greatest power over the practice's financial position but know little about finance, and creditors, who also have great power over the practice's financial condition, even though they know little about medicine. Practice managers who perform these tasks well make the practice efficient and effective, and by doing so, earn promotion and job security.

Practice managers are in a unique position to make medical personnel financially aware, and to make creditors aware of the practice's strengths that the accounting system might not capture. Practices compete for patients, contracts, and capital. Financially efficient and sound practices are better able to compete than inefficient ones. Practice managers are in a position to encourage physicians to be efficient and to make creditors aware of the practice's financial strengths. Bankruptcy is very real in today's medical market. Medical practices themselves may go bankrupt or they may be involved in the bankruptcies of related organizations, including hospitals, managed-care organizations, and practice management companies.[1] Practice managers are in a position to keep their practices out of bankruptcy and away from affiliations that contribute to bankruptcy.

In the past, practice managers were a buffer between outside parties and the medical staff. Practice managers could take care of the finances so that the medical staff could practice medicine. This luxury is much less possible today. Practice managers should know enough about financial accounting to speak the language of accountants, creditors, lenders, and regulators. On the managerial side, the practice manager must know enough about finance and financial systems to ensure they serve the needs of the practice effectively. The practice manager also must be able to present financial information very simply so that medical personnel can understand it and realize how it affects what they do and how they do it.

The Relationship Among the Practice Manager, the CPA, Auditors, and Potential Lenders

The practice manager also is the interface between the medical staff and the certified public accountants (CPAs) who prepare the financial statements, prepare the taxes, and conduct any audits or reviews. The practice manager benefits the practice by translating what medical staff does into what the CPA needs, and vice versa. The practice

Table 9-1	Comparison of Financial and Managerial Accounting	
	Financial	**Managerial**
Audience	Creditors and investors	Members of the practice
Major uses	Financial statements	Budgets, business decisions, and performance reports
Ultimate authority	PCAOB (publicly traded companies); FASB (other companies)	None, although the IMA is an importance resource for developments
Requirements	Specified in GAAP	None
Focus on each practice's unique characteristics	Limited; the goal is to enable comparisons between practices	Extensive, because the goal is to guide practice decisions

manager must know enough about how to prepare financial statements and how to audit them to work effectively with accountants and auditors. Effective cooperation usually means faster preparation and lower fees to prepare financial statements, and faster, more favorable, and less expensive audits.

On the managerial side, the external CPA may be 100% correct in the presentation, but 100% wrong in describing the finances in a way in which the managers can use the information to manage the practice effectively. Practice managers are also the critical link between the practice and potential lenders who need important information not usually included with the financial statements, including age of the medical staff and trends in patient volumes, factors that can result in a lower interest rate for borrowing. Potential lenders usually require this information as part of their due diligence, but practice managers can take the lead, and thus present this information in a way that best serves the practice.

Principles of Financial Accounting: The Generally Accepted Accounting Principles

GAAP (Generally Accepted Accounting Principles) refers to the rules or protocols that govern how financial information is presented. GAAP is arbitrary and therefore may not present the complete picture of the practice's financial condition. However, GAAP enables financial information to be compared between medical practices.

Healthcare presents unique circumstances that GAAP may not address in a way acceptable to most healthcare providers. Contractual adjustments and charity care are two examples. Hospitals traditionally showed gross revenues and then contractual adjustments as a reduction in revenues to arrive at net revenues. GAAP now requires hospitals to show only the net revenues on the face of their financial statements. Hospitals previously indicated charity care as an expense or as an offset to revenue. GAAP now permits hospitals to show charity care as a footnote only.[2] Although physicians have more flexibility in how they disclose contractual adjustments and charity care in financial accounting, that flexibility could disappear.

Principles of Accounting Information and GAAP

This section summarizes the principles of accounting information and GAAP, especially what these principles mean for practice managers in terms of their

responsibilities to physicians and to the financial community. The following sections describe the basic objectives of accounting, the requirements for good financial information, the standards for good financial information related to recognition and measurement, and the elements of the major financial statements.

Basic Objectives of Accounting Information and Financial Reporting

The *Statement of Financial Accounting Concepts No. 1* states that:

> Financial reporting should provide information that is useful to present to potential investors and creditors and other users in making rational investment, credit, and similar decisions. The information should be comprehensible to those who have a reasonable understanding of business and economic activities and are willing to study the information with reasonable diligence.[3]

The *Statement* also states that financial reporting should:

- Provide information to help investors, creditors, and others to assess the amounts, timing, and uncertainty of prospective net cash inflows to the related enterprise because their prospects for receiving cash from investments in, loans to, or other participation in the enterprise depend significantly on its cash flow prospects.
- Provide information about the economic resources of an enterprise, the claims to those resources (obligations of the enterprise to transfer resources to other entities and owners' equity), and the effects of transactions, events, and circumstances that change resources and claims to those resources.
- Provide information about an enterprise's financial performance during a specific time period. Investors and creditors often use information about the past to help in assessing the prospects of an enterprise in the future. Thus, although investment and credit decisions reflect investors' and creditors' expectations about future enterprise performance, those expectations are commonly based at least partly on evaluations of past enterprise performance.
- Provide information about how an enterprise obtains and spends cash; about its borrowing and repayment of borrowing; about its capital transactions, including cash dividends and other distributions of enterprise resources to owners; and about other factors that may affect an enterprise's liquidity or solvency.

- Provide information about how management of an enterprise has discharged its stewardship responsibility to owners (stockholders) for the use of enterprise resources entrusted to it.
- Provide information that is useful to managers and directors in making decisions in the interests of owners.[3]

Less technically, the goal of financial accounting is to provide information that is (1) useful to those making investment or credit decisions who have a reasonable understanding of business and economic activities; (2) helpful to recent and potential investors and creditors and other users in assessing the amount, timing, and uncertainty of future cash flows; and (3) about economic resources, the claims upon those resources, and changes in them.[4]

Implications for Practice Managers. Accounting professionals presume that people who use accounting information have a reasonable understanding of business and economic activities, which excludes many laypeople. Practice managers, however, must realize that many users of the practice's financial information, such as physicians, will lack these skills and that they need to have sufficient accounting knowledge to act as an intermediary between accounting professionals and the practice's governance.

Primary and Secondary Qualities of Good Financial Information
The fundamental concept of accounting information is that it should communicate the appropriate information in an understandable fashion.[3,5-7]

The profession has defined primary and secondary qualities for information in order to make it useful for decision making. The primary qualities are:

- *Relevance:* Will have an impact on a decision
- *Reliability:* Repeating the measurements yields the same data

To be relevant, the information should be timely and should predict the outcome of an event, or confirm or reject a prior event. To be reliable, the information should be accurate, and should not be slanted either positively or negatively. Reliability also means that other investigators would obtain the same information if they replicated what the first investigator did.

The secondary qualities for understandable information are:

- Comparability across organizations
- Consistency with previous years

Implications for Practice Managers. Practice managers should know the financial decisions that the accounting information will be used to support. The financial statements of a practice seeking a major loan will read differently than those from a practice whose members are seeking to retire. Practice managers can reduce audit costs and make their financial data easier to understand if they maintain financial data in the same way from year to year and are aware of how other practices report financial information.

The Standards for Good Financial Information Related to Recognition and Measurement
The profession has developed standards related to revenue recognition and measurement. They include the "basic assumptions" and the basic principles of accounting.[6] The basic assumptions are:

- *Economic entity separate from owners:* The practice's assets and liabilities are separate from the owners'.
- *Going concern:* Assets and liabilities are valued with the assumption that the practice will continue. This assumption usually means that the assets and liabilities include accruals, prepaid expenses, and assets that are valued at historical cost rather than replacement cost or current cost.
- *Monetary emphasis:* Accounting information emphasizes what can be measured in money such as physical assets or owed expenses.
- *Periodicity:* Financial information is measured at the same time every year, usually the end of the calendar or fiscal year.

Implications for Practice Managers. Practice managers should be aware of each of these assumptions. Regarding the economic entity, the practice manager must clarify which assets belong to the practice and which belong to the owners. It can be easy to commingle assets. For example, a physician may use his or her personal computer for the practice's business. Some emergency physician groups have a physical office that is located in a physician's home. Although the partnership or practice agreement can help clarify which assets belong to the practice, the manager must keep these agreements current and supplement them when needed. These concerns become especially important if the practice becomes unable to pay its bills or payments to member physicians depend on assets donated.

The going concern assumption is important because if it cannot be assumed that the practice will continue, then it becomes necessary to revalue the practice's assets to what they can be sold for, and to revalue the practice's liabilities to their current market values. Receivables and sometimes payables are usually settled for much less than their face value if the practice is no longer a going concern.

The monetary emphasis is especially important to practice managers because much of the information important to creditors and lenders is not measurable in monetary terms. This information includes the age distribution of the physicians and the practice's market share. Practice managers should have this nonmonetary information available and take the initiative to share it with creditors and lenders. Although managers can expect creditors to demand this information as part of the due diligence process, managers can profit from taking the initiative.

Basic Principles of Financial Accounting

These principles help guide how to record financial transactions, given the accounting assumptions described in the previous sections. The transaction principles are:

- *Historical cost:* Assets are recorded on the books at their purchase price, rather than their current cost or replacement cost. The accounting profession prefers historical cost to replacement cost because historical cost is factual whereas replacement cost is an estimate.
- *Revenue recognition (realized and earned):* A practice can recognize or record revenue when it has been earned, but not before.
- *Matching revenue and expense to achieve income:* Expenses are matched against the revenues they produce to compute net income. The matching principle is one argument for depreciation because depreciation annually reduces (or matches) the revenues the asset produces.
- *Full disclosure:* The practice must disclose all material information. "Inadequate disclosure of material fact" is grounds for both civil and criminal action.

Implications for Practice Managers. The historical cost principle has two important implications for practice managers. First, managers should maintain records of the purchase price and current depreciation for all assets. These records are especially crucial in the practice's first audit. Second, practice managers should also help physicians understand that using historical cost can lead to wrong business decisions if the asset's replacement cost differs from its historical cost.

Practice managers should not recognize revenue prematurely. For example, suppose a practice signs a 3-year capitated contract. Unless the contract guarantees to pay the practice regardless of any conditions (which is very unlikely), the manager should recognize the revenues at the end of each month—after the services have been provided. Physicians may wish to treat the 3 years of revenue as if it were earned on the first day of the contract. That is incorrect. The revenues are recognized as they are earned; this addresses the possibility of the practice closing before the 3-year contract is over.

Practice managers should know the source of revenues and where the expenses are incurred to achieve these revenues. This information supports both financial accounting and internal decision making. Although matching expenses and revenues can be difficult—the depreciation expense for equipment may support more than one service, for example—practice managers need to know where the revenues come from and how much they cost to earn.

Practice managers should ensure full disclosure. Legally, it can be as wrong to hide information as it is to falsify it. What information has to be disclosed changes in response to market conditions and government initiatives. Creditors tend to look harder at financial reports during economic slumps, and the government can change its emphasis between administrations. Managers should know what financial information has become important and what previously important financial information has become less so. Managers might make it a policy to discuss this issue with their accountant annually in order to have all important information ready.

Constraints

The accounting profession recognizes that accounting information is not free to collect or share. The information is collected subject to four constraints:

- *Cost-benefit:* Accounting information should not be collected if it costs more to collect than it yields in benefits.
- *Materiality:* Accounting information should not be collected if it does not have a "material" impact on financial decisions.
- *Industry practices:* Accounting information is not collected philosophically or in a vacuum. Most industries have established ways to collect and report accounting information. The accounting profession believes that historic industry practices should be respected, even if they conflict with pure accounting theory.
- *Conservatism:* If there are two equally valid ways to measure a revenue or expense, or to value an asset, then the method that yields the lowest net income should be selected. This constraint does not mean

that income must always be reduced, but that when there are two equally valid accounting methods, err on the side of caution.

Implications for Practice Managers. Practice managers control all administrative costs, including the cost to collect and report financial information. They are also responsible for collecting and reporting all material financial information. Therefore, practice managers should keep abreast of what financial information is important and what information is likely to become important in the future.

Regulators and the courts are very willing to disregard industry accounting practices and disclosure customs. The current concerns that industry practices in mutual funds have hidden fraud echo earlier concerns that industry practices in healthcare hid Medicare abuse.

Therefore, practice managers should know industry practices in order to satisfy current auditors, but they must also know which industry practices are likely to change. Again, an annual discussion with the practice's accountant can be very helpful.

The Financial Accounting Standards Board (FASB) has also defined the elements of financial statements,[7] as shown in **Table 9-2**.

Implications for Practice Managers. Practice managers must know how to read a financial statement and know the meaning of each account in a financial statement. They must also know the difference between accounts like revenues and gains, or expenses and losses so that they can communicate effectively with their CPA, the auditor, their creditors, and their own staff.

Table 9-2 **Elements of Financial Statements**	
Element	**Definition**
Asset	Probable future economic benefits obtained or controlled by a particular entity as a result of past transactions or events.
Liabilities	Probable future sacrifices of economic benefits arising from present obligations of a particular entity to transfer assets or provide services to other entities in the future as a result of past transactions or events.
Equity	Residual interest in the assets of an entity that remains after deducting its liabilities. In a business enterprise, the equity is the ownership interest.
Investments by owners	Increases in the net assets of a particular enterprise resulting from transfers to it from other entities of something of value to obtain or increase ownership interests (or equity) in it. Assets are most commonly received as investments by owners, but may also be services, satisfaction, or conversion of liabilities of the enterprise.
Distributions to owners	Decreases in net assets of a particular enterprise resulting from transferring assets, rendering services, or incurring liabilities by the enterprise to owners. Distributions to owners decrease ownership interests (or equity) in an enterprise.
Comprehensive income	Change in equity (net assets) of an entity during a period from transactions and other events and circumstances from nonowner sources. It includes all changes in equity during a period except those resulting from investments by owners and distributions to owners.
Revenues	Inflows or other enhancements of assets of an entity or settlement of its liabilities (or a combination of both) during a period from delivering or producing goods, rendering services, or other activities that constitute the entity's ongoing major or central operations.
Expenses	Outflows or other using up of assets or incurrences of liabilities (or a combination of both) during a period from delivering or producing goods, rendering services, or carrying out other activities that constitute the entity's ongoing major or central operations.
Gains	Increases in equity (net assets) from peripheral or incidental transactions of an entity and from all other transactions and other events and circumstances affecting the entity during a period, except those that result from revenues or investments by owners.
Losses	Decreases in equity (net assets) from peripheral or incidental transactions of an entity and from all other transactions and other events and circumstances affecting the entity during a period, except those that result from revenues or investments by owners.

Cash and Accrual Accounting, and Modified Accrual Accounting

Cash and accrual accounting present two different views of the same question: what was earned and what was spent? Cash accounting recognizes income when cash is collected and recognizes expenses when cash is paid. Accrual accounting recognizes income when it is earned (rather than when the cash is collected) and recognizes expenses when they are incurred (rather than when they are paid). The goal of cash accounting is to answer the question "How much cash does the practice have?" The goal of accrual accounting is to answer the question "How much income did the practice earn?" Accrual accounting therefore includes receivables (income earned but not collected) and payables (expense incurred but not yet paid). Accrual accounting also recognizes several other categories of accounts that do not exist in cash accounting: expenses such as depreciation that do not involve cash payments, receivables, payables, and prepaid expenses and revenues.

The following example illustrates the major differences between cash and accrual accounting. A medical practice provided a physical examination last year for $100 and spent $10 in supplies for that physical. The practice paid $5 of these expenses last year. This year, the patient finally paid, which enabled the practice to pay the rest of the expenses. The first three accounts in the example are accrual accounts and show accrual income. By definition, "net income" means net income on an accrual basis. The last three accounts are cash accounts, and the final account, net cash, is the cash basis income.

Account	Entry last year	Entry this year
Accrual accounts		
Accrual income	$100	$0
Accrual expenses	$10	$0
Net income	$90	$0
Cash accounts		
Cash received	$0	$100
Cash disbursed	$5	$5
Net cash	$5	$95

Accrual accounting recognized the revenue last year when it was earned. Cash accounting recognized the inflow this year when it occurred. Similarly, suppose a capitated practice is paid on January 1 for an entire year of services. Cash accounting recognizes the entire cash payment of January 1. Accrual accounting would recognize the revenues evenly over the course of the year, or perhaps as services were provided.

Depreciation is a major difference between cash and accrual accounting that is especially important to practice managers. Depreciation is "the rational and systematic allocation of the cost of a capital item to the revenues it produces over its useful life." Less technically, depreciation matches the cost of a capital item to the revenues it produces. Suppose a practice has an x-ray machine that costs $1,000, has an expected life of 5 years, and has no scrap or salvage value. For simplicity's sake, assume that that machine produces revenues of $2,000 each year and costs $50 to run. It is paid in Year 4.

The accrual and cash accounting for this machine are shown in **Table 9-3**.

Table 9-3	**Cash and Accrual Accounting Principals**				
Year	**1**	**2**	**3**	**4**	**5**
Revenues	$2,000	$2,000	$2,000	$2,000	$2,000
Depreciation*	200	200	200	200	200
Other expenses	50	50	50	50	50
Net income (accrual)	**$1,750**	**$1,750**	**$1,750**	**$1,750**	**$1,750**
Cash in	$2,000	$2,000	$2,000	$2,000	$2,000
Cash out	1,050	50	50	50	50
Net cash	**$950**	**$1,950**	**$1,950**	**$1,950**	**$1,950**
*Technically, straight-line depreciation					

Practice managers should be aware of the cash implications of buying and replacing the machine. They should also know how much revenue the machine generates each year and how much expenses are involved. Probably, the machine generates less revenue but costs more to run each year. Practice managers should also realize the difference between accounting depreciation and tax depreciation. The purpose of accounting depreciation is to measure net income. That is not the purpose of tax depreciation. Tax depreciation can permit an asset to be depreciated in 1, 3, or 5 years, or permit the asset to be expensed in the year purchased. These options are not relevant to measuring income, and practice managers should be aware that confusing tax and accrual depreciation may result in bad decisions for the practice.

Practice managers should know the advantages of both cash and accrual accounting, and when to use them. Cash accounting measures cash. Practice managers should know how much cash the practice has in order to pay bills. During bad economic times, potential creditors and lenders tend to focus more on cash than on accruals. Cash may be the only important factor if the practice must deal with financial distress. Managers of primarily fee-for-service practices may find cash accounting more realistic than accrual accounting because these practices earn accrual revenues long before the cash is received, and therefore may incur expenses before they have the cash to pay them. From a tax standpoint, cash accounting means the practice pays taxes only on the cash it has collected. Physicians may also be more able to understand cash accounting than accrual accounting.

On the other hand, accrual accounting is consistent with GAAP, especially with the matching principle, because accrual accounting matches revenues and expenses. If the practice can assume it will collect its receivables and pay its payables, which is realistic during prosperous times, then accrual accounting provides a more realistic picture of financial performance than cash accounting. In the simple example shown earlier, the practice earned $90 last year rather than $95 this year. Accrual accounting also avoids the distortions to income that can occur when a large amount of cash is collected or when a large number of bills are paid. Accrual accounting makes it easier to compare practices for this reason and makes it easier to keep track of discounts and offsets for managed care. The MGMA chart of accounts, for example, permits the following accrual:

Gross charges − Adjustments = Net revenue

It can be more difficult to keep track of adjustments under a cash basis because only the cash received is recorded.

Capitated practices will find it advantageous to use accrual accounting for two reasons. First, capitated practices tend to receive cash before services are provided and before expenses are incurred. Cash income therefore may be unrealistically high. Accrual accounting is more realistic because it includes expenses that are incurred but not reported (often referred to as IBNR), which have to be paid and should influence decision making, even though they have not been reported, much less paid. For this reason, practice managers in heavily capitated practices may want to emphasize accrual accounting when discussing the practice's financial condition with the physician members.

Modified Cash Accounting

Modified cash accounting (sometimes called modified accrual accounting) uses the cash basis to compute cash income but includes accounts receivable and long-term equipment as assets. However, the receivables are not recognized as revenue until they are collected, and the depreciation is not recognized as an expense until it is paid. Modified cash accounting has an advantage over accrual accounting in that it does not recognize revenues until they are collected. However, it has the corresponding disadvantage of not recognizing expenses until they are paid. The MGMA chart of accounts lists the accrual accounts used in modified cash or accrual accounting.

■ Methods of Depreciation

As discussed in the previous section, depreciation is "the allocation of the cost of tangible assets to expense in a systematic and rational manner to those time periods expected to benefit from the use of the asset." Less technically, depreciation from a financial accounting perspective reflects the wearing out of capital assets (starting with their purchase prices) as they are used to generate income. While many accountants describe depreciation as "the cost of the capital assets used up." Depreciation indeed spreads the asset's cost over its useful life. It does not however measure the actual decline in market value due to the asset's being used. Depreciation is a noncash or accrual expense that reduces income just as if it were a cash expense. It is important to measure depreciation accurately in order to compute income accurately. An inaccurately large depreciation expense understates income, whereas an inaccurately small depreciation expense overstates income. The greater depreciation expense is as a percentage of total expenses, the more attention auditors give to depreciation, and the more attention practice managers should give to depreciation in order to compute net income fairly. While there are several ways to compute depreciation, all of them require an estimate of the asset's useful life or how long it can be used (how long it will last) and its residual or scrap value (what it will be worth as scrap when it can no longer be used for its original purpose).

This section discusses:

- The principal ways to compute financial accounting depreciation: straight-line method, activity unit method, and accelerated methods
- Using different methods of depreciation for different classes of assets
- Group and composite depreciation
- Modifying depreciation expense due to a change in the asset's estimated useful life
- Changing methods of depreciation
- Accounting for sales of depreciable assets

Principal Methods of Depreciation

Straight-Line Depreciation

Straight-line depreciation assumes that assets wear out or become obsolete evenly over their useful lives, regardless of how often or how much they are used. Many accountants prefer straight-line depreciation to other methods because it makes the fewest assumptions about how assets wear out. If we assume that an MRI lasts for 10 years and has salvage or scrap value of $1,000, straight-line depreciation is computed as follows:

Historical cost:	$10,000
Less: Salvage value	1,000
Depreciation base:	$9,000
Divided by 10 years	$900 depreciation expense per year

The major challenges to using the straight-line method are estimating the asset's expected useful life and estimating its residual or salvage value. Practice managers should know industry guidelines in order to make these decisions fairly. Although MGMA does not have guidelines for the expected useful lives of depreciable assets, practice managers should discuss this issue with their CPA, know industry practices, and be consistent in estimating the useful lives of depreciable assets.

Activity Unit Depreciation

The activity unit method assumes that assets wear out as they are used. In this sense, activity unit depreciation directly matches depreciation expense with the revenues each use produces. If an MRI is good for 1,000 uses, then activity-based depreciation per use is:

Historical cost:	$10,000
Less: Salvage value	1,000

Depreciation base:	$9,000
Divided by 1000 uses	$9 per use

The major challenges to using activity unit depreciation are estimating the number of units an asset can reasonably produce and estimating the asset's scrap value.

Accelerated Depreciation

Accelerated depreciation methods assume that assets wear out more quickly during their first years of life than they do later, or at least they are much more efficient during their first years of life than they are later. Automobiles are a good example of the logic of accelerated depreciation. It is generally believed that an automobile loses more of its value during its first year than it does during its fifth year.

The two most commonly used methods of accelerated depreciation for financial accounting are declining-balance method and the sum-of-the-year's-digits method and the.

Declining Balance Method. The declining balance method uses some multiple of the straight-line rate to compute an annual depreciation expense. The most commonly used declining balance method is the double declining balance method which uses twice the straight-line rate to compute annual depreciation expense. The multiple remains the same and is applied each year to the remaining book value rather than to the depreciation base. The declining balance method ignores scrap value to compute annual depreciation expense; however, depreciation expense stops once scrap value is reached. An example of triple declining balance is shown in **Table 9-5**.

Sum-of-the-Years'-Digits Method. The sum-of-the-years'-digits method is not commonly used currently, although it was used in the past. The sum-of-the-years'-digits method computes a decreasing depreciation charge based on a decreasing fraction of the asset's depreciation base. The decreasing fractions are based on the sum of the digits in the number of years in an asset's useful life. The numerator of the fraction is the number of years, starting with the highest.

The sum-of-the-years'-digits depreciation for the MRI is computed as follows:

Historical cost:	$10,000
Less: Salvage value	1,000
Depreciation base:	$9,000

If the asset lasts 10 years, then the denominator of the fraction is:

$$10 + 9 + 8 + 7 + 6 + 5 + 4 + 3 + 2 + 1 = 55$$

Table 9-4 Sum-of-the-Years'-Digits Method of Depreciation

Year	Depreciation Base	Remaining Useful Life (yrs)	Depreciation Fraction	Depreciation Expense	Remaining Book Value
1	$9,000	10	10/55	10/55 × $9,000 = $1,636.36	$7,363.64
2	$9,000	9	9/55	9/55 × $9,000 = $1,472.73	$5,890.91
3	$9,000	8	8/55	8/55 × $9,000 = $1,309.09	$4,581.82
4	$9,000	7	7/55	7/55 × $9,000 = $1,145.45	$3,436.36
5	$9,000	6	6/55	6/55 × $9,000 = $981.82	$2,454.55
6	$9,000	5	5/55	5/55 × $9,000 = $818.18	$1,636.36
7	$9,000	4	4/55	4/55 × $9,000 = $654.55	$981.82
8	$9,000	3	3/55	3/55 × $9,000 = $490.91	$490.91
9	$9,000	2	2/55	2/55 × $9,000 = $327.27	$163.64
10	$9,000	1	1/55	1/55 × $9,000 = $163.64	$0.00
Total		55	55	$9,000	

The denominator of the fraction is literally the sum of the years' digits (in this example, 55). The numerator of the fraction is the year itself. **Table 9-4** shows how to compute the sum-of-the-years'-digits depreciation for the MRI.

Federal and state governments prescribe depreciation methods for tax purposes that can differ from those used in financial accounting. Practice managers should know the depreciation method used for tax accounting and should be able to reconcile tax depreciation with financial accounting depreciation.

Using Different Methods of Depreciation for Different Types of Assets

Practice managers can use different methods of depreciation for different types of assets, as shown in **Table 9-6**.

For example, the manager can use straight-line depreciation for buildings, activity unit depreciation for some assets, and accelerated methods for other assets. Practice managers can also group assets into classes and apply the same method of depreciation and the same depreciation rate to all assets in that class. This step can make it easier to compute depreciation compared to having a separate depreciation schedule for each depreciable asset. Regardless of the methods used, practice managers should make it clear why they selected a particular method of depreciation for each asset or class of assets, and they should document how they computed the depreciation expense for each asset or group. The more complicated the methods of depreciation and the more methods of depreciation used, the more complicated the

Table 9-5 Triple Declining Method of Depreciation

Year	Book Value at Beginning of Year	Depreciation Rate	Depreciation Expense	Accumulated Depreciation	Book Value at End of Year
1	$10,000	0.30	$3,000.00	$3,000.00	$7,000.00
2	$9,000	0.30	$2,100.00	$5,100.00	$4,900.00
3	$9,000	0.30	$1,470.00	$6,570.00	$3,430.00
4	$9,000	0.30	$1,029.00	$7,599.00	$2,401.00
5	$9,000	0.30	$720.30	$8,319.30	$1,680.70
6	$9,000	0.30	$504.21	$8,823.51	$1,176.49
7	$9,000	0.30	$176.49*	$9,000.00	$1,000.00

*Limited to $176 to prevent end-of-the-year book value from being less than scrap value of $1,000. Many companies shift to straight-line depreciation in the latter years of an asset's useful life to spread the remaining depreciation over the last years.

Table 9-6	**Comparing Methods of Financial Depreciation**			
Method	**Assumptions**	**Advantages**	**Disadvantages**	**Common Uses**
Straight line	Asset declines constantly over time	Easy to compute Generally recognized Constant effect on income	Ignores declines not due to constant decline over time, such as technological obsolescence	Buildings
Activity unit	Asset declines constantly with each use	Reflects wear and tear due to use Effects on income depend on how much the asset is used	Ignores declines over time not due to use, such as deterioration	Some equipment
Accelerated	Asset declines most rapidly during first years of use	Frequently reflects business reality	Hard to explain Can be hard to justify If straight-line depreciation is appropriate, accelerated depreciation may understate income in early years and overstate income in later years	Some equipment

audit becomes and the more difficult it can be to explain a practice's net income.

Group and Composite Depreciation

Practice managers can also collect assets and depreciate the entire collection together rather than depreciating each asset separately. Managers of large practices may find this option desirable rather than computing depreciation on each asset separately. A collection of similar assets is called a "group" and the depreciation is called "group depreciation." A collection of dissimilar assets is called a "composite" and the annual depreciation is called "composite depreciation."

As an example, a practice has MRIs worth a total of $100,000 that are expected to last 3 years and be worth $5,000 at disposal. It also has x-ray machines worth a total of $25,000 that are expected to last 10 years and be worth

$1,000 at disposal. The group or composite depreciation rate is computed as shown in **Table 9-7**.

Composite depreciation rate = annual depreciation ÷ historical costs

or $57,566 ÷ $125,000 = 46.05%

Composite life* = depreciation base ÷ annual depreciation

or 190,000 ÷ $57,566 = 2.07 years

*Also called depreciable life

Changing Estimated Useful or Depreciable Life

Estimates of an asset's useful life are just that—estimates—and the accounting profession recognizes that estimates may need to be revised. An asset's estimated useful life may need to be lengthened or shortened. Lengthening an

Table 9-7	**Rate of Depreciation**				
Asset	**Historical Cost**	**Disposal Value**	**Depreciation Base**	**Estimated Useful Life (yrs)**	**Annual Depreciation (straight line)**
MRIs	$100,000	5,000	$95,000	3	$31,666.67
X-rays	25,000	1,000	24,000	10	$25,899.00
Total	$125,000		$119,000		$57,565.67

asset's estimated useful life reduces annual depreciation expense whereas shortening an asset's estimated useful life usually increases depreciation expense. Both changes are handled "currently and prospectively," which means the new annual depreciation expense is used this year and in the future. There is no need to change the previous years' depreciation expenses or the total amount in accumulated depreciation.

It is important to distinguish between reducing an asset's expected useful life and an asset's suffering a "permanent impairment in value." The former is a change of estimate whereas the latter reflects a significant event such as a fire loss or a major technological change. Suppose the MRI becomes obsolete but is still usable in year 3 and will be useful for another 2 years rather than another 7 years. Because of the technological change, the MRI is now worth $5,000. The MRI had been depreciated using straight-line depreciation and $100 scrap value. At the end of year 3, before the impairment, the MRI had a book value of $7,300 ($10,000 historical cost – 3 years* × $900 depreciation per year).

*The gain on the sale is computed as the difference between cash + accumulated deficit less historical cost.

The entry to record the permanent impairment that reduced the MRI's value to $5,000 is:

Loss due to technological obsolescence: $5,000
    Accumulated depreciation-equipment: $5,000

The annual depreciation expense for the remaining 2 years of useful life is $4,000 ÷ 2 = $2,000. The depreciation base is $4,000 rather than the $5,000 book value because of the scrap value of $1,000.

Changing Methods of Depreciation

Practice managers may change the method of depreciation for an asset or a class of assets. Auditors generally want to know the reasons for the change. GAAP includes rules for how to show the change in method in the financial statements. Practice managers should discuss with their CPA who prepares the financials the nature of the change in method and the reasons so that the financials can be prepared accurately.

Accounting for the Sales of Depreciable Assets

The accounting is straightforward if an asset is sold for cash. The cash received, the asset, and the related accumulated depreciation are removed from the books, and gain or loss is recognized as the difference between the cash received and the asset's carrying value at the time of sale.

If the MRI were sold at the end of year 5 for $8,000, assuming straight-line depreciation and 10-year life, the entry to record the sale is:

Cash	$8,000
Accumulated depreciation (MRI) – $4,500	
	($900/year × 5 years)
MRI	$10,000 (historical cost)
Gain on MRI sale	$ 2,500*

To record the sale of an MRI for cash. No similar asset was acquired.

*The gain on the sale is computed as the difference between cash + accumulated deficit – historical cost.

The accounting becomes more complicated if the MRI is exchanged for a newer MRI (a similar asset) or a dissimilar asset (such as land), or if the MRI is exchanged for another asset (either similar or dissimilar) and cash. The practice manager should consult with a CPA regarding the financial accounting treatment of these exchanges. The sale or exchange of an asset being depreciated as a group or a composite is not treated as a regular sale or exchange and should be brought to the attention of a CPA.[8]

Implications for Practice Managers

Practice managers are responsible for the financial aspects of their practice's depreciable assets. At a minimum, they need to know the accounting methods used for depreciable assets, how that depreciation affects income, the expected useful lives of assets, and how the alternative methods of depreciation would affect the practice's income and decisions. These responsibilities become even more important as depreciable assets become a larger percentage of total assets, and as depreciation becomes a larger percentage of total expenses. Practice managers should ensure that the practice's CPA and auditor understand and agree with the practice's depreciation policies. The practice manager must also ensure that the CPA and auditor know enough about medicine to provide guidance in this area. Practice managers should also ensure that the practice's management and principal physicians understand the practice's depreciation policies and how they affect income.

Practice managers have some discretion in selecting the depreciation method and how they group assets. Practice managers of newer practices, especially those not expected to show substantial income during their first years of existence, might decide not to use accelerated depreciation in order to "save" depreciation expense for later years when the practice may need to shield income from taxation. On the other hand, managers might find it advantageous to choose accelerated depreciation if the practice is currently profitable but may see lower profits if key physicians plan to retire soon. Managers can also select accelerated depreciation if the practice usually disposes of assets before the end of their useful life, but might find it more logical to select straight-line depreciation if the practice tends to hold assets until they are no longer useful. These choices are considered legitimate business decisions. However, managers who change depreciation methods frequently in order to reach a "target income" invite extensive scrutiny by auditors and tax officials and can find their decisions causing more trouble than benefit.

Chart of Accounts

The chart of accounts is the basis of any accounting system, either cash or accrual. The chart of accounts is the list of accounts the accounting system uses to record the practice's financial condition. The practice cannot track any revenue or expenses not listed in the chart of accounts. However, the more accounts the practice uses, the more costly the accounting system becomes. The selection of which accounts to use is an example of the need for accounting information to be relevant. Practice managers should know the chart of accounts and select those accounts the practice needs. Smaller practices usually need fewer accounts than larger practices, and practices must usually expand the number of accounts they use as they grow.

The MGMA Chart of Accounts

The *MGMA Chart of Accounts* provides the framework for a medical practice's financial system.[9] Unlike many other charts of accounts, the *MGMA Chart of Accounts* is specifically designed for the financial needs of a medical group practice. It includes the accounts needed to describe a group practice's financial life, and its accounts flow logically into the financial statements a group practice has to produce. The *MGMA Chart of Accounts* was first published in 1978 and has had four subsequent revisions to accommodate changes in accounting rules and to reflect the evolving healthcare environment. The fifth edition of the *MGMA Chart of Accounts* was published in February 2011.

The *MGMA Chart of Accounts* classifies financial transactions into nine major categories and assigns a four-digit coding number to each. The nine major categories are ordered in the way they appear on the practice's financial statements. The major categories and their codes are shown in **Table 9-8**.

The first three categories relate to the balance sheet or statement of financial position. The remaining categories relate to the statement of income and to the order in which they appear on the statement of income. However, GAAP requires that gains or losses from discontinued operations, extraordinary gains and losses,

Table 9-8 **Major Categories and Codes**

Account Numbers	Description
1000	Assets
2000	Liabilities
3000	Owners' Equity Accounts
4000	Operating Revenue
5000	Operating Expenses—Support Staff
6000	General and Administrative Expenses
7000	Clinical and Ancillary Services
8000	Physician- and Nonphysician-Related Expenses
9000	Nonoperating Revenue and Expenses and Provision for Conversion to Cash Basis Accounting

and the cumulative effects of accounting changes must be shown separately on the statement of income, rather than where they would appear if they were part of normal operations.

The adjustments and allowances category begins with a 4 (the category for revenues) rather than a 6 (services and general expenses) because allowances and adjustments must be treated as offsets to revenue rather than as expenses.

Small practices may need only these accounts. Larger practices can take advantage of the other features of this coding system. The two most important features are the subcategories of the nine major categories and using the last two digits of the coding number. The *MGMA Chart of Accounts* subdivides each major category into subcategories, as shown in **Table 9-9**. The subcategories for each category can be "rolled up" to equal the total for that category. For example, for assets, total assets (account 1,000) equals the sum of all the subaccounts, 1,100 through 1,900.

The numeric coding system used in the fifth edition of the *MGMA Chart of Accounts* has four fields. Each field represents a different purpose of accumulating financial information and is designed to accommodate the varying degrees of financial sophistication present in medical groups. The chart of accounts starts with the four-digit basic field just discussed, which provides the complete set of financial accounts and accommodates a limited degree of cost allocation and cost tracing. If a practice's financial information needs are not met with the basic field, the following three additional fields

Table 9-9	Subcategories
Account Numbers	**Description**
1000	**Assets**
1100–1500	Current Assets
1600	Investments—Long-Term Receivables
1700–1800	Noncurrent Tangible Assets
1900	Intangible and Other Noncurrent Assets
2000	**Liabilities**
2100–2300	Current Liabilities
2400	Long-Term Liabilities
3000	**Owners' Equity Accounts**
4000	**Operating Revenue**
4100	Gross Charges
4200	Adjustments to Fee-for-Service Charges
4300	Cash Received
4400	Bad Debt Recovery
4500	Patient and Payer Refunds
4600	Third-Party Settlements
5000	**Operating Expenses—Support Staff**
5100–5200	Employee Salaries and Bonuses
5300	Employee Benefits
5400	Temporary Staff Expenses
6000	**General and Administrative Expenses**
6100–6800	Facility and Administrative
6900	Bad Debt Expense
7000	**Clinical and Ancillary Services Expenses**
7100–7700	Clinical, Ancillary Services, and Research Expenses
7800	Purchased Professional and Medical Services
7900	Cost of Goods Sold
8000	**Physician- and Nonphysician-Related Expenses**
8100	Physician Compensation
8200	Physician Benefits
8300	Nonphysician Provider Compensation
8400	Nonphysician Provider Benefits
8500	Residents, Fellows, and Postdocs Compensation
8600	Residents, Fellows, and Postdocs Benefits
8700	Distributions to Nonphysician Owners
9000	**Nonoperating Revenue and Expenses and Provision for Conversion to Cash Basis Accounting**
9100	Nonmedical Revenue
9200	Nonoperating Expenses
9300–9600	Taxes and Assessments
9900	Provision for Cash Basis Conversion

are available to accommodate the specific needs of the practice:

1. *Entity field:* Allows a practice with multiple legal entities that has the chart of accounts to "roll up" consolidated financial reports with great ease
2. *Responsibility center field:* Allows data to be accumulated by specific administrative cost centers, ancillary services centers, clinical departments, or locations
3. *Provider field:* Accommodates collecting revenue or expense information for specific providers

The four fields can be illustrated as follows:

Entity Field	Basic Field	Responsibility Center Field	Provider Field
00	0000	00	000

This design allows for any practice to use the same four-digit basic field with up to 99 different legal entities, 99 separate responsibility centers, and 999 providers. These four fields provide the flexibility needed to accommodate the information needs of virtually every type of medical group.

Flow of Financial Information

This section describes how financial information flows from the chart of accounts to the financial statements. Practice managers should ensure that this information is accurate, is gathered efficiently, and serves both the practice and its creditors.

The financial statements are a final product of the financial information system. The system is diagrammed as shown in **Figure 9-1**.

Journals

The word "journal" comes from the Latin word for "day." Journals are a chronological record of financial activities. Journals are like a diary of what happened in the life of the practice. For example, at 9 am the practice collected revenues; at 10 am it accrued revenues; at 11 am it paid some bills. Journals therefore describe what happened each day.

Small practices may find it possible to record all transactions in one journal, called the general journal. Larger practices usually have a separate journal for cash receipts and cash disbursements, and may have a separate journal for equipment and for classes of patients such as Medicare patients. A separate journal makes it easier to keep track of a particular activity. For example, a

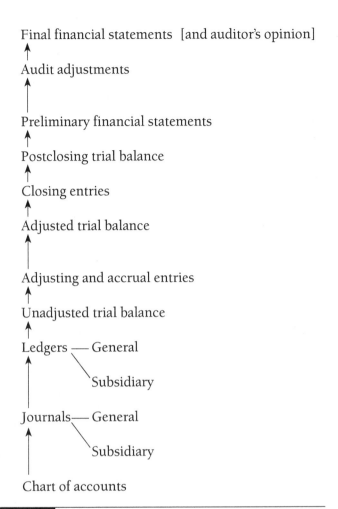

Final financial statements [and auditor's opinion]

↑

Audit adjustments

↑

Preliminary financial statements

↑

Postclosing trial balance

↑

Closing entries

↑

Adjusted trial balance

↑

Adjusting and accrual entries

↑

Unadjusted trial balance

↑

Ledgers —— General

        ＼Subsidiary

↑

Journals—— General

        ＼Subsidiary

↑

Chart of accounts

Figure 9-1 Financial information system.

cash receipts journal makes it easier to answer questions about the cash received. However, each subsidiary journal makes the financial system more complicated and more costly. The practice managers should decide which financial activities warrant their own subsidiary journal.

Ledgers

The word "ledger" means "line." A ledger has one line for every account and gives the current value of that account. Ledgers summarize the journals. For example, on one day there might be five activities that involve receiving cash. The ledger summarizes the five entries into one entry that is the total amount of cash the practice has. Ledgers and journals give different information about the practice's financial condition. The ledgers answer, "How much do we have?" and "How much do we owe?" Journals describe the individual financial transactions that add up to what the practice owes and owns. The process of transferring information from the journals to the ledgers is called "posting." Most automated computer

systems automatically post the journal information to the appropriate ledgers and subsidiary ledgers. These systems are called "one-write systems" because one entry into the journal automatically adjusts all other relevant financial records.

Example of the Accounting Process and the Flow of Financial Information

This section illustrates key aspects of the accounting process. It shows how the chart of accounts is the foundation of the accounting system; how the journals flow into the ledgers; how the ledgers are adjusted; how the adjusted ledgers are used to prepare the financial statements; and how an auditor might view the entire process. Only a small number of accounts are used in this example to make it easier to see the accounting process.

Community Health Partners is a single-specialty partnership practice that consists of two physicians, both owners, and is organized as an S corporation. The founding agreement that started the practice said that Physician A owned 60% of the practice and Physician B owned 40%. The partners do not receive a salary or any interest on their contributed capital. The practice contracts for a part-time receptionist for $1,000 a month and pays on the fifteenth and end of the month. It pays $2,000 each month for office space. It tracks payments from Medicare separately from other payments. It has one cash account, one general checking account, and a payroll checking account. The practice transfers $1,000 from the cash account to the payroll checking account on the fifteenth of each month. (Businesses generally create a separate account for payroll rather than using the general cash account.) Each partner pays his own malpractice insurance. The practice pays $100 each month for electronic patient billing services. At year end, the practice pays $300 for each physician's professional memberships and $300 towards each physician's license fees. The practice is on an accrual basis.

The following events occurred during the practice's first year.

To start the practice on January 1, the partners (owners):

◾ Contributed a total of $10,000 cash (Partner A contributed $6,000 and Partner B contributed $4,000)

This contribution is recorded in the cash receipts journal.

Debits: Cash receipts journal/Amount (All debits in the cash receipts journal are to Cash, Account 1111.)

    1111   Cash $10,000

Credits: Account/Amount

    3010 Contributed Capital Partner A $6,000

    3011 Contributed Capital Partner B $4,000

- Contributed office equipment worth $5,000 with 10-year expected life and $100 scrap value

This contribution is recorded in the general journal.

Debits: Account/Amount

1751 Furniture and Fixtures $5,000

Credits: Account/Amount

    3010 Contributed Capital Partner A $3,000

    3011 Contributed Capital Partner B $2,000

- Prepaid 3 years of fire insurance for $3,000

This transaction is recorded in the cash disbursements journal; all credits in the cash disbursements journal are to cash.

Debits: Account/Amount

1950 Fire insurance paid in advance $3,000

Credits (All credits are to the cash account, Account 1111.)

    Cash $3,000

On January 10, the practice saw a Medicare fee-for-service patient. The gross professional charge was $120 and the allowable charge was $100. The patient had already satisfied the Medicare deductible, meaning that the practice needed to collect only the 20% copay of $20. The patient's ID number is ABC.

This activity is recorded in the cash receipts journal because cash was collected.

Debits: Account/Amount

1111 Cash $20

1303 Receivables: Medicare $80

    Credits: Account/Amount

    4521 Adjustments: Medicare $20

    4121 Medicare Gross Revenues $100

Pt ABC Procedure Gross charge $120; Medicare allowable charge $100; $20 patient copay collected

On January 15, the practice paid the receptionist half a month's salary of $500.

This activity is recorded in the payroll checking account (1112), which flows through the cash disbursements journal because cash was disbursed.

Debit: Account/Amount

    5001 Contracting fee: receptionist $500

    Credit: Account/Amount
    1112 Payroll checking accounts $500

To record payment of contract fee for receptionist for one half month

On January 31, the practice paid the monthly charge of $1,000 rental on the office space and $100 for patient billing services.

6120	Building and facility rent/lease	$2,000	
1111	Cash		$2,000

To record monthly rental payment on office space

6358	Patient billing services	$120	
1111	Cash		$120

To record monthly charge for the electronic patient billing service

On March 1, Medicare paid the claim for the services rendered on January 10.

This activity is recorded in the cash receipts journal because cash was received.

For this service, the accounts in this patient's subsidiary ledger are:

Patient number: ABC	
Date of service	1.10.20XX
Payer	1303—Medicare
Procedure 1	1234
Gross charge	$120
Discount or adjustment	$20
Net charge to insurer	$80
Copayment	$20
Copayment date	1.10.20XX
Date insurer billed	1.20.20XX
Date insurance payment received	3.1.20XX
Amount received	$80
Amount remaining from insurer	$0

The practice manager can use the information in the ledgers to monitor how long it takes to bill the insurer, how long it takes to receive payment, how efficiently the practice collects copayments, how promptly each insurer pays, and how completely each insurer pays.

During the rest of the year, the practice billed $500,000 in allowable charges, all from discounted fee-for-service payers. These charges were also recorded in Account 4110 since both Medicare and the commercial insurers paid on a fee-for-service basis. The practice recorded $100,000 of contractual adjustments (Account 4210) and recorded the difference ($400,000) as AR: fee-for-service, Account 1310.

This account (1310) includes both the amount due from the patient and the amount due from the insurance company. The practice, however, may want to create a subaccount for each. If we assume that patients pay 20% of allowable charges, then Account 1310.1 (AR—third parties) would have a balance of $320,000 and Account 1310.2 (AR—patients) would have a balance of $80,000.

The practice collected $300,000 from these patients and insurance companies, which it recorded in Account 1111, cash.

Adjusting Entries

Adjusting entries are made on the last day of the reporting period to recognize and record revenues that have been earned but not received in cash and expenses that have been incurred but not paid in cash. These revenues and expenses would have been recorded already had cash been received or paid. These adjusting entries make the financial records more complete and therefore the financial statements more accurate. Adjusting entries usually correct both the balance sheet and the income statement. Common adjusting entries are depreciation and the allowance for bad debt. Depreciation estimates the expense of using up equipment to produce revenues, and the allowance for bad debt estimates the expense of doing business on credit. Neglecting to record depreciation would not show the wear and tear on equipment, and not recording the allowance for bad debt would show receivables as being completely collectible.

To continue the example from the previous section, annual depreciation expense on the furniture and fixtures are calculated as:

Purchase price	$5,000
Less: Scrap value	100
Depreciable base	$4,900
Divided by 10 yrs	$490 per year

The practice records:

6210 Depreciation expense—furniture and fixtures $490

1820 Accumulated depreciation—furniture and fixtures $490

Prepaid insurance was used for a year. Therefore insurance expense is recorded for a year even though no additional cash was paid.

6716 Insurance expense $1,000
1512 Prepaid insurance $1,000

At year end, $4,500 of the remaining receivables from third-party payers were estimated to be uncollectible (Account 1323) and $500 of patient accounts receivable were uncollectible (Account 1321).

The practice's only payable at year end is the receptionist's half-month salary of $500. The practice acknowledges an estimate of $10,000 for claims incurred but not reported. However, the partnership does not record this expense because malpractice is each partner's personal responsibility rather than the partnership's.

Debits: Account/Amount Cash receipts journal (All debits are to cash, Account 1111)
Credits: Account/Amount 1303 Receivables—Medicare $80

To record collection of Medicare payment for patient ABC for service rendered on January 10

The practice also keeps a subsidiary record for each patient. The accounts in this record are:

- **Patient name: ABC**
  - Date of service
  - Patient insurer
- **Procedure 1 number**
  - Procedure 1 gross charge
  - Procedure 1 discount or adjustment
  - Procedure 1 net charge
  - Procedure 1 copayment
  - Procedure 1 copayment date
  - Procedure 1 date insurer billed
  - Procedure 1 amount received from insurer
  - Procedure 1 amount remaining from insurer
- **Procedure 2 number**
  - Procedure 2 gross charge
  - Procedure 2 discount or adjustment
  - Procedure 2 net charge
  - Procedure 2 copayment
  - Procedure 2 copayment date
  - Procedure 2 date insurer billed
  - Procedure 2 amount received from insurer
  - Procedure 2 amount remaining from insurer
- **Procedure 3 number**
  - Procedure 3 gross charge
  - Procedure 3 discount or adjustment
  - Procedure 3 net charge
  - Procedure 3 copayment
  - Procedure 3 copayment date
  - Procedure 3 date insurer billed

- Procedure 3 amount received from insurer
- Procedure 3 amount remaining from insurer

The practice's year-end general ledger and unadjusted trial balance are shown in **Table 9-10**.

The accrual adjustments to the unadjusted trial balance are:

The practice records:

6210 Depreciation expense—furniture and fixtures $490

1820 Accumulated depreciation—furniture and fixtures $490

To record depreciation expense on furniture and fixtures

6561 Fire insurance expense $1,000

1950 Prepaid fire insurance $1,000

To record one year's fire insurance expense

5001 Contracting fee—receptionist $500

2261 Accrued contracting fees payable $500

To record accrued contracting fees of the receptionist

The adjusted trial (preclosing) balance is shown in **Table 9-11**.

Closing involves closing the revenue, contractual adjustments, expense accounts, and the dividend or drawing accounts (the "temporary" accounts into the capital accounts, and then computing the new values of the capital accounts). As discussed before, revenue, expense accounts, and dividend/drawing accounts have zero beginning balance because they measure revenues, expenses and dividend/drawing accounts during the reporting period, not since the practice started. The account income summary is a temporary account that serves as a bucket that revenues are poured into and expenses are drained out of. Net income is the remainder. Temporary accounts are created during the closing process and have zero value when the closing is completed.

The practice use Account 9998 for Net Fee-for-Service Revenue (the net of accounts 4110 Gross Charges—Fee-for-Service—Professional and Technical and 4210 Contractual Adjustments—Fee-for-Service—Professional

Table 9-10 Unadjusted General Ledger

Community Health Partners
Unadjusted General Ledger
December 31, 20XX

Number	Account	Debits ($)	Credits ($)
1111	Cash	269,200	
1112	Payroll Checking Accounts		500
1310	Accounts Receivable—Fee-for-Service	100,000	
1321	Allowance for Bad Debts—Patients		500
1333	Allowance for Bad Debts—Third-Party Payers		4,500
1721	Furniture and Fixtures	5,000	
1821	Accumulated Depreciation—Furniture and Fixtures		490
1950	Prepaid Expenses—Noncurrent Portion (for fire insurance)	2,000	
3010	Contributed Capital—Partner A		9,000
3010	Contributed Capital—Partner B		6,000
4110	Gross Charges—Fee-for-Service—Professional and Technical		500,120
4210	Contractual Adjustments—Fee-for-Service—Professional and Technical	100,020	
5311	Salaries—Medical Receptionist	12,000	
6120	Building and Facilities Rent/Lease	24,000	
6210	Furniture, Fixtures, and Equipment Depreciation	490	
6358	Patient Billing Services	1,200	
6716	Insurance, Fire, Theft, and Other Casualty Insurance Related to Occupancy	1,000	
6910	Accounts Receivable Write-Offs (Third Party Payers)	4,500	
6920	Collection Agency Write-Offs (Patients)	500	
8247	Physician Professional Development—Dues and Memberships	600	
8248	Physician Professional Development-Licenses	600	
	Total	$521,110	$521,110

	Table 9-11	**Adjusted General Ledger**		

Community Health Partners
Adjusted General Ledger
December 31, 20XX

Number	Account	Debits ($)	Credits ($)
1111	Cash	269,200	
1112	Payroll Checking Accounts		500
1310	Accounts Receivables—Fee-for-Service	100,000	
1321	Allowance for Bad Debts—Patients		500
1333	Allowance for Bad Debts—Third-Party Payers		4,500
1721	Furniture and Fixtures	5,000	
1821	Accumulated Depreciation—Furniture and Fixtures		490
1950	Prepaid Expenses—Noncurrent Portion (for fire insurance)	2,000	
3010	Contributed Capital—Partner A		9,000
3010	Contributed Capital—Partner B		6,000
4110	Gross Charges—Fee-for-Service—Professional and Technical		500,120
4210	Contractual Adjustments—Fee-for-Service—Professional and Technical	100,020	
5311	Salaries—Medical Receptionist	12,000	
6120	Building and Facilities Rent/Lease	24,000	
6210	Furniture, Fixtures, and Equipment Depreciation	490	
6358	Patient Billing Services	1,200	
6716	Insurance, Fire, Theft, and Other Casualty Insurance Related to Occupancy	1,000	
6910	Accounts Receivable Write-Offs (Third Party Payers)	4,500	
6920	Collection Agency Write-Offs (Patients)	500	
8247	Physician Professional Development—Dues and Memberships	600	
8248	Physician Professional Development—Licenses	600	
	Total	$521,110	$521,110

and Technical) and Account 9999 for the Income Summary. Closing revenues and expenses into the income summary account (Account 9999) are shown in **Table 9-12**. The journal entries are:

		Debits ($)	Credits ($)
9998	Net Fee-for-Service Income	400,100	
9999	Income Summary		400,100
9999	Income summary	44,890	
5311	Salary expense receptionist		12,000
6210	Dep expense furn fix		490
6210	Rental lease payments		24,000
6358	Patient billing services		1,200
6716	Fire and cash ins exp		1,000
6910	AR write offs		5,000
8247	Prof dues		600
8248	Licenses		600

Income summary has a credit value of $355,210, the practice's net income for the year.

The last step in the closing process is to close the income summary account into the partners' capital accounts in the ratio the partners agreed to: 60% to partner A and 40% to partner B.

The journal entry (account/amount) and the explanation are as follows:

9999 Income summary $355,210
3010 Partner A Capital $213,126
3011 Partner B Capital $142,084

To close the income summary account into the capital accounts in the ratio agreed to (Partner A—60%; Partner B—40%)

Table 9-12	Schedule to Close Revenues and Expenses into Income Summary	

Community Health Partners
Schedule to Close Revenues and Expenses into
Income Summary December 31, 20XX

9998	Net Fee-for-Service Income	$400,100
	Total additions (credits) to Income Summary	$400,100
5311	Salaries—Medical Receptionist	$12,000
6120	Building and Facilities Rent/Lease	24,000
6210	Furniture, Fixtures, and Equipment Depreciation	490
6358	Patient Billing Services	1,200
6716	Insurance, Fire, Theft, and Other Casualty Insurance Related to Occupancy	1,000
6910	Accounts Receivable Write-Offs (Third Party Payers)	4,500
6920	Collection Agency Write-Offs (Patients)	500
8247	Physician Professional Development—Dues and memberships	600
8248	Physician Professional Development—Licenses	600
	Total subtractions (debits) from Income Summary	$44,890
9999	Income Summary (Net Value)	$355,210
9999	Income summary	
5311	Salary expense receptionist	$12,000
6210	Dep expense furn fix	$490
6210	Rental lease payments	$24,000
6358	Patient billing services	$1,200
6716	Fire and cash ins exp	$1,000
6910	AR write offs	$5,000
8247	Prof dues	$600
8248	Licenses	$600

Table 9-13	Postclosing General Ledger (Permanent accounts only)		

Community Health Partners
Postclosing General Ledger
December 31, 20XX

Number	Account	Debits ($)	Credits ($)
1111	Cash	269,200	
1112	Payroll Checking Accounts		500
1310	Accounts Receivables— Fee-for-Service	100,000	
1321	Allowance for Bad Debts—Patients		500
1333	Allowance for Bad Debts—Third-Party Payers		4,500
1721	Furniture and Fixtures	5,000	
1821	Accumulated Depreciation— Furniture and Fixtures		490
1950	Prepaid Expenses— Noncurrent Portion (for fire insurance)	2,000	
3010	Contributed Capital— Partner A		222,126
3010	Contributed Capital— Partner B		148,084
	Total	$376,200	$376,200

The postclosing general ledger is shown in **Table 9-13**.

The balance sheet (technically, the statement of financial position) is made from the postclosing trial balance and is shown in **Table 9-14**. Note that the statement of financial position is a snapshot of the practice as of a certain date, and therefore is dated as of that specific date.

The income statement (technically, the statement of income) is made from the adjusted trial balance rather than the postclosing trial balance because the revenues and expenses have been "closed" into the partners' equity accounts as part of the closing process. Note that the statement of income describes an entire year (and hence is dated "For the Year Ending"). See **Table 9-15**.

This simple example illustrates only operating income and expenses. A larger practice would have nonoperating revenues and expenses. It may also have net gains or losses from discontinued operations, extraordinary events, and cumulative effects of accounting changes. Each of these is shown separately, and the last three are shown net of any taxes. This simple example shows only the balance sheet and income statement. It does not show the statement of cash flows.

Possible Auditor's Comments

It is unlikely that an auditor would propose any major adjustments in the financial statements themselves. An

Table 9-14	Statement of Financial Position	
Community Health Partners *Statement of Financial Position* *December 31, 20XX*		
Assets		
Cash		$269,200
Accounts Receivable	$100,000	
Less: allowance for bad debts	5,000	
Net accounts receivable		95,000
Prepaid expenses		2,000
Total current assets		$366,200
Office furniture	$5,000	
Less: accumulated depreciation	490	
Net office furniture		4,510
Total assets		$370,710
Liabilities and equity		
Liabilities		
Contracted service fees payable		$500
Total liabilities		$500
Equity		
Partner A Capital	$222,126	
Partner B Capital	148,084	
Total equity		$370,210
Total liabilities and equity		$370,710

Table 9-15	Statement of Income	
Community Health Partners *Statement of Income* *For the Year Ending December 31, 20XX*		
Revenues		
Gross discounted fee for service revenues	500,120	
Less: contractual allowances	100,020	
Net discounted fee for service revenues		400,000
Total net revenues		$400,100
Expenses		
Rent	$24,000	
Salaries	12,000	
Bad debt expense—third-party payers	4,500	
Electronic billing expense	1,200	
Fire insurance expense	1,000	
Physician memberships	600	
Physician license fees	600	
Bad debt expense—patient accounts	500	
Depreciation expense—furniture and fixtures	490	
Total expenses		$44,890
Net income		$355,210

auditor may question showing both net and gross revenues from discounted fee-for-service payers and Medicare in favor of showing only the net revenues. The justification might be that showing gross revenues is misleading because hardly anyone pays them and the practice has decided to accept the discounted price. Practice managers should know current financial reporting standards for their type of practice and prepare their financial statements accordingly. An auditor might also want a schedule of depreciation for all depreciable assets. This schedule becomes more important the more depreciable assets the practice has.

Internal Control

The practice manager is responsible for the practice's system of internal controls. The Committee of Sponsoring Organizations (COSO), which includes the Institute of Internal Auditors, has defined internal control as[10]:

A process, affected by an entity's board of directors, management, and other personnel, designed to provide reasonable assurance regarding the achievement of objectives in the following categories:

- Effectiveness and efficiency of operations;
- Reliability of financial reporting; and
- Compliance with applicable laws and regulations.

Thus, it is clear that internal control involves the entire organization and that the processes permeate the activities of all members of the organization. Internal control cannot be delegated to any specific element of the organization, but must be part of the organization's culture to be effective.

Less technically, a strong system of internal control generally means that the financial statements are more likely to be accurate, the practice is efficient, and the practice complies with the law. Because billing questions usually involve medical information, compliance with laws and regulations includes compliance with the Health Insurance Portability and Accountability Act (HIPAA). In a medical practice, internal control demands the practice manager and the senior physicians to be good stewards of the practice's resources. The stewardship issue becomes especially important when physicians begin to suspect each other or believe that the senior or most powerful physician has structured the practice for his or her benefit, rather than for the benefit of the entire practice.

A strong system of internal controls is crucial for auditors, external accountants, government regulators, creditors, lenders, and even members of the practice. A weak system of internal controls may require an auditor to expand the audit, which makes the audit more costly and time consuming. The more the auditor can rely on internal controls, the less he or she must rely on his or her own testing. Medicare and Medicaid officials now expect a strong system of internal controls, and a failure to have such a system can jeopardize future funding. Most practices eventually make a mistake in their Medicare or Medicaid billing. A strong system of internal controls can help convince the Medicare or Medicaid officials that the mistake was only a mistake, rather than a systemic weakness that must be fixed before the practice can continue to participate in federally funded programs. Section 404 of the Public Company Accounting Reform and Investor Protection Act (Sarbanes-Oxley) requires management to acknowledge its responsibility for internal control and to assess how well those controls have worked during the past year. The same section requires the auditor to issue an "attestation report" on management's internal control assertions. Although the Sarbanes-Oxley act currently applies to publicly traded companies, it is possible that the act will be extended to nonpublic companies, and some states are taking action in this regard.

The practice manager can establish (and achieve the benefits of) strong internal controls by: (1) developing standard procedures, (2) ensuring separation of responsibilities in those procedures, (3) training staff in these procedures, (4) testing these procedures regularly, and (5) establishing mitigating controls when necessary.

Standard Procedures

Every practice needs procedures (preferably written procedures) about financial matters. Every practice should make it clear who is responsible for greeting the patient, verifying insurance coverage, collecting any copays, recording collection of any copays, and depositing those copays. Every practice should determine who is responsible for billing the insurance company, collecting payments from the insurance company, investigating denials from

the insurance company, and reconciling cash deposits with payments from the insurance company. Information about how promptly and completely each insurance company pays is not only valuable to the physicians, but also crucial to effective and efficient operations.

On the billing side, every practice should determine who is responsible for coding and billing, and who is responsible for identifying services that are not covered by the patient's insurance and for collecting from the patient. It is highly advisable for every practice to have a charity care policy, to communicate that charity care policy, and to enforce that policy. On the expense side, every practice should determine who can authorize an expense, how vendors are selected, who is authorized to pay an expense, and how expenses are recorded.

Separation of Functions

Separation of functions is crucial to internal controls. For example, good internal control requires that:

- The same person does not authorize an expense, receive the benefits of the expense, and record the expense.
- The same person does not decide the amount of revenue, receive the revenue, and record the revenue.

For example, a physician should not be able to decide to purchase a piece of equipment, order the equipment, receive the equipment, and then pay for the equipment. This situation makes it more likely that not all physicians in the group would have approved the purchase, that the price is higher than necessary, that the practice does not list the piece of equipment as one of its assets, and/or that the practice did not pay for equipment in a timely manner. Similarly, the same person should not determine the copay, collect the copay, and then deposit the copay. This situation makes it more likely that the practice can collect an incorrect copay, credit it to the wrong account, and/or fail to deposit the copay promptly.

Good internal controls might require that all capital expenses be budgeted, that the practice obtains competitive bids for all equipment, that the manager receives all equipment before it is put into use, and that a depreciation schedule be established for all equipment before it is received.

Training Staff

Internal controls are useless if staff (including physicians) do not know about them. The practice manager must ensure that staff is trained. This training is especially important regarding Medicare and Medicaid. The federal government can demand a corporate compliance agreement or corporate integrity agreement for the practice to continue to participate in federally funded programs. These agreements almost always require staff training.

Testing

The practice manager needs to test the system of internal controls. The testing can include tracing a patient's visit through the recordkeeping system and comparing this year's expenditures to last year's (analytical reviews). The practice manager should be ready to share these tests with the auditor to demonstrate the strength of the internal control system.

Mitigating or Compensating Controls

Every system of internal controls has weaknesses. The practice manager should know what these weaknesses are and take steps to mitigate the potential effects of these weaknesses, to ensure they do not result in accidental error or deliberate error (fraud). The manager should share these mitigating controls with auditors and regulators.

For example, it may be impractical in a small group practice to have separate people determine a patient's copay, collect the copay, record the copay, and (if cash) deposit the copay. As already stated, mitigating controls are those steps the practice takes to ensure that weaknesses in internal controls do not result in error or fraud. So if the same person determines and collects the copays, the manager should investigate unusually large or small copays, especially cases where there is no copay. If the same person collects the copay, records the copay, and deposits the copay, the practice may encourage payment by credit card and use a one-write system to compensate for this internal control weakness. Many smaller practices do not accept credit cards because of the fees credit card companies charge. In these cases, the practice should have a policy to issue the patient a receipt, to deposit cash and checks daily, and to compare cash collections to cash deposits.

■ Budgeting for Practice Managers

Budgeting in medical practices is closely associated with the practice's planning process. The budget defines the resources expected to be available to attain the short-term and long-term goals and objectives established for the practice. The budget also functions as a controlling element, enabling management to assess the amount of resources devoted to an activity as well as the return to the practice from the activity.

Purposes and Functions

Ernest J. Pavlock, in *Financial Management for Medical Groups*, identified six distinct purposes for budgets[11]:

- Aid in making and coordinating short-range plans and in communicating plans to all managers
- Serve as a means to motivate managers to achieve the goals of their responsibility centers by providing target indicators
- Provide an authorization for staff to use and acquire resources
- Enable managers to anticipate the expected environment in order to take advantage of favorable conditions or to minimize the impact of unfavorable conditions
- Establish benchmarks to control ongoing activities
- Set criteria for evaluating managerial performance

Steven A. Finkler and David M. Ward, in *Cost Accounting for Health Care Organizations*, describe how budgets serve the important function of communicating to an organization's staff the goals of the organization and how the organization will achieve its goals. Finkler and Ward consider budgets as having three significant roles[12]:

- Forcing managers to plan ahead and consider alternatives
- Improving organizational communications and coordination
- Providing a basis for evaluation of unit and managerial performance

Relationship Between Budgets and Accounting Systems

Budgets relate closely to the organization's accounting system, but are very distinct from accounting, because budgeting does not have the established rules and regulations of the accounting industry. The GAAP governs how financial information is presented, whereas the budget involves processes that are determined solely by the organization and does not have to comply with external rules or regulations. The budget is similar to an organization's accounting system in that it allows the structuring of a large amount of financial data and illustrates the interrelationships of the data, and also provides for the orderly presentation of financial information for management decision making. However, whereas financial accounting is designed to present data that is both comparable across organizations and consistent with previous years, a budget is unique to each organization and, by its nature, is designed to address only a specific time period.

Budgets also differ considerably from the accounting system in how they function. The accounting system addresses financial performance in a retrospective manner, describing what has occurred. The organizational budget functions both prospectively as it delineates a plan and retrospectively when it compares actual performance to the plan. The two systems are interdependent. The budget cannot exist without accounting information as input and to assess the organization's performance in the context of the budget; however, accounting information, by itself, has very limited managerial uses.[13]

Type of Budgets

Although organizations generally use the term "budget" as implying a single activity, in reality, an organization uses several different budgets to address its specific needs. The organization's mission, structure, and approach to management are what determine the different types of budgets for the organization. Additionally, unlike financial statements, budget formats do not have to comply with external requirements. Consequently, budgets can be tailored to the needs of the organization and its management functions.

Although the specific structure and design of budgets differ with the needs of each organization, medical groups need to use several different types of budgets.[14,15]

Comprehensive or Master Budget
A medical practice needs several different types of budgets that relate, one to another, to accomplish the objective of defining the revenues and expenses associated with providing health services during the defined time period(s). One budget defines the volume and types of services the practice will provide, another estimates the revenue associated with the volume of service, another examines the expenses, and still another aggregates expenses and revenues into a single forecast of profit and loss for the entire practice. Another budget focuses on the flow of cash into and out of the practice while yet another considers the purchase or replacement of capital equipment and facilities. All of these budgets are brought together in the organization's comprehensive or master budget.

The comprehensive budget has both informal projections and formal statements that flow one to another, and in combination forecast the practice's financial future. The components of the comprehensive budget, the interrelationship of each part of the budget, and the flow of information from one budget part to another are illustrated in **Figure 9-2**.

The different components of the comprehensive budget can be classified into three major parts:

1. Forecasts of volume and the earning expectations of the practice's physicians
2. Cash-flow planning and systems to manage short-term resources

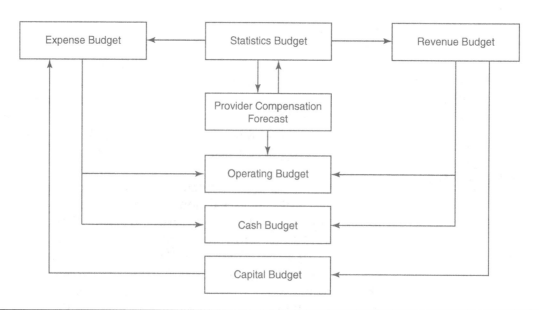

Figure 9-2 The comprehensive budget.

3. Formal documents that parallel the structure and format of the practice's financial statements and describe capital expenditures, change in balance sheet position, and a projected financial positions statement

Statistics Budget

The statistics budget is the foundation for all other budgets. It states the expected volume of services and makes key assumptions. It provides the general guidance needed to establish all other budgets used by the organization.

In a smaller, less sophisticated practice, the statistics budget can be incorporated into the organization's operational budget. The advantage of having a separate statistics budget is that it requires all forecasting in the organization to have the same set of assumptions for volume of services, types of services, rate of inflation, and so on.

Accurate volume estimates are critical to the potential success of the entire budget process. Unfortunately, volume forecasts are difficult to predict because the number and types of patients is dependent on many factors, some within the control of the practice and some outside its control. Marketing campaigns, new managed-care contracts, termination of managed-care contracts, area business expansion, and business personnel layoffs are only some of the activities that affect practice volumes. Overestimating volume creates excess capacity in the practice, which substantially increases practice overhead expenses and therefore reduces practice net income. Underestimating volume may have almost as severe a consequence. If demand for services exceeds the capacity of the practice, patients will migrate to competitors and be lost to the practice, while operating costs will increase due to staff overtime and inefficiencies caused by overcrowding.

Provider Compensation Forecast

Physician-owned medical group practices can be organized as sole proprietorships, professional corporations, or partnerships. These organizations compensate the physician owners/shareholders/partners from the pool of revenue available after operating costs and the salaries of nonphysician providers and salaried physicians are paid. The specific methodology of distributing this pool varies for each practice, with some organizations using an equal distribution of this pool, other practices paying physicians proportionally based on their collections or production, and other practices using still other methods. Regardless of the method of distribution, the amount of total owner/shareholder/partner compensation is limited to the amount that practice revenue exceeds the expenses the medical group pays.

This limitation in the amount of physician compensation does not necessarily affect medical groups that are part of larger integrated delivery systems or that are owned by a parent corporation. These organizations may receive subsidies from their parent that can be used to offset operating costs or to pay physicians.

Along with the volume prediction in the statistics budget, forecasting the amount of profits available to pay physicians is an essential aspect of developing the practice's budget. Physician-owned practices need to forecast the amount of revenue that will be available for physician income. Likewise medical groups that are subsidiaries of larger organizations need to forecast both the amount of physician compensation and the amount of operating subsidy.

Practices organized as professional or business corporations have the option of retaining earnings in the corporation and not distributing all revenue to the shareholders. If the practice has a retained earnings policy, the amount of retained earnings is also part of the provider compensation forecast.

Expense Budget

Information from the statistics budget also determines the expense budget, which estimates the costs of providing the services that were the basis for the revenue budget. The expense budget addresses each expense category in the practice, support staff salaries and fringe benefits, fixed assets (building and capital equipment), consumable supplies, contracts, and purchased services. Usually, expenses in the budget are separated into fixed and variable costs to allow the practice to understand the effect of changes in the volume of services on the cost of providing the services.

Revenue Budget

The volume information from the statistics budget is combined with reimbursement information to create the revenue budget. Reimbursement estimates, the mix of services, and the mix of payers combined with predictions on the practice's ability to collect accounts receivable create the revenue budget. In addition to the amount of revenue available to the practice, the revenue budget also needs to forecast when the revenue will be received.

Operating Budget

The operating budget combines the revenue and expense budgets to predict profit or loss at the level of service specified in the statistics budget.

In larger, more complex organizations, each major department creates an operating budget to forecast the positive or negative contribution from the department to the larger organization, with the organization's operating budget being the aggregation of the operating budgets of its organizational parts.

In smaller, less complex organizations, the revenue budget, the expense budget, and the operating budget are frequently combined in a single document, predicting the financial performance of the entire practice.

Cash Budget

The cash budget provides management with a forecast of the organization's short-run solvency and its need for supplemental cash in the form of a loan or line of credit to meet predicted expenses. The cash budget translates the operating budget into a prediction of the flow of cash into and out of the practice on a monthly, weekly, or daily basis. The cash budget is the cornerstone for short-term cash management in the practice.

Capital Budget

The capital budget is used to plan for the purchase of assets that have lives greater than 1 year. The greater cost of capital items and their long lives call for both different budgeting techniques and different accounting methods. The cost of capital equipment or a building is depreciated at a predetermined rate, regardless of the actual expenditure of cash by the practice for its purchase. The budgeting techniques used to determine whether a capital purchase has an appropriate return on investment are, likewise, very different from the techniques used in other types of budgets.

■ The Budget Process

Budgets can be created in isolation within the medical group or in a coordinated manner. The most efficient process necessitates synchronizing the various budgets so the output of one budget provides input to another. Likewise, if the practice creates separate budgets for subordinate entities, such as satellite or branch clinic sites or departments, the budgets for the subordinate entities are prepared concurrently with the organizational budget.

Before the statistical budget can be prepared, the organization needs to establish its goals and objectives for the time period of the budget. The planning process is a responsibility of the medical group's governance. In larger practices, the governance is a board of directors for the medical group, elected by the physician partner/shareholders as representative leaders. In smaller practices, all physicians equally share the governance responsibility. The planning process also needs to have input and involvement of the practice's administrative staff and key managers.

Creating the budget can be described as a five-step process, involving each layer of governance and management.

Step One

The medical group's governance establishes the overall goals and objectives for the organization, defines budgeting responsibilities, confirms the activity levels stated in the statistical budget, and assesses changes in level of physician or nonphysician provider staffing. The practice's governance also makes the provider compensation forecast, determining the pool of revenue after operating costs that will be used to compensate physicians.

Step Two

Practice administration refines the objectives in operational terms and prepares working documents for any satellite or branch clinic sites and department managers. The documents state the overall practice activity level, guidance for changes in activity levels for various components of the practice, information on changes in reimbursement levels, and other assumptions needed for the subordinate entities to prepare their budget input.

Step Three

Satellite or branch clinic sites and department managers use the guidance from administration to project activity levels in their areas, determine staffing needs, and draft a revenue budget and expense budget for their entity.

Step Four

The practice manager aggregates the revenue and expense budgets from the satellites, branches, and departments to create a draft practice revenue budget and expense budget. Based on the amount established in the provider compensation forecast, the practice manager refines the revenue and expense budgets for the subordinate entities in order to determine the provider compensation forecast. If the amount established in the provider compensation forecast cannot be attained by controlling costs or increasing administrative efficiency, the practice's administration cannot complete the budget, and must request that the practice governance either increase the statistics budget (thereby increasing practice productivity) or reduce the provider compensation forecast in order to balance the amount of total expenses with the amount of total practice revenue.

After the subordinate revenue and expense budgets are accepted, the administration aggregates the budgets into the practice's operating budget. Based on the practice's aggregated revenue budget and expense budget, the cash budget is prepared, as are projected statements of financial position.

Step Five

The operating budget, cash budget, and capital budget are presented to the medical group's governance in the context of the comprehensive budget. The governance reviews, amends, and eventually approves the comprehensive budget.[11]

The Role of the Practice Manager

The majority of responsibility for budget development and execution falls upon the practice manager and the medical group's administrative staff. Some actions, such as establishing the goals and objectives of the practice, establishing the key values stated in the statistics budget, or determining the amount of the provider compensation forecast must be made by the physicians who govern a private medical group, or the senior managers in an integrated delivery system. Although these issues must have the consent and approval of the organization's governance, the practice manager has to ensure that the practice's governance addresses these issues and that definitive guidance is given. The practice manager also has to assess the overall feasibility of the budget and must be ready to bring issues back to the practice's governance for review and revision, if the expense or revenue budgets cannot support the volume of services expressed in the statistics budget or the provider compensation forecast.

The practice manager is also the messenger who carries the budget guidance from the practice's governing physicians or executives to the administrative, clinical, and ancillary managers who will develop their portions of the budget.

Lastly, the practice manager has to ensure that the practice's physicians agree with the budget and will follow the budget's guidance. This latter role can be very difficult because it can entail directing a recalcitrant physician to abide by a group decision. In these situations, the practice manager should enlist physicians from the group's governance or who have more seniority in the practice to deliver the message of the importance of the budget to the practice's economic future, rather than risk personal harm that could occur if the manager confronted the physician.

■ Creating the Statistics Budget

Forecasting the amount and type of services is, perhaps, the most critical aspect of establishing a budget for the medical group. Patient volume along with the mix and relative complexity of the services affect every aspect of the budget. The amount of operating revenue for the practice that is stated in the revenue budget is directly related to the services provided by the group; some expenses, such as medical supply costs, will increase or decrease proportionally with changes in patient volume.

The statistics budget does not provide specific detail on the use of resources, such as changes in staffing levels, but offers general guidance on key values that are used to create the various components of the comprehensive budget. The statistics budget establishes the key values that are used by multiple entities within the medical group to develop their respective portions of the budget and ensures that each portion of the budget uses the same assumptions and volume estimates.

Key values that should be included in the statistics budget include:

- Total professional service gross charges or total professional service work relative value units (RVUs)
- Total laboratory service gross charges or total laboratory service RVUs
- Total radiology service gross charges or total radiology service RVUs
- Total contractual adjustments
- Total patient encounters
- Percentage increase/decrease in Medicare conversion factor
- Percentage increase/decrease in reimbursement by other payers

Some of the values expressed in the statistics budget are aggregates that apply to the entire practice, whereas some of the values should be computed for each provider. The most important value that applies to each provider is the measure of provider production chosen for the budget (i.e., professional service gross charges or RVUs). By estimating each provider's total production for the year, the provider compensation forecast is an easy computation. All that is required is to apply a gross collection ratio or the estimate of provider compensation per RVU to the production value, and the provider's compensation is easily forecast. Likewise, computing the revenue budget for the practice is very straightforward, because it is a simple calculation involving the production information expressed in the statistics budget.

The amount of services in the statistics budget can be estimated using several techniques:

- Past activity
- Calculation based on an estimate of demand
- Calculation based on scheduled provider time

Past Activity

The easiest method to estimate future volume is to assume that it will be similar to what happened in the past. Assuming that the external environment has not changed significantly, it is reasonable to assume that the number and type of services the practice will deliver in the next year will be the same as those provided in the most recent time period. Unfortunately, the environment is not always stable. For example, new physician practices may come into the market area, local employers may shift health insurance plans to carriers whose provider panels do not include the practice's physicians, or the practice may make decisions to add or delete services. In many instances, past performance can be used as a starting point in predicting future service volumes. For example, if the medical group adds a new physician, and has not made other fundamental changes, the total service volume can be estimated by simply adding the number of and type of services that the new physician will provide.

Calculation Based on an Estimate of Demand

Medical groups entering a new market, establishing a branch facility, creating a new ancillary service, or adding a different physician specialty may not have adequate historical information to estimate service volume. In this instance, the demand for services can be estimated using several techniques. The most common process is to use demographic information describing the population in the new market area compared to the demographic profile of the population in the practice's other locations along with the known volume and service information for the practice in the existing markets to estimate the service demand in the new market. If the market area is particularly underserved, a market share approach could be used to estimate the volume of services that will be provided.

Calculation Based on Scheduled Provider Time

A third technique uses known provider production levels and scheduled provider time to estimate service volume. Again, past production is the basis for the estimate. Although this methodology can be quite complex, in its most basic form, input consists of the number of available days for each provider (usually by month), the total services for each provider for the time periods, and the number of projected days that each provider will work in the future time periods. One advantage of this process is the involvement of each provider in scheduling available days. The workload information can be extremely helpful in scheduling support staffing levels to coincide with peak workload months, or to accommodate planned absence for vacation or continuing education.

Regardless of the methodology used to create the values for productivity, it is extremely important that the involved individuals and departments agree with the estimate. Each provider must agree to the amount of professional service gross charges or RVUs that he or she is expected to produce. Likewise, if the practice has a laboratory director and radiology director they would need to concur with the production levels expected for their ancillary services.

The amount of total contractual adjustments is computed by applying the estimated values of percentage increase/decrease in Medicare conversion factor and percentage increase/decrease in reimbursement by other payers to the historical amount of adjustments to gross charge estimates. Knowing the amount of contractual adjustments in the current time period, and the predicted changes by the Centers for Medicare and Medicaid Services and the practice's other major payers, the computation of total contractual adjustments is very straightforward.

■ Creating the Provider Compensation Forecast

In physician-owned practices, the provider compensation forecast aligns the income expectations of the physician owners with the reality of the practice budget. Practices that are hospital-owned or part of larger organizations also need to create a provider compensation forecast to project the amount of provider compensation and to assess any subsidy paid to the practice by the parent organization. All practices need to assess whether the budget will include an amount for retained earnings.

The provider compensation forecast uses the patient volume information developed in the statistics budget to validate the level of provider compensation. It is important to relate the amount of budgeted provider compensation to the patient workload developed in the statistics budget. By doing so, providers are made aware that the amount of their compensation is dependent on the practice meeting the production forecast.

Projecting the provider compensation forecast employs the same techniques as for the statistics budget. Historical compensation levels can be used in the same way as past activity is used to project the volume and types of patient services. An alternative method is to calculate the ratio of physician compensation to gross charges in the current time period and to use this ratio with the predicted amount of gross charges established in the statistics budget.

If the amount computed for the provider compensation forecast is assessed to be insufficient to retain or appropriately reward the group's providers, the first action the practice should consider is to increase the volume of services stated in the statistics budget. If the amount of services increases, the amount of practice revenues may also increase sufficiently to compensate the providers. If it is not practical to increase service volume, then the practice has only two other strategies that can provide the desired increase in provider compensation. The revenue budget can reflect better collections on accounts receivable or the expense budget can be structured to decrease costs. If revenues cannot be increased at the same level of patient volume or if costs cannot be lowered, then the provider compensation estimate has to be reduced to a realistic level.

Because the amount of provider compensation is directly related to the amount of provider production stated in the statistics budget, the two budgets are interactive, because changes in one affect the other.

■ Creating the Expense Budget

The statistics budget established the volume information that, in large part, determines the expense budget. The expense budget must forecast each significant expense category for the practice. With the information in the statistics budget and historical information, each expense can be estimated.

Some expenses are fixed and do not vary with volume. Examples of fixed costs in a medical group include building lease cost/depreciation, equipment lease cost/ depreciation, or a service contract with a CPA to provide accounting advice and to complete required tax filings. Regardless of the number of patient encounters for the practice, these costs do not change. Other costs are variable and are directly proportional to patient volume. Examples include medical supply costs or a contract for transcription of physician dictation to the medical record, which change as patient volume changes. Some expenses function in a "step-fixed" manner, which do not change for a specific range of patient volume, but increase if volume increases beyond the range, or is reduced if volume is less than the range. A good example of this cost behavior is the practice's staff. If patient volume changes substantially from the estimate, then the practice either has to hire additional staff members or has to pay overtime to staff members who work longer hours.

The number of patient encounters is fundamental to determining staffing levels for the practice. If the statistics budget forecasts an increase in patient encounters, the practice needs to assess whether staffing levels will be affected. In some instances, new equipment or technologies may allow the existing staff to be more efficient and there will not be a need to hire additional staff or to pay overtime. In other instances, the expense budget needs to include the costs associated with an increase in staff. Regardless, the expense budget must include cost-of-living adjustments, merit pay increases, programmed bonus payments, or other increases in compensation. Changes in the cost of employee fringe benefits must also be programmed, such as the cost of employee health insurance, disability insurance, life insurance, and continuing education expenses.

Medical supply costs can be forecast based on historical costs, increased by estimates for price increases by suppliers and the patient volume estimate from the statistics budget. A similar method can be used to predict consumable supply costs in the radiology and clinical laboratory, based on the amount of radiology and clinical laboratory services stated in the statistics budget.

Fixed costs can be included in the budget by line item. In most instances, the amount is known due to long-term lease contracts or depreciation schedules. In other cases, estimates from suppliers or contractors along with historical costs are the source of information.

The first version of the expense budget is seldom an accurate expression of future costs. In almost every instance the expense budget undergoes multiple refinements as staff changes are considered and either accepted or rejected, or as projects that seemed promising are either included in the budget or excluded. Changes in staffing levels have the largest impact on the expense budget and should receive the greatest scrutiny by management.

■ Creating the Revenue Budget

Because the statistics budget defines the amount of production for the practice as well as key changes in reimbursement, the revenue budget centers on the business office operations. Specifically, the revenue budget includes estimates for bad debt and the predicted change in accounts receivable that will occur during the year. These values can be expressed individually, or the net effect can be stated as the adjusted collection percentage for the practice.

The statistics budget contained the amount of provider and ancillary services production and the contractual adjustment needed to estimate potential cash collections, excluding the effect of bad debt. The estimate for bad debt is included in the revenue budget. Closely related is the amount of change in accounts receivable that occurs during the year. If the practice's business office improves the collection process and reduces the amount of accounts receivable, or if the business office reduces the amount of bad debt, then total revenue increases.

The revenue budget is therefore computed as:

Total gross charges – Total contractual adjustment – Bad debt + Change in A/R = Total projected revenue

The revenue budget also predicts when revenue is received, based on monthly estimates of production, the time required to bill third-party payers and patients, and the time needed to collect and post payments for billed services. The timing of when revenue is received is an important input to the cash flow budget.

The previous computations presume that the practice is reimbursed on a fee-for-service basis. If the practice has contracts with health maintenance organizations (HMOs) that reimburse on a capitation basis, the revenue budget is developed differently. Capitation contracts specify that the practice is reimbursed a fixed amount for each HMO beneficiary assigned to the practice. This amount is usually referred to as the capitation rate, or a prospective payment per member per month. The revenue budget for capitation contracts is computed as the capitation rate for each HMO contract times the number of HMO beneficiaries covered under the contract. Medical groups with capitation contracts should establish a separate responsibility center to track expenses and revenues for each capitation contract and the services (usually measured in fee-for-service equivalent charges) provided to HMO plan members.

Creating the Operating Budget

The operating budget combines the revenue and expense budgets to predict profit or loss. In larger, more complex organizations, each major department creates an operating budget to forecast the positive or negative contribution from the department to the larger organization, with the organization's operating budget being the aggregation of the operating budgets of its organizational parts. In smaller, less complex organizations, the operating budget reflects the overall financial performance of the entire practice.

After the preliminary operating budget is prepared, the practice manager has to assess the feasibility of attaining the budgeted amounts and whether the budgeted amounts are acceptable to the practice.

Ideally, if the practice is physician owned, and it does not have a policy of retained earnings, the completed operating budget indicates that total revenue minus operating expenses, minus provider compensation equals zero. If the resulting value is positive, the positive amount can be used to increase the provider compensation forecast, or it can be reserved to accommodate unexpected expenses. In the more common instance, the resulting value is negative. In this instance, the manager can reassess whether practice revenue can be increased by better business office operations, expenses can be decreased, provider compensation can be reduced, or production can be increased to bring the budget in balance.

Practices that are hospital owned or part of an integrated delivery system will have a targeted amount for the operating budget, as opposed to an expectation that the operating budget will show a zero net amount. However, the evaluation process is the same, as well as the options to increase or lower the net amount of the operating budget.

Creating the Cash Budget

It is important that the revenue budget predicts the timing of cash receipts, at least on a monthly basis, for the full time period of the budget. This is critical input to the cash budget, which forecasts the medical group's short-run solvency and its need for supplemental cash in the form of a loan or line of credit to meet predicted expenses.

The cash budget is part of the comprehensive budget, but separate from the practice's operating budget. It predicts anticipated sources and uses of cash and cash flow into and out of the practice. The cash budget should provide a detailed forecast of cash receipts and operating expenses for each day in the upcoming 2 weeks, each week for the upcoming 2 months, and each month for the next year. These time periods are crucial to managing both predictable expenses such as payroll or a single premium insurance payment and discretionary expenditures such as staff bonuses, physician income reconciliation bonuses, or prepayment of loans.

Proper use of the cash budget can enable the medical group to minimize the need for short-term loans or use of a bank line of credit to cover predictable expenses. It is also the first predictor of the accuracy of the operating budget. Because the cash budget is a series of trial balances of the medical group's revenue and expenses, a forecast of successive negative cash flows is a leading indicator that the operating budget was too ambitious.

In short, the cash budget is the cornerstone for short-term cash management in the practice.

Creating the Capital Budget

The capital budget, like the cash budget, is independent of the operating budget, because it plans for the purchase of assets that have useful lives greater than 1 year. The greater cost of capital items and their long lives call for both different budgeting techniques and different accounting methods than the operating budget.

The cost of capital equipment or a building is depreciated on a predetermined rate, regardless of the actual expenditure of cash by the practice for its purchase. The depreciation rate is determined by the expected life of the capital asset as described in the earlier part of this chapter, and is governed by both accounting rules and the U.S. tax code.

The techniques used to determine whether a capital purchase has an appropriate return on investment apply the concept of the time value of money (as it applies to the purchase price or depreciated cost of the asset) and the expected revenues from its use. The time value of money is the concept that a dollar of cash in hand today is worth more than a dollar of cash to be received at any time in the future. The two concepts used to express the time value of money are future value and present value. Future value is the amount to which a given amount of cash will grow at the end of a given period of time when compounded at a specified interest rate. Present value is the reverse concept, which expresses the value of a cash flow that will be received in the future, discounted to the present.[13]

The decision to purchase or lease a capital asset needs to be based first on medical necessity. Certain equipment items are required for essential medical services or for patient safety and are required, regardless of the financial return to the practice. For example, a cardiology practice may purchase an automatic external defibrillator, hoping that it would not need to be used, but it must be available if a patient experiences cardiac arrest.

Other decisions should be based on the potential economic benefit to the practice. Using the concepts of future value and present value, the cost of the asset can be compared to the expected return to the medical group for use of the asset. By discounting every future cash flow as well as the initial purchase price and future operating costs in terms of its present value, a true rate of return can be calculated. Knowing the rate of return allows the medical group to make a more informed decision on the purchase of capital assets. Because medical groups are generally undercapitalized, the decision to purchase capital equipment needs to be made with an understanding of maximizing the return to the group for its investment.

Zero-Based Budgeting

The comprehensive budget is designed as an incremental or traditional budget. Budgets for the previous time period are the starting point for developing the projections for this time period. The service volume projections specified in the statistics budget are usually based on the medical group's experiences in the most recent past. Likewise, the prediction for changes in reimbursement is based on a change from the current time.

The zero-based budget, as its name suggests, starts each time period anew. Each segment of the budget begins at the lowest possible level and builds each assumption for volume, cost, or income independent of past performance.

Zero-based budgeting is much more complex than the incremental budget that builds on past experience. At the same time, a zero-based budget provides substantial insights into practice expenditures and revenues. Zero-based budgeting techniques can be used when a new service or new location is contemplated. Starting from scratch can be an effective strategy when creating the budget for a proposed activity, because it requires the managers and physicians involved in the new activity to thoroughly evaluate service volumes, fixed and variable expenses, and potential revenue.

Fixed Versus Flexible Budgeting

The design of the comprehensive budget focuses on the volume predictions that are made in the statistics budget. Although the budget is prepared in a static fashion, with predicted levels of patients and services, the reality is that actual volumes will be different. A flexible budget assumes that actual performance will be different from the original budgeted amounts and adjusts the initial budget to accommodate the different volume of services. Essentially, it provides a retrospective view of what would have been the predicted budget amounts if the volume of services expressed in the statistics budget were different, assuming that all of the other budget assumptions remained the same.

In order to create a flexible budget, the practice needs a careful assessment of fixed and variable costs and an understanding of the variable costs that are attributed to the specific changes that the practice experienced. For example, the portions of the expense budget that address capital asset depreciation or professional liability insurance are not affected by an increase in the number of patients, but medical supply expenses, administrative costs, and staff costs could be affected as the practice expends additional supplies, pays staff overtime, or hires new staff.

Creating a flexible budget is a significant commitment in additional work for the practice's administrative staff members. A flexible budget has substantial benefits in its ability to assess the performance of various parts of the practice and to more accurately predict the financial future of the medical group, but these benefits are achieved at a substantial cost in time and effort.

Using the Comprehensive Budget as a Management Tool

The comprehensive budget is the practice manager's most important tool. The various budgets that compose the comprehensive budget provide information that allows the manager to forecast financial success or difficulty for the practice.

The statistics budget has the key assumptions of patient volume, provider production, and reimbursement. These values are important because they predict the future of the medical group. If patient volume is lower than predicted, or if provider production is less, the manager needs to assess the potential impact on practice revenue that will occur in the near future. Because medical groups normally require 30 or more days to collect accounts receivable from the best payers, a decrease in production will not be recognized immediately. The statistics budget is an early warning system for the administrator to predict potential financial problems.

The expense budget has a similar opportunity. Tracking how close actual expenses follow the predictions in the budget enables the practice manager to understand whether operating costs are being properly managed, and whether a particular expense is in line with the budget expenses or out of control. By identifying specific areas that exceed the budget, the manager can place explicit controls on just the expenses that need more control. In a similar fashion, the expense budgets prepared by the various satellite or branch facilities or departments in larger medical groups can provide a comparison of general performance for the facilities and departments, allowing the practice administrator to assess the performance of subordinate managers and provide additional guidance and counseling where needed.

The revenue budget gives the practice manager an assessment of the performance of the business office staff. Allowing for differences in volume from the statistics budget, the ability of the business office to collect accounts receivable is expressed directly in the revenue budget. If patient volume and provider production meet or exceed the statistics budget, the revenue budget will have a commensurate increase, provided that the business office is performing properly.

The cash budget is the short-term assessment of performance for the medical group. Using its predictions allows the manager to prepare for the changes in revenue and expenses that occur each month. Using the cash budget, a manager can ensure that the practice has sufficient cash in bank accounts to cover predicted expenditures such as payroll, insurance premiums, or property tax assessments. The cash budget predicts when the practice will need a short-term loan, which gives the manager time to obtain the loan at a more favorable interest rate.

The capital budget ensures that the practice obtains the best return for its equipment investment, and allows the practice manager to evaluate whether equipment has the volume of services that was assumed when it was purchased. Information on service volume not only provides insight into the financial return for the equipment, but also gives insight into potential wear that could cause early replacement or whether changes in technology have caused a change in medical services and the device is becoming obsolete.

The most important budget tool for the manager is the information available in the provider compensation forecast. In physician-owned medical groups, the medical group's physicians employ the practice manager. If physician personal income does not meet expectations, the doctors will not be pleased with the performance of their practice manager. Displeasure arising from lower-than-expected compensation can lead to the physicians deciding to change practice managers in the hope of having higher incomes. Because the provider compensation forecast is determined for each provider in the group, the practice manager can compare actual physician compensation to the predicted amount in order to adequately inform any provider who will earn less than the forecast.

References

1. American Medical Association. Bankruptcies in healthcare: a physician's guide. Accessed at http://www.amaassn.org/ama1/pub/upload/mm/368/bankruptcies_final.pdf
2. American Institute of Certified Public Accountants. Audits of providers of health care services; 1996.
3. Financial Accounting Standards Board. *Statement of financial accounting concepts no. 1. Objectives of financial reporting by business enterprises.* Norwalk, CT: FASB; November 1978.
4. Kieso DE, Weygant JJ. *Intermediate accounting* (5th ed.). New York: Wiley; 1986:27.

5. Financial Accounting Standards Board. *Statement of financial accounting concepts no. 2. Qualitative characteristics of accounting information.* Norwalk, CT: FASB; May 1980.

6. Financial Accounting Standards Board. *Statement of financial accounting concepts no. 5. Recognition and measurement in financial statements of business enterprises.* Norwalk, CT: FASB; December 1984.

7. Financial Accounting Standards Board. *Statement of financial accounting concepts no. 6. Elements of financial statements.* Norwalk, CT: FASB; December 1985. Norby WC. Accounting for financial analysis. *Financial Analysts Journal.* March–April 1982:22–23, 29–80.

8. American Institute of CPAs. Accounting for nonmonetary transactions. APB opinion no. 29. May 1973. In: *Accounting standards: original pronouncements.* Jersey City, NJ: AICPA; 2003. Pub no. 005123.

9. Piland N, Glass K (eds.). *Chart of accounts for health care organizations.* Englewood, CO: Medical Group Management Association; 1999.

10. Committee on Sponsoring Organizations of the Treadway Commission. COSO definition of internal control. Accessed at http://www.coso.org/key.htm

11. Pavlock EJ. *Financial management for medical groups: a resource for new and experienced managers* (2nd ed.). Englewood, CO: MGMA Center for Research; 2000:381–382, 387–388, 554–560.

12. Finkler SA, Ward DM. *Cost accounting for health care organizations* (2nd ed.). Gaithersburg, MD: Aspen; 1999:348–349.

13. Center for Research in Ambulatory Health Care Administration. *The organization and development of a medical group practice.* Englewood, CO, Center for Research in Ambulatory Health Care Administration 1976:217–218.

14. Gapenski LC. *Cases for healthcare finance.* Health Administration Press; 1999:213–214.

15. Cleverley WO, Cameron AE. *Essentials of health care finance.* Gaithersburg, MD: Aspen; 2002.

CHAPTER

10

Financial Management and Reporting

Lee Ann H. Webster, MA, CPA, FACMPE

To understand the financial performance of a physician practice, one needs a firm understanding of the practice's financial statements. Benchmarking and financial analysis are powerful tools the practice executive can use to take the performance of the practice to the next level. In order to properly use these tools, however, a manager must have a solid understanding of the elements of financial statements, bases of accounting, and the level of service provided by the accountants issuing the financial statements. Even a leader who does a superior job motivating people and managing resources cannot achieve optimal financial performance unless he or she understands how to read and analyze financial statements.

When an independent Certified Public Accountant (CPA) reports on financial statements, his or her report may reflect one of three levels of service—audit, review, or compilation. The amount of work and the procedures performed by the accounting firm in preparing financial statements based on one of these three levels varies significantly (see **Table 10-1**). In analyzing financial statements, it is important to understand the work ordinarily performed by the accountant and the degree of assurance provided by each level of service.

All levels of service require the accountant to have sufficient knowledge of the accounting principles of the industry in which the entity operates. This understanding enables him or her to perform the designated level of service for financial statements that are appropriate for an entity operating in that industry. This requirement does not prohibit an accountant without experience in a particular industry, such as the medical practice industry, from accepting an engagement for a client in that industry. The standards allow the accountant to gain knowledge through methods such as studying American Institute of Certified Public Accountants (AICPA) or industry publications or consulting with individuals knowledgeable in the industry. All levels of service require that the accountant have an understanding of the client's business. The level of understanding required of both the industry and the client's business operations will generally increase with the level of service.

■ Audits

Audited financial statements reflect the highest level of service provided by an independent CPA. In performing an audit, a CPA must follow generally accepted auditing

Table 10-1	Comparison of Audit, Review, and Compilation Services		
	Audit	**Review**	**Compilation**
Opinion, assurance	Opinion and assurance	No opinion, limited assurance	No opinion, no assurance
Read financial statements	Yes	Yes	Yes
Perform inquiries and analytical procedures	Yes	Yes	No
Obtain written representations from management	Yes	Yes	No
Obtain corroborative evidence	Yes	No	No
Perform an assessment of internal control and the related risk	Yes	No	No
Engagement designed to detect fraud	No	No	No
Usual cost	Highest	More than compilation, but less than audit	Lowest
Notes to financial statements (disclosures)	Required	Required	May omit substantially all disclosures
Accountant independence	Required	Required	Not required, but must disclose the fact that accountant is not independent

standards (GAAS) issued by the Auditing Standards Board. An audit is the only level of service in which the CPA examines the financial statements. In doing so, the auditor performs certain tests and analytical procedures of the accounting records and financial statements. He or she will corroborate the financial information through such procedures as confirmation of bank balances and accounts receivable, inventory observation, and other methods of inquiry and observation. An audit will generally include an evaluation of the client's system of internal control.

Based on this examination, the accountant issues an opinion as to whether the financial statements present fairly the financial position, results of operations, and cash flows (if applicable) of the entity in accordance with generally accepted accounting principles (GAAP) or other comprehensive basis of accounting (OCBOA). (See the discussion of GAAP and OCBOA later in this chapter.) An audit is the only level of service in which the accountant's report is an opinion. This opinion will be unqualified, qualified, adverse, or a disclaimer. An unqualified opinion is the best opinion an auditor can give, indicating he or she believes the financial statements are in accordance with GAAP or an OCBOA. A qualified opinion means the auditor believes the statements are generally in compliance with GAAP or an OCBOA, but has a reservation

about something in the financial statements that prevents him or her from issuing an unqualified opinion. The auditor's report will explain this matter. An adverse opinion indicates that the financial statements contain material differences from GAAP or an OCBOA and explains these differences. A disclaimer means the auditor cannot obtain enough information to issue an opinion.

Although an audit provides the highest level of assurance regarding the financial statements, this is normally the most costly form of financial statement, both in dollars and in the amount of internal resources that the practice must dedicate to work with the auditors. Many practices that have an audit do so because a bank or governmental agency requires the audit. Even for practices with significant bank debt, a bank may not require an audit if the physicians are personally guaranteeing the debt. Consequently, many practices elect to have compiled or reviewed financial statements (discussed later in this chapter) rather than an audit.

Audit Misconceptions

People sometimes confuse an audit of the financial statements with other engagements referred to as "audits" that are essentially operational in nature, such as billing or operational audits. As described earlier, an audit of financial statements is an audit performed in accordance with GAAS. To avoid any misunderstanding regarding the nature and scope of any audits, both the accountant and the practice should obtain an engagement letter—an understanding in writing of the services to be performed by the accounting firm.

Currently, the primary purpose of an audit is not to search for fraud. The auditors' responsibility is to obtain reasonable assurance that the financial statements are free of material misstatement, including material misstatement caused by fraud. That said, in reaction to some of the frauds uncovered in recent years, the Auditing Standards Board released several Statements on Auditing Standards that assist auditors in understanding and fulfilling their responsibility for fraud in an audit of the financial statements. Perhaps the best known of these, Statement on Auditing Standards (SAS) No. 99, "Consideration of Fraud in a Financial Statement Audit," provides guidance to auditors to improve the likelihood that they will detect material misstatements caused by fraud. Among the changes included in this pronouncement are the addition of a brainstorming session by the audit team regarding fraud risks, increased emphasis on professional skepticism, procedures to address management override of internal control, and a presumption that revenue recognition is a fraud risk.[1]

Reviews

In performing a review engagement, an accountant performs more work than he or she would typically perform in a compilation engagement, but less work than in an audit engagement. The Accounting and Review Services Committee of the AICPA determines the standards for these services, and the related pronouncements are called Statements on Standards for Accounting and Review Services (SSARS).

The purpose of the review engagement is to provide limited assurance that no material modifications to the financial statements are necessary in order for them to be in conformity with the applicable accounting framework,[2] such as GAAP or an OCBOA.

A review requires that the accountant perform inquiry and analytical procedures. Examples of analytical procedures include comparison of current year financial statements with comparable prior year statements and budgets or forecasts, and financial ratios to industry norms.[2] Inquiries would concern items such as actions taken at board of directors meetings, unusual transactions, subsequent events, and changes in the entity's business activities or accounting practices. The accountant

would also inquire as to questions that may have arisen during the conduct of the engagement.[2]

In performing a review, the accountant obtains written representations from management as to its responsibility for the fair presentation of the financial statements, the system of internal control, the prevention and detection of fraud, full and truthful response to all inquiries, completeness of information, and knowledge regarding subsequent events. The chief executive officer, the chief financial officer, and other members of management who the accountant believes are responsible and knowledgeable, directly or through others in the organization, about the matters covered in the letter, should sign this letter.[2]

A review does not require the accountant to obtain an understanding of the client's system of internal control or an assessment of the related risk, to obtain corroborative evidential matter (i.e., confirm accounts receivable or observe inventory), and certain other procedures normally performed during an audit. However, the accountant should perform additional procedures when he or she becomes aware that information he or she receives may be incorrect or unsatisfactory.[2]

Compilations

A compilation is the lowest level of service that an independent CPA may provide when he or she reports on financial statements. As with review engagements, the AICPA Accounting and Review Services Committee establishes the professional standards for these engagements.

The amount of work required of an accountant in a compilation engagement is significantly less than the amount required in an audit or a review. The objective of a compilation is to assist management in presenting financial information in the form of financial statements. In performing a compilation, SSARS require that an accountant read the financial statements before issuing his or her report and consider whether they are appropriate in form and free from obvious material errors. In this context, the term "error" refers to mistakes such as clerical or mathematical errors made in preparing the financial statements, or mistakes in the application of accounting principles, such as inadequate disclosure.

In connection with performing a compilation, an accountant does not express an opinion or any other form of assurance on the financial statements. Consequently, the accountant is not required to make inquiries or perform other procedures to verify, corroborate, or review information supplied by the entity.[2] The accountant is only required to read the financial statements for appropriateness and errors in the manner discussed previously.

Of course, many accountants performing a compilation do more work than this. SSARS require an accountant to consider other procedures that may be necessary to report on compiled financial statements, such as adjusting the entity's books or consulting on accounting matters. Particularly with small practices, accounting firms may actually maintain the client's general ledger and prepare financial statements for the client. SSARS also require an accountant to make inquiries or perform other procedures if he or she becomes aware of or suspects that the financial statements may be incomplete, incorrect, or otherwise unsatisfactory. SSARS further state that if the client refuses to provide additional or revised information, the accountant should withdraw from the engagement.[2]

Although an accountant who is not independent with respect to the client may not perform an audit or review engagement, he or she may perform a compilation. The fact that the accountant is not independent must be disclosed in the final paragraph of the accountant's report.[2]

■ In-House Statements

Financial statements prepared for internal purposes by practice personnel (even those who have CPA certificates) should not be confused with financial statements reported on by an outside, independent accountant. First, by definition, internal financial personnel are not "outside," and thus are not independent. The reporting standards and procedures for compilation, review, and audit engagements do not apply to these statements. Although formal internal financial statements and the related accounting records would generally follow the accounting standards for whatever basis of accounting the practice uses for external reporting, other internal statements and special use analyses may be prepared in whatever format the entity deems useful for decision-making purposes.

■ The Accountant's Report

When an accountant performs services in connection with financial statements intended for third parties, the statements must include a report. The report identifies the level of service. Each page of the related financial statements and notes should refer to this report. The following are examples of reports for the three different levels of service.

Audit Report: Unqualified Opinion, Accrual Basis[3]

To the Board of Directors
West Side Multispecialty Group, P.C.

We have audited the accompanying balance sheets of West Side Multispecialty Group, P.C., as of December 31, 20X2 and 20X1, and the related statements of income and retained earnings, and cash flows for the years then ended. These financial statements are the responsibility of the management of West Side Multispecialty Group, P.C. Our responsibility is to express an opinion on these financial statements based on our audits.

We conducted our audits in accordance with auditing standards generally accepted in the United States of America. These standards require that we plan and perform the audit to obtain reasonable assurance about whether the financial statements are free of material misstatement. An audit includes examining, on a test basis, evidence supporting the amounts and disclosures in the financial statements. An audit also involves assessing the accounting principles used and significant estimates made by management, as well as evaluating the overall financial statement presentation. We believe that our audits provide a reasonable basis for our opinion.

In our opinion, the financial statements referred to above, present fairly, in all material respects, the financial position of West Side Multispecialty Group, P.C., as of December 31, 20X2 and 20X1, and the results of its operations, changes in retained earnings, and cash flows for the years then ended in conformity with accounting principles generally accepted in the United States of America.

Firm's Signature
Date

Review Report: Accrual Basis[2]

To the Board of Directors
West Side Multispecialty Group, P.C.

We have reviewed the accompanying balance sheets of West Side Multispecialty Group, P.C., as of December 31, 20X2 and 20X1, and the related statements of income, retained earnings, and cash flows for the years then ended. A review includes primarily applying analytical procedures to management financial data and making inquiries of company management and owners. A review is substantially less in scope than an audit, the objective of which is the expression of an opinion regarding the financial statements as a whole. Accordingly, we do not express such an opinion.

Management is responsible for the preparation and fair presentation of the financial statements in accordance with accounting principles generally accepted in the United States of America and for designing, implementing, and maintaining internal control relevant to the preparation and fair presentation of the financial statements.

Our responsibility is to conduct the reviews in accordance with Statements on Standards for Accounting and Review Services issued by the American Institute of Certified Public Accountants. Those standards require us to perform procedures to obtain limited assurance that there are no material modifications that should be made to the financial statements. We believe that the results of our procedures provide a reasonable basis for our report.

Based on our reviews, we are not aware of any material modifications that should be made to the accompanying financial statements in order for them to be in conformity with accounting principles generally accepted in the United States of America.

Firm's Signature
Date

Compilation: Income Tax Basis, Substantially All Disclosures Omitted[2]

To the Board of Directors
West Side Multispecialty Group, P.C.

We have compiled the accompanying statements of assets, liabilities, and equity—income tax basis of West Side Multispecialty Group, P.C. as of December 31, 20X2 and 20X1, and the related statements of revenues, expenses, and retained earnings (deficit)—income tax basis, for the years then ended. We have not audited or reviewed the accompanying financial statements, and accordingly, do not express an opinion or provide assurance about whether the financial statements are in accordance with the income tax basis of accounting.

Management is responsible for the preparation and fair presentation of the financial statements in accordance with the income tax basis of accounting and for designing, implementing, and maintaining internal control relevant to the preparation and fair presentation of the financial statements.

Our responsibility is to conduct the compilation in accordance with Statements on Standards for Accounting and Review Services

issued by the American Institute of Certified Public Accountants. The objective of a compilation is to assist management in presenting financial information in the form of financial statements without undertaking to obtain or provide assurance that there are no material modifications that should be made to the financial statements.

Management has elected to omit substantially all of the disclosures ordinarily included in financial statements prepared on the income tax basis of accounting. If the omitted disclosures were included in the financial statements, they might influence the user's conclusions about the Company's assets, liabilities, equity, revenues, and expenses. Accordingly, these financial statements are not designed for those who are not informed about such matters.

Firm's Signature
Date

Bases of Accounting

The two basic accounting methods used in medical practice financial statements are the accrual method and the cash method. Because financial statements prepared on these two bases of accounting differ significantly, and both methods are frequently used for medical practice financial statements, a practice executive should have a basic understanding of both methods of accounting and their differences. Some practices utilize both methods—using accrual basis accounting for tax and financial statement purposes, while computing compensation (including bonuses) on the cash basis. According to the Medical Group Management Association's *Cost Survey for Single-Specialty Practices: 2010 Report Based on 2009 Data*, 60.54% of medical practices used the cash method and 39.46% used the accrual method for tax reporting. For internal management reporting, 56.93% used the cash method and 43.07% used the accrual method.[4]

A practice executive must also have a thorough understanding of the method of accounting used in preparing the financial statements she or he is using. Failure to do so can lead to faulty analysis and poor decision making.

Accrual Basis of Accounting
Accrual basis financial statements include transactions when they occur regardless of when the related cash changes hands. These statements recognize income when it is earned, rather than when the practice receives the related cash. Accrual basis financial statements recognize expenses when they are incurred as opposed to when they are paid. They report assets, liabilities, and equities when

they become an economic reality, regardless of when the related cash is exchanged. Thus, if an accrual basis medical practice incurs transcription services in Year 1 and pays for them in Year 2, these expenses would be included as an expense and a liability in the financial statements for Year 1. These practices record fee-for-service income and the related receivable when the physician sees the patient, rather than when they collect fees for the related services. For medical practices, this timing of revenue recognition is probably the most significant difference between cash and accrual basis accounting.

Generally Accepted Accounting Principles. The accrual basis of accounting is the foundation for financial statements prepared in conformity with GAAP. The AICPA publishes an *Audit and Accounting Guide for Health Care Organizations* annually. The guide states, "Financial statements of health care organizations should be prepared in conformity with generally accepted accounting principles."[3] This guide applies to medical practices, as well as to other healthcare organizations. Until recently, GAAP consisted of a hierarchy of accounting rules and literature, with pronouncements of the Financial Accounting Standards Board at the top of the hierarchy and prevalent industry standards at the bottom of the hierarchy. Effective September 15, 2009, a new codified version of GAAP called "FASB ASC" (Financial Accounting Standards Board—Accounting Standards Codification) became effective, replacing the former GAAP hierarchy. FASB ASC is not meant to change GAAP; it is intended to reduce the complexity of GAAP by having one source of GAAP, thus making it easier to research and determine authoritative accounting standards. The Governmental Accounting Standards Board (GASB) also governs accounting and financial statement presentation for medical practices that are governmental entities.

Cash Basis of Accounting

The cash basis of accounting requires that revenues be included in income when they are actually or constructively received and expenses be deducted when they are paid, regardless of when they are incurred. Assets, liabilities, and equities are also recognized when the cash is actually or constructively received. Thus, if a cash basis medical practice incurs transcription services in Year 1 and pays for them in Year 2, these expenses would be included as an expense in the financial statements for Year 2. The liability is never recognized in the financial statements. Fee-for-service income is recognized when the cash is received, regardless of when the physician performs services for the patient. Although cash basis practices spend considerable time and effort keeping up

with their accounts receivable, this receivable is never recognized for financial statement purposes.

Under the "pure" cash basis of accounting, the financial statements reflect only transactions that increase or decrease cash or cash equivalents. Because the pure cash basis is rarely used in practice, the term "cash basis" is frequently used to describe financial statements that are actually prepared using the "modified" cash basis of accounting. The modified cash basis of accounting is defined as the pure cash basis incorporating "modifications . . . having substantial support."[5(pp 16)] For a medical practice, these modifications generally include capitalizing fixed assets, depreciation, and the accrual of retirement plan contributions and payroll taxes. One problem with the modified cash basis is that the modifications to the pure cash basis that have substantial support have not been clearly defined in accounting literature. Excessive modifications to the pure cash basis may result in financial statements that are essentially GAAP financial statements that contain departures from GAAP.[5]

Income Tax Basis of Accounting

The income tax basis of accounting is the accounting method an entity uses or expects to use to file its income tax return, and is usually based on the federal tax laws found in the Internal Revenue Code (IRC). Most medical practices that purport to utilize the cash or modified cash basis of accounting are actually on the "income tax basis" of accounting; that is, their modifications to the cash basis of accounting are actually those prescribed by tax regulations for cash basis taxpayers. Consequently, many accountants prefer income tax basis rather than modified cash basis financial statements for these entities. The income tax basis of accounting is based on a specific set of regulations (those of the IRS) and is therefore better defined than the modified cash basis.[5] Thus, the term "income tax basis" will be used to refer to the modified cash basis financial statements presented as examples in this chapter.

Other Comprehensive Bases of Accounting

In 1981, the AICPA Special Committee on Accounting Standards Overload recommended that small businesses be allowed to present their financial statements on the same basis they use for their income tax returns, thus acknowledging that GAAP financial statements may not be suitable for all entities. Compliance with GAAP can be expensive and time consuming for smaller businesses, and many users of financial statements are satisfied with financial statements prepared on the cash basis, income tax basis, or some other basis prescribed by a regulatory agency. Authoritative accounting literature refers to these other accounting methods as other comprehensive bases of accounting (OCBOA). The AICPA Accounting and Review Services Committee permits compiled and reviewed financial statements using OCBOA,[2] but they must include a description of the OCBOA.[2] Audited financial statements may also be prepared in accordance with an OCBOA if that basis of accounting is properly disclosed and is one of the following:

- The basis of accounting used to comply with requirements of financial reporting provisions of a governmental regulatory agency to whose jurisdiction the entity is subject
- The basis of accounting used by the entity for income tax purposes
- The cash receipts and disbursements basis of accounting, and modifications thereof having substantial support (i.e., depreciation)
- A definite set of criteria having substantial support that is applied to all material items appearing in financial statements, such as price-level basis of accounting[6]

Thus, the modified cash and income tax bases of accounting meet the definition of an OCBOA. An outside accountant may issue compilation, review, or audit reports for practices using these accounting methods.

Factors Determining Choice of Accounting Method

Factors affecting a practice's choice of accounting method include the size of the practice, legal form of entity, operating characteristics, tax laws, and the requirements of owners, creditors, or regulators. The income tax (cash) and accrual methods of accounting can produce markedly different financial statements, and some practices may utilize both methods. Practice executives should understand both methods to effectively analyze their financial statements.

The primary advantage to accrual basis financial statements is that they present the most accurate picture of the practice's financial situation. Accrual basis financial statements properly match revenues with the expenses used to generate those revenues and display the related balance sheet amounts. Bankers, other creditors, outside investors, or regulatory agencies may require accrual basis financial statements. Practices that are not permitted to use the cash basis for tax purposes must use accrual basis accounting for their financial statement presentation, unless a regulatory agency requires another method of accounting. The accrual basis is more appropriate for practices with complex financial situations or significant

operating liabilities, such as those for payments to other providers under capitated contracts.

The modified cash or tax basis of accounting is appropriate for practices that prepare their income tax returns on the cash basis. Most physician-owned practices meet the IRS definition of a "qualified personal service corporation" and are allowed to use the cash method for tax reporting regardless of their volume of cash receipts.[7] Practices that do not qualify as personal service corporations may use the cash basis if they have cash receipts of less than $10 million ($5 million for C corporations or partnerships with a C corporation partner) and are not otherwise required to use the accrual basis of accounting.[8]

In 2002, the IRS issued Revenue Procedure 2002-28, which allows an increased number of taxpayers to compute their taxable income on the cash basis. This law allows some smaller entities with inventories or significant supplies on hand (such as an inventory of eyewear in an ophthalmology practice) that were previously required to use the accrual basis of accounting to use the cash method.[8] Consequently, some practices that did not qualify for the cash method in the past do now.

Because the cash basis of accounting does not recognize fee income until it is collected, many practices recognize significant tax savings by using the cash basis for income tax reporting. Section 446(a) of the IRC requires that taxable income be determined on the same basis of accounting the taxpayer regularly uses to compute its income in keeping its books.[9] Thus, in order for a practice to take advantage of the tax savings offered by using the cash basis of accounting for tax purposes, the practice must generally keep its books and prepare its financial statements on the cash basis. Certain exceptions to this rule exist. Due to the potential adverse consequences of maintaining books and tax returns on different bases of accounting, a practice should consult a tax professional for guidance in this area.

The modified cash/income tax basis of accounting is usually less expensive and less cumbersome than the accrual method. Thus, financial statements can be generated in a timely and less costly manner. Physician–owners of a practice are often primarily interested in the entity's cash flows and the related distributions of income in the form of salaries, bonuses, and retirement plan contributions. Because modified cash or tax basis financial statements closely mirror these amounts, physician–owners usually understand these statements better than accrual basis statements.

The major drawback to the cash or income tax basis of accounting is that because it is based on cash flow rather than a true matching of revenues and expenses, the statements may not realistically reflect the practice's financial situation. For example, a practice that is experiencing cash flow difficulties may be behind in paying its vendors. Thus, the related expenses would not appear in the cash basis income statement, giving the impression that the practice's financial condition and performance are better than the actual scenario.

Management and other users need to be aware that in performing financial analysis and benchmarking, adjustments to cash basis financial statement data may be necessary in order for these techniques to be useful. Supplemental data regarding accounts receivable and accounts payable would be necessary to compute accounts receivable and liquidity ratios. Additional information regarding other financial statement amounts may be necessary. A modified cash/income tax basis practice can minimize these potential differences if the timing and amount of expenses paid and revenues received follow a consistent annual pattern.

In summary, the two major accounting methods used by medical practices are the accrual method and the cash method. The accrual method recognizes income and expenses when they are incurred. The cash method recognizes revenues and expenses when they are received or paid. Accountants usually prefer income tax basis financial statements for cash method practices, because their modifications to the pure cash basis of accounting are traditionally those prescribed by federal income tax laws, which are better defined than the modified cash basis of accounting.

■ Financial Statements

The basic GAAP financial statements are the balance sheet (or statement of financial position), the income statement (or statement of operations), the statement of changes in equity (net assets), and the statement of cash flows. The statement of changes in equity/net assets is often combined with the income statement. Except in the case of compiled financial statements that omit substantially all disclosures, a formal set of financial statements will also include Notes to Financial Statements, which contain certain disclosures required by GAAP or OCBOA. Annual financial statements are usually presented on a comparative basis, including the current year and the prior year.

The titles of OCBOA financial statements will vary from those listed in the previous paragraph, and assist the user in identifying the basis of accounting. For example, an income tax basis balance sheet may be called "Statement of Assets, Liabilities and Equity—Income Tax Basis." An income tax basis income statement might be called "Statement of Revenue and Expenses—Income Tax Basis."

OCBOA financial statements are not required to include a statement of cash flows.[5] Financial statements will usually combine the balances of related general ledger accounts into one line item. For example, a practice may have several accounts for cash, but only list the total amount of cash on the balance sheet. A practice may wish to consider using the *MGMA Chart of Accounts*, published by the Medical Group Management Association (MGMA). This chart of accounts, originally published in 1976, has been updated five times, with the most recent edition being published in 2011. This chart of accounts is considered to be the standard chart of accounts for medical practices, and is adaptable to the cost surveys published by the MGMA.

Included in this chapter are the financial statements of West Side Multispecialty Group, P.C. ("West Side"). West Side is a fictitious medical practice, and any resemblance to the financial information of any actual practice is purely coincidental. For illustrative purposes, both accrual basis and income tax basis statements are presented, as well as a worksheet detailing the adjustments necessary to convert from the accrual basis (GAAP) to the income tax basis (Table 10-6).

Balance Sheet

The balance sheet (or statement of financial position) gives a snapshot of the entity's financial position at a point in time. The basic equation for a balance sheet is:

$$\text{Assets} + \text{Liabilities} = \text{Equity}$$

This statement shows the entity's assets (what it owns), its liabilities (what it owes), and its equity or net assets (what it is worth). A balance sheet presents the accounts in order of their liquidity—the rate at which they convert to cash. Financial statements are prepared on a historical cost basis with certain adjustments in accordance with GAAP or OCBOA. Consequently, the balance sheet should not be used as a valuation tool to determine the market worth of the practice.

Both the accrual and income tax basis balance sheets of West Side Multispecialty Group, P.C., are shown in **Tables 10-2** and **10-3**.

Current Assets

Current assets are those the practice expects to convert to cash within 1 year.

Cash

Because cash is the most liquid asset, it is shown first on the balance sheet. If certain cash accounts are restricted to nonoperating uses that go beyond 1 year, consideration should be given to including these balances in the investments section.

Table 10-2 Balance Sheets as of December 31, 20X2 and 20X1

	20X2	20X1
Assets		
Current Assets:		
Cash	$1,250,000	$1,266,000
Marketable securities	234,000	190,000
Patient accounts receivable, net of allowance for doubtful		
accounts of $205,000 in 20X2 and $180,000 in 20X1	6,300,000	5,300,000
Accounts receivable–other	13,000	8,000
Deferred tax debits—current	6,000	-
Prepaid expenses	105,000	99,000
Total current assets	7,908,000	6,863,000
Investment:		
Land held for future clinic site	500,000	500,000
Property and equipment, at cost:		
Leasehold improvements	682,000	655,000
Equipment	7,881,000	7,631,000
	8,563,000	8,286,000
Less: Accumulated Depreciation	3,520,000	2,120,000
Property and equipment, net	5,043,000	6,166,000
Other Assets:		
Goodwill	600,000	600,000
Total Assets	$14,051,000	$14,129,000
Liabilities and Stockholders' Equity		
Current Liabilities:		
Notes payable	$335,000	$237,000
Current maturities of long-term debt	1,020,000	930,000
Accounts payable	250,000	300,000
Accrued payroll, benefits, and taxes	1,560,000	1,395,000
Claims payable	163,000	173,000
Claims payable—incurred but not received	82,000	75,000
Income taxes payable	159,000	21,000
Deferred taxes	-	5,000
Total current liabilities	3,569,000	3,136,000

(continues)

Table 10-2 Balance Sheets as of December 31, 20X2 and 20X1 (continued)		
	20X2	20X1
Long-Term Liabilities:		
Long-term debt, less current maturities	2,850,000	3,870,000
Deferred taxes	521,000	420,000
Total long-term liabilities	3,371,000	4,290,000
Total Liabilities	6,940,000	7,426,000
Stockholders' Equity:		
Common stock, $1 par, authorized 200,000 shares: issued and outstanding 100,000 shares	100,000	100,000
Contributed capital in excess of par	1,400,000	1,400,000
Retained earnings	5,611,000	5,203,000
Total stockholders' equity	7,111,000	6,703,000
Total Liabilities and Stockholders' Equity	$14,051,000	$14,129,000

Cash overdrafts are not an asset. They are a liability, and should be shown in the current liabilities section of the balance sheet.

Practice executives should ensure that their organizations establish effective internal control over cash. The AICPA has cautioned that large amounts of cash payments received for medical services can create an opportunity for embezzlement. Given a lack of sufficient internal control or management oversight, the potential misappropriation can be covered up through bad debt, contractual, or other write-offs.[10]

Marketable Securities and Short-Term Investments

This category includes items such as certificates of deposit and marketable debt and equity securities, such as government bonds and stocks listed on the New York Stock Exchange (NYSE), that are traded regularly and can be converted to cash. GAAP financial statements report these items at fair market value.[3] OCBOA financial statements prepared on the income tax basis report these amounts at cost.[11]

The marketable securities in West Side's GAAP financial statements are shown net of a $16,000 unrealized investment loss (see Table 10-6 later in this chapter.) Because income tax laws do not recognize investment gains or losses until they are realized, adjustment (A) was necessary to eliminate this loss in the income tax basis statements. This entry also records the $15,000

income tax basis gain realized in 20X2 that was previously recorded as an unrealized gain on the 20X1 GAAP financial statements.

Accounts Receivable

Accounts receivable represent the balances due from patients, Medicare, Medicaid, insurance companies, HMOs, and other third parties for services and sales to patients and other customers. Although physicians often anticipate receiving less than the full fee schedule rate for their services, the accounts receivable is usually recorded in the general ledger account at the full fee schedule rate. A separate allowance account is set up for the estimated difference between the fee schedule amount and the anticipated payment. GAAP financial statements report this accounts receivable amount net of the related allowances for anticipated contractual adjustments, bad debts, and other write-offs.[3]

West Side Multispecialty Group, P.C., has the following accounts receivable and related allowance accounts as of December 31, 20X2:

Accounts Receivable (Fee schedule amount of charges due)	$7,786,000
Allowance for Contractual Adjustments	(1,252,000)
Allowance for Charity Care	(29,000)
Allowance for Bad Debts	(205,000)
Net Amount	$6,300,000

Table 10-3	Statement of Assets, Liabilities, and Equity—Income Tax Basis As of December 31, 20X2	
		20X2
Assets		
Current Assets:		
Cash		$1,250,000
Marketable securities		250,000
Accounts receivable—other		13,000
Total current assets		1,513,000
Investment:		
Land held for future clinic site		500,000
Property and equipment, at cost:		
Leasehold improvements		682,000
Equipment		7,881,000
		8,563,000
Less: Accumulated Depreciation		5,294,000
Property and equipment, net		3,269,000
Other Assets:		
Goodwill		400,000
Total Assets		$5,682,000
Liabilities and Stockholders' Equity		
Current Liabilities:		
Notes payable		$335,000
Current maturities of long-term debt		1,020,000
Accrued payroll, benefits, and taxes		450,000
Income taxes payable		-
Total current liabilities		1,805,000
Long-Term Liabilities:		
Long-term debt, less current maturities		2,850,000
Deferred taxes		-
Total long-term liabilities		2,850,000
Total Liabilities		4,655,000
Stockholders' Equity:		
Common stock, $1 par, authorized 200,000 shares: issued and outstanding 100,000 shares		100,000
Contributed capital in excess of par		1,400,000
Retained earnings (deficit)		(473,000)
Total stockholders' equity		1,027,000
Total Liabilities and Stockholders' Equity		$5,682,000

The net amount of the accounts receivable ($6,300,000) is reported and the allowance for bad debts ($205,000) is disclosed on the balance sheet.

Because the modified cash/tax basis of accounting does not recognize revenue until it is collected, trade accounts receivable are not included in OCBOA financial statements prepared on these bases. "Trade" accounts receivable are those that arise in the normal course of an entity's trade or business, such as the provision of medical services or sales of related supplies in a medical practice. Accordingly, the user needs to perform any analysis of these accounts from other financial records, such as the medical practice management (revenue cycle) reports. Users will most likely want to see supplemental schedules to analyze accounts receivable for GAAP practices as well, because GAAP financial statements normally do not show sufficient detail to perform an analysis of the accounts receivable.

The accounts receivable balance is a factor of a practice's net charge volume and collection rate. Assuming a practice maintains a fairly consistent collection effort, a change in fee-for-service revenue would cause a similar percentage change in the accounts receivable balance. The accrual basis financial statements of West Side show accounts receivable of $6,300,000 at December 31, 20X2, as compared to $5,300,000 at December 31, 20X1—an increase of $1,000,000 or 18.86%. By contrast, net fee-for-service revenue increased only 7.27% from $55,000,000 to $59,000,000 for the corresponding years (see Table 10-4 later in this chapter). Thus, West Side's accounts receivable balance increased significantly more than indicated by the increase in fee revenue. The increased accounts receivable balance points to a slowdown in cash flow and requires immediate attention from management.

Accounts receivable can be subject to both misappropriation and material misstatement. As discussed in the "Cash" section, when sufficient internal controls are absent, an employee might embezzle cash receipts and hide this defalcation in the accounts receivable allowance accounts. As discussed in the "Revenues" section later in this chapter, the fact that the allowances for contractual adjustments, charity care, and bad debts are accounting estimates can put revenues and the related accounts receivable at risk for material misstatement. Because accounts receivable is usually one of the larger items on an accrual practice's balance sheet, a material misstatement in accounts receivable can cause the financial statements as a whole to be materially misstated. Practice executives need to take the necessary steps to ensure that the organization has sufficient internal controls over accounts receivable and properly computes the related allowance accounts.

Adjustment (B) eliminating accounts receivable is necessary for West Side to convert from GAAP to the income tax basis, because cash basis taxpayers do not recognize income until it is received. The beginning 20X2 balance of $5,300,000 is adjusted to retained earnings, because that difference was attributable to prior years. Only the current year change in accounts receivable affects the current year income. For West Side and many other practices, the change in accounting for accounts receivable creates the largest difference between accrual and income tax or cash basis financial statements.

Those receivables that do not result from the normal business operations of the organization, such as those due from employees or related parties, should be listed separately from the trade receivables discussed in this section. These amounts should be reported at net realizable value, and classified as current or long-term according to their terms or expected date of collection. Both GAAP and OCBOA financial statements may contain these types of accounts.

Inventories and Supplies on Hand

Supplies usually consist of medical and surgical supplies, pharmaceuticals, linens, uniforms, housekeeping, maintenance, and office supplies. In many cases, the amounts of these supplies on hand will not be significant, and the practice can expense them as they are acquired. Material amounts of supplies on hand should be shown in the current asset section of the balance sheet for both GAAP and tax basis financial statements.

In addition to providing services to patients, some practices sell merchandise to their patients or the general public. For example, an ophthalmologist may sell eyeglasses and contact lenses; a dermatologist may sell skin care products. For these practices, the unsold merchandise on hand would appear as inventory in the current asset section of the balance sheet. Both GAAP and income tax basis financial statements would include inventory on the balance sheet. GAAP requires the inventory be valued at the lower of cost or market. Tax basis financial statements would value inventory using the method the entity uses for tax purposes, which could be the lower of cost or market or some other permitted method. For income tax basis practices, the inclusion of inventory on the balance sheet is an example of a modification to the pure cash method of accounting.

Inventory is usually not a significant line item in physician practice financial statements, and many practices do not carry inventory. Like other businesses with inventory, practices that do maintain inventory should pay considerable attention to internal control over inventory. Items that are small, easy to steal, and have value either for an employee's personal use or for resale are susceptible to theft. Practices that carry a significant amount of drug or medical supply inventory, such as oncology or pediatric practices, should consider using a computerized inventory system to allow for better management of these assets. The AICPA has cautioned that, in the healthcare industry, a pharmaceutical inventory with a high street value or that is in high demand has an increased risk of misappropriation.[10]

Prepaid Expenses

One of the principles of accrual accounting is the matching principle. Expenses must be properly matched with the revenues used to earn such revenue. Some expenses, such as rent, taxes, and insurance, may actually be paid before they are incurred. Just as expenses incurred but not paid are set up as a liability, expenses paid but not yet incurred are shown as an asset on the balance sheet, rather than as an expense on the income statement. Amounts that will be expensed within 1 year are classified as current assets. Those that will be realized in future periods beyond 1 year are classified as other assets.

The cash basis of accounting recognizes expenses when they are paid. This is generally true for entities on the cash method for income tax reporting, except that taxpayers may not take deductions for expenses that will be incurred beyond the end of the following tax year. Cash or income tax basis practices may have prepaid income taxes if they overpaid their estimated income taxes. In addition, cash basis taxpayers may not deduct prepaid interest.[11] Therefore, except for interest and taxes, cash basis taxpayers on the income tax basis of accounting would ordinarily not have significant prepaid expenses.

To convert West Side from GAAP to the income tax basis, adjustment (C) is necessary to eliminate prepaid expenses. Only the $6,000 current year increase affects current year income tax basis earnings. The beginning balance is adjusted through retained earnings because it occurred in prior years.

Other

This category includes current assets not included in any other category. Examples include, but are not limited to, short-term deposits and deferred charges, such as deferred taxes. Deferred taxes result from the difference between income taxes computed on taxable income and those computed on GAAP income. Deferred taxes may be debits (assets) or credits (liabilities) and may be either current or long-term.

Investments

This long-term asset classification is used to report investments other than the marketable securities and short-term investments included in the current assets section of the balance sheet. Unlike marketable securities and short-term investments, investments reported in this category are generally not available to finance current operations.

Debt securities that the practice intends to hold to maturity would be included in this category. It is important to note that the same bonds could be classified as either current or long-term, depending on the intent of management. If management intends to use the bonds as a source of funds for current operations, then the bonds are classified as current assets and valued accordingly. If management intends to keep the bonds for a longer period of time and use them for some other purpose, such as retiring debt or purchasing a building, they would be included in this long-term category.[3]

Equity securities that do not have a ready market are included here, as well as investments in affiliates, partnerships, and certain oil and gas interests. An investment in land or other assets not currently used in the practice's operations would also be included in this section. For example, West Side's investments include land held for a future clinic site.

For-profit entities generally report these long-term investment amounts at cost, whether they use GAAP or OCBOA. GAAP financial statements present debt securities at amortized cost; that is, the investment is initially recorded at cost, and a ratable portion of any discount or premium is recognized as an increase or decrease in expense each year. Not-for-profit and governmental entities report all debt and equity investments with readily determined values at fair value.[3]

Long-Term Receivables

This category is used to report receivables that are due in 1 year or more. Generally, these receivables do not result from operations. An example would be a loan to a physician or affiliate with a maturity greater than 1 year. All such receivables should be reviewed for impairment and reported at net realizable value.

Property and Equipment

Tangible assets the practice uses in its operations that have a useful life of greater than 1 year are included in this category. Examples are land, land improvements, buildings, building improvements, leasehold improvements, equipment, furniture, and construction in progress. The allowance for depreciation on fixed assets other than land is also included in this presentation. Both GAAP and OCBOA income tax basis financial statements will include these items, but valuation of the assets and the related depreciation accounts may vary due to differences between GAAP and federal income tax regulations.

GAAP requirements for capitalizing leased property are generally stricter than federal income tax regulations. Consequently, in some instances, leased property may be treated as a capital lease for GAAP purposes, but qualify as an operating lease for tax purposes. In this case, GAAP financial statements would show this property on the balance sheet as an asset and depreciate it. OCBOA income tax basis financial statements would not include this asset on the balance sheet—instead the lease payments would appear as an expense on the income statement.

GAAP requires that assets contributed by an owner be reported at fair market value. Tax regulations allow the entity to value this property at the donor's adjusted tax basis. Consequently, if a physician owner contributes property to the practice, GAAP and OCBOA valuations may differ.[3]

Fixed assets have a useful life of more than 1 year, but (except for land) are expected to have a finite life. Thus, depreciation spreads the cost of these assets over their expected useful lives. Different methods of depreciation result in differing net asset and expense values. The straight-line method recognizes an even amount of expense each year of the asset's life. Accelerated methods recognize higher amounts in the early years of an asset's life and smaller amounts in the later years. The units-of-production method expenses an amount proportionate to the amount an asset is actually used during the year.

Tax depreciation rules vary from those prescribed by GAAP. The most common difference is due to the accelerated depreciation allowed on tangible personal property by federal tax regulations, whereas GAAP depreciation is usually computed on either a straight-line or less aggressive accelerated method. Recent tax legislation has increased the allowable accelerated depreciation, further increasing this difference. These accelerated depreciation methods result in significantly higher first-year depreciation for tax purposes than that computed according to GAAP. This process would reverse in the later years of asset life, with GAAP providing the higher depreciation expense in those years. GAAP depreciation generally provides for more even depreciation over the asset's life than tax depreciation. This difference also results in a higher net asset value for GAAP financial statements in the early years of an asset's life.

For West Side, current year tax depreciation exceeds GAAP depreciation by $574,000, and adjustment (D) reduces income tax basis earnings by this amount. Prior years' cumulative differences are $1,200,000, which is taken to retained earnings. The entire difference increases accumulated depreciation on the balance sheet.

Other Assets

This section includes noncurrent assets that do not fit into any of the other categories. Intangible assets are generally included in this section. These include, but are not limited to, goodwill, franchises, copyrights, patents, trademarks, and trade names. Because the IRC allows most intangible assets acquired after August 10, 1993, to be amortized over a 15-year period, income tax basis financial statements include the related amortization expense, and intangible assets are reported net of accumulated amortization.[3]

GAAP treatment of an intangible asset varies depending on whether its life is finite or infinite. GAAP prohibits amortization of goodwill and other intangibles with an indefinite useful life, and instead requires that they be tested for impairment at least annually. Other assets are amortized on the straight-line method over their useful lives.[3]

Income tax basis financial statements include organization and business start-up costs net of any related amortization in this section. Tax regulations require that these costs be capitalized. Taxpayers may elect to amortize these costs over a period of not less than 60 months using the straight-line method. GAAP generally requires these costs be expensed as incurred. Consequently, GAAP financial statements do not include organization or start-up costs as assets.[3]

West Side has $600,000 goodwill as the result of acquiring another practice 5 years ago. For GAAP purposes, this amount has not been amortized. For income tax purposes, it is being amortized over a 15-year period, at a rate of $40,000 per year. Adjustment (E) records the current year amortization of $40,000 and the prior years' effect of $160,000 to retained earnings.

Examples of other amounts included in this section would be noncurrent deposits and deferred charges, such as those for deferred taxes.

Current Liabilities

Current liabilities are those obligations the entity has incurred and is obligated to pay within 1 year.

Accounts Payable

Accounts payable include trade obligations that have been incurred and are payable within 1 year. Trade obligations are those amounts due to vendors that are incurred in the entity's normal course of business. Examples of such expenses for a medical practice include, but are not limited to, laundry and linens, medical supplies, pharmaceuticals, office supplies, and bills for professional services. GAAP balance sheets include accounts payable. Because cash basis taxpayers do not recognize these expenses until they are paid, these entities generally do not include accounts payable in their financial statements.

West Side has accounts payable of $250,000 for administrative supplies and services, medical supplies, and drugs. Because cash basis taxpayers do not recognize expenses until they are paid, it is necessary to eliminate this liability (adjustment F) in converting to tax basis financial statements. The beginning balance of $300,000 increases retained earnings, and the net difference of $50,000 decreases current year expense and, therefore, increases current year net income.

Claims Payable

Amounts payable to other providers under capitation agreements would be included in this section for GAAP financial statements. Because cash basis taxpayers cannot deduct these items until they are paid, most practices heavily involved in these types of arrangements file tax returns on the accrual basis and use GAAP for financial reporting.

Claims Payable Incurred but Not Reported (IBNR)

Practices that reimburse other providers under capitation arrangements incur the liability to the other provider when the service is performed. Because of the normal time lag between the provision of services and the filing of a claim, an estimated amount is accrued for these services.[12] When applicable, this amount appears on GAAP financial statements but not on income tax basis OCBOA statements for cash basis taxpayers. As explained under "Claims Payable," most practices with significant involvement in these types of arrangements are on the accrual basis.

Cash basis taxpayers cannot deduct the amounts accrued as claims payable and claims payable IBNR until they are paid. Thus, adjustment (H) is necessary to eliminate West Side's GAAP basis accrual, taking the current year change to the income statement, and the beginning balance to retained earnings.

Notes and Loans Payable

Any short-term notes or loans should be included in the current liabilities section of the balance sheet.

Current Maturities of Long-Term Debt

The portion of long-term debt that is due within 1 year also appears as a current liability.

Payroll and Pension Liabilities

For most practices, payroll is a significant expense. The practice also has certain liabilities related to payroll, such as salaries earned but not paid and the related payroll taxes and benefits. An accrual basis statement shows these liabilities as well as those for vacation pay, sick pay, and other compensated absences that have been earned but not taken. In addition, any postretirement benefits for which the organization is obligated, such as health insurance, should be included as a liability on the balance sheet, and properly classified as to current or long term.[3]

Cash basis taxpayers utilizing the income tax basis of reporting generally include payroll taxes and other amounts withheld from the employees (such as insurance premiums) in this section. Other accrued items such as salaries and wages, sick pay, vacation pay, postretirement benefits, and the employer portion of insurance premiums are expensed as paid and, thus, not included on the balance sheet.

The balance due to employee retirement plans is generally accrued as a current liability in financial statements of both GAAP and income tax basis OCBOA financial statements. Federal tax laws allow both cash and accrual basis taxpayers to accrue contributions to qualified plans so long as they are paid by the due date (including extensions) of the applicable tax return. The ability to accrue these qualified retirement plan contributions is a beneficial cash management tool for corporate cash basis practices, which typically pay out a large percentage of their potential profits in order to legally avoid corporate income taxes.

West Side's GAAP balance sheet shows accrued payroll, benefits, and taxes of $1,560,000. Of this amount, $450,000 represents payroll withholdings and accrued retirement plan contributions, which are deductible for cash basis taxpayers. The difference of $1,110,000 cannot be deducted for a cash basis taxpayer until paid. Adjustment (G) reduces current year expense by the current year increase of $165,000 and reduces retained earnings by the $945,000 for beginning of the year difference.

Deferred Revenue

Sometimes practices collect fees from patients before their physicians perform the related services. For example, an obstetrician may collect a global fee for pregnancy care including delivery of the baby prior to the delivery. Modified cash/income tax basis practices report these fees as income when they are received. Because accrual basis accounting recognizes income when it is earned, amounts of these prepayments not yet earned would be shown as deferred revenue.

Other

For GAAP financial statements, other obligations that have been incurred but not paid, but that will be paid or otherwise settled within 1 year, should be shown in the current liabilities section. Accrued expenses other than those mentioned previously should also be accrued. These include accrued taxes, rent, insurance, or any other expense that has been incurred but not reported. Also included in current liabilities is the amount of any current deferred income tax credits. Cash basis taxpayers generally do not include any of these amounts on OCBOA tax basis statements.

Long-Term Liabilities

Both GAAP and OCBOA financial statements should present long-term debt, net of current maturities, as a long-term liability in the balance sheet. Long-term debt includes, but is not limited to, notes, mortgages, and capital lease obligations with maturities of greater than 1 year.

A GAAP basis practice should accrue any other expenses that it has incurred but are not due for more than a year and present them as long-term liabilities in the balance sheet. Long-term deferred tax credits would also be included in this section.

Adjustment (I) eliminates both the current tax accrual and the deferred tax debits and credits that appear on West Side's GAAP financial statements. In the cash basis version of its financial statements, West Side has a net tax loss and a cumulative net deficit, so no taxes are due. On the GAAP basis, this practice had net income that resulted in both current and deferred income taxes. Although practices reporting GAAP basis financial statements most likely file their tax returns on the accrual basis, they can still have a significant difference between taxes computed on GAAP income and accrual basis taxable income. The deferred taxes in this example are the result of the timing differences arising primarily from the use of accelerated depreciation methods and recognition of investment gains and losses.

Equity

The final section of the balance sheet is the equity section. This section shows the net worth of the practice after deducting the liabilities from the assets. The format and captions in this section will vary somewhat depending on the type of legal entity—C corporation, S corporation, limited liability company (LLC), partnership, sole proprietorship, or not-for-profit.

The presentation is similar whether the statements are prepared using GAAP or an OCBOA. The amounts can be substantially different, as is the case with West Side. In 20X2, West Side shows total GAAP retained earnings of $5,611,000 as compared with a deficit of $473,000 on the income tax basis—a difference of $6,084,000.

Contributed Capital

Contributed capital represents the amount contributed to the entity by the owners. For both C and S corporations, the contributed capital accounts include the different classes of stock at their par or stated value. The statements should disclose the number of shares authorized, issued, and outstanding. The statement lists the different classes of stock in their order of preference upon liquidation. For example, preferred stock comes before common stock. After listing the various classes of stock, a corporation shows the amount of contributed capital in excess of par or stated value.

Sole proprietorships, partnerships, and limited liability entities show as contributed capital the amounts invested and profits retained in the business by the owner(s). Although only the total amount of capital normally appears on the financial statement, partnerships and limited liability entities need to keep separate subaccounts for each owner.

Distributions and Retained Earnings

At the end of the year, the entity's income, along with the various distributions to the owners, is usually closed to retained earnings (for corporations) or the appropriate capital account for noncorporate entities. The various components that make up the changes to the accumulated earnings are detailed in the Statement of Changes to Retained Earnings (or Net Assets, Members' Capital, etc.). Frequently, this statement is combined with the income statement.

Both C and S corporations accumulate the dividends and distributions paid to the shareholders throughout the year in one or more "dividends paid" or "distributions paid" account and close these accounts to retained earnings at the end of the year. The annual net profit or loss is also closed to retained earnings at the end of the year. The amount reported on the balance sheet as retained earnings at the end of the year is usually the net total of these amounts. Appropriated and unappropriated retained earnings should be stated separately.

Sole proprietorships, partnerships, and LLCs accumulate the various owner, partner, or member draws throughout the year and close these accounts to the capital account at the end of the year. Net income or loss is also closed to the capital account at this time.

A not-for-profit entity closes its current surplus or deficit for the year to its net assets account. The practice should maintain separate net assets accounts for unrestricted net assets, temporarily restricted net assets, and permanently restricted net assets. These amounts should also be listed separately on the financial statements.

Income Statement

The income statement shows the results of operations (income, expenses, and net profit or loss) for a period of time. The year (12 months) is the standard period for measuring the results of operations, and the related financial statements are the annual financial statements. On occasion, an entity may have a reporting period of less than a year. This could happen for the first or last year of operations, due to a change in ownership or form of entity, or due to a change in reporting year (such as a change from a fiscal year to a calendar year). Statements for periods less than a year (other than those for a short year as described earlier) are referred to as interim statements.

The basic equation for the income statement is:

$$\text{Revenues} - \text{Expenses} = \text{Net Income or Loss}$$

The relationship between the income statement and balance sheet is that the net income or loss from the income statement is added to the equity section of the balance sheet. This is necessary in order for the balance sheet to "balance"; that is, assets do not equal liabilities plus equity, unless current earnings are added to equity.

The income statement shows operating revenues and expenses separately from nonoperating revenues and expenses. In addition, this statement shows net income from operations as well as overall net income.

The income statements in this chapter use groupings from the *MGMA Chart of Accounts*. These groupings allow for separate subtotals for support staff costs, nonphysician provider (NPP) costs, and physician costs. Having these subtotals makes it easier for the practice to evaluate these costs and compare them against industry benchmarks. This format also provides subtotals for "Total medical revenue after operating cost" and "Total medical revenue after operating cost and NPP cost." These are profitability indicators commonly used for medical practices and help allow for comparisons against industry benchmarks. Finally, this format allows for better profitability and expense comparisons among different types of entities, because physician costs are reported similarly for corporate and noncorporate entities.

The GAAP and income tax basis income statements of West Side Multispecialty Group, P.C., are shown in **Tables 10-4** and **10-5**.

Revenues

This section shows the net operating revenues for the practice. The three typical categories of revenue for a medical practice are fee-for-service revenue, capitation revenue, and other medical revenues, such as sales of medical supplies, grant revenue, expert witness fees, and medical director fees. If it is significant, the income statement should report net capitation revenue separately from other net patient service revenue.[3]

Table 10-4 **Statements of Income and Retained Earnings for the Years Ended December 31, 20X2 and 20X1**

	20X2	20X1
Revenues:		
Fee-for-service revenue (net of contractual allowances and discounts)	$59,000,000	$55,000,000
Less: Provision for bad debts	(770,000)	(690,000)
Net fee-for-service revenue less provision for bad debts	58,230,000	54,310,000
Capitation revenue	5,100,000	5,500,000
Other	1,900,000	1,200,000
Total medical revenue	65,230,000	61,010,000
Operating Cost:		
Support Staff Cost:		
Staff salaries	15,250,000	14,500,000
Payroll taxes	1,315,000	1,250,000
Employee benefits	2,985,000	2,750,000
Total support staff cost	19,550,000	18,500,000
General Operating Cost:		
Information technology	950,000	890,000
Malpractice insurance	1,000,000	1,200,000
Drug supply	2,800,000	3,000,000
Medical and surgical supply	880,000	950,000
Depreciation	1,400,000	1,100,000
Building and occupancy	3,500,000	3,500,000
Administrative supplies and services	810,000	990,000
Professional and consulting fees	360,000	332,000
Clinical laboratory	1,400,000	900,000
Radiology and imaging	600,000	560,000
Promotion and marketing	230,000	226,000
Other general and administrative	1,500,000	1,900,000
Total general operating cost	15,430,000	15,548,000
Total operating cost	34,980,000	34,048,000
Total Medical Revenue After Operating Cost	30,250,000	26,962,000
Less: NPP cost	2,750,000	2,450,000
Total Medical Revenue After Operating and NPP Cost	27,500,000	24,512,000
Less: Physician cost	26,500,000	24,200,000
Net Income (Loss) After Provider-Related Expenses	1,000,000	312,000
Other Income (Expense):		
Interest expense (net)	(341,000)	(257,000)
Income from long-term investments	20,000	30,000
Unrealized gains and (losses) on investments	(16,000)	15,000
Gain on disposal of equipment	-	500,000
Other Income (Expense), Net	(337,000)	288,000

(continues)

Table 10-4 Statements of Income and Retained Earnings for the Years Ended December 31, 20X2 and 20X1 (continued)	20X2	20X1
Income Before Provision for Income Taxes	663,000	600,000
Provision for (reduction of) Income Taxes	255,000	240,000
Net Income (Loss)	408,000	360,000
Retained Earnings, Beginning of Year	5,203,000	4,843,000
Retained Earnings, End of Year	$5,611,000	$5,203,000

An accrual basis practice reports the net revenues actually earned during the year, regardless of when they are collected. Fee-for-service income is generally considered earned when the services are provided to the patient. Capitation income is generally considered earned when coverage is provided to an enrollee.[3] The practice should accrue any revenue that has been earned but not billed as of the financial statement date.

Charity care is the provision of healthcare services to patients with a demonstrated inability to pay. Bad debts are charges the practice theoretically should be able to collect, but does not for various reasons such as inaccurate demographic data, billing errors, or patient failure to pay. The practice should differentiate charity care from bad debt expense in accordance with its internal criteria; this requires judgment. The level of charity care and management's policies regarding charity care should be disclosed in the financial statements. This disclosure is usually made in the notes to financial statements.[3]

In the past, the amount of net fee-for-service revenue reported for all accrual basis nongovernmental practices consisted of gross charges less contractual write-offs and charity care. The provision for bad debts was included in operating expenses, rather than being subtracted from net fee-for-service revenue. During July 2011, the FASB issued Accounting Standards Update 2011-07 (ASU 2011-07). This standard requires healthcare entities that recognize significant amounts of patient service revenues at the time of service without assessing the patients' ability to pay to record the provision for bad debts as a contra revenue account, rather than as an operating expense (as is the case for most accrual basis businesses).[13] The accrual basis statements for West Side are presented using the new format; that is, with the provision for bad debts subtracted from fee-for-service revenue. Accrual basis nongovernmental health care entities that do assess patient ability to pay in connection with recording patient service revenue should continue to classify the provision for bad debts related to patient service revenue as an operating expense. GASB Statement No. 4 requires governmental healthcare entities to report fee-for-service revenues net of the provision for bad debts.[3]

Practice executives whose financial statements are on the accrual basis need to ensure that the amount of net revenue recognized in their financial statements is a reasonably accurate representation of the amount the practice will ultimately collect. For accrual basis practices, these amounts are especially subject to misstatement because they involve accounting estimates. As a result of Statement on Auditing Standards (SAS) No. 99's requirement that auditors presume revenue recognition is a fraud risk, auditors scrutinize these amounts more carefully with the increased professional skepticism this standard also requires. The AICPA's *Audit Risk Alerts: Health Care Industry Developments 2003–04* indicates a potential risk of material misstatement when bonuses or incentive compensation are tied to operating results,[10] as is often the case in medical practices. The AICPA's *2010/11 Audit Risk Alert: Health Care Industry Developments* also warns auditors about accounting estimates, citing the current economic climate as warranting additional skepticism.[10] Even practices that do not have audits need to devote sufficient resources to ensure that their financial statements are properly accrued revenues. Several individuals and groups that have studied fraudulent reporting schemes concluded that the vast majority involved improper recognition of revenues. Even when fraud is not a factor, bad estimates can create revenue amounts and financial statements that are materially misstated. This computation should not be done just on historical data, but requires analysis of changes in the practice's fee schedule, payer mix, coding patterns, payer reimbursement policies, charity care, and other relevant factors. Failure to adequately compute these amounts may impact more

Table 10-5 **Statement of Revenue, Expenses, and Retained Earnings—Income Tax Basis for the Years Ended December 31, 20X2**

	20X2
Revenues:	
Net fee-for-service revenue	$57,230,000
Capitation revenue	5,095,000
Other	1,900,000
Total medical revenue	64,225,000
Operating Cost:	
Support Staff Cost:	
Staff salaries	15,250,000
Payroll taxes	1,315,000
Employee benefits	2,985,000
Total support staff cost	19,550,000
General Operating Cost:	
Information technology	950,000
Malpractice insurance	1,000,000
Drug supply	2,825,000
Medical and surgical supply	890,000
Provision for bad debts	-
Depreciation	1,974,000
Amortization	40,000
Building and occupancy	3,500,000
Administrative supplies and services	825,000
Professional and consulting fees	360,000
Clinical laboratory	1,400,000
Radiology and imaging	600,000
Promotion and marketing	230,000
Other general and administrative	1,506,000
Total general operating cost	16,100,000
Total operating cost	35,650,000
Total Medical Revenue After Operating Cost	28,575,000
Less: NPP cost	2,750,000
Total Medical Revenue After Operating and NPP Cost	25,825,000
Less: Physician cost	26,335,000
Net Income (Loss) After Provider-Related Expenses	(510,000)
Other Income (Expense):	
Interest expense (net)	(341,000)
Income from long-term investments	35,000
Unrealized gains and (losses) on investments	-

(continues)

Table 10-5	Statement of Revenue, Expenses, and Retained Earnings—Income Tax Basis for the Years Ended December 31, 20X2 (continued)	
		20X2
Gain on disposal of equipment		-
Other income (expense) net		(306,000)
Income Before Provision for Income Taxes		(816,000)
Provision for (reduction of) Income Taxes		-
Net Income (Loss)		(816,000)
Retained Earnings, Beginning of Year		343,000
Retained Earnings (Deficit), End of Year		$(473,000)

than the financial statements. For example, if a practice computes physician bonuses on the accrual basis using overstated revenue amounts, it could encounter a cash shortage when lower amounts are actually collected.

A cash basis taxpayer reporting on the tax basis shows only the revenues that were actually collected during the year, regardless of when they were earned. Fee-for-service income, capitation income, and other sources of revenue are reported when the cash is actually or constructively collected. Because contractual adjustments, charity care, and bad debts are never collected, a cash basis practice reports revenue net of all these amounts and does not need to make the related accounting estimates that an accrual basis practice makes.

Capitation revenue is reported net of any amounts paid or payable to other providers under subcapitation agreements. Adjustment (H) is necessary to record the effective of the current year accruals for claims payable and claims payable incurred but not received.

In summary, medical practices include fee-for-service, capitation revenue, and other medical revenue in the revenue portion of their income statement. Both accrual and cash basis practices report fee-for-service revenues net of contractual adjustments and charity care. All cash basis practices and accrual basis governmental practices will also report these revenues net of the provision for bad debts. Depending upon when they assess patient ability to pay, accrual basis nongovernmental practices will either subtract the provision for bad debts from the fee-for-service revenues or include this cost in operating expenses. For a cash basis practice, revenue amounts reflect actual cash receipts. For an accrual basis practice, these amounts are based on accounting estimates. Because misstatement of net revenues could result in misleading financial statements, an accrual basis practice should invest the resources necessary to make a reasonably accurate estimate of these amounts.

Operating Expenses

This section reports the expenses incurred by the organization in earning medical revenue. Within this category, the entity may classify and subclassify these expenses in a natural or functional matter.[3] Thus, the practice has some discretion in the manner in which it reports operating expenses on its financial statements.

Income statement reporting for GAAP and OCBOA tax basis practices is similar. The amounts vary due to differences in the timing and method of cost recognition. As discussed under "Revenues," GAAP financial statements currently include bad debt expense as an operating expense, whereas OCBOA income tax basis financial statements of cash basis taxpayers will not include this item.

The income statement discloses the total operating expenses and the net income or loss from operations.

Salary and Fringe Benefits

This section includes all payroll and related expenses for employees other than physicians and mid-level providers. Employees in this category include, but are not limited to, nurses, transcribers, receptionists, administrative employees, and employees providing ancillary services. Expenses for employees in this category include salaries, payroll taxes, retirement plan contributions, health and other employee insurance, professional development expenses, telephones, beepers, licenses, vehicles, and travel.

General Operating Cost

This category includes services and general expenses other than purchased services and/or payroll and related benefit costs. Office and administrative expenses are included in this category. Examples include equipment rental, telephones, postage, security, office supplies, business insurance, malpractice insurance, billing expenses, forms, business licenses, depreciation on tangible personal property, and professional services. As previously discussed, some accrual basis nongovernmental practices will include their provision for bad debts in this section rather than subtracting it from fee-for-service revenue in the revenue section of the income statement. Clinical expenses included in this category include costs of drugs and medications, medical supplies, laundry and linen, maintenance and depreciation of clinical equipment, biohazardous waste removal, medical records expenses, and the clinical portion of telephone and postage expenses. This section would also include occupancy costs such as rent, utilities, property taxes, depreciation of building, and leasehold improvements.[12]

Total Medical Revenue After Operating Cost

This subtotal reflects the practice's profit after subtracting all support staff and general operating cost, but before paying physicians and nonphysician providers. This is a measure of the practice's profitability for its operations before paying its providers.

Nonphysician Provider Cost

This section includes all costs associated with nonphysician providers, such as salaries, payroll taxes, retirement plan contributions, health insurance costs, continuing education, and other benefit costs. These costs are shown in the aggregate in West Side's income statement, but might also be listed separately, as is shown for the support staff above.

Total Medical Revenue After Operating and NPP Cost

This subtotal reflects the practice's profit after subtracting all support staff, general operating cost, and nonphysician provider cost, but before paying the physicians. This is a measure of the practice's profitability from its operations before paying its physicians.

Physician Cost

Costs related to all physicians, whether owners or employees, are included in this section. The practice should maintain subaccounts in its general ledger to keep a separate accounting of the costs and distributions to owner and nonowner physicians.

Net Income After Provider-Related Expenses

This subtotal measures the practice's income after paying its providers but before consideration of nonoperating income and expense.

Other Income and Expense

This category is used to report revenues and expenses that are not related to the practice's operations. Interest income, dividend income, gain or loss on investments, and other investment income and losses are included in this category. Interest expense and charitable contributions are also reported here.

Income Before Provision for Income Taxes

This section shows the practice's income before income taxes.

Income Taxes

The financial statements of for-profit entities include line items for income before the provision for income taxes, provision for income taxes, and then net income.

GAAP financial statements include the provision for income taxes as computed on GAAP income. As discussed earlier, this amount probably differs from the actual amount of income taxes computed on the organization's income tax returns. Those cumulative differences appear on the balance sheet as deferred tax debits and credits and are shown as assets or liabilities on the balance sheet, and further classified as to current or long term.

Cash basis practices record the provision for income taxes in the period in which the income taxes are paid.

Net Income

The final item on the income statement is net income.

For West Side, the difference between GAAP and income tax basis net income is significant. West Side reports net income of $408,000 on the GAAP financial statements, while reporting an $816,000 net loss on the income tax basis financial statements—a material difference of $1,224,000. The contrasting net income amounts represent the same practice with the same assets, liabilities, and operations—the difference is the basis of accounting. **Table 10-6** shows the worksheet that details the adjustments necessary to convert West Side's GAAP financial statements to the income tax basis for 20X2.

For West Side Multispecialty Group, P.C., the most significant difference between its GAAP and income tax basis net income was the accrual of accounts receivable (Adjustment B) which resulted in the recognition of $1,000,000 additional net income in 20X2 on the accrual basis that was deferred to future years for the income tax (cash) basis. This deferral of revenue recognition from accounts receivable is the primary reason many physician-owned practices use the cash basis for income tax purposes and, thus, have income tax basis financial statements. For a practice whose annual charges and related accounts receivable balance are continuously increasing, use of the cash basis results in significant income tax savings. The effect of this tax savings is even larger when one considers that over the cash basis entity's history the entire net accounts receivable balance ($6,300,000 for West Side) has not been subject to income taxes, whereas an accrual basis entity would have paid taxes on this amount. Even when a practice has a year in which a decrease in its

Table 10-6 Accrual to Cash Conversion 20X2

	Accrual		Dr		Cr	Cash
Cash	1,250,000					1,250,000
Marketable securities	234,000	(A)	16,000			250,000
Accounts receivable (patients)	6,300,000			(B)	6,300,000	0
Accounts receivable (other)	13,000					13,000
Deferred tax debits - current	6,000			(I)	6,000	0
Prepaid expenses	105,000			©	105,000	0
Land held for future clinic site	500,000					500,000
Leasehold improvements	682,000					682,000
Equipment	7,881,000					7,881,000
Accumulated depreciation	(3,520,000)			(D)	1,774,000	(5,294,000)
Goodwill	600,000			(E)	200,000	400,000
Note payable	(335,000)					(335,000)
Current maturities of long-term debt	(1,020,000)					(1,020,000)
Accounts payable	(250,000)	(F)	250,000			0
Accrued payroll, benefits, and taxes	(1,560,000)	(G)	1,110,000			(450,000)
Claims payable	(163,000)	(H)	163,000			0
Claims payable IBNR	(82,000)	(H)	82,000			0
Income taxes payable	(159,000)	(I)	159,000			0
Deferred taxes - current	0					0
Long-term debt, less current maturities	(2,850,000)					(2,850,000)
Deferred taxes - long term	(521,000)	(I)	521,000			0
Common stock	(100,000)					(100,000)
Contributed capital	(1,400,000)					(1,400,000)
Retained earnings	(5,203,000)	(B)	5,300,000	(B)		(343,000)
		(A)	15,000			
		(D)	1,200,000	(F)	300,000	
		(E)	160,000	(G)	945,000	
		©	99,000	(H)	250,000	
				(I)	419,000	
Net fee-for-service revenue less provision for bad debts	(58,230,000)	(B)	6,300,000	(B)	5,300,000	(57,230,000)
Net capitation revenue	(5,100,000)	(H)	250,000	(H)	245,000	(5,095,000)
Other revenue	(1,900,000)					(1,900,000)
Support staff salaries	15,250,000					15,250,000
Payroll taxes	1,315,000					1,315,000
Employee benefits	2,985,000					2,985,000
Information technology	950,000					950,000
Drug supply	2,800,000	(F)	245,000	(F)	220,000	2,825,000
Medical and surgical supply	880,000	(F)	30,000	(F)	20,000	890,000
Malpractice insurance	1,000,000					1,000,000
Depreciation	1,400,000	(D)	574,000			1,974,000
Amortization		(E)	40,000			40,000
Building and occupancy	3,500,000					3,500,000

Table 10-6 Accrual to Cash Conversion 20X2 (continued)

	Accrual		Dr		Cr	Cash
Administrative supplies and services	810,000	(F)	25,000	(F)	10,000	825,000
Legal and other professional	360,000					360,000
Promotion and marketing	230,000					230,000
Clinical laboratory	1,400,000					1,400,000
Radiology and imaging	600,000					600,000
Other general and administrative	1,500,000	©	105,000	©	99,000	1,506,000
Nonphysician providers	2,750,000					2,750,000
Physician salaries and benefits	26,500,000			(G)	165,000	26,335,000
Interest expense	341,000					341,000
Investment income	(20,000)			(A)	15,000	(35,000)
Unrealized gains and losses on investments	16,000			(A)	16,000	0
Gain on disposal of equipment						0
Provision for income taxes	255,000			(I)	255,000	0
Net Income (Loss)	0					
			16,644,000		16,644,000	0

accounts receivable yields a higher cash basis net income, the cumulative deferral of taxes on accounts receivable remains a powerful reason to continue to file income taxes on the cash basis.

The next largest difference between the two bases of accounting is the larger depreciation balance (Adjustment D) claimed on the income tax basis statement. This difference was the result of the more aggressive early depreciation and write-off of fixed assets allowed for tax purposes. In the later years of an asset's life, the difference reverses with GAAP depreciation being higher than the tax basis depreciation. Accelerated depreciation methods are generally not an incentive for practices to choose the cash method over the accrual method, because accrual basis taxpayers may also use accelerated depreciation for income tax purposes. The difference between GAAP and tax depreciation results in a timing difference in expense recognition, with deferred taxes being accrued on the difference. These current year deferred taxes of $90,000 are part of the total income tax expense of $255,000 (Adjustment I) that makes up the next largest difference between the GAAP and tax basis net income.

Differences between the amount of expenses incurred and paid represent another difference between the methods of accounting (Adjustments C, F, G, H). When the amount of accounts payable and accrued expenses increase, an accrual basis taxpayer can deduct these amounts whereas a cash basis practice cannot. As in the case with accounts receivable, the cumulative amount of deductions for expenses incurred but not paid is often significant. Because the amount of payables is usually less than the amount of receivables, this additional deduction for accrual practices does not usually persuade practices eligible for cash basis tax reporting to adopt the accrual method.

Other differences between West Side's GAAP and tax basis net income result from amortization of goodwill and differences in recognizing investment income. The amortization of goodwill (Adjustment E) is a permanent difference, because GAAP does not recognize this expense. A GAAP expenditure for impairment could be booked should the goodwill become worthless or lose value. The differences in investment income (Adjustment A) are timing differences and will even out over the life of the investments.

In summary, net income reported for the same practice with the same operations can vary significantly depending on whether the practice uses the GAAP or income tax–modified tax basis of accounting. The practice's income tax liability can also vary significantly depending on the basis used for tax purposes. A practice executive needs to be aware of these differences when performing financial analysis or tax planning.

Analytical Procedures Applied to Income Statement Data

As previously discussed in this chapter, accounting and auditing standards require that independent accountants perform analytical procedures when performing an audit or review of financial statements. Analytical procedures are a powerful tool for understanding and evaluating financial statements. Auditors identify a greater number of material audit adjustments by performing analytical procedures than by doing any other type of procedure. Some experts contend that auditors would have detected some of the more notorious financial reporting scandals sooner had they properly used some simple analytical procedures. In addition to discovering financial misstatements, accountants find that performing analytical procedures gives them an increased understanding of a client's business, thus dramatically improving their operational recommendations to the client.[14]

Practice executives can use these same analytical procedures to better understand their own financial statements and find ways to improve their practice's operations. Analytical procedures consist of a study of the relationships among financial and nonfinancial data, and range from simple comparisons to complex models. Examples of frequently used analytical procedures include:

- Comparing current-period financial information with comparable prior-period information
- Benchmarking current financial data against industry data
- Comparing current-period financial information with budgets, forecasts, or other estimated results
- Performing ratio analysis on financial and/or nonfinancial data
- Studying the relationships among financial data for the period

The following discussion demonstrates analytical procedures comparing current and prior-period financial statements. Because an income statement represents transactions over a period of time and the balance sheet represents amounts at a point in time, relationships among income statement data are generally more stable than among balance sheet data.[14] Thus, this discussion focuses on income statement data.

Table 10-7 **Comparative Income Statement Analysis for the Years Ended December 31, 20X2 and 20X1**

	20X2	%	20X1	%	Net Change Amount	$
Revenues:						
Fee-for-service revenue (net of contractual allowances discounts)	$59,000,000	90.45%	$55,000,000	90.15%	$4,000,000	7.27%
Less: Provision for bad debts	(770,000)	−1.18%	(690,000)	−1.13%	(80,000)	11.59%
Net fee-for-service revenue less provision for bad debts	58,230,000	89.27%	54,310,000	89.02%	3,920,000	7.22%
Capitation revenue	5,100,000	7.82%	5,500,000	9.01%	(400,000)	−7.27%
Other	1,900,000	2.91%	1,200,000	1.97%	700,000	58.33%
Total medical revenue	65,230,000	100.00%	61,010,000	100.00%	4,220,000	6.92%
Operating Cost:						
Support Staff Costs:						
Staff salaries	15,250,000	23.38%	14,500,000	23.77%	750,000	5.17%
Payroll taxes	1,315,000	2.02%	1,250,000	2.05%	65,000	5.20%
Employee benefits	2,985,000	4.58%	2,750,000	4.51%	235,000	8.55%
Total support staff cost	19,550,000	29.97%	18,500,000	30.32%	1,050,000	5.68%
General Operating Cost:						
Information technology	950,000	1.46%	890,000	1.46%	60,000	6.74%
Malpractice insurance	1,000,000	1.53%	1,200,000	1.97%	(200,000)	−16.67%

Table 10-7 Comparative Income Statement Analysis for the Years Ended December 31, 20X2 and 20X1 (continued)

	20X2	%	20X1	%	Net Change Amount	$
Drug supply	2,800,000	4.29%	3,000,000	4.92%	(200,000)	−6.67%
Medical and surgical supply	880,000	1.35%	950,000	1.56%	(70,000)	−7.37%
Depreciation	1,400,000	2.15%	1,100,000	1.80%	300,000	27.27%
Building and occupancy	3,500,000	5.37%	3,500,000	5.74%	0	0.00%
Administrative supplies and services	810,000	1.24%	990,000	1.62%	(180,000)	−18.18%
Professional and consulting fees	360,000	0.55%	332,000	0.54%	28,000	8.43%
Clinical laboratory	1,400,000	2.15%	900,000	1.48%	500,000	55.56%
Radiology and imaging	600,000	0.92%	560,000	0.92%	40,000	7.14%
Promotion and marketing	230,000	0.35%	226,000	0.37%	4,000	1.77%
Other general and administrative	1,500,000	2.30%	1,900,000	3.11%	(400,000)	−21.05%
Total general operating cost	15,430,000	23.65%	15,548,000	25.48%	(118,000)	−0.76%
Total operating cost	34,980,000	53.63%	34,048,000	55.81%	932,000	2.74%
Total Medical Revenue After Operating Cost	30,250,000	46.37%	26,962,000	44.19%	3,288,000	12.19%
Less: NPP cost	2,750,000	4.22%	2,450,000	4.02%	300,000	12.24%
Total Medical Revenue After Operating and NPP Cost	27,500,000	42.16%	24,512,000	40.18%	2,988,000	12.19%
Less: Physician cost	26,500,000	40.63%	24,200,000	39.67%	2,300,000	9.50%
Net Income (Loss) After Provider-Related Expenses	1,000,000	1.53%	312,000	0.51%	688,000	220.51%
Other Income (Expense):						
Interest expense (net)	(341,000)	−0.52%	(257,000)	−0.42%	(84,000)	32.68%
Income from long-term investments	20,000	0.03%	30,000	0.05%	(10,000)	−33.33%
Unrealized gains and (losses) on investments	(16,000)	−0.02%	15,000	0.02%	(31,000)	−206.67%
Gain on disposal of equipment	−	0.00%	500,000	0.82%	(500,000)	−100.00%
Interest expense (net)	(337,000)	−0.52%	288,000	0.47%	(625,000)	−217.01%
Income Before Provision for Income Taxes	663,000	1.02%	600,000	0.98%	63,000	10.50%
Provision for (reduction of) Income Taxes	255,000	0.39%	240,000	0.39%	15,000	6.25%
Net Income (Loss)	408,000	0.63%	360,000	0.59%	$48,000	13.33%
Retained Earnings, Beginning of Year	5,203,000		4,843,000			
Retained Earnings, End of Year	$5,611,000		$5,203,000			

Table 10-7 shows the worksheet that analyzes the income statement line item balances for 20X2 and 20X1 according to their percentage of revenue, change in amount, and percentage change.

In reviewing these numbers, some people may express concern that the practice's total operating cost increased by $932,000 (2.74%) and nonphysician provider costs increased $300,000 (12.24%), even though it had the same number of physicians (88) both years. Certainly, good business sense dictates that a practice should avoid unnecessary overhead. In some situations, however, added overhead can help generate more revenue and increased profit. For a physician-owned medical practice, the goal is to generate more income per physician. West Side certainly did generate more income; total medical revenue was up $4,220,000 or 6.92%. Total medical revenue after operating and NPP cost (a measure of profitability) increased a total of $2,988,000 (12.19%) or $33,954 per physician.

This West Side example demonstrates that, in some circumstances, additional overhead can boost physician income. In this situation, the practice added ancillary services, thus increasing expenses for support staff, clinical laboratory, and depreciation from the related asset additions. It also added some nonphysician providers to provide support to the physicians and generate some charges of their own. Because of the added ancillary services and nonphysician providers, West Side was able to increase its revenues by more than it increased its costs.

Also contributing to West Side's increased profitability was a staffing reorganization in which the practice terminated some lower-paid employees and replaced them with a smaller number of more skilled employees (including the nonphysician providers just discussed). Although the more skilled employees commanded higher wages, they were more productive. A reduction in turnover, which had been particularly high in the pediatrics division, also contributed to the increased profitability. Management is especially proud of the decreases in other general and administrative expenses (21.05%), administrative supplies and services (18.18%), drug supply cost (6.67%), and medical and surgical supply cost (7.37%). These decreases resulted from restructuring the purchasing function and incorporating some employee suggestions. As a result of one employee suggestion, the practice began locking the supply cabinets and giving keys only to several designated employees who were responsible for distributing supplies to the other employees. The practice also began taking competitive bids from its suppliers and initiated an approved vendor list; management was surprised at the price reductions they realized. The decreases in medical and surgical supply cost and drug cost were especially impressive; because these are variable costs (increasing or decreasing directly with volume), the practice would have expected to see an increase in this amount. The practice even reduced its malpractice insurance by shopping around for professional liability coverage.

Management could not stop increases in certain expenses. The group is currently analyzing the 6.74% increase in information technology to determine ways to control those costs. Rising health insurance premiums for the group's employees were a contributing factor to the 8.55% increase in employee benefits. The rising health insurance premiums have been a problem for businesses in general. The practice continues to look for solutions.

Although West Side's clinical staff exhibited increased productivity in 20X2, the billing department's performance suffered. The provision for bad debts increased 11.59%. This increase combined with the 18.86% increase in accounts receivable discussed previously in this chapter are strong indicators that management needs to spend time addressing billing and collection issues in order to further improve profitability and cash flow.

Practice executives obtain greater benefit from analytical procedures by performing them on a monthly rather than annual basis. Analysis of data by location and specialty may also yield better information. AICPA training materials indicate that analytical procedures will be more effective in detecting material misstatements when performed on a disaggregated basis. Thus, comparisons on a monthly basis, by location, or by line of business can be more effective in identifying certain issues than those made on an annual or company-wide basis. For example, an analysis of annual sales data for Mattel, Inc. versus its competitors would not have raised suspicions of an existing fraud, whereas the analysis of the same data prepared on a monthly basis would have indicated unusual fluctuations.[14]

Similarly, an executive who analyzes data more frequently and on a smaller scale will garner more timely and detailed information about his or her practice. He or she is better positioned to initiate action to correct problems or take advantage of opportunities than a practice executive who analyzes only year-end data. MGMA Cost Survey data indicates that better performing practices in the area of profitability and cost management continually monitor and track financial performance, regularly compare practice performance to external benchmarks, and compare actual expenses to budget on a monthly basis.[15] Thus, both AICPA and MGMA data indicate more analysis is better; analytical financial procedures are more powerful when performed throughout the year, as opposed to annually.

Statement of Changes in Equity

The statement of changes in equity explains the changes that occurred in these accounts during the reporting period. Depending on the form of entity, this statement might also be called the statement of changes in stockholders' equity, partners' capital, owner's equity, members' capital, or net assets.

This statement may be combined with the income statement. Generally, entities with simple changes to equity, such as the increase in retained earnings from net income, would combine this statement with the income statement. This is the case with West Side, whose accrual basis statements include the Statements of Income and Retained Earnings and whose income tax basis statements include the Statement of Income and Retained Earnings (Deficit)—Income Tax Basis. Entities with more complicated changes, such as the issuance of additional capital stock, would use a separate statement to show these changes.

Statement of Cash Flows

The statement of cash flows explains how the organization obtained and used cash during the accounting period. This statement analyzes cash inflows and outflows from operating activities, investing activities, and financing activities, and also discloses significant noncash investing and financing transactions.

This statement is important because many users want to understand how the entity generates and uses cash. GAAP income may differ significantly from cash flow.

A practice with rapidly growing GAAP income may have a negative cash flow because of the lag in collecting its accounts receivable. Another practice may show a net loss, but have positive cash flows because it borrowed money.

As mentioned previously in this chapter, a statement of cash flows is not required for OCBOA financial statements. A practice using OCBOA may want to consider including this statement. A statement of cash flows is not the same thing as a modified cash basis income statement. Although an income statement prepared on the modified cash basis will usually more closely resemble cash flow than one prepared using GAAP, it still differs from an OCBOA income statement because of the various modifications to the pure cash basis of accounting. Physician owners often want to know why income statement amounts differ from the amount of cash available for distributions to physicians. The statement of cash flows for the West Side Multispecialty Group, P.C., shown in **Table 10-8**, answers this question.

Table 10-8 **Statements of Cash Flows for the Years Ended December 31, 20X2 and 20X1**

	20X2	20X1
Cash Flows from Operating Activities:		
Net Income (Loss)	$408,000	$360,000
Depreciation	1,400,000	1,100,000
(Gain) on disposal of equipment	–	(500,000)
Unrealized gains and losses on investments	16,000	(15,000)
Deferred income taxes	90,000	195,000
Changes in assets and liabilities:		
(Increase) decrease in accounts receivable	(1,000,000)	100,000
(Increase) in accounts receivable (other)	(5,000)	(2,000)
(Increase) decrease in prepaid expenses	(6,000)	21,000
Increase (decrease) in accounts payable	(50,000)	60,000
Increase (decrease) in payroll, benefits, and taxes payable	165,000	(50,000)
Increase (decrease) in claims payable	(10,000)	19,000
		(continues)

Table 10-8 Statements of Cash Flows for the Years Ended December 31, 20X2 and 20X1 (continued)

	20X2	20X1
Increase (decrease) in claims payable IBNR	7,000	(6,000)
Increase (decrease) in income taxes payable	138,000	21,000
Net cash flows from operating activities	1,153,000	1,303,000
Cash Flows from Investing Activities:		
Purchase of marketable securities	(250,000)	(175,000)
Sales of marketable securities	190,000	400,000
Purchase of leasehold improvements	(27,000)	(25,000)
Sale of equipment	–	500,000
Purchase of land for future clinic site	–	(500,000)
Purchase of equipment	(250,000)	(310,000)
Net cash flows from investing activities	(337,000)	(110,000)
Cash Flows from Financing Activities:		
Net increase (decrease) in notes payable	98,000	(370,000)
Repayment of long-term debt	(930,000)	(200,000)
Proceeds from issuance of common stock	–	–
Net cash flows from financing activities	(832,000)	(570,000)
Increase (decrease) in Cash	(16,000)	623,000
Cash at Beginning of Year	1,266,000	643,000
Cash at End of Year	$1,250,000	$1,266,000

Cash Flows from Operating Activities

The first section of the statement of cash flows shows the cash flows from the practice's business operations. These include cash receipts from medical services and related activities, such as the sale of medical supplies or pharmaceuticals. Examples of cash disbursements from operations include payments for salaries and benefits to clinic physicians and staff, medical supplies and pharmaceuticals, rent, office supplies, laundry and linens, and payment to other providers.

This section can be shown using either the direct method or the indirect method. The direct method lists the gross amounts of the various types of operating cash receipts and disbursements such as cash receipts for medical services, cash payments for salaries, cash payments for medical supplies, and so on. The advantage of this method is that it is intuitively logical. The FASB recommends the direct method as the preferred method for presenting cash flows from operating activities.

Even though the direct method is preferred by the FASB, the indirect method of presenting cash flows from operations is more popular.[16] The indirect method begins with net income as reported on the income statement, then displays the following adjustments:

- Deduct increases in current asset accounts.
- Add decreases in current asset accounts.
- Add increases in current liability accounts.
- Deduct decreases in current liability accounts.
- Add back noncash expenses and losses such as depreciation.
- Deduct noncash revenues and gains, such as gains on sales of equipment.

Note that these adjustments apply only to items affecting operating activities. Changes in items such as marketable securities and dividends payable are not included here because they are considered investing and financing activities, respectively.

The advantage of the indirect method is that it provides an analysis of the differences between cash flow from operations and net income from operations. It is also generally easier and less time consuming for the accountant to prepare.

Cash Flows from Investing Activities

Investing activities usually involve the purchase or disposal of long-term assets. An example would be the purchase or sale of investment property, such as bonds. A purchase or sale of a fixed asset, such as computer equipment, a building, or office furniture, would also be considered an investing activity.

Cash Flows from Financing Activities

Financing activities are those that relate to the debt or equity financing of the practice. Examples of cash flows from financing activities include the receipt of cash proceeds from a loan or the repayment of a loan. The contribution of capital by the practice's physician owners can also be a financing activity, as would the payment of dividends.

Noncash Investing and Financing Activities

When an entity enters into a significant noncash investing or financing activity, it should be disclosed in a separate schedule at the end of the statement of cash flows. An example of such a transaction would be a physician exchanging a piece of land for corporate stock. Another such situation would be the acquisition of a building or other fixed asset in exchange for a mortgage or loan payable.

■ Notes to Financial Statements

GAAP stipulates that financial statements must include certain disclosures in order for them to be complete. When OCBOA financial statements contain items that are the same as or similar to those included in GAAP financial statements, the OCBOA statements must also include these disclosures. In practice, most OCBOA financial disclosures are almost identical to GAAP disclosures.[5] Some disclosures may appear on the face of the financial statements, but most will appear in the Notes to Financial Statements.

The potential number of disclosures that may be included in financial statements is very large. The following discussion includes some of the disclosures typically found in the financial statements of a practice. The disclosures in a particular practice's financial statements may vary.

The notes include summary information regarding the organization's business operations and accounting policies, such as basis of accounting (if an OCBOA), depreciation methods, recognition of fee-for-service and capitation revenue, and charity care. A discussion regarding concentrations of credit risk is also included. Healthcare entities usually have a geographic risk because their patients are primarily local residents and a payer risk because a large amount of revenue usually comes from only a few payers. The notes also disclose information regarding related party transactions.

The notes will include additional information regarding certain financial statement line items such as investments, property and equipment, and long-term debt. Information regarding leasing arrangements, prepaid healthcare arrangements, and retirement plans are also included.

Other items with potentially significant impact on the entity's financial position generally must be included in the notes. These include, but are not limited to, subsequent events, commitments and contingencies, going concern issues, and accounting changes. Examples of such items include uninsured malpractice claims and a contract to purchase a new clinic building.

For compilation engagements only, an entity may elect to omit substantially all disclosures. An accountant is not allowed to omit disclosures if he or she is aware of an intent to mislead reasonably expected financial statement users.[2]

■ Conclusion

Practice executives can lead their practices to better financial performance by using analytical financial procedures to locate areas of potential financial improvement and opportunity. Those executives who perform these procedures on a monthly basis and on disaggregated data (such as by location or specialty) can garner better information than those who use these procedures only on year-end practice-wide data.

In order to use these powerful analytical financial tools, the executive must first have a good understanding of financial statements, bases of accounting, and the tax regulations affecting his or her practice. To better utilize outside accountants, he or she needs an understanding of the different levels of services they perform. A practice executive who does not understand these items cannot effectively perform or interpret the financial analyses that he or she needs to rely on in leading his or her practice and improving its financial performance.

References

1. Ramos M. *Fraud detection in a GAAS audit: SAS no. 99 implementation guide.* New York: American Institute of Certified Public Accountants; 2003:5–9.

2. American Institute of Certified Public Accountants. *Codification of statements on standards for accounting and review services. Numbers 1 to 20.* New York: AICPA; January 2011:§90.04.

3. American Institute of Certified Public Accountants. *Accounting and auditing guide: health care entities.* New York: AICPA; June 1, 2010.

4. Medical Group Management Association. *Cost survey for single-specialty practices: 2010 report based on 2009 data.* Englewood, CO: MGMA; 2010:11.

5. Ramos M. *Preparing and reporting on cash and tax basis financial statements.* New York: American Institute of Certified Public Accountants; 1998.

6. American Institute of Certified Public Accountants. Author Section 623. Sections .02–.04. Accessed April 30, 2011, at http://www.aicpa.org/Research/Standards/AuditAttest/DownloadableDocuments/AU-00623.pdf

7. Internal Revenue Code. §448(b)2.

8. Internal Revenue Procedure 2002-28.

9. Internal Revenue Code §446(a).

10. American Institute of Certified Public Accountants. *Audit risk alerts: health care industry developments—2003/04.* New York: AICPA; 2003:76.

11. Holton S, O'Dell J, Lindsey S, Eason S. *Guide to cash, tax and other bases of accounting,* Fort Worth, TX: Practitioner; 2003.

12. Piland N, Glass PH, Glass K. *Chart of accounts for health care organizations.* Englewood, CO: Center for Research in Ambulatory Care Administration; 1999:52.

13. Accounting Standards Update 2011-07. Financial Accounting Standards Board. Accessed January 7, 2012, at http://www.fasb.org/cs/BlobServer?blobcol=urldata&blobtable=MungoBlobs&blobkey=id&blobwhere=1175822797036&blobheader=application%2Fpdf

14. American Institute of Certified Public Accountants. Analytical review procedures in an audit engagement. Jersey City, NJ: AICPA; 2004.

15. Medical Group Management Association. *Performance and practices of successful medical groups: 2003 report based on 2002 data.* Englewood, CO: MGMA; 2003.

16. Edmonds T, McNair F, Milam E, Edmonds C, Schneider N. *Fundamental financial accounting concepts.* New York: McGraw-Hill; 2003.

CHAPTER

11

Practice Benchmarking

Elizabeth Woodcock, MBA, FACMPE, CPC

Benchmarking is the process of measuring and comparing data to identify opportunity for improvement and to achieve a higher level of performance. The goal is to reach best performance for the process or outcome that is being compared by identifying variances, evaluating how higher performance is achieved, and applying the lessons learned. The management of a medical practice can use benchmarking for financial and operational issues. Benchmarking provides the data and the road map for achieving best practices.

The management of a medical practice handles a range of information about its finances and operations. Using benchmarking, complex volumes of data can be summarized for comparison. Faced with hundreds of reports and thousands of data points, management can focus on key indicators to administer the business of a medical practice. The comparison may be made to internal data (physician to physician), historical data (the previous quarter to the current quarter), external data (available from professional associations or from another industry), or a combination of all three.

Data can be extracted from a variety of sources, but often come from the practice management system, including billing, coding, registration and scheduling information, and the practice's financial statements.

Most benchmarks are retrospective, such as a gross collection rate, so it is important for management to collect data, benchmark, and take action in a timely manner. In addition to timeliness, benchmarking is not static; to be useful, benchmarking needs to be an ongoing process.

Benchmarking does require commitment from management, because the process requires time to develop, report, and make use of the results. The process itself is simple, however, compared to the level of dedication needed from all stakeholders to improve the process or outcome when benchmarking has identified an opportunity for performance enhancement. Prior to committing time and energy to benchmarking, ensure that stakeholders are engaged for the long term.

Benchmarking can be used for all aspects of the practice. This chapter summarizes the key financial and operational benchmarks used by practices to identify opportunities for improvement and to achieve a higher level of performance.

Included in this chapter are examples of benchmarking used by West Side Multispecialty Group, P.C. ("West Side").

West Side is a fictitious medical practice; any resemblance to the finances or operations of any particular practice is purely coincidental.

Financial Benchmarks

Benchmarks regarding the financial performance of a practice can assist management with complex business decisions. Management can use a range of financial benchmarks; this section highlights benchmarks for revenue, productivity, accounts receivable, expenses, profitability, and liquidity.

Revenue

The income statement of a practice reports its revenue, typically including sources such as "fee-for-service," "capitation," and "other." There are, however, numerous benchmark-related revenues that are commonly used by management.

Gross Collection Rate

A practice establishes a common price or fee schedule for each service it performs. The practice provides services to patients who are covered by an insurance company or payer that has contracted with the practice to pay a certain rate for each service (an allowable), or, in the absence of a contract, a predetermined fee is considered payment. If the patient does not have insurance, he or she is his or her own payer, and, absent of any discounts, is expected to pay the practice's full price.

The practice's fee schedule is equal to or higher than payments for its services. Thus, the practice's revenue is lower than the sum of its prices. The ratio of collections to charges is the gross collection rate (GCR). (It is of note that the example assumes that management has calculated the value of its capitated charges into gross charges. If not, then management would need to calculate the gross fee-for-service collection rate, and only use fee-for-service [FFS] collections and FFS charges.)

Because charges can be arbitrarily set and changed by the practice, as can the average allowable by the payer, the GCR is an imprecise and broad measure of collection effectiveness. Due to the variability of charges and allowables between practices even of the same specialty, benchmarking against external data sources does not allow management to draw any conclusions regarding performance. The adjusted collection rate, to be discussed later in this chapter, is a more precise measure because it factors out the monies to which a practice is not entitled (the contractual allowance) or will not collect (bad debt), regardless of how it sets and changes its fees and the allowables it receives.

The gross collection rate is calculated by dividing net collections by gross charges:

$$\text{Calculation: } \frac{\text{Net collections}}{\text{Gross charges}}$$

Example:

	20X2	20X1
Net collections*	$63,330,000	$59,810,000
Gross charges	$80,215,326	$77,806,687
Gross collection rate	78.95%	76.87%

*Net collections equals net fee-for-service revenue less provision for bad debts plus capitation revenue, both reported on the income statement.

The management of West Side was encouraged to see an improvement in the practice's GCR. No conclusions could be drawn about the performance of the practice, however, because the management noted that changes had been made to West Side's fee schedule at the end of 20X1 and that several payers had discontinued reimbursement for some frequent services offered by West Side. In addition, intensive coding training had been conducted for all providers in the first quarter of 20X2, which resulted in higher coding levels and, thus, more charges than in 20X1. With these significant influences on its gross charges, the management of West Side cannot draw any conclusions about this positive change in its GCR.

Adjusted Collection Rate

To track the internal management of payments, management should also express its collections as a percentage of the payer's obligation (the allowable). The net or adjusted collection rate (ACR) offers management a revealing indicator of financial performance. The ACR equals net collections divided by net charges. Net charges are those monies that the practice is obligated to receive, either through a contractual relationship (e.g., allowables) or an otherwise predetermined expectation (e.g., a self-pay patient to pay full charge). If the practice's billing system lacks the ability to automatically calculate the monies that the practice is obligated to receive, add net fee-for-services collections to all bad debt and noncontractual adjustments to calculate net charges. In order to assure accuracy, management must define a process for and train its staff on identifying all noncontractual adjustments, which is discussed later. The adjusted collection rate should be close to 100%; any less is considered a loss for bad debts or noncontractual write-offs.

The percentage is calculated exclusively for fee-for-service revenue and charges because capitated payments are made based on a utilization rate, not by charge.

It is of note that this computation may not be meaningful when performed on data from a short period of time (e.g., 1 month). Instead, the ACR should be calculated based on an annual, or 12-month rolling average, basis.

$$\text{Calculation: } \frac{\text{Net fee-for-service collections}}{\text{Net fee-for-service charges}}$$

Example:

	20X2	20X1
Net fee-for-service collections*	$58,230,000	$54,310,000
Net fee-for-service charges	$60,061,887	$5,966,612
Adjusted collection rate	96.95%	97.04%

*Net fee-for-service collection equals net fee-for-service revenue less provision for bad debts.

The management of West Side was disappointed in the declining ACR. To analyze the root cause of the change in performance, a more detailed analysis was conducted.

For further analysis, management can analyze a detail of the bad debt and other noncontractual write-offs that were written off. Write-offs are often a result of the practice's inability to collect from patients (bad debt and charity care) or meet payers' claims filing deadlines, or are the result of internal administrative mistakes. Standard industry practice is to include accounts sent to a collection agency to pursue payment as a bad debt.[1] If collected, the write-off is reversed, and the revenue posted. Although a minimal amount of write-offs is expected, write-offs resulting from poor administrative processes or personnel should be identified, analyzed, and fixed.

Calculation: Amount ($) by write-off category

Example:

Bad debt	$200,000
Charity care	$150,000
Timely filing deadline	$225,000
Registration errors	$152,000
Coding/bundling errors	$64,000
Other	$146,000
TOTAL	$937,000

In this example, the management of West Side determined that the decline in the ACR was a result of failing to meet the claims filing deadlines of several payers. An internal audit was conducted to determine the root cause of the missed deadlines, which was a problem with the interface between West Side and its claims clearinghouse. The write-off analysis allowed management to address the situation before it caused further problems.

It is of note that the balance sheet, which lists an allowance for doubtful accounts, does not offer management the level of detail necessary to identify the nature of and responsibility for the write-off. In order to benchmark noncontractual write-offs, the practice should establish codes in its billing and accounting software to differentiate these write-offs, by type of write-off, from contractual allowances.

Collection Rate by Payer

Each payer offers a different rate of reimbursement for the services provided to its beneficiaries, who are patients receiving services at the practice. The reimbursement per procedure code is called an allowable; the sum of the allowables divided by the practice's charges for those services can be calculated as the payer's collection rate. In addition to the GCR for the practice, management can determine and evaluate a collection rate for each payer.

$$\text{Calculation: } \frac{\text{Net collections by payer}}{\text{Gross charges by payer}}$$

Example:

Payer	GCR
Medicare	87%
Medicaid	63%
Commercial	94%
Patient/self-pay	52%
Other	74%

The collection rate by payer proves particularly beneficial if the practice establishes its fee schedule according to a consistent scale (for example, Medicare's resource-based relative value scale [RBRVS]). Thus, comparing payer collection rates allows management to determine a rank order of payers. In this example, West Side recognizes that its commercial payers reimburse at much higher rates than all other payers. A more detailed analysis by payer, and payer plan, offers management the ability to rank and monitor payers.

Each payer offers a different reimbursement rate for the services rendered by the practice on behalf of its beneficiaries—the patients—so it is important for management to understand and measure the percentage that each payer contributes to the practice's business.

Payer Mix

The source of payment can be summarized in a practice's *payer mix*, which defines the sources of payment as a percentage of its business. Standard industry definition is the percentage of payment from a payer expressed as a percentage of prices or charges, although value can also be derived from expressing the payer mix as a percentage of revenue.

$$\text{Calculation: } \frac{\text{Gross charges by payer}}{\text{Total gross charges for practice}}$$

Example:

Payer	Percentage of Charges
Medicare	34%
Medicaid	8%
Commercial	41%
Patient/self-pay	11%
Other	6%

Measuring and monitoring payer mix over time allows management to evaluate changes in its business. Applying a weighted average analysis to its payer mix and the GCR for each payer, the practice can estimate the financial impact of a shift in the payer mix. Depending on the results, management can make efforts to avoid, alter, or further the impact.

Example:

Current

Payer	Percentage of Charges	GCR
Medicare	34%	85%
Medicaid	8%	49%
Commercial	41%	90%
Patient/self-pay	11%	51%
Other	6%	58%
Gross collection rate		**78.95%**

Shift and Impact

Payer	Percentage of Charges	GCR
Medicare	30%	87%
Medicaid	17%	51%
Commercial	36%	88%
Patient/self-pay	11%	53%
Other	6%	77%
Gross collection rate		**76.87%**

In this example, the management of West Side can see that its business has shifted to Medicaid. Even though Medicaid had increased its reimbursement during the same period, it does not make up for the transfer of business to this payer. West Side can make efforts to improve its collection rate by negotiating higher allowables from its payers, or alter its patient population by offering new services and sites, or through marketing. Because the payment rates to the practice vary by payer, evaluating changes in the payer mix over time can reveal important revenue trends.

It is of note that the GCR is dependent on the gross charges of the practice. Gross charges can be impacted by changes in volume, coding practices, and the practice's prices or charges. A change in GCR, therefore, cannot lead management to conclude that reimbursement has improved or declined. The adjusted or net collection rate is a more precise index for collection effectiveness.

Reimbursement by Service Line

In addition to monitoring reimbursement by payer, management should identify and monitor revenue by each service line. The service lines depend on specialty, but ancillaries, procedures, surgeries, office encounters, hospital encounters, and any other services provided should be included. Comparing volume by service line to reimbursement by service line allows management to evaluate the relative contribution of each service line, as shown in **Figure 11-1**. Thus, decisions can be made about adding, extending, retracting, or even discontinuing services.

$$\text{Calculation: } \frac{\begin{array}{c}\text{Volume measurement}\\\text{(encounter, RVU, etc.) by service line}\end{array}}{\text{Volume measurement for total practice}}$$

$$\text{Calculation: } \frac{\text{Revenue by service line}}{\text{Total practice revenue}}$$

Example:

Through the analysis demonstrated in Figure 11-1, West Side's Division of Family Medicine determined that its in-house laboratory services were limited in their contribution to the business. In-house labs represented a high volume, but a limited revenue opportunity. The opposite conclusion was made for procedures, preventive visits, and imaging, all of which represented low volume services but high revenue. The management of the division chose to target the services with high collections for further growth, although it was recognized that some of its services would have to remain loss leaders. Family Medicine would have to continue some basic laboratory services, for example, to ensure that quality care was delivered in a timely manner and patient expectations were met.

Practices with surgeons and proceduralists should also measure surgical or procedure revenue as a percentage of total revenue, as shown in **Figure 11-2**. The contribution of these services—the surgical yield—to the bottom line should also be benchmarked.

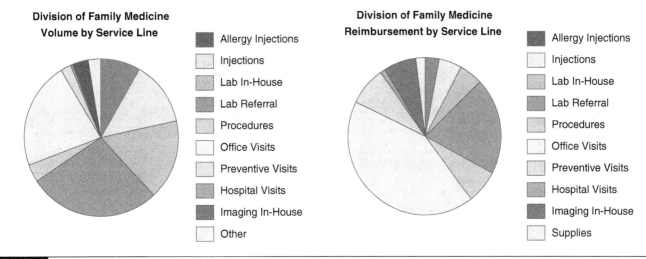

Figure 11-1 Relative contribution of each service line—Division of family medicine.

Calculation: $$\frac{\text{Revenue derived from surgeries or procedures}}{\text{Total revenue}}$$

In this example, West Side's Division of General Surgery recognized that its revenue derived from surgeries as a percentage of total revenue was declining. The source was determined to be a retiring surgeon, but the data alerted the division to the fact that it was necessary to replace this position in short order. The period between the retirement phase and the new hire was quantified, and the division addressed the revenue shortfall. The percentage increased and remained at consistent levels after the new surgeon was hired and fully credentialed to provide and bill for her services.

Reimbursement per Procedure Code

In order to better identify revenue trends, management should understand and analyze information about what each payer is expected to pay—and what they actually do—to the most detailed level.

Management should identify its top 20 to 25 procedure codes by specialty, and the rates of payment for these codes by payer (see Table 11-1), directly from the contract with the payer and/or its stated fee schedule. Absent of that, the rates should be collected from explanation of payments received from the payer by the practice, although this is certainly not a fail-safe method. For the majority of specialties, the top 25 codes will define 80% of the practice's revenue stream.

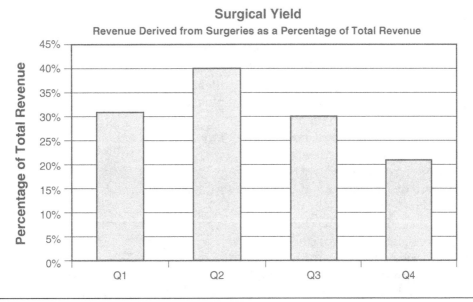

Figure 11-2 Surgical yield example, Division of General Surgery, West Side.

Table 11-1	Reimbursement per Procedure Code					
CPT(R)	Description	Medicare	Medicaid	Commercial A	Commercial B	Commercial C
11200	Removal of skin tag	$83.58	$70.19	$94.76	$73.70	$112.31
99201	Office/outpatient visit, new, level 1	$41.11	$32.55	$45.69	$37.41	$58.96
99202	Office/outpatient visit, new, level 2	$71.01	$64.59	$73.22	$61.36	$103.35
99203	Office/outpatient visit, new, level 3	$102.95	$95.96	$104.91	$91.16	$153.53
99204	Office/outpatient visit, new, level 4	$158.33	$135.53	$162.36	$128.76	$216.86
99205	Office/outpatient visit, new, level 5	$197.06	$172.13	$199.88	$163.52	$275.40
99211	Office/outpatient visit, est., level 1	$19.71	$14.56	$21.54	$20.22	$34.05
99212	Office/outpatient visit, est., level 2	$41.45	$37.71	$41.96	$35.83	$60.34
99213	Office/outpatient visit, est., level 3	$68.97	$52.65	$71.07	$50.01	$84.23
99214	Office/outpatient visit, est., level 4	$102.27	$82.14	$110.89	$78.04	$131.43
99215	Office/outpatient visit, est., level 5	$137.60	$119.11	$141.23	$113.15	$190.57
99221	Initial hospital care, level 1	$97.17	$96.51	$101.42	$86.95	$123.36
99222	Initial hospital care, level 2	$132.17	$111.27	$150.21	$89.01	$178.02
99223	Initial hospital care, level 3	$194.01	$154.95	$209.18	$123.96	$247.92
99231	Subsequent hospital care, level 1	$38.39	$33.23	$44.86	$26.58	$53.17
99232	Subsequent hospital care, level 2	$69.31	$54.89	$74.10	$43.91	$87.82
99233	Subsequent hospital care, level 3	$99.55	$78.04	$105.35	$62.43	$124.86
99235	Observ./hosp. same date	$172.26	$181.46	$244.97	$145.17	$290.34
99239	Hospital discharge day	$101.25	$95.21	$128.53	$76.17	$152.34
99304	Nursing facility care	$88.00	$87.82	$89.66	$78.26	$156.52
99305	Nursing facility care	$123.67	$120.97	$124.56	$96.78	$193.56
99307	Nursing fac. care, subseq	$42.13	$39.65	$44.52	$50.48	$45.66
99308	Nursing fac. care, subseq	$64.89	$58.89	$65.89	$69.00	$68.97
99316	Nursing fac. discharge day	$79.84	$72.54	$82.11	$73.48	$84.52

Rates are sample only. CPT codes and descriptions are copyright 2012 American Medical Association.

Management can utilize the procedure code analysis to identify payers that are paying lower-than-market rates, as well as to ensure that all payments being posted are equal to the agreed-upon rate. After the Division of Internal Medicine reviewed this analysis, it was decided that management would develop a targeted marketing campaign to the employers who offered the PPO and Commercial A plans to their employees. The management set up meetings with the benefits officers at these employers to discuss ease of access and quality of care. The meetings proved valuable, because the Division of Internal Medicine saw an influx of patients covered by these two payers—and a corresponding increase in revenue.

The detailed reimbursement per procedure code analysis is an excellent resource; however, the payment rate for each payer can be summarized as a percentage of Medicare or RBRVS according to the actual services rendered for this payer's beneficiaries by the practice.

Expressing each payment rate as a percentage of RBRVS allows the practice to compare the contribution of each payer to its financial success.

Underperforming payers can be approached for higher allowables, to renegotiate the terms of the contract, or to discontinue the relationship.

$$\text{Calculation:} \quad \frac{\text{Collections by payer}}{\substack{\text{Collections by Medicare (expressed at} \\ \text{100\% of the Medicare allowable)}}}$$

Example:

Medicare	100%
Medicaid	83%
Blue Cross/Blue Shield	112%
Commercial A	104%
Commercial B	96%
Commercial C	138%

The payment rate also can be expressed at the overall practice level as a percentage of RBRVS, such as 121% of RBRVS. The management of West Side monitors this ratio carefully from year to year, because a decline in the overall practice reimbursement level requires immediate action to renegotiate allowables, alter the payer mix, and decrease expenses. As noted, the shift to Medicaid had resulted in a decrease in the overall payment rate. West Side was responding through its efforts to improve its infrastructure, reduce its costs, and increase the services it provides in-house in order to reduce its subcapitation payments to external providers.

Productivity

Because the U.S. reimbursement system rewards a practice for volume, a strong revenue stream is dependent on the productivity of its personnel. Measuring, monitoring, and benchmarking the productivity of the individuals in a practice is fundamental to financial management.

Productivity of Providers

There are numerous productivity measurements for physicians and physician extenders; the main ones are highlighted here.

Charges. This is the sum of the fees charged for the services provided to all patients seen during a specified period of time. Fees depend on the practice's fee schedule, which varies by practice, so benchmarking with external data has limited application.

Revenue. This is the sum of the money collected during a specified period of time for services provided to patients. Revenue depends on the practice's payer mix, which varies by practice and often among the providers within a practice. Measuring productivity by revenue causes providers of patients covered by higher-paying payers to appear more productive when, in reality, they may not be.

Encounters. The sum of the billable, face-to-face visits with patients during a specified period of time. Encounters are often tracked by place of service, including office, outpatient clinic, and inpatient hospital. Measuring productivity by encounters is limited by its inability to account for the work involved in the encounter. This simple count of visits does not measure the intensity of the encounter, which may consume 2 minutes or 2 hours, and may be reimbursed at $15 to $1500. Moreover, there is no industry standard for the definition of an encounter; if used for internal benchmarking, management must decide on the definition in advance.

Relative value units. This is the sum of the relative value units (RVUs) associated with the encounters with patients during a specified period of time. RVUs are "nonmonetary, relative units of measure that indicate the value of health care services and relative differences in resources consumed when providing various procedures and services."[2] Several such systems exist, but the industry standard and the one used most frequently is the Resource-Based Relative Value Scale (RBRVS). RBRVS RVUs measure the value of the physician work, practice expense, and malpractice expense for each procedure code relative to the other codes.

In RBRVS, which is the scale utilized by Medicare and many other payers to establish their allowables for each procedure code, RVUs are expressed either as a total or by component, to include work, malpractice, and practice expense. The component most useful in measuring productivity is work. As a measure of clinical productivity, work RVUs are the best benchmark to use, particularly if external data comparisons are made. The scale is the same for all providers; fee schedules and the mix of payers are irrelevant. RVUs inherently measure the work associated with the encounter.

Management can calculate RVU production, and compare production internally with peers or externally with industry data. Conclusions regarding the relative productivity of providers can be made, and efforts to improve productivity, including peer pressure simply from seeing the data, can be introduced.

There are limitations of using RVUs, for which management should account. If management uses RVUs to benchmark productivity, it is important to realize that the scale changes annually. Moreover, caution should be used if benchmarking is performed between specialties because the scale has historically placed more value on procedures and surgeries.

Finally, there are no RVUs (total or work) for nonclinical activities or some clinical services. To utilize RVUs for nonclinical activities, management should calculate an average RVU per hour by each specialty. Physicians can track their time and apply this average RVU per hour to the time at the full rate, or some agreed-upon discounted value rate by activity.

Calculation:
$$\frac{\text{Total work RVUs}}{(\text{Clinical work RVUs divided by hours worked}) \times \text{Hours worked in nonclinical activities}}$$

Example:

Physician A

Practice RVU value rate (based on clinical effort)	
Clinical	100%
Teaching	100%
Research	75%
Administration	95%

Table 11-2	Physician A Report Card	
Clinical		
Average work RVUs produced per week		109
Average clinical hours worked per week		30
Average work RVUs per clinical hour		3.63
Nonclinical		
Average teaching hours worked per week		4
Average work RVUs for teaching per week (Calculation: $4 \times 3.63 \times 100\%$)		14.52
Average research hours worked per week		15
Average work RVUs for research per week (Calculation: $15 \times 3.63 \times 75\%$)		40.84
Average administration hours worked per week		1
Average work RVUs for administration per week (Calculation: $1 \times 3.63 \times 95\%$)		3.45
Total		
Average work RVUs produced per week—all activities (Calculation: $109 + 14.52 + 40.84 + 3.45$)		167.81
Average work RVUs produced per year—all activities (Calculation: 167.81×46) (based on 46 weeks worked per year)		7,719

Because West Side contracted with its local medical school to provide teaching services to its students, management used this calculation for its physicians involved in this contract. In addition, several physicians in each division were assigned to administrative duties. This time was also valued. Thus, West Side is able to produce a comprehensive and fair productivity analysis for all of its physicians such as the example provided in **Table 11-2**.

To determine RVUs for clinical services not assigned values (such as some laboratory and anesthesia services), management should calculate the average charge per RVU and compare it to the average charge per procedure code for the service it wishes to impute an RVU value.

Example, determining total RVUs for procedure code 12345[*]:

Total gross charges	$1,519,652.00
Total RVU production	15,432.00
Average charge per RVU	98.47
Charge for procedure code 12345	$435.00
Estimated total RVUs	4.42

[*]Sample only.

The management of West Side used this methodology for services provided by its anesthesiologists and pathologists, as well as to value the multiple procedures and surgeries provided by its proceduralists and surgeons.

By using standard protocols for determining RVUs for nonclinical time and services without RBRVS units, productivity comparisons utilizing RVUs can be extremely valuable for management.

With the exception of encounters, a provider's coding patterns can influence all of the productivity measures. For example, a provider who spends the same time with every patient but is better educated and equipped to document and appropriately code to the highest level of the service will likely have higher charges, revenue, and RVUs.

In addition to measuring the productivity of physicians, the practice should develop productivity benchmarks for its physician extenders that are consistent with the indicator chosen for physicians (e.g., encounters). It is of note that a practice employing a physician extender who is billing "incident to" the physician's services may not record the extender's productivity. To do so, management should establish a code for both the physician practicing alone and the physician practicing with said extender. (Both codes can be programmed to print the physician's identification number on the claim form, so they are really just for internal tracking purposes.) A code can also be established for the extender him- or herself, if billing separately from the physician. The sum of the services incurred under "incident to" and stand-alone equals the extender's productivity.

Finally, the provider must be present to produce services, so the provider's time is an important factor to consider when calculating productivity. Most providers do not work 4 to 8 weeks per year as a result of continuing medical education (CME), vacation, and other leave time. Thus, when comparing productivity during a specified period of time, management should account for leave by reporting the productivity measurement based on half-day sessions or days worked. Moreover, management should define a session or a day based on the actual hours worked.

In addition to the providers, productivity measurements can be applied to staff functions. Tracking the unit of service per full-time equivalent (FTE) staff, as well as the expenses associated with them, allows management to evaluate staff efficiency.

Example:

	20X2	20X1
Total RVU production	542,500	522,964
FTE staff	550	586
RVUs per FTE staff	986	892

The management of West Side measured its RVUs per FTE staff to evaluate the results of overall staffing reductions, improvements in human resources management, more qualified (and higher paid) staff, as well as workflow enhancements during the last quarter of 20X1. The results were exceptional; less staff produced 10% more than the previous year. The new infrastructure produced more units of work—at a higher profit margin.

In addition to measuring RVUs per FTE staff, a more detailed analysis can be conducted by function, including nursing, front office, ancillaries (by service), and billing office. Tracking RVUs (or another appropriate unit of work such as "claims processed" for the billing staff) per FTE staff by function over time allows management to evaluate staff performance and the appropriateness of staff allocations based on work.

Management also can use RVUs to measure the productivity of each encounter by calculating RVUs per encounter. This is an excellent benchmark for internal comparisons among providers because it measures the provider's output per unit of work. Maintaining a higher RVU per encounter may indicate higher—or better—coding, as well as the ability to produce more reimbursable work in the same period of time. A related benchmark is revenue per encounter, which reflects a provider's payer mix as well as his or her service line and its relative reimbursement.

Example, Division of Gastroenterology:

	Dr. A	Dr. B	Dr. C	Dr. D
Total work RVUs	6,430	7,950	8,460	9,430
Total revenue	$545,600	$594,600	$685,700	$705,000
Total encounters	3,580	3,950	4,250	4,480
Work RVUs per encounter	1.80	2.01	1.99	2.10
Revenue per work RVU	$84.85	$74.79	$81.05	$74.76

Through the analysis demonstrated in the example, the management of the Division of Gastroenterology recognized that Dr. A was producing at lower levels of RVUs per encounter, yet achieved the highest revenue per work RVU. An audit was conducted (to include a bell curve analysis, which is described in the example), and it was determined that Dr. A was undercoding for his evaluation and management services based on his documentation, but was fortunate enough to maintain a more lucrative payer mix than his associates. The analysis prompted management to intervene with coding training for Dr. A, who promptly increased his work RVUs per encounter by accurately documenting and coding the services he was performing, which increased his revenue even further beyond his associates.

In addition to benchmarking productivity, the actual services performed by each provider can be measured and compared both internally and externally. Management can benchmark evaluation and management (E/M) codes by analyzing a provider's bell curve. The bell curve is a pictorial depiction of the volume of the new and established office visits produced by the practitioner.

Through the analysis demonstrated in **Figure 11-3**, management determined that the Division of Family Medicine was undercoding its new patient visits, and training was commenced to address the services and documentation to support coding at higher levels.

A related but more detailed analysis can be conducted with all procedure codes billed by each provider. Variations among providers with a similar patient base can be analyzed for opportunities.

Accounts Receivable

One of the most important assets that a practice maintains is accounts receivable (A/R). Reported on the balance sheet, A/R are amounts due from patients, insurance companies, and other customers (e.g., a law firm if expert witness work is performed). These monies represent the majority, if not all, of the practice's future revenue. Due to the complex nature of the U.S. healthcare reimbursement system, the management of billing and collections activities is the core administrative function in a practice. Even if a practice maintains a lucrative payer mix and superior productivity, the collection of the practice's revenue depends on is ability to measure—and manage—this process.

Because of its importance, several benchmarks are commonly presented and analyzed for A/R. These benchmarks are total A/R, days receivables outstanding (DRO), and aged trial balance (ATB). A discussion regarding the importance of analyzing credit balances and bad debt follows. Finally, tracking and evaluating denials is highlighted.

Total A/R

The amount of all monies owed to the practice is referred to as its total A/R. Although often viewed as a management concern, having a large amount of A/R is not a negative reflection on the management of this asset. A/R reflects the physicians' productivity; the more patients seen, the higher the A/R. Although trends in total A/R over time can be revealing, its existence at any point in time is not. Thus, to benchmark A/R, management should evaluate the DRO and the ATB.

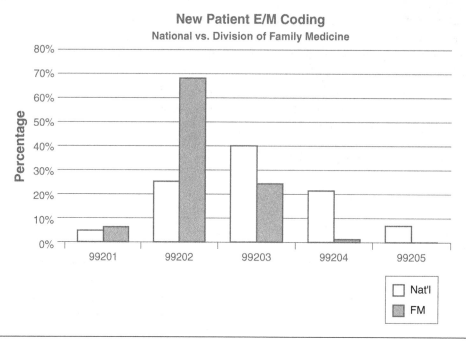

Figure 11-3 Example, Division of Family Medicine, West Side: New patient E/M coding.

An accrual basis balance sheet reports accounts receivable on a net basis, but industry benchmarks reflect gross A/R.[3] Following industry definition, this section uses the practice's gross A/R when calculating benchmarks; however, management should recognize that the actual value of the A/R is much lower than what is reported in management reports, and should not be relied on for cash flow or financing.

Days Receivables Outstanding (DRO)

By accounting for volume and time, the calculation of DRO (often referred to as "days in A/R") reveals the practice's ability to manage this asset. The standard industry definition is to divide total A/R by the practice's average daily charge during the past year.[4]

$$\text{Calculation: } \frac{\text{Total A/R}}{(\text{Total annual gross charges} / 365)}$$

Example:

	20X2	20X1
Total accounts receivable	$7,786,000	$6,054,000
Average daily charge	$180,065	$167,840
DRO	43.24	36.07

The management of West Side was discouraged about the increase in its DRO from 36 to 43 days. DRO, which normally ranges from 30 to 45 for medical practices, depending on the specialty and the market, can be influenced by external forces, such as payers' reimbursement policies or administrative practices, as well as internal processes, such as the practice's ability to capture accurate patient demographic and insurance information at registration. With further analysis, West Side discovered that its decrease in performance was a result of both external and internal issues. In 20X2, payers had shifted more financial burden to their beneficiaries, and West Side was not equipped to effectively handle time-of-service collections. Thus, patient receivables rose, and the DRO increased. The management of West Side was able to target intervention, and improve time-of-service collections and its DRO.

It is of note that although the industry standard is the average daily charge over a year, this method can lead to misleading fluctuations in DRO for practices with seasonal variability in production (e.g., an allergy practice). To control for the fluctuation, management can use the average daily charge based on the last 1 to 3 months.

DRO reveals the time in which a practice can convert this asset into cash. It is of note that most practices maintain their internal A/R records on a gross basis; that is, the A/R is based on the practice's charge or fee schedule, not the percentage the practice expects to receive. If a valuation is necessary, a discount rate, which can be estimated by the practice's GCR—adjusted for changes in payer mix, anticipated bad debt, and other current reimbursement conditions—should be calculated and applied.

A similar ratio can be applied to accounts payable (A/P), the monies that a practice owes to its creditors. The days in A/P reveals the average payment period for a practice.

$$\text{Calculation: } \frac{365 \times \text{average accounts payable}}{\text{Annual purchases on credit}}$$

The days in accounts payable should be less than the DRO in order for the practice to optimize its cash flow.

Aged Trial Balance (ATB)

The principle of the time value of money reveals that a dollar in hand is more valuable than a dollar in the future. Thus, monies outstanding, or A/R, should be as young as possible. The ATB is the practice's total A/R, presented by age: current (0–30 days outstanding), 31–60, 61–90, 91–120, and over 120 days.

At the practice's initiation, all of the A/R begins as current. As the practice matures, the A/R stabilizes and the ATB offers an excellent financial indicator regarding the management of A/R.

Calculation: $\dfrac{\text{A/R by category of age (per 30-day period)}}{\text{Total A/R}}$

Example:

Category	A/R	Percentage of Total
Current	$3,023,000	38.83%
31–60	$1,595,000	20.49%
61–90	$774,000	9.94%
91–120	$698,000	8.96%
Over 120	$1,696,000	21.78%
Total	$7,786,000	100.0%

The management of West Side used the ATB to evaluate the patient receivables problem identified in the example. Indeed, the percentage of A/R over 120 days, which is normally 10–12%, had risen to 21.78% in 20X2 due to West Side's inability to effectively manage its patient receivables.

For a more detailed analysis, management can analyze the ATB of monies owed by each financially responsible party—Medicare, Medicaid, commercial, patients, and so forth. A detailed ATB allows management to identify areas of concern and target resources in the billing office.

Example:

This example reveals a concern regarding outstanding Medicaid and patient receivables. Upon investigation, West Side management identified an internal Medicaid administrative error that was fixed after communicating with the Medicaid office, and a realization that, in addition to poor time-of-service collections, patient statements had not been transmitted for 60 days, which was immediately corrected.

Credit Balances

In addition to collecting on its A/R, a practice receives monies that are paid by customers as a result of a mistake at the practice (e.g., submitting a duplicate claim for the same service) or of a customer (e.g., a patient paying more than he or she owes on his or her account). These overpayments should be processed appropriately in a timely manner; however, for a period of time, they are carried by the practice as negative A/R. Some practices also carry numerous other credit balances in their A/R resulting from unapplied cash, payment posting errors, and old unresolved overpayments from customers and payers. When reporting A/R benchmarks, a large amount of old credit balances can artificially deflate the A/R. A practice with an underperforming billing office may report positive A/R indicators unless the credit balances are removed. Management should benchmark the A/R net of only the legitimate credit balances that are anticipated to be refunded to the appropriate party (versus old unresolved credits or those created by internal posting errors).

Bad Debt

A practice may choose to declare part of its A/R as "uncollectible," and outsource the collection of those accounts to a collection agency. It is standard industry practice to write those accounts off of the A/R.[5] If utilizing accrual accounting, management is required to disclose the amount of bad debts the practice anticipates on its balance sheet under "accounts receivable" in its current assets, as is demonstrated in West Side's balance sheet, presented in Chapter 10, which notes "net of allowance

Days	Medicare A/R	Medicare Percentage of Total	Medicaid A/R	Medicaid Percentage of Total	Commercial A/R	Commercial Percentage of Total	Patient A/R	Patient Percentage of Total	Total A/R	Total Percentage of Total
Current	453,222	61.0%	68,932	14.3%	1,164,512	43.9%	1,336,334	34.2%	$3,023,000	38.83%
31–60	168,098	22.6%	86,844	18.0%	725,687	27.3%	614,371	15.7%	$1,595,000	20.49%
61–90	58,933	7.9%	96,522	20.0%	301,112	11.3%	317,433	8.1%	$774,000	9.94%
91–120	49,861	6.7%	75,681	15.7%	268,752	10.1%	303,706	7.8%	$698,000	8.96%
Over 120	12,544	1.7%	155,244	32.1%	194,899	7.3%	1,333,313	34.1%	$1,696,000	21.78%
Total	$742,658	100.0%	$483,223	100.0%	$2,654,962	100.0%	$3,905,157	100.0%	$7,786,000	100.0%

for doubtful accounts of $205,000 in 20X2 and $180,000 in 20X1." This allowance is an estimate of the amount of bad debts currently in accounts receivable. In addition, the management must also report the "provision for bad debts," which represents both actual and estimated bad debts for the entire year, on its income statement as either a contra-revenue account or as an operating expense, depending upon how generally accepted accounting principles (GAAP) apply to its accounting practices. West Side's income statement reports $770,000 and $690,000 as contra-revenue items in 20X2 and 20X1, respectively. The bad debt ratio expresses the bad debt as a percentage of net fee-for-service collections.

$$\text{Calculation: } \frac{\text{Bad debt}}{\text{Net fee-for-service collections}}$$

Example:

	20X2	20X1
Bad debt	$770,000	$690,000
Net fee-for-service collections	$58,230,000	$54,310,000
Bad debt ratio	1.32%	1.27%

The management of West Side recognized that the bad debt of 20X2 would be higher than the previous year due to the write-offs that had to be taken for missed claims filing deadlines as well as uncollectible patient receivables.

If the practice chooses to outsource the management of additional accounts due to internal resource constraints or exceptional results from a collections agency, accounts that are still considered collectible should not be ignored, even though they were sent to an agency. For benchmarking purposes, the practice should maintain the amount of accounts sent to a collection agency, and evaluate its DRO and ATB with and without these monies. Although standard industry definition is to exclude these accounts, it is important for management to monitor them. Furthermore, for financial reporting purposes, A/R should be listed at "net realizable" value. Thus, if an outsourcing strategy that involved an agency earlier in the collections cycle was deployed, management should establish a parameter to determine the point at which the collection potential diminishes. Depending on the outsourcing arrangement, this may be 30 days after outsourcing, or even longer.

Denials

In order to detect problems before they become noncontractual write-offs, management should monitor the reasons for denials of claims from insurance companies. Denials are often a result of registration issues, such as lack of eligibility or coverage for the services rendered. If management monitors the number of and reasons for denials, the practice can intervene and prevent denials from occurring in the future.

Benchmarks include the number of claims denied as a percentage of the total submitted, as well as the reasons for those denials. Tracking the reasons can be done manually through tallying the denials received on the explanations of benefits (EOB) received from the payers, or automated through the establishment and utilization of denial codes during the payment posting process.

Example:

Reason for Denial	Number	Percentage
Applied to deductible	18	11.61%
Patient not eligible	21	13.55%
Noncovered services	36	23.23%
Copayment/coinsurance	17	10.97%
Invalid/incomplete authorization	4	2.58%
Invalid/incomplete information (noncoding)	5	3.22%
Coding	48	30.97%
Other	6	3.87%
Total Front End	**155**	**100.00%**
Info requested from patient	8	4.60%
Physician not in network	42	24.14%
Duplicate	62	35.63%
Claim pending	9	5.17%
Timely filing	37	21.26%
Other	16	9.20%
Total Back End	**174**	**100.00%**
Other/unknown (repricing)	14	60.87%
System errors	9	39.13%
Total other	**23**	**100.00%**
Grand Total	**352**	**100.00%**

By identifying problem areas, personnel involved in creating the denial can be educated on preventing the denial—and the cost of working it to get paid.

Expenses

Practice expenses are expressed on the financial statement, but the measurement of the practice's ability to convert those expenses into revenue is a critical benchmark used by management.

Overhead Rate

The overhead rate is defined as total operating cost divided by total medical revenue. Standard industry definition is to include all nonprovider expenses as operating expenses. These expenses include, but are not limited to, personnel, facility, supplies, and marketing.

Calculation: $\dfrac{\text{Operating expenses}}{\text{Total medical revenue}}$

Example:

	20X2	20X1
Total operating cost	$34,980,000	$34,048,000
Total medical revenue	$65,230,000	$61,010,000
Overhead rate	53.63%	55.81%

The management of West Side religiously tracks its overhead rate every year, and was pleased to see a decline from the previous year. West Side attributed the decline to the increase in revenue that resulted from the staffing and work redesign, as discussed earlier. However, more revealing data can be found by measuring overhead rates for each of the practice's divisions, which West Side measures every quarter.

Overhead rates vary by specialty. Surgical practices maintain lower staffing expenses (because their support staff in the operating room is employed by the hospital) and higher reimbursement per service. Thus, the overhead rate for surgical practices, which ranges from 40% to 55%, is often lower than for their colleagues in medical specialty (45% to 60%) or primary care practices (55% to 65%). Multispecialty practices, such as West Side, range from 55% to 65%, although large practices have been successful in reducing overhead by several percentage points. For further analysis, each major expense category can be expressed as a percentage of revenue. Ratios can also be developed and monitored for key expense categories, such as occupancy, support staff, and malpractice expenses as a percentage of revenue.

Because support staff costs represent the majority of operating expenses in most practices, the support staff overhead cost, or payroll ratio, is an important indicator to measure and monitor. To calculate, divide the support staff cost by total medical revenue.

Calculation: $\dfrac{\text{Support staff cost}}{\text{Total medical revenue}}$

Example:

	20X2	20X1
Support staff cost	$19,550,000	$18,500,000
Total medical revenue	$65,230,000	$61,010,000
Payroll ratio	29.97%	30.32%

The management of West Side monitored its payroll ratio during its staffing reductions and performance improvement initiative. Its goal was achieved: Invest in less but better staff (at slightly higher levels of income); for every dollar invested in personnel, more revenue should be achieved. The payroll ratio decrease from 30.32% to 29.97% demonstrated their accomplishment.

In addition to the payroll ratio, another important ratio to evaluate support staff management is the employee turnover ratio. That ratio can be measured by the number of employees who have left during a specific period of time versus the total employed. It is industry standard to measure the employee turnover ratio on an annual basis, and to utilize full-time equivalents instead of a head count. A high employee turnover ratio adds material cost to the practice due to the cost of recruiting and training a replacement, as well as the loss of productivity for the position as it is being filled. Finally, high employee turnover can also represent a lack of employee morale and loyalty, which has a negative impact on productivity.

Calculation: $\dfrac{\text{Total FTEs who have left the practice}}{\text{Total FTEs employed by the practice}}$

Example, Division of Pediatrics:

	20X2	20X1
Employee turnover ratio	33.9%	20%

The management of West Side became concerned about its employee turnover in its Division of Pediatrics, which was particularly problematic due to the seemingly positive change in human resources management for the practice. The turnover ratio for the Division of Pediatrics exceeds 33%, which is well above West Side's average of 15%. The turnover represents significant costs to West Side, because they had to recruit, train, and orient more than a third of the Division of Pediatrics staff. Upon further investigation, discussions with employees revealed that the work environment was not positive, despite West Side's human resources initiative. Expectations for job performance and output were not clear, tools and resources to accomplish their jobs were lacking, and supervisors used intimidation as the primary management tactic. West Side management stepped in to improve the situation, and the turnover subsided and the productivity of the division increased by the last quarter of 20X2.

Benchmarking overhead can reveal the practice's ability to turn expenses into investments. It is of note that the ratio can be lowered without reducing any costs. If revenue—which is the denominator—is raised without any change to the operating infrastructure, the overhead rate can be lowered.

Cost Accounting

For a more detailed benchmarking analysis of expenses, management can use cost accounting. Cost accounting provides a methodology to allocate costs to units of work, thus allowing management to determine the relative value of services offered.

Cost is defined as "a resource sacrificed or forgone to achieve a specific objective."[6] Accounting measures costs as monetary amounts. In many situations, determination of a particular cost is easy and straightforward. For example, a practice can determine its legal costs by adding up the various invoices for legal services. Other costs, such as the total cost of providing a particular service to a patient or the cost of sending out a bill, are more difficult to determine and must be computed using various methods of analysis and allocation.

Cost accounting is the process of measuring and reporting both financial and nonfinancial resources incurred to acquire or utilize commodities or services within an organization.

Management can use any measure of work to perform cost accounting, but RVUs offer the most value in understanding practice costs. Because the majority of insurance companies reimburse physicians for services on a per-RVU basis, management can use the cost per RVU to measure the relative value of each contract.

Using total RVUs, as opposed to the work component only, is recommended for cost accounting because the total RVU includes components for physician work, practice expense, and malpractice. All of these factors are important when measuring and comparing practice costs. RVUs can simplify much of the work in practice cost accounting. The fact that these values are based on extensive research of work in a medical practice; embraced by the government, national physician organizations, and many commercial payers as the national standard; and are readily available eliminates the need for practices to compute them. Management can use RVUs to determine the cost of providing a particular service, as follows:

1. Add up all the practice's costs, including provider costs.
2. For each procedure code, multiply the number of procedures performed by the practices by the RVU for that procedure code. Add the amount for all procedure codes to calculate the total RVUs performed by the practice.
3. Divide the total practice costs by the total RVUs to calculate the practice's cost per RVU.

4. For each procedure, multiply the RVU for that procedure code by the practice's cost per RVU to calculate the practice's cost for that procedure.

Example, Division of Otolaryngology, 99213:

Costs	$2,350,000
RVUs	40,000
Cost per RVU	$58.75
RVU for 99213	2.03
Cost per 99213	$119.26

The management of West Side's Division of Otolaryngology calculated its cost per 99213 to be $119.26. This can be measured over time to reveal trends in expenses, as well as to evaluate the reimbursement for procedure codes and relative contribution per payer.

RVUs also can be used to allocate common costs to the different departments in preparing departmental income statements. Although some costs, such as rent, may be best allocated by floor space, and human resources management costs may be best allocated by staff FTEs, RVUs provide a vehicle for allocating other administrative and general practice costs, as follows:

1. Calculate the total RVUs for each department and the total practice RVUs.
2. For each department, compute the percentage of RVUs for that department to the total practice RVUs.
3. Multiply the department RVU percentage by the total allocable overhead amount for the practice to get each department's share of overhead.

Example, West Side has $600,000 of overhead to allocate to its divisions:

	Total Department RVUs	Percentage of Total	Overhead Allocated to Department
Medicine/Surgery	82,000	82.00%	$492,000
Radiology	12,000	12.00%	$72,000
Pathology	6,000	6.00%	$36,000
Total	100,000	100.00%	$600,000

Cost accounting can assist management in understanding and comparing internal costs among specialties and functions, as well as providers. In addition, benchmarking to revenue allows management to understand the extent to which reimbursement is contributing to its profitability—if at all.

Profitability

The net income or profit of a practice is the excess of revenues over operating expenses, as reported on the income statement of the practice. The net income of many practices is negligible if not zero, however, because the income is distributed throughout the fiscal year in income and bonuses to the physicians. Although some money is held as retained earnings, for benchmarking purposes, the profit of a practice is its physicians' income.

Physician Income

The income distributed to physicians reflects the practice's ability to generate and collect revenue for the physicians' services using the infrastructure created and paid for by the practice. Benchmarks for physician income are available from multiple sources, and are reported for starting salaries, as well as by region, percentage of managed-care penetration, practice size, and structure of practice.

In addition to benchmarking income, management should evaluate income as it relates to the work output of the physicians. This ratio of income to work can be defined as income per unit of work, such as work RVUs.

Calculation: $\dfrac{\text{Total funds available for income distribution}}{\text{Total work RVUs produced}}$

Example, Division of Gastroenterology:

Total funds available for income distribution	$1,820,000
Total work RVUs produced	32,270
Income per work RVU	$56.40

The management of West Side's Division of Gastroenterology measured its income per work RVU every year. The ratio helped management determine if the level of income received by the division was within market rates for the amount of work produced, which compares favorably to the industry median of $53.93 for gastroenterology.[7] The ratio was always calculated prior to recruiting, and provided to candidates, to assure new recruits that West Side was providing competitive income for the level of work produced.

If income comparisons reveal a variance from normative data, which ranges from $35 to more than $150 per work RVU,[8] depending on specialty and geographical location, a comparison of the income-to-work ratio is in order. If the physicians' income is lower than the median, but the income-to-work ratio is similar, the physicians

are being compensated appropriately for the work they're performing. If they want to achieve a higher level of income, then they must work harder. However, because the infrastructure in most practices consists primarily of fixed expenses, the incremental work can be disproportionately more profitable.

If the income-to-work ratio is lower than the median, management should evaluate reimbursement for services performed, the service lines offered, and its internal collections processes. If the income-to-work ratio is higher than the median, the physicians are compensated at a higher level than their peers for working the same or less. The latter may be a function of the practice's payer mix and reimbursement levels, the service lines offered, or simply operating a better business.

Breakeven

At some point during the year, the physicians perform reimbursable work that is adequate to cover the cost of the practice's infrastructure. This is the breakeven point, and a breakeven analysis is an important computation for any practice.

In order to perform a breakeven analysis, one must first analyze cost behavior patterns and classify costs as either fixed or variable. A fixed cost remains the same (over a wide range of potential volume) regardless of the activity level. For example, the rent on the practice's building remains constant no matter how many patients the physicians see. A variable cost changes in proportion to the activity level. For example, more patient encounters result in a proportionately higher cost of medical supplies.

To explain the concept, let's assume that West Side hired a new physician in the Division of Geriatrics. Each encounter, the new physician produced an average of $50 in revenue. The variable cost per visit (linen, administrative supplies, and medical supplies used per visit) was calculated at $5. The $5 per visit is based on the total variable costs incurred during the months in review divided by the number of visits during that month. The fixed costs (office rent, insurance premiums, administrative staff salaries, equipment leases, etc.) were $120,000 annually.

The new geriatrician sees 500 patients per month, and the management of West Side wants to know if this is adequate to break even.

- Revenue per visit: $50 per visit
- Total visits: 500 per month
- Total revenue: $25,000 ($50 × 500) per month
- Desired physician income: $12,500 per month (or $150,000 per year)

- Fixed costs: $10,000 per month
- Variable costs: $2,500 ($5 per visit × 500 visits) per month

The total costs that the Division of Geriatrics needs to cover are the fixed costs plus the new physician's income, which together equal $22,500 per month. Because some of the revenue per visit, which is $50, must be used for variable expenses, which are $5 per visit, management can use $45 per visit to allocate toward the desired expense base. This $45 is the "contribution margin" expressed on a unit-of-service basis. The $45 is referred to as "unit contribution margin" because it is the units (i.e., encounter) contribution covering the practice's fixed costs. Management divides the total fixed cost (including income target) of $22,500 by the $45 unit contribution margin, which equals 500 patient visits—the breakeven volume.

With 500 patient visits per month, the new geriatrician covers his current costs, as well as his annual income.

The management of West Side also receives a call from another new physician in the Division of Physical Medicine and Rehabilitation, who maintains an equal amount of infrastructure, but who wants to increase her income from $150,000 to $240,000. Management needs to determine the number of patient visits that this physiatrist needs to meet her stated income goal.

Including her income goal, the fixed expenses for the practice will be $360,000 per year, or $30,000 per month. The variable costs are still $5 per visit. If the reimbursement remains at $50 per visit, the physician has $45 left over to pay for her fixed expenses and income.

To calculate the number of visits the physician needs to see per month, management divides the $30,000 in fixed costs and physician income by $45 and arrives at 667 visits per month.

- Fixed cost ($10,000 per month) + physician income ($20,000 per month) = total fixed cost
- Revenue per visit ($50) – variable expense per visit ($5) = unit contribution margin per visit ($45)
- Fixed expense ($30,000 per month) ÷ the unit contribution margin per visit ($45) = visits needed per month (667)

Management responds to the new physiatrist who desires an income of $240,000: "Without changing the infrastructure or the revenue per visit, you need to see 667 visits per month, or 8,000 per year."

Figure 11-4, the cost-volume-profit (CVP) graph, pictorially describes the relationship among cost, volume, and profit in a practice.

Liquidity

The availability of cash, or near-cash assets, provides a practice with the resources to operate and invest to further its business. The indicator of this availability is liquidity. Liquidity benchmarks are used by bankers and other creditors when evaluating the credit worthiness of a practice desiring a loan.

The liquidity of the practice is affected by the economy and market, as well as internal operations. If, for example, the practice experiences a time period in which its payer mix shifts from a lucrative payer to patients without

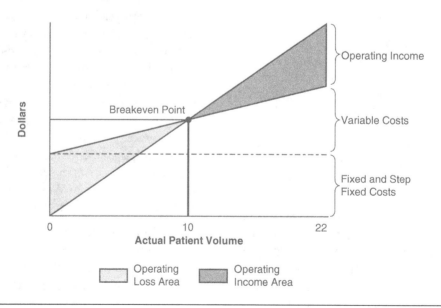

Figure 11-4 Cost-volume-profit (CVP).

insurance, its assets will decrease and its liquidity will fall. Liquid resources provide a practice with the financial flexibility to operate as an ongoing business concern.

The factor of time is important in measuring liquidity. The practice may be able to meet its financial obligations in 2 years, but not tomorrow. Thus, the benchmarks for liquidity include short-term and long-term measurements.

The short-term ratios—current ratio and quick ratio—assess a practice's ability to meet its current financial obligations. The long-term ratios—long-term debt ratio and debt–equity ratio—evaluate a practice's ability to meet its financial responsibilities for interest and principal payment on its maturing long-term debt. In sum, the current and quick ratios measure short-term liquidity, and the long-term debt and debt–equity ratios measure long-term liquidity.

Current Ratio

A measure of short-term liquidity, the current ratio is the sum of current assets divided by the sum of current liabilities. Current assets are those available within 1 year of the balance sheet date; current liabilities are obligations requiring cash in that same period.

Calculation: $\dfrac{\text{Current assets}}{\text{Current liabilities}}$

Example:

	20X2	20X1
Current assets	$7,908,000	$6,863,000
Current liabilities	$3,569,000	$3,136,000
Current ratio	2.22	2.19

Quick Ratio

Another measure of short-term liquidity, the quick ratio includes only the fraction of current assets that a practice can quickly convert to cash. The quick ratio, which is also referred to as the "acid test ratio," offers a summary of the practice's financial position at a given point in time. The numerator includes cash, marketable securities, and A/R; the denominator remains current liabilities.

Calculation: $\dfrac{\text{Cash, marketable securities, A/R}}{\text{Current liabilities}}$

Example:

	20X2	20X1
Cash, marketable securities, and A/R	$7,784,000	$6,756,000
Current liabilities	$3,569,000	$3,136,000
Quick ratio	2.18	2.15

It is preferable for the current and quick ratios to be at or greater than 1; as in the examples, however, the ratios can be misleading. In a poor economy, a practice may use its cash to pay its current liabilities, thereby increasing the ratio. A decrease in the ratio may accompany an improving economy as the practice conserves assets by delaying payment of current liabilities. Management can delay purchases until near the end of a financial term to manipulate the current ratio.

In sum, current and quick ratios are an important financial benchmark to measure short-term liquidity, but should be accompanied by other indicators prior to any conclusion being made about the practice's operations.

Long-Term Debt Ratio

The long-term debt ratio is the total long-term debt divided by the sum of total long-term debt and stockholders' equity.

Calculation: $\dfrac{\text{Long-term debt}}{\text{Long-term debt and stockholders' equity}}$

Example:

	20X2	20X1
Long-term debt	$3,371,000	$4,290,000
Long-term debt and stockholders' equity	$10,482,000	$10,993,000
Long-term debt ratio	0.32	0.39

Debt–Equity Ratio

Another commonly reported indicator is the debt–equity ratio. This ratio is reported by dividing total liabilities (current and noncurrent) by total equities (total liabilities and stockholders' equity).

Calculation: $\dfrac{\text{Total liabilities}}{\text{Total liabilities and stockholders' equity}}$

Example:

	20X2	20X1
Total liabilities	$6,940,000	$7,426,000
Total liabilities and stockholders' equity	$14,051,000	$14,129,000
Debt–equity ratio	0.49	0.53

In general, the lower the ratios, the greater the likelihood that the practice will be able to meet its debt payments in the future. Following the initial start-up period, a practice should maintain stable earnings and cash flow. Thus, a mature practice may carry a high debt ratio that is safe.

It is of note that financial analysts use different variations and definitions of the liquidity indicators. It is important for management to agree upon and use a consistent definition.

All of the liquidity ratios depend on the accuracy of the data reported on the financial statements. None can be utilized alone to draw a conclusion about the practice as a business; they should be used as indicators to draw management's attention to investigate certain aspects of the business. When comparing ratios across time, management should account for changing conditions, such as economic and market changes, or internal changes such as the retirement of a physician.

When applying for a loan or otherwise evaluating a practice, bankers analyzing a practice's liquidity often request additional detailed information about the practice's receivables, given its importance to the revenue stream. Because A/R is not included on a cash basis financial statement, bankers generally add an A/R amount adjusted to discount for contractual and noncontractual allowances in performing these analyses. Bankers generally realize that practices pay out all or most of their earnings in compensation to physicians and thus have low net worth per the financial statements. However, a heavily indebted practice is a concern. To mitigate their risk, bankers also look at the historic earnings by the physicians and the individual physicians' creditworthiness.

■ Operational Benchmarks

Benchmarks regarding the operations of a practice can assist management with complex decisions regarding provider, staff, and space allocations, as well as patient access and service. Benchmarks include supply and demand indicators, space, and customer satisfaction.

Supply and Demand

Finding and maintaining a balance of provider supply and patient demand is important to managing an efficient and service-oriented practice. If supply exceeds demand, the volume of patients seen may not produce enough revenue to cover the infrastructure. If demand exceeds supply, the practice erects barriers to access. These barriers create inefficiency and diminishing margins as staff work daily to deflect patient demand.

In order to understand and benchmark supply and demand, management should focus on access indicators. The first set of indicators is appointment availability. The time to next available established patient appointment and the time to next new patient appointment should be tracked and monitored (see **Figure 11-5**). Management should take into consideration any contractual obligations (e.g., managed-care contracts may require same-day access for their beneficiaries), as well as competitors (e.g., the appointment availability of a similar specialist in the same market).

Calculation: Time to next available new patient appointment, as measured in calendar days

Calculation: Time to next available established patient appointment, as measured in calendar days

The management of West Side evaluated the time to next available appointments for each of its divisions. Access for new and established patients was monitored closely, because West Side operates in a highly competitive market. If access exceeded 30 days in any division, management met with the division administrator to discuss plans to improve access. Discussions were held around improving efficiency and productivity, hiring a new provider, and decreasing patient demand by evaluating payer contracts with low reimbursement.

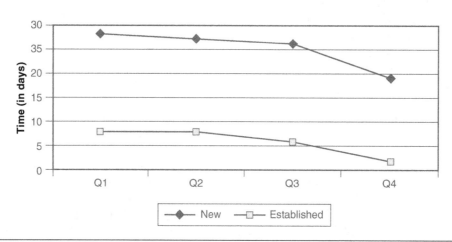

Figure 11-5 Example, West Side: Time to next available appointment by patient type.

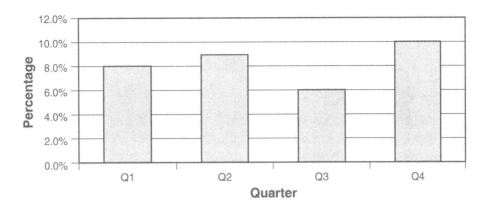

Figure 11-6 Example, West Side: Appointment no-show rate.

If these indicators are longer than a patient is willing to wait because of his or her own need for care, or access to a competitor, the patient is more likely to fail to present for a scheduled appointment. The appointment no-show rate is defined as the number of patients who did not present for their scheduled appointment divided by the total number scheduled. Because no-shows represent lost revenue, without any contribution to overhead, they should be monitored closely, as shown in **Figure 11-6**.

$$\text{Calculation: } \frac{\text{Appointment no-shows}}{\text{Total scheduled appointments}}$$

West Side monitored its appointment no-show rate for each of its divisions to ensure that increases in no-shows were addressed immediately. For example, the Division of Ophthalmology experienced a no-show rate of 15% during one quarter. Upon further analysis, it was discovered the division had also experienced a 2-month wait for patient appointments. By placing telephone calls to patients who had not presented for their appointments, the division realized that these patients had moved their care to a competitor. The issue was addressed immediately by improving access through opening early morning office hours, hiring a mid-level provider, and beginning the search for a new ophthalmologist.

Closely related to no-shows are appointment cancellations. Although cancellations are more manageable, if unfilled they have the same financial impact as do no-shows. Thus, management should monitor the number of cancellations that convert to appointments versus remaining unfilled. The rate is called the cancellation conversion rate (see **Figure 11-7**).

$$\text{Calculation: } \frac{\text{Cancellations converted to appointments}}{\text{Total cancellations}}$$

The management of West Side monitored its cancellation conversion rate by division. Management expected the rate to be 100%. When the Division of Rheumatology dipped to 77% during Q2, management stepped in for an evaluation. It was discovered that the division's appointment scheduler was not converting any cancellations that occurred after 2 PM, at the request of a physician. Management intervened, and discussions were held with the new physician about productivity expectations and inappropriate personnel management. Improvements were being made, and by the end of Q4, the rate was resuming to its previous levels.

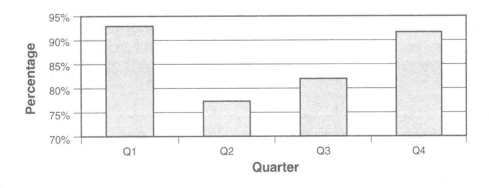

Figure 11-7 Example, Division of Rheumatology, West Side: Cancellation conversion rate.

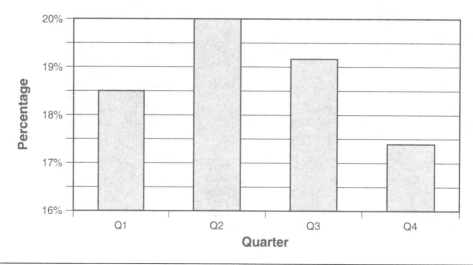

Figure 11-8 Example, Division of Neurosurgery, West Side: New patient appointments as a percentage of total appointments.

Another access indicator is new patient appointments as a percentage of total appointments, as shown in **Figure 11-8**. The percentage should be maintained or increased to ensure a practice's growth.

$$\text{Calculation:} \quad \frac{\text{New patient appointments}}{\text{Total scheduled appointments}}$$

The management of West Side monitored its new patient appointments as a percentage of its total appointments for each division. The statistic was particularly important for its surgical divisions. The Division of Neurosurgery was surprised to see its new patient appointment rate drop in Q4. Management evaluated the situation, and determined that a large group of community orthopedic surgeons who had traditionally been referring patients with spine problems to West Side had hired its own spine surgeon. Immediate effort was made to meet with the group to discuss the division's quality of care and service, and a referring physician campaign was commenced for referring physicians. The drop in referrals prompted the Division of Neurosurgery to initiate a 24-hour turnaround for referring physician correspondence, as well as a consult nurse who facilitated all referrals immediately. Referring physicians responded positively to the division's performance improvement, and the percentage of new patient appointments rose.

A final indicator for all practices is the size of the patient panel being actively managed. Active patient panel is defined as the number of unique patient account numbers seen within the last 2 to 3 years, depending on specialty. If a patient was seen four times in the last 2 years, that patient would still count as one. Of course, when a

physician starts a practice, the panel is zero. As the practice grows, so does the panel. Monitoring the panel size, as well as the access indicators, is important to determine if and when demand exceeds supply. At the point that patient demand exceeds supply, management needs to decide to recruit another physician or physician extender, manipulate demand by closing all or some of the practice, and/or increase the efficiency of the practice.

Benchmarking a ratio of productivity (discussed previously) to appointment access can assist management in deciding if efficiency is the concern (see **Figure 11-9**). Physicians in the lower-left quadrant, such as Physician A, should be new physicians. If they have been in practice for several years, yet continue to produce at low levels

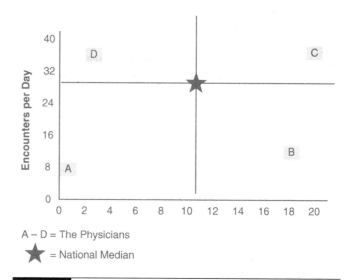

A – D = The Physicians

★ = National Median

Figure 11-9 Example, Division of Allergy, West Side: Time to next available new patient appointment.

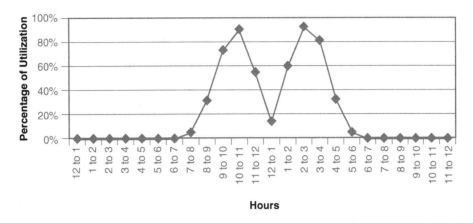

Figure 11-10 Example, Division of Urology, West Side: Space utilization by hour of day.

despite the fact that patients can enjoy fast access, this reveals that patient demand may be a concern. In other words, there are simply not enough patients for this established physician to render medical services. Physicians in the lower-right quadrant, such as Physician B, reveal a problem. These physicians are low producers with limited appointment availability. The appointment availability reveals that they are unwilling or unable to accommodate additional patient demand, yet are not producing at the level of their peers. Physicians in the upper-left quadrant, such as Physician D, reveal the ideal situation—high productivity, but ease of access. Physicians in the upper-right quadrant, such as Physician C, have likely switched to deflecting demand. Already producing at higher levels than their peers, it is important to discuss limiting access or increasing the supply.

West Side's Division of Allergy determined that the average of all of its physicians plotted in the upper-right quadrant. West Side intervened to not renew a contract with a payer with fees that were lower than the division's

cost per RVU, and began recruiting a mid-level provider to assist with access for patients with acute clinical needs.

Space

A key determinant of efficiency is the amount of functional space in which to practice, as well as how it is utilized. Management can benchmark the number of exam and procedure rooms, as well as the functional square footage.

Having the space is important, but utilizing it is a better operational indicator. Utilization of the practice's space capacity can be measured in different time frames: hour of the day, day of the week, and month of the year. Management can gather and plot data for the average volume of encounters during each of these time frames.

When the Division of Urology approached the management of West Side with a request to move to new space, citing space constraints in its existing office, management commenced a capacity study to evaluate the urology clinic's volume by hour of the day, day of the week, and month of the year, as shown in **Figures 11-10**, **11-11**, and **11-12**.

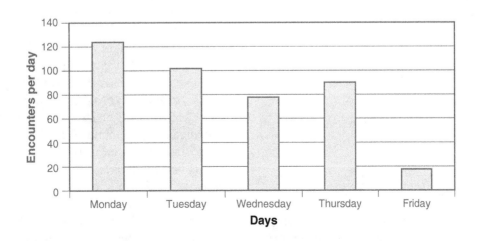

Figure 11-11 Example, Division of Urology, West Side: Space utilization by day of week.

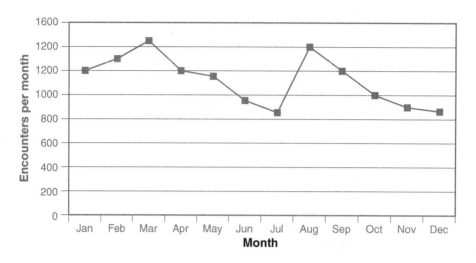

Figure 11-12 Example: Space utilization by month office encounters.

When West Side presented the analysis to the Division of Urology, it was determined that a new space—with a cost exceeding $500,000—was not needed. The division responded by changing its office hours to 7 AM to 7 PM, moving several physicians to Friday clinics (after coordinating operating room schedules with the local hospital), and offering staff the opportunity to work four 10-hour days. With these changes, the space "problem" resolved itself immediately.

Because most practices pay for and can utilize their space 24 hours a day, 7 days a week, benchmarking utilization as a percentage of capacity reveals opportunities for improvement. Management can alter demand through changes in the appointment schedule or scheduling processes, or shift physician and staff resource allocation to improve the utilization of the existing space.

In addition to the utilization of space, management can evaluate productivity according to space. An excellent benchmark is the number of total RVUs produced per square foot.

$$\text{Calculation: } \frac{\text{Total RVUs}}{\text{Total square feet}}$$

Example, Division of Urology, West Side:

	20X2	20X1
Total RVUs	26,895	24,689
Square feet	7,500	7,500
Total RVUs per square foot	3.59	3.29

A year after West Side's Division of Urology implemented its new space utilization plan, its productivity per square foot had increased significantly. By using its space more wisely, the division was able to improve its revenue, without increasing its infrastructure costs.

Customer Satisfaction

A practice has a wide variety of customers, including patients and referring physicians. Benchmarking their level of satisfaction with the practice is an important measurement of the service, access, convenience, and operations that the practice is offering.

Patient satisfaction surveys can be used either for specific projects, such as a performance improvement initiative regarding the telephones, or distributed and measured on a periodic basis. Maintaining consistent questions can prove beneficial to measuring improvement over time.

In addition to patient satisfaction, specialists who rely on other physicians to refer patients should monitor referring physician satisfaction. Factors should include quality of care, communication, access, and patient satisfaction. Again, using consistent questions allows management to monitor progress.

The management of West Side uses a patient satisfaction survey that is consistent for all of its divisions. Data are summarized and reported to each division every quarter. In addition to a practice questionnaire, West Side always develops a satisfaction survey specific to any performance improvement initiatives that it conducts. The survey is distributed to patients and/or referring physicians before, during, and after the initiative is implemented in order to track its success.

Satisfaction surveys reflect the voice of the customer. Practices should use surveys to ensure that their operation is meeting the needs of their patients and referring physicians.

■ Conclusion

In this chapter, a multitude of benchmarks is presented for the finances and operations of a medical practice. Each benchmark has value, but it is important to recognize that conclusions cannot be drawn by a single indicator. Indeed, the value of benchmarking is to monitor the finances and operations of the practice by measuring a range of indicators. Management must decide on benchmarks that have comparability, relevance, predictability, and consistency over time.

The benchmarks chosen may depend on the specialty and size of the practice. For example, the surgery yield is a critical indicator of revenue for a surgical practice, but has little value to a primary care practice. Perhaps the most important consideration in choosing benchmarks to measure and monitor is that management must be able to take action. Utilizing indicators that are not actionable derives no value for the practice.

The following is a sample dashboard of benchmarks:

Adjusted collection rate

Reimbursement as a percentage of RBRVS

Work RVUs per FTE physician

Total RVUs per FTE mid-level provider

Total RVUs per FTE support staff

Days receivables outstanding

Percentage of total A/R over 120 days outstanding

Bad debt ratio

Overhead rate

Payroll ratio

Cost per total RVU

Income per work RVU

Time to next available appointment

No-show rate

New patients as a percentage of total appointments

Benchmarking is an important tool for management to monitor and analyze its finances and operations. By measuring data across time, internally among different people and processes, as well as against external normative data, the management of a practice can develop a clear road map for process improvement and achievement of best practice.

References
1. Medical Group Management Association. Bad debts due to fee-for-service activity includes accounts assigned to collection agencies. In: *Cost survey: 2011 guide to the questionnaire.* Englewood, CO: Medical Group Management Association.
2. Glass KP. *RVUs: applications for medical practice success* (2nd ed.). Englewood, CO: Medical Group Management Association; 2008.
3. Medical Group Management Association. Amounts owed to the practice by patients, third-party payers, employer groups and unions for fee-for-service activities before adjustments for anticipated payment reductions, allowances for adjustments or bad debts. In: *Cost survey: 2011 guide to the questionnaire.* Englewood, CO: Medical Group Management Association.
4. Medical Group Management Association. Days of gross fee-for-service charges in accounts receivable equals total A/R divided by the multiplication of gross charges times 1/365. In: *Cost survey for multispecialty practices: 2011 report based on 2010 data.* Englewood, CO: Medical Group Management Association.
5. Horngren CT, Datar SM, Foster G. *Cost accounting: a managerial emphasis.* Upper Saddle River, NJ: Prentice Hall; 2003.
6. Centers for Medicaid and Medicaid Services. 2011 non-facility total relative value unit, national. Accessed October 2, 2011, at https://www.cms.gov/PhysicianFeeSched/
7. Medical Group Management Association. *Physician compensation and production survey: 2011 report based on 2010 data.* Englewood, CO: Medical Group Management Association.
8. Medical Group Management Association. *Physician compensation and production survey: 2011 report based on 2010 data.* Englewood, CO: Medical Group Management Association.

■ Acknowledgments

My sincere appreciation to Lee Ann Webster, who provided guidance and support for this chapter.

Health Information Technology for Medical Group Practices

Margret Amatayakul, MBA, RHIA, CHPS, CPHIT,
CPEHR, CPHIE, FHIMSS

Use of information technology in healthcare is not new. Many practices, especially large ones, have used computers for business applications, such as general ledger, payroll, and accounts payable, for a long time. However, despite the fact that the concept of the electronic health record (EHR) will be 50 years old when Medicare incentives end and reimbursement sanctions begin to be imposed in 2015 for those not making meaningful use of certified EHR technology,[1] health information technology (HIT) is not as widely deployed for clinical purposes and represents a much more significant undertaking than traditional "back office" applications. Whether considering HIT in general (referring to use of computers for any application unique to healthcare, such as billing, patient scheduling, medical records, telemedicine, or health information exchange) or EHR in particular, there are important strategies for deploying these projects successfully.

Many practices recognize that the federal government's incentives, and even sanctions, under the American Recovery and Reinvestment Act (ARRA) Health Information Technology for Economic and Clinical Health (HITECH),[1] are only a temporary and partial reason for taking on the transformative change required to achieve

success with HIT. It is no mistake that the real wake-up call for building a better health *system* was the Institute of Medicine (IOM) report *To Err Is Human*,[2] which focused the nation's attention on patient safety and quality of care—using, among other system elements, HIT.

This chapter is intended to guide the medium to large, often multispecialty and/or multisite, and potentially academic-based, medical group practice through assessing readiness, planning, acquiring, implementing, maintaining, and optimizing use of HIT in general and EHR in particular. It offers tools and techniques for whatever stage a practice is in with respect to HIT and EHR.

■ Scope

Most practices identify cost—including being capital poor and concerns for loss of productivity—as the most significant barrier to HIT. As a result, the federal government has sought to incentivize meaningful use of EHR, demonstrate best practices, increase the HIT workforce, and provide consultative support (although primarily for small, primary care practices) to promote adoption specifically of EHR. Yet financial incentives are not the only driver for adoption of HIT today. Recognizing national, organizational, and personal restraining forces and driving forces for HIT can be a useful exercise in assessing a practice's readiness for EHR and other HIT. Then, setting in motion critical success factors can help ensure that whatever the scope of the EHR project or wherever a practice may be on its HIT migration path, it will have a solid chance for achieving value.

Drivers for Adoption of Health Information Technology

Product maturity has held many back from acquiring HIT. It is much more difficult to develop EHRs than information systems for most other industries because EHRs are not about "crunching numbers." In fact, they are not even about automating paper, but rather are about enhancing the utility of health information in patient care.[3] Change, most often in workflow, is a second major barrier. Many who approach adoption of EHR do not fully appreciate the level of change needed to take full advantage of HIT. Robert McDonald, a physician champion in the process of selecting an EHR, observed in a conversation that "my colleagues understand EHR at the intellectual level, but they don't 'get it' at the intestinal level." Workflow certainly includes the sequence of steps taken to pull a chart and record patient care events. More importantly, workflow is about using the system's information processing capabilities to aid in differential diagnosis, selecting an appropriate drug, remembering to offer preventive care services, or making other such decisions. These are mental processes that often cannot be visualized, but are a significant change for people when first using an EHR.

It is the clinical transformation that a mature product affords that leads to perhaps the biggest reason why most providers will not return to paper records after acquiring an EHR. Many note that on a day-to-day basis, patient safety and quality of care are things one takes for granted—until an event occurs where the EHR truly makes a difference. Such anecdotes are only now beginning to be quantified, but they are real and powerful motivators. Administrative simplification is a second strong force that underlies adoption of EHR. Administrative simplification embodies everything from helping address reimbursement complexity to reducing everyday hassles of lost charts or missing labs.

Several other driving and restraining forces are illustrated in **Figure 12-1**. EHR has become a competitive advantage in certain markets. A series of television ads for an integrated delivery network tells viewers that "You're empowered by the nation's most advanced electronic medical records systems."[4] The movement toward patient-centered medical homes (PCMHs) and accountable care organizations (ACOs) created under the Patient Protection and Affordable Care Act of 2010 depend on HIT to exchange information across the continuum of care. Managing in a value-based purchasing environment will depend not only on productivity improvements that can accrue from EHRs if implemented properly, but on the ability to share data across the continuum of care[5,6] and to measure, report on, and improve upon the quality of care delivered in an organization.[7,8] It is often said, "You can't manage what you can't measure." Without tools to help track quality of care, a practice can lack direction in where it needs to focus its improvement efforts. When an ACO puts a practice at risk for not assuring quality care, a practice must have the tools to help every step of the way. In addition, revenue enhancement and cost savings are possible after the learning curve has been mastered, especially for large practices.

Additional restraining forces include concerns about vendor viability, access to technology-savvy staff, and potential patient reactions. Although the legality of an EHR has been questioned in the past, it is much less of an issue currently; however, liability issues surrounding reliance on clinical decision support are a growing concern.

DRIVING FORCES	RESTRAINING FORCES
Incentives/Sanctions	Cost/Productivity
Patient Safety	Product Maturity
Administrative Simplification	Change
Competitive Advantage	Vendor Viability
PCMH/ACO	Tech-Savvy Staff
Revenue Enhancements	Patient Reactions
Cost Savings	Legal and Liability

Figure 12-1 Forces impacting adoption of HIT.

Source: Reprinted with permission, © Margret\A Counseling, LLC.

Yet the root cause of these concerns is almost always demonstrated to be incomplete or poor implementation of the EHR. In these instances, workflow and process redesign are insufficiently or not at all addressed, often leading to partial implementations, which have been found to be worse than no implementation.[9–11]

Critical Success Factors for Health Information Technology

Just as there are the five rights of medication administration—right patient, right drug, right dose, right route, and right time—there are also five rights for HIT success and five rights associated with effective patient care that should be supported by an EHR.

The five rights for HIT success are right hardware, right software, right people, right policies, and right processes.[12] HIT is obviously about *right hardware* and *right software*, but many believe the 80/20 rule applies. The right hardware and software probably only contribute about 20% to successful HIT use. So long as the software acquired is mainstream and meets user requirements and the hardware reflects what is optimally needed to run the software, the remaining 80% of a successful adoption of HIT relates to people, policies, and processes. This is not to suggest that clear articulation of user requirements or acquisition of optimal technology is easy. It is just that there are now sufficient numbers of products from which to choose that these steps are often easier than addressing more internally facing issues. Dr. Adler similarly describes the three T's—team, tactics, and technology—needed for success.[13]

Right people include the right practice leadership, physician champions, and project manager; involvement by all stakeholders (providers, nursing staff, administrative and IT staff); and vendor support staff working as a team. *Right policies*, which may be formal or informal directions that guide decision making in the face of uncertainty, include the ability to manage change, set expectations and goals, communicate effectively, and plan thoroughly. When asked what they would do differently if they could, many who have implemented HIT cite the need for more upfront planning and attention to the human and organizational aspects of HIT. Adler notes that "Dysfunctional organizations are likely to have dysfunctional [EHR] implementations. Excellent communication, clear lines of authority, and an explicit decision-making process promote success."[13] Finally, *right processes* are the tactical elements that define the five rights that an EHR should support for effective patient care. As first described by Dr. Kremsdorf, these rights are right clinical data, right presentation, right decisions, right work processes, and right outcomes.[14]

Right clinical data refers not only to the need for all applicable data to be available, but also that the data are collected accurately by the right person, at the right time, and in the right form and format. Right data collection includes utilizing both patients or their caregivers and staff at the appropriate level of their credential to support data entry. For instance, computer-acquired patient histories capture data at the right time—when patients have access to their medicine cabinet or when the pain occurs. Right form and format include the need for a robust clinical vocabulary, mapped to applicable code sets for further use. For example, a proprietary vocabulary may be more user-friendly, but because the meaningful use incentives require the problem list to be standardized and encoded using the *International Classification of Diseases*, 9th revision, Clinical Modification (ICD-9-CM) or SNOMED-CT,[1] the proprietary vocabulary must be mapped to either or both of these standardized vocabularies. (Other standard vocabularies for EHRs include the Logical Observations Identifiers Names and Codes [LOINC] for laboratory results and other observational data,[15] and RxNorm,[16] which provides normalized names for clinical drugs and links to drug vocabularies commonly used in pharmacy management and drug interaction software, including First Databank, Micromedex, MediSpan, Gold Standard Alchemy, and Multum.)

Right presentation goes hand-in-hand with right clinical data. For computers to process data, such as for a drug-allergy alert, the data must be structured. But structured data are not necessarily user-friendly. Free text must be permitted to help tell the patient story.[a] The IOM observes that a key capability of an EHR system is enabling structured data to be reformatted into narrative information, and narrative information converted to structured data (via natural language processing).[17] Right presentation includes data collection templates that are easy to navigate and context-sensitive, following a logic pattern that varies with user and patient needs. Right presentation also refers to how and when data are displayed to the user. It does little good for a clinician to be presented with a reminder when he or she opens the chart that the patient presenting with upper respiratory infection is due for colon cancer screening; a better time might be when documenting the patient's assessment and plan and the

---

a. See the Health Story Project at http://www.healthstory.com or the HL7Wiki that describes data standards for the flow of information between common types of healthcare documents and EHRS at http://wiki.hl7.org/index.php?title=Health_Story:_Integrating_Narrative_Notes_and_the_EHR_(formerly_CDA4CDT).

patient is more amenable to agreeing to such preventive care services.

Right decisions are computational processes performed on the right data and presented in the right manner to support right processes and ultimately achieve right outcomes. Kremsdorf observes that

> Clinical medicine is inherently challenging due to the complexity of the human body and how it responds to disease. Our understanding of illnesses and what is optimal diagnosis and therapy is continually changing, and doing so faster than ever. Even so, in spite of all the sophisticated testing now used, clinical decisions are fundamentally only considered judgments, weighing an array of facts and hunches.[14]

In researching computational technology for effective healthcare, the National Research Council observes that

> Persistent problems [in healthcare] do not reflect incompetence on the part of health care professionals—rather, they are a consequence of the inherent intellectual complexity of health care taken as a whole and a medical care environment that has not been adequately structured to help clinicians avoid mistakes or to systematically improve their decision making and practice.[11]

Kremsdorf concludes that "computer-based tools can organize information to reflect advances in understanding and present the best protocols to optimize care."[14]

Right processes are the manifestation of right decisions being implemented correctly. Classic business process improvement has as its goals to decrease rework, lower defect rates, eliminate waste, reduce number of steps, shorten cycle time/response time, lower cost, improve quality, enhance customer service and satisfaction, and so on. These are all laudable, and most apply to improving the healthcare value proposition through use of EHR. Right processes, however,

are more fundamental. As noted earlier, processes are often not visible. Right processes not only address changes in medication refilling, telephone messaging, patient check-in, test resulting, referrals, and the like, but also include recognizing the value of information and knowledge in direct medical practice.[18] There are ways to more rapidly get answers to questions[19] while potentially valuing a slower EHR process that saves time downstream.[13]

Right outcomes are obviously the purpose of adopting EHR. Because of the fragmented nature of healthcare today, it is very difficult to determine whether there have been right outcomes for patients. EHRs not only will support processes that help assure right outcomes, but also make quality measurement, reporting, and improvement more feasible.

Scope of Health Information Technology

Health information technology (HIT) is a broad concept of applying information technology to healthcare. Although the focus currently is on EHR, which can be considered a subset of HIT, EHR might be best viewed as a convening process in which information from multiple sources (1) is brought together at the point of care to provide clinical decision support, (2) provides the ability to capture and query information relevant to healthcare quality, and (3) enables exchange of health information with other providers.

The terms "electronic medical record" and "electronic health record" sometimes are used synonymously. In 2008, however, the federal government commissioned the National Alliance for Health Information Technology (NAHIT) to reach industry consensus on definitions for these terms,[20] which are provided in **Figure 12-2**. NAHIT also provided a definition of personal health record (PHR), which can be integrated with, or completely separate from, an EHR.

The functions to be performed by an EHR, although becoming more standardized, are still open to interpretation.

Electronic Medical Record	Electronic Health Record	Personal Health Record
An electronic record of health-related information on an individual that can be created, gathered, managed, and consulted by authorized clinicians and staff within one healthcare organization.	An electronic record of health-related information on an individual that **conforms to nationally recognized interoperability standards** and that can be created, managed, and consulted by authorized clinicians and staff **across more than one healthcare organization**.	An electronic record of health-related information on an individual that conforms to nationally recognized interoperability standards and **that can be drawn from multiple sources while being managed, shared, and controlled by the individual**.

Figure 12-2 Definitions of EMR, EHR, and PHR

Source: National Alliance for Health Information Technology. 2008. Defining key health information technology terms.

In its 2003 *Letter Report on Key Capabilities of an Electronic Health Record System*, the IOM identified eight key capabilities for EHR[17]:

1. Health information and data
2. Results management
3. Order entry/management
4. Decision support
5. Electronic communication and connectivity
6. Patient support
7. Administrative processes
8. Reporting and population health management

The IOM's *Letter Report* formed the basis for the development of an EHR System Functional Model by Health Level Seven (HL7).[21] HL7 is the predominant organization that creates standard protocols for exchange of health information across clinical applications. (The American National Standards Institute [ANSI] Accredited Standards Committee [ASC] X12 creates standard protocols for exchange of financial and administrative data for claims, eligibility verification, electronic remittance advice, and the like. The National Council for Prescription Drug Programs [NCPDP] creates standard protocols for retail pharmacy applications, including electronic prescribing. Digital Imaging and Communications in Medicine [DICOM] produces standards to exchange digital x-rays and other images.) When the Certification Commission for Health Information Technology (CCHIT) first formed, it used the HL7 EHR System Functional Model and other applicable standards in developing its extensive list of criteria for EHR product certification.[22]

Most recently, the federal government created standards, implementation specifications, and criteria for which EHR technology must be certified in order for providers to earn incentives.[23] These drew from the standards work already cited. Note, however, that the regulations governing product certification indicate that the certification criteria represent the minimum capabilities EHR technology needs to include.[24] This does not preclude EHR developers from including additional capabilities that are not required for purposes of certification, and organizations—whether or not they are recognized as Office of the National Coordinator-Authorized Testing and Certification Bodies (ONC-ATCB)—are free to develop additional, voluntary certifications to reflect such enhanced criteria. However, the minimum criteria include functions, such as the ability to automatically generate a clinical summary and report quality measures, that have not previously been included in most EHR offerings.

Typically, HIT applications that are not considered a part of an EHR used in an ambulatory setting, but that may complement—and even be integrated with—an EHR, include the following elements:

- Practice management system (PMS)
- Document imaging and management system (DIMS) or electronic document management system (EDMS)
- Personal health record (PHR)
- Health information exchange (HIE) applications that provide support for the exchange of information across multiple participants
- Ancillary systems, such as laboratory information systems (LISs), radiology information systems (RISs), or picture archiving and communication systems (PACSs)
- Medical devices, or "smart peripherals," that collect information
- Utilities, such as clinical decision support beyond that found within an EHR application
- Registries for collection and processing of a predefined data set, such as a tumor registry, a diabetes registry, and many others
- Clinical data warehouse (a relational database optimized for online analytical processing)

■ Planning for Health Information Technology

Planning is a process of creating and maintaining the steps necessary to achieve a goal. Although planning is considered a fundamental property of intelligent behavior, the terms "plan," "step," and "goal" associated therein are often considered akin to "four-letter words" by many providers. And unfortunately, because the timeline for adopting EHR to achieve the meaningful use incentives is short, many who might otherwise have considered planning will find the need to rapidly acquire EHR is a good excuse not to plan. But according to those who have previously implemented HIT, planning is an essential step. It does not need to take a long time, but it is needed to initiate the change management process vital to success.

Planning for HIT should include envisioning what life will be like with an EHR, goal setting, and readiness assessment. For large practices, planning may entail compiling a migration path, or roadmap, that sets out the sequence of HIT applications to be implemented. Planning also requires identifying and organizing the team of people to work on the HIT project(s) and to provide for ongoing maintenance of the HIT program.

Visioning and Goal Setting

Visioning generates common goals, offers a possibility for fundamental change, gives people a sense of control, and generates creative thinking and passion.[25] Although it is often used in improving communities, many have found a visioning exercise useful for building a community of passionate EHR users. David Blumenthal, MD, National Coordinator for Health Information Technology from 2009 to 2011, observed the following in discussing EHR:

> It's not the technology that's important, but its effect. Meaningful use is not a technology project, but a change management project. Components of meaningful use include sociology, psychology, behavior change, and the mobilization of levers to change complex systems and improve their performance.[26]

A good visioning exercise is for a practice to reflect on one of its worst days in the life of the practice. As the group considers what happened, they should then think about how that day might have been different with an EHR. As the group envisions a better day, they can think about what its members might say to the people they encounter (e.g., a professional colleague, a retired member of the practice, a patient, a government official, a representative of a business in the community). Group members can write these statements down and comment on them. At that point, the practice is ready to craft a common vision statement. It is important to consider all points of view—from a file clerk who pulls charts to the chief medical officer as well as everyone in between who may ultimately be touched by an EHR, including billing staff, nursing staff, trainees, practice administrators, and physicians. Everyone can relate to whatever their "pain points" were that day, and everyone needs to understand their place in the new world with EHR.[27]

From that visioning exercise, more specific goal statements should arise. Initially, goals will be stated as generalities: improve patient care, reduce wait time, avoid medication errors, reduce risk and improve revenue, and so on. Ultimately, however, goal statements need to be specific, measureable, achievable, realistic, and time-based (i.e., SMART). For example: "Using templates and being guided by one-on-one end user support, we want to reduce provider transcription by 50% within 1 year of adopting EHR and by 85% within 2 years of adopting EHR to ensure structured data for earning meaningful use (MU) incentives and to reduce organizational expense."
Table 12-1 provides a structure to help a practice construct its goals.

Table 12-1 Writing SMART Goals

Goal Elements	Sample Scenario	A Practice's Example
Specific	Reduce provider transcription to ensure structured data for earning MU incentives and reduce organizational expense	
Measurable	by 50%	by 85%
Achievable	using templates	
Realistic	with one-on-one end user support	
Time-based	by Yr 1	by Yr 2

Source: Reprinted with permission. Health IT Certification, LLC.

One issue with setting SMART goals is that many healthcare organizations are reluctant to commit to specific metrics. It will be necessary to reassure all stakeholders that, although goals are important, they are not cast in concrete. The organization needs to be committed to achieving its goals and must help everyone in the process; however, goals can be changed if they seem to be too ambitious after the fact. The intent is not to punish people for not achieving a goal, but to applaud success and help reach the desired level of success. A root cause analysis is often needed to determine why a goal is not being met. There are many potential reasons: need for more training, redesign of workflow, additional system configuration, or external factors that make the goal infeasible. As health reform shifts the payment system from one that rewards volume and intensity to one that promotes value (improved care at lower cost), very specific goals—for all aspects of the practice—are needed for the local accountability that is being imposed by the accountable care organization or other constructs.[28]

Readiness Assessment

Practices will vary in how ready they are to take on HIT. Sometimes groups are not as ready as they think they are. Readiness is needed in leadership, user attitudes and beliefs, computer skills, information technology resources, and financial resources. An honest appraisal of these factors can help considerably in making incremental changes to a practice before the enormity of the EHR change occurs.

Leadership commitment is essential to support any HIT project. Adler was quoted earlier in the chapter, describing the need to address dysfunctional organizations.[13] It can be useful to conduct a leadership assessment. Many are available on the Web, such as one developed by the Dartmouth-Hitchcock Medical Center and promoted by the Institute for Healthcare Improvement.[29]

User attitudes and beliefs need to be understood and addressed in a way that will help achieve interest in and desire for HIT. A team readiness assessment is a way to take the pulse of the group with respect to EHR. A standardized form[12] or one the practice compiles can provide necessary insights for where future awareness building, education, and communications are needed to overcome barriers to using HIT.

Computer skills are important to assess because many physicians, nurses, and other clinicians may have minimal experience using computers. This can be a paper-and-pencil survey of what potential users of HIT know how to do on a computer (e.g., open a file, copy and paste text, save a document)[12] or what they need help with, or an online test, many of which are available on the Web as freeware.

Information technology resources include both identifying staff skills and taking an inventory of current hardware and software. Even though a HIT project for a large practice may include adding IT staff, it is important to understand what skills are available within the practice. Include persons who may not be "IT staff" but have a keen interest and could become super users. Similarly, new and/or additional hardware and telecommunications support may be necessary and software currently used may need replacing and/or updating. Inventorying these can help a practice anticipate costs and level of change. Again, starter inventories are widely available on the Web.[30]

Financial resource evaluation is part of planning. This should take the form of understanding both the practice's current financial position and the cost/benefit of the HIT under consideration. With respect to financial position, a practice needs to understand whether retaining earnings is feasible and their tax ramifications; identify existing lines of credit; determine its ability to take out a loan; and evaluate its experience with winning grants. Anticipating the total cost of ownership (TCO) of an EHR and what potential financial benefits may accrue can solidify financial planning into a business case a practice can take to the bank. A study conducted in 2005 by the Medical Group Management Association (MGMA) and the University of Minnesota found that practices experience on average a 24.8% cost overrun from the vendor's cost estimates.[31] Often this is due to not anticipating total cost, including items such as an upgrade needed for the LIS to share

structured lab results with the EHR, office furnishings or construction such as installing swing arms for monitors or keyboard drawers to make it easier for end users to use the EHR at the point of care, and a dedicated project manager (and additional staff depending on the size of the organization). Potential financial benefits should also be anticipated. These can be in cost avoidance, cost savings, increased revenue, and enhanced profitability. Productivity improvements are feasible after the learning curve is completed, although most often these lead to other forms of financial benefits or better quality of care and reduced hassles.

Migration Path

For many small practices, acquiring HIT may be only a one- or two-step process in which a practice management system (PMS) and EHR are acquired—individually over time or together as an integrated package. For large practices, and even some small practices that want to ease into HIT, a migration path may be desired or necessary. **Table 12-2** provides a structure for plotting a migration path.

A migration path identifies the applications and technology a practice plans to acquire over time and the dependencies among them. For instance, an organization may approach its HIT acquisition by first acquiring a billing system, then a fully functional PMS, and next a digital dictation system to support the electronic feed of transcription and print images of lab results into an EDMS. Data may get abstracted or scanned into one or more registries. A common occurrence when acquiring an EHR is the need to upgrade ancillary systems. For instance, viewing a print image of a lab result is often sufficient for physicians prior to adopting EHR. But once a practice acquires an EHR that can plot a trend line of lab results, compare lab results to different medications or doses of a medication, and perform drug-lab checking (e.g., is this drug contraindicated for this patient who has poor liver function?), the LIS may need an upgrade or it may need to be replaced in order for it to generate structured data in a form acceptable to the EHR.

A migration path also illustrates dependencies between applications and operations. Dr. Blumenthal, as previously quoted, notes that "meaningful use is not a technology project. . ."[26] Operational elements of people, policies, and processes must be considered. For example, a practice tightly affiliated with a hospital may want to access hospital applications through a provider portal, but finds it does not have the bandwidth to support such an exchange of data. The hospital may also require stricter adherence to Health Insurance Portability and Accountability Act

Table 12-2	HIT Migration Path Structure			
	Current	**Phase 1**	**Phase 2**	**Phase N**
Applications: Financial/administrative Ancillary Core clinical Specialty Utilities Knowledge resources Personal health records Health information exchange				
Technology: Servers Human–computer interfaces Network devices and telecom Interfaces Security Database(s)				
People: Project governance Physician champion Project manager Domain teams Support staff				
Policy: Communication Compliance Standards Documentation Data integrity Quality measurement				
Process: Workflow Process redesign Change management Risk management Privacy				

Source: Reprinted with permission, © Margret\A Consulting, LLC.

(HIPAA) security policies prior to providing access to its applications. An e-prescribing system will also require more bandwidth and networking redundancy, as well as a health information exchange participation agreement. Somewhere along the HIT path the practice may want to move to real-time eligibility verification and electronic remittance advice, especially as the transactions standards are being upgraded to version 5010 and the health reform legislation is requiring adoption of standard operating rules to improve the transactions' utility. If so, the practice will find it needs to work with its health plans to ensure comprehensive return of information in these transactions. Most importantly, each EHR must be customized to meet each practice's needs. For a multispecialty practice, each specialty must convene a group to review and identify modifications needed in generic templates. Likewise, current workflows and processes need to be understood so that changes can be made that consider the practice's needs and the product requirements.

Acquiring an EHR may not even be the last step in the migration path. More robust registries, clinical decision support utilities, data warehousing, and new applications that may be required for participants in accountable care organizations or other structures may need to be acquired subsequently. Instead of acquiring these in a haphazard manner, a migration path serves as a strategic plan that the practice can agree upon and only modify thoughtfully.

Organizing the Team

It should go without saying that a project of the scope of HIT requires a project committee and project manager, as well as staff to support the implementation. It is worth repeating again, however, Dr. Blumenthal's observation that "meaningful use is not a technology project. . .".[26] IT staff are critical to success, but potentially more important are executive leadership, a physician champion, and representatives of all stakeholders in the EHR.

Initially, a practice may convene a *project committee* to evaluate the feasibility of undertaking an EHR or other HIT project. Many large practices have a standing IT committee or project management office (PMO) that could spawn such a focused project committee.

Once the decision is made to undertake a comprehensive EHR or HIT selection process, a *selection committee* forms with representatives from all stakeholder groups as well as an executive sponsor, procurement officer, chief financial officer, legal counsel, and human resources and/ or labor relations. Selecting the system that best meets the functional requirements of the clinical community depends on multiple stakeholder input, including nurses and other clinicians as well as a physician champion and other representative physicians. (It can be helpful to add a "curmudgeon" physician to the group who can represent resisters and pave the way for converting these to committed users.) Although the physician community may be paying for the system, it should be recognized that other clinical staff will be using the system in support of physician work, potentially for an even greater proportion of time than the physicians. These individuals have important insights that physicians may not always recognize. Preparing for significant changes in workflows and processes may also require changes in job descriptions and even union negotiations or attention to civil service rules. Obviously, negotiating the contract will be

a significant undertaking that can be aided by people who have experience making large investments.

Early in the selection process, the committee also needs to understand the nature of the decision making required to go forward through each step of the process: Who has authority to approach vendors? Does the board sign off on requesting a final offer from a vendor or does this require a vote of all members of the practice? Who approves contract signing? Because of the direct impact on providers, many practices extend the approval process to all partners or even all providers.

Once HIT is selected, a *steering committee* may be formed. As a clinical project, the steering committee may be led by a physician champion, again with input from nurses and other clinicians, and potentially a representative of the patient community at appropriate points in the project. An academic-based practice may want to include student representatives and researchers. A multispecialty practice will want to form domain teams. The steering committee will also oversee the implementation, and should be delegated authority to make decisions concerning project standards, changes to critical components of the applications (including setting the sensitivity of alerts and recommending policies on documenting rationale for overriding alerts), rollout strategy, and myriad other elements.

Maintaining the HIT Program

Once the HIT is implemented, the "project" becomes a "program," requiring ongoing maintenance and support. Many practices convene a *health informatics committee* that provides program governance and support for enhancements, best practices, monitoring goal achievement, and even recommending internal sanctions where applicable.

■ Workflow and Process Mapping

Workflow and process issues may be the number one impediment to EHRs being widely accepted and adopted. Unfortunately, many practices do not perform the upfront work of understanding and redesigning workflows and processes. They may not recognize the importance of visualizing current workflows and processes during the selection period. Staff may not know how to map workflows and processes at the needed level of detail. Finally, many vendors do not support workflow and process redesign, so the result is often that the vendor's workflow is forced on the practice even if it may not be suitable.

Reasons for Addressing Workflows and Processes

There are a number of important reasons for addressing workflows and processes throughout the EHR project:

- Mapping current workflows and processes helps make them visible, and therein helps people recognize the need for improvement, creating interest in and motivation for an EHR.
- Issues associated with current workflows and processes may be able to be addressed before HIT is implemented, so change occurs gradually and yields early wins.
- Understanding current workflows and processes reveals the nature of functions performed in the practice, enabling a comprehensive set of functional requirements to be developed as criteria for selecting an EHR.
- Comparing current workflows and processes with how a vendor's product addresses them helps narrow the field of vendors to only those who address a practice's specific needs. Any functionality that is missing becomes a point of negotiation—both in recognizing compromises the practice may have to make and in seeking a solution from the vendor that is documented in the contract.
- During implementation, variances in current workflows and processes can be used to customize the product. This is not to suggest that a practice should mimic its current workflows and processes with the EHR, but that the practice should redesign workflows and processes to best meet each specialty's needs with the EHR.
- Using the maps of current and redesigned workflows and processes can help in training new users and in monitoring how effectively each person uses the new EHR, and enables the root cause of issues to be identified more quickly.
- Maps of redesigned workflows and processes serve as documentation of procedures for ongoing training of new staff and providers.

Workflow and Process Mapping

Process is the manner in which work needs to be completed in order to achieve a particular result. Workflow is the sequence of steps, decisions to be made, and handoffs taken to perform work. Mapping is the documentation of the nature of these processes and workflows. Some practices hire consultants to map their processes for them, although individuals who actually perform the work and know it best are actually in the best position to do the

mapping. An organization may adopt a formal workflow and process improvement program, such as Lean[32] or Six Sigma,[33] or simpler structures focusing on information systems process improvement[34] may be deployed just as well.

When mapping workflows and processes associated with using information, the tool most often used is the systems flowchart, the basic structure of which is illustrated in **Figure 12-3**. Ovals designate process boundaries. To avoid mapping too large a process at one time, boundaries help assure the pieces "fit" together—one process starting where another leaves off. Rectangles explain the process. "Who does what" should be described. Credentials (RN, LPN, or MA) or functional titles (receptionist) should be used instead of names of people. This keeps the map generic and removes the potential for bias or blame, especially when studying current workflows and processes that may contain workarounds or other opportunities for improvement. Diamonds are decision points and should reflect a question (e.g., Can RN approve refill?). Decision points are often the most difficult for new mappers to identify because they are frequently not visible. Any process, however, that entails alternatives or choices should be depicted as a decision point. The decision symbol must have at least two branches (e.g., Yes and No; or equal to/greater than and less than) and may have more (e.g., Refer to nurse triage, Refer to MD, Refer to pharmacy). Each branch then must have an action that follows. The action may be a process, another decision point, or a boundary (i.e., end point).

An easy way to approach process mapping with the systems flowchart is to replicate the basic symbols of process and decision with "sticky notes," where the process is

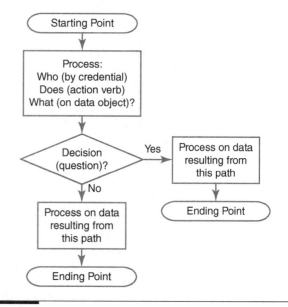

Figure 12-3 Basic systems flowchart.
Source: Used with permission, © Margret\A Consulting, LLC.

the note placed horizontally and the decision is the note placed at an angle. These can be placed on a wall or large sheet of paper (rolls of examining room table sheets work very well). Once the basic structure for a given process is depicted, the sticky notes can be moved around if elements of the map are missed. Different color sticky notes can be used to illustrate variations.

At the macro level, the workflows and processes to be mapped are those that will be impacted by the HIT being acquired. Typical workflows and processes in ambulatory care practices are listed in **Table 12-3**, although these can be added to, deleted from, or modified based on a specific practice's needs.

At the micro level, each macro-level process may be performed differently by different persons, different specialists, and different practices. For instance, a family physician may need to document much more data than a surgeon, and a surgeon may spend the most time with an EHR viewing images. When mapping current processes, the level of detail should be sufficient to identify all potential functions to be performed by an EHR (e.g., for renal specialists, calculating glomerular filtration rate [GFR] and staging kidney disease may be very important functions to look for in an EHR).

Workflow and Process Redesign

Once a workflow and process map seems complete, redesign requires looking for bottlenecks, sources of delay, rework due to errors, role ambiguity, duplication, unnecessary steps, and cycle time. For each step in the process, some key questions to consider include:

- *Why is it done? Is it necessary?* For example, dictating a separate referral letter may be unnecessary if a copy of a progress note may include more complete information.
- *Why is it done at this location?* For example, a patient may be in a better position to identify medications being taken when at home rather than at the clinic.
- *Why is it done at this time?* For example, patients may prefer to have scheduled lab work performed in advance of a visit so results can be discussed on a more timely basis.
- *Why is it done by this person?* For example, many refill requests can be handled by nurses.
- *Why is it done this way?* For example, a mother may prefer to pay out-of-pocket for an e-visit than to take time off from work to bring Johnny to the office for yet another earache.

Redesigning workflows and processes may best be enabled by a consultant or someone in the practice who is knowledgeable about healthcare, but not involved directly in the process. This person can help "push the envelope," where those closer to the process may be unable or unwilling to see a better way. When redesigning processes, the level of detail may need to be greater than when mapping current processes (e.g., identifying the source of all data necessary to stage chronic kidney disease and to create an action plan for compliance with Kidney Disease Outcomes Quality Initiative [KDOQI] guidelines).

Practitioners must be open to suggestions for change. Dr. Zaroukian notes that willingness to strive may be the key factor in successfully implementing an EHR.[35] A key element in workflow and process redesign is for those involved to remember that they are not just creating a

Table 12-3	Common Ambulatory Care Workflows and Processes	
Visit-Related Processes	**Nonvisit Processes**
Previsit registration, scheduling, eligibility verification	Lab results review and management
Check-in	Prescription refill/renewal requests
Patient intake	Other phone calls
Chart review	Patient follow-up
Diagnosis and problem list maintenance	Release of information: forms completion, clinical summaries, referral letters
Care planning/prior authorization	Chronic disease management
Prescribing and medication list maintenance	Quality measurement, reporting, and improvement
CPOE/staff tasking	Required reporting
Procedure	Pay for performance/ incentives management
Lab/x-ray ordering	Research/analytics
E&M coding	
Charge capture and billing	
Referral management	
Patient instruction	
Visit summary	
Check-out	

Source: Used with permission, © Margret\A Consulting, LLC

new way or their way or the vendor's way, but the right way that will ensure practice efficiency and effectiveness. The redesigned processes must then be translated into the design of templates, clinical decision support logic, practice guidelines, and the like.

■ EHR Considerations

If a practice is one of the approximately 50% of very large or hospital/health system–owned practices[36] or 75% of other practices that do not yet have an EHR,[37] it is likely to be contemplating acquisition in the near future. In addition to the planning and workflow/process mapping steps described in the previous sections, the practice will want to understand the EHR and HIT marketplace, the meaningful use incentive criteria, what technology will be necessary to exchange data within an accountable care organization, and other factors relative to what it is planning to buy prior to undergoing a formal selection process.

Understanding the Marketplace and Meaningful Use Incentive Criteria

In 2006 when the first HIT product certification was initiated by CCHIT, Dr. Mark Leavitt, then chair of CCHIT, estimated that there might be over 200 products on the market calling themselves EHR, with just under half of all ambulatory products (and about two-thirds of hospital products) certified.[38] At the conclusion of the first round of product certification in 2008, approximately 150 products had been certified by CCHIT. As of the writing of this chapter, over 700 ambulatory EHR products were certified by the ONC-ATCB certification process,[39] over 300 of which were "modular." Under the Standards and Certification Criteria Final Rule, a *complete EHR* is one that has been certified to meet all the mandatory certification criteria applicable to the practice setting. For ambulatory EHR products, there are 23 general criteria and 10 criteria specific to ambulatory care that must be met. *EHR modules* are those technologies that are certified to at least one and often many, but not all, of the certification criteria.[23] The certification criteria include the requirement to generate quality measures, but do not require that all potential quality measures from which a practice may choose to report are enabled.

Clearly, the number of certified products and the fact that the certification criteria represent the minimum capabilities EHR technology needs to support the meaningful use incentives means that providers have considerable work to do in making informed choices about which products to consider. A process of "triangulating" information

from multiple sources can be used to reach a short list, perhaps of 10–12 products to consider initially:

1. A practice should only look at and acquire an ONC-ATCB certified product (or suite of modularly certified products). This may seem bold, but it gives a practice the latitude to earn or not earn the meaningful use incentives as it wishes. It provides a wide-open field and will not likely limit a search unduly.

2. The practice should consider products most commonly used in its community—by other practices of similar size and type as well as the ambulatory product offered by its local hospital's vendor. If a practice anticipates joining an accountable care organization, it will want to consider how well the products in the community are able to communicate or whether there is an existing health information exchange organization to support the necessary sharing of information across the continuum of care. Even though a practice may not consider all of the products used in the community, at least it will have people its members can speak with about the products, their implementation experiences, and their record of ongoing support services.

3. The practice should review product lists produced by specialties in its practice. If it is a large multi-specialty practice, it will need to triangulate these to see which products occur on most of the lists.

4. Finally, the practice should include the EHR product supported by its incumbent PMS. Even if the practice chooses to replace its PMS with a more integrated PMS-EHR, it will have at least satisfied its curiosity with respect to what some believe is an "easier choice," even though it generally ends up being less than ideal. (Again, another bold assumption may be that if the PMS vendor's EHR is so great, why would the practice not have already acquired it?)

Practice Management Integration

Many practices dread the thought of replacing their tried and true PMS. However, a fully integrated PMS and EHR system often is far superior to what is currently in place, the incremental cost of the PMS component is not that great, and even the work effort to replace the PMS is manageable. There are several considerations here:

■ *Appointment scheduling and patient follow-up:* These can be enhanced with an integrated system (and it is not against HIPAA regulations to allow scheduling staff access to the additional limited information needed to make scheduling go more smoothly). Patients will appreciate being able to have needed studies performed in advance of their visit and the practice may be able to generate more revenue by more regular follow-up.

■ *Claims processing, eligibility verification, remittance advice reconciliation, prior authorizations, and other HIPAA transactions and code sets:* These requirements can be facilitated by an integrated product, especially now that many health plans are beginning to adopt standardized operating rules[39] (which will be required under the Affordable Care Act [ACA]) that will make it much easier to adopt real-time transactions directly with the health plan.[b] This could potentially reduce or even eliminate the need for billing services and/or clearinghouses and their associated fees. Easier and more accurate eligibility verification will increase cash flow and reduce denials and collections.

■ *Adoption of newer versions of the HIPAA transactions and code sets:* Although the v5010 was required by January 1, 2012, the ACA legislation requires more frequent updating of these standards which should be easier to facilitate with a newer PMS. Likewise, adoption of ICD-9-CM diagnosis codes in the EHR to meet the meaningful use criteria for problem lists will put a practice in a better position to adopt the ICD-10-CM diagnosis codes for claims requiring them after October 1, 2013.

■ *E&M coding and charges:* These can more directly move from the EHR to claims, facilitating faster turnaround, virtually no lost charges, and fewer denials.

■ *Data conversion:* For patient demographic data this is very feasible, although most practices opt to manually build payer files, procedure and fee schedules, provider appointment templates, and other maintenance files for a fresh start.[40]

■ *Single database of PMS-EHR:* This enables more simplified and powerful reporting capabilities.

■ *E-visits:* These are facilitated by an integrated PMS-EHR product. Some health plans are starting to pay for these,[41] and several medical societies have provided guidance,[42] including a CPT code.

Sequencing the implementation of an integrated PMS-EHR usually entails implementing the PMS component first, although it is feasible—if unconventional—to reverse these if necessary to earn the meaningful use incentives. Another consideration relating to the PMS-EHR implementation is that of converting data from an old PMS to the new. Although it will likely be necessary and generally feasible with some clean-up activity to convert patient demographic data, most practices do not convert their schedule or their accounts receivable. This is because they generally find that the older PMS is so vastly different that the clean-up required after the conversion is more cumbersome, time-consuming, and costly than the data conversion itself. This is especially true for accounts receivable, where maintaining the old system until the accounts are paid or selling the accounts may be far more cost effective.

Relationship of EHR to Other HIT

A final consideration prior to plunging into a formal selection process is to evaluate what HIT the practice may already have and how that will or will not fit with a new PMS and/or EHR. Practices may well have e-prescribing, a provider portal to their hospital and other providers such as an imaging center, reference lab, registries to which they contribute data, e-visit functionality via a patient portal, a personal health record offering, research databases, telemedicine, and connectivity with a health information exchange organization (HIO). They may also have various ancillary applications, such as an LIS, an RIS, a surgery scheduling system, a DIMS or EDMS, and a digital dictation or speech recognition system. At a minimum, an inventory of these products, versions, and capabilities should be made available as part of what the practice provides to an EHR vendor upon which to base a quote for interfaces and potential upgrades or replacements.

If a practice does not have these applications and desires some or all of them, they should be inventoried in the requirements specifications. Some, such as e-prescribing, may be an integral part of a new EHR; others, such as DIMS or EDMS, may require an additional or separate purchase. Inventorying these will also help the practice stage them in its migration path—some may be better acquired prior to EHR and others after.

In addition to applications that the practice may have or could have acquired prior to EHR, members of the

---

b. See Letter Report to the Secretary of the Department of Health and Human Services on Affordable Care Act, Administrative Simplification: Operating Rules for Eligibility and Claims Status Transactions, September 30, 2010, from the National Committee on Vital and Health Statistics as an example: http://www.ncvhs.hhs.gov/100930lt2.pdf

practice may also find it desirable to add utilities to the EHR. These include a number of different types of clinical decision support applications, data capture aids, and data warehousing/data mining/analytics products.

Finally, the practice may also need to consider acquiring a specialty EHR. Unfortunately, although one product can generally be customized to satisfy most medical specialty needs, it is unlikely that a single product will also be able to adequately support behavioral health, dentistry, home care, and other such healthcare practice settings.

■ HIT Selection

Whether acquiring a new EHR or add-on applications to an existing EHR, or even undertaking a reselection, a formal selection process should be used. Many practices agonize over what product to select or even whether to buy. In addition to the purposeful planning already described, a formal selection process ensures proper due diligence and garners trust that the product selected best meets practice needs.

A HIT selection process should include specifying functional requirements; determining the appropriate acquisition strategy for the practice; agreeing to a vendor selection code of conduct; performing vendor due diligence, including issuing a request for proposal, receiving product demonstrations, conducting site visits, and performing reference checks; and contract negotiation.

HIT Functional Requirements Specification

Many times a practice finds that it does not have a full enough understanding of EHR to create its own comprehensive list of functional requirements, let alone to identify those that may be unique to the practice, and which will differentiate one product from another. With the meaningful use incentive criteria, many practices also wonder why it is necessary to create their own functional requirements list.

The process of defining unique functional requirements makes for a more informed consumer and provides confidence in a practice's ability to select the right product. Such an understanding is best gleaned from studying current workflows and processes and viewing demos for educational purposes. A practice should not undertake an EHR selection process without more fully understanding the functionality and its implications for the practice.

Although every ONC-ATCB certified product does have a common set of functionality, there are significant differences in the additional functionality offered by vendors as well as how the functionality performs (i.e., usability). To better understand the practice's needs, practice members should compare the results of the practice's current workflow and process mapping with standard lists of functional requirements. These lists are widely available, as suggested earlier in the discussion of understanding the marketplace, and include the IOM key capabilities for EHR, the HL7 EHR System Functional Model, the CCHIT Certified 2011 Ambulatory EHR Certification Criteria (which are more comprehensive than the meaningful use incentive criteria),[43] and/or vendor lists published by medical specialty societies. If a functionality identified from the workflow and process mapping is not on one of these lists, it may truly be unique or simply described differently. In any event, that functionality should be on the practice's "short list" of desired functions, at least until such time as it understands differences in terminology that may cause the practice to remove the function from its list.

HIT Acquisition Strategy

How to acquire the software and hardware should also be an early consideration in the selection process. There are three general categories of software acquisition to consider, each with variations depending on who manages the hardware and where it is located. **Table 12-4** provides a summary of the HIT acquisition strategies.

An important distinction to make in evaluating different HIT acquisition strategies is to recognize that to *install*

Table 12-4 **Summary of HIT Acquisition Strategies**

Strategy	Who runs?	What applications?	On whose computers?	With whose data?
Straight licensure	Practice	Practice	Practice	Practice
Service outsourcing	Vendor	Practice	Practice	Practice
Hardware hosting	Vendor	Practice	Vendor	Practice
ASP/SaaS	Vendor	Vendor	Vendor	Practice
Community offering	Hospital/IDN	Hospital/IDN	Hospital/IDN	Shared

refers to simply loading software onto hardware, whereas to *implement* means to configure the software to a practice's needs and specifications. Implementation generally also includes data conversion, interface development, testing, training, and go-live support (even though some of these services may be priced separately and some or all of them may be outsourced by the primary vendor).

Another important distinction is the difference between client/server and service-oriented architectures. *Client/ server (C/S)* architecture uses a primary server computer (or set of servers) to house software and data; the client computers—sometimes with minimal processing and storage capability of their own (then called "thin clients")—are used to access and enter data processed by the server(s). *Service-oriented architecture (SOA)* uses tools designed for use on the World Wide Web to provide software services and house data within the "cloud" (i.e., via a secure Internet connection). SOA may be referred to as "cloud computing," offering "on-demand" software services.

Straight licensure is the classic approach to acquiring an EHR. It uses a C/S architecture, where the practice pays a license fee up front for the software and then a percentage of that for ongoing maintenance and access to upgrades. The software is generally the most customizable, and may include tools that enable users to perform some of their own customization. Initial implementation services are generally bought from the software vendor, whereas subsequent upgrades and customization may be performed by the practice's staff or outsourced to an IT management company. Although the practice may also buy hardware from the software vendor, it can buy it independently. The practice may have the software vendor install the hardware, hire someone to install it, or install the software itself. The practice also may choose to use a *hosted* environment, in which an IT management company installs the practice's software on its own hardware. Straight licensure not only entails an upfront investment, but also requires paying directly for outsourcing, hosting, or internal IT staffing.

An *application service provider (ASP)* and *software as a service (SaaS)* are approaches to acquiring HIT software and hardware that are more like a rental agreement, where the practice's software and data are housed at a vendor location and are accessed through a secure telecommunications service or Internet connection. The practice may pay a modest service charge up front for configuration of the software, and then pay a monthly service fee for use of the software and maintenance. Although some vendors use the terms "ASP" and "SaaS" synonymously, there are important differences:

- The ASP model is an older one. Typically the vendor utilizes a C/S architecture with a Web front

end. The ASP model also is more customizable, potentially more expensive, and more conducive to the constant online transaction processing that is characteristic of EHR use.

- The SaaS model requires the practice to use the software more as-is, "out of the box," and is more commonly used for occasional online analytical processing, such as end-of-month reporting or special projects.

In both models, the practice supplies its own input devices, has minimal IT staffing requirements, and needs a strong service-level agreement with the vendor. It also needs full redundancy in connectivity services and/or the ability to work locally during any downtime, which means thin clients are not possible. Some providers have hesitated to adopt one of these models because of concerns over security and control of data. In general, however, such vendors often have stronger security controls than what many provider organizations have because that is their business and they build those controls into the cost of the products. Ownership of data must be specified in the contract, but often the primary concern is being able to access the data in the event the vendor goes out of business. In reality, moving from one vendor to another is difficult whether the data is maintained in-house or not.

Community offering, for want of a better term, is a provisioning model that has recently been initiated by a few major EHR vendors. In this model, the vendor provides software licenses to a large hospital or integrated delivery network (IDN), then allows the hospital or IDN to roll out the product to affiliated groups. The hospital or IDN effectively becomes the affiliate's vendor, providing (usually minimal) customization and support. A key factor in this offering is that it is based on a single Active Directory, where data across the hospital or IDN and its affiliates are shared with each other, within the parameters of logical access controls. Some affiliates find this is an excellent way to acquire a product they might not otherwise be able to afford and believe the ability to share patient data across the continuum contributes to better healthcare. Others, however, prefer not to be tied so closely to a given hospital or IDN and/or may have concerns that the logical access controls are insufficient to prevent the hospital or IDN from gaining unauthorized access to their patients' and practice-proprietary data.

HIT Vendor Selection Code of Conduct

A final step before plunging directly into performing due diligence on selecting a vendor is to consider adopting a vendor selection code of conduct. HIT is a major investment, made in a highly competitive environment, with vendors highly protective of their intellectual property rights. Many practices have found it helpful to ensure that proper protocol is followed so that bias is not introduced into the project and the process is performed in a manner that protects everyone's confidentiality. Such a code of conduct usually addresses formality of process, communications, use of selection criteria, acceptance of vendor gifts, equal treatment, confidentiality of the process, protection of vendor trade secrets and intellectual property, and sanctions for noncompliance with the code.

HIT Vendor Selection Due Diligence

The process for selecting a HIT vendor can be likened to a funnel (see **Figure 12-4**), where the universe of vendors enters the funnel and the field narrows continuously to the single vendor of choice. The funneling process usually begins with narrowing the field to a reasonable number of vendors (10 to 12) to perform an initial screen that will result in 5 or 6 vendors to whom to send a request for proposal (RFP). The practice will then conduct an analysis of RFP responses to narrow the field to three or four vendors who will perform structured product demonstrations. Members will then perform visits to view vendor products, and ultimately will identify the one vendor of choice. Throughout this process, reference checks may be performed to aid in narrowing the field at each step.

Initial Screening

As suggested in the earlier section on understanding the marketplace, it will generally be fairly easy to identify 10 to 12 vendors on which to perform an initial screening process. These will be ONC-ATCB certified vendors used by others

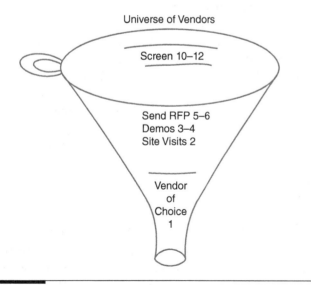

Figure 12-4 Narrowing the field of vendors.

in the community, those commonly found on multiple specialty lists, any incumbent PMS vendor that has an EHR product, and potentially a hospital's vendor if it offers an ambulatory care product (whether it has a community offering or not). To screen these, it is advisable that steering committee members informally engage in conversations with users, visit trade shows to speak with attendees at vendor booths, and attend the incumbent vendors' users' group meeting. Steering committee members (and others) may use the websites of these vendors to view demos, read product reviews, and peruse white papers. (When signing up for demos or acquiring a white paper, the practice should use a generic e-mail account so as not to be bombarded by salespersons.) Steering committee members should reach consensus on vendors to whom to send an RFP.

Request for Proposal

The RFP is a formal request for a vendor to provide a practice with an offering for the product it seeks, including providing a price proposal and contract that outlines terms and conditions. There may be any number of forms of RFP, but typically the following elements are included:

- Introduction and purpose.
- Instructions for response.
- Background information on the practice, including volume of patients, number of locations, specialties represented, case mix, staffing (including number of physicians, number of physician extenders, and number of other staff), and any milestone dates to which the practice wishes to adhere (e.g., when to start earning meaningful use incentives).
- Vendor profile seeking information about the vendor on the history of the company, partnerships, product versioning history, financial performance, customer information, certifications, recognitions and awards, and a request for references.
- Functional requirements (see the following discussion).
- Technical requirements outlining the nature of the practice's computing environment, request for optimal hardware configuration (and pricing for same if expecting to buy from the software vendor), security controls, telecommunications requirements, contingency plan (data backup, redundancy, business continuity plan, disaster recovery plan), and the vendor name, product name, and version number/date of any applications for which the practice may want an interface to be developed.
- Implementation, including a sample plan outlining typical timeframes for each major milestone, qualifications of staff, description of practice staff

expectations for system configuration, how customization requirements are communicated to the vendor, how workflow and process redesign is addressed, issues management and escalation process, and risk management.

- Testing and training requirements, including requirements for separate testing and production environments, types of testing and dress rehearsal expectations, number of anticipated super users, sandbox capabilities for new users to "play" with using the EHR prior to go-live, end user training, and one-on-one support.
- Documentation of owner's manual.
- Ongoing support/maintenance outlining service levels.
- Copy of contract and any contractual considerations.
- Sealed price quote as a separate electronic file and/or in a sealed envelope that details the cost for all hardware, software, training (including location and number of days), implementation and testing (including travel expenses for implementers), ongoing support, maintenance agreement, and/or service-level agreement, as applicable. The purpose of this separation is to avoid having all members of the selection committee review the price proposal, which often creates bias, especially because price is always subject to negotiation.

Functional requirements may be as detailed or general as desired. Given the state of the marketplace today, practice variation, and inability to rely on any certification to address unique needs, it is recommended that a practice include, at a minimum, the functional requirements that are unique to the practice. Others prefer not to leave anything to chance and provide a comprehensive list of functionality. The practice should request the vendor to supply an objective indication of its capabilities to address

Functionality Requirements: Indicate how your proposed solution makes available the following features and functions. Information supplied here will be expected to serve as a contractual obligation in any contract we may enter into for this product. Describe availability as:

4 = installed in one or more sites
3 = installed in one or more sites, but not available for general release until (specify date)
2 = Planned for future release (specify timeframe)
1 = Not available, but will develop for additional fee (provide on price proposal)
0 = Not available, no current plans to develop

Functions	Availability	Description of How Product Performs This Function
...		
2. Data capture functions		
a. Capture and record current and active diagnoses for problem list that is encoded in ICD-9-CM or SNOMED.		
...		

Figure 12-5 Portion of an RFP functional requirements table.

Source: Used with permission, © Margret\A Consulting, LLC.

each requirement and a brief narrative description of how it provides the capabilities. **Figure 12-5** provides a portion of the functional requirements section of an RFP with such a table.

In addition to a functionality table, some practices include a performance scenario or request for use case. This is a description of a patient visit with key questions seeking information on how the product performs the functionality at each step in the visit. The scenario is typically of a fairly complicated patient and may span several pages of the RFP. This scenario is also very effective for any subsequent product demonstrations. **Table 12-5** provides a partial example of this scenario. In the example, the range of responses could be anything from having the

Table 12-5	**Portion of a Performance Scenario**
What the Practice Wants to Do	**How the System Performs the Function**
...	
11. Medical assistant wants to retrieve data on patient's blood sugars in range of 104–122, review current medications including any that are new from the previous visit, and check patient's exercise diary and diet record.	
12. Medical assistant wants to notify physician that patient is ready to be seen.	
...	

Source: Used with permission, © Margret\A Consulting, LLC.

medical assistant call up individual blood sugar results, call up the chart's medication list, and review notes where the physician may have recorded information on exercise and diet, to having the medical assistant request a trend line of specified blood sugars, retrieve the medication list updated by an e-prescribing information exchange service, and view the patient's personal health record for exercise and diet history. Clearly the former response does not reflect as sophisticated a product as the latter response.

Review Responses to RFP

The responses received from the vendors will be large, multipart documents. The project manager should do a cursory review to make sure the responses are complete and potentially divide up the task of review so that clinicians review functionality, IT staff review technology, and others review implementation and business aspects.

Although some practices attempt to score either the entire RFP response or at a minimum the functionality, it can be easier and more meaningful to create a separate vendor analysis tool (as illustrated in **Table 12-6**). Ideally this should be a single-page document (or spreadsheet) in which key differentiators are prioritized. Creation of such a tool while waiting for responses to the RFP can be yet another aspect of the selection committee's educational process. As objective a scoring scale as possible should be adopted that everyone understands and uses consistently.

The table can be constructed not only for review of the RFP responses from each vendor, but also to document findings from subsequent forms of due diligence for each vendor as applicable. In the example, four vendors—A, B, C, and D—were issued an RFP, but further due diligence is planned only for vendors A and D. Notice in the table that some of the cells are grayed out, indicating that for the specific differentiator, that form of due diligence may not be most suitable. For instance, although some elements of implementation may be gleaned from the RFP that the vendor will address in questions during a product demonstration, for other elements of implementation, site visits and reference checks will give better information.

Table 12-6 Portion of a Vendor Analysis Tool

Key Differentiators Scoring scale: 4 = Exceeds 3 = Meets 2 = Marginal 1 = Future 0 = Does not meet	Vendor A RFP	Vendor B RFP	Vendor C RFP	Vendor D RFP	Vendor: B Total RFP	Total Demo	Total Site Visit	Total Ref. Checks	Overall Total Vendor: D
Functionality									
1. CDS									
2. Quality measures									
...									
...									
Usability									
1. Use of screen real estate									
Technology									
...									
Implementation									
...									
Vendor									
1. Clinical staff									
2. R&D %									
...									

Source: Used with permission, © Margret\A Consulting, LLC.

Additional Due Diligence

As the practice progresses through its due diligence, it should be able to further narrow the field of vendors.

At the conclusion of RFP response review, a portion of the vendors may be asked to supply a formal product demonstration. Even if the practice has had previous product demonstrations, this one should be attended by all selection committee members and afford ample time for questions. Typically it is at least 1 day in length. It is a good idea to ask the vendor to provide a short version of its "typical" demo, during which selection committee members ask no questions but take notes on elements that seem to be missing or unclear. (These are likely to be elements of weakness.) Then request that the vendor demo the performance scenario the practice has created, during which selection committee members should ask as many questions as they can possibly consider, including those that focus on potential weaknesses or missing functions. Finally, many practices have the vendor demo the product in a "vendor fair" type of situation, where "stations" are set up so that all members of the practice are able to attend short (10- to 15-minute) demos. Selection committee members circulating through the fair can glean important insights into practice concerns as well as have an opportunity to get some hands-on experience and ask follow-up questions to verify key points in their demo. During this time, the vendor's IT staff may be meeting with the practice's IT staff, the implementation specialist with the practice's project manager, and potentially the primary salesperson with the practice's chief financial officer.

Once the field of vendors is narrowed further, the practice may wish to conduct site visits. The vendor will arrange these and will be present. A sufficient number of selection committee members should be present so that one is always available to occupy the salesperson while the rest speak with different members of the host site. The discussion should not be limited to only one individual at the site—visitors should attempt to talk randomly to as many people as possible so different viewpoints are obtained. A site visit may be able to provide some hands-on experience and is an excellent source for tips on implementation strategies. Do not expect the host to reveal any "dirty laundry," and do not be surprised that the host is compensated for the visit in some form. However, in both the site visit and reference checks, there are ways to ask questions that can provide telling answers:

- What do you like the most about this product and what do you like the least about this product? (This question can lead off the discussion; then ask it again at the end of the conversation after greater

rapport has been established. This might provide a more straightforward response.)
- What would you do differently if you had a chance to do it again?
- What budgetary considerations did you miss in planning?
- How long did the system take to implement and what problems did you encounter?
- How long did it take physicians to return to full productivity?
- What are you hoping to see in the next release of the product?
- Why did you select this product over others you considered?
- Irrespective of the product, do you have suggestions for things we should do or not do?

Corporate site visits are an additional consideration. If a vendor believes a practice is very serious about its product, it may invite members of the practice to corporate headquarters to meet the chief executive officer, the chief technology officer, and others. Such a site visit can help members understand the corporate culture of the vendor, gain access to more comprehensive financial information, and learn more about the company's research and development efforts, including future product plans.

Reference checks have not been listed as a separate step in the due diligence because reference checks can be useful throughout the entire due diligence process—to anticipate any issues during a demo, to follow up on demo questions, in advance of a site visit, in appreciation for the site visit, and with others randomly chosen who might have special insights. Some vendors supply virtually a complete list of references suitable to the size and type of practice; others provide a more limited offering. A good way to identify additional references is to collect business cards at trade shows and conferences practice members attend, peruse the Web for testimonials of persons who can be contacted, and attend any user group meeting to which the vendors extend an invitation. In evaluating every aspect of the due diligence, consider any outlier as a potential red flag for further follow-up, but avoid making a snap judgment. It is possible that a practice had a poor implementation or has a disgruntled user irrespective of the product itself.

Contract Negotiation

Once consensus is reached on the vendor of choice, the practice may wish to advise other vendors that it is no longer interested in their offerings. There is no need to provide further explanation, but a firm request for no further contact may be necessary. It can be a good idea to keep a "number two" vendor at bay; and some practices negotiate with two vendors simultaneously if they truly believe they are equal in functionality. All contracts are negotiable and must be negotiated.

Request a best offer from the vendor of choice. Many practices hire a HIT contract specialist as well as have their attorney review the contract. As a first step, be sure practice members completely understand what they are buying—including any third-party software, in-bound and out-bound interfaces, customization, service level, data conversions, and the like. As the responsible practice member attaches the response to the RFP to the contract, he or she should make sure that anything the practice wants that the vendor does not currently offer but has "promised" is in writing and compensation is afforded in the event the promise is not kept in a timely manner or falls short.

An issues letter should be included addressing everything, including price, payment schedule, and terms. Most vendors will negotiate on price fairly easily, but will want payments made on a timetable rather than project milestones. Do not give up on the payment schedule to get a lower price, because paying everything before the system goes live does not allow for any leverage thereafter. Also be cautious that price discounts are not made up for in subsequent maintenance fees, implementation charges, or other items. Make sure reasonable caps are put on travel expenses, other variable costs, and increases for additional licenses, additional modules acquired later, and maintenance fees. So long as the practice agrees to pay maintenance fees and accept product upgrades on a regular basis, ensure it does not pay for any upgrades associated with regulatory requirements. Beware of end-of-year or end-of-quarter offerings—they are often made to avoid having the practice address terms, although if the practice can act swiftly they may warrant consideration.

Finally, most vendor contracts need terms to be made mutual. For example, many contracts include a clause that the practice cannot hire the vendor's staff; but the vendor also should not be able to hire the practice's staff for some period of time or without consent.

■ HIT Implementation

Depending on the product the practice acquires, the implementation process can be lengthy (and cost more than the license itself). As previously noted, an ASP or SaaS model will permit less customization than straight licensure of a client/server model, require significantly fewer in-house IT staff, and therefore take less time to implement. Still,

there is a fairly significant work effort and definitely a period of learning. Because of the scope of the project for large practices, vendors may utilize a consulting company. Whatever the vendor and/or its consultant does for the practice, however, the practice should have its own project manager, physician champion, domain teams, super users, application/data analyst, and sufficient IT staff to manage whatever technology will be the practice's responsibility. Ideally these individuals should have been identified during and participated in the selection process. The following description of implementation assumes a client/server model. Implementations for an ASP or SaaS model will be less complex but require the same elements.

Steps in implementation usually include establishing a project management infrastructure, hardware selection and installation, site preparation, chart conversion, system configuration, data conversion, interface development, workflow and process redesign, testing, training, turnover and roll-out strategies, and go-live.

Project Management Infrastructure

A project that is the scope of an EHR or other major HIT requires a detailed project plan, budget, resourcing plan, communications plan, issues management, change control, and risk management. Typically the first step a vendor will take with the practice is to review the implementation plan and establish parameters for issues reporting, escalation, and resolution.

Although the vendor will have its own detailed project plan, the practice also needs a project plan that incorporates the vendor's milestones and delineates additional activities for which it is responsible. If not performed during the selection process, a project plan gap analysis should be performed to identify what the vendor might not do during implementation and to make sure the practice acquires sufficient resources to fill those gaps.

The project plan should incorporate a communications plan to ensure that all participants are kept up-to-date on the project's progress and applicable individuals are aware of issues. A communications plan should help the project manager make sure that the right messages are delivered by the right persons at the right time to the right people using the right media. This may include such detail as a reminder to the chief executive to say thank you to a design team. Also important are messages that reassure staff they will not be replaced by the EHR, or that plans have been made to transition staff in the event of layoffs.

Project planning software may be used to construct the work breakdown structure. If used, such software will likely include budget and resource leveling tools. The budget should be drawn from the total cost of ownership that was initially projected, modified with the final contract price list and payment schedule. Resource leveling refers to the allocation of staff to activities in order to accomplish the work within the scheduled time and budget.

Issues management is an extremely important element of project management. As with the project plan, the vendor will have an issues management process, but the practice will also want its own as well. An issues management process should include identification of all issues, large and small; when and how they occurred; when they expect to be resolved; who is responsible for their resolution; and the date resolved and nature of resolution. If an issue is not able to be resolved on first pass, escalation is necessary. Part of the vendor's initial planning with the practice should identify to whom the practice should escalate issues. The practice should also have its own internal escalation process.

Whether an issue brings about a change or a planned customization results in a change, the vendor will typically log the change into a change control database. Large practices will do some of their own customization, at least on an ongoing basis, so it is a good idea to also have a change control process. Change control refers to managing requests for change, ensuring changes are made only as applicable and on a timely basis, that they are tested and documented, and that users are trained on them. Changes should not be made to a system unless there is a formal request (and usually prioritization), an investigation of the nature of the change, and approval for the change. This is particularly true for clinical applications, where a change in a single data element (such as making a required field an optional field) can have a ripple effect that impacts clinical decision support and potentially impacts actual clinical decision making. Documentation of the change should be maintained as part of the practice's records retention program, because it can be subject to discovery in a legal proceeding.

A final step in gearing up for a HIT implementation project is risk management, which is a process of identifying, assessing, prioritizing, and controlling the probability and/or impact of any factor that could cause the project harm. Risk management may also recognize where the practice can take advantage of opportunities that present themselves. An important source of identifying potential risk is the issues log. Risk management, however, should be an ongoing and proactive process in which potential risks are anticipated so their occurrence can be avoided or diminished in severity.

Hardware Selection and Installation

Although hardware selection for the HIT applications may be performed concurrently with the application selection process, the selection of human–computer (input devices) interfaces frequently is performed at the beginning of the implementation process. If a practice is acquiring its own servers, network devices, and other peripherals, it should ensure they meet the vendor's optimal hardware requirements for running the application and it should expect that the vendor will require a suitability review and provide approval.

Selection of human–computer interfaces is often a more complicated process. Providers new to EHR may not be able to make definitive choices about what they want to use until they have tried out different devices. This is particularly true for mobile devices (e.g., tablets) in a wireless environment; providers often come to find they prefer wired desktops. It can be helpful to acquire a sampling of devices and allow new users to try them out prior to making decisions across the board. There are significant challenges associated with device speed, potential Wi-Fi interference, battery life, weight, ruggedness, infection control, and other issues. Although one size does not fit all and often one size does not even fit one person in all situations, it is still necessary to settle on a minimum number of device types and a single operating system platform for economies of scale and easier maintenance.

Hardware installation may also entail upgrading or adding wireless to network capabilities and enhancing broadband capacity. Here a vendor's initial optimal requirements may even be insufficient, because providers often want more documents scanned than are probably needed (see the later discussion on chart conversion), greater access to digital images, more refined imaging techniques, and sophisticated analytics capabilities (see the later discussion on data analytics).

All hardware and network enhancements need to be tested prior to use.

Associated with hardware installation must be contingency plans, including backup plans, full server and network redundancy, business continuity, and disaster recovery. Often associated with hardware installation is implementation of applicable security controls. Many providers balk at access controls and strong authentication requirements, but not only are they (and audit logging) mandated by the HIPAA regulations, they also are essential elements of healthcare documentation. Constantly logging in and out each time a healthcare professional accesses an application is especially onerous. Biometrics or proximity tokens associated with role-based access controls and break-the-glass emergency mode procedures are essential to garnering clinician acceptance.

Site Preparation

In a client/server environment, hardware installation may require creation or enhancement of a data center, or location where servers and other computer hardware are maintained under appropriate temperature, humidity, power, and fire-safety controls. Site preparation, however, can also relate to the need for placement and use of human–computer interfaces. New furniture, kiosks, swing arms, electrical outlets, docking stations, battery charging stations, and even a "parking lot" for mobile carts with computers may need to be added or created.

Chart Conversion

Although not necessarily the next task to be performed in the implementation sequence, chart conversion is often a topic of concern to providers, even prior to selection. Chart conversion refers to making information in current paper-based medical records available in an EHR. Physicians agonize over potentially not having instantaneous access to old records, only to find that they rarely access them online if they are scanned in as images. Today's strategies now entail a combination of abstracting key data for entry into the EHR as structured data prior to the first time a patient is seen with the EHR, and scanning a very limited number of documents chosen by the provider after the patient is seen the first time with the EHR. Which data to abstract will vary by specialist, but at a minimum the active problem list, current medication list, and allergies are common to all. Recent lab results are also very important. Another potential strategy is for the provider to dictate a more comprehensive note at the time the patient is last seen prior to go-live. This note may then be the only document that needs to be scanned or electronically fed into the EHR as an image and is more readily retrievable than having to open a multitude of documents to find one piece of information.

Advanced planning and reassurance that paper records will be available when requested is needed. Paper records should not be destroyed until the state statute of limitations and other retention requirements have run out. Alternatively, if the practice wants to reduce all costs associated with paper record storage and plans to scan records as a means to archive these records and then destroy the paper, the strategy to abstract and enter key selected data is still an important way for new users to begin their use of the EHR.

System Configuration

Also called system build, system configuration refers to the loading of master files and tables specific to the practice. Much like selecting a preferred font type and size, letter and memo templates, toolbar design, and other elements that make it easier to use a word processing application, system configuration includes myriad details to be preloaded into the system to make first use of the system easier for end users. These include things such as the names of all staff, their credentials, National Provider Identifiers for providers, DEA numbers for physicians, patient scheduling rules, names of lab tests ordered from different laboratories, commonly used telephone or fax numbers, names and locations of local pharmacies, and so on. Some of these data can be acquired from predefined directories or libraries; however, even when such data may reside in an old practice management system or other business application, most practices find the exercise of updating the lists and hopefully streamlining some of the processes can be very beneficial. Vendors will supply "workbooks" for the practice in which to record their configuration requirements. It is strongly advised that end users be involved in this aspect of system setup.

System configuration for an EHR will also entail creation and/or review of "favorite" diagnoses names and codes for each provider, "favorite" medication lists, clinical templates, standing orders, decision support rules, and other elements of structured data entry and retrieval. At this time the sensitivity of clinical decision support rules should be set, if adjustable within the product. Some practices turn off all rules except for a very small number that are agreed to be those relating to potentially fatal events. Slowly other rules are added as desired. These more clinically oriented configurations should be performed by the applicable domain teams.

Data Conversion

Data conversion is an inexact process due to the proprietary nature of most vendors' software. Except for very large patient demographic files that typically include fairly standard data structures, most practices opt to enter data directly into a new PMS or EHR.

Despite issues with data conversion, it is critical when a practice is reselecting an EHR. Some vendors are acquiring a fair amount of experience conducting data conversion for practices who reselect. If the vendor being considered does not have such experience, a third party who specializes in data conversion may well be worth the investment. The expectation should still be that not all data will convert completely correctly. These should be identified and workaround databases potentially created.

Interface Development

An interface is software specially written to exchange data between two disparate systems, such as an LIS and an EHR (or an old PMS and a new EHR). For an interface to be written, each system should comply with the same standard protocol. For health information, this protocol most commonly is HL7; for picture archiving and communication systems (PACS) the protocol is the DICOM standard. But even when the two systems comply with the same version of the standard, because of the degree of optionality in the standards, the process is still one of negotiation. As a result, interfaces are costly to write, are written to exchange only the minimum data necessary, and may only be written to send data in one direction (unidirectional), or one direction at a time (bidirectional). In addition, any time a change is made to one of the systems being interfaced, the impact of the change to the interface itself must be checked. Very large practices with multiple ancillary systems can have many interfaces where an "interface engine" may be required to help manage the interfaces.

Although it would be ideal to at least have different applications sold by the same vendor based on the same architecture, such an environment is not universal. Practices should be aware that just because two applications come from the same vendor does not necessarily mean they are based on the same architecture. Some vendors are known for developing their own applications so they are integrated, but other vendors are equally well known for simply acquiring other products and developing a "strong" interface between the new product and their existing products. When using such products it is very clear that they do not have the same "look and feel" and therefore are only interfaced and not integrated. Consider Microsoft Office, where the look and feel of Word and Excel are similar but not exactly the same, and some not-so-intuitive steps have to be taken sometimes to move Word files into Excel or vice versa. In the same way, the ability to exchange structured data with other applications is critical.

Workflow and Process Improvement

As described in the section on "Workflow and Process Mapping," once an EHR is acquired and being implemented, it is vital to evaluate current workflows and processes and determine how they should best be redesigned to take advantage of the EHR. End users must be involved in this process, although as commonly reported, "most practices do not go to the source for their crucial input."[44] Underestimating workflow changes is the top listed "worst mistake" to make when considering an EHR investment.[45]

Workflow and process improvement should be addressed during implementation; however, it is very likely that once users begin actually using the system they will come to better appreciate the need to address workflow and process improvement, and will have better ideas about how they would like to see the workflows and processes addressed.[46]

As users engage in workflow and process redesign, it is important to ensure that they do not attempt to change workflows and processes back to how things worked in the paper environment. Because data entry is always a challenge, physicians often revert back to dictating or request more comment fields in an attempt to type notes, increasing their frustration even more. And, of course, not capturing structured data for use in clinical decision, information exchange, and quality measurement support removes from the EHR its main values for the physician.

A key question to ask in workflow and process improvement is, who should enter what data and when? An interesting editorial by Steele observes that "most people fail to recognize that the sophisticated computers and systems that power American industries and streamline operations rely upon data entry performed by a workforce of minimum or near-minimum wage earners. . . . Highly compensated corporate executives . . . are not taking on the tasks of data entry."[47] Although this editorial was written to question "government-enforced EHR," it did support use of EHR—but called for "flexible, creative, and incremental thinking" to resolve the "burdens of EHR data entry."[47]

Dr. Bachman notes that in 1968, the *Mayo Clinic Proceedings* published a pioneering article "Toward Automating the Medical History." He cited the following strengths of medical history capture software: It allows more data to be captured; gives the patient more time to complete an interview; uncovers more sensitive information; provides more adaptability to non-English-speaking patients, patients with hearing impairment, or patients who are illiterate; and provides structured information for research. Dr. Bachman also observed the following weaknesses in such software: it may generate false-positive responses, may not be accepted by a minority of patients, is unable to detect nonverbal behavior, and requires changes in workflow. However, he further notes that "with the advent of EHR, the gathering of history and documentation from patients is increasingly important . . .".[48] A more recent study of patients who used a computer interview at the University of Wisconsin-Madison in 2004 found that 88.8% were willing to use the computer interview for minor conditions and 81.1% for other medical complaints.[49]

Today, several EHR products incorporate a medical history interviewing utility, or it can be acquired separately and used via a personal health record, patient portal, or kiosk in the waiting room or examining room. Because these now embed logic structures, they can be set to capture the desired amount of data. The questions can be presented to the patient in lay language and returned to the provider in a manner that allows validation of key points during the on-site visit.

As suggested by Steele, in addition to patients reducing the data entry burden for providers, staff should be expected to enter certain data. Dr. Kleeberg has observed that many providers do not use their office staff to their full credentials. If staff are not trusted to do data entry, they should be retrained or replaced.[c]

Another element important to improving workflows and processes is that although they will vary by physician specialty,[50] there is value in achieving as much standardization as possible, at least within a specialty and to the extent feasible across specialties. Appropriate standardization improves the ability to learn the system and hence improve productivity with use of the system. Adoption of standard vocabularies ensures effective data collection, for both the one specialist and all others who may be treating the patient, as well as better use of data downstream of the patient care visit, including for subsequent visits, referrals, and follow-up. Approaching workflow and process improvement with an eye toward achieving standardization also helps ensure that standards of care are practiced—even if the workflow and process vary by user preference.

Testing

Although rarely cited among common EHR mistakes, testing the system prior to go-live, other than for interfaces, is often not performed to the extent it should be. A test plan should be constructed that identifies the type of testing to be performed at each step in the implementation and who is responsible for performing the testing and approving results. As each individual application is configured, a unit and function test should be performed. This reviews screen design, report layouts, and basic clinical decision support logic. Interface testing ensures that all interfaces exchange the appropriate data among the applications to which they apply. As all applications and their interfaces come together, integrated system testing determines how well the applications generate the right data for display, for reports, and for clinical decision support. Performance and stress testing checks system response time. Such testing may need to be performed at the vendor's lab where peak volumes can be simulated. If the configuration cannot be tested in this manner, at a

minimum checking on system response times during site visits and in reference checks with organizations similar to the practice's is a suitable substitute.

"Acceptance testing" is a term that has multiple meanings. According to many EHR vendor contracts, "acceptance" of a system means that the licensee has taken delivery of the software and "accepts" it as satisfactory. This is not the more typical meaning of acceptance testing in most software engineering circles, where acceptance testing is performed on a *completed* system—either by the vendor prior to delivery of the completed system (factory acceptance testing) or by the user after configuration has been performed (user acceptance testing). User acceptance testing is a process run against user-supplied input data or an acceptance test script. A few EHR vendors have adopted these latter meanings, and even extend it to operational acceptance testing, which includes a "walk-through" where the system is evaluated in the context of the processes and procedures in which it is used.

The key to testing of the EHR, then, is to ensure the practice understands the terms being used in the contract, and to assure that unit, interface, and integrated system testing will be performed after configuration to the desired specifications. Testing should not be considered a part of end user training, dress rehearsal, or go-live—although sadly that is the case for many EHR vendors. Testing at such times puts the new user at a significant disadvantage and can cause distrust in the system. Ideally, an operational acceptance test is performed 30, 60, or 90 days after go-live and triggers the final milestone payment. Although there should be testing of system configuration and any interfaces developed for an ASP or SaaS model of software acquisition, the more limited amount of configuration generally does not require as extensive testing.

Training

Training occurs at several points during implementation. Super users are typically trained early in the implementation process so they learn how to perform some of the configuration themselves, including making changes to templates, creating reports, and adjusting the sensitivity of clinical decision support. Super users will also guide the workflow and process redesign and assist in end user training and support.

A training plan can be helpful. Often it includes everything from orientation, general education, and briefings about HIT and EHR to skills building, specific instruction, coaching, and refresher training. A database may be maintained that identifies everyone who requires any form of training, when it should be performed, that it has been performed, and whether any required competency

---

c. Paul Kleeberg, MD, FAAFP, FHIMSS, Clinical Director, REACH—Regional Extension Assistance Center for HIT. Personal interview. July 2010.

has been achieved. The training plan may also denote the training approach and modalities to be used. Although its initial implementation of computerized provider order entry (CPOE) was not successful, Cedars-Sinai found that pairing types of training with types of clinical users was imperative. Physicians do best with focused group sessions, one-on-one training, and just-in-time support; in contrast, nurses and other clinicians prefer classroom instruction and reference material. Not surprisingly, (younger) house staff preferred computer-based training.[51]

However training is conducted, there are two absolutes with respect to EHR training: (1) do not skimp on training and (2) everyone must be trained. Training is often last in a long list of items on a price list, and some practices decide they can manage it on their own with their super users. This is never the case because the super users will still be fairly new users and will be very busy participating in the implementation. Another risk area is not requiring training for physicians who think the system should be so intuitive that they can learn it on their own. They may well learn basic tasks on their own, but may not learn more than that so will not be taking full advantage of the system. They also do not learn the "right" way to use the system and associated workflows and processes that have been redesigned. Many new users focus exclusively on screen layout and data input. They often do not consider how they are positioned in association with the patient, how to talk with the patient at the same time as performing data entry or look-up, or how to reassure the patient that the new system will not lose their data, is secure, confidentiality is maintained, and so on.

Some vendors conduct a dress rehearsal, where those going live are brought through a near-live simulation of using the system, often with administrative staff playing the role of patients so that nursing staff and providers can practice in advance of the first real use. This has proven to be invaluable for those doing it, and can easily be replicated by anyone, whether the vendor supports it or not.

Turnover and Rollout Strategies

Turnover strategy refers to whether duplicate processing will be continued for a period of time after the first go-live of a system. Turnover strategies may be parallel or straight. In parallel turnover, the current process will continue for some period of time as the new process is rolled out. The purpose is often to ensure that the new system is working properly. In straight turnover, the old process is not used after the new process begins. Parallel turnover is sometimes considered when implementing a new practice management system (PMS). More often than not, however, the two PMSs are so different in their capabilities that

comparing the output of the processes running in parallel is virtually impossible. (Although, many practices will continue to work down their accounts receivable in the old PMS, retaining their license for 6 to 12 months, after which they generally can sell remaining accounts or write them off.) Duplicate data entry into paper charts and EHR is unrealistic. In fact, it is very important to "close" paper charts from data entry after the EHR goes live. A hybrid record situation where it is not clear whether recent labs or notes are in the paper chart or in the EHR is a hassle, and a potential risk to patient care.

Rollout strategy refers to whether the practice goes live in phases or all at once (a big bang). Although small practices may consider a big bang approach, most large practices use a phased strategy. There are several ways to approach phasing: by physical location (e.g., site, floor, pod, etc.), organizational unit/specialty (e.g., urgent care, all pediatricians, family practice-A, etc.), functionality (e.g., e-prescribing, look-up only, messaging, full documentation), and transitioning (e.g., first two patients first morning, first five patients second morning, etc.; only "easy" patients first 2 days, "more complicated" patients next 2 days, etc.). The decision table in **Table 12-7** illustrates these options. Additional rollout considerations include: selecting "light" months to go live, scheduling only follow-up visits for the first 2 weeks, adding 15 minutes to comprehensive exams, shifting open access to other physicians who have already gone live or have not yet gone live, and keeping the practice open for longer hours or additional days of the week so there is no overall impact of productivity loss on the practice.

When using a phased rollout strategy, the hybrid record situation can be avoided by scanning paper and

Table 12-7 Phased Rollout Strategies

	Functionality		
	All	Some	Transitioning
Physical	Y	N	Y
	Y	N	N
	N	Y	Y
	N	Y	N
Organizational Unit/Specialty	Y	N	Y
	Y	N	N
	N	Y	Y
	N	Y	N

Source: Used with permission, © Margret\A Consulting, LLC.

electronically feeding other documents into the EHR until all users are up on the EHR. If practices have little cross-over of patients by site or specialty they may be able to avoid such scanning. They can designate dates when each unit goes live and expect others to remember these dates when they have occasional need to access their records.

Go-Live

Go-live is the action of using the HIT in a production environment for the first time. This is a critical milestone not only for users, but also for the payment schedule, where go-live triggers a milestone payment.

To prepare for go-live, the practice should use a go-live checklist to make sure everything is ready. Such a checklist includes everything from making sure the first users have been trained and have participated in a dress rehearsal to checking that every device is plugged in or fully powered. Vendors may have their own go-live checklist, but it is a good idea for a practice to have its own with respect to its own responsibilities.

During go-live, staff must be readily available to provide end user support. One organization describes the need to "swarm users with support." All hands must be on deck. Support staff must be visible at all times (often wearing unique clothing to distinguish themselves for quick access), sometimes literally being "at the elbow" of new users. In addition to the traditional help desk, a large practice may consider setting up a special hotline in the event trained personnel are not immediately available. The telephone number of the hotline should be put on a sticky note on every computer.

Go-live should also include some form of communication to patients. Some vendors supply "under construction" signs; some practices prepare a pamphlet that describes their new EHR, introduces the staff wearing red jackets as physician computer helpers, reassures patients of its privacy and security, and requests their patience as the practice rolls out its new EHR. In general, most patients are very understanding; many may have undertaken a similar event in their own work environment. Younger patients may offer tips to help! Even older patients appreciate the move to a digital world. After all, the fastest-growing group of users of the Internet is those over 65 years of age,[52] and the most frequent use of the Internet by "silver surfers" is for health information,[53] although there are increasing concerns about consumers' understanding of health information on the Web.[54,55] In fact, many physicians have more concerns about how patients will react to their use of EHR in the examining room than patients actually have such concerns, especially after the first month of use and with appropriate

training.[56] It is important, however, for the provider to communicate with the patient about use of the EHR—it is new, it is secure, it helps keep better track of everything. They should position themselves in a manner that enables them to see the patient and the computer simultaneously, and to become accustomed to using the computer as an educational tool with the patient.

Go-live should be monitored closely and adjustments made as quickly as possible, especially if it is found that providers are not able to keep up with their patient load. Productivity loss is a significant concern. It can be overcome, however, especially by engaging providers throughout the EHR project and abstracting key data in advance so that new users are not presented with a "blank screen" on first use. A recent study found that once providers achieved 6 months of experience with the EHR, they were able to see 9 more patients per month, achieved a 22% increase in monthly charges, and had an increase of 12 RVUs per provider per month.[57]

At the conclusion of the first day, or even at lunch of the first day, there should be a go-live assessment. Support staff should be queried for feedback. New users should be asked how things went. The Regenstrief Institute advises holding bagel breakfasts and pizza lunches for user feedback.

Celebration is an important part of go-live. Celebration should ensure appropriate appreciation is expressed to all, including new users. Executive management should be highly visible. One hospital's chief executive officer spent the entire first day of CPOE implementation on the nursing unit, to be available to anyone who wanted to discuss anything and to demonstrate how important the hospital felt successful adoption was. A gold star placed on a new user's badge is often worn proudly. A "progress-o-meter" showing the growing number of users who make it through the first day, or the first day without loss of productivity, is not trivial. (Why do you think the United Way uses such symbols all over America?) But even just a pat on the back, shake of the hand, or mention in a house organ instills a sense that the hard work of HIT pays off.

■ HIT Optimization

There is life after HIT go-live! But this life will be different, and that expectation should be set far in advance of implementation. Life after go-live also has to be regularly monitored. Keeping the bagel breakfasts and pizza lunches going on a regular basis affords a forum for both fielding complaints and getting good ideas. Rounding is essential.

At one academic medical center, a new chief information officer conducted his first rounds to the clinics—only to find that fewer than half were barely using the EHR that supposedly had been fully implemented over a year prior. He also found that it was taking screens 45 to 75 seconds to load per screen, with users stating they didn't know the system could be faster, so they hadn't complained—they simply stopped using the system. These situations must be avoided. Some specific areas that can be planned or anticipated for optimization include formal benefits realization study, informal monitoring of goal achievement, retraining, workflow and process redesign, reconfiguration of templates and clinical decision support, ongoing system maintenance and upgrades, system enhancements, and new technologies.

Formal Benefits Realization Studies

Formal benefits realization studies may include return on investment, quality improvement assessment, patient and user satisfaction, and awards. Not all practices conduct all such studies in a formal manner, but many large groups find a formal benefits realization study an important part of their overall mission.

Return on investment follows directly from the original cost/benefit analysis, including total cost of ownership, developed during planning. Although it can be challenging to put boundaries on time and factors contributing to costs and benefits for HIT, even gross approximations can be helpful to reassure new users that productivity is improving, the project met budget, and goals are being met. If the practice did not conduct a formal benefits analysis, there may be prior cost reports that can be reviewed.

Quality improvement and patient safety are an important benefit of HIT. Almost every practice that implements HIT and EHR can point to anecdotal evidence of such. Once again, however, formal studies are often performed in limited circumstances and often by academic practices who are more accustomed to research methodology. However, others may find that a more formal approach to quality improvement establishes important expectations. Monitoring quality of care will be a key ingredient in successful risk sharing within an accountable care organizational structure.

To evaluate the impact of HIT on quality, predefined metrics and baseline data are helpful to determine the scope of improvement. Where practices have not collected baseline data, perhaps because it was too cumbersome in a paper environment, effective quality improvement studies can be performed after HIT is implemented to determine whether there is a trend of improvement

following go-live. Quality measurements might begin with participating in the Physician Quality Reporting System (PQRS). Certainly, the incentives for meaningful use of EHR incorporate quality reporting, although not yet with a focus on improvement. State-based programs also exist. An interesting phenomenon has occurred in Minnesota, where MN Community Measurement, an independent nonprofit community organization, started a healthcare quality reporting program in 2002. Its purpose was to assist patients in making informed choices about providers, give providers information to deliver the right care for their patients, and help purchasers of healthcare obtain information about the value they are getting for their healthcare dollars. Although it is not clear whether patients are using the site as intended, the significant increase in improvement on health scores each year clearly suggests that clinics and medical groups are watching the scores closely and making changes.[58]

A key component of quality improvement is not only using HIT to its fullest extent, but also adopting a culture of quality improvement. There is an important intersection between HIT and healthcare quality, where quality measures, clinical guidelines, and decision support tools must come together.[59] Many practices adopt the IOM's six dimensions of quality patient care (safe, patient centered, effective, efficient, timely, and equitable).[60] The National Priorities Partnership's priorities are also important to consider in focusing a quality culture. Priorities it identified in 2008 contributed to the creation of the meaningful use incentive criteria, and were updated in 2010 to include patient and family engagement, safety, care coordination, palliative and end-of-life care, equitable access, elimination of overuse, population health, and infrastructure supports.[61]

Patient and user satisfaction surveys are easy to conduct and can be quite insightful. Providers are often concerned that patients won't like the EHR, and a survey can put that myth to rest (so long as skilled trainers work with providers during their EHR training to address positioning and communications with patients). This is another opportunity to communicate with the patient about the EHR. User satisfaction survey results also are often a surprise to those thinking no one likes the EHR. Both surveys should be structured so that an honest assessment of both an EHR's potential strengths and weaknesses can be made. Both surveys should be conducted more than once, perhaps a month after go-live and then again 3 and 6 months thereafter, and then as needed.

Award seeking is not something most healthcare organizations do frequently, but can be an important element in the HIT project. It was previously noted that a celebratory atmosphere includes appreciation for hard work. An internal award system can recognize and relieve the stress of system configuration, testing, training, and go-live. Seeking external awards can also contribute to the desire for optimal performance. For instance, since 1994 the Nicholas E. Davies Award of Excellence, now administered by the Healthcare Information and Management Systems Society (HIMSS), has recognized excellence in the implementation and value from health information technology, specifically EHRs.[62] The National Quality Forum is another opportunity to demonstrate outcomes associated with quality efforts, including those supported by HIT.[63] The National Committee for Quality Assurance (NCQA) accreditation can demonstrate successful accomplishment of its principles of the patient-centered medical home and contribute to success within an accountable care organization.

Informal Monitoring of Goal Achievement

Whether a formal study is performed or not, monitoring goal achievement is vital. There then needs to be visible action taken wherever goals are not being met, including not only retraining, redesign of workflows, and/or reconfiguration of templates and clinical decision support as applicable, but also a review of the organization's quality culture as noted earlier and the goals themselves. Are the goals SMART enough for the organization? There are a few goals that most organizations include, at least in their early thinking, that are vital or can be a surrogate for more advanced benefits realization studies. Such studies also support the "user acceptance test" that signals a final payment after go-live. But these studies should be ongoing, at least until such time that they level off to acceptable performance.

Productivity monitoring is vital, and extra support should be given to any provider not reaching par within the milestone timeframes set. Such support should not include allowing users to return to old ways, but truly helping individuals make the transition and then "freezing" the new way.[d]

Reduction in transcription is often an excellent measure to determine whether providers are using structured templates. The amount of transcription will go down if users are entering data directly into the EHR. If feasible, transcription should be measured by number of lines per user so that individual counseling can be applied.

Quality of the data entry should also be monitored. Especially as new users begin to better navigate the system, shortcuts will be found. These can be very helpful,

but can also become a documentation compliance issue if not performed correctly. For instance, "copy and paste" shortens documentation time, but if the material copied is not changed to reflect the actual patient, the documentation will be erroneous and all documentation will begin to look exactly the same. In addition, such notes do not contribute structured data for clinical decision support. Also ensure that every use of drop-down menus and checkboxes/radio buttons is appropriate for the encounter. For example, many drug names are very similar, so ensuring that the one chosen is the one desired is important. Some of these issues can be overcome by the system actually learning the user's favorite selections and putting them at the top of a list. However, the correct choice must be made initially. Overuse of comment fields is another issue for new users. Often fearing that the checkbox is insufficient to explain their patient's story, new users will type extensive notes into these fields, often without checking the appropriate box, leading to the inability of the system to provide clinical decision support because it does not have structured data. Finally, many EHR systems include conversion of structured data into narrative notes that are more user friendly. Clinicians should be involved in reviewing these during system configuration; however, post go-live, these should be reviewed for their relevancy and that they are not becoming too rote.

Ongoing System Maintenance and Enhancements

A HIT system must be maintained such that users will find it always accessible and responsive, and trust the information derived from it. This means that hardware, connectivity, and software must be maintained on a regular basis.

System upgrades and enhancements are inevitable in a HIT environment. Depending on their scope, the practice may find it has the equivalent of another "mini-HIT project" on its hands with some upgrades. Practices should be aware that upgrades must be accepted within the timeframe specified in the contract or they may be subject to paying for back-loading desired upgrades. Most vendors distinguish upgrades (which are covered in the maintenance agreement subject to the previously mentioned qualification) from enhancements (often new components or modules).

Enhancements, in particular, further support the care delivery process.[64] If a personal health record or patient portal was not part of the initial EHR implementation, this can be a huge factor in reducing the data entry burden. Encouraging chronically ill patients to maintain a health diary can promote better compliance with the treatment

---

d. See "Lewin's freeze phases" and other change management tools at http://ChangingMinds.org/index.htm

regimen. Secure messaging with patients and other providers can aid follow-up and reap many benefits, from customer satisfaction to improvements in patient safety and quality of care that can now be measured. (Better data may also be received on whether patients have had their prescription filled, are taking their medication, following their diet, getting their immunizations at the retail pharmacy, and so on.) Direct patient monitoring may be an enhancement to an existing telemedicine program, or the start of a new telemedicine program. Smart peripherals, such as automated blood pressure cuffs, scales, and the like, can both reduce the data entry burden and ensure greater accuracy.

Research can be enhanced with access to more comprehensive—and more standardized, hence accurate—disease registries and sophisticated data warehousing and analytics capabilities. Most HIT and EHR vendors do not supply a data warehouse or advanced analytics as part of their HIT or EHR. However, some vendors are starting to provide such support on a subscription basis. Large practices may want to acquire these tools separately, or interface to those they already have.

It is no mistake that the federal government's meaningful use incentive program includes criteria for providing patients with automated forms of instructions, copies of their health information, and clinic visit summaries in the Continuity of Care Record (CCR) format[e] or Continuity of Care Document (CCD) format.[f,g] These

and similar requirements to exchange health information electronically among referring physicians, with public health departments, and for bio-surveillance are keys to moving toward patient-centered medical homes, accountable care organizations, or other structures that promote care across the continuum.

New Technologies

The federal government also has invested large sums of money in promoting health information exchange organizations (HIO)[h] and a nationwide health information network (NHIN).[i] Although still in their early stages, such structures promote the ability not only to obtain access to needed information for patient care across the continuum, but also to support programs to access community service support programs, organ donors, clinical trials, and patient/caregiver support groups.

■ Future Directions in HIT

Who knows what the future may hold—but the future starts with what the Institute of Medicine described as "essential technology for healthcare" some 25 years ago when it formed the Committee on Improving the Patient Record, and 5 years later, in 1991, released its first patient record study report.[60]

Large practices not only have an obligation to acquire HIT and EHR in support of their patient care services, but also have a history of being innovative and able to carry out the research that continues to be needed to reduce unintended consequences of EHRs, that empowered consumers have accurate and easy-to-understand information, and that Medicine 2.0 is only one of many next steps towards advancing healthcare.

In summary, Dr. Blumenthal's observation that patient care, not technology, will drive meaningful use of HIT is a powerful message. EHRs are not a technology project, but a clinical transformation intended to make the U.S. healthcare system work better for patients and providers. This means that it is the providers themselves that must be informed consumers—achieved through engagement in the HIT program throughout its course from beginning to ongoing optimization.

---

e. ASTM. E2369 - 05e2 Standard Specification for Continuity of Care Record (CCR) is an XML-based core data set of the most relevant administrative, demographic, and clinical facts about a patient's healthcare, covering one or more healthcare encounters. It may be prepared, displayed, and transmitted in paper or electronically in a browser, as an element in an HL7 message or Clinical Document Architecture (CDA) complaint document, in a secure email, or as a PDF file, HTML file, or word processing document. See: http://www.astm.org /Standards/E2369.htm

f. Corepoint Health. 2009. The Continuity of Care Document (CCD) provides a consolidated, single standard for clinical documents that harmonizes the content of the ASTM CCR and HL7 Clinical Document Architecture (CDA): http://www .corepointhealth.com/sites/default/files/whitepapers /continuity-of-care-document-ccd.pdf

g. Health Level Seven (HL7). Clinical Document Architecture (CDA) Release 2.0 provides an exchange model for clinical documents that renders both document format and machine-readable coded semantics: http://www.hl7.org /implement/standards/cda.cfm

---

h. See HHS State Health Information Exchange Program information at http://healthit.hhs.gov/portal/server .pt?open=512&objID=1488&mode=2

i. See HHS Nationwide Health Information Network: Background and Scope at http://www.hhs.gov/healthit /healthnetwork/background/

References

1. Medicare and Medicaid Programs; Electronic Health Record Incentive Program; Final Rule. 42 *Federal Register* 412, 413, 422, et al. (July 28, 2010):44314–44588.

2. Institute of Medicine. *To err is human: building a safer health system.* Kohn LT, Corrigan JM, Donaldson MS, eds. Washington, DC: National Academies Press; 1999.

3. Institute of Medicine. *The computer-based patient record: an essential technology for health care.* Dick RS, Steen EB (eds.). Washington, DC: National Academies Press; 1991.

4. NorthShore University HealthSystem. TV ads. Accessed at http://www.northshore.org/about-us/press/advertising/tv-ads.aspx

5. Cabana MD, Jee SH. Does continuity of care improve patient outcomes? *Journal of Family Practice.* 2004;53(12):974–980.

6. Agency for Healthcare Research and Quality. *The roles of patient-centered medical homes and accountable care organizations in coordinating patient care* (AHRQ Pub. No. 11-M005-EF). Rockville, MD: AHRQ; 2010.

7. National Committee for Quality Assurance. *NCQA patient-centered medical home 2011.* Washington, DC: NCQA; 2011.

8. American Academy of Family Physicians, American Academy of Pediatrics, American College of Physicians, American Osteopathic Association. *Joint principles of the patient-centered medical home.* Washington, DC: Patient-Centered Primary Care Collaborative. Accessed at http://www.pcpcc.net/content/joint-principles-patient-centered-medical-home; 2007.

9. American Academy of Family Physicians Center for Health Information Technology. *Brief report of the AAFP's EHR pilot project: key learnings from six small family practices.* Leawood, KS: AAFP. Access at http://www.centerforhit.org/PreBuilt/chit_pilotresults.pdf; 2005.

10. Casalino LP, Dunham D, Chin MH, et al. Frequency of failure to inform patients of clinically significant outpatient test results. *Archives of Internal Medicine.* 2009;169(12):1123–1129.

11. National Research Council. *Computational technology for effective health care: immediate steps and strategic directions.* Stead WW, Lin HS, eds. Washington, DC: National Academies Press; 2009.

12. Amatayakul M. *Electronic health records: transforming your medical practice* (2nd ed.). Englewood, CO: Medical Group Management Association; 2010.

13. Adler KG. How to successfully navigate your EHR implementation. *Family Practice Management.* 2007;14(2):33–39.

14. Kremsdorf R. The five rights of effective patient care. *Informatics Review.* 2005. Accessed at http://www.informatics-review.com/thoughts/5rights.html

15. Regenstrief Institute. Logical Observations Identifiers Names and Codes (LOINC®). Accessed at http://www.loinc.org

16. U.S. National Library of Medicine, National Institutes of Health. RxNorm. Accessed at http://www.nlm.nih.gov/research/umls/rxnorm/

17. Institute of Medicine, Tang PC. *Key capabilities of an electronic health record system: letter report.* Washington, DC: National Academies Press; 2003.

18. Zakim DN, Braun PF, Alscher MD. Underutilization of information and knowledge in everyday medical practice: evaluation of a computer-based solution. *BMC Medical Informatics and Decision Making,* 2008;8(50). Accessed at http://www.biomedcentral.com/content/pdf/1472-6947-8-50.pdf

19. Ely JW, Osheroff JA, Chambliss ML, et al. Answering physicians' clinical questions: obstacles and potential solutions. *Journal of the American Medical Association.* 2005;12:217–224.

20. National Alliance for Health Information Technology. Defining key health information technology terms. 2008. Accessed at healthit.hhs.gov.

21. Health Level Seven. EHR system functional model. 2007. Accessed at http://www.hl7.org/documentcenter/public/standards/EHR_Functional_Model/R1/EHR_Functional_Model_R1_final.zip

22. Certification Commission for Health Information Technology. Ambulatory 2007 EHR certification. 2007. Accessed at http://www.cchit.org/certify/2007/ambulatory-2007-ehr-certification

23. Health Information Technology: Initial Set of Standards, Implementation Specifications, and Certification Criteria for Electronic Health Record Technology; Final Rule. 45 *Federal Register* 170 (July 28, 2010):44590–44654.

24. Establishment of the Temporary Certification Program for Health Information Technology; Final Rule. 45 *Federal Register* 170 (June 24, 2010):36188.

25. World Resources Institute. How to conduct a "visioning" exercise. 2000. Accessed at http://www.gdrc.org/ngo/vision-dev.html

26. Blumenthal D. Presentation to the American Medical Informatics Association. December 27, 2009. Reported in: http://www.informationweek.com/blog/healthcare/229204271?printer_friendly=this-page The Ohio State University Extension. Building dynamic groups: a values and visioning exercise. 2009. Accessed at http://www.ag.ohio-state.edu/~bdg/pdf_docs/e/E05.pdf

27. Engelberg Center for Health Care Reform at Brookings. *Issue brief: accountable care organizations: reforming provider payment—moving toward accountability for quality and value.* Lebanon, NH: Dartmouth Institute for Health Policy & Clinical Practice; 2009.

28. Johnson JK. Clinical microsystem assessment tool, Dartmouth-Hitchcock Medical Center. 2003. Accessed at http://clinicalmicrosystem.org/materials/worksheets/microsystem_assessment.pdf

29. Stratis Health. Health information technology toolkit for physician offices. 2010. Accessed at http://www.stratishealth.org/expertise/healthit/clinics/clinictoolkit.html

30. Gans D, Kralewski J, Hammons T, et al. Medical groups' adoption of electronic health records and information systems. *Health Affairs.* 2005;24(5):1323–1333.

31. Chalice R. *Improving healthcare using Toyota lean production methods: 46 steps for improvement* (2nd ed.). Milwaukee: ASQ Quality Press; 2007.

32. Barry R, Murcko A, Brubaker C. *The Six Sigma book for healthcare: improving outcomes by reducing errors.* Chicago: Health Administration Press; 2002.

33. Cassidy A, Guggenberger K. *A practical guide to information systems process improvement.* Boca Raton, FL: CRC Press; 2001.

34. Zaroukian MH, Sierra A. Benefiting from ambulatory EHR implementation: solidarity, Six Sigma, and willingness to strive. *Journal of Healthcare Information Management.* 2006;20(1): 53–60.

35. Merrill M. Survey: hospital-owned practices lead EHR adoption. *Healthcare IT News.* October 25, 2010. Accessed at http://www.healthcareitnews.com/news/survey-hospital-owned-practices-lead-ehr-adoption

36. Merrill M. Sunny outlook for small practice EMR adoption, meaningful use cloudy. *Healthcare IT News.* March 29, 2010. Accessed at http://www.healthcareitnews.com/news/sunny-outlook-small-practice-emr-adoption-meaningful-use-cloudy

37. Office of the National Coordinator for Health Information Technology. Certified health IT product list. Accessed December 28, 2010 at http://onc-chpl.force.com/ehrcert/EHRProductSearch?setting=Ambulatory

38. Leavitt M. Health IT initiatives: Not magical, just practical. *Health Affairs.* August 19, 2008 http://healthaffairs.org/blog/2008/08/19/health-it-initiatives-not-magical-just-practical/

39. CAQH. CORE overview. Accessed at http://www.caqh.org/CORE_overview.php

40. Nelson R. Successful ways to implement a practice management system and EHR. MGMA In Practice blog. Accessed at http://blog

.mgma.com/blog/bid/33018/Successful-ways-to-implement-a-practice-management-system-and-EHR

41. Gearon CJ. Take two and e-mail me at your convenience. America's Health Insurance Plans. 2008. *AHIP Coverage* (July/August 2008). American Academy of Family Physicians. E-visits. 2008. Accessed at http://www.aafp.org/online/en/home/policy/policies/e/evisits.html

42. Certification Commission for Health Information Technology. CCHIT certified 2011 ambulatory EHR certification criteria. 2010. Accessed at http://www.cchit.org/certify/2011/cchit-certified-2011-ambulatory-ehr

43. Pennell U, Fishman E. Known pitfalls and proven methods for a successful EMR implementation. 2005. Accessed at http://www.emrconsultant.com/emr_pitfalls.php

44. Dolan PL. Before buying an EMR system, learn from others' mistakes. *American Medical News.* 2009. Accessed at http://www.ama-assn.org/amednews/2009/06/22/bica0622.htm

45. Fahy J. Automating clinical workflow with EHR: an ongoing process. PedSource. 2010. Accessed at http://www.pedsource.com/print/15474

46. Steele E. EHR implementation: who benefits, who pays? *Health Management Technology.* (July 27, 2006);7:43–44.

47. Bachman JW. The patient-computer interview: a neglected tool that can aid the clinician. *Mayo Clinic Proceedings.* 2003;78:67–78.

48. Smith PD, Grasmick M. Computer interviewing in a primary care office: the patients are ready. *Studies in Health Technology and Informatics.* 2004;107(Pt 2):1162–1165.

49. Bhargava H, Sweeney J. UC Davis study finds e-medical records have varying effects on productivity. UC Davis News and Information. December 26, 2010. Accessed at http://www.news.ucdavis.edu/search/printable_news.lasso?id=9665&table=news

50. Brisset PR, Gilman CS, Morgan, MT et al. Who are your CPOE users and how do you train them? Lessons learned at Cedars-Sinai Health System. *MEDINFO 2004.* International Medical Informatics Association. Amsterdam: IOS Press. 2004.

51. Pew Internet and American Life Project. Change in Internet use by age group, 2000-2009. Accessed at http://www.pewinternet.org/Infographics/2010/Internet-acess-by-age-group-over-time.aspx

52. Atkinson NL, Saperstein SL, Pleis J. Using the Internet for health-related activities: findings from a national probability sample. *Journal of Medical Internet Research.* 2009;11(1). Accessed at http://www.jmir.org/2009/1/e4/

53. McQuillan L. Study finds critical challenges to consumers' understanding and use of evidence-based health care. American Institutes for Research. June 30, 2010. Accessed at http://www.air.org/news/index.cfm?fa=viewContent&content_id=851

54. Jessen W. Medicine 2.0 and participatory medicine. June 6, 2010. Accessed at http://www.walterjessen.com/medicine-2-0-and-participatory-medicine/

55. Hsu J, Huang J, Fung V, et al. Health information technology and physician-patient interactions: impact of computers on communication during outpatient primary care visits. *Journal of the American Medical Informatics Association.* 2005;12:474–480.

56. Cheriff AD, Kapur AG, Qiu M, Cole CL. Physician productivity and the ambulatory EHR in a large academic multi-specialty physician group. *International Journal of Medical Informatics.* 2010;79(7):492–500. Accessed at http://www.ncbi.nlm.nih.gov/pubmed/20478738

57. MN Community Measurement. Minnesota HealthScores. Accessed at http://www.mnhealthscores.org

58. National Quality Forum. Wired for quality: the intersection of health IT and healthcare quality. *Issue Brief NQF.* March 2008;8.

59. Institute of Medicine, Committee on Quality of Health Care in America. *Crossing the quality chasm: a new health system for the 21st century.* Washington, DC: National Academies Press; 2001.

60. National Quality Partnership. *Input to the Secretary of Health and Human Services on priorities for the 2011 national quality strategy.* Washington, DC: National Quality Forum; 2010. Accessed at http://www.qualityforum.org/Setting_Priorities/Addressing_National_Priorities.aspx

61. Healthcare Information Management and Systems Society. HIMMS Davies award. Accessed at http://www.himss.org/davies/index.asp

62. National Quality Forum. Awards. John M. Eisenberg Patient Safety and Quality awards. Accessed at http://www.qualityforum.org/Events/Awards/Awards.aspx

63. Turisco F, Rhoads J. Beyond e-health records: technologies that enhance care delivery. 2010 CSC Papers winner from CSC Leading Edge Forum. 2010. Accessed at http://www.csc.com/cscworld/publications/56901/57009-beyond_e_health_records_technologies_that_enhance_care_delivery

CHAPTER

13

Office Practice Risk Management

Geraldine Amori, PhD, ARM, CPHRM, DFASHRM

Office-based risk management is increasingly important because more care is being rendered in the office and less in inpatient facilities. Historically, office practice risk management was not a primary management concern. The lawsuits with the greatest jury awards were those based on in-patient events and claims. Surgery and obstetrics were key targets of claimants and attracted the attention of administrators because they represented the greatest financial losses. Nonetheless, errors do occur in the practice setting and can have significant medical and financial impact.[1-3]

Changes in the last 15 years have shifted the focus of care from the inpatient to the outpatient setting. With that, administrators have become more aware of the inherent risk in office-based practices:

- Traditionally, managed care has encouraged the office-based primary care treatment of patients who at one time might have been hospitalized. With the introduction of patient-centered medical homes, pay for performance, and accountable care organization regulations, the model of healthcare delivery is constantly evolving.

- Consistent with that trend, pressure has increased to hospitalize patients later in the course of treatment (when compared to past trends) and for the shortest period of time. This results in greater pressure on the office practice to monitor prehospitalization and posthospitalization status.

- Media coverage of fraud and abuse has raised patient awareness of billing issues and appropriate management of care.

These factors contribute to the fact that risk management in the office practice is a complex and different activity than risk management in the inpatient facility. Confounding the identification and prevention of losses in the office setting is the nature of the office-based provider–patient relationship. In the inpatient setting, an event related to potential litigation is generally known prior to discharge of the patient. Conversely, in the outpatient setting, the care that generates the potential litigation and the doctor's awareness of the alleged potential harm may be separated by hours, days, and in some cases years. For example, an adverse reaction to a prescription may not be known to the doctor for several days. Further, an inpatient's condition is monitored constantly, unlike that of the patient seen in the office. Consequently, the doctor's office may not be aware that an event has occurred until the complaint is served, or an attorney requests patient records. Even then, the nature of the event may be difficult to define. The record reflects the last interactions, which may have been appropriate and do not reveal any indication of potential adverse outcomes. In addition, there may be years between the last visit and the notice of claim. Patients who are angry tend to stop seeing the offending provider. Furthermore, a missed diagnosis or misdiagnosis may not become apparent until long after the last visit. Finally, the irritation or injury from the care may not become suit-worthy in the potential claimant's mind until time and expense exacerbate the effects of the outcome on the quality of patient life.

This chapter provides an overview of the risk management process as it applies to the medical office practice. The risk management process is explained and risk management techniques are discussed. Finally, the most common risk exposure considerations are pointed out for each of the major risk management categories of the medical office practice.

■ The Risk Management Process

The business of healthcare is the delivery of clinical services. Consequently, the delivery of clinical care is the first risk exposure focus for most administrators. Although it is true that much of the liability the practice faces is because of perceived or actual failure to fulfill clinical duties, it is short-sighted to limit the risk management process to clinical risk management. Other exposure areas can result in losses that can be equally, if not more devastating to the business.

It becomes clear to the experienced risk manager that most risk originates in communication processes and systems. Just as is true in the context of patient care, it is also true in each process in a physician practice. In spite of how much they assist the practice from a data processing or technological perspective, communication systems such as telephones, tablet computers (e.g., iPads), digital phones with photo and video capabilities, computers, and on-call systems also can create exposures to risk. The billing process, starting with the gathering of personal and insurance information through the billing and collection process, presents exposures. The processes for banking, the procurement and maintenance of property, the purchase of supplies, and the employment of full-time and agency staff each presents an opportunity for risk exposures that should be managed.

Even those risks that appear unrelated to communication, such as property destruction or loss as a result of natural disasters, have at their core the need for effective coordination and communication. Together, the issues of exposure for the business are known as the practice's total risk or enterprise-wide risk management. The concept of enterprise-wide risk management addresses this idea of exposures being evaluated independently of each other, as well as how they interrelate with every other aspect of the business.

The six primary categories of risk exposure in the office practice are:

1. Professional exposures (liability)
2. Personnel exposures
3. Property exposures (general liability and safety)
4. Financial exposures
5. Exposures from technology and its uses
6. Legal/regulatory exposures

Losses in any one of these categories can have a severe financial impact to the practice. When losses include more than one category, the exposures can be exponential. In order to address each of these areas of risk, the administrator or risk manager must carefully identify and analyze each aspect of the business operations. The risk management process consists of five steps:

1. Identify risk exposures.
2. Assess hazards to evaluate the risks.
3. Evaluate different techniques and combinations of techniques for loss control.
4. Select the best technique with the information available and implement it.
5. Monitor consistently to improve and refine techniques.

The application of these steps to each system and area of exposure generates the risk management plan for the practice.

Ultimately, the risks about which a practice should be most concerned are those that affect the ability of the practice to perform its functions and to remain fiscally viable. There are two kinds of losses that have the potential to adversely influence the practice. The first kinds of losses are those that occur frequently, resulting in many small losses and cumulative expense. The second kinds of losses are those that occur infrequently, but result in significantly larger unique losses. Consequently, although some perfunctory operations may appear to carry little risk, it is important that the individual conducting the risk assessment be willing to ask the question "What if?" at every level of operation.

The Five Steps of the Risk Management Process

The risk management process is a management process designed to identify and address potential risk exposures. Generally, risk exposures are thought to be events, conditions, or situations that could result in financial loss to the organization. The process for addressing risk is logical and systematic: identification of exposure, assessment of potential impact based upon frequency or severity, identification of potential ways to mitigate potential impact, selecting and applying identified techniques, and finally monitoring the efficacy of selected techniques.

Step 1: Risk Identification

Methods for identifying and assessing risks vary from practice to practice. Typical methods include flowcharting of processes to identify where problems can occur, proprietary or standardized questionnaires, and reviews of financial records showing where losses have occurred in the past or where there have been great fluctuations in financial stability. In addition, interviews with staff and consultation with experts can be informative. Each of these methods can identify areas where process failure can lead to communication breakdown and creation of exposure.[4] Each of these methods can be applied in the six categories of risk: professional, property, personnel, financial processes, information technology, and legal/regulatory compliance.

In each of the six categories of losses, a thorough analysis should be conducted. First, each major process within the category should be identified. For example, in the financial area, the processes of payroll, accounts receivable, and billing may be the initial processes that are analyzed. The analysis begins by flowcharting the process, then having discussions with staff, perhaps discussions with experts, or conducting a thorough review of the literature. The financial data for several years should be analyzed to determine the factors that have contributed to fluctuations or unanticipated expenses. The data from this process will expose potential failure points in the process. Interestingly, the analyst may find that similar exposures occur in many different processes. The comparison of data across processes may create patterns demonstrating the comparative strength of loss exposures.

In the clinical arena, the processes may be identified differently. A patient visit should be analyzed, starting with the initial phone call, which can identify areas of potential process disruption. The system for taking messages and conveying information to the clinicians should be analyzed. The process for ordering, receiving, reviewing, and recording diagnostic test results should be reviewed. Next, the processes for implementing and ensuring adherence to treatment guidelines can be identified for the major diagnostic categories that are treated in the practice. The analyst will find that processes do not function reliably in many areas. In addition, points where processes convene are significant areas for system breakdown. A simple tool such as a patient satisfaction survey can help a risk manager identify areas of possible risk exposures as well as opportunities to improve patient service in general.

Although this process analysis may sound similar to those used in quality improvement methodologies, there are differences. In quality improvement, the goal is to improve the process so there is less opportunity for error. The ultimate goal is to improve patient care and to ensure that waste and rework are negated to the extent feasible. Improving patient care is clearly related to reduction of loss; however, that is not the direct goal of the quality process. In addition, based on the extent to which money spent on waste and rework is money that is not available for other purposes, it also can be considered a loss exposure. Instead, process analysis for the purpose of risk assessment focuses specifically on potential system failures that can lead to errors, omissions, commissions, or other acts that will require remediation. These failures can cost the practice actual or potential resources that otherwise could be used to grow the business. They are therefore considered loss exposures.

Step 2: Risk Assessment

The next phase of the risk identification process is the analysis of the identified exposures to determine the potential severity of the exposure. Given the complexity of the healthcare business, there will be many more risks than time and money to address them. Consequently, exposures must be prioritized in terms of their impact on the overall ability of the practice to remain fiscally sound. Some risks are inherent in the work. Other risks might best be transferred to others via contract or delegation, or not assumed at all. Exposures identified in the initial phase of the process must be evaluated against the strategic goals and objectives of the practice. A practice's mission or goals may lead it to accept a risk that another practice may not. A charitable foundation with a mission of service to underserved minorities of a community would not decide to reduce a potential loss exposure by limiting the types of insurance or payment it accepts. By the same token, a practice that specializes in cosmetic surgery may choose to require payment in advance for procedures in alignment with its goal of fiscal responsibility to its shareholders. Furthermore, each exposure must be evaluated in terms of its frequency of occurrence and the severity of loss incurred.

Bariatric surgery, for example, is a growth industry.[5] Comorbidities and the potential for significant complications render morbidly obese patients high risk. A practice experiencing three bariatric professional liability suits in 5 years is likely to experience costly ramifications. Three suits may not be high frequency if the practice has successfully performed 20 such surgeries, 15 of which were highly successful. Nonetheless, the cost of loss may be notable. By the same token, if the practice has experienced 10 "delay in diagnosis" suits in 5 years that resulted in much smaller claims, the total cost of loss may still be significant. Often the expense of defense and staff time involved in defending a claim may be greater than any judgment awarded the plaintiff. Cost of loss includes the expenses associated with preventing ultimate awards. Consequently, frequency and severity are factors of the analysis that must be considered when deciding how to approach loss control. Finally, it is tempting to assume that although a large loss has the potential to occur, it has not "happened here," therefore it is unlikely to occur at all. The temptation to be lulled into a false sense of security must be avoided.

Step 3: Evaluating Techniques and Technique Combinations for Loss Control

The next phase in the risk management process consists of evaluating the feasibility of alternative techniques for controlling the frequency and severity of losses. In this step, alternative approaches are considered for each significant exposure. Risk exposures take many forms and require unique approaches. Hypothetical examples of situations that could arise include:

■ Certain small banks in the locale accept Internet transmission of direct deposit, although it is not their strongest service. The transmission software systems between contracted payroll vendor and the bank used by some local employees has been identified as having compatibility problems, resulting in delayed or missed transmission. Employees believe they have funds when they may not. Whose risk is this? What are the practice's responsibilities and options?

■ An employed physician performs office-based surgery that requires specific supplies, and the medical supplier is across the river. Significant weather prohibits delivery of supplies needed for the week's surgeries. Does the practice cancel scheduled surgeries? What is the backup plan?

■ The computer system is backed up on a server maintained in the basement because it is the coolest area of the building. The dam up the river breaks, resulting in unprecedented flooding. Does the practice have a plan for ensuring that there is no loss of important data?

■ The chief operating officer is a 42-year-old athletic female. She goes on vacation and is involved in an accident. Is the practice prepared for temporary and possibly permanent replacement?

■ The highest-producing physician in the practice has a heart attack and dies suddenly. How is the practice going to replace this revenue?

■ A senior physician is accused of Medicare fraud. What is the practice's plan regarding involvement, defense, and public relations management?

■ The practice undergoes a third-party payor audit. The payor's position is that the practice owes $250,000 in overpayments due to erroneous coding.

For each risk exposure identified in the practice, the choices are the same: accept the risk, find methods to finance potential losses and methods to reduce the frequency or severity of loss, transfer the risk contractually, or avoid the risk completely.

Accepting Risk and Applying Loss Control Techniques. Many risks in healthcare are accepted and covered financially through commercial insurance as part of the cost of doing business. Automobile, property, directors and officers, key person, business interruption, and other specific types of insurance coverage can insure those unforeseen, infrequent, and costly exposures. Those exposures that are more expected and inherent in the practice of medicine and business, such as worker and patient safety, patient care liability, and office practices, lend themselves to loss prevention or reduction techniques. These are the types of exposures where communication breaks down, handoffs are unstable, and consistency and process reliability are a necessity. Loss control techniques that are effective include checklists, forced behavior processes that cannot proceed unless the steps are followed precisely, and feedback loops to reduce reliance on individual memory. Furthermore, these are the areas where staff education, guidelines, and leadership are essential to ensure that processes do not revert to less structured, less effective methods of operation. Loss control for physical property or systems relies on methods such as duplication or segregation of assets. The value of backed-up data is diminished if that backup is maintained in close physical proximity to the original data being protected. Data loss through heat, flooding, theft, or other damage to the premises is negated if both sources of information are damaged.

Contractual Risk Transfer. A common, and often desirable, approach to loss control is contractual risk transfer. Practices that utilize outside services may choose to transfer the risk for liability related to the functions being performed to those service providers through contractual language such as indemnification clauses. This allows the practice to be relieved of liability while enjoying the benefits of having the services.

Interestingly, commercial insurance is a form of contractual transfer of risk. For the price of the premium, the insurer assumes the contractually agreed-upon risks for losses incurred by the practice. The caveat is that premiums may be affected by the accumulated losses the practice experiences both as an individual entity and as a member of a risk class. In other words, increased risk exposure will result in increased cost of premiums. The underwriting of commercial insurance is a fascinating discussion that is beyond the scope of this chapter.

Risk financing is a vital part of the total approach to risk management that must be considered by the office practice. A variety of financing options exist to address those risks that must be assumed and for which no amount of loss control can guarantee elimination of exposure. Although commercial insurance may be the easiest to manage, it is also the most expensive. Underwriting techniques do not evaluate any individual entity, but use the practice loss information in conjunction with aggregated data from a variety of sources to determine a potential for loss. In addition, the insurer's need to ensure its own economic viability results in significant additional fees to the insured. Other forms of risk financing, including current expensing of losses, funded and unfunded reserves, borrowing, trusts, and captives, each represents an approach that must match the laws of the state and the type of loss exposure. Frequent low-cost exposures may be accounted for in operational budgets or unfunded reserves; in other words, pay losses as incurred through operational dollars. High-cost or low-frequency losses may be accounted for through a line of credit or unfunded reserves. For each category of risk, each exposure is analyzed and the appropriate mechanism for risk control, transfer, or financing must be applied.

Trusts, captive insurance companies, and risk retention groups have become the professional liability insurance vehicles of choice for any practice that has sufficient funds and ongoing revenues to support the financial requirements. Self-insurance for professional liability has the benefit of being impervious to the market fluctuations in the commercial insurance industry. Premiums and overhead costs are based on the actual loss costs of the participants rather than industry trends. Furthermore, effective loss control and loss reduction efforts directly affect the participating practices through an effect on cost. The benefits are straight and robust. Of course, there are drawbacks to this type of mechanism. Although groups insured through self-insurance mechanisms are fortunate to be unaffected by temporary insurance increases that may be due to hard market conditions, they also do not benefit from the savings represented through soft market conditions, with one exception. Self-insured organizations do benefit from the reduced rates on umbrella and other layers, as do the commercially insured. When commercial insurance is abundant and inexpensive, the self-insured groups continue to set aside funds based on actual costs and experience. It is tempting to liquidate funding at these times in order to take advantage of the short-term savings on commercial premiums. Consequently, the use of self-insurance vehicles must be viewed as long-term approaches. Over time, the investment in a self-insurance program and solid loss-control initiatives will result in significant savings over the market-driven fluctuations of the commercial market.

Step 4: Selecting and Applying Techniques for Managing Potential Risks (Loss Control Alternatives)

The selection of a technique for managing potential risks is based on the individual organization's appetite for risk, resources, and the impact of those choices on other aspects of the organization's operation. It is impossible to say that the same approach to managing risk will apply in every organization and for every situation.

Every organization should assign the responsibility of risk management to a team of personnel. The role of a risk management team to is look at the exposures identified and the level of risk posed to the organization. Taking into consideration the extent to which the organization is risk averse, and the potential unintended consequences of each strategy, choices can be made from the strategies identified in Step 3 of the process.

Step 5: Monitoring Selected Risk Control Techniques

Once the approach or combination of approaches to address each exposure has been selected and implemented, the effective risk manager monitors for the effectiveness and continued reliability of those methods. The risk management technique most appropriate for a practice in a time of growth may not be valid at a later time in the practice's development. The risk management process is, by definition, a continuing process. New exposures develop through new types of business, changes brought about by legislative or regulatory requirements, changes in information technology systems, new medications, or changed telephone systems. The practice must be constantly reevaluated to identify new risk exposures. This will result in tighter risk controls and ensure that the quality of business systems is consistently monitored.

The remainder of this chapter will identify and discuss some of the most common risk exposures in the office setting: professional liability, personnel, property, and financial exposures.

■ Office Practice Exposures

Professional liability arises out of the patient, staff, and provider relationship. The premise for professional liability is simple: Patients seek to create a relationship with a provider for certain services. The provider agrees to that relationship by seeing the patient and commencing care. This bilateral acceptance of the relationship establishes a duty to deliver services. Patients have expectations about those services in terms of the standard by which those services are provided. When those services fail to meet those expectations, there is a perceived breach of that duty. If that breach falls below the standard of care and there is an injury directly related to the failure to perform that duty, then the behavior may constitute negligence, and the provider would be exposed to liability for the negligent treatment.

Risk Exposure: The Relationship with the Patient

The relationship with the patient is at the core of a physician practice, as well as the crux of potential clinical risk. It is also the most fragile aspect of the work performed by a medical practice. Literature has demonstrated repeatedly that communication breakdown is the most frequent factor leading to a professional liability allegation.[6-9] It is not just the communication about care that falters. Communication with patients takes many forms. There is the written material given to patients to educate them about a condition or treatment. There is the sound of staff on the phone, and on the electronic answering equipment. There is the communication about the level of concern the practice has for patients. That concern is conveyed through the complexity of the appointment-making process, wait times, follow-up, and billing systems. There is the appearance and care of the practice's facility and grounds. Finally, there is the communication that occurs face to face, telephonically, or electronically with practitioners. It is comforting to consider these aspects of communication primarily a patient satisfier. In reality, these aspects of patient interaction convey an overall sense of attention to the needs of patients and families. The patient's perception built upon these elements is projected into other areas of the patient relationship. A patient who perceives that the practice is careless about how patients are treated will relate that to his or her own experience should he or she feel that the practitioner has not given sufficient time or information. Lawsuits based on breakdown of communication are rarely based on a single interaction, but a host of exchanges that culminate in a final experience the patient associates with a negative outcome and harm to themselves.

There are three types of communication that contribute to potential litigation. The communication directly with the patient about the care; the communication about the patient that pertains to care, such as test results and referral information; and finally, the information about the practice and policies that do not directly affect patient care. These elements of communication establish the tone of the relationship with the patient. None of these types of communication results in litigation in and of itself. Each of them, however, contributes to potential litigation when paired with an unexpected outcome. The patient with whom the provider had dissatisfactory or misinterpreted interpersonal communication about care is likely to sue if there is a bad outcome because of feelings of frustration or anger. The patient who suffers a breakdown in communication regarding test results or other processes that led to a delay in diagnosis or belated treatment is likely to sue if he or she feels that the communication breakdown is reflective of the provider's attitude toward patients. Finally, the patient whose expectations are not met because of statements made in marketing materials or because of billing policies is likely to sue in the face of an unexpected outcome because of feelings of being misled or insufficiently advised about the practice. Effective communication does not prevent suits; however, ineffective communication can be the determining point for whether litigation is pursued.

Each major component of risk exposure related to professional liability ultimately ties back to communication. Even in situations in which there is legitimate clinical liability, the manner in which a practice has communicated with the patient who has been injured can influence the outcome of litigation.

Risk Exposure: Communication with the Patient About Care

Appointments: New Patients
Communication scripting should be provided for appointment staff so that they do not hint of express warranty

or satisfaction. For example, patients may ask, "Will I like Dr. Jones?" Staff, in an effort to be supportive to the patient may respond, "I know you'll like Dr. Jones, all his patients do." This type of innocent and intentionally helpful statement can set an unrealistic expectation for patients and subsequent allegations of being misled. This perception will result in mistrust of the system. A better response may be, "It would be difficult for me to know if you will like him; however, many of his patients say nice things about him." Similarly, patients could ask, "Can Dr. Lopez help me?" A response of "I'm sure Dr. Lopez will be able to make you feel better" might be perceived as a guarantee of cure at worst, and acceptance of the patient for treatment at best. Better ways to approach these types of questions would be for the appointment staff to respond, "Dr. Lopez will be able to examine you and help you decide what your next steps should be." This response allows Dr. Lopez to be able to decide during the examination and interview process whether she is both able and willing to work with this patient.

Complicating the determination of relationship is the emerging trend towards having patients contact the practice and make appointments online. The opportunity for a claim of relationship potentially exists prior to the first visit unless the practice is very clear on its website that establishing the first appointment is for the purpose of evaluation only and does not constitute a therapeutic relationship. It is recommended that office practices seek legal guidance to ensure their website wording is in compliance with statutes and regulations applicable in the organization's jurisdiction.

Establishing the Relationship: The First Appointment

At the first appointment, patients should be told the expectations of the practice as well as their rights. It is not enough to provide patients with a Health Insurance Portability and Accountability Act of 1996 (HIPAA) statement and a brochure about the practice. This approach assumes that the patient and family can read, that they will read the material, and that they will understand and assimilate the material.

A 5-minute conversation that is documented in the record establishes the parameters for the relationship and sets the tone for honest, two-way expectations and interactions. Patients should be advised about:

- Practice expectations about appointments, cancellations and no-shows, and payments
- Systems or services in place to help meet financial hardship
- How and to whom to direct any questions, concerns, or complaints

Furthermore, patients and families should be evaluated in terms of their willingness to participate as a partner in care. During the discussion, the practitioner can explain:

- Care is a two-way process. If the patient finds he or she is unable to follow provider recommendations, he or she should speak up without fear of recrimination, so the care plan can be adjusted.
- The practitioner will be more upset if the patient acquiesces to recommendations and does not follow them than if the patient speaks up about his or her inability or unwillingness to adhere to recommended treatment.
- If medication is too costly so that the patient does not take it as prescribed, the practitioner must be advised.
- The patient should take specific steps in the event of an emergency, including a reaction to the treatment.
- Medicine is an imperfect science. The practitioners, for all their efforts, may make errors. Consequently, it is important that the practitioner and the patient work together toward the desired outcome. The patient should call, speak up, or come for another visit if the recommendations are not working.

Occasionally patients arrive for their first visit with a complete medical record in hand. Clearly, in this case, it is impossible for the provider to carefully review the entire record within the context of an initial visit. In this situation, the taking of the patient history is very important, including the question about any significant abnormal test results. The practitioner should also be clear with the patient about the purpose of the current visit and ask about significant events of the past. In the case of a complex medical history, it would behoove the provider to review the record in more detail later for any information that might prove pertinent to the care.

Although this type of discussion appears burdensome and risky for an initial visit, it sets the tone for care. It also assures that patients have been educated about the expectations of the practice. This provides the parameters for decisions the practice may unfortunately decide it needs to make later to terminate the relationship. The establishing of parameters, setting of expectations, and delimiting of boundaries together form a framework for the practitioner–patient relationship that supports honest communication and limits potential allegations of lack of communication.

Appointments: Returning Patients

The risk does not end with the first appointment. Care must be taken to put processes in place to address the needs of a patient who returns to the practice for care.

To what extent are patient scheduling needs accommodated for acute care or routine visits? How are patients who regularly demand special treatment handled? What are the policies about cancellations, no-shows, failure to copay, waiting room behavior, and children in the waiting room of adult care areas?

A prime example of how the appointment system can be the first step in a string of failures is how scheduling conflicts are handled. What is the practice process for resolution if the practitioner asks the patient to return in a specific time period and there are no available appointments? Similarly, the patient who calls and is very concerned about an issue but is asked to wait to be seen may have an acute problem he or she failed to describe adequately. The policy issue and risk exposure in these instances relate to the practice guidelines regarding staff instruction for handling these specific types of events. If policy dictates that when there is a conflict between the practitioner-requested return and the schedule, the staff has authorization to address it in a way that is acceptable to the practice, then the risk is addressed.

Consent and Disclosure

Informed consent and disclosure of unanticipated outcomes are central concerns in patient-centered care.[10-12] Consent, although theoretically considered the approach to discussion, rather than a piece of paper, was historically invoked when significant risks or invasive procedures were involved. New ways of thinking about patient involvement in care create a new approach to consent in the office practice that goes beyond traditional risks and benefits of invasive procedures.[12,13]

Assuming that malpractice litigation is correlated more with ineffective communication than solely with outcomes,[6] consent should become part of the way care is delivered on a daily basis. This type of process utilizes routine query of the patient's ability and willingness to engage in a recommendation or treatment approach. Rather than saying, "I want you to exercise three times a week," the aware practitioner will ask "Are you willing to exercise three times a week? How will you fit this into your schedule?" The care interaction is changed from one of the patient as a passive recipient of care to that of an active participant in care. The difference becomes more significant when the potential allegation that, "The doctor never told me I had to take this medication with food," is countered with the documented, "The patient said he would take the medication at dinner." Further, by questioning how the patient plans to integrate recommendations into his or her daily life, there is an increased probability that the patient may

question the recommendations, increasing the potential for compliance.[14,15]

An additional benefit to this approach is in the treatment of those patients who request significantly greater amounts of narcotic medications than practitioners believe are appropriate. Clear written agreements between patients and providers about how narcotic drug requests are to be handled (i.e., frequency of refills, etc.) will document practitioner efforts to provide reasonable pain relief while promoting limited reliance on potentially addicting medications This particular issue has expanded in importance in recent years with the increasing incidence of prescription drug abuse. It is crucial that the practice has clear policies about narcotic use and that patients are informed early of the terms of prescription care.

Related to ongoing consent is the issue of disclosure. In its hospital accreditation standards, the Joint Commission has established the patient safety standard that organizations will advise patients of unanticipated outcomes.[16] Although this standard specifically applies to inpatient facilities, the concept of disclosure is one that has merit in the office practice as a component of care transparency. With honest communication as a standard for the care delivery process, the likelihood of runaway jury verdicts is reduced.[14,17]

Disclosure, like other methods of communication, occurs daily in healthcare. Practitioners disclose diagnostic test results, diagnoses, and prognoses. The Joint Commission patient safety standard specifically applies to sharing with patients outcomes of treatment that differ significantly from care expectations. Unanticipated outcomes may result from errors, complications, or other unanticipated individual responses to care. The disclosure of unanticipated outcomes can be a highly debated topic among physicians and insurance companies because of concerns related to admission of error versus efforts at transparency.

Termination of Care

Deciding to terminate a patient relationship is a difficult and serious decision. It is also one of those areas of care that is almost entirely unique to the outpatient office setting. Issues of abandonment are always a consideration.

Most providers come to this type of decision when a patient has failed to comply with office policy regarding cancellation of appointments or payment. Other reasons for termination include patient behavior that intimidates or endangers staff or other patients, or significant and consistent noncompliance with treatment plans that have been agreed to by the patient.

The conditions under which a provider may consider terminating the patient relationship include:

- The patient does not have a current, active condition for which the provider is the only practitioner who can treat in a reasonable radius.
- The practitioner provides emergency care for a reasonable amount of time until the patient can initiate care with another appropriate provider.
- The practitioner provides sufficient medication or other treatment resources until such time as the patient has initiated care with the subsequent provider.
- The practitioner supplies the patient with names of other providers or a resource to identify other providers who may assume his or her care.
- The practitioner provides a copy of the patient's medical records to the new provider.

The difficulty arises when the practitioner, ready to terminate the patient, is confronted by a patient or family that alleges that the unacceptable behavior had never been discussed or explained. Therefore, the patient alleges that the act of termination is one of abandonment, and possibly discrimination.

In the communication approach described thus far, the patient would have had practice expectations explained at the first appointment. This would have been reinforced by simple reading material outlining the role of the patient in their care as well as the resources available through the practice. Subsequently, the patient would have been engaged in the treatment process and have participated in the routine decisions about treatment approach. If care had not gone as planned, an open discussion would have occurred addressing both the practitioner's concerns and those of the patient. Finally, should the practitioner conclude that the relationship is putting the practitioner or the office at risk through the patient's behavior, the practitioner has substantial documentation that every effort has been made along the continuum of the relationship to communicate clearly and effectively with the patient.

The standard risk management approach to letters of termination includes using a standard letter that terminates the relationship, gives the patient 30 days to find a new provider, refers the patient to the local medical association that provides referrals, and describes a process for emergency care.

Complaints and Grievances

Unless a practice is attached to a hospital and bills using the hospital's Medicare number, it is not subject to the Centers for Medicare and Medicaid Services (CMS) Conditions of Participation for Hospitals. Nonetheless, the office practice would be best served by a formal and respectful method for handling patient complaints similar to that outlined for hospitals by CMS. Patients' perception of care or business methods provides the practice an opportunity to view itself from a different perspective. That perspective provides a unique point of view on various risk exposures. By managing complaints and grievances effectively, the practice has the ability to proactively apply loss control techniques to previously unseen potential failures in the system. In addition, the practice can identify means to improve internal communication, communication with patients, and communication with the community.

Loss Control Techniques for Managing Complaints. The practice policies and procedures for managing complaints should reflect the practice philosophy about complaints. Ideally, the practice will perceive complaints as opportunities to identify actual and potential failures in the communication processes of the practice. The wording of the policies and procedures is key to communicating this philosophy. The complaint management process should include the following:

- Identify who should respond to complaints, assuming that complaints should be handled at the lowest possible level in the practice.
- Empower staff to respond to complaints at a reasonable level with which they are comfortable.
- Identify to whom a complaint, whether resolved or not, should be reported. This should be the person who has the ultimate responsibility for monitoring the progress of the complaint to resolution.
- Create guidelines for written follow-up to patients and families after a complaint.
- Create guidelines for responding to a complaint for which there exists no possible resolution that will satisfy the patient.
- Create guidelines for responding to physical or verbal threats or unacceptable language.

Billing Procedures

Although it might be argued that billing procedures reflect potential financial risk exposure, they also reflect potential exposures related directly to patient communication and interactions. Patients may not advise the practice of dissatisfaction with service or care until receipt of the bill triggers resentment. At that point, any previous negative experiences become exacerbated and can erupt into full-fledged patient relations issues. They can also be the tipping point that leads the patient or family to seek out an attorney for compensation.

An Example: No Communication Until We Heard from the Collection Agency

We heard nothing from either the hospital or the physician after our son died of what clearly was a medication error in the hospital. We were prepared to forgive them. Our son had been very ill. The next thing we heard, however, was a call from the billing office 8 weeks later saying that we were being sent to a collection agency. At that point we couldn't contain our anger. We might not have minded paying, even if somebody, anybody, had acknowledged what had happened to us. But they didn't. So we went to an attorney. We didn't really want money. They couldn't give us back our son. But we wanted them to understand how much they had hurt us by not caring.

Loss Control Techniques for Communication Regarding the Billing Process. Policies and procedures surrounding the billing process should address:

- Methods for early and clear communication with patients and families about the billing process and patient responsibility. Communication should be in writing as well as verbally addressed in the first appointment.
- Methods for simple and nonthreatening communication with patients about the status of accounts before turning them over to a collection agency. Ensure that misunderstandings are clarified and addressed before turning accounts over.
- A selection process for identifying billing vendors and collection companies that use methods in alignment with the practice philosophy, mission, and values.
- Methods for ensuring that billing vendors and collection companies adhere to HIPAA regulations and have a plan if a potential or actual breach occurs.
- Contractual stipulation with billing vendors and collection companies such that the practice retains ultimate control over all patient accounts including decisions to stop the collection process. Furthermore, ensure that the agency cannot pursue legal action against a patient without permission from the practice.
- A process whereby any patient who is ultimately sent to collections has their chart reviewed to see if there could be liability exposure in the care provided.
- Consultation with legal counsel before waiving or reducing any account for any reason other than reasons of financial hardship, and before signing any third-party or other significant contracts.

Risk Exposure: Communication About the Patient Related to Care

Communication breakdowns within the system about the patient often contribute to allegations of professional liability. Communication processes that can contribute to missed diagnosis or incorrect diagnosis include appointment tracking, medical record documentation, tracking and communicating test results, medication renewal and prescribing practices, referral follow-up (both into and out of the practice), after-hours coverage, and medication prescribing policies.

System failures in medical record documentation can occur in a variety of ways. An electronic medical record is convenient and drives appropriate documentation. However, the practice assumes the exposure of electrical failure, computer failure, software failure, hacking, and people who manage to bypass system safeguards.

The tracking and communication of diagnostic test results is a common area of systems failure. Too often procedures in the office practice rely on practitioner memory to review results. The system should be built such that test results cannot be missed or forgotten and communication to the patient is an automatic process. Missed diagnosis and late diagnosis are the major categories of malpractice allegation in the office practice.[1] These are directly correlated with the systems in the practice for managing the flow of diagnostic information.

System breakdowns in medication prescribing and renewal practices, including prescribing by covering providers after hours, can present huge liability concerns. The practice should evaluate the classes of medications for which it will require more stringent renewal policies and educate patients. Questions about liability have occurred when patients, not advised about practice policies, have gone without medications assuming prescriptions had been called to mail-order pharmacies. In other situations, patients may be angry because they have gone without pain medication because they failed to adhere to practice policies stating that narcotic medications will not be prescribed after hours. Education and explanation are key to patient adherence to practice policies.

Finally, the practice system for accepting and making referrals represents a communication process fraught with potential for information to be lost and for patient care to lapse. The practice should be clear in setting patient and provider expectations surrounding referrals. Timelines, referral outcomes, and subsequent treatment steps should be clearly communicated and documented. This area represents a fragile aspect of the care continuum where checklists and automatic reminders can help prevent system failure.

Risk Exposure: Written Materials in the Practice

Written materials about the practice constitute one of the most basic forms of communication with patients. Patients frequently may see marketing materials prior to meeting with a provider and may even seek out a provider because of these materials. Promises perceived by patients who read the brochures or billboards regarding the practice may be interpreted by patients as a form of guarantee. Marketing assertions regarding being the "best," providing the "best" services, assuring satisfaction with procedures or outcomes, or comparisons to competitors have the potential to be used as part of a suit as the claimed standard. Careful wording is advised to convey the practice's qualities and standards without rendering a promise of results. Many physician professional associations have guidelines relating to acceptable representations that should be made by a practice.

Similarly, written information related to patient care must be written in a way that can be understood by a wide range of patients. Medical literacy research advises that a full 48% of the public, including high school graduates, are unable to accurately read and interpret a bus schedule.[18] Health literacy has been shown in numerous studies to have an effect on care. Studies of Medicare enrollees have found that nearly half the patients surveyed did not understand written instructions, such as "Take medicine every 6 hours," and just over 25% did not understand or could not identify their next appointment. Furthermore, the studies found that health literacy decreased with age and contributed to increased utilization of healthcare services.[19] Compounding this, the cultural diversity of U.S. society renders written communication a difficult task. Cultural diversity in this framework is not only ethnic diversity, but also generational differences, socioeconomic and educational differences, and gender and religious considerations.[20] Any of these characteristics of any individual patient will affect his or her ability to assimilate and interpret accurately the variety of written material regularly provided to patients and families. Written material provided to patients and families includes:

- Information about practice expectations of patients
- Billing information
- Information about specific conditions and medications
- Information about procedures (consent forms)
- Privacy information

Ideally, this type of information should be reviewed by a panel or advisory group made up of patients. Their feedback can provide the practice valuable data about what patients are interpreting, and possibly misinterpreting, relating to the information they are being provided. Recommendations for written material include:

- Target language at a fifth-grade level.
- Utilize high contrast in the color of the background and lettering (both in brochures and pamphlets and for signage).
- Utilize a large, simple font. (This is not only for those with impaired eyesight, but also for those for whom English may be a second language.)
- Define words that are medically related.
- Use diagrams and illustrations whenever appropriate.
- Any information posted on the wall should be set for the eye level of the primary patient group (understanding that cultural groups may vary in height).[18,19]

It is important to know the language needs of the practice's patient base, and to supply the necessary materials in those languages.

Risk Exposure: Sample Medications

Sample medications in the office setting are both a benefit for patients and a risk exposure. From the perspective of patient care, sample medications allow the practitioner to have the patient try a medication prior to asking them to purchase a complete prescription. Also, samples facilitate immediate initiation of treatment. Samples let the practitioner help patients who are financially constrained either begin the medication regimen or reduce the amount of prescription drugs needed to be purchased. Patients appreciate sample medications and often perceive them as a gesture of kindness by providers.

On the other hand, once a patient has begun a regimen using a brand-name drug, he or she may be reluctant to take a generic formulation out of a worry about loss of efficacy. Furthermore, if the patient has a negative reaction to the medication, the physician has a responsibility for having provided medication education prior to administration. Finally, if there is a lot or product recall, the office has full responsibility to ensure that all of the drug is removed and managed appropriately.

Despite the exposures, sample medications are often seen as a service to patients. With appropriate controls, they can be considered by the practice.

Loss Control Techniques for Sample Medications

Among the loss control processes that should be included:

- Sales representatives:
  - Limited access to physicians and staff to avoid practice disruption

- Limits on access to patient demographics or data
- Limits on the types of tangible and intangible gifts that pharmaceutical companies or their representatives are permitted to give the practice, providers, and staff

■ Medications themselves:
  - Limits on which personnel can receive the sample supply from the pharmaceutical representative
  - Limits on the volume of the inventory, which is tightly monitored and regularly reviewed (weekly is recommended)
  - Proper disposal of outdated drugs (including return to pharmacy representatives for disposal)
  - Limited access to the supply by specified personnel, maintained in a controlled, locked access area
  - Strict process for drug dispensing including documentation requirements for patient education, and the lot, dose, type, and amount of every drug recorded in the individual patient record and in the inventory log
  - Labeling of all samples with patient name, medication name, route, dosage, times, and so on
  - Dispensing of patient education materials on dosage and potential reactions along with samples

Loss Exposure: Patient Privacy

HIPAA, as defined by its final rule published February 2003 in the *Federal Register*, protects patients against the "unauthorized use or disclosure" of individually identifiable medical information.

HIPAA applies to any health plan, healthcare clearinghouse, or provider who transmits any health information in an electronic form in connection with a "transaction." By the definition provided in the rule, a transaction is an electronic communication about[2]:

■ Enrollment or disenrollment in health plans
■ Eligibility for a health plan
■ Premium payments
■ First report of injury
■ A health claim or encounter, including status, attachment, payment, or remittance advice
■ Referral authorizations or certifications

Given that not all providers transmit information electronically, not all providers fall under the HIPAA regulations. At the same time, all covered entities must ensure that their "business associates" also comply with the regulation.[21] Business associates are those parties who provide services that the practice would have to do itself including such services as transcription, medical record copying, utilization review, and claims processing. Part one of the rule applies to how information is transmitted between covered entities and their business associates.

Part two of the rule, the Privacy Rule, applies to how patient information can be used and disclosed, and must be protected. This portion of the rule applies to use of the patient information by the business associates. This part of the rule also has a major impact on how daily business is conducted in the office practice. It encompasses much of what has traditionally been considered best practices for confidentiality of patient information.

The type of information protected under this rule is known as protected health information (PHI). PHI includes information that can identify or be easily linked with the patient such as diagnosis, birth date, address or phone number, Social Security number, or images of the patient.[22] The definition is intentionally very broad. Consequently, internal practice processes must be carefully analyzed to ensure they are in compliance with the rule. Furthermore, staff must be regularly educated and reminded about subtleties of compliance with the rule.

Among the rights of patients under the Privacy Rule are the right of patients:

■ To inspect and have copies of their PHI
■ To request corrections to the record
■ To request restrictions to the use of the information
■ To an accounting of any and all releases and uses of the information
■ To be educated about the uses of their information

Patients must be given written notice of their rights and obligations under the act. The written notice must contain the rights, duties, and complaint procedures for perceived breach of this rule. It must be written in clear language and it must contain a description of the types of uses for which the entity does not need patient approval.[23]

Loss Control Techniques for Privacy

Many of the conditions of the privacy rule, although sounding burdensome, are no different than best practices for confidentiality that have been accepted for a number of years; however, practices now are faced with regulation and civil penalties for noncompliance. Ultimately, practices must balance the rights of patients as delineated in the rule with reasonable ability to provide care. Reaction to the rule has led some practices to an over-restriction on use of information that, in fact, impedes the ability to provide coordinated and effective treatment to patients. Recognizing that civil penalties are a significant loss exposure for which no commercial risk financing is satisfactory, carefully evaluated and designed loss control strategies are essential to address HIPAA considerations.

Beyond the concerns about HIPAA, concerns about patient privacy arise from a pragmatic perspective. Care needs to be taken when leaving phone messages with appointment dates, times, and so on so as not to breach any PHI protections. Unless the practice is familiar with a patient's domestic situation and has express permission to leave explicit information at a specific phone number, care must be taken.

To address the rule, consider the following:

- Consult with privacy specialists knowledgeable of the HIPAA transaction rule.
- Have outside reviewers (perhaps patients themselves) review and edit the HIPAA statement for patients, evaluating for appropriate reading level and clarity.
- Ensure staff receive regular and ongoing training.
- Ensure that HIPAA training is part of orientation for all staff.
- Conduct a privacy audit of all aspects of the practice where PHI is collected, stored, used, or released for adherence with the rule.
- Assess internal systems for assuring capability to comply with patient requests regarding restriction of use or release of PHI.
- Assess tracking systems for potential failures in the audit system.
- Assess the practice complaint and grievance process to ensure fair and respectful management of breach of privacy allegations.

Risk Exposure: Medical Devices

The Safe Medical Devices Act (SMDA) of 1990 requires that any serious injury related to a device should be reported to the Food and Drug Administration (FDA) through the MedWatch program or directly to the manufacturer. Although the SMDA applies to hospitals, nursing homes, and ambulatory surgical facilities, as well as other inpatient facilities, it does not apply to physician offices under most circumstances. It also does not apply to chiropractors, school nurses, or dentists. However, if the physician office implants devices, the practice should contact the manufacturer.[23,24] Some implantable devices, even when the procedure is performed in the office practice, fall under the jurisdiction of the SMDA.[25]

Physician practices are not required to report to the FDA except for those specified devices. Nonetheless, the FDA does encourage physician offices to participate. Physicians who implant devices have a responsibility to find out from either the FDA or the manufacturer if the device is subject to the SMDA.[26] The FDA uses the information gathered through MedWatch to monitor the safety of medications, medical devices, some nutritional supplements, and radiation-emitting machines. Information about laser machines, ultrasound machines, and radiological equipment could contribute significantly to the efforts of the MedWatch program.

Loss Control Techniques for Purchasing Equipment

The practice should have clearly delineated procedures for purchasing any medical equipment, nutritional supplements, and medical supplies, including a prepurchase assessment of potential risks and benefits, equipment maintenance by qualified technicians, staff training, a plan for managing recalls, and a plan for managing and reporting any injuries.

Loss Control Technique: Policies and Procedures

There have been numerous references in this chapter to the necessity of having written policies and procedures for processes related to clinical care and patient interactions. Sometimes procedures targeting patient interactions are viewed as important in the hospital setting, yet an unnecessary burden in the office practice setting. Although it is common to create procedures related to human resource or safety issues, policies and procedures for everyday interactions with patients may be overlooked. It is assumed that all employees have been oriented in the proper methods for communicating with patients, and the need for written documentation is perceived as redundant and possibly as troublesome fodder for attorneys.

Policies and procedures in the office practice, can, however, be the practice's ally in allegations of liability. Written documentation of the accepted practice within the office, so long as it is followed, can support decisions made by practitioners and staff members during the course of care. Furthermore, solid written procedures can serve as support for impartial treatment of patients when that impartiality is called into question. Policies and procedures generally should not be more stringent than required under any applicable law. If they are, there is a greater burden on the practice to ensure that these policies and procedures are followed. If the practice is audited by a governmental agency, for example, that agency may review the more stringent procedures and hold the practice to a higher audit standard. Finally, well-documented policies and procedures can be used to train staff about acceptable behaviors in the practice, and provide them with support should patients or families challenge their behavior or requests. Examples of the benefits of written policies that are followed by staff follow.

An Example: Discrimination Allegation

A risk manager in a large multispecialty practice had been supporting the creation of a written policy that carefully mirrored the state regulation about reporting suspected abuse or neglect of minors. Providers argued that the law spoke for itself and a policy would be redundant. Nonetheless, the policy was crafted and clearly delineated the specific conditions for reporting, a statement about nondiscrimination in their adherence to the regulation, and practice-specific procedures for following the regulation and recording their compliance. Several years after the policy was implemented, the practice reported a woman for suspected neglect. The woman filed a claim of racial discrimination alleging that she would not have been reported had she been of the predominant race of the community. Because the practitioners had followed their internal policy, the case was dismissed by the judge.

An Example: Alleged Failure to Refer

A large multispecialty practice group had a uniform written policy for the documentation of cancelled appointments. Because of a patient's symptoms, the primary care provider had urged her to see a specialist. The primary care provider documented offers on multiple occasions to make appointments for the patient. The patient refused, alleging she would make the appointments herself. The patient made and cancelled one appointment. She never made another. She furthermore cancelled subsequent scheduled visits with the primary care physician. She failed to see the primary care physician for 2 years. The next time she saw the primary care provider, she was quite ill. At that point it was discovered she had advanced-stage cancer. She died shortly afterward. The patient's brother, an attorney, sought judgment against the primary care physician for failure to refer for treatment. The carefully documented appointment cancellations as well as the offered facilitation of the referral resulted in a verdict for the defense.

Examples of Beneficial Policies and Procedures from the Loss Control Perspective

Some of the patient care processes that benefit from written and followed policies and procedures include:

- Appointment-making policies, including walk-in policies, resolution of conflict when the physician requests a return for which there are no available slots, and so on.
- Billing and payment procedures

- After-hours coverage
- Documentation of after-hours calls and conversations
- After-hours narcotic prescribing
- Narcotic prescribing guidelines
- Termination of patient relationship guidelines
- Release of medical records (not just to whom, but timeliness and how requests are processed and legal charges associated with record provision—usually state specific)
- Treatment of minors (including clear definition of emancipated minors)
- Inclement weather office closing and hazard removal
- Documentation guidelines
- E-mail and Internet usage for personal use and communication with patients
- Managing inappropriate patient, family, or physician or staff behavior
- Appropriate access to medical information, online or hard copy
- Referral policies
- Sample medications (acceptance, distribution, documentation, and monitoring)
- Storage of medications
- Storage of hard copy medical records
- Storage of electronic data
- How to handle past medical records unaffiliated with current care—either relevant or irrelevant to current provider relationship
- Handling of medical emergencies on site
- Reporting of patient events in the office, patient complaints, and reported patient events that occur outside the office relative to the care that is provided
- The use of clinical guidelines and office accepted best practices
- Bloodborne pathogens
- Response to fire, flood, water or electrical outage, or other natural disasters
- Emergency preparedness for community disasters
- Bioterrorism preparedness
- Procedures for responding to police or other representatives of the law
- Procedures for responding to unannounced federal investigators
- Procedures for responding to unannounced state investigators
- HIPAA
- Procedures for communicating test results
- Access to material safety data sheet (MSDS) information and hazardous material handling

This list is not all-inclusive, but exemplifies the types of policies that function as potentially effective loss control aids when properly documented and followed. Ideally, every process that has been identified in the risk exposure analysis should have documented statements about the practice's operating philosophy, and guidelines for procedures.

The inherent caveat for written policies and procedures is that they must be crafted carefully. A policy that reflects an ideal standard, to which no practitioner or staff will adhere because of the confining and constricting parameters it delineates, is a potentially harmful policy. That policy is one that puts the practice in jeopardy should a lawyer use it as the standard against which actual behavior in a case is being measured. They also must be followed consistently. For example, if the policy states records will be purged every year following certain parameters and the policy has not been specifically followed, the practice could be accused of spoliation of evidence.

From a risk management perspective, a well-written policy should include[27]:

- A policy statement that includes the purpose, objectives, and philosophy of the policy. Ideally, a policy purpose should reflect the norms of the practice. A positively worded policy, designed to teach the culture of the practice to staff, will be a valuable teaching tool as well as a positive reflection on the practice.
- Definitions for key terms included in the policy even if some are perceived to be obvious. For example, terms that are often assumed to be universal such as "inclement weather," "patient complaint," "parent," and "family member" can lead to confusion because of different staff members' beliefs about the definition of those terms.
- Criteria for when the policy applies and, likewise, does not apply.
- The procedure or guideline for applying the policy. A well-written procedure should state the conditions and allowances for variability in behavior. Each situation is unique. Although a procedure guides the staff or provider through the most appropriate actions, those actions may not fit the circumstances at some point in time. Providers or staff should be encouraged to use judgment when appropriate; however, documentation of the decision to deviate from the procedure should be strongly encouraged.
- A process for resolving any conflicts that might arise in either the application or the interpretation of the policy. Usually the conflict resolution policy would include consultation with an administrator or professional colleague. Also, documentation of the conflict and its resolution should be strongly encouraged.
- Dates and process for review. Generally, policies and procedures should be reviewed no less than every 3 years to ensure that they continue to reflect the current laws, regulations, philosophies, and actions that apply.

Loss Control Technique: Use of Patient Safety Techniques in the Office Practice

Although policies and procedures may serve to force the analysis of acceptable practice in the group, to orient staff, and to document procedures, there is an additional benefit to thinking through all organizational processes, both clinical and operational. That benefit falls into the area of patient safety.

With the 1999 Institute of Medicine (IOM) report, *To Err Is Human*, patients became aware of the frequency and nature of medical errors. Although the office-based practice may seem to have few opportunities for actual patient injury during a visit, there are opportunities for error to occur and patient injury in the course of care beyond the missed and incorrect diagnosis of professional liability fame.

Medication error can happen even when no procedures exist in the office. In settings where conscious sedation, topical anesthesia, or clinical procedures occur, the risk for medication error is clear. Nonetheless, in the typical office practice, sample medications are dispensed, and prescriptions are written and renewed. Each of these activities creates the opportunity for improper interpretation and dispensing of medication.[28] The Institute for Safe Medication Practices (ISMP) recommends the use of only standard abbreviations because of the propensity for misreading and misinterpretation.[29] The Joint Commission has echoed that concern through its patient safety goals.[30] This list has become the standard for how to write prescriptions and medication information in such a way as to reduce the likelihood of medication error. Furthermore, the office group needs to address through its policies and procedures the acceptable methods for taking information from patients and validating it for prescription renewal, for verifying that information has been accurately received by the pharmacy, and for documenting the transaction in the patient record.

An Example: The Generic Substitution

A rural office practice typically accepted requests for prescription renewal from patients over the telephone. Staff who took the call customarily wrote the information on a piece of paper, called the pharmacy, and then placed the paper in a basket to be filed. On this particular occasion a patient called for a prescription to be called in for his diabetes medication. This patient had been taking both an anticoagulant and diabetes medication for several years. The patient was noncompliant in the consistent taking of his medications. Consequently neither the office nor the pharmacy could rely on the amount of medication dispensed being a valid predictor of when he would need a prescription renewed. The patient was renewed and the patient, believing the medication to be for his diabetes (because it was the same color that his diabetes medicine had always been), took it as he always had. Shortly thereafter the patient became very ill and was hospitalized. The patient returned home and within a week was readmitted. At this point the physician requested that the patient bring all his medications with him. It was discovered that the prescription provided was a generic version of the anticoagulant. The patient, believing it to be for his diabetes because the color and shape were the same, confusingly took it as well as the anticoagulant.

Other issues that involve an element of risk may include sterilization of equipment used for procedures, infection control measures, storage of medication and equipment, and processes for managing the safety of office procedures. Although the risk is more obvious in inpatient procedures and only those procedures perceived to have minimal risk are performed without the support of emergency medical services, an increasing amount of risk is being assumed by office practices.

Safety science has contributed significantly to the delivery of healthcare services. James Reason has become renowned for his work showing that latent errors occur in every process in every system.[31] A proactive culture of safety encourages the reporting and analysis of situations where injuries may or may not yet have occurred in order to reduce the likelihood of events occurring. The important considerations for the office practice include:

- A culture of safety must be developed; it does not happen automatically. Physicians, staff, and patients must be included in the process. Leadership has the responsibility to set the tone through commitment in strategic planning and reinforcement in regular meetings that awareness of potential safety hazards is the job of each

individual. Reporting of potential and actual problems must be reinforced and rewarded through recognition. Furthermore, these risk exposures must be addressed.

- An easy-to-use incident reporting system must be in place. If providers or staff do not believe that action is taken on issues reported, reporting will diminish. Feedback is essential to reinforce continued participation.

- Patients and families must be included in the effort to recognize actual and potential safety issues. Current efforts focus on including the patient and family as partners in care.[32] Although this is laudable from the perspective of respecting the patient's autonomy and rights, there is an additional intangible benefit to the practice. The patient who advises that she did not receive her laboratory result callback in the time promised, that she had difficulty with the appointment system, or that the ice on the sidewalk is hazardous is making the practice aware of the potential for a serious system failure that could result in allegations of liability. This information goes beyond patient satisfaction into the realm of essential management knowledge.

The tools of patient safety can be applied as easily in the office practice as in the hospital setting. Potential liability can be mitigated by awareness of safety science concepts such as[33]:

- Human factors issues:
  - Recognize that heat, cold, noise, chaos, over- or underlighting, and other environmental factors can lead to increased error.
  - Staff and practitioner fatigue, illness, hunger, and other individual factors can lead to increased errors.
  - Components of medical equipment that are interchangeable can lead to increased error.
- Guidelines in the form of checklists that are simple and available can decrease reliance on memory, vigilance, and calculation, all of which can lead to error.
- Recognize that increasingly complex systems have exponentially increased opportunities for error.

By evaluating systems for risk exposures, the opportunity occurs to simplify care delivery systems, identify guidelines and best practices, create policies and procedures to support the use of those guidelines, and create checklists to ensure that staff and practitioners are easily able to comply.

The Ultimate Loss Control Technique: Medical Record Documentation

Quality medical record documentation is probably the ultimate loss control for most allegations of professional liability. Documentation provides an account of the practitioner's care process. It is evidence of the steps taken to determine a diagnosis, including diagnostic tests. It records practitioner thought processes, including all diagnoses considered and rejected. It notes important interactions in the care process, including discussion of alternative treatments, risks and benefits of treatment, and actions taken by the practitioner when the patient's actions are different from the agreed-upon treatment program.

Documentation can serve as an instrument for legal defense; however, that is not the only reason for ensuring complete and balanced records. Documentation in the office practice serves four primary functions:

1. It provides clinical communication with any practitioner who may see the patient for current or future care. It records the care chronologically and supports treatment. Additionally, practices are increasingly providing patients with copies of visit notes. Consequently, documentation can be considered a valuable tool for communicating with patients as well as increasing the concept of transparency in the system.

2. Documentation is the basis for billing charges. Compliance with billing criteria is an area of risk with significant implications for the practice. Although every insurer has its own standards for documentation sufficiency, the criteria established by the Centers for Medicare and Medicaid Services constitute the standard that is accepted by most payers. Noncompliance with CMS criteria is the basis for federal fraud and abuse allegations for organizations that receive federal funding. The CMS criteria are complicated and specific to the service being provided. Discussion of those criteria is beyond the scope of this chapter; however, the practice must ensure that coders and billing staff understand the need for appropriate billing practices. Physicians must also understand the criteria for billing and for supervision of residents or allied health personnel.

3. It helps maintain compliance with regulations and standards. A variety of regulations and standards apply to documentation depending upon the setting of care and the applicable accreditation, regulatory, and statutory bodies. In general,

federal regulations are those promulgated by CMS. Standards for documentation depend on the care being rendered and the setting. It is incumbent on the practice to know the appropriate documentation standards for the type of care rendered. In addition, HIPAA privacy regulations require documentation of tracking of protected health information. In addition to federal regulations, individual states may have statutes that may address such issues as contents, retention, and disposal of medical records. Professional practice standards for professionals performing services in the practice may dictate specific aspects of care that must be documented. Groups such as the American Nursing Association, Health Insurance Association of America, and American Health Information Systems Society have standards for documentation that apply within the profession. Finally, any organization that is accredited by the Joint Commission will have standards based on the setting in which care is given.[34]

4. Documentation is a risk management tool to support the clinical actions and decision making of the provider. If a lawsuit occurs, the documentation in the record is the evidence of actions and clinical considerations. A general truth is that the practitioner should imagine medical record entries projected onto a screen about 12 feet wide in front of a full courtroom. This is the risk management aspect of documentation that is addressed in this chapter.

There are five aspects of medical record documentation that produce effective risk management support for care. Records that create the best evidence for clinical decision making and action are:

- Complete and accurate
- Reflective of thought processes including decisions that are ruled out or eliminated
- Consistent
- Objective
- Able to be understood by the layperson

Complete and Accurate

The medical record that will provide the best risk management is one that is complete and accurate. The types of information that should be included are:

- *Date and time of all entries:* Date and time entries provide evidence that information was not entered after the fact and made to appear within an earlier sequence of events.

- *Date and time of telephone calls:* Telephone calls reflect official communication outside of the office visit. The patient's and the provider's perception of practitioner instructions and attention to symptom seriousness may be altered with outcome. Documentation of actual phone conversations is the only evidence of actual communication as well as the timing of the conversation in the course of events.

- *Signature, including the first and last names and professional designation:* Some practices use the convention of initials and professional designation. This has fallen out of favor because it is difficult to identify staff and providers years after care is rendered. Particularly in the treatment of minors, there may be a long time between an event and litigation. Clear documentation will have the staff name in full along with professional designation. Should the practice still use the initial protocol, ensure that there is a key in each chart designating the initials and the appropriate providers.

- *Examination results that are within normal limits as well as those outside the normal range:* Elimination of normal results can elicit questions about whether the exam was conducted. Documentation of both types of results presents a complete picture of the evaluation process.

- *Complexity of clinical problems:* Unless the complexity of clinical problems is addressed in the record, assumptions can be made about the simplicity of problems, and hence the apparent simplicity of medical decision making. Documentation of factors contributing to the difficulty of the decision process provides evidence of the potential for a variety of approaches or the indirect route to the ultimate treatment plan.

- *List of all medications and herbal supplements:* With the rise in popular use of herbal supplements and teas, it is increasingly important that the record list all over-the-counter or herbalist-dispensed tinctures, teas, and pills that patients consume. Many patients may not recognize the interactions of these medications with prescription drugs. Other patients erroneously believe that natural substances found in supplements are categorically not harmful. The psychopharmacological effect of many over-the-counter supplements may, in fact, affect diagnosis as well as treatment.

- *Dosage, amount, and number of authorized refills of prescriptions given:* A common problem is that the number of authorized refills is undocumented. Documentation of dose, amount, and number of refills provides evidence that the practitioner has a plan to reevaluate the need for medication, as well as the type and efficacy of the medication at a given point in the treatment. The lack of this evidence can elicit questions about the care with which the practitioner is monitoring the course of treatment and side effects of medications.

- *Sample medications given including amount and lot number:* In the office practice, responsibility for identifying patients who have received recalled drugs is the responsibility of the practice. If a patient should have an adverse reaction to a medication and allege that the reaction was due to a defective drug administered by the practice, the lot number is the documentation that will support verification with the manufacturer.

- *Site and intensity of pain:* Intensity of pain is subjective. Furthermore, it changes over time and in historical perspective. Recording the patient's subjective report of site and pain intensity at each interaction/visit may be the only defense against future allegations about practitioner attention to the severity of symptoms. Any noncompliance with pain medications or multiple providers should be explored and well documented. Pill counts and the like may be appropriate depending on the if there is a question of drug stockpiling or emerging drug dependency. Whenever possible, quote the patient in the record on the specifics of their pain levels.

- *Time and site of injections:* Recording the time of injections as well as the site provides important data should the patient have a drug reaction. Medications differ in time action. A patient who alleges a reaction to a medication that is outside the expected range may, in fact, be responding to different stimuli. Proper recording of time of injection can prove timely response to drug reaction, and possibly support other clinical interventions when it is clear that symptoms are not caused by the drug administered.

- *Date that consultation and other reports are received:* Although most reports have the date they are written or dictated on them, this supports only the timeliness of the report generation. As the receiving practitioner, it is essential that reports are documented with the date received to support the timeliness of action taken after report receipt. It would not be good risk management to be held accountable for time lost in report transition through electronic or other mechanisms.

- *Consent properly documented:* Consent for treatment is not necessarily a form, but a process of communication. Regardless of whether documentation involves use of a form, the general aspects of consent that must be documented include:

- The specific condition for which treatment or a procedure is being recommended
- The nature of the proposed treatment or procedure
- The risks and benefits of the treatment/procedure
- Alternatives to the proposed treatment or procedure (including the alternative of no treatment)
- Risks and benefits to the alternatives (including the risks of no treatment)
- Statements supporting that the patient received adequate opportunity to ask questions and to receive explanations (a notation of some of the more significant questions and responses is preferred)
- Statements supporting that the patient was given the opportunity to make the decision without undue influence and without fear of prejudice on future care

Recommendations for follow-up appointments or other referral: The responsibility to recommend a follow-up appointment or a referral lies with the provider. Although the patient has the responsibility to follow through with recommendations, memory can be selective in the face of a bad outcome. The provider's defense that referral or recommendation was made is often only the medical record documentation.

Cancellation of appointments and practice efforts to follow up on missed appointments: Similar to the referral, inaction on the part of the patient can result in allegations of malpractice in a bad outcome. The record of appointment cancellations and recorded efforts to follow up with patients who do not show up for appointments documents the provider's effort to ensure proper and timely care to the patient.

Patient verbal or written statements of dissatisfaction or satisfaction with care: There are two times when documentation of patient statements is important. One is when the patient makes statements of dissatisfaction with any aspect of care. Documentation of both the statement and the practitioner's efforts to address the dissatisfaction are evidence that the dissatisfaction was not ignored. Patient complaints about issues not related to care should be documented other places than in the medical record. However, careful documentation is recommended

in case future complaints about care allude to other types of dissatisfaction with the practice. The second situation in which patient comments about care are important is when the patient makes positive statements about the care received. This is important because family members often influence a patient to bring suit when an outcome is less than expected. In the face of family pressure, the patient may forget the positive aspects of care. Recorded statements can support clinical decisions made with the patient and the tenor of the course of treatment. Even holiday cards with positive comments about the patient–practitioner relationship or care would be evidence of the nature of the relationship if it were called into question during legal proceedings.

Unanticipated turns in the course of the illness, reactions to medications, or treatment outcomes: All unanticipated outcomes should be recorded as factually as possible. The layperson may be tempted to regard unanticipated outcomes as a failure by the practitioner or the system. Accurate, complete, and factual recording of the sequence of events leading to the unanticipated outcome may serve as the only evidence of proper clinical action and decision making on the part of the practitioner.

Laboratory and other test results: Failure to follow up on and notify patients of test results has prompted lawsuits, as has the failure to order appropriate testing. Usually those suits occur when a late diagnosis results in a preventable outcome. In order to avoid judgments for claims where there was proper notification, ensure that the record includes documentation that:

- Laboratory and other test results were received, including the date received
- Patients have been notified of the results, including the mechanism by which they are notified
- Patients know what to do in response to the consultation and test results

Changes in symptoms: The medical record should clearly document what a patient is told to do if symptoms should worsen or change. It should also record how the patient indicated they understood the instruction.

Corrections made in a manner that does not raise suspicion of information cover-up: The techniques for making corrections appropriately include:

- Use black (preferably) or blue ink only. (Pencil fades. Blue sometimes does not copy well. Black is the preferred ink for long-term legibility.)

- Write legibly, or dictate. Illegible handwriting makes documentation impossible to use in a courtroom. Illegible handwriting makes orders, instructions, and prescriptions difficult to follow. Furthermore, if the jury cannot understand the note, it is as if the note didn't exist as evidence.
- To make corrections on a hard copy record:
  1. Draw a single line through the entry so that the underlying error can be seen.
  2. Write "error," date, time, and initial the correction so that it is clear that the practitioner knew it was an error and when during the course of treatment the error was corrected.
  3. If possible, the person who made the error should write the correction.
  4. Write or type the correction in the next available space, dated and timed in chronological sequence of care, not where the original error occurred.
- In order to avoid the appearance that the record is being altered to support information after a complaint or unexpected outcome, avoid:
  - Tracing over notes
  - Using carets (^) for inserts
  - Using correction fluid, erasing, or blackening out text
  - Removing pages with errors
  - Making revisions once a lawsuit is filed
- When a patient requests a change to the record, follow the HIPAA policies of your practice. In general, the organization has a right to request that the patient request changes to the record in writing. The organization also has a right to deny those changes; however, that, too, should be in writing. In any case, the record should note the date any change is made and the patient's letter requesting the change should be kept in the record whenever possible.
- Be aware that all changes made to electronic medical records (EMR) have embedded metadata that will document the date and time that information was added or changed. It is important that when you date the entry you are recording the information accurately to avoid the appearance of creating discrepancy to deceive should there be litigation.

Reflective of Thought Processes

The medical record that will best support a practitioner in a complex medical situation resulting in a bad outcome will be the one that reflects the thought process of the provider. Those thought processes include rule-outs—determination of tests to order as well as tests eliminated because of the limited potential information yield. General rules for recording processes particularly useful in complex situations include documenting:

- Any diagnosis, treatment, or plans that are ruled out
- Any medication the patient requests and reasons for rejecting or accepting his or her suggestion
- The working diagnosis on which initial treatment decisions are made
- Warnings provided to patients about procedures, medications, treatments, herbal supplements, activities, noncooperation with treatment plans, and so on
- Questions the patient or family asks about the medication, treatment, or other aspects of care and the answers provided to them
- Requests for consultation or referrals made on behalf of the patient

Consistent

A medical record needs to be consistent to support continuous attention to the process of care in the face of an adverse outcome. Techniques for ensuring the record presents a constant and careful approach to care will:

- Ensure that when a new complaint is mentioned, it is asked about and a response recorded at the next visit
- Ensure that when a patient is complaining about a recurring problem, the record has documented it at a previous time

Objective

Objective documentation is free of personal bias. It reflects the course of care and is not a vehicle for expounding points of view not related to the patient's health. Techniques for objective documentation include the avoidance of statements that:

- Are derogatory of the patient or the patient's family
- Are abbreviations of derogatory phrases
- Use statements such as "malpractice" or "negligent"
- Are discriminatory or subjective
- Criticize the care or clinical decisions of others

Able to Be Understood by the Layperson

Laypeople, by and large, compose juries. Furthermore, most patients are laypeople. In an era when patient access to records is understood, misunderstanding about care can be prompted as easily as it can be stopped by the medical record. As has been discussed earlier in this chapter, laypeople have a different understanding of terms than medical practitioners. It is essential to remember that the record is not the sole property of the practice, but will be seen by many without the medical framework in which to interpret it. As a communication tool, it is incumbent upon the practitioner to ensure that a patient, another provider, or a jury can equally well read the documentation and have a basic understanding of the course of care.

Finally, do not change the record once you are aware of possible care issues. At the time of care, it is acceptable to amend with a single line out and a new entry. After care is complete, without notice of suit or issue, an addendum is appropriate. But once there has been an indication of a potential claim, make no further corrections or amendments to the record.

■ Personnel Exposures

Employees are the practice's greatest asset; they are also a significant source of risk exposure. The relationship between employer and employee is complex. In exchange for pay, benefits, and a safe environment, employees are expected to exert their best effort toward accomplishing their assigned tasks. In order to protect employees from unfair expectations or unsafe working conditions, employers are governed by federal and state statutes and regulations designed to promote safe, respectful, and nondiscriminatory treatment. Employer risk exposure is related to the fulfillment of those obligations under the law.

Significant Employment Statutes

There are certain statutes important to the employment relationship with which every employer must be familiar:

- *National Labor Relations Act of 1935:* This act defines the unfair labor practices regarding employers and employees and provides for hearings based on complaints in these areas.
- *Labor Management Reporting and Disclosure Act of 1959:* This act defines the relationship between unions and their members. It also requires that organizations report any monies spent to influence the way employees exercise their rights under penalty of illegal activity if it is not disclosed.
- *Fair Labor Standards Act (FLSA):* This act requires employers to pay all nonexempt employees at no less than the state minimum wage. States may

have supplemental state laws. It also requires that those employees receive pay for work greater than 40 hours at 1.5 times the minimum rate.
- *Equal Pay Act of 1963:* This act prohibits differences in pay between men and women who perform "substantially equal jobs" unless those differences are due to some factor other than gender such as merit pay, seniority, or training.
- *Title VII of the Civil Rights Act of 1964:* This act prohibits discrimination on the basis of race, color, religion, sex, or national origin in hiring, discharge, compensation, and any terms, conditions, or privileges of employment.
- *Age Discrimination in Employment Act of 1967:* This act protects employees over the age of 40 from age-related discrimination in regard to hiring, discharge, compensation, and other terms and conditions of employment.
- *Occupational Safety and Health Act (OSHA) of 1970:* This act established the OSHA administration, which is responsible for promulgating standards and conducting inspections to ensure safe work environments.
- *Equal Employment Opportunity Act of 1972:* This act amends the Civil Rights Act of 1964 by prohibiting discrimination in hiring on the basis of sex, age, religion, race, color, or national origin. This act applies to private employers and state and local governments.
- *Rehabilitation Act of 1973:* This act applies to all institutions that receive federal funds and has as its goal the protection of handicapped employees.
- *Americans with Disabilities Act of 1990:* This act prohibits discrimination against an individual when that discrimination is based on the individual's disability. Disabilities for which an employer must make reasonable accommodation if the individual is otherwise qualified for the job are defined as major life impairments, such as hearing disabilities or visual disabilities. Effective March 25, 2011, the Americans with Disability Act has been expanded to include conditions such as bipolar disorder, diabetes, epilepsy, and multiple sclerosis. Practices need to understand what reasonable accommodation means. Resources are available at http://www.eeoc.gov/facts/adahandbook.html.
- *Family Medical Leave Act of 1993:* This act requires private-sector employers of 50 or more employees to provide employees up to 12 weeks of unpaid job-protected leave for medical reasons. Employees must have worked 1,250 hours over the past 12 months for the act to apply.

- *Employee Polygraph Protection Act:* This act prohibits employers from requiring or using, accepting, or referring to a polygraph test on any employee or potential employee.
- *Uniformed Services Employment and Re-employment Rights Act (USERRA):* This act provides job and benefit protection that allows members of the uniformed services to take up to 5 years of leave for active duty, duty training, or absence for a physical.
- *Weingarten Rights:* This act originally applied to unionized employees and offered them the right to have a representative present during an investigative interview that might result in disciplinary action. In 2000, the National Labor Relations Board (NLRB) ruled that nonunion employees were entitled to essentially the same right. All employees have the right to request that a coworker be present during any investigative interview from which disciplinary action may arise. However, the employer is not obligated to go beyond reasonable effort to accommodate the schedule of the requested worker and is not required to postpone interviews until a time that is "convenient" for the coworker.
- *Workers' compensation laws:* These laws vary among states. However, in all states, workers must be provided prompt and reasonable medical benefits and income for injuries incurred on the job. Furthermore, the laws are designed to provide a single remedy so that in return for appropriate and timely care of the employee, the employer is relieved of personal injury litigation.

Loss Control Techniques for Human Resources Issues

The office practice can minimize the opportunities for loss through carefully delineated employment processes to which they strictly adhere. Employment issues tend to be highly charged and sensitive issues. Those areas most responsive to risk management intervention include:

- *The hiring process:* Jobs should be well defined, highlighting the essential functions of the job, and not the method for carrying out the job. Advertising must be fair and not discriminate against any group of individuals. The job application should only ask for information that is essential for determining the qualifications of the applicant to perform the job functions. The interview should be nonbiased, and free of disability-related or other prohibited questions, and should avoid making misleading or inaccurate statements.

- *Background investigation:* Whenever possible, criminal checks should be conducted on all employees, and a sexual predator database search run on any employee who works with children or has access to confidential patient or financial information.
- *Employee handbooks:* Handbooks should spell out both employer expectations and the rights of employees. They should also state clearly and in an obvious placement that they do not constitute a contract of employment.
- *Formal employee orientation:* Orientation should be formal, as well as specific to the job for which the individual has been hired. An orientation checklist should be used, which delineates each aspect of the practice for which the employee has been trained. Adequate training in HIPAA, OSHA, emergency preparedness, sexual harassment, and other aspects of the practice should be authenticated with a signature of the orienting supervisor.
- *Clear process:* The employee disciplinary and grievance process should be clearly defined and the procedure delineated.
- *Clear standards:* Employee performance standards should be clearly described, and the process for documenting unacceptable performance should be delineated, as well as the steps for lodging a grievance.
- *Invasion of privacy policy:* There should be a clear understanding of what constitutes invasion of privacy, and policies/practices should be consistent with that understanding.
- *Harassment policy:* The practice's harassment policy should be clear. There should be evidence of ongoing and regular staff training in each employee's file.
- *Personnel records:* Only supervisors, human resource professionals, and the employee should have access to personnel records.
- *Drug and alcohol testing:* Federal contractors and recipients of federal grants may be subject to the Drug-Free Workplace Act, which mandates a policy statement and drug-free awareness program. Other employers may implement drug testing programs in concert with the applicable laws of the state.
- *Safety program:* Compliance with OSHA regulations and safety procedures not only reduces the likelihood of state investigations, fines, and liability losses, but also serves to reduce the likelihood of workers' compensation claims.
- *Termination:* Voluntary or involuntary termination should include a termination interview to gather

information on the employee's work experience at the practice. From the risk management perspective, the interview serves as a loss control device. It allows the employer to determine if there are any unknown issues, such as harassment or discrimination, that are creating a work environment that is unacceptable to the departing employee. In addition, the exit interview gives the practice the opportunity to tell the departing employee of benefits such as the Consolidated Omnibus Reconciliation Act (COBRA) and any other termination policies of the practice. In the case of an involuntary termination, the practice should ensure that supporting facts are accurate and are documented in a fair and nondiscriminatory manner according to company policy. Ensure that all pertinent federal and state statutes have been followed. Finally, care should be taken to ensure that the employee departure from the facility is handled in a respectful manner while addressing the safety needs of both the departing employee and the remaining staff.[25,35]

Property and Facilities Exposure

The category where office practices are most likely to see losses from accidental causes is in the area of property and facilities. Risk exposure for property is not static. Property risk exposure changes with acquisition, movement, and wear and tear. Long-term effects of weather can change risk to the property itself. When people use property, or are present on the property, they create safety issues. Examples of how the interaction of people and property create risk include access to the office, safety in reception areas, the potential for violence on the property, and examination room safety. All of these are property- and facilities-related risk exposures as well as general liability exposures. The effective risk management process will regularly evaluate the current safety status of the practice. There are risk control techniques to address general liability concerns as well as those that may have regulatory implications.

Safety of Patients on the Premises

The safety of patients and staff entering and leaving the building should be of primary concern to the practice. Common issues include crime in the parking area, trips and falls, and emergency communication. An International Association for Healthcare Security and Safety (IAHSS) survey of crime in healthcare facilities published in 2010 found that violent crimes such as rape,

sexual assault, simple assault, robbery, and aggravated assault had increased 200% from 2004.[37] The practice should ensure that parking areas are well lit and that procedures are in place to protect staff and patients who may have to go into parking areas when light is low or when weather conditions may reduce the safety of walkways. Injuries to patients, visitors, and staff can be costly. Not all general liability commercial insurance policies provide medical coverage for injuries on the property. The practice should ensure that risk financing mechanisms are in place and that policies address the management of patient/visitor/employee injuries. Employee injuries are generally covered by workers' compensation once the worker is on the employer's property.

Loss control techniques for access include:

- Accessibility of parking area, walkways, and practice entrances by those with mobility difficulties
- Sufficient lighting so that all hazards and dangers can be seen by those with any sight impairments
- Stair height and depth appropriate for the patient population
- Walkways, parking areas, and hallways free of trip hazards, including ice, snow, and pools of water
- Color contrasts used for signage and directions appropriate for those with sight impairments in dim conditions
- Emergency call system from outside the office for any individual injured who is accessing or leaving the building
- Policies that address patient or staff injury outside of the immediate office area
- Clear areas of ingress and egress during periods of snow, ice, flooding, construction, and the like

Reception Area

Although the waiting area may not seem fraught with risk exposure, injuries in the reception area are due primarily to unanticipated behaviors or a lack of match between the furnishings of the area and the patient population. Furniture must be appropriate to the patient population to avoid injury from falls. Solid, stable chairs that support patients who have difficulty with mobility and are not easily tipped by children are the best selection for most offices. Fish tanks or other environmental enhancements should be secure and unable to be tipped, run into, or provide the opportunity for electrical hazards. Children's play areas should not have surfaces with pointed edges (such as tables or shelves), toys that present choking hazards, or toys that have not been properly sterilized, thereby creating an infection exposure. The office should stay current with child product recalls to ensure that any safety concerns are identified, and should have procedures for ensuring that toys are maintained in a safe state. Broken toys should be removed from the office to prevent harm. Finally, parents should be made aware both verbally and through signage that staff cannot be responsible for watching children in the office and that the parent retains that responsibility.

Plants add to the welcoming atmosphere of the office, and in most situations are not problems. However, in offices where children are likely to be present, consideration should be given to ensuring that no poisonous plants are accessible to children. Furthermore, blooming plants may be a problem for allergic or asthmatic patients and staff. The best loss control measure for the office practice is to refrain from having blooming plants and to ensure that no plant in the office is poisonous if consumed.

Violence

Violence is a reality of our society. The practice may not be held legally responsible for the acts of a violent person on the premises; however, it may be held liable for not providing sufficient security or for lack of proper procedures for managing potential violence. Violence in the office practice can come from many sources: a person who is angry with a patient or staff member, a person in a state of chemical imbalance, a disgruntled employee, or a person who desires to steal medications or other office items.

Risk control techniques to address the potential for violence might include (where feasible and appropriate)[25,38]:

- Controlling access to the office
- Phones for patient use in the waiting area
- Sufficient lighting both inside the waiting area and in access ways
- Staff ability to visually monitor the entire waiting area with a camera or mirror coverage for areas not directly visible
- Secured windows and doors
- Limited amounts of lightweight furniture that could potentially be used as weapons by an angry person
- Sufficient trained staff to manage and de-escalate an emergency
- 911 programmed into the telephone or a panic button linked directly to the police
- A plan for staff to summon help inside the practice
- Locked storage for patient valuables
- Secure access to pharmaceuticals, sharps, and other potentially desirable supplies
- Written policies and procedures for action in the face of potential violence
- Signage advising that weapons cannot be brought into the practice

Loss Control Techniques for Examination Room Safety

Examination rooms should be designed and maintained with safety, security, and privacy in mind. Loss control techniques for maintaining safety in the examination room might include:

- Ensuring that the room is set up so the egress is not blocked by the examination table or other equipment
- Ensuring that windows are secure
- Ensuring that sharps containers are mounted so that children cannot easily reach into them
- Ensuring that nothing sharp is left unattended when the provider is not in the room
- Ensuring that prescription pads and sample medications are maintained out of patient areas and locked when not in use
- Ensuring that equipment controls are not within easy access of patients
- Ensuring that water temperatures are set to 120 degrees or less
- Ensuring that electrical outlets are secured with child protection devices and that electrical cords do not create a trip hazard

Other Types of Premises Liability

There are other safety considerations in the office practice that may involve patients, but are more specifically focused on the safety of the premises. Electrical cords and extension cords can contribute to both trip hazards and fire hazards. The storage of cleaning agents and sterilization agents can contribute to both fire hazards and accidental poisoning. Other types of facility safety include fire, emergency preparedness for natural or other disasters, air quality, and underground storage tanks. The risk exposure analysis must include a complete evaluation of every room in the practice and must look at the variety of places where an accident could happen.

Fire Safety

The National Fire Protection Agency (NFPA) Life Safety Code addresses the safety of both occupants and buildings. The practice should be familiar with this code and the implications for risk management. The practice should have a plan to evaluate and segregate as much as possible the elements required for a fire. In addition, policies and procedures should delineate the process for managing the fire and for ensuring the safety of patients and staff should a fire occur.

Fire requires three elements, known as the fire triangle: heat, oxygen, and fuel. Office practices have many sources of heat, from computers and space heaters to lasers. By ensuring the sources of heat are contained and safe, the next step is to ensure that those sources of heat are not provided fuel for combustion. Fuel can be in the form of volatile substances such as acetone, alcohol, and other chemicals, or flammable materials such as paper. Electrical fires occur when there are faulty or worn power connections, wires overheat, or the heat from wires ignites flammable materials. Employees should be discouraged from using personal equipment that is not Underwriters Laboratory (UL) approved. Outlets should be reviewed regularly for overloading and equipment checked for frayed or damaged connections.

The presence of patients and families, many of whom are ill or experiencing difficulty in mobility, increases the complexity of an emergency evacuation plan. Nonetheless, the NFPA recommends the use of the RACE Plan. Race stands for Rescue people from the fire; Activate the alarms; Control the fire by closing doors and windows on the way out; Extinguish the fire if you feel safe, and Evacuate.[25,38]

Emergency Preparedness

Emergency preparedness is an area of loss control that covers a gamut of unanticipated potential hazards. The Joint Commission requires that hospitals have an emergency preparedness plan. Although the office practice may not be held to such a standard, state laws may require a plan. Additionally, being prepared to manage potential property loss and community disaster is good business. After a disaster, the practice will have to deal with such issues as utilities failures, water purity and shortages, and operational integrity of the building.

Experts agree that the best way to be prepared for a disaster is to have a comprehensive yet flexible plan in place and to practice implementing it.[25] Components of a disaster plan should include:

- Evacuation routes and alternatives posted in all patient rooms
- Postemergency meeting place
- Methods for assisting patients and others with limited mobility
- Communication structure for maintaining inter-staff contact during the emergency
- Details of leadership decision authority for deciding when and how to return to the office
- Policies for reopening for business

Loss control mechanisms can be initiated to reduce the severity of losses from natural disasters. Designing the office so that key information is stored where breaking pipes or flooding will not destroy important documents is essential. Loss control methods may include duplication of information or segregation of parts of the information from the main office area. Noting the placement of key operational equipment or information in relation to windows, flammable materials, and heat sources is also key in planning. Large, clearly described evacuation procedures, battery-lit emergency exits, flashlights with working batteries, blankets for carrying patients from the building, and a battery-operated radio are all preparations the practice can take to ensure the safety of providers and patients.

■ Financial and Business Operations

In some ways this is the most complex and most subtle of the categories. It encompasses a variety of activities and issues that can affect the financial stability of the entity. Required adherence to federal and state statutes and regulations constitutes an area where noncompliance results in exposure to the entity.

Key Laws and Regulations That Affect Office Practice Risk Management

Although it would be impossible to cover all the key legislation and regulation that pertains to office practice risk management, a few noteworthy regulations can create tremendous legal and financial exposure for the office practice. Some of these pieces of legislation pertain to interactions with patients during the course of care. Some were not discussed earlier because the loss is of a more financial nature in the forms of fines and penalties rather than professional liability. Nonetheless, it is essential that the practice be knowledgeable and observant of these particular statutes and regulations in the course of providing patient care.

- *False Claims Act (31USC§§ 3729-3733):* This act permits lawsuits by the government or any individual against someone who submits a false claim to the government. Claims for services to Medicare, Medicaid, or any other government-funded health plan that are proven to be false or fraudulent can be subject to personal or practice fines. False claims can also be filed as a criminal offense with a potential penalty of imprisonment up to 5 years, and fines of $250,000 per count personally and $500,000 per count for the organization.

- *Ethics in Patient Referral Act (42 USC § 1395NN):* This is also known as the Stark law. This act prohibits physicians from specific types of financial arrangements with referral sources if the referral involves certain types of health services. If an entity is among those specified health services, and the physician or his or her family has a financial relationship with it, the physician cannot make a referral to that entity.
- *Safe Medical Devices Act of 1990 (SMDA):* As described earlier, this act applies only to those physician offices where implantable medical devices are used. It is the practice's responsibility to contact the manufacturer to determine whether the device is among those affected by the SMDA.
- *Mammography Quality Standards Act of 1992 (later amended by the Mammography Quality Standards Reauthorization Act of 1998):* This act applies to any practice that is certified, or plans to be certified, under the act to provide mammography services. The act also applies to any practitioner, facility, or employee who provides breast cancer treatment, diagnosis, and screening.
- *Medicare-Medicaid Antikickback Statute (42 USC § 1320a-7b):* This act establishes that any person or entity that "knowingly or willfully" seeks or receives a bribe, kickback, or rebate for a referral for a program, service, or reimbursable item is subject to criminal charges as well as a civil monetary penalty.
- *Patient Protection and Affordable Care Act (PPACA; Public Law 111-148):* This act contains various provisions to curb fraud and abuse in federal healthcare programs and makes changes to the False Claims Act (FCA) and the Stark and antikickback laws.
- *Exclusion statute (42 USC § 1320a-7):* This excludes individuals and entities convicted of certain types of criminal offenses from participation in all federal healthcare programs.
- *Civil monetary penalties law (42 USC § 1320a-7a):* This authorizes the imposition of civil monetary penalties and sometimes exclusion from participating in federal healthcare compliance programs for various activities that violate certain federal laws.
- *RAC audits:* In 2006, CMS was authorized to perform audits on all Medicare Part A, B, and C and Medicaid providers. These audits allow electronic analysis of all provider claims and specifically look at use of proper codes, duplicate claims, and number of units billed.
- *Health Insurance Portability and Accountability Act (HIPAA):* As discussed earlier, this act applies to organizations that transmit protected health information (PHI) electronically for specified purposes. It establishes processes for using PHI, and civil as well as criminal penalties for nonadherence. It also addresses an individual's rights regarding their ability to access and/or modify their medical record. This act further allows a patient to request to receive communications by alternative means, to inspect and copy their protected health information with some exceptions, to request corrections and amendments to their protected health information, to request restrictions on use of their protected health information, to receive an accounting of disclosures of their protected health information, and to revoke authorization for release of protected health information. The organization should maintain separate policies and procedures specifically to address the privacy aspect of HIPAA.
- *Title XIII of the federal Health Information Technology for Economic and Clinical Health (HITECH) Act:* Enacted as part of the American Recovery and Investment Act of 2009, this act made revisions to the HIPAA privacy and security rules and made business associates subject to the HIPAA health information security rule. The HITECH Act requires business associates to implement written security policies and procedures with respect to the protected health information they handle and imposes other legal requirements with regard to electronic health information. As of February 17, 2010, "business associate agreements" with covered entities must contain provisions that reflect their legal obligations under the HITECH Act.
- *Sarbanes-Oxley Act of 2002:* This act applies to public companies required to file periodic reports to the Securities and Exchange Commission (SEC). This statute establishes that public companies cannot extend or arrange for personal loans or other forms of credit to directors and executive officers.
- *Newborns' and Mothers' Health Protection Act of 1996 (NMHPA):* This act applies to health plans, and states that health plans may not limit a mother and infant's hospital benefits to less than 48 hours for a normal vaginal delivery, nor to less than 96 hours following a caesarean section.
- *Clinical Laboratory Improvement Amendments (CLIA):* These amendments apply to laboratories and establish quality standards. CLIA sets up

three categories of covered tests: waived complexity, moderate complexity, and high complexity. In order for a laboratory to provide any level of test greater than waived complexity, it must apply for CLIA accreditation and meet the quality standards for proficiency, patient test management, quality control, personnel qualifications, and quality appropriate for the level of testing the laboratory performs.

■ *Protection of Human Research Subjects regulations (45 CFS part 46 et. seq.):* These regulations apply only if the practice is involved in conducting research. Should research be part of the office practice, the practice should become familiar with these regulations and connect with the local institutional review board (IRB).

■ *Child abuse and neglect/elder abuse:* Statutes are found in every state of the union regarding neglect and abuse. Adherence to these statutes is a key responsibility for the practice. Failing to do so can lead to fines and possibly legal action.

Contracted Services

Practice management in today's environment comprises a host of activities that the majority of practices cannot staff with full-time employees. In this environment, outsourced and contracted services are common and expected. Contracted relationships benefit the practice to the extent that risks can be transferred. However, risks may inadvertently be assumed for employees over whom the practice has little control if the contract is not worded most carefully.

Typical specialists with which a practice might contract include transcriptionists, medical record personnel, medical record copying services, billing and collection services, payroll services, laundry services, accounting/bookkeeping services, building cleaners, ice and snow removal, and temporary services. The issues may be different depending on the sensitivity of the work being conducted; however, basic issues remain the same. The practice will want the service provider to assume responsibility for adequate and appropriate training of its staff on issues of privacy and confidentiality, infection control, work safety, and ergonomics. The practice will want to contractually transfer liability to the vendor for any negligent acts of its employees and for the vendor to hold the practice not liable ("hold harmless") for any conditions that may arise out of the relationship. Further, the practice will want to contractually ensure that the vendor will reimburse or "indemnify" the practice for any

expenses it incurs from negligence of the vendor. The practice will want to ensure that the vendor provides certificates of insurance proving, for at least the date of the inception of the contract, that the vendor is covered for important coverages including but not limited to workers' compensation, professional liability (where appropriate), automobile (where appropriate), and documentation of bloodborne pathogen training and HIPAA training (where appropriate).[39]

Other types of financial contracts are common in the office practice. Relationships with health plans, third-party administrators if self-insured for health insurance benefit or workers' compensation, and banks are among the most common.

Managed-care contracts pose a unique and complex set of risks for the practice. Not only are the issues of financial viability of the arrangement at issue, but also questions about the differences among contracts that might lead to the "favoring" of one set of patients over another, leading to allegations of unequal treatment among patients. Health plans require careful consideration and planning prior to entering an agreement. The practice should plan through risk financing techniques how it will minimize financial loss if patient care should exceed the contractual allowances, and how it will plan for any unplanned financial demise of the plan. The practice should also evaluate each new plan relative to other plans it accepts in order to ensure that it does not set up a situation in which providers are encouraged to discriminate on the basis of payment.

Unique considerations must be given to contractual relationships with medical service providers. Radiology, laboratory, or durable medical equipment services may be housed within the facility or adjacent to the facility to provide convenience to patients. Although the intention may be value-added service and assurance that clinical recommendations will not be ignored because of difficulty accessing services, these types of relationships involve many of the same issues as contracts with vendors. More importantly, these types of contracts must be reviewed to ensure there are no violations of federal legislation such as the Stark law mentioned in the previous section, the federal antikickback legislation, or, if they are working with the practice to conduct research, the Protection of Human Subjects regulations.

Finally, the organizational structure of the practice itself must be evaluated for exposures. Each type of structure will have inherent risks. Careful consideration, planning for the inevitability of dispute surrounding those issues, and a legally sound basis for addressing the issues are essential. The types of issues that need to be addressed through either corporate structure or contractual relationship with physicians include:

- Definition of the relationships with hospitals with whom clinicians have privileges
- Delineated methods whereby associated physicians become incorporated into the group
- What are the financial and employment status arrangements with the providers in the group?
- If there are partners in the practice, what are the financial arrangements?
  - How are funds distributed?
  - How are investment decisions made?
  - Who determines the method for arranging the financial structure (such as CDs, checking, or money market arrangements of the group)?
  - How are insurance decisions made?
- How will treatment of provider family members be managed?
- How are the financial requests or needs of partners addressed?
- How are conflicts of interest identified and addressed? (For example, what if a practice partner invests in a business that might create a legal conflict?)

It is never wise to enter into a contractual relationship without the counsel of an attorney. Subtleties in wording can generate an unrecognized risk exposure costing the practice significant unplanned costs. The best risk management in these situations is careful evaluation of the risk before entering into the situation, and establishing the parameters of the relationship in such a way that risk is minimized.

■ Summary

Risk management in the office practice encompasses each aspect of the daily operation of the practice. An effective risk management program will identify risk exposures in each aspect of the business. Methods for identifying and analyzing risk include a thorough evaluation of each business and care process; an audit of the property and facility for safety exposures; a thorough review of policies and procedures to ensure they are accurate, clear, and easily followed; questionnaires; and assessments by consultants. Identified risk exposures then should be addressed by implementing strategies to reduce the frequency or the severity of loss. Additional preparation for potential losses includes risk financing for losses that may occur.

There are five primary categories in which risk exposures occur in the office setting. The most familiar one, professional liability, is strongly correlated with communication failures. Creating procedures that address communication with the patient and about the patient that utilize the best practices of safety science can mitigate the potentially expensive losses that professional liability incurs.

The second category of risk exposure is the area of human resources and personnel. Care must be taken to ensure that employees are protected from injury, harassment, and discrimination. Human resources policies and procedures must be structured such that federal and state statutes and regulations are addressed. Furthermore, employee safety and well-being must be ensured through appropriate safety and security measures

The third major category of risk exposure in the office setting is property and safety. Losses to the property itself through natural disaster or destruction can be costly. Furthermore, safety considerations, such as protections against violence, fire, natural disasters, and injury to patients, visitors, and employees, require ongoing monitoring and reevaluation to mitigate potential losses.

Business operations constitute the fourth category of potential risk exposure. Inherent in that aspect of risk is the dynamic tension between risk-taking for growth and risk minimization to reduce the likelihood of losses. Loss control techniques address the application of statute and regulation to the daily operation of the practice, the evaluation of contractual relationships to avoid unwanted assumption of risk, and the careful structuring of the practice itself so that it does not inadvertently create business situations that can lead to lawsuits and alleged violations of federal legislation.

The fifth category of risk exposure is related to the other four. Information technology provides unique opportunities for identity theft, breach of privacy, business interruption, and expanded opportunities for discovery in litigation. It is essential that technology systems be sound, safe, redundant to protect against loss of data, and standardized. Staff and providers must use good judgment in all Internet-based interactions, and systems must be encrypted wherever feasible for protection.

Losses will occur despite the best loss control efforts. Risk financing is an essential part of any risk management program to ensure that the practice's operations are not disrupted by the financial burden. Risk financing may take a variety of forms. The easiest and the most expensive is purchasing commercial insurance. The physician office practice may want to purchase insurance for professional liability, business interruption, general liability, automobile and nonowned automobile, property, employment liability, workers' compensation, directors and officers, and property. Other forms of risk financing, such as funded or unfunded reserves, borrowing, or self-insurance vehicles such as trusts, risk retention groups, and captives, may be appropriate depending on the financial strength and loss history of the practice.

Risk management strategies require constant monitoring because the legal and financial environment in which healthcare business is conducted is dynamic. A multitude of healthcare reform efforts have been implemented, and the future holds many more. Reform efforts encompass everything from reimbursement changes to access realignment. Regardless of specific modalities, reform efforts all focus on getting more healthcare resources to patients across the United States, and motivate improved patient safety efforts with performance-based compensation to providers. Although it is impossible to tell exactly what forms those changes will take, a resurgence of the alignment of medical practices with larger healthcare organizations is occurring. Accountable care organizations and patient-centered medical homes are beginning to proliferate with an emphasis on effective and efficient care.[40] The future of the stand-alone medical practice office is in question, but there will always be a need for office-based care.

Although risk management is an accepted component of healthcare delivery in the inpatient setting, its value in the office practice cannot be overemphasized for its importance to every aspect of the business.

References

1. Fischer G, Fetters MD, Munro MA, Goldman EB. Adverse events in primary care identified from a risk-management database. *Journal of Family Practice.* 1997;45(1):40–46.
2. Fetters MD. Medical error in primary care. In: Rosenthal MM, Sutcliffe KM, eds. *Medical error: what do we know? What do we do?* San Francisco: Jossey-Bass; 2001:60–61.
3. Manoogian D. Risk management in the managed care context. In: Kavaler FK, Spiegel AD, eds. *Risk management in health care institutions: a strategic approach.* Sudbury, MA: Jones and Bartlett; 2003.
4. Head G, Horn S. *Essentials of risk management.* Malvern, PA: Insurance Institute of America; 1991:11.
5. Alt SJ. Bariatric surgery programs growing quickly nationwide. *Health Care Strategic Management.* 2001;19(9):1.
6. Ambady N, Laplante D, Nguyen T, et al. Surgeons' tone of voice: a clue to malpractice history. *Surgery.* 2002;132(1):5–9.
7. Beckman HB, Markakis KM, Suchman AL, Frankel RM. The doctor–patient relationship and malpractice: lessons from plaintiff depositions. *Archives of Internal Medicine.* 1994;154(12):1365–1370.
8. Vincent C, Young M, Phillips A. Why do people sue doctors? A study of patients and relatives taking legal action. *Lancet.* 1994;343(8913):1609–1613.
9. Hickson GB, Clayton EW, Githens PB, Sloan FA. Factors that prompted families to file medical malpractice claims following perinatal injuries. *Journal of the American Medical Association.* 1992;267(10):1359–1363.
10. Witman AB, Park DM, Hardin SB. How do patients want physicians to handle mistakes? *Archives of Internal Medicine.* 1996;156:565–569.
11. Mazor KM, Simon SR, Yood RA, et al. Health plan members' views about disclosure of medical errors. *Annals of Internal Medicine.* 2004;140(6):409–418.
12. Allshouse K. Treating patients as individuals. In: Gerteis M, Edgman-Levitan S, Daley J, eds. *Through the patient's eyes: understanding and promoting patient-centered care.* San Francisco: Jossey-Bass; 1993:29.
13. Amori GH (chair). *Disclosure of unanticipated events: the next step in better communication with patients* (Part 1 of 3 parts). ASHRM Monograph. Chicago, Illinois: American Society for Healthcare Risk Management, 2003.
14. Ellers B. Innovations in patient-centered education. In: Gerteis M, Edgman-Levitan S, Daley J, eds. *Through the patient's eyes: understanding and promoting patient-centered care.* San Francisco: Jossey-Bass; 1993:107.
15. Amori G. Communicating with patients and other customers. In: Carroll R, ed. *Risk management handbook for health care organizations.* San Francisco: Jossey-Bass; 2003:824.
16. Joint Commission on the Accreditation of Healthcare Organizations. *Comprehensive accreditation manual for hospitals. The official handbook.* Oakbrook Terrace, IL: JCAHO; 2001:RI., 1.2.2.
17. Popp PL. How will disclosure affect future litigation. *Journal of HealthCare Risk Management.* 2003;23(1):5–9.
18. National Institutes of Health. Clear and to the point: guidelines for using plain language at NIH. Accessed at http://www.od.nih.gov/execsec/guidelines.htm
19. Moore C. Health care literacy and patient safety: the new paradox. In: Youngberg BJ, Hatlie MJ, eds. *The patient safety handbook.* Sudbury, MA: Jones and Bartlett; 2004:243.
20. Spector RE. *Cultural diversity in health and illness.* Upper Saddle River, NJ: Pearson Education; 2004:20.
21. 45 CFR §164.103.
22. Glitz R, Stanton C. The Health Insurance Portability and Accountability Act (HIPAA) of 1996. In: Carroll R, ed. *Risk management handbook for health care organizations.* San Francisco: Jossey-Bass; 2003:1135–1140.
23. Kavaler FK, Spiegel AD. *Risk management in health care institutions: a strategic approach.* Sudbury, MA: Jones and Bartlett; 2003.
24. Cohen M. Statutes, standards and regulations. In: Carroll R, ed. *Risk management handbook for health care organizations.* San Francisco: Jossey-Bass; 2003:1052–1056.
25. Epstein AL, Harding GH. Risk management in selected high risk hospital departments. In: Kavaler FK, Spiegel AD, eds. *Risk management in health care institutions: a strategic approach.* Sudbury, MA: Jones and Bartlett; 2003:356.
26. ECRI. *Special report: physician office safety guide.* Plymouth Meeting, PA: ECRI; 1998.
27. Amori GH (chair). *Disclosure of unanticipated events: creating an effective patient communication policy* (Part 2 of 3 parts). ASHRM Monograph. 2003.
28. Cohen M, ed. *Medication errors.* Washington, DC: American Pharmaceutical Association; 1999.
29. Institute for Safe Medication Practices. ISMP medication safety alert. *ISMP List of Error-Prone Abbreviations, Symbols, and Dose Designations.* 2003;8(24):3–4.
30. Joint Commission. Accessed on February 15, 2012, at http://www.jointcommission.org/assets/1/18/Official_Do_Not_Use_List_6_111.PDF
31. Spath PL, ed. *Partnering with patients to reduce medical errors.* Chicago: Health Forum; 2004.
32. Reason J. *Human error.* Cambridge, UK: Cambridge University Press; 1999.

33. Ternov S. The human side of medical mistakes. In: Spath P, ed. *Error reduction in health care.* San Francisco: Jossey-Bass; 2000:97–138.

34. Pozgar GD. *Legal aspects of health care administration.* Sudbury, MA: Jones and Bartlett; 2004.

35. Johnson SK, Kicklighter L, Para P. Documentation and the medical record. In: Carroll R, ed. *Risk management handbook for health care organizations.* San Francisco: Jossey-Bass; 2003:265–285.

36. White PJ. Employment practices, legal issues. In: Carroll R, ed. *Risk management handbook for health care organizations.* San Francisco: Jossey-Bass; 2003:853–881.

37. International Association for Healthcare Security and Safety. IAHSS survey reveals healthcare statistics. Accessed June 24, 2011, at http://www.pr.com/press-release/256209

38. Kavaler FK, Spiegel AD. Assuring safety and security in health care institutions. In: Kavaler FK, Spiegel AD, eds. *Risk management in health care institutions: a strategic approach.* Sudbury, MA: Jones and Bartlett; 2003:198–201.

39. Curran ML. Organizational staffing. In: Carroll R, ed. *Risk management handbook for health care organizations.* San Francisco: Jossey-Bass; 2003:911–937.

40. Gorszkruger D. Perspectives on healthcare reform: a year later, what more do we know? *Journal of Healthcare Risk Management.* 2011;31(1): 24–30.

Bibliography

Ambady N, Laplante D, Nguyen T, Rosenthal R, Charmeton N, Levinson W. Surgeons' tone of voice: a clue to malpractice history. *Surgery.* 2002;132(1):5–9.

Amori GH (chair). *Disclosure of unanticipated events: the next step in better communication with patients* (Part 1 of 3 parts). ASHRM Monograph. Chicago, Illinois: American Society for Healthcare Risk Management, 2003.

Amori GH (chair). *Disclosure of unanticipated events: creating an effective patient communication policy* (Part 2 of 3 parts). ASHRM Monograph. Chicago, Illinois: American Society for Healthcare Risk Management, 2003.

Amori GH (chair). *Disclosure of unanticipated events: what works now and what can work even better* (Part 3 of 3 parts). ASHRM Monograph. Chicago, Illinois: American Society for Healthcare Risk Management, 2004.

Beckman HB, Markakis KM, Suchman AL, Frankel RM. The doctor-patient relationship and malpractice. Lessons from plaintiff depositions. *Archives of Internal Medicine.* 1994;154(12):1365–1370.

Carroll R, ed. *Risk management handbook for health care organizations.* San Francisco: Jossey-Bass; 2003.

Clinical Skillbuilders. *Better documentation.* Springhouse, PA: Springhouse; 1992.

Cohen M, ed. *Medication errors.* Washington, DC: American Pharmaceutical Association; 1999.

ECRI. *Special report: physician office safety guide.* Pennsylvania: ECRI; 1998.

Fischer G, Fetters MD, Munro MA, Goldman EB. Adverse events in primary care identified from a risk-management database. *Journal of Family Practice.* 1997;45(1):40–46.

Frampton SB, Gilpin L, Charmel PA. *Putting patients first: designing and practicing patient-centered care.* San Francisco: Jossey-Bass; 2003.

Gerteis M, Edgman-Levitan S, Daley J, et al. *Through the patient's eyes: understanding and promoting patient-centered care.* San Francisco: Jossey-Bass; 1993.

Head G, Elliott MW, Blinn J. *Essentials of risk financing.* Malvern, PA: Insurance Institute of America. 1996.

Head G, Horn S. *Essentials of risk management.* Malvern, PA: Insurance Institute of America; 1991.

Hickson GB, Clayton EW, Githens PB, Sloan FA. Factors that prompted families to file medical malpractice claims following perinatal injuries. *Journal of the American Medical Association.* 1992;267(10):1359–1363.

Institute for Safe Medication Practices. ISMP medication safety alert. *ISMP List of Error-Prone Abbreviations, Symbols, and Dose Designations.* 2003;8(24):3–4.

Institute of Medicine. *To err is human.* Washington, DC: National Academies Press; 1999.

Kavaler FK, Spiegel AD. *Risk management in health care institutions: a strategic approach.* Sudbury, MA: Jones and Bartlett; 2003.

Kraman SS, Hamm G. Risk management: honesty may be the best policy. *Annals of Internal Medicine.* 1999;131(12):963–967.

Mazor KM, Simon SR, Yood RA, et al. Health plan members' views about disclosure of medical errors. *Annals of Internal Medicine.* 2004;140(6):409–418.

Merry A, Smith AM. *Errors, medicine and the law.* Cambridge, UK: Cambridge University Press; 2003.

National Institutes of Health. Clear Communication: An NIH Health Literacy Initiative. Accessed on February 15, 2012, at http://www.nih.gov/clearcommunication/plainlanguage

Pozgar GD. *Legal aspects of health care administration.* Sudbury, MA: Jones and Bartlett; 2004.

Reason J. *Human error.* Cambridge, UK: Cambridge University Press; 1999.

Rosenthal MM, Sutcliffe KM, eds. *Medical error: what do we know? What do we do?* San Francisco: Jossey-Bass; 2002.

Schryve DL, ed. *An assessment manual for medical groups.* Englewood, CO: Medical Group Management Association; 2002.

Seare J. *Medical documentation.* Salt Lake City, Utah: Medicode; 1993.

Spath PL, ed. *Error reduction in health care.* San Francisco: Jossey-Bass; 2000.

Spath PL, ed. *Partnering with patients to reduce medical errors.* Chicago: Health Forum; 2004.

Spector RE. *Cultural diversity in health and illness.* Upper Saddle River, NJ: Pearson Education; 2004.

Vincent C, Young M, Phillips A. Why do people sue doctors? A study of patients and relatives taking legal action. *Lancet.* 1994;343(8913):1609–1613.

Witman AB, Park DM, Hardin SB. How do patients want physicians to handle mistakes? *Archives of Internal Medicine.* 1996;156;2565–2569.

Youngberg BJ, Hatlie MJ. *The patient safety handbook.* Sudbury, MA: Jones and Bartlett; 2004.

Essential Knowledge for Contemporary Management

Legal Issues Associated with Medical Practices and Business Arrangements in the Healthcare Industry

Bruce A. Johnson, JD, MPA
Jennifer L. Weinfeld, JD

An understanding of the legal issues associated with medical practice business arrangements requires an understanding of the nature of medical practices, their operations, and their relationships with third parties in the context of the nation's larger healthcare delivery and payment systems. As a general matter, medical practice–related legal issues will tend to arise in connection with the medical practice's operations and in the relationships that the medical practice, its physicians, and other providers create and maintain with third parties, including other providers and provider organizations, and with payers of healthcare services.

Examples of the types of legal issues that will be explored in this chapter relating to medical practice operations and relationships include the following:

- Issues related to the proper legal organization and operation of a medical practice, including the application of state laws dealing with the licensing of physicians and other healthcare providers, and state "corporate practice of medicine" and similar laws and rules that impact who can own and operate a medical practice.

- Arrangements to ensure that a medical practice and its individual providers can receive payment for the healthcare services they furnish to patients, including requirements governing enrollment and participation in the Medicare and other third-party payer programs generally, and reimbursement rules that govern whether and how a medical practice can deliver and receive payment for the services it provides.

- The various external structural relationships that are frequently created by medical practices in the context of the broader delivery system, including the formation and operation of larger provider organizations and the establishment of other relationships with participants in the healthcare delivery system. These external relationships will potentially implicate various federal and state laws and rules, including those governing antitrust, fraud and abuse, and others.

Our reference to relationships as providing the context for legal issues must be viewed solely as a useful rule of thumb rather than as a definitive rule of law. Many legal issues tend to arise in the context of relationships (e.g., a professional liability claim arises in the context of a relationship between a physician and an individual patient). However, in some cases the actions of a single participant (e.g., a physician, a hospital) can be sufficient to raise legal issues and result in the imposition of legal liability. Accordingly, it is important to note that in a strict legal sense, the existence of two or more participants is not always required for a legal violation to occur.

As a practical matter, numerous relationships and interactions occur between and among the various participants in the heathcare delivery system. With the advent of healthcare reform, numerous arrangements are being considered and established involving physicians and medical practices, institutional providers such as hospitals and other healthcare facilities, and other provider organizations. Likewise, as systems of accountable care are used with increasing frequency, numerous other relationships are being created involving physicians and medical groups, employers, commercial insurers, and other payers of healthcare services.

Today's regulatory environment is also becoming more complex. As a result, new relationships are also being developed between and among various regulatory bodies with the goal of coordinating compliance and enforcement activities as they relate to medical practices and other healthcare providers. The regulatory bodies include the Centers for Medicare and Medicaid Services (CMS), which is responsible for administering the Medicare payment and reimbursement system; the U.S. Department of Health and Human Services Office of Inspector General (OIG), which focuses on enforcing federal fraud and abuse laws that are associated with the payment and delivery of healthcare services; the U.S. Federal Trade Commission (FTC) and Department of Justice Antitrust Division, both of which are involved in antitrust law enforcement; and the exempt organization branch of the Internal Revenue Service (IRS), which is responsible for the enforcement of laws governing tax-exempt organizations such as hospitals, health systems, and many large medical groups. These activities and relationships present a range of potential legal issues to medical practices and their participants, which are illustrated in the discussion that follows.

■ Legal Issues Related to Medical Practice Organization and Operation

Numerous legal issues impact the organization and operation of a medical practice. Laws and rules governing business organizations generally apply to medical practices.

These include laws governing the legal entities that can be used to operate a business (e.g., corporation, limited liability company, partnership), laws and rules governing the relationship between employers and employees (e.g., wage and hour laws, benefit programs, and others), state and federal tax laws governing the payment of taxes by business enterprises, and numerous others. Given that numerous laws can affect the operational aspects of a medical practice, our primary focus is on laws and rules that are specific to healthcare, or that have a major impact on the medical practices involving the services of physicians and other individual healthcare providers.

For the purposes of this chapter, a "medical practice" refers to the organizational and operating structure through which medical (i.e., physician) services are furnished, without regard to its particular legal form or operating format. The term "medical group" is used generically to refer to any number of structural configurations of medical practices involving physicians and other individual healthcare providers. A medical group may be physician-owned and operated, hospital-owned or affiliated, a single or multiple legal entities, or involve other structural variations. These concepts of a medical practice, medical group, and other commonly used terms that are associated with the organization, operation, and delivery of medical care involve functional as opposed to legal definitions.

In contrast, the law does set forth specific legal definitions for certain key medical practice organizational and operating formats. For example, the term "group practice" has a highly technical legal definition found in the federal physician self-referral or Stark law. Before delving into specific legal definitions and details, the next section will provide perspective on some of the legal issues impacting the functional and operational aspects of medical practices and medical groups operating today.

Medical Practice and Medical Group Structural Variations

As noted, a medical practice may be operationally defined as the organizational structure through which medical services are provided by physicians and other licensed healthcare providers. Medical groups might be further defined operationally as involving a group of medical practices that furnish patient care to a population of patients who are involved with a common organizational structure, operational systems, and culture. Thus, a medical group practice can be conceived as consisting of numerous medical practices that share common attributes, but not all medical group practices are structured, organized, or operated in exactly the same manner.

Medical groups can certainly involve a single, physician-owned legal entity that serves as the employer of substantially all the group's physicians and other providers. The legal and organizational structures of many medical groups, large and small, including single and multispecialty group practices, fit this "traditional" structural model involving a physician-owned and operated practice. This structure is also generally consistent with the hundreds of medical group practices that comply with the definition of a group practice under the Stark law.

Yet today many other structures are being created, operated, and referred to as "medical groups," including hospital/health system–affiliated medical groups, independent practice associations (IPAs) or network medical groups, and others. These medical groups share some, but not necessarily all, of the attributes of the more traditional medical groups.

For example, a hospital/health system–affiliated medical group may, but need not, use a single legal entity that is used exclusively as the employer entity for hospital-affiliated physicians and the operation of their medical practices. Some hospital-affiliated medical groups use the hospital legal structure itself as the employing entity, such that there is no single legal platform that is solely designed to house and operate physician practices. Other hospital-affiliated medical groups may consist of multiple legal and/or organizational structures that collectively comprise the medical group enterprise.

Likewise, IPA model medical groups and the medical practices aligned with other network organizations frequently view themselves as involving "medical groups"— even though they have legal and structural dimensions that are very different from those described earlier. IPAs and other special-purpose provider networks (collectively "networks") are enterprises that bring together otherwise separate providers (usually physicians and/or other individual healthcare providers) in an affiliated manner to deliver healthcare services.

In a network, individual healthcare providers or provider groups typically establish ownership and/or contractual relationships with the network organization pursuant to which the individual providers agree to provide healthcare services to health plan beneficiaries under network-sponsored contracts. Networks customarily do not provide services directly to consumers. Rather they coordinate or arrange for the provision of healthcare services to consumers by the network's participating providers. Some network-type programs are operated by payer organizations such as indemnity insurance companies or Blue Cross/Blue Shield organizations. In such programs the payers establish independent contractual relationships with providers and market preferred provider organization (PPO) or IPA-type healthcare delivery products without the intervening involvement of a provider-sponsored network entity.

Physician–hospital organizations (PHOs) are cooperative enterprises that bring physicians and hospital providers together in a separate, vertically integrated business enterprise; they constitute networks and may involve network model medical groups. As with other networks, the PHO legal entity does not directly deliver healthcare services, but generally coordinates the provision of services through the PHO's participating physician and hospital providers. PHOs are composed of physicians and medical practices that take on various structural forms (including a large complement of hospital-employed physicians), but the PHO's medical practice participants are tied together through a network organization that may be viewed as involving a medical group. In such network model medical groups, truly independent medical practices of various sizes and characteristics continue to exist—meaning each will commonly have its own legal entity, offices, systems, and infrastructure. Nonetheless, the network still constitutes a "medical group" because the medical practices in the network share patients, a common structure, and at least some attributes of a common medical practice culture.

In today's emerging accountable care system of healthcare delivery and financing, it is likely that accountable care organizations (ACOs) will have their own medical group participants. As with other commonly used terms and concepts in the healthcare delivery system, there is not currently a legally precise definition for what constitutes an ACO, although the Medicare program has proposed a legal definition for purposes of participation in shared savings arrangements under the Patient Protection and Affordable Care Act (PPACA) health reform legislation. Section 3022 of PPACA established numerous legal, structural, operational, and other requirements that would apply to an ACO. In April 2011, CMS published a proposed rule that defined an ACO as a legal entity composed of certain eligible ACO participants who work together to coordinate care for Medicare fee-for-service beneficiaries. The agency set forth various proposals related to who could participate in the ACO (including medical groups, hospitals, and others), and how the ACO would interact with providers, payers of healthcare services, and patients. Additional information on the structure and operation of ACOs under the proposed rule is provided later in this chapter in connection with the discussion of medical practice external relationships, and to illustrate the potential application of various laws discussed in this chapter.

Other organizational structures may also be involved in healthcare delivery in a particular community or marketplace, including what are commonly referred to as "medical foundations" or other structures that effectively combine physicians and hospitals and/or hospital systems into a single organization for the delivery of healthcare services through the foundation's affiliated physician providers. Other organizational forms include management services organizations (MSOs) that are jointly owned and/or sponsored by physicians, hospitals, or others to provide management and administrative support services to physicians, their medical practices, and medical groups. MSOs do not actually deliver healthcare services, but are organized to provide various forms of practice support services to healthcare providers, such as billing and collection services, management information services, and other components of infrastructure and services that must be acquired and used by healthcare providers under an accountable care delivery environment system.

A definitive summary of the universe of provider organizations or the range of vertical and horizontal integration strategies is beyond the scope of this chapter. Moreover, what an organization may be called and created to do in one particular community may be vastly different from what an organization with the same name does in another community. In addition, enterprises in various communities increasingly have "blended" functions.

Medical Practice Ownership and Operation

State laws governing the licensing of physicians and other healthcare providers commonly impose restrictions on who may be licensed to engage in the practice of medicine and what types of organizations may employ physicians and other licensed professionals to furnish medical services to the general public. State licensure laws combined with corporate laws governing the formation and operation of legal entities within a particular state will commonly impact the form of legal entity that is used for a single medical practice or medical group, and the identity of the parties who own and operate that enterprise. Virtually all states permit medical professionals to organize, operate, and own a medical practice using a corporate form of organization. Most states permit licensed physicians to use other legal forms in connection with their medical practices, including limited liability companies (LLC), partnerships, and others. Many states require that the legal entity used for the medical practice must be organized and operated as a professional variation of one of these (e.g., PLLC, PLLP, etc.), and that only licensed professionals may organize and own the practice.

Related to, and frequently a component of, state licensure statutes are requirements prohibiting what is commonly called the "corporate practice of medicine."[a] The corporate practice of medicine doctrine generally forbids physicians from practicing medicine on behalf of, or in concert with, any person or organization other than a physician-owned entity. Several policy concerns underlie the doctrine, including the desire to: (1) avoid layperson control over professional medical judgment; (2) prevent commercial exploitation of the practice of medicine; and (3) prevent any conflict between a physician's duty of loyalty to his or her patient, and to his or her employer. In many states, physicians who violate the prohibition on the corporate practice of medicine are subject to disciplinary action including potential loss of their medical license. Because licensure laws are set forth in 50 separate bodies of state law, the existence and application of the corporate practice of medicine doctrine varies from state to state. Many states have no such a provision, thereby permitting medical practices to be owned and operated by persons who do not hold a medical license. Other states have watered down the corporate practice of medicine prohibition to allow nonprofit hospital service corporations, health maintenance organizations, and other enterprises to employ physicians and operate a medical practice. In some jurisdictions, hospital employment of physicians may be authorized on the ground that the delivery of medical care is consistent with the hospital's mission. Some states permit hospitals to own a separate legal entity (i.e., a wholly owned or partially owned subsidiary) that itself operates a medical practice. Many states also allow employers to hire physicians to provide medical services to their own employees and dependents at company-sponsored clinics, but not to the public generally.

Even where the corporate practice of medicine prohibition has been relaxed, professional licensure laws still typically require physicians to exercise independent professional judgment in their care of patients. The precise scope of the prohibition on the corporate practice of medicine varies from state to state, so the legal rules associated with the practice of medicine must be closely examined in connection with the formation and operation of any new medical practice to promote the development of a legally sound structure.

Enrollment in, Payment of, and Reimbursement for Medical Services

Beyond the basic legal structure of a medical group or practice lies the fundamental question of how the medical

---

a. See, e.g., Col. Corp. Code §§ 13401, 13401, 13401.5. Colo. Rev. Stat. § 12-36-134, and N.Y. Bus. Corp. Law § 1501 et seq.

practice and its physicians and other providers will get paid for the services they provide. Medical professionals are required to be qualified and licensed to provide medical and other healthcare services under state licensing laws. Yet medical licensure is a necessary but not a sufficient basis to permit individual physicians and their practices to receive payment from third-party payers for the services they furnish to patients. In order to receive reimbursement from such third-party payers, individual physicians and their medical practice entities must generally be enrolled in the underlying third-party payer's payment program.

Each payer organization has its own enrollment requirements and processes; this chapter will examine the requirements imposed on enrollment under the Medicare program. The Medicare program enrolls clinics, group practices, and certain eligible professionals as individual suppliers to permit such enrolled entities to bill and receive reimbursement from Medicare for covered services. (Enrollment for such a freestanding clinic is conducted through the use of CMS-855B, which generally permits enrollment by clinics/group practices and certain other suppliers under the Medicare program.) Hospitals and certain other institutional providers are separately enrolled and referred to as "providers" under Medicare. Under federal laws that provide the statutory basis for the Medicare program, eligible professionals include physicians, physical therapists, speech therapists, occupational therapists, audiologists, and certain other practitioners.[1] Certain other individual practitioners who commonly work in medical practices and medical groups are also eligible to separately enroll in the Medicare program and receive Medicare payments, including physician assistants, nurse practitioners, certified nurse specialists, and other professionals.[2] In general, Medicare provides that where persons in these (and certain other) categories are licensed under state law, they may enroll in Medicare in order to receive payment for covered medical and other services that are furnished within the scope of their license.

Where a physician or other supplier is enrolled in Medicare, that enrollment generally permits the receipt of payment or reimbursement for covered healthcare services furnished to a patient by the individual healthcare provider enrollee. That individual provider may receive payment directly, or more commonly, "reassign" the individual provider's right to payment to the provider's employer or another organization.[3] Payment and enrollment by Medicare and other third-party payers is made by reference to unique identification numbers: the NPI and the PTAN. The National Provider Identifier (NPI) number is a unique 10-digit identification number issued to healthcare providers by CMS and assigned by the National Plan and Provider Enumeration System. Obtaining an NPI is required by the Health Insurance Portability and Accountability Act of 1996 (HIPAA) for all healthcare providers (as defined in HIPAA). Although issued by CMS, obtaining the NPI does not by itself establish eligibility for Medicare reimbursement. The Provider Transaction Account Number (PTAN), sometimes referred to as the Medicare Identification Number, is a generic term for any number other than the NPI that is used to identify a Medicare supplier. Only Medicare-eligible providers may obtain a PTAN to bill Medicare, and a PTAN is required for providers to receive reimbursement from Medicare. Both the physician (or nonphysician practitioner) and his or her medical practice or group legal entity will have an NPI and a PTAN. By virtue of their enrollment, each Medicare-enrolled physician, clinic, or other supplier agrees to, and is obligated to, the Medicare program's various laws and rules.

Medicare Reimbursement

The Medicare program also imposes numerous complex rules and requirements on the reimbursement of covered medical and other healthcare services. These rules define the basis for payment of services (e.g., as services paid for under Medicare Part A, Part B, or otherwise), the level of reimbursement, as well as special payment restrictions and rules based on the type of service, the site of service, and other factors.

For example, the Medicare program provides payment under Medicare Part B for covered medical and other health services,[4] including those that are furnished "incident to" the services of physicians and certain other healthcare providers.[5] Among other things, these rules impose requirements on what services will be paid for, and on how the services must be furnished and supervised (e.g., by requiring, in the case of incident to services, direct supervision and imposing other requirements).

Specific rules govern services paid for by Medicare. For example, Medicare has specific rules governing the furnishing and reimbursement of diagnostic tests such as x-rays, advanced imaging procedures (e.g., MRI, CT), and others, where the tests are furnished by a medical practice or other supplier. The Medicare "anti-markup rule"[6] imposes a limitation on the amount Medicare will pay for diagnostic tests (including the professional component [PC] and the technical component [TC] of such tests) under certain circumstances. The anti-markup rule imposes a limitation on payment where the performing physician does not "share a practice" with the billing physician or other supplier. Under the rule, the performing physician will share a practice with the billing physician or other supplier under two alternative scenarios[7]:

- The performing physician furnishes substantially all (at least 75%) of his or her professional services *through* such billing physician or other supplier.
- The performing physician is an owner, employee, or independent contractor of the billing physician or other supplier, and the TC or PC is performed in the office of the billing physician or other supplier (with certain additional requirements imposed upon certain physician organizations).

As this example illustrates, Medicare rules governing reimbursement impose specific, highly detailed, and complex requirements on how Medicare-covered services are furnished, including requirements that impact the organization, operation, and means by which the services are provided by a medical practice.

Adding to this complexity is the fact that today, many of the same types of healthcare items and services may be furnished through different enrolled entities, and in various settings under the Medicare program. For example, the Medicare antimarkup rule applies to the furnishing of diagnostic testing services in medical practices and clinics, but it also applies to other entities that are enrolled and able to furnish and receive reimbursement for the same types of diagnostic testing services, namely entities that are separately enrolled as independent diagnostic testing facilities (IDTF). Where IDTF enrollment is used, separate IDTF enrollment is required for each diagnostic testing facility location, and each location must meet the Medicare IDTF enrollment standards. The standards include requirements related to billing for diagnostic tests, prohibitions on the sharing of space with another Medicare-enrolled supplier, and others.[8]

The same types of diagnostic testing services (e.g., x-ray, CT, MRI) that may be furnished by a medical practice or IDTF supplier under Medicare may also be furnished and paid for under the Medicare program as services that are furnished by a hospital, in a provider-based or hospital outpatient department (HOPD) setting. Thus, diagnostic tests that in some settings are delivered as services ancillary to a physician-owned and operated medical practice may be furnished by an IDTF, or furnished and paid for as hospital services. The key distinction in this example relates to the enrolled entity and site of service through which the services are furnished and billed (i.e., through an entity enrolled in Medicare as a clinic, through an IDTF, or in an HOPD), as opposed to the particular type of healthcare service (diagnostic testing services) provided.

Provider-Based Reimbursement

Ambulatory clinics operated by medical groups may be operated in what are commonly referred to as freestanding clinics, or through provider-based clinics[9] that are operated under the license of a hospital provider. In the case of provider-based clinics, the clinical space in which patients are seen is subject to the hospital's licensure, ownership, and control.

Obtaining provider-based status allows a hospital to bill Medicare a facility fee under the outpatient prospective payment system, with the facility fee designed to pay the cost of the overhead associated with the operation of the provider-based clinic. Hospitals often seek provider-based status for some of their ambulatory clinics so they can realize aggregate financial gains by billing for the facility fee. Where services are furnished in a provider-based facility, the Medicare reimbursement for physician and professional services is reduced because of a site-of-service differential (provider-based vs. freestanding clinic setting), but the total compensation paid through the combination of the facility fee and the payment for professional services is commonly greater than a payment for professional services furnished in nonhospital or freestanding clinic settings.

Medicare standards applicable to provider-based clinics or departments are numerous and complex. Specific requirements are imposed on provider-based facilities that are on-campus (generally defined as facilities that are within 250 yards of a hospital's main buildings) and those that are off-campus. Provider-based departments must generally meet specific requirements, regardless of whether they are located on or off the hospital campus, including that the provider-based department and the hospital must be operated under the same hospital license, the department must be clinically integrated with the hospital (e.g., professional staff of the department must have clinical privileges at the hospital), and the hospital must have monitoring and oversight of the department in the same manner as with other hospital departments.

Provider-based departments also must be financially integrated with the hospital, as evidenced by shared income and expenses, and they must be held out to the public and to other payers as part of the hospital such that when patients enter the department, they must be aware that they are entering the hospital and will be billed accordingly. Provider-based clinics or departments must also comply with the applicable antidumping requirements of the Emergency Medical Treatment and Active Labor Act (EMTALA). Physician services provided within the provider-based department must be billed with the correct site of service code (hospital outpatient department) so that appropriate payment for physician and other practitioner professional services can be made, and provider-based departments and services must be furnished in accordance with numerous other requirements.

Freestanding Clinic Models
The mere existence of a hospital in the operating structure of a practice does not necessarily mean the services of a hospital-affiliated practice or medical group are themselves furnished and billed as provider-based services. Today, the majority of physician services continue to be furnished in freestanding clinic settings that are not hospital-based (i.e., they are not furnished in a provider-based/HOPD facility). Freestanding clinics may be operated by a physician-owned medical practice, or as a hospital-owned practice that is not operated as part of the hospital itself (e.g., not as a provider-based or HOPD clinical facility). (Enrollment for such a freestanding clinic is conducted through the use of CMS-855B, which generally permits enrollment by clinics/group practices and certain other suppliers under the Medicare program.) Put otherwise, in hospital-owned freestanding clinic settings, the clinical facility operates independently from the hospital and is not subject to the aforementioned provider-based rules, and the services provided by practitioners furnishing services in the clinic are not considered services that are furnished in a hospital. Where a freestanding clinic is operated by a hospital, the hospital does not receive a facility fee payment, nor is reimbursement for physician or other professional services that are furnished in the setting reduced for the hospital site-of-service differential. Instead, physician services are paid under the Medicare physician fee schedule with an "office" site of service.

As illustrated earlier in this discussion, numerous legal issues can arise in connection with the organization and internal operation of medical practices and medical groups. Those issues will, themselves, frequently vary depending on the structure used to operate the medical practice, the services the practice provides, the particular setting for the practice and services, and other variables. Many of the legal issues referenced previously, including those governing licensure under state law, scope of practice, enrollment, and the like, have additional implications in the context of medical practice external business and operational relationships, as described in the following section.

Legal Issues Impacting Medical Practice External Relationships

The laws and rules governing the external relationships and activities of medical practices and groups are also numerous. "External relationships" refers to a range of business activities that are undertaken by the medical practice and its providers in today's healthcare delivery system, including their participation and external relationships in that delivery system. In general, the applicable legal issues and restrictions are grouped into three broad categories.

First, provisions of the federal Medicare and Medicaid law impose a variety of restrictions designed to prohibit fraud and abuse. These include the federal physician self-referral or Stark law, which applies to physician financial and referral relationships with entities that furnish designated health services.[10] This also includes other fraud and abuse prohibitions such as the antikickback statute,[11] the Medicare civil monetary penalty statute,[12] and the False Claims Act, which deals with activities such as submitting false claims for reimbursement, false representations, and other fraudulent activities. These laws apply to the operational activities of many medical practices, as well as to the relationships that the practices and their physicians have with payers, other healthcare providers, and others involved in the healthcare delivery system.

Second, federal and state antitrust laws may also impact medical group operations and relationships, in particular in today's environment involving the creation and operation of large medical group practices, networks, integrated delivery systems, and care organizations.[b] These laws impact the size, relationships, and operations of the numerous enterprises being created today to participate in the accountable care system of healthcare delivery.

Finally, a host of other state laws, including those governing the business of insurance, state antifraud laws, and others, often impact the external relationship and activities of medical practices.

This section will begin with a review of antifraud laws, focusing on the Stark law and its application to medical practice internal operations and external relationships.

The Stark Law
The federal physician self-referral prohibition, also known as the Stark law, is one of numerous laws and

---

b. See, for example, 15 U.S.C. § § 1,2 (Sherman Act § 1,2); 15 U.S.C. § (Clayton Act § 7); and 15 U.S.C. § 45 (Federal Trade Commission Act § 5).

ethical prescriptions that govern physician referrals to organizations with which the physician has a financial relationship.[10] The Stark law gets its short-form name from the law's chief sponsor, U.S. Representative Fortney (Pete) Stark (D-Calif). The law was first enacted in 1989 (Stark I), and amended effective in 1995 (Stark II). The law has been in force for many years, with the interpretive rule-making process lagging over time. Initial, proposed, and final rules governing Stark I and II were published in 1995, 1998, 2001, 2004, and 2007. Additional revisions to the basic regulatory structure have occurred in connection with the publication of other rules under the Medicare program. This tortured process, over a period of years, highlights the challenges CMS has faced in implementing a complex law, while considering the increasingly divergent interests and demands of different segments of the healthcare industry. The Stark law applies to physicians and their referrals and financial relationships, although the law is also broadly applied to other healthcare providers and organizations. The Stark law generally prohibits physician referrals for certain ancillary healthcare services (defined as designated health services or DHS) to entities with which the physician (or a member of the physician's immediate family) has a financial relationship, *unless* an exception to the law applies. Each of these elements has its own specific meaning and highly specific requirements, as summarized in the following paragraphs.

Specifically, the Stark law applies to "physicians,"[13] as defined by Medicare program payment rules as a doctor of medicine or osteopathy, a doctor of dental surgery or dental medicine, a doctor of pediatric medicine, a doctor of optometry, or a chiropractor as defined by Medicare. Where a DHS referral is made by anyone other than a person qualifying as a physician professional (e.g., by nonphysician providers such as nurse practitioners or physician assistants), then the referral is not subject to the Stark law.

A referral is defined broadly under the Stark law, and it generally includes a request by a physician for any DHS for which payment may be made by the Medicare program.[13] This includes the ordering, certifying, or recertifying of the need for any such service. A referral does not include any designated health services personally performed by the physician him- or herself. In practical terms, a physician makes a referral under the Stark law whenever he or she requests a procedure, test, item, service, or supply that is classified as a designated health service, but the physician does not personally perform the service him- or herself.[13] For such purposes, "personal performance" has a literal and narrow meaning, such that if any person other than the physician is involved in performing the service, then the physician has not *personally performed* the service.

(Note that certain additional requests for services ordered by pathologists, radiologists, and radiation oncologists are also excluded from the definition of a referral.)

Under the Stark law, an entity or DHS entity[13] to which the prohibition on physician referrals applies includes virtually any organization that performs or furnishes DHS, and to which CMS makes payment for those services, either directly or under assignment. This means that for Stark law purposes, an entity includes a physician's solo practice or a practice of multiple physicians, including any other corporation, partnership, limited liability company, or other enterprise that performs or furnishes DHS (e.g., a hospital, outpatient rehabilitation facility, clinical laboratory, IDTF, or similar organization that receives referrals from physicians for DHS, and that bills and receives payment from Medicare for those services). CMS expanded its original definition of an entity to include any person or entity that actually *performs the DHS*. For example, a physician makes a referral to an entity that will implicate the Stark law when he or she refers a patient to a hospital *or* to a separate company that performs services that are subsequently billed by the hospital "under arrangements."[13]

The Stark law only applies to referrals for designated health services, which are or may be payable in whole or in part by the Medicare program. In general, this means services that are eligible for payment by Medicare, in whole or in part, to the patient or to the provider of the service (e.g., physician, group, independent laboratory, hospital, etc.) are DHS. The law defines both the professional and technical components of a particular service as designated health services.[13]

The law applies to the following specific categories of designated health services, and CMS has provided general or specific descriptions of which specific services in individual categories constitute DHS. Those categories and general descriptions consist of the following[c]:

- Clinical laboratory services (generally identified using Current Procedural Terminology [CPT] and Healthcare Common Procedure Coding System [HCPCS] codes, including all CPT codes in the 80000 series).
- Physical therapy, occupational therapy, and speech-language pathology services (generally including certain CPT codes in the 97000 series).

---

c. The final rule provides that the specific services defined as DHS in certain categories will be identified by CPT/HCPCS codes. Such codes are listed in, and updated through, the annual publication of the Medicare physician fee schedule.

- Radiology and certain other imaging services, including the professional and technical components of diagnostic tests and procedures using x-rays, ultrasound, or other imaging services; computerized axial tomography (CAT) scans; magnetic resonance imaging (MRI); dexascan services; and nuclear medicine services.
- Radiation therapy services and supplies (generally consisting of CPT codes in the 70000 series, including planning related to radiation therapy and treatment procedures involving protons, plus certain other radiation therapy services and therapeutic nuclear medicine procedures).
- Durable medical equipment and supplies (DME), prosthetics, orthotics and prosthetic devices and supplies (POS) (generally defined as such in applicable Medicare fee schedules).
- Home health services.
- Outpatient prescription drugs (defined generally as all prescription drugs and biologicals covered by Medicare Part B or Part D).
- Inpatient and outpatient hospital services (defined by reference to payment and coverage provisions of the Medicare laws and rules). Inpatient hospital services are those furnished either by the hospital or by others under arrangement with a hospital. Outpatient hospital services are defined by reference to existing Medicare coverage and payment laws and rules; such services include therapeutic, diagnostic, and partial hospitalization services; outpatient services furnished by a psychiatric hospital; and outpatient critical-access hospital services.

The Stark law defines financial relationships to generally include ownership and investment interests and compensation arrangements between a physician (or a member of the physician's immediate family) and an entity that performs or furnishes DHS.[14] Such arrangements and the associated financial relationships may be either direct or indirect. Ownership or investment interests include those in which a physician owns, directly or indirectly, shares of stock or other equity interests in an organization that furnishes or performs DHS. Compensation arrangements include those involving an exchange of any remuneration between a physician or a member of a physician's immediate family and an entity that furnishes DHS. The Stark law and final rule provide an expansive definition of remuneration by providing that it means any payment or other benefit made directly or indirectly, in cash or in kind, but with certain narrow exceptions.

A financial relationship is direct for purposes of the Stark law if remuneration passes between the referring physician (or a member of his or her immediate family) and the DHS entity, but the remuneration *does not* pass through any intervening persons or organizations. Direct financial relationships would include, for example, a physician member's ownership of stock in a professional corporation legal entity that houses the physician's medical practice and furnishes designated health services. Similarly, a physician's direct receipt of compensation from a hospital or other DHS entity under a medical director or similar arrangement would also constitute a direct financial relationship.

Indirect financial relationships generally involve uninterrupted ownership or compensation arrangements that pass through another entity or person between the referring physician and DHS entity—meaning that there is an unbroken chain of ownership or investment interests, compensation relationships, or both between the referring physician (or immediate family member) and the DHS entity. Although indirect ownership arrangements are relatively easy to understand (i.e., an unbroken chain of ownership interests, with each link in the chain involving an ownership interest), indirect compensation arrangements are less so, and the regulatory requirements governing indirect compensation arrangements continue to evolve. Under early versions of the Stark law's implementing regulations, there were many circumstances in which no indirect compensation relationship would be present, in which case the Stark law did not apply to a particular arrangement. Because of this, CMS subsequently adopted a largely all-inclusive approach to determining whether an indirect compensation arrangement exists, and it clarified the requirements of the Stark law exception that would govern such indirect compensation arrangements.

In addition, over time CMS has made additional changes to narrow the circumstances in which an indirect compensation arrangement will exist, to provide that where a physician organization is involved in what would otherwise be characterized as an indirect compensation arrangement, the physician owners, employees, and independent contractors to that physician organization will be deemed to "stand in the shoes" of the physician organization. In such circumstances, the organization must comply with a Stark law exception applicable to *direct* (as opposed to indirect) compensation arrangements. This new provision effectively converts otherwise indirect compensation arrangements (due to the presence of an intervening entity between the physician and the DHS entity) into compensation arrangements that must comply with an exception to the Stark law governing direct compensation arrangements. For purposes of the stand-in-the-shoes provision, a physician organization is defined as a physician (including a professional corporation of which the physician is the sole owner), a physician practice, or a group practice that complies with the Stark law's highly technical definition of a group practice.

Stark Law Exceptions

Where all conditions required for the application of the Stark law are present (i.e., physician referral to an entity for DHS, where the physician or an immediate family member has a financial relationship with the DHS entity), an exception under the Stark law must apply or the law will be violated. The law's exceptions are therefore of significant importance given the breadth of the law and its potentially wide application to a variety of relationships between physicians and organizations that provide designated health services.

The Stark law affects physician practices—including solo practice physicians and those practicing in physician-owned medical group practices—in different ways depending on whether the financial and referral relationships are internal or external to the physician practice entity.

Where designated health services such as x-ray, physical therapy, outpatient prescription drugs, or others are furnished and billed for through a physician's medical practice entity, then the Stark law will apply to these "within practice" or *internal* DHS financial and referral relationships, and the practice must comply with an exception under the law. The Stark law's in-office ancillary services exception[15] and the employment exception[16] are most commonly used to permit such within physician practice DHS referrals.

The Stark law also affects physician financial and referral relationships that are outside of or *external* to the physician's own medical practice entity. These include lease and service arrangements established between physicians and/or their medical practices with hospitals and other DHS entities, medical director and other relationships with DHS entities that are outside of the physician practice entity, and potentially many other financial and referral relationships that will implicate the law and require compliance with an exception. Moreover, because the law defines remuneration in a way that will trigger the law's application broadly (i.e., as virtually any payment, in cash or in kind), exceptions are required for many financial and referral relationships.

Many exceptions are available under the law, with different exceptions available to address ownership or compensation arrangements, or both, including those dealing with the following:

- Physician ownership and compensation arrangements relating to DHS furnished through a bona fide group practice,[17] referred to as the in-office ancillary services exception[15]
- Compensation associated with employment relationships
- Compensation paid in connection with professional service arrangements including medical directorships with hospitals and other DHS entities
- Leases of office space and equipment
- Financial arrangements associated with physician recruitment and/or retention
- Medical practice acquisition transactions
- Relationships within academic medical centers and practice plans
- Investments in public companies that furnish DHS
- Access to and use of health information technology, electronic health records, and similar technology from other organizations
- Incidental benefits and support that physicians might receive from hospitals and other organizations (such as medical staff benefits, referral services, obstetrics malpractice subsidies, and other benefits)
- Arrangements that comply with certain safe harbors to the antikickback statute
- Other relationships that physicians or their family members may have with DHS entities

The in-office ancillary services and employment exceptions that are commonly used in the context of internal or within medical practice referrals are reviewed in the following sections, as are the exceptions for personal services arrangements, and space and equipment leases that are commonly used in connection with physician DHS referrals to external organizations.

The Stark In-Office Ancillary Services Exception

The in-office ancillary services exception[15] is used frequently by medical practices because it allows physicians in medical group practices to make referrals for certain DHS within the medical practice, furnish those DHS to practice patients, and bill Medicare and Medicaid for the services without violating the Stark law. The in-office ancillary services exception has several highly specific requirements and restrictions that can be grouped into four broad categories.

First, the exception imposes requirements on who furnishes the designated health services that are provided through the medical practice and how they are provided. It also deals with the issue of who supervises nonphysician personnel and what level of supervision those personnel receive when designated health services are furnished through the group. More precisely, designated health services provided through a medical practice under the in-office ancillary services exception *must* be furnished personally by any one of the following[16]:

- The referring physician him- or herself
- Another physician who is a member of the same group practice as the referring physician
- An individual who is supervised by the referring physician, or if the referring physician is in a group practice, by another physician in the group practice, as long as the supervision complies with all other applicable Medicare payment and coverage rules for the services

The in-office ancillary services exception to the Stark law also imposes requirements related to where a medical practice furnishes designated health services to the patient. Specifically, medical practices can furnish designated health services under the in-office ancillary services exception in two possible locations[17]:

- In the same building in which the physician making the DHS referral or another physician who is a member of the same group practice furnishes physician services unrelated to the furnishing of DHS payable by Medicare, any other federal healthcare payer, or a private payer (with the same building generally being defined as having the same U.S. Postal Service address)
- In a centralized building that is used by the group practice for the provision of some or all of the group practice's designated health services

The third essential requirement of the in-office ancillary services exception relates to how the designated health services are billed, commonly referred to as the billing test. To comply with the billing test, designated health services provided via the in-office ancillary services exception must be billed by any of the following[18]:

- The physician performing or supervising the designated health service
- The group practice of which the performing or supervising physician is a member, under a billing number assigned to the group practice, or by the group practice if the physician supervising the furnishing of designated health services is a physician in the group practice under a billing number assigned to the group practice

- An entity that is wholly owned by the performing or supervising physician, or by that physician's group practice under the wholly owned entity's billing number, or under a billing number assigned to the physician or group practice
- An independent third-party billing company acting as an agent of the physician, group practice, or entity referenced above, under a billing number assigned to the same, and under a billing arrangement that meets an exception to the Medicare prohibition on reassignment

Compliance with each of these options also requires compliance with underlying Medicare requirements related to billing and reassignment.[19]

Lastly, to furnish designated health services through a medical practice through the use of the in-office ancillary services exception, the medical practice (other than a true solo practice) must meet the Stark law's highly complex and specific requirements as a bona fide group practice,[17] with those specific requirements relating to the following:

- The group's legal organization and number of physicians providing services through the group practice
- The services provided by the group's members
- The amount of services provided through the group by member physicians
- The means by which the group distributes revenues and costs
- The group's operation as an integrated, unified business
- The physician–patient encounters requirement
- The means by which physicians in the group practice are compensated by the group (i.e., the compensation test)

Importantly, a medical group must meet *all* of the other requirements of this definition for it to constitute a bona fide group practice under the Stark law.

Exception for Bona Fide Employment Relationships

A separate exception to the Stark law is available to permit referrals associated with compensation arrangements involving bona fide employment relationships.[16] This exception will typically be relied upon to permit DHS referrals between a physician and a hospital or other organization that both employs the physician and furnishes DHS. This exception may also be relied upon in the context of group practice relationships with the group's physician employees, although the in-office ancillary services exception is more typically used when the employing organization involves a bona fide group practice due to the greater flexibility in physician compensation arrangements permitted under the in-office ancillary services exception.

Where the bona fide employment exception to the Stark law is used, it will apply to any amount paid by an employer to a physician (or immediate family member of a physician) who has a bona fide employment relationship with the employer for the provision of services. The employment exception's specific requirements include[16]:

- The employment arrangement must be for identifiable services, meaning the services must be known and identified in connection with the employment arrangement.
- The amount of the remuneration under the employment relationship must be consistent with the fair market value of the services, and not be determined in a manner that takes into account (directly or indirectly) the volume or value of any DHS referrals by the referring physician or other business generated between the parties.
- The compensation is provided under an agreement that would be commercially reasonable even if no referrals were made to the employer.

Personal Services Arrangements Exception

The Stark law exception for personal services arrangements covers remuneration from a DHS entity under a single arrangement or multiple arrangements with a physician, an immediate family member of the physician, or a group practice.[22] This exception may be used for internal arrangements within medical groups, or more commonly in relationships such as medical director arrangements involving physicians and hospitals or other DHS entities. The following conditions must be met to comply with the Stark law's personal services arrangements exception:

- Each personal services arrangement must be in writing, signed by the parties, specifying the services covered by the arrangement.
- The arrangement must cover all of the services to be furnished by the physician (or an immediate family member of the physician) to the entity (with this requirement met if all separate arrangements between the entity and the physician and the entity and any family members incorporate each other by reference or if they cross-reference a master list of contracts maintained and updated centrally and available for review).
- The aggregate services contracted for must not exceed those that are reasonable and necessary for the legitimate business purposes of the arrangements.

- The term of each arrangement is for at least 1 year (and if an arrangement is terminated during the term with or without cause, the parties may not enter into the same or substantially the same arrangement during the first year of the original term of the arrangement).
- The compensation to be paid over the term of each arrangement must be set in advance, it must not exceed fair market value, and it cannot be not determined in a manner that takes into account the volume or value of any referrals or other business generated between the parties.
- The services to be furnished under each arrangement must not involve the counseling or promotion of a business arrangement or other activity that violates any state or federal law.

The final rule governing personal services arrangements permits a "holdover" personal service arrangement for up to 6 months following the expiration of an agreement of at least 1 year that met the conditions listed previously so long as the holdover personal services arrangement is on the same terms and conditions as the expired agreement. For purposes of the personal services exception, a physician or family member can furnish services through employees whom they have hired to perform the services, through a wholly owned entity, or through locum tenens physicians, except that the regular physician need not be a member of a group practice.[22]

As illustrated, the Stark law has broad application to medical practices and physicians, including with respect to the medical practice's internal structure, services, and operating format, as well as with respect to the financial and referral relationships that the practice's physicians have with other DHS entities. Some of the exceptions that are commonly relied upon to permit physician financial and referral relationships outside of the medical practice are reviewed in the following sections.

Exception for Space Leases

The Stark law and final rule provide an exception for compensation arrangements involving payments for office space made by a lessee to a lessor.[23] This exception is available for compensation arrangements in which the physician (or immediate family member) or a physician organization directly establishes a space-rental arrangement with a third party—as either a tenant or a lessor. Under this exception, the rental or lease agreement for real estate (e.g., office or other space) must meet the following requirements[23]:

- A written agreement must be signed by the parties and specify the leased premises.

- The term of the agreement must be for at least 1 year. If the agreement is terminated within the term, with or without cause, the parties may not enter into a new agreement during the first year of the original term.
- The space rented may not exceed that which is reasonable and necessary for the legitimate business purposes of the tenant. The space also must be used exclusively by the tenant, who does not share it with any person or entity related to the tenant (with fair market value payments permitted for the use of common areas).
- The rental charges over the term of the agreement must be set in advance and must be consistent with fair market value.
- The rental charges over the term of the arrangement must not be determined in a manner that takes into account the volume or value of any referrals or other business generated between the parties.
- The agreement must be commercially reasonable even if no referrals were made between the lessee and the lessor.

Equipment Rental Lease Exception

Requirements applicable to the Stark law exception governing equipment rental arrangements are similar to those applicable to space rental arrangements.[24] Lease arrangements may exist when either the physician or the entity is lessor or lessee (i.e., a physician leases equipment to a provider of designated health services, or the DHS provider leases equipment to an individual physician). This exception could also be used when a solo-practice physician establishes a lease relationship through his or her practice or a wholly owned legal entity, or where a physician stands in the shoes of his or her physician organization. Where a compensation arrangement involving equipment rental implicates the Stark law, compliance with the exception applicable to equipment leases requires the following:

- The rental or equipment lease agreement must be in writing, signed by the parties, and specify the equipment it covers.
- The equipment rented or leased must not exceed that which is reasonable and necessary for the legitimate business purposes of the lease or rental, must be used exclusively by the lessee, and must not be shared with or used by the lessor or any person or entity related to the lessor.
- The agreement must be for a term of at least 1 year (with this requirement met if the agreement is terminated during the term, with or without cause, as long as the parties do not enter into a new

agreement during the first year of the original term of the agreement).
- The rental charges over the term of the agreement must be set in advance, consistent with fair market value, and not determined in a manner that takes into account the volume or value of any referrals or other business generated between the parties.
- The agreement must be commercially reasonable even if no referrals were made between the parties.

The exceptions for both space and equipment leases also allow for a "holdover" month-to-month rental for up to 6 months immediately following an agreement with a term of at least 1 year, as long as the rental is on the same terms and conditions of the immediately preceding agreement providing for the rental arrangement.[24]

It is common for business relationships engaged in by medical practices and their physicians to implicate the application of the Stark law so as to require compliance with an applicable exception to the law to permit specific financial and referral relationships.

Because of the potentially expansive application of the Stark law, coupled with the sanctions associated with Stark law violations—essentially nonpayment of services, required refunds, and other potential liability[d]—attention to Stark law compliance is essential for medical practices themselves, and for hospitals and other entities that furnish designated health services resulting from physician referrals. Although compliance with the Stark law is essential, Stark law compliance is assessed independently of compliance with other applicable fraud and abuse laws, including the antikickback statute and others, many of which have significantly broader potential application to a range of healthcare business relationships involving medical practices and physicians.

Federal Antikickback Statute

The federal antikickback statute[25] provides for the imposition of criminal penalties on anyone who knowingly and willfully offers, pays, solicits, or receives any remuneration—effectively, anything of value—directly or indirectly, overtly or covertly, in cash or in kind, in return for referring an individual to a person for the furnishing or arranging for the furnishing of an item or service for which payment may be made under the Medicare or Medicaid programs, or in return for or recommending the purchase, lease, order, or arrangement for any good, facility, service, or item for which payment may be made under the Medicare or Medicaid programs. Violation of the antikickback law is a felony, punishable by fines, imprisonment,

---

d. See 42 C.F.R. § 411.353(b) and (c).

or both. An individual or entity also can be excluded from the Medicare and Medicaid programs for violations of the law. Analogous state laws impose similar requirements, though this discussion is limited to the federal statute.

The antikickback statute was originally enacted by Congress to eliminate Medicare and Medicaid abuses that increase program costs. The law was written, and has been interpreted by courts and administrative bodies, to have broad application to many healthcare business activities. Courts have held, for example, that a violation of the law occurs if any portion of a payment to a physician is intended to induce referrals, regardless of whether the physician is also providing professional services in exchange for the payment. The Internal Revenue Service has also stated that an organization's tax-exempt status may be jeopardized if the facility violates the provisions of the antikickback law.

The application of the antikickback statute can be illustrated by the facts of several well-known prosecutions under the statute. The 1985 case of *U.S. v. Greber*[26] involved an osteopathic physician (Dr. Greber) who was the founder and president of Cardiomed, a company that provided cardiac diagnostic services, including Holter monitors that were used to collect data on cardiovascular activities. As part of its normal routine, Cardiomed processed data collected on the Holter monitors, billed Medicare for the diagnostic services, and forwarded a portion of the reimbursement it received from Medicare to the referring physician as an interpretation fee. Prior to giving the data to the referring physicians, Dr. Greber actually evaluated the information collected.

The court convicted Dr. Greber for violating the antikickback statute and found that Cardiomed's payment of "interpretation fees" to the referring physicians was, in fact, the payment of remuneration prohibited under the antikickback law. The court held broadly that if even one purpose of the fee is to induce referrals, then a violation of the antikickback statute occurs, notwithstanding the surrounding clinical circumstances.

Another seminal antikickback statute case was the 1989 case of *U.S. v. Bay State Ambulance Company*,[27] which involved a hospital administrator (Mr. Felsi) who was a member of a committee with responsibility to award an ambulance service contract. The facts revealed that Mr. Felsi developed a close relationship with an ambulance company (Bay State) over the years, and had traveled to out-of-state conferences, and received new cars, money, and other benefits from Bay State. Following his participation in the ambulance service bid review process, Bay State received the contract. Mr. Felsi was convicted of violating the antikickback statute because he received remuneration in exchange for referrals of healthcare business reimbursed under the Medicare program.

A third illustrative antikickback statute prosecution, *Hanlester Network v. Shalala*,[28] involved several limited partnerships in a clinical laboratory including various physicians. The labs were managed by an outside management company, which was paid under a preset compensation formula. The U.S. Department of Health and Human Services (DHHS) Office of Inspector General challenged the arrangement and sought to exclude the labs from Medicare participation for allegedly violating the antikickback law by offering and paying prohibited remuneration to the physician investors to induce their referrals to the labs, and on other grounds.

After extensive review and appeal, the highly publicized case came before the U.S. Court of Appeals for the Ninth Circuit for review. The court in the Hanlester Network decision concluded that the antikickback statute requirement of "knowing and willful" solicitation or receipt of remuneration means that an individual does not violate the law unless he or she: (1) knows the law prohibits certain conduct, and (2) engages in the conduct with the specific intent of violating the statute. This is a much narrower interpretation of the law than the courts reached in the earlier Greber or Bay State cases, and it has been criticized as too lenient by some law enforcement officials.

The Hanlester Network case involved facts widely different from those involved in either Greber or Bay State, each of which involve naked agreements or payments made by a person seeking referrals to a person in a position to make them. The Hanlester Network decision involves a more complex factual situation that does not as clearly illustrate the scope of the antikickback statute. It does, however, provide an additional indicator of the manner in which the antikickback statute can potentially enmesh joint ventures involving healthcare providers.

In both the Greber and Bay State cases, the courts held that illegal remuneration—money, cars, or other items of value—were conveyed in exchange for referrals that were paid for under Medicare or state healthcare programs.[e]

---

e. Information is provided on Bay State, Greber, and the Hanlester Network enforcement actions to illustrate the types of fact patterns that can result in challenges on antikickback statute grounds. Numerous other enforcement actions are documented, each with its own unique fact patterns. See, e.g., *United States v. Starks*, 157 F. 3rd 833 (11th Cir. 1998); *United States ex rel. Drakeford v. Toumey, d/b/a Toumey Healthcare System*, No 3:05-CV-02858-MJP (D.S.C., Mar. 29, 2010), jury verdict March 29, 2010. Alleged violations of the antikickback statute and other antifraud provisions are also addressed in enforcement actions that do not go to trial, or are not reported in appellate court decisions, but that result in the provider organization (medical group, hospital, etc.) becoming subject to a corporate integrity agreement or similar form of governmental oversight.

It is important to note that the antikickback statute itself applies not only to remuneration intended to induce referrals, but also to any payments intended to induce the lease, purchase, ordering, or arranging for any good, service, or item paid for by the Medicare or Medicaid programs. Accordingly, the law has wide possible application in healthcare delivery and related activities, including many relationships that are created and maintained by medical practices and physicians in their normal day-to-day business activities.

Safe Harbor Regulations

Because of the antikickback statute's potential breadth, the law has possible application to a broad range of relatively common commercial activities in healthcare. Thus, in 1991, the DHHS Office of Inspector General promulgated "safe harbor" regulations intended to clarify the legal status of several healthcare business relationships and ventures that may be relatively innocuous or even beneficial in nature, but that might technically fall within the scope of the antikickback statute's prohibitions.[29] The safe harbor regulations specify a number of business arrangements that are afforded protection or a safe harbor from the antikickback statute's sanctions, and additional safe harbors have been promulgated over time.

Safe harbors have been promulgated for specific transactions or arrangements, including[29]:

- Certain investment interests, including those in publicly traded entities, ambulatory surgical centers, and others
- Arrangements involving the rental of space or equipment
- Personal service and management contracts
- Bona fide employment arrangements
- Transactions involving the sale of physician practices
- Referral services
- Certain transactions involving group purchasing organizations
- Certain activities involving increased coverage, reduced cost-sharing amounts, or reduced premium amounts offered by health plans
- Certain price reductions offered by providers to health plans

The antikickback statute safe harbors tend to contain several common threads that can be applied to business arrangements that may not fall squarely within a particular safe harbor. Those common threads include a requirement that business arrangements be set forth in advance, be documented in writing, and be in existence for at least 1 year. Moreover, the safe harbors indicate a requirement that business transactions not involve payments that are "volume sensitive" or in which compensation varies based on the value of business referred. Also, any payments must be consistent with genuine fair market value and otherwise be commercially reasonable in nature.

Some of the most relevant safe harbors in the medical practice context include the following.

Employment Relationships Safe Harbor. The antikickback statute will not apply to an amount paid by an employer to an employee under a legitimate employment relationship in connection with furnishing any item or service paid for under the Medicare or Medicaid programs. More precisely, under the employment safe harbor, remuneration does *not* include any amount paid by an employer to an employee, who has a bona fide employment relationship with the employer, for employment in the furnishing of any item or service for which payment may be made in whole or in part under a government healthcare program.[30] The term "employee" under the safe harbor has the same meaning as it does for purposes of 26 U.S.C. § 3121(d)(2) (any individual who, under the usual common law rules applicable in determining the employer–employee relationship, has the status of an employee). The employment safe harbor does not, by its terms, impose an explicit requirement that the compensation earned must be consistent with fair market value (FMV) or that the parties enter into a written employment agreement.

Personal Service and Management Contracts Safe Harbor. In general, such contracts could apply to a variety of arrangements such as management agreements, medical directorships, or other payments from a principal to his or her agent for services.[31] The arrangement must be in a written document that specifies the services and is signed by the parties, have a minimum 1-year term, and include compensation equal to the fair market value set in an arm's-length negotiation. In addition, the safe harbor contains the requirement that the purpose of the agreement may not be to counsel or promote a business arrangement or other activity in violation of any law. Special provisions also apply if the services are to be provided on a periodic, sporadic, or part-time basis.

Space Rental Safe Harbor. Lease arrangements for the use of space (such as office space) will be acceptable so long as: (1) the arrangement is set out in writing and executed by the parties; (2) the lease specifies the premises covered; (3) if other than on a full-time basis, the lease specifies the intervals and rent for such periods; (4) the term is for not less than 1 year; and (5) the aggregate rental charge is set in advance, is consistent with fair-market value in an arm's-length transaction, and is not determined in a manner that considers the value or amount of referrals or business between the parties.[32] These various structural requirements also tend to be found in other comparable safe harbors involving other business transactions.

Although the safe harbors under the antikickback statute have elements that are frequently the same as or similar to the requirements applicable to exceptions under the Stark law, compliance with the two laws must be assessed separately. Moreover, to comply with a Stark law exception, strict and complete compliance with every element of the exception is required. In contrast, although compliance with an antikickback safe harbor is advised, it is not required, and even partial or substantial (but not full) compliance promotes compliance with the antikickback statute.

Advisory Opinions

The OIG also issues advisory opinions on compliance with the antikickback statute. These advisory opinions are available to the public, but are binding only on the Secretary of the Department of Health and Human Services and the party requesting the opinion. Nonetheless, advisory opinions provide additional guidance on the structure and permissible features of financial arrangements involved in quality-based compensation relationships.

False Claims Act

The U.S. Civil False Claims Act (FCA) prohibits false claims from being submitted to the U.S. government. Under the FCA, any person who knowingly presents a false claim to the U.S. government, or otherwise engages in certain activities with the intent to defraud the government, is liable for civil penalties, plus three times the amount of damages incurred, unless certain exceptions apply. When the FCA is used in the context of healthcare claims, this means that civil money penalties can potentially be imposed for each item on the healthcare claim form, plus a penalty equal to three times the amount of improper charges. Needless to say, under the FCA the money penalties in what would appear to be a relatively small case can quickly turn into a massive financial judgment. Moreover, because the FCA involves a civil, as opposed to criminal, action, the U.S. government has a lesser burden of proof than that required in a criminal prosecution, thus making a verdict in favor of the government more likely. This lesser burden of proof, combined with the potentially massive awards, has resulted in an increasing number of FCA prosecutions.

Although the FCA has been in existence for many years, there has been increased application of the act in the context of healthcare, combined with certain unique whistleblower provisions in the statute, raising the importance of the FCA to healthcare providers, including medical practices, hospitals, and others. The FCA expressly provides that, in addition to the U.S. government, private parties may bring civil actions for violations of the act. Such private prosecutions are typically called "qui tam" actions. The FCA's qui tam provisions are designed to encourage whistleblower actions in helping to ferret out fraudulent activities that affect governmental programs. Under the FCA's qui tam provisions, the private party who brings the action (or assists the government in bringing the action) stands to gain from any money judgment and recovery. Qui tam plaintiffs can receive, under certain circumstances, up to 30% of the award of civil money damages and penalties in a successful suit. Thus, the qui tam provisions serve as a potent incentive to self-interested insiders and others who have knowledge of activities that might be in violation of the FCA.

The qui tam provisions of the FCA have historically been used by private individuals in connection with healthcare fraud. Under the FCA and the qui tam actions, private parties and/or the government can bring suit against medical practices, physicians, other healthcare providers, and organizations such as suppliers, alleging fraud in their practices. However, in addition to these past applications, whistleblowers have brought qui tam suits under other federal laws, including the antikickback statute and Stark laws.

By illustration, under such suits, the qui tam plaintiff typically asserts that physicians or other providers referred patients to companies that have offered remuneration to the physicians in exchange for referrals—activities that would be in violation of the antikickback statute. In effect, the position is that a violation of the antikickback statute constitutes fraud against the United States, and as such, is a false claim subject to the FCA. Similar allegations are commonly brought based on alleged violations of the Stark law. Under this legal theory, alleged violations of the antikickback, Stark, and other laws are "boot-strapped" into FCA violations, and as such allow for qui tam actions that are rooted in violations of the antikickback, Stark, and other laws. Qui tam actions may thus be brought under a host of antifraud laws, with the practical effect being to expand the risk of healthcare liability under the FCA and the fraud and abuse laws more generally.

Civil Monetary Penalty Statute

The Medicare Civil Monetary Penalty (CMP) statute is also potentially implicated in any number of healthcare business transactions in the emerging system of accountable care healthcare delivery and financing. The CMP law prohibits a hospital from knowingly making a payment, directly or indirectly, to a physician as an inducement for the physician to reduce or limit items or services furnished to Medicare or Medicaid beneficiaries under the physician's direct care. It also prohibits a physician from knowingly accepting such payment.[33]

The CMP law is potentially implicated in any number of existing and emerging relationships involving physicians. These include so-called "gainshare" arrangements in which hospitals seek to enlist physicians in managing hospital costs for certain high-cost items, including devices and supplies, and then seek to share a portion of the cost savings with the physicians as part of such arrangements. Gainshare arrangements were generally proposed in the late 1990s, and initially rejected in a number of advisory opinions on CMP grounds. New versions of gainshare programs were subsequently developed and have been approved, provided that such programs incorporate a number of important safeguards to promote compliance with the CMP and other statutes. As hospitals and physicians establish closer business relationships under systems of accountable care, the CMP law is also potentially implicated in any number of compensation relationships, including arrangements in which hospitals seek to pay physicians to assist with quality, cost, or other goals. More precisely, the law will potentially be implicated for a particular compensation incentive payment if the payment could induce physicians to reduce or limit items or services furnished to Medicare and Medicaid patients.

The fraud and abuse provisions referenced in the previous sections are sufficiently expansive that they have potential application to a wide range of healthcare business relationships involving physicians and medical practices in a variety of contemporary settings. The interplay of multiple laws directed at fraud and abuse can be illustrated in a recent enforcement action. The case of *Toumey Healthcare System*[34] involved allegations of improper conduct and violations of the Stark law and the FCA. In the Toumey case, Toumey Hospital entered into part-time physician employment contracts with 18 physicians for the purpose of practicing medicine and providing services at the hospital's outpatient surgical center. A qui tam action was brought against Toumey Hospital by a physician in the community who declined to enter into a part-time employment contract. The government intervened in the qui tam matter and alleged violations of the Stark law and FCA, but it did not allege violations of the antikickback statute.

In the Toumey case, the government alleged that the compensation arrangements did not meet the Stark law's exception for employment arrangements because the compensation paid exceeded fair market value, the contracts were not "commercially reasonable," and the agreements and compensation took into account referrals and other business between the hospital and physicians. The government also took the position that by submitting claims to the Medicare program for services that were referred by the physicians under arrangements that did not meet an exception to the Stark law, the hospital also violated the FCA. The case went to a jury trial, and the jury found that although there was no violation of the FCA, the compensation arrangements with the part-time physicians did not comply with a Stark law exception and therefore violated the Stark law, resulting in a $44.9 million damage award by the court.

Toumey and other cases, including those that do not result in written decisions but that frequently result in corporate integrity agreements and similar forms of governmental oversight relating to fraud and abuse violations, illustrate the importance of these antifraud laws to healthcare business activities, including those of medical groups and physicians. Each of these laws, and others, including those set forth in state antifraud statutory schemes, must be considered in connection with the operation of medical group practices, and in connection with the creation of financial and other relationships involving physicians and their medical practices operating today. In addition to the laws governing healthcare fraud and abuse, other laws with more general application, including federal and state laws governing antitrust, have potential implications for healthcare business operations and relationships in today's changing delivery system.

Antitrust Laws

Federal and state antitrust laws are designed to promote a vigorous competitive environment on the theory that free market competition will produce new products and services, lower prices, and other efficiencies.[f] Antitrust laws protect competition, not competitors. Accordingly, although individual competitors may have concerns with the "fairness" of particular activities, the primary antitrust question will be whether the activities have a negative impact on competition, to the public's presumed detriment. Two primary antitrust-related questions arise in the context of medical group formation and operations.

Market Power

Antitrust laws are generally concerned with whether a medical group or other entity is so large and powerful in

---

f. See, for example, 15 U.S.C. §§ 1, 2 (Sherman Act § 1, 2); 15 U.S.C. § 18 (Clayton Act § 7) and 15 U.S.C. § 45 (Federal Trade Commission Act § 5).

the relevant market that it will be able to dictate prices or otherwise act in an anticompetitive manner. These types of market power concerns require close attention to the existence of "substitutes" in the particular product and geographic markets. More precisely, the question is whether a third party (e.g., a third-party payer of healthcare services) will have substitutes from whom it may obtain products or services in the event that the medical group or other organization under question seeks to raise prices or refuses to deal with the purchaser.

The existence of market power essentially hinges on two threshold definitions related to: (1) the relevant product or service, and (2) the relevant geographic market for the particular product or service. Other variables, such as the ease of market entry, the presence of regulatory or other barriers to entry, and the relative availability of substitute providers, may also be important factors in assessing a medical group's or other organization's market power. An organization's business practices will often be subject to heightened legal scrutiny if market power is found to exist.

Joint Action

Antitrust laws also are concerned with ensuring that ventures are sufficiently "integrated" to promote rather than impair the competitive process. Section 1 of the Sherman Antitrust Act prohibits contracts, combinations, and conspiracies "in restraint of trade"; in doing so, the law prohibits price fixing, concerted refusals to deal, and similar forms of joint action by individual competitors within the healthcare industry. This means, for example, that agreements by physicians, medical practices, or groups that are not adequately integrated financially or clinically can be deemed illegal per se under the antitrust laws. A classic example of such improper behavior involves the seminal case of *Arizona v. Maricopa County Medical Society*,[35] in which agreements regarding the prices that physicians would charge third-party payers were facilitated by a local medical society, and were condemned as illegal because the physicians were not integrated in any adequate manner.

Joint action concerns can be mitigated by achieving financial and/or clinical integration. When such integration is achieved, antitrust law evaluates otherwise forbidden collective provider behavior under the antitrust "rule of reason," which may permit quality, cost, and related efficiencies to offset otherwise problematic joint behavior by competitors. Financial integration consists of true financial risk sharing through which the parties share opportunities for profit and risk of financial loss. Financial risk sharing can be provided in medical groups or other

settings through the use of a single legal entity coupled with business integration and shared risk. Where a medical group involves multiple legal entities (i.e., network medical groups), financial integrations can be achieved through contracts with third-party payers involving partial and full capitation, and other payment methods that are negotiated and administered by the network itself. Thus, arrangements involving financial integration can be achieved through a joint venture entity such as an IPA, or, more commonly, a group practice legal entity through which participating physicians and other providers bill and collect for professional services and from which they are compensated.

Importantly, physicians and medical practices can also become clinically integrated for antitrust compliance purposes by investing sufficient human and other capital into systems, processes, and activities that actively focus on clinical care delivery in order to improve quality and/ or reduce the cost of care. Clinical integration represents a relatively new means of achieving antitrust compliance for medical groups and other healthcare organizations, and only recently has substantial guidance been provided by the government to clarify how clinical integration can be achieved successfully from practical and operational perspectives.

Recent advisory opinions of the Federal Trade Commission (FTC) in the matters of Tri-State Health Partners[36] in Maryland and the Greater Rochester Independent Practice Association[37] (GRIPA) now provide useful guidance illustrating how otherwise separate providers in a community can organize themselves to deliver services in a clinically integrated manner, without undertaking true structural integration through a combination or merger of otherwise separate practices. Although every provider community will involve its own facts and circumstances, other keys to achieving clinical integration will likely include the delivery of care in a coordinated, interdependent manner, often emphasizing principles of evidence-based medicine; data collection and benchmarking involving participants in the venture; and an overall commitment by physicians to verifiably improved patient outcomes.

In assessing antitrust variables, it should be emphasized that the law focuses attention on substance as well as form. Legal precedent has historically established that a single organization cannot "conspire with itself" (i.e., a single legal entity that is structurally, economically, and otherwise truly integrated cannot engage in prohibited joint action). However, merely creating a single legal platform for a medical group without acting and operating in an integrated manner, whether financially, clinically, or both, may not be sufficient to pass antitrust muster. For example, in the matter of Surgical Specialists of Yakima, PLLC,[38] the U.S. Federal Trade Commission concluded that despite the existence of structural integration in the form of a medical group composed of a single legal entity, the Yakama surgical group was not sufficiently integrated in its actual operations to be protected against charges of violating the antitrust laws. Thus, form will not trump true substance concerning combinations or mergers of previously separate medical practices.

Antitrust Safety Zones

Because of the impact of the antitrust laws on health-care business activities, the principle federal agencies responsible for enforcement of federal antitrust laws—the U.S. Department of Justice (DOJ) and the FTC—jointly issued six statements of antitrust enforcement policies in the healthcare area. The policy statements addressed a variety of healthcare-related transactions including hospital mergers, hospital joint ventures involving high-technology or other expensive medical equipment, physicians' provision of information to purchasers of healthcare services, hospital participation in exchanges of price and cost information, joint purchasing arrangements involving healthcare providers, and physician network joint ventures. The policy statements were designed to provide guidance to the healthcare community, and to address perceived uncertainty concerning the enforcement agencies' policies and the potential negative impact that enforcement policy had on pro-competitive mergers, joint ventures, or other activities that could lower healthcare costs.

The original safety zones were issued in 1993 and subsequently revised and expanded in 1994 to add policy statements[39] addressing hospital joint ventures involving specialized clinical or other expensive healthcare services, providers' collective provision of fee-related information to purchasers of healthcare services, and analytical principles relating to a broad range of healthcare provider networks (i.e., IPAs, PHOs, and other multiprovider networks), and to expand the several other statements and safety zones. The enforcement agencies have periodically revised some or all of the statements based on their additional experience and ongoing changes in the healthcare field, with recent revisions focusing on the enforcement policy statement on physician network joint ventures and the multiprovider networks.

The safety zones generally present the DOJ's and FTC's approach to the analysis of all types of healthcare provider networks under general antitrust principles, including those dealing with market concentration or power, and

integration as discussed earlier. The safety zones set forth a set of principles, combined with illustrations, with the goal being to help provide structure and guide decision making by participants in the healthcare delivery system. Akin to the aforementioned regulatory safe harbor regulations under the antikickback statute, the antitrust safety zones describe conduct that the federal enforcement agencies will generally not challenge under the antitrust laws. Also, akin to the antikickback safe harbors, although the antitrust safety zones describe facts and circumstances that generally will not be challenged absent extraordinary circumstances, this does not mean that conduct falling outside the safety zones is likely to be challenged by the agencies. To the contrary, given that antitrust analysis is, by its nature, fact-dependent, it is entirely possible that conduct or facts that are outside of the safety zone will not also be subject to antitrust scrutiny.

For example, the statement governing physician network joint ventures addresses physician-controlled ventures in which the network's physician participants collectively agree on prices or price-related terms and jointly market their services. The statement sets forth the enforcement agencies' approach to the analysis of such physician network joint ventures, as well as safety zones that describe physician network joint ventures that agencies deem unlikely to raise competitive concerns. As noted, a physician network joint venture's failure to fall within the safety zone does not mean the joint venture is unlawful under the antitrust laws, but merely that the network will not receive the benefits of safety zone compliance, and may therefore require a closer review of the applicable facts.

The safety zone for physician network joint ventures distinguishes between ventures that are exclusive (e.g., the network's physicians are restricted in their ability to contract or affiliate with other network joint ventures or health plans) and those that are nonexclusive (e.g., the network's physician participants are permitted to independently affiliate with other network health plans). As a general matter, in the case of joint ventures that are exclusive in nature, the enforcement agencies will generally not challenge an exclusive physician network joint venture whose physician participants share substantial financial risk and comprise 20% or less of the physicians in each practice specialty in the relevant geographic market.

The safety zone for nonexclusive network joint ventures is similar in that it requires a sharing of substantial financial risk, and permits up to 30% or less of the physicians in each physician specialty who practice in the relevant geographic market. Issues of exclusivity or nonexclusivity are evaluated based on the facts in the particular marketplace, as opposed to merely reviewing contractual arrangements. As a result, factors beyond the underlying contracts, such as the actual existence of competing networks in the area, and actual actions by physicians to contract and earn revenues outside of the network arrangements, are considered in evaluating exclusivity. The safety zones also describe and provide examples of financial risk-sharing activities.

The antitrust policy statements and safety zones provide useful guidance to physicians, medical practices, and their advisors with respect to federal antitrust enforcement policy. As such, the policy statements can assist participants in the healthcare delivery system in evaluating potential activities to assess antitrust risk. In overall terms, the antitrust laws require attention to various activities and arrangements that could be detrimental to competition, including the operation of medical groups that are so large and powerful that they can stifle competition, and the combination of otherwise separate medical practices in a manner that is not sufficiently integrated. Each analysis is, and must be, undertaken in light of specific "facts on the ground" in a local community. However, in general, where there are few, if any, substitute providers and/or integration (financial, clinical, or both) is weak, then close consideration of the rationale for the combination is in order. Conversely, where the medical groups collectively comprise a mere subset of the provider population in the relevant markets, and they are truly engaging in financial risk sharing, investing human and other capital to change clinical care, or both, then the venture is more likely to be deemed pro-competitive and appropriate, if challenged, from an antitrust perspective.

Antitrust concerns also can arise where other restrictions on competition are imposed, including some exclusivity requirements, improper information exchanges of price or wage data, and other allegedly anti-competitive arrangements. Potential antitrust concerns may also arise in connection with the enforceability of noncompete covenants in contractual arrangements and otherwise in connection with other actions and/or restrictions that have a potential impact on the competitive marketplace.

Tax-Exempt Organization Concerns

Many healthcare organizations such as large medical group practices, faculty practice plans, hospitals, medical foundations, and community clinics enjoy an exemption from federal income taxation pursuant to § 501(c)(3) of the Internal Revenue Code (IRC). Tax-exempt status confers a number of benefits on organizations, including the ability to use tax-exempt bonds as a beneficial means of financing, the treatment of contributions made to the organization as deductible to the contributing party, and others.

To obtain and retain their tax-exempt status, § 501(c)(3) tax-exempt organizations must engage exclusively in charitable and other exempt activities, and must comply with a number of other requirements. Section 501(c)(3) of the IRC defined certain types of organizations that may be granted tax-exempt status. Among other things, the law limits the award of exempt status to:

> Corporations . . . , organized and operated *exclusively* for religious, charitable, . . . or educational purposes, . . . no part of the net earnings of which inures to the benefit of any private shareholder or individual. . . . [emphasis added]

It should also be noted that the granting of tax-exempt status by the IRS is often distinct from the separate state-law process of incorporation as a nonprofit corporation. It is entirely possible, and sometimes desirable, to charter a business entity as a nonprofit but fully taxable organization. Moreover, the receipt of exemption from federal taxation does not automatically confer exemption from state tax laws.

IRS § 501(c)(3) states that tax-exempt organizations must be organized and operated for charitable and other exempt purposes. In the healthcare arena, hospitals are the most common form of tax-exempt healthcare enterprise, although other organizations such as community clinics, faculty practice plans, and others may also be eligible and receive an exemption. In almost every case, such organizations derive their tax-exempt status because they are deemed to be engaged in charitable activities of benefit to the community as defined by the law governing charities.

Indications of charitable purposes of hospitals meeting this "community benefit" standard include that (1) the organization has a governing board broadly representative of the community as opposed to "merely" the interests of physicians, administrators, or others with private interests; (2) the hospital has a medical staff open to all qualified physicians in the area; (3) the hospital operates an emergency room open to all people without regard to ability to pay; and (4) the hospital provides nonemergency care for persons in the community able to pay the cost of such care, either through private insurance, through public programs such as Medicare and Medicaid, or otherwise. Variations of these same concepts apply to other organizations that are tax-exempt and participate in the healthcare delivery system.

Private Inurement and Private Benefit

Tax-exempt organizations must also comply with the so-called prohibitions on private inurement and private benefit to obtain and retain their exemption from taxation. In general, the private inurement prohibition requires that the exempt organization ensure that no part of the organization's net earnings inure, in whole or in part, to the benefit of private shareholders or individuals.

Private shareholders and individuals are generally defined to include those "insiders" who have professional or private interests in the activities of the organization, as opposed to members of the public or the charitable organization's other intended beneficiaries. There is no de minimis exception in connection with a finding of prohibited private inurement; even the slightest amount of prohibited inurement is sufficient to violate the rules underlying tax-exempt status.

In the context of healthcare organizations, for example, private individuals or insiders of a hospital or other healthcare-affiliated organization would typically include physicians and others on the organization's staff. The generic terms and the prohibitions on private inurement are intended to prevent insiders from siphoning off the organization's charitable income or assets for their own use.

Overall, any transaction between a tax-exempt organization and a private individual in which the individual appears to receive a disproportionate share of the benefits in the exchange relative to the charity or exempt activity served may present an inurement issue. Common transactions in which such issues may arise include compensation arrangements, sales or exchanges of property, commissions, rental arrangements, gifts, and contracts to provide goods or services to the exempt organization. As a general guideline, the IRS has historically tended to conclude that if a transaction is consistent with ordinary business practices in similar circumstances, then prohibited inurement will likely not be present. On the other hand, to the extent that the transaction departs from what is otherwise "commercially reasonable," prohibited inurement may be found.

The concomitant restriction on private benefit shares common elements with the prohibition on private inurement, but must be addressed independently. Under the private benefit prohibition, any benefit conferred on private individuals must be merely incidental to the overall public benefit. To comply with this requirement, the benefit must be both qualitatively and quantitatively incidental. For example, a tax-exempt hospital effectively confers private benefits on certain physicians as individuals, because the hospital permits physicians to use the hospital's facilities. This is generally acceptable, however, because the hospital could not further its own charitable purposes of providing healthcare to the community without allowing physicians to use the hospital's facilities in support of their medical practices and the delivery of patient care, so the private benefit conferred is viewed as qualitatively incidental.

For private benefit to be quantitatively incidental, the benefit conferred by the activity must be insubstantial in relation to the overall public benefit of the particular activity. In essence, this means that the benefit received by the public from having a hospital facility greatly exceeds the relatively insubstantial or small benefit that is conferred to physicians and other private parties by having such a facility.

The prohibitions on private inurement and private benefit do not represent insurmountable barriers to a tax-exempt healthcare organization's reasonable participation in healthcare-related joint ventures and cooperative activities involving hospitals and physicians. As with compliance with the antikickback and Stark prohibitions, a key requirement is that such involvement must be in a "commercially reasonable" fashion (i.e., the exempt entity participates on terms that are generally consistent with those that would be offered to the venture by outside, non-tax-exempt or conventional organizations).

As a practical matter, the apparent similarities between the restrictions imposed by an organization's tax-exempt status and those of the antikickback prohibitions are not simply coincidental. In a significant informal regulatory pronouncement known as the Thornton letter, the potential linkage between the two prohibitions was made clear. The Thornton letter was a 1992 letter from the then-chief fraud and abuse law enforcement official in the Inspector General's Office in the Department of Health and Human Services, D. McCarthy Thornton, to T.J. Sullivan, the then-head of the IRS Exempt Organization Branch, the division responsible for oversight of tax-exempt enterprises such as hospitals. In that letter, Mr. Thornton expressed concern about the potential antikickback law implications of hospital purchases of physician medical practices, suggesting in general that if the payment for a practice exceeds an objective determination of the fair market value, "it can be inferred that the excess amount paid over the fair market value is intended as payment for the referral of Medicare/Medicaid program-related business."[40]

The linkage between the antikickback and private inurement/private benefit prohibitions is underscored in the body of other available IRS materials, such as those commenting on the tax-exempt status of medical foundations, integrated delivery systems, or other provider organizations, as well as those dealing with physician–hospital joint ventures. Although such regulatory communication may conclude overall that the enterprise will be granted tax-exempt status, the maintenance of such tax-exempt organization status has been expressly conditioned on the organization's compliance with the antikickback statute.

Intermediate Sanctions Law

In addition to the general prohibitions related to private inurement and private benefit that apply to tax-exempt healthcare organizations, Section 4958 of the Internal Revenue Code, commonly known as the "intermediate sanctions" law, allows the Internal Revenue Service (IRS) to impose sanctions on certain persons who receive or approve excessive economic benefits from tax-exempt organizations. The law was enacted to provide the IRS with sanctions short of revoking the tax-exempt status of an organization itself, but instead to permit the IRS to impose "excise taxes" on the individuals involved in the prohibited excess benefit transactions. Section 4958 provides for the imposition of personal excise taxes on disqualified persons who benefit from excess benefit transactions, as well as taxes on the organization managers who approve such excess benefit transactions under certain circumstances.

In general, an excess benefit transaction occurs when an exempt organization provides an economic benefit to a disqualified person, and the organization receives less than the value of the benefit from the disqualified person in return. Transactions that are reasonable and consistent with FMV will not constitute excess benefit transactions. Common excess benefit transactions include the payment of compensation for services that is in excess of FMV. However, other transactions can involve exchanges of property such as rent or loan arrangements between an exempt organization and a disqualified person that involve terms that are not consistent with FMV.

Disqualified persons who are involved in an excess benefit transaction may be subject to personal excise taxes at two levels. One level of tax may be imposed on the difference between the amount received and FMV of the value actually provided. A second personal excise tax may be imposed in the event that the excess benefit transaction is not repaid or "corrected." Importantly, the law also allows for the imposition of a tax on organizational managers who knowingly approve an excess benefit transaction under certain circumstances.

Notably, not every physician will be classified as a disqualified person under the law, because the law generally only classifies disqualified persons as those who are in a position of leadership or significant influence in the tax-exempt organization. Nonetheless, the combination of the general requirements applicable to tax-exempt organizations related to private inurement and private benefit and the requirements of the intermediate sanctions law tends to increase the compliance focus of exempt-organization leadership on ensuring all business relationships with physicians, other healthcare professionals, and their organizations are on FMV, commercially reasonable terms.

Other Issues Related to Tax-Exempt Status

A variety of other rules apply to the operation of tax-exempt organizations in addition to those listed in the previous sections, many of which will have implications for medical practice business arrangements. By illustration, where tax-exempt bonds are used to finance property used in connection with healthcare operations (e.g., hospital construction), rules governing the private use of the bond-financed property apply. Under Revenue Procedure 97-13, the tax-exempt organization must ensure that arrangements with third parties (e.g., physicians, medical practices, or others who are themselves not tax-exempt) do not result in prohibited private use of the property in a manner that could negatively affect the exempt status of the tax-exempt bonds or, in some instances, impact the organization's tax-exempt status. In light of these concerns, tax-exempt hospitals and other organizations generally have arrangements in place to ensure compliance with various "safe harbor" arrangements described in Revenue Procedure 97-13 (as modified by Revenue Procedure 2001-39).

Similarly, tax-exempt law also affects the structure and operating format of joint venture arrangements involving tax-exempt hospitals and similar organizations, including in connection with the formation of network organizations (e.g., PHOs, ACOs, etc.) or other provider enterprises (e.g., joint venture ambulatory surgical centers). In particular, the *St. David's Health Care System v. U.S. case*[41] applied other tax guidance[42] to hold that when a tax-exempt organization is a participant in a nonexempt joint venture, then the tax-exempt organization must maintain sufficient control over the joint venture to ensure that the joint venture works in furtherance of the tax-exempt organization's charitable purposes. This guidance has implications for the participation of tax-exempt hospitals, clinics, and other organizations in joint venture enterprises, and in the overall governance structure of the joint venture organization (including with respect to voting rights, quorum, reserve powers, and similar mechanisms), as well as operational processes and practices that permit the tax-exempt organization to promote and protect its charitable mission.

Overall, where a medical practice is itself operated through a tax-exempt organization (as is commonly the case in hospital-affiliated medical practice organizations, including those in academic medical centers and other hospital-affiliated organizations), or where a physician or medical practice is creating business relationships with a tax-exempt enterprise, a range of legal issues including those referenced earlier will be potentially implicated and need to be addressed.

State Insurance Laws

The insurance laws of all 50 states impose certain requirements on organizations engaged in various aspects of the business of insurance. The laws are intended, in part, to provide a certain minimal level of protection to those who contract with insurance companies. These state insurance laws typically require, for example, (1) the maintenance of financial reserves to provide protection against insolvency, and (2) contracts that contain certain statutorily defined terms and include certain key information. State insurance laws typically impose specific requirements on commercial insurance companies and other organizations that participate in the delivery and/or financing in the state, in particular where the organization is deemed to assume actuarial risk.

State insurance laws may apply to the activities of medical groups and provider organizations under a number of different theories. These include that: (1) the organization is engaged in the business of insurance and, therefore, must comply with laws governing insurance companies; (2) it must be licensed as an insurance company, health maintenance organization, or similar enterprise due to the types of business activities in which it engages (e.g., acceptance of capitated reimbursement); or (3) because there is a contractual or other relationship between a licensed organization such as an indemnity insurer and a medical group or other provider organization, it should be subjected to regulatory scrutiny to protect the public interest from a consumer protection perspective.

Insurance laws are embedded in state statutory schemes and are enforced by state administrative agencies. Therefore, just as there are 50 different bodies of insurance law, there are also many different interpretations of what constitutes the "business of insurance" for insurance regulation purposes, effectively leaving the actual determination to the courts for decision. Courts have historically evaluated the existence of several different features

in an organization's business activities before finding the enterprise to be engaging in the business of insurance, so as to subject the organization to state insurance laws. Key criteria used to ascertain whether an arrangement constitutes the business of insurance and the establishment of an insurance contract include the existence of an insurable interest combined with a risk of loss, the assumption of risk of loss by another party, the spreading and payment of a premium for the assumption of the loss, and other factors.

The U.S. Supreme Court has examined the question of what constitutes insurance in the context of healthcare-related provider agreements. In its 1979 decision in *Group Life and Health Insurance Co. v. Royal Drug*,[43] the Court identified three key criteria deemed relevant to decide whether a practice constitutes the business of insurance, so as to be exempted in that context from the reach of antitrust laws under the McCarran-Ferguson Act exemption.[44] In general, the McCarran-Ferguson Act exempts the business of insurance from various forms of federal legislations including aspects of federal antitrust low to a limited extent. Those criteria are:

1. Whether the practice has the effect of transferring or spreading policyholders' risk
2. Whether the practice is an integral part of the policy relationship between the insurer and insured
3. Whether the practice is limited to entities in the insurance industry

The Court held that certain pharmacy provider agreements did not constitute or involve the underwriting or spreading of risk. Rather, the agreements were characterized as involving merely the purchase of goods and services, not the business of insurance, and the arrangement was deemed subject to antitrust scrutiny in the absence of the statutory exemption.

It is often thought unlawful under the insurance and HMO laws of many states for an entity (including a medical group, physician, hospital, or other provider organization) to accept actuarial risk without being licensed as an appropriately regulated insurance entity, HMO, or similar enterprise. Regulators in various states have differing views regarding whether the acceptance of capitated payments under different circumstances constitutes the acceptance of actuarial risk. Some regulators view such activities as involving acceptance of risk because they obligate the entity to provide all of the required services in exchange for a fixed monthly payment. State insurance laws tend to be relevant to provider organizations such as medical groups, IPAs, PHOs, and others (to potentially include accountable care organizations) because the provider organization may be viewed in the eyes of state insurance regulators as offering to provide programs or benefits that may be deemed to involve the business of insurance under state law.

State insurance laws directed at risk-bearing provider organizations tend to emphasize consumer protection by regulating benefit schemes, the comprehensiveness of the provider organization's benefit package, and limiting copayment and deductibles obligations. The laws also tend to focus on the financial solvency and stability of the enterprise by imposing periodic financial reporting and examination requirements, along with financial reserve and deposit requirements. From the perspective of individual and institutional healthcare providers who are forming organizations to participate in an accountable care environment, the existence of licensing requirements that impose net worth and other obligations can stand as a significant regulatory hurdle to the development of the enterprise.

■ Illustration of Application of Legal Issues to Accountable Care Organizations

In many communities accountable care organizations (ACOs) are being established in order to participate in changing models of healthcare delivery and financing. No two ACOs will be structured or operated in the same manner. Nonetheless, the proposed rule governing ACOs under the Medicare program provides a useful description of the legal and operational characteristics of an ACO enterprise, and a useful example of how various laws and rules, including those governing payment and reimbursement, fraud and abuse, antitrust, and other issues, may be implicated in the design and operation of such organizations. The following reviews many of the major themes of the proposed rule for ACOs published on March 31, 2011 and finalized on November 2, 2011, and illustrates the application of the various laws reviewed prior to ACOs and changing approaches to healthcare financing and delivery that encourage enhanced value through systems of accountable care.

ACOs in General

An ACO refers to a legal entity composed of certain eligible ACO participants that work together to coordinate care for Medicare fee-for-service beneficiaries. Section 3022 of PPACA established numerous eligibility and governance requirements for ACOs; the

rule outlines the parameters for the organization in greater detail.

Under the rule, several groups of providers and provider organizations are eligible to participate in the ACO shared savings program, including (1) ACO professionals (including physicians and other practitioners) in a group practice arrangement; (2) networks of individual practices of ACO professionals; (3) partnerships or joint venture arrangements between hospitals and ACO professionals; and (4) hospitals employing ACO professionals. (In this context, "hospital" is limited to acute care hospitals paid under the inpatient prospective payment system, although critical access hospitals are on the list of eligible ACO entities.) Eligible entities in these categories would be allowed to form ACOs independently or in collaboration with each other.

ACO Legal Entity

Under the rule, an ACO would generally require a separate legal entity structured as a corporation, partnership, LLC, foundation, or any other entity permitted by state law. The legal entity must be capable of receiving and distributing shared savings; repaying shared losses; establishing, reporting, and ensuring ACO compliance with program requirements such as the monitoring and reporting of quality performance; and performing other statutory ACO functions. The ACO entity must have a tax identification number (TIN), and although the ACO entity need not be enrolled in Medicare, each individual participating entity (i.e., the ACO's participating medical groups and other ACO participants) must be enrolled. The rule would permit an existing legal entity that otherwise qualifies as an eligible ACO not to form a new separate entity for purposes of this program, so long as the entity operates the ACO independently; however, if the entity wants to include other providers and suppliers as part of its ACO who are not a part of its existing legal structure, it must establish a separate entity with a separate TIN.

ACO Governance

Within the ACO's legal structure, the rule requires the ACO to demonstrate a shared governance mechanism that provides all ACO participants (even those who are not independently eligible) with proportionate control over the ACO decision-making process. According to the rule, the governing body must have the authority to execute the statutory functions of an ACO (e.g., defining processes to promote evidence-based medicine) and may include a board of directors, board of managers, or any other governing body that allows for shared decision making among all participants. CMS required that ACO participants must have at least 75% control of the ACO's governing board, and that each participant be represented by the governing board members. If the ACO is composed of a self-contained, financially and clinically integrated entity with a pre-existing governing body, no separate governing body is required.

The rule also prescribed criteria related to the ACO's leadership, operations, and systems. Among other requirements, the rule requires ACO operations to be managed by an executive, officer, manager, or general partner who is appointed and may be removed by the governing body. Clinical management within the ACO would be directed by a senior-level medical director who is a board-certified physician, licensed and present in the state in which the ACO operates. The ACO participants, providers, and suppliers would be required to have a meaningful financial or human investment in the ongoing operations of the ACO. The ACO must have a physician-directed committee to oversee the quality assurance and process improvement program, and it is required to develop and implement evidence-based medical practice or clinical guidelines for delivering care, specifically covering diagnoses with significant potential to achieve quality and cost improvements, as well as related infrastructure that allows for the collection and evaluation of ACO data for all providers/suppliers.

Pursuant to a statutory mandate, CMS required that an ACO provide documentation regarding how it would promote evidence-based medicine, including the development and periodic revision of evidence-based guidelines; how it would promote patient engagement; and the processes to be used to report quality and cost measures and care coordination through the use of telehealth, care coordinators, and transition of care programs.

Program Integrity Requirements

To minimize the potential for fraud and abuse, CMS also imposed a series of program integrity measures. Among other things, the rule requires all ACOs to have a compliance plan in place, the ACO must mandate full compliance with the 3-year agreement in all of its ancillary contracts with ACO participants, and it is required to have a conflicts-of-interest policy applicable to all members of the governing body.

Shared Savings Methodology

The rule provides for an initial 3-year agreement period for ACOs participating in the basic shared savings program. Under the shared savings arrangements, the ACO would share in savings on healthcare costs for the ACO's assigned beneficiaries in relation to a benchmark. Under

what CMS called a "one-sided" shared savings model, the ACO would share in savings without being held accountable for repaying any losses if actual expenditures exceed the benchmark. Alternatively, an ACO could participate in a two-sided shared savings model, which would allow the ACO to share in savings *and* be held accountable for repaying any losses if actual expenditures exceed the benchmark. The rule provides that ACOs that elect to enter into the shared savings program under the two-sided model will be eligible for higher sharing rates than are available under the one-sided model.

Coordination with Other Laws and Enforcement Agencies

The formation and operation of ACOs and the activities of medical groups and others in connection with ACOs and shared savings programs has the potential to implicate many of the laws and rules discussed previously in this chapter. Because of this, in conjunction with the proposed rule, the principle federal regulatory agencies with responsibility for administering and enforcing many such laws collaborated to issue additional information regarding how ACOs would be considered under other regulatory schemes. For example, in addition to the final rule issued by CMS, the OIG concurrently issued guidance with respect to the antikickback statute and civil monetary penalties statutes as applied to certain aspects of the formation and operation of ACOs, and the IRS also provided its perspective with respect to the application of tax-exempt organization laws as applied to ACOs and their participants. Likewise, the FTC and Department of Justice antitrust divisions provided perspective with respect to the antitrust-related implications of ACOs and their operation. A brief review of some of the means by which ACOs would potentially implicate these laws, and a review of the compliance-related strategy taken by these agencies, follows.

Stark Law Implications for ACOs

By their very nature, the formation and operation of ACOs would likely create various direct and indirect financial relationships between physicians and other entities that perform and furnish designated health services that are subject to the Stark law's self-referral prohibitions. Each of these financial and referral relationships would therefore require compliance with an applicable exception to the law under a legally appropriate arrangement. For example, in physician–hospital-owned ACO legal entities, each participant is likely to provide funding for the ACO's development and operation. Likewise, the ACO will likely distribute savings that it receives from CMS under the shared savings program. Moreover, individual physicians and others will likely create a number of contractual, service, lease, and potentially other relationships with the ACO and with other ACO participants in connection with the ACO's formation and operation, many of which would implicate the Stark law.

Under an interim final rule also published on November 2, 2011, where an ACO is established that meets the specific requirements set forth in the proposed rule related to ACO structure, operations, oversight, and otherwise, the Secretary of the U.S. Department of Health and Human Services will waive application of the provisions of the Stark law to defined financial arrangements. Specifically, such waivers would apply to distributions of shared savings received by an ACO from CMS under the shared savings program to or among ACO participants during the year in which the shared savings were earned by the ACO. Waivers would also be granted for activities that are reasonably related to the purposes of the shared savings program under a "pre-participation" waiver or a "participation" waiver, both of which relate to the ACO's participation in and operations under the shared savings program. Such waivers would not provide protection for other financial relationships with referring physicians that are outside of the ACO, meaning that all such financial and referral relationships would need to meet an existing exception under the Stark law (e.g., the personal services, indirect compensation, or another applicable exception). Similarly, all other financial relationships (other than distributions of shared savings) involving physicians (or their immediate family members) or entities participating in the shared savings program that implicate the Stark law would need to satisfy an existing exception to the Stark law. Other waivers were also finalized, including one which applies when arrangements fully comply with applicable exceptions to the Stark law and others.

Antikickback Statute

As noted previously, although the Stark and antikickback statutes are similar, compliance is assessed independently. As a result, the same or potentially different arrangements between or among the ACO participants that are discussed with respect to the Stark law could implicate the antikickback statute. By illustration, the creation of a joint venture entity as the legal platform for the ACO organization (e.g., a limited liability company) that is jointly owned by physicians, medical groups, hospitals, and/or others could potentially implicate the antikickback statute, as could the distribution of shared savings amounts that are received by the ACO and distributed to the ACO participants.

In conjunction with the CMS publication of the interim final rule governing ACOs, the Secretary of DHHS also proposed to waive application of the provisions of the antikickback statute with respect to distributions of shared savings received by an ACO from CMS under the shared savings program to or among ACO participants, ACO providers/suppliers, and individuals and entities that were ACO participants or ACO providers/suppliers during the year in which the shared savings were earned by the ACO for activities necessary and directly related to the ACO's participation in and operations under the shared savings program. The pre-participation and participation waivers referenced prior would also apply to permit antikickback statute compliance as would the waiver applicable to financial relationships between or among the ACO, ACO participants, and ACO providers/suppliers necessary for and directly related to the ACO's participation in and operations under the shared savings program that implicates the Stark law and fully complies with an exception to the Stark law.[g] Other financial arrangements outside the ACO would need to fit in a safe harbor or otherwise comply with the antikickback statute. Failure to qualify for one of the waivers under the antikickback statute would not mean that an arrangement is illegal under the antikickback statute. To the extent that the antikickback statute is implicated by a financial arrangement that is not subject to a waiver, the financial arrangement would need to comply with the law itself.

Civil Monetary Penalties Law

The Secretary will also waive application of the Civil Monetary Penalties law provision addressing hospital payments to physicians to reduce or limit services with respect to the following two scenarios:

- Distributions of shared savings received by an ACO from CMS under the shared savings programs where the distributions are made from a hospital to a physician, provided that
  - The payments are not made knowingly to induce the physician to reduce or limit medically necessary items or services

---

g. Ordinarily, compliance with the Stark law does not operate to immunize conduct under the antikickback statute, and arrangements that comply with the Stark law are still subject to scrutiny under the antikickback statute. CMS and the OIG finalized a limited exception to that general rule for those financial relationships between and among the ACO, its ACO participants, and its ACO providers/suppliers that relate closely to the ACO's operations.

- The hospital and physician are ACO participants or ACO providers/suppliers, or were ACO participants or ACO providers/suppliers during the year in which the shared savings were earned by the ACO
- Any financial relationships between or among the ACO, its ACO participants, and its ACO providers/suppliers necessary for and directly related to the ACO's participation in and operations under the shared savings program that implicates the Stark law and fully complies with an exception to the Stark law or one of the other applicable waivers.

Antitrust Policy Statement

In conjunction with the publication of the final rule governing ACOs, the FTC and DOJ issued an antitrust safety zone for ACOs. Under the safety zone, ACOs meeting CMS's eligibility standards under PPACA would be deemed clinically integrated, thereby permitting joint negotiations undertaken by the ACO with private payers to receive some favorable treatment during the ACO's participation in the shared savings program.

The ACO safety zone also addressed other key issues related to potential market power by an ACO by providing information regarding how the FTC and DOJ would look at ACOs and their organizations. Specifically, under the final safety zone for ACOs, ACO participants providing a common service would need to have a combined market share of 30% or less in their primary service area (PSA; with a PSA defined as a contiguous area from which 75% of the ACO's patients are drawn) in order to fall within the safety zone. Nonrural ACOs exceeding 50% PSA threshold are not subject to mandatory DOJ/FTC review to gain CMS approval to participate in the shared savings program representing a change from the proposed safety zone. ACOs with PSAs that are in excess of 30% but outside of the safety zone and below 50% PSA may still be lawful and precompetitive. The proposed safety zone also required that hospitals and ambulatory surgical centers must be nonexclusive to ACOs, whereas physicians may be exclusive.

■ Conclusion

As this chapter's discussion illustrates, a myriad of legal issues are or can be implicated in connection with medical practice business operations and relationships. These range from state and federal laws and rules of general application that apply to the activities of medical and nonmedical business enterprises, to a wide variety of healthcare-specific legal and regulatory requirements that apply to physicians, medical practices, and other organizations. With the advent of healthcare reform, the body of applicable laws and rules, already vast, continues to grow and change at a rapid rate.

For nonlawyer medical practice professionals, key skills in helping to promote appropriate legal compliance include an ability to identify the general practices and relationships involved in a particular business activity and relationship, so as to identify, at a high level and in a general manner, the potential issues that may be implicated. That type of issue spotting can then be augmented by practical consideration of the key facts related to the actual or potential situation (e.g., what parties are involved, what are the business goals and objectives, what financial and/or referral relationships might be present, what individuals and/or entities would be paid and for what services, etc.), with the full body of facts submitted to appropriate healthcare legal counsel for consideration and guidance. The type of background understanding and analysis related to medical practices, their operations, and relationships with third parties in the context of the nation's larger healthcare delivery and payment systems can help to equip medical practice professionals with the tools to guide their organizations and their own actions, to remain out of harm's way, and to structure and operate the medical practice in an appropriate, legally compliant manner.

References
1. 42 U.S.C. § 1395w-4(k)(3).
2. 42 U.S.C. § 1395u(b)(18)(C).
3. 42 C.F.R. § 424.80.
4. 42 U.S.C.S. § 1395x(s).
5. 42 U.S.C.S. § 1395x(s)(2)(A).
6. 42 C.F.R. § 410.33.
7. 42 C.F.R. § 414.50(a)(2)(ii) and (iii).
8. 42 C.F.R. § 410.53; Medicare Program Integrity Manual, Chapter 10, section 4.19.1.
9. 42 C.F.R. § 413.65.
10. 42 U.S.C. § 1395nn.
11. 42 U.S.C. § 1320a-7b(b).
12. 42 U.S.C. § 1320a-7a(b).
13. 42 C.F.R. § 411.350.
14. 42 C.F.R. § 411.354.
15. 42 C.F.R. § 411.355(b).
16. 42 C.F.R. § 411.357(c).
17. 42 C.F.R. § 411.352.
18. 42 C.F.R. § 411.355(b)(1).
19. 42 C.F.R. § 411.355(b)(2).
20. 42 C.F.R. § 411.355(b)(3).
21. 42 C.F.R. § 424.80(b)(5).
22. 42 C.F.R. § 411.357(d).

23. 42 C.F.R. § 411.357(a).

24. 42 C.F.R. § 411.357(b).

25. 42 U.S.C. § 1320a-75(b).

26. *United States v. Greber*, 760 F.2d 68 (3d Cir.), *cert. denied*, 474 U.S. 988 (1985).

27. *U.S. v. Bay State Ambulance and Hosp. Rental Service, Inc.*, 874 F.2d 20 (1st Cir. 1989).

28. *Hanlester Network v. Shalala*, 51 F.3d 1390 (9th Cir. 1995).

29. 42 C.F.R. § 1001.952.

30. 42 C.F.R. § 1001.952(i).

31. 42 C.F.R. § 1001.952(d).

32. 42 C.F.R. § 1001.952(b).

33. 42 U.S.C. § 1320a-7a.

34. *United States ex rel. Drakeford v. Toumey, d/b/a Toumey Healthcare System*, No 3:05-CV-02858-MJP (D.S.C., Mar. 29, 2010), jury verdict 3/29/10.

35. *Arizona v. Maricopa County Medical Society*, 457 U.S. 332 (1982).

36. *TriState Health Partners, Inc. Advisory Opinion*, Federal Trade Commission (April 13, 2009).

37. *Greater Rochester Independent Practice Association, Inc. Advisory Opinion*, Federal Trade Commission (Sept. 17, 2007).

38. In the Matter of Surgical Specialists of Yakima, PLLC, 136 F.T.C. 840 (2003).

39. Federal Trade Commission. Statement of Department of Justice and Federal Trade Commission enforcement policy on physician network joint ventures. Accessed at http://www.ftc.gov/bc/healthcare/industryguide/policy/statement8.htm

40. December 22, 1992 letter to T. J. Sullivan, Technical Assistant, Office of the Associate Chief Counsel, Internal Revenue Service from D. McCarthy Thornton, Associate General Counsel, HHS Office of Inspector General. Accessed January 24, 2012, at http://oig.hhs.gov/fraud/docs/safeharborregulation/acquisition122292.htm

41. *St. David's Health Care System v. U.S.*, 349 F. 3rd 232 (5th Cir. 2003).

42. Rev. Rul. 98-15.

43. *Group Life and Health Ins. Co. v. Royal Drug Co.*, 440 U.S. 205 (1979).

44. 15 U.S.C § 1011-1015.

Labor and Employment Laws Applicable to Physicians' Practices

Peter D. Stergios, JD
John M. McKelway, JD
Jennifer Itzkoff, JD

The healthcare industry has been characterized by significant technological and scientific changes during the past century. Technological and scientific breakthroughs are becoming almost a routine part of medical practice. By understanding this evolution one can better appreciate how far the industry has advanced and, in certain situations, predict future technological and scientific changes.

The labor and employment laws that regulate the healthcare field also have evolved because of legislative enactments and judicial rulings over the same period, sometimes driven by these changes in medical practice. As well, doctors (along with the American Medical Association) are contemplating unionization as a means of dealing with large healthcare organizations, insurance companies, and complex governmental regulations. Doctors may be acting in restraint of trade in violation of federal antitrust laws if they combine to set prices, which has led them (in situations where they can claim employee status) to consider using unions and the labor laws under the protection of the National Labor Relations Act (NLRA) to bargain with healthcare corporations as a means of obtaining a lawful exemption from coverage under the antitrust laws. Doctors, as well as others in the medical profession (again, to the extent that they are employees within the meaning of the applicable federal, state, or local human rights laws), assert claims relating to their race, religion, sex, sexual preference, age, disability, or other protected status if they are victims of discriminatory treatment in the workplace.

Motivated by practice and economic pressures growing within the industry, many doctors and nurses, who are regarded as professionals, are actively litigating the right to be represented by labor organizations. Even as the healthcare industry has seen growth and change, so too have unions experienced greater success in obtaining status and recognition under the NLRA. To advance their representation interests, unions have marketed themselves as advocates for healthcare employees seeking redress for perceived breaches of employment discrimination laws, such as Title VII of the Civil Rights Act of 1964; workplace protection and safety laws, such as the Occupational Safety and Health Act (OSHA); antiretaliation or "whistleblower" laws; the Family and Medical Leave Act (FMLA); and a plethora of other worker protection laws.

Some healthcare employers have begun to consider mandatory arbitration of these kinds of statutory disputes. The Supreme Court of the United States has expanded the ability to use final and binding arbitration of statutory rights as a substitute for federal or state court litigation, subject to certain rules that provide due process and other protections that the courts are beginning to establish in their decisions. Lower federal courts and state courts have created standards by which such arbitration agreements can be enforced, which can vary significantly from one jurisdiction to another.

The one constant in the healthcare workplace is change, manifested not only in technology and science, but also in the law and the nature of workforce rights and remedies. This, as well as economic forces, contributes to the shifting environment in which management must deal with its workforce.

Further, in response to changes in the industry, large practices are growing through merger and acquisition; some now have over 100 physicians and hundreds of employees. This size places these practices in a very vulnerable position in terms of compliance with labor law. It is incumbent upon these large emerging practices to ensure that they comply.

Although the statutes reviewed in this chapter generally apply to physicians' practices, a careful analysis should always be undertaken to determine whether an employer–employee relationship exists. Often, an engagement between an individual and an entity, such as a hospital or physician practice group, is not an employer–employee relationship but something else entirely—most commonly, an independent contractor relationship. Many of the statutes discussed here do not extend protections to persons engaged as independent contractors (see, for example, the subsequent sections on "State Wage and Hour Laws" and "Employment Eligibility Verification"). Therefore, before deciding on a course of action regarding a particular individual who provides services to the organization, a careful manager must consider the character of the relationship between the organization and the individual—whether he or she is an employee or an independent contractor. Laws vary significantly from state to state, and misclassification of employees as independent contractors carries with it the prospect of significant exposure and penalties.

This chapter is not by any means exhaustive, but instead provides an overview and an analysis of the basic substantive provisions of labor and employment laws regulating the healthcare industry. As physician practices continue to get larger as a result of consolidation, a knowledge of labor law becomes more of an imperative.

■ Federal and State Civil Rights Laws

Federal Protections

Various federal, state, and local laws prohibit discrimination in the workplace on the basis of race, color, national origin, sex, disability, religion, or age. Additionally, several states and municipalities have enacted laws protecting an individual from discrimination on account of sexual orientation, marital status, criminal record, or recreational activities. The unifying theme behind these laws is that an employer should not treat individuals differently because of personal characteristics unrelated to job performance (i.e., race, sex, disability, age, etc.). In general, an employer should hire, promote, advance, discipline, or discharge an individual on the basis of that individual's job skills and work performance. Moreover, an employer should treat employees with similar job skills and performance records similarly.

Race, Color, and National Origin

Federal law, as embodied in Title VII of the Civil Rights Act of 1964[1] and similar state and local laws, make it unlawful for an employer to discriminate against an employee on the basis of race, color, or national origin (as well as sex and religion, as discussed later in the chapter) by: (1) failing to hire, discharging, or otherwise discriminating with respect to an employee's terms and conditions of employment; (2) depriving an individual of employment opportunities; or (3) retaliating against an employee who opposed discrimination. Title VII generally applies only to employers that employ 15 or more employees for each working day in each of 20 or more weeks in the current or preceding calendar year.[2] State and local laws may provide broader coverage.

Under Title VII, an individual may prove discrimination under one of two theories. First, an individual may show that he or she suffered disparate treatment discrimination, which consists of intentional discrimination directed at the individual specifically. In a disparate treatment case, the focus is on whether the individual (or group of individuals, referred to as a "class") suffered intentional discrimination. The pertinent question is whether the employer treated the individual differently or less favorably than another similarly situated individual because of the individual's personal characteristics. Disparate treatment claims also encompass complaints asserting a hostile work environment or harassment.

Another method by which an individual may prove discrimination is by demonstrating a disparate impact (or adverse impact), which refers to neutral practices that affect members of a protected group more severely than others. In a disparate impact claim, the individual does not need to demonstrate an intent to discriminate. In either a disparate treatment or a disparate impact case, the employee bears the burden of proof to establish discrimination.

An employer may defend against discrimination charges by demonstrating that it engaged in nondiscriminatory practices or that its actions were justified. General defenses include a legitimate, nondiscriminatory business reason; a bona fide seniority or merit system; a professionally developed test that is job-related to the position and consistent with business necessity; or a bona fide occupational qualification (not applicable with respect to race and limited applicability with respect to sex).

An individual claiming discrimination may initiate a formal complaint in one of several ways, depending on the locality in which he or she lives. An individual may initiate a discrimination claim by filing a charge of discrimination with the federal Equal Employment Opportunity Commission (EEOC), or by filing a discrimination complaint with a state or local fair employment practice agency. Additionally, in some jurisdictions an individual may file a complaint directly in state court. No litigant may file a complaint directly in federal court without first having instituted a proceeding before a fair employment practices agency and allowing that agency to handle the charge. If the fair employment practices agency declines to handle the charge, then an individual may file a complaint in federal court, but only after the individual receives what is known as a "right to sue" letter from the EEOC.

A successful claimant may be entitled to one or more remedies: instatement to the position sought, back pay, front pay, emotional distress damages, punitive damages, attorney's fees, or other relief that a court deems appropriate.[a]

Sex, Sexual Harassment, and Pregnancy

Under federal law and various state and local laws, discrimination against an employee on the basis of sex is prohibited. Like claims for race, color, and national origin discrimination, sex or gender discrimination claims can arise in several ways. A litigant may file for disparate treatment including hostile work environment or harassment, or may file a claim for disparate impact. Employers also must take care not to discriminate on the basis of sex with respect to compensation.[3] On January 29, 2009, President Obama signed the Lily Ledbetter Fair Pay Act, amending Title VII to provide that the statute of limitations starts anew with each discriminatory paycheck.[4]

Sexual harassment can manifest itself in two ways. First, in so-called "quid pro quo" harassment, an employee may claim that she or he was pressured or induced to provide sexual favors to someone in authority to obtain an employment-related benefit in return. Second, in a "hostile work environment" claim, the employee asserts that the employer has created a work atmosphere so offensive or unpleasant that it amounts to an adverse work condition. In a hostile work environment claim, the harassment may involve verbal, physical, or visual conduct, and the harassing conduct may be committed by a supervisor, coworker, or even a nonemployee.

Under certain circumstances, even if the victim employee was subjected to harassment, an employer may be able to defend against the charge. First, however, employers automatically will be liable for sexual harassment by supervisors that culminates in a tangible employment action against the employee, such as discharge, demotion, failure to promote, or significant loss of benefits. On the other hand, an employer may escape liability for alleged discrimination by a supervisor if no tangible job action was taken against the employee who was the subject of the alleged discrimination, so long as the employer provided a means of redress and the employee failed to take advantage of the opportunities the employer provided.[5,6] If the harassing behavior was not committed by a supervisor but by a coworker, then the employer may defend itself by showing that the employee failed to demonstrate that it knew or should have known of the harassment or, if it had notice, that it took immediate and corrective actions.

Furthermore, for purposes of employment, discrimination on the basis of pregnancy is considered discrimination on the basis of sex. It is a violation of Title VII to deny a woman employment because she is currently pregnant or might become pregnant, or to terminate her employment because she is pregnant.[b] Moreover, if an employee requests leave because of pregnancy or childbirth, covered employers are urged to check whether the request falls within the FMLA, which allows eligible employees up to 12 weeks of unpaid leave for the birth of a child, or other applicable law. The EEOC has also issued comprehensive guidelines addressing discrimination against individuals who care for children, the disabled, and the elderly.[7] Employers should also consult the laws in their states or municipalities for other laws covering sex discrimination and pregnancy.

---

a. Individuals subject to race discrimination may also bring suit under the Civil Rights Acts of 1866 and 1871, which give all persons the same right "to make and enforce contracts, to sue, be parties, give evidence, and to the full and equal benefit of all laws and proceedings." Procedurally, courts treat lawsuits under these statutes similarly to suits brought under Title VII, although there is no prerequisite that an individual must file an administrative charge with a fair employment practices agency.

---

b. See also Pregnancy Discrimination Act of 1978, 42 U.S.C. § 2000e(k).

Disability

Title I of the Americans with Disabilities Act (ADA) prohibits discrimination against qualified individuals with disabilities.[8] The definition of a disability, although seemingly simple, is the subject of extensive discussion by courts and fair employment agencies, and was expanded effective January 1, 2009.[9] In brief, the ADA defines a person with a disability as an individual who has a physical or mental impairment that substantially limits a major life activity (or has a record of an impairment or is regarded as having an impairment). To affect a major life activity, the impairment must substantially limit an individual's ability to perform key functions, such as caring for him- or herself, performing manual tasks, walking, hearing, seeing, speaking, breathing, learning, or working. Minor or temporary impairments cannot constitute a disability, nor can personal characteristics or cultural traits.

Often, an employer will be asked to make a reasonable accommodation for an individual with a disability. A reasonable accommodation is a change in the work environment or in the way things are customarily done that enables an individual with a disability to enjoy equal employment opportunities. Employers must be aware that the ADA prohibits discrimination against qualified individuals with a disability who can perform the essential functions of the position with or without a reasonable accommodation.

Generally, accommodations are made on a case-by-case basis, because the nature and extent of a disabling condition and the requirements of the job will vary. The principal test in selecting a particular type of accommodation is that of effectiveness (i.e., whether the accommodation will enable the person with a disability to perform the essential functions of the position). A reasonable accommodation may include job restructuring, part-time or modified work schedules, or reassignment to a vacant position. An employer should keep in mind, however, that it does not have to provide an accommodation that causes an "undue hardship" (i.e., significant difficulty and expense in providing the accommodation).

If the employee makes a request for a reasonable accommodation, the employer should initiate the "interactive process" in which the employer meets with the employee to discuss the employee's request and available alternatives if the request is too burdensome. Generally, the employer may ask for certain limited information about the disability, such as the nature, severity, and duration of the impairment; the activity that the impairment limits; and the extent to which the impairment limits the employee's ability to perform the activity or activities. In considering a reasonable accommodation, the company does not have to eliminate or reassign an essential function of the position, lower production standards, or create a new job as a reasonable accommodation.

The ADA also prohibits employers from requesting a medical examination of a prospective employee prior to extending an offer of employment. However, an employer may require that an individual submit to a medical examination after the job offer has been extended as a condition of employment, as long as the employer requires all new employees hired to that position to submit to an examination, keeps the results confidential, and does not use the results to discriminate on the basis of a disability.

Like Title VII, the ADA generally applies only to employers that employ 15 or more employees.[10] As with other fair employment laws, several states and localities have disability laws, many of which may be different in their scope and coverage than the ADA.

Religion

Federal law under Title VII prohibits discrimination based on religion, and it also imposes an affirmative duty upon a covered employer (one with at least 15 employees) to reasonably accommodate an applicant's and employee's religious beliefs, observances, and practices, unless the requested accommodation would cause an undue hardship to the employer's business. Additionally, many states and municipalities have laws containing provisions that address religious accommodation in the workplace.

Although, in general, an employer does not have to bear more than a minimal cost to accommodate an employee's religious need, in practice, responding to requests for religious accommodation can often be difficult. For instance, if an employee requests time off for a religious reason and this request creates a scheduling conflict, the employer should attempt to accommodate the request by finding a voluntary substitute or arranging a flexible work schedule, although an employer may not discriminate against one employee to satisfy the religious accommodation request of another. Similarly, if an employee requests a religious accommodation to be excused from performing a certain task, the employer generally should attempt to accommodate the request, unless the request consists of a major portion of the employee's work. Employers often face difficult questions about accommodating an employee's request to engage in religious practices during the workday. Again, the question is whether the request infringes upon the workplace and the rights of other employees or whether the request may be accommodated with little or no cost.

Age

The Age Discrimination in Employment Act[11] (ADEA) prohibits employers from discriminating against persons age 40 years or older because of their age. The ADEA protects employees in all aspects of employment, including hiring, promotion, and discharge. The general question in an age discrimination case is whether age was a "determining factor" in the employment decision. At issue is how the complaining party's performance and treatment compared to younger, similarly situated employees and the reasons offered by the employer for the challenged action. Additionally, employers should take care to avoid making comments that indicate a bias against older workers. An exception to the ADEA permits the compulsory retirement of any employee who has reached age 65 and who, for the 2-year period immediately before retirement, is employed in a bona fide executive or high policymaking position, if such employee is entitled to an immediate nonforfeitable annual retirement benefit from a plan of the employer that equals at least $44,000.[12]

The ADEA applies to employers that have 20 or more employees for each working day in each of 20 or more weeks in the current or preceding calendar year.[13] As with all fair employment practices laws, employers should check their state and local laws, which may also prohibit discrimination on the basis of age and may extend coverage to smaller employers.

State and Local Protections

Although federal law prohibiting discrimination is quite extensive, federal law does not ban certain forms of workplace behavior, such as discrimination based on sexual orientation or marital status. However, several states and municipalities have enacted laws banning discriminatory conduct in these areas. Similarly, many states and localities have enacted laws prohibiting discrimination because of a criminal record or recreational activities. In general, an employer is advised to check the laws in the employer's state and municipality regarding questions in these areas.

Sexual Orientation
Title VII's prohibition against discrimination because of sex prohibits employment discrimination on the basis of gender, but it does not cover claims on the basis of sexual orientation (e.g., homosexuality). However, several states do ban sexual orientation discrimination, as do several municipalities, including New York City[14] and San Francisco.[15]

Marital Status
Federal law does not prohibit an employer from using marital status as a factor in making employment decisions, as long as the employer applies this factor in the same fashion to all employees, whether male or female.

Again, though, several states and localities have passed fair employment laws prohibiting an employer from using an employee's marital status as a factor in employment. Similarly, federal law does not prohibit nepotism policies or practices that either favor or disfavor the hiring of family members of current employees. These employment policies must be scrutinized, however, to ensure that they are not used as pretexts to exclude women or members of minority groups.

Criminal Record
Several, if not most, states have enacted laws prohibiting an employer from discriminating against an employee on the basis of an arrest or conviction. These laws restrict an employer's ability to request and use an individual's arrest or conviction record as a condition of employment. In general, employers may not inquire about prior arrests, but under certain circumstances may inquire about prior convictions when they are job-related. In the healthcare context, laws governing prior arrests and convictions can vary, but in almost all cases the laws governing this area are more relaxed to permit healthcare institutions flexibility to avoid having employees with certain types of convictions (e.g., violent crimes) working with certain patient populations (e.g., children). Indeed, some jurisdictions have background check procedures that must be followed prior to hiring a new employee who will work in the healthcare field.

Recreational Activities
Several states have enacted statutes prohibiting discrimination against employees for off-duty conduct. The general thrust of the statutes is to prohibit employers from discriminating against an employee for engaging in certain types of lawful conduct outside of the workplace and during nonworking hours. Conduct covered by these statutes may include political activities, use of consumable products (such as alcohol and tobacco), recreational and leisure activities, and membership in a union.

■ Affirmative Action: Federal Contractor Requirements

Federal affirmative action requirements are based on Executive Order 11246, issued by President Johnson in 1965, which requires all businesses with substantial federal government contracts to take affirmative action to ensure that all individuals have an equal opportunity for employment, without regard to race, color, religion, sex, national origin, disability, or status as a Vietnam-era or special disabled veteran.[16,c] Healthcare providers may be considered federal contractors based on their receipt of federal moneys.

The U.S. Department of Labor's Office of Federal Contract Compliance Programs (OFCCP) is responsible for enforcement of federal affirmative action requirements. The OFCCP has taken the position that healthcare organizations that provide services to federal employees will be subject to its jurisdiction. The OFCCP requires a contractor, as a condition of having a federal contract, to engage in a self-analysis to discern the existence of any barriers to equal employment opportunity. A contractor in violation of affirmative action mandates may have its contracts canceled, terminated, or suspended in whole or in part, and the contractor may be declared ineligible for future government contracts.[16]

In December 2000, the U.S. Department of Labor issued new regulations that changed the format and content of affirmative action plans and altered the manner in which federal contractors must provide information. [16,d] Nonconstruction contractors with 50 or more employees and government contracts of $50,000 or more are required, under Executive Order 11246, to develop and implement a written affirmative action plan for each establishment. The plan must identify those areas, if any, in the contractor's workforce that might reflect underutilization of women and minorities.[16] The regulations define underutilization as having fewer minorities or women in a particular job group than would reasonably be expected by their availability. When determining availability of women and minorities, contractors consider, among other factors, the presence of minorities and women having requisite skills in an area in which the contractor can reasonably recruit.[16] Based on this analysis and the availability of qualified individuals, the contractor must then establish goals to reduce or overcome the underutilization, which may include expanded efforts in outreach, recruitment, training, and other activities to increase the pool of qualified minorities and females.[16]

---

c. The Office of Federal Contract Compliance Programs is responsible for enforcing Executive Order 11246, as amended, as well as other federal laws banning discrimination and requiring federal contractors and subcontractors to take affirmative action to ensure that all individuals have an equal opportunity for employment, without regard to race, color, religion, sex, national origin, disability, or status as a Vietnam-era or special disabled veteran.

d. See also 41 C.F.R. §§ 60-1 and 60-2, which revise the OFCCP regulations originally issued in 1978.

■ Individual Employment Rights

Whistleblowers

"Whistleblowing" is a term often used to describe an employee's dissemination of information critical of, or reflecting adversely on, an employer, typically for the purpose of correcting or preventing some violation of the law or other harm.[17] More than a dozen federal laws attempt to protect whistleblowing employees from retaliation in many areas of private sector activity where public health and safety are at stake.[17]

Of particular importance for healthcare providers are the antiretaliation provisions of the False Claims Act (FCA),[18] which prohibits any person or company from filing a false claim against the federal government. The FCA is intended to deter companies from fraudulently procuring federal funds.[19] Under the FCA, a private citizen may file suit against an alleged violator on behalf of the U.S. government. This is referred to as a qui tam action, and the private citizen is the qui tam relator or whistleblower.[19] Under the FCA, any employee who is discharged, demoted, suspended, or otherwise adversely affected in the terms and conditions of employment by his or her employer because of lawful acts done by the employee in furtherance of an action under the FCA, including investigation or initiation of, testimony for, or assistance in an action, is entitled to appropriate relief to make that employee whole, including back pay and other damages.

The FCA has been referred to as the "centerpiece of the health care antifraud effort."[20(p. 182)] Its provisions have been applied not only to situations involving misrepresentations of the facts surrounding the services for which federal payment is requested, but also to alleged violations of Medicare and Medicaid quality of care requirements.[20(pp 182–4),e]

Additionally, many states have enacted whistleblower protection legislation, often specifically addressed to the healthcare industry. For example, the New York State legislature expanded the scope of its general whistleblower protection law to specifically prohibit a healthcare employer from taking retaliatory action against

---

e. For example, in *United States ex. rel. Aranda v. Community Psychiatric Centers*, 945 F. Supp. 1485 (Western District of Oklahoma, 1996), a psychiatric hospital was accused of failing to provide Medicaid patients with the "reasonably safe environment" required by federal law. In that case, the government argued an implied certification theory (i.e., that by billing Medicaid for its services, the hospital had implicitly certified that it was in compliance with the program's quality requirements).

an employee because of that employee's threat to disclose, or actual disclosure of, a practice of the employer that the employee reasonably believes constitutes improper quality of patient care, or because of an employee's refusal to participate in any activity, policy, or practice that the employee in good faith reasonably believes constitutes improper quality of patient care.[21,f]

In order to offer employees an outlet for internal whistleblowing activities, an effective compliance and reporting program should be instituted. Such a program can help identify weaknesses in internal systems and management, demonstrate to employees and the community the employer's commitment to obeying the law, create a centralized source for the distribution of information on fraud and false claims, develop better communications between management and employees, and enhance the ability to initiate immediate and appropriate corrective action.[19]

Fair Credit Reporting Act

Employee background checks should be considered an essential element in the hiring process of all healthcare employees. A thorough background check can reveal instances of dishonesty, incompetence, and unreliability, and under certain circumstances limit an employer's liability in a claim of negligent hiring.[8] However, in certain situations an employer's background check may subject it to burdensome federal and state regulations. The employer must take special care either to comply with applicable requirements or to take actions to ensure that the requirements are not applicable, especially with respect to credit and criminal record reports.

The Fair Credit Reporting Act (FCRA)[22] governs the collection, dissemination, and use of an individual's credit information. The statute has specific provisions in regard to the furnishing and use of consumer reports for employment purposes.[22] Its main impact on healthcare employers governs the acquisition of background checks on current and potential employees. In most cases, for a covered employer legally to receive background information on an employee or applicant from a third party, such as a credit reporting agency, that employer must comply with the comprehensive regulations set forth under the FCRA.

Generally, in order to acquire reports on employees, the employer must meet special eligibility, disclosure, and use requirements. This includes certifying to the credit reporting agency that it is eligible to receive such reports, making a disclosure of the background check to employees and applicants, and following specific procedures before taking adverse actions against employees. If an adverse action, such as firing or refusing to hire an employee, is based in whole or in part on a consumer credit report, the employer must provide the individual a copy of the report and a statement of one's rights under the FCRA.

If an employer wishes to avoid the onerous requirements imposed under the FCRA, it may limit its background checks to information that it obtains directly from public entities, without the assistance of a third party. In general, information that is obtained by an employer directly from a federal, state, or local record repository is not a "consumer report" subject to FCRA regulations, because the repository (such as a courthouse or a state law enforcement agency) is not normally a "consumer reporting agency."

The Fair and Accurate Credit Transaction Act of 2003 (FACT)[23] amended the FCRA, partly in response to a series of opinion letters in which the Federal Trade Commission's staff interpreted the FCRA to apply to an employer's use of a third party to investigate employee complaints of sexual harassment and discrimination.[h] This interpretation, although not binding on the courts, would have made the use of a human resource consultant or law firm to investigate such claims subject to the FCRA's notice and compliance procedures. This obligation would create an obvious tension between an employer's duty to fully investigate and keep confidential workplace discrimination claims, and employee rights under the FCRA.[i] FACT excludes from the definition of a consumer report those communications provided to an employer in conjunction with an investigation for suspected

---

f. See also Ohio Rev. Code Ann. § 4723.33 (prohibiting retaliation against nurses and dialysis technicians who report healthcare violations); Cal. Health and Safety Code §1278.5 (prohibiting retaliation against physicians who advocate for medically appropriate healthcare for patients); and 210 ILS. 45/3-608 (same re: Nursing Home Care Act).

g. See, e.g., Fla. Stat. Ann. § 768.096.

---

h. See, e.g., Meisinger Letter, fn. 1 (August 31, 1999), at FTC website, http://www.ftc.gov/os/statutes/fcra/index.htm

i. But see *Hartman v. Lisle Park District*, 158 F. Supp. 2d 869, 876 (Northern District of Illinois, 2001) (rejecting argument that FCRA abrogated the attorney–client or work-product privileges in regard to workplace misconduct investigation, and finding that a report prepared by an attorney about an employee's transactions or experiences with the attorney's client—the employer—qualified as a report containing information solely as to transactions or experiences between the consumer and the person making the report within the meaning of the FCRA, even though the report was prepared by an entity other than the employer).

employee misconduct relating to employment.[24] After taking adverse action based on the information contained within a communication for this purpose, FACT requires that an employer provide the consumer with a summary of the nature and substance of the communication upon which the adverse action is based.[24] The employer will not, however, be required to disclose the sources of information.[24]

Failure to comply with the FCRA may result in state or federal enforcement actions, as well as private litigation. In addition, any person who knowingly and willfully obtains a consumer report under false pretenses may face criminal prosecution. In order to help safeguard against liability under the FCRA, an employer should either avoid adopting practices that would trigger the requirements of the FCRA or institute reasonable procedures in order to assure compliance. Generally, if a company can establish that it has maintained reasonable procedures to assure compliance, it can set forth an affirmative defense to liability.

Employee Polygraph Protection Act

The Employee Polygraph Protection Act of 1988 generally makes it unlawful for an employer to directly or indirectly require, request, suggest, or cause any employee or prospective employee to take or submit to any lie detector test.[25] Violators of the act can be assessed civil penalties of up to $10,000 and incur civil damages in suits brought by affected employees. However, for a healthcare employer, numerous exceptions may apply. The act does not apply with respect to any state or local government, or any political subdivision of a state or local governmental employer.[26] Additionally, a limited exemption exists for polygraph tests administered in connection with an ongoing investigation involving economic loss or injury to an employer's business (such as theft, embezzlement, or misappropriation), provided that the employee had access to the property that is the subject of the investigation, that there is a reasonable suspicion that the employee was involved in the incident, and that certain pretest notifications are provided to the employee. The economic loss must relate to the business of the employer; therefore, a theft committed by one employee against another employee of the same employer would not satisfy the requirement.[k]

Another exemption exists in regard to drug security, drug theft, or drug diversion investigations.[28] Employers authorized to manufacture, distribute, or dispense certain controlled substances can administer polygraph tests if the test is administered to a prospective employee who would have direct access to the controlled substances, or if the test is administered in connection with an ongoing investigation of misconduct involving the controlled substances and the employee had access to the property that is the subject of the investigation.

WARN Act

The Worker Adjustment and Retraining Notification Act (WARN) was passed by Congress in 1988.[25] WARN requires certain employers (generally those with 100 or more employees, excluding part-time employees) to provide notice to affected employees, their union (if any), and state and local officials 60 calendar days in advance of a plant closing or mass layoff.[25,l] Advance notice is required to provide workers and their families with time to adjust to the prospective loss of employment, to seek and obtain alternative jobs, and, if necessary, to enter skill training or retraining that will allow these workers to successfully compete in the job market. WARN also provides for notice to state dislocated worker units, so that dislocated worker assistance can be provided.[29] In addition to WARN, state and local laws may place additional notice requirements upon employers, including smaller employers, planning a mass layoff or plant closing. The penalties for failing to comply with WARN's notice requirements include up to 60 days' back pay and civil penalties of up to $500 for each day of the violation. WARN can be triggered when there is either a permanent or temporary closing of a single site of employment or at one or more facilities or operating units that affects 50 or more employees during any 30-day period. A mass layoff is one that results in an employment loss at a single site of employment during any 30-day period for (1) at least 33% of the employees and at least 50 employees, or (2) at least 500 employees.

WARN does contain exemptions from the notice requirements, and, in some cases, provisions that allow for reduction in the amount of notice required.[30] The act provides for a shortened notice period under a faltering company exception when the employer was actively seeking capital, and that capital, if obtained, would have enabled it to avoid or postpone a closing, and the employer reasonably believed that giving the 60-day notice would have jeopardized its opportunity to obtain the capital. Other justifications for providing shortened notice may arise when unforeseeable business circumstances preclude such notice, or when a natural disaster is the cause

---

k. See, e.g., *Lyle v. Mercy Hospital Anderson*, 876 F. Supp 157 (Southern District of Ohio, 1995).

l. See also 20 C.F.R. § 639.1.

of the shortened notice. A complete exemption from the notice requirement is provided when the closing or layoff constitutes a strike or lockout not intended to evade the requirements of the act, or when the closing or layoff is the result of the completion of a particular project or undertaking, and the affected employees were hired with the understanding that their employment was limited to the duration of that project or undertaking.[31]

Wage and Hour Laws

The Fair Labor Standards Act (FLSA) establishes minimum wage, overtime, and record-keeping requirements for most public and private employers. However, many employees are exempted from the FLSA's requirements. Difficult issues often arise in determining whether an employee qualifies as exempt under the FLSA. This chapter addresses some common issues that arise under the FLSA, particularly in the healthcare setting.

The FLSA's requirements apply only to employees, not to independent contractors. It is, therefore, important to understand whether a worker is an independent contractor or an employee. Courts generally conduct a fact-specific inquiry on this issue and consider five factors to determine whether an independent contractor is in reality an employee:[m]

1. The degree of control exerted by the alleged employer over the worker (e.g., who sets the worker's hours, provides tools and working materials, uniforms, transportation, expenses, etc.)
2. The worker's opportunity and risk for profit and loss
3. The worker's investment in the business
4. The permanence of the working relationship
5. The degree of skill required to perform the work

Although a written consulting agreement may constitute evidence of contractor status, it is not determinative. Because independent contractor laws vary greatly from state to state, it is prudent to seek legal counsel before entering into such arrangements.

Many healthcare providers rely on the services of volunteers. Under some circumstances, however, a provider could incur liability under the FLSA for failing to compensate volunteers at least the minimum wage. Courts typically employ an "economic reality" test and consider a "true" volunteer to be one who donates his or her services to a charitable, educational, or religious organization and performs a service normally thought of as voluntary or charitable.[32] A volunteer ordinarily must not be displacing an employee or performing services that are customarily performed by an employee. Thus, although a traditional "candy striper" in a hospital setting would ordinarily meet the test of a volunteer, a person who performs services in a hospital's gift shop or services for a for-profit corporation that do not constitute "charitable activities" may not be a true volunteer.

Minimum Wages and Overtime

Generally, under the FLSA, employers must pay not less than the federal minimum wage for each hour worked by an employee.[33] (Note, however, that state law may set a higher minimum wage rate than that established under the FLSA. Employees in such states must receive the higher rate established by applicable state law.) Under the FLSA, an employee's workweek spans seven consecutive 24-hour periods. Under certain circumstances, an employer may average an employee's earnings over the workweek, and if the average hourly earnings for non-overtime hours equal at least the minimum wage, the minimum wage requirement is considered satisfied for that week. Of course, hourly wages below the minimum in one workweek may not be offset by wages above the minimum in another.

Under the FLSA, a nonexempt employee also must be paid one and one-half times his or her regular hourly rate for hours worked over the maximum hour standard.[34] The maximum hour standard, and in turn an employee's overtime compensation, is generally figured on a weekly basis. For most employees, the maximum number of hours an employee may work in 1 week without being paid overtime is 40 hours.[34,n] However, for certain workers in hospitals and residential care establishments, overtime pay may be calculated on either a 7-day, 40-hour workweek basis or on a 14-day, 80-hour basis. Specifically, hospitals or institutions primarily engaged in the care of resident patients may use the 14-day work period to calculate overtime compensation if an agreement or understanding exists between the employer and employee prior to performance of the work. Overtime compensation is paid for hours worked in excess of 80 hours during the 14-day period and in excess of 8 hours in any workday.[35]

---

m. See, e.g., *Doty v. Elias*, 733 F.2d 720, 722 (10th Cir. 1984).

n. Note, however, that the FLSA's regulations contain many exceptions to this rule, such as for employees who hold positions with inherently irregular hours of work ("Belo" plans), fluctuating workweeks, union contracts with guaranteed hours, and so on.

White Collar Exemptions

There are many statutory exemptions under the FLSA, the most common of which are those that apply to certain executive, administrative, and professional employees, and certain outside sales employees, among others (the so-called "white collar" exemptions). The executive, administrative, professional, and computer professional exemptions are discussed here.

An exemption allows an employer to avoid the FLSA's overtime pay requirements with respect to the exempt employee. For any of the white collar exemptions to apply (with the exception of computer professionals), the employee in question must satisfy various "tests" under the FLSA. First, the employee must be paid a predetermined weekly salary that does not vary based on the quantity or quality of the employee's work (the "salary basis" test). Deductions or docking of pay for disciplinary reasons, poor performance, partial day absences, and other reasons may jeopardize an employee's exempt status because such deductions are inconsistent with the salary basis test.[36,o]

An employee's duties also must be considered to ensure that they are in accord with one or more of the white collar exemptions. For example, to satisfy the exemption for executive employees, the employee generally must manage an enterprise or department, regularly direct two or more employees, and have primary duties that relate directly to management policies or general business aspects, such as interviewing, selecting, training, directing, recommending employees for promotions, disciplining, or delegating work, among others.[37] Officers and high-ranking employees of a hospital or corporation ordinarily will meet the requirements of an exempt executive employee.

To satisfy the requirements for the administrative employee exemption, an employee generally must, in addition to the salary basis test, primarily perform work related to management policies or general business operations, and exercise discretion and independent judgment in the performance of his or her duties. In addition, an exempt administrative employee must have the authority to make independent choices without immediate supervision.[38] Examples of employees who generally qualify as administrative employees are executive assistants, department heads, and managers.

Employees who satisfy the FLSA's white collar exemption for professionals generally include doctors, registered nurses, certain registered (or certified) medical technologists,[39,p] and other highly skilled employees who spend most of their time doing work requiring advanced knowledge that is acquired by a specialized course of study. An exempt professional generally must, in addition to being paid on a salary basis, perform original and creative duties in work requiring scientific or specialized study and the exercise of independent judgment.[40] One court of appeals ruled in 2000 that home care nurses were exempt from the FLSA's overtime provisions as professionals.[41] The Wage and Hour Administrator of the U.S. Department of Labor has stated that employees classified as physician's assistants may meet the test for the professional exemption.[42] On the other hand, the Wage and Hour Administrator also stated that the position of medical assistant was not exempt, on the basis that the educational prerequisites of the position did not involve a "prolonged course of specialized intellectual instruction and study," as required for a professional exemption.[43]

The computer professional exemption applies to highly skilled employees, generally not computer technicians or operators. Although computer professionals usually have a bachelor's degree or higher, no specific degree is required. The level of skill necessary to be considered a computer professional may be gained through education and field experience.[44] To qualify for the computer professional exemption, an employee must be highly skilled in computer systems analysis, programming, or related software functions, and must primarily: (1) apply systems analysis techniques and procedures, including technical support functions, and (2) design, develop, analyze, create, test, or modify computer or machine operating systems. Rather than a predetermined weekly salary, computer professionals must be paid a specified hourly rate to qualify for the exemption.

---

o. Note, however, that a disciplinary deduction from an exempt employee's pay is permissible if it is for the infraction of a "safety rule of major significance." 29 C.F.R. § 541.602(b)(4). Although the issue has not been squarely addressed by the courts, the Wage and Hour Administrator of the U.S. Department of Labor has taken the position that a registered nurse's violations of his or her employer's rules "relating to patient well-being and job performance are not the type of deductions that would be permitted by section 541.602(b)(4) of the regulations." See Wage and Hour Administrator's Opinion Letter No. 90-42NR (March 29, 1991). See also *Klein v. Rush-Presbyterian-St. Luke's Med. Ctr.*, 990 F.2d 279 (7th Cir. 1993).

p. A registered or certified medical technologist is considered an exempt professional if he or she has successfully completed "three academic years of preprofessional study in an accredited college or university plus a fourth year of professional course work in a school of medical technology approved by the Council of Medical Education of the American Medical Association . . . ." See 29 C.F.R. § 541.301(e)(1).

Whether an employee is exempt from the requirements of the FLSA is not always easy to determine. An employee's job title alone does not make the employee exempt. Rather, an employer must examine the employee's actual job duties and individual circumstances. The FLSA's exemptions are narrowly construed, and the employer bears the burden of proving that its employees are exempt. Should the determination that an employee is exempt be made erroneously, back pay and penalties could be assessed by the Department of Labor.

Joint Employment Under the FLSA

An important consideration in the healthcare field is the effect of a finding of "joint employment" under the FLSA. Two or more employers may be considered joint employers under the FLSA, which would require aggregating all hours worked for the two employers for purposes of the act's overtime pay requirements. Aggregation of all hours worked for two employers may dramatically increase the joint employers' liability for overtime pay for affected employees.

The determination of whether an individual's employment by two or more employers constitutes joint employment for purposes of the FLSA depends on all the facts of a particular case. If two or more employers are acting "entirely independently of each other and are completely disassociated" with respect to an individual's employment, each employer may disregard all work performed for the other in considering its obligations under the FLSA.[45] However, if the facts establish that the employee is employed jointly by two or more employers [i.e., that employment by one employer is not completely disassociated from employment by the other employer(s)], all of the employee's work for all of the joint employers during the workweek is considered as one employment for purposes of the act.[45]

The effect of a finding of joint employment of an individual is that all such joint employers are responsible, both individually and jointly, for compliance with all applicable provisions of the FLSA, including overtime, with respect to the individual's entire employment for the particular workweek.[45]

A joint employer relationship generally will be considered to exist: (1) where there is an arrangement between the employers to share the employee's services, as, for example, to interchange employees; (2) where one employer is acting directly or indirectly in the interest of another employer in relation to the employee; or (3) where the employers are not "completely disassociated" with respect to the employment of a particular individual and may be deemed to share control of the employee, directly or indirectly, by reason of the fact that one employer controls, is controlled by, or is under common control with the other employer.[45,q]

Family and Medical Leave Act

The Family and Medical Leave Act of 1993 (FMLA) is a federal law that generally requires private sector employers of 50 or more employees to provide up to 12 workweeks of unpaid, job-protected leave, within any 12-month period, to eligible employees for certain family and medical reasons.[46,47] Covered employers are also required to maintain eligible employees' preexisting group health insurance coverage during the leave and to restore eligible employees to the same or an equivalent position at the conclusion of the FMLA leave.[48,49] Many states have also enacted family and/or medical leave laws that may apply different or stricter standards than the FMLA.

To be eligible for FMLA benefits, an employee must[50,51]:

- Work for a covered employer
- Have worked for the employer for at least 12 months
- Have worked at least 1250 hours for the employer over the previous 12 months
- Work at a location in the United States or in any territory or possession of the United States where at least 50 employees are employed by the employer at a single worksite, or at multiple worksites within a range of 75 miles

Eligible employees may be entitled to take FMLA leave for any of the following reasons: the birth and care of a newborn child of the employee; the placement with the employee of a child for adoption or foster care; to care for an immediate family member (spouse, child, or parent) with a serious health condition; or when the employee is unable to work because of his or her own serious health condition.[52,53]

FMLA Notice Requirements

Both the employer and the employee have notice requirements under the FMLA. Specifically, employees seeking to use FMLA leave are required to provide 30-day advance notice of the need to take FMLA leave when the need is foreseeable and such notice is practicable. The notice from the employee can be verbal. However, the employer may request that employees comply with its customary and usual notice and procedural requirements for requesting leave.[54,55]

---

q. But see *Ling Nan Zheng v. Liberty Apparel Co.*, 355 F3d 61, 71 (2d Cir. 2003) (adopting a broader "economic realities" test for assessing joint employer status under the FLSA).

Employers also may require employees to provide medical certification supporting the need for leave because of a serious health condition, second or third medical opinions (at the employer's expense) and periodic recertification, and periodic reports during FMLA leave regarding the employee's status and intent to return to work.[56,57] Employers also must provide notice to the employee as to whether he or she is eligible for FMLA leave within 2 days of making the eligibility determination and prior to the date the requested leave is to begin.[58,r]

Other Notable FMLA Provisions

Spouses employed by the same employer are jointly entitled to a combined total of 12 workweeks of family leave for the birth and care of a newborn child, for placement with the employees of a child for adoption or foster care, and to care for a parent who has a serious health condition.[59,60] Under some circumstances, employees may take FMLA leave intermittently—which means taking leave in separate blocks of time, or by reducing their normal weekly or daily work schedule.[61,62]

Although most employees are entitled to be returned to the same or an equivalent position at the conclusion of their FMLA leave, employers can deny job restoration to a salaried employee who is among the highest paid 10% of the employer's workforce, if that person is considered a "key employee." However, this designation must occur at the time the leave is designated.[63,64]

State Wage and Hour Laws

Although the FLSA imposes no limit on the number of hours an employee may work per day or week, so long as he or she is appropriately compensated for hours worked on a minimum wage and overtime basis, certain states' laws do restrict the number of hours an employee may work per day and per week.[s] Similarly, although the FLSA does not require that an employer provide meal periods for employees, some states' laws do.[t]

Many states have enacted laws dictating when an employer is allowed to withhold or make deductions from an employee's wages. Some typical state laws restrict an employer from withholding or diverting any portion of an employee's wages unless: (1) the employer is required to do so under state or federal law (e.g., Social Security or income tax deductions); (2) the employee has given the employer written authorization for the withholding; or (3) there is a reasonable good faith doubt as to the amount of wages set off or amount owed by the employee to the employer.[u]

Other states have enactments that are more strict, prohibiting an employer from making deductions from wages unless it has obtained prior written authorization from the employee, and such deductions are for specific items, as defined by the law.[v] Other states are stricter still, permitting an employer to make only those deductions required by law, or expressly authorized in writing by the employee, so long as such deductions are "for the benefit of the employee," such as for group health or life insurance, 401(k) contributions, and union dues.[w] In such states, an employer is prohibited from making wage deductions for spoilage or breakage, cash shortages or losses, or fines or penalties for lateness, misconduct, or quitting without notice.

Some states may also permit an employer to withhold wages from a terminated employee's final paycheck for the value of any property belonging to the employer that is not returned by the employee.[x] However, under no circumstances should any such withholding cause a nonexempt employee's wages to be reduced below the applicable minimum wage for that pay period.

Employers must also consider whether state law requires any particular time for or method of payment of wages. For example, some states require wages to be paid no less frequently than monthly, semimonthly, or weekly.[y] Many states also require that terminated employees receive all wages due within a certain number of days following termination of employment.[z]

Many states also regulate the method of payment of employees' wages, such as requiring payments in cash or check, with appropriate time off for employees to cash paychecks. With the increasing popularity of direct deposit of wages by electronic funds transfer, some states also have enacted laws restricting employers from directly depositing the wages of nonexempt employees without the employee's advance written consent.[aa]

---

r. The U.S. Supreme Court has rejected the Department of Labor's position that an employee whose employer had failed to give the employee timely notice of designation of FMLA leave was entitled greater than the 12 weeks of leave mandated by the FMLA. See *Ragsdale v. Wolverine Worldwide, Inc.*, 122 S.Ct. 1155 (2002).

s. See, e.g., California Labor Code §§ 1810, et seq.; Nev. Rev. Stat. § 608.018.

t. See, e.g., New York Labor Law § 162.

u. See, e.g., Arizona Revised Statutes § 23-352.

v. See, e.g., California Labor Code §§ 200, et seq.

w. See, e.g., New York Labor Law § 193.

x. See, e.g., Arizona Revised Statutes § 23-352 (3).

y. See, e.g., New York Labor Law § 191; Ariz. Rev. Stat. § 23–351.

z. See, e.g., New York Labor Law § 191; Cal. Lab. Code § 201; Ariz. Rev. Stat. § 23-353.

aa. See, e.g., New York Labor Law § 192.

Employee Benefits in the Healthcare Industry

The range and variety of benefits available to employees of healthcare entities are similar to those available for employees in other industries. For those entities that are tax-exempt organizations,[65] however, special rules and exceptions may apply. Generally, these benefits are subject to two comprehensive federal laws: the Employee Retirement Income Security Act of 1974 (ERISA)[66] and the Internal Revenue Code (Code). Through piecemeal legislation, Congress has added a number of additional requirements for group health plans.[bb] Moreover, significant amendments to the Code and ERISA were made by the Consolidated Omnibus Reconciliation Act of 1985 (COBRA), which also has had an impact on group health plans.

Deferred Compensation

Many employees are attracted by the potential retirement benefits offered in the healthcare industry. Those benefits fall into three categories: (1) qualified retirement plans under Section 401(a) of the Code, (2) tax-deferred annuities under Section 403(b) of the Code, and (3) unfunded deferred compensation plans under Section 457 of the Code. The sections contain numerous requirements for participation, vesting, funding, and distributions.

Qualified Retirement Plans

These plans must satisfy specific statutory and extensive regulatory requirements.[cc] The two types of plans most often utilized are pension and profit-sharing plans.

A defined benefit pension plan provides participants with a fixed or determinable retirement benefit at normal retirement age, based on a formula set forth in the plan.[dd] The formula may provide for a monthly or yearly benefit, which often is based on the participant's length of service and compensation. Employers sponsoring such plans must make minimum and maximum contributions each year in accordance with an actuarial determination.

A money purchase pension plan provides the participant with a fixed contribution each year. The contribution is based on a fixed percentage of annual compensation or a fixed amount per hour, week, or other unit of work, and the employer is obligated to make that contribution regardless of profits. These plans have been less popular in recent years because they guarantee a retirement benefit, or at least a fixed level of contributions.

A defined contribution pension plan, often some form of profit-sharing plan, has become more popular for tax-exempt organizations since 1980, when the Internal Revenue Service determined that they could maintain such plans.[67] Such a plan has individual accounts, and the number of retirement benefits will depend on the value of the account investments upon retirement or termination of employment.

A recently popular variation to this type of plan is the cash or deferred arrangement (CODA) plan, also known as the 401(k) plan, which permits employee salary deferrals on a pretax basis and employer matching contributions, which are usually limited to a percentage of salary reduction. Salary deferrals are capped on an annual basis and are adjusted for cost-of-living increases on an annual basis. These types of plans usually are designed as participant-directed accounts under ERISA Section 404(c), thereby removing fiduciary liability from employers or their designated fiduciaries who administer the plans. Tax-exempt employer sponsors have only been permitted to offer CODAs since 1997.[68]

The benefits under 401(k) plans for highly compensated employees (HCEs) also are limited by nondiscrimination requirements, which limit HCEs from contributing or matching contributions in excess of a certain percentage of the contributions for nonhighly compensated employees (NHCEs).[69,70]

Tax-Deferred Annuities Under Section 403(b)

Prior to 1997, an alternative similar to the 401(k) plan was the 403(b) plan, which could be adopted by tax-exempt organizations only.[71] These types of retirement plans contain similar participation, vesting, distribution, and other requirements as for qualification under Section 401(a) of the Code.

The Economic Growth and Tax Relief Reconciliation Act of 2001 (EGTRRA)[72] contains a number of reforms that enhance the benefits provided under all types of plans. These include increases in the annual deferred contribution and defined benefit contribution and compensation limits, elective deferral limits, and a new provision for catch-up contributions for individuals over age 50.

Unfunded Deferred Compensation Plans

Unfunded deferred compensation plans (or Section 457 plans) are permitted by the Revenue Act of 1978, which was codified as Section 457 of the Code. In 1986, Congress extended to private tax-exempt organizations

---

bb. See, e.g., Health Insurance Portability and Accountability Act of 1996 (HIPAA), Public Law No. 104-191; Mental Health Parity Act of 1996 (MHPA), ERISA § 712, I.R.C. § 9812, 4980D; Newborns and Mothers' Health Protection Act of 1996 (NMHPA), ERISA § 711, I.R.C. § 9811; and Women's Health and Cancer Rights Act of 1998 (WHCA), ERISA § 713.

cc. See Treasury Regulations §§ 1.401(a), et seq.

dd. Treasury Regulations § 1.401-1(b)(1)(i); see also Revised Rules 79-90, 1979-1 CB 155.

the ability to maintain Section 457 plans.[73] There are two types of plans—eligible[74] and ineligible.[75] Although an eligible Section 457 plan can offer immediate 100% vesting, the unfunded status of the plan makes its benefits susceptible to economic downturns, which could result in nonpayment of benefits.

Welfare Benefits

The term "welfare benefit plan" generally refers to any employee benefit plan that does not provide for deferral of contributions.[76] These plans are heavily regulated by the Code and ERISA. In recent years, other laws, especially the Health Insurance Portability and Accountability Act (HIPAA), have had a serious impact on the administration of these plans by, among other things, implementing privacy and related requirements with respect to personal health information of plan participants.[77]

Favorable tax treatment for employees (e.g., noncludable income) under the Code and avoiding incurring excise taxes is of primary importance to the tax-exempt organization. Accordingly, a welfare benefit plan must abide by various rules under the Code. In addition, ERISA imposes reporting and disclosure requirements, fiduciary duties, and claims administration procedures on employers sponsoring such plans.[78] Most welfare benefit plans are subject to ERISA because of the broad definition of the term "welfare benefit plan,"[79] but certain benefits are excepted.[80,81] A group health plan subject to ERISA also must comply with ERISA Parts 6 (COBRA) and 7 (portability, access, and renewability requirements under HIPAA).

The specific types of welfare benefit plans subject to ERISA's requirements that most often are adopted by employers are as follows:

- Group term life insurance (Section 79 of the Code)
- Health and disability benefit plans (Sections 105 and 106 of the Code, and for group health plans, COBRA, HIPAA, Medical Secondary Payer Requirements, and related laws)
- Disability income plans (Section 105 of the Code)
- Educational assistance benefits (Section 117 of the Code for tuition reimbursement programs and Section 127 for educational assistance plans)
- Group legal services plans (Section 120 of the Code)
- Cafeteria plans (Section 125 of the Code)
- Dependent care assistance programs (Section 129 of the Code)
- Fringe benefits (Section 132 of the Code)
- Adoption assistance programs (Section 137 of the Code)
- Long-term care insurance (Sections 7702B and 106 of the Code)

Funding arrangements similar to those utilized for non-tax-exempt organizations include the following:

- Voluntary employee benefit association (VEBA) (Section 501(a)(9) of the Code)
- Supplemental unemployment compensation benefits trust (Section 501(a)(17) of the Code)
- Section 501(c)(3) supporting organizations for charities
- Grants or trusts (Sections 671–677 of the Code)

Related Significant Legal Requirements

In order to qualify to comply with various sections of the Code and ERISA, health industry employers must be aggregated under Section 414(b) and (c) (parent–subsidiary group and brother–sister group of employers) of the Code (incorporating Code Section 1563 with respect to "controlled groups"). The Internal Revenue Service has taken the position that nonstock corporations are subject to Sections 414(b) and (c). Similar aggregation rules apply under Section 414(m) of the Code (service organizations), Section 414(n) (leased employees), and Section 414(o) (all other potential employee benefit requirements). Aggregation would result in treating employers of the aggregated employees as if they were a single employer for (1) nondiscrimination requirements and (2) funding requirements.

The administration of employee benefit plans is also subject to civil rights in employment laws, including the ADEA, Titles VI and VII of the Civil Rights Act of 1964, the ADA, the FMLA, the Rehabilitation Act of 1973, and the Equal Pay Act.

■ Privacy Issues in the Workplace

Few areas of the law have undergone such significant change as the area of workplace privacy, driven in large part by technological advances. Previous generations of employers were not faced with questions concerning computer usage, electronic mail, voice mail, the Internet, social media, and personal mobile devices. Concurrently, it has become increasingly possible for employers to learn more about their employees and prospective employees, which is tempting in light of publicity around reports of workplace violence and concerns about employer liability. Employers must seek to balance their legitimate business interest in obtaining information about an employee or applicant against an employee's right to privacy. In the healthcare industry, an employer also owes to its patients the careful balancing of these competing interests.

The issue of employee privacy may arise in a variety of contexts within the employment relationship, including background checks of applicants, employee surveillance, and monitoring of employee communications. The legal standards applicable may depend on a number of factors, including the nature of the activity at issue, the nature of the employer, and the work environment. Employee privacy rights may arise from a number of sources, including federal or state constitutions; federal, state, or local statutes; and the common law. For example, the Fourth Amendment to the U.S. Constitution extends certain privacy rights to government employees in the public workplace, but not to employees of the private sector. Some state constitutions also provide additional privacy protections.[ee]

In addition, federal and state statutes may extend certain privacy protections to employees. For example, the Omnibus Crime Control and Safe Streets Act, as amended by the Electronic Communications Privacy Act (ECPA),[82] restricts employer monitoring of employee telephone calls. Also, some states recognize certain common law torts that address violations of employee privacy, including intrusion upon seclusion and public disclosure of private facts. These different sources of law may overlap to provide varying degrees of employee privacy protection, depending on the nature of the employer, the state in which the workplace is located, and the kind of conduct at issue.

Privacy in the Hiring Process

Privacy issues may arise even before the commencement of the employment relationship. Employers have an obvious need to investigate the qualifications and trustworthiness of potential employees for a number of reasons, not the least of which is the need to avoid potential liability to third parties for the tort of negligent hiring or retention. At the same time, however, this need for information is tempered by the danger of potential liability for claims of invasion of privacy or violation of other federal or state protections. In this regard, employers should be cautious when reviewing information on social media sites of prospective applicants.

As part of the hiring process, employers should require all applicants to complete an application form. The application should elicit information relating to past employment, references, education, licenses, and criminal convictions (being mindful that some state laws may restrict this line of questioning and may limit an employer's ability to use a criminal conviction as an absolute bar to employment). The application materials also should include a written consent and release of liability allowing an employer to contact former employers and references and to conduct a background check. Inclusion of a statement regarding the consequences of the falsification of an application and the failure to provide complete responses, as well as an affirmation of the truthfulness of the application, will leave little doubt in the applicant's mind that the employer will conduct a thorough background check. Employers should verify the information provided and create a written record that demonstrates verification and details the results of any investigation.

As described earlier, in order for an employer to legally receive background information from a third party, the employer must comply with the provisions of the Fair Credit Reporting Act (FCRA).[83] An employer may obtain different reports, and for each there are different levels of requirements. A consumer report includes any written, oral, or other communication of information by a consumer reporting agency bearing on a consumer's creditworthiness, credit standing, character, general reputation, personal characteristics, or mode of living that is used for employment purposes. To acquire a consumer report an employer must meet requirements discussed in the previous section. Additional notice requirements must be followed when an employer procures an "investigative consumer report," which the FCRA defines as a consumer report in which the information is obtained through personal interviews with neighbors, friends, associates, or other acquaintances of the consumer. As a result of the complex requirements of the FCRA, employers should consult with counsel to ensure compliance.[ff]

Electronic Surveillance and Monitoring of Employees

Privacy issues continue after the employment relationship begins. Advancements in technology provide both increased opportunity and added responsibility for employers to monitor the activities of their employees. One avenue for employee monitoring is video surveillance. Silent video surveillance (recorded audio on a videotape may run afoul of the federal and state wiretap laws, as detailed below) usually is considered lawful when the employees or others under surveillance have no reasonable expectation of privacy, such as when cameras are placed in hallways, lunchrooms, and other public areas. However, employers are well advised to take care in conducting this type of monitoring, because it may raise constitutional

ee. See, e.g., California Constitution, Article I, § 1; Florida Constitution, Article I, § 23; Illinois Constitution, Article I, § 6.

ff. For a more detailed discussion of the FCRA, see pp. 18–20.

issues for public employers and invasion-of-privacy issues for private employers. Monitoring restrooms or locker rooms, for example, absent extremely unusual circumstances and specific warnings that the areas are under video surveillance, likely will lead to claims of invasion of privacy or intentional infliction of emotional distress. Unionized employers may be obligated to bargain over the issue of employee surveillance.[84]

In addition to video surveillance, employers increasingly monitor the electronic communications of their employees. Although a number of states have wiretap laws that limit monitoring of employee communications, including criminal statutes, electronic and telephone surveillance also are governed by the federal Omnibus Crime Control and Safe Streets Act, as amended by the ECPA. The ECPA prohibits the intentional interception, use, and disclosure of oral, electronic, and wire communications, which includes communication via telephone, voice mail, and electronic mail.

There are a number of exceptions to the ECPA. For example, the "consent" exception allows monitoring when at least one party to the communication consents, either expressly or implicitly. (Note, however, that some state laws require two-party consent.) Because the issue of implied consent is very fact-specific, it is safest to obtain written consent from the employee prior to monitoring. The "service provider" exception allows an employee of the owner of a communication system to monitor communications if it is done within the normal course of his or her employment and the interception occurs as a result of necessary activity or in order to maintain and protect the rights and property of the service provider. The "business extension" exception includes monitoring with telephone equipment or components furnished to the user by a provider in the ordinary course of business and that are being used by the subscriber in the ordinary course of business. This exception potentially allows an employer to monitor an employee's telephone calls through the use of a standard telephone extension provided in the ordinary course of business.

The ECPA also protects "stored" communications (as opposed to communications in transit, as discussed earlier). However, the ECPA provides a broad exception that allows employers access to stored communications, if accessed pursuant to authorization by the entity providing the service. This exception should allow employers to access e-mail on computer systems provided by the employer.

Although monitoring of an employee's Internet use or computer files does not necessarily fall within the protective scope of the ECPA, there may be restrictions based on state laws and common law privacy claims. To minimize claims, employers should reduce employees' expectation of privacy through a clear and well-publicized Internet, e-mail, and social media use policy, and be consistent in exercising their right to manage the workplace in a legitimate, business-related manner. In light of the expanded use of digital medical records, such policies should be coordinated with policies addressing HIPAA and similar regulations.

Searches in the Workplace

On occasion, a healthcare employer may wish to search employer-provided lockers, desks, offices, or even personal items brought into the workplace. Because the Fourth Amendment's prohibition on unreasonable searches and seizures applies to government agencies and officers, public entities face some restrictions on their right to conduct workplace searches. Private employers, however, may conduct searches (if not acting in conjunction with police or government agents) without violating the U.S. Constitution. However, employers still must be careful, because state constitutions, statutes, and common law may limit the nature and scope of permissible searches.

Liability for employer searches turns in large part on the reasonableness of the employee's expectation of privacy and the reasonableness of the search. To minimize liability, employers should post notices and otherwise make clear to employees that their and the employer's property may be subject to searches and that the employer's request that they submit to a search is not an accusation of wrongdoing. In addition, employers should make efforts to limit the intrusiveness and potential for embarrassment of the search. The search should be kept confidential to the extent possible. Employers should notify employees that assigned desks, offices, or lockers may be searched; that the employer will keep an extra key; and that refusing to consent to a search may result in discipline. Persons who conduct the search should never physically touch the employee.

■ Safety in the Workplace

The Occupational Safety and Health Act (OSHA) is the primary workplace safety statute.[85] Under OSHA, employers have two primary duties: compliance with the health and safety standards promulgated by the Occupational Safety and Health Administration and compliance with the "general duty clause," which requires employers to provide a place of employment free from recognized hazards that are likely to cause death or serious physical harm.

OSHA mandates additional record keeping and reporting requirements as well.

There are a number of health and safety issues specific to the healthcare industry, including blood-borne pathogens and biological hazards, potential chemical and drug exposures, waste anesthetic gas exposures, ergonomic hazards, laser hazards, hazards associated with laboratories, needle-stick hazards, latex allergy, and radioactive materials and x-ray hazards, just to name a few. OSHA specifically addresses many of the hazards in the healthcare workplace. Because of the broad spectrum of potential risks to employee health and safety and the numerous regulations managing those risks, employers are advised to seek counsel's assistance in maintaining compliance.

Drug and Alcohol Testing

Drug and alcohol testing is an area full of potential legal pitfalls and may involve a number of legal issues, including the ADA, common law privacy protections, and, for public employers, state and federal constitutional issues. Even so, due in large part to the costs of substance abuse in the workplace, including lost productivity, absenteeism, and workplace accidents, employers are increasingly testing their employees and applicants. Moreover, failure to test, considering the safety-sensitive nature of most healthcare jobs and the general acceptance of drug testing by employers, may increase the possibility of liability for those employers who choose not to test. In addition, many federal contractors and grant recipients must take specific measures to ensure a drug-free workplace under the Drug-Free Workplace Act of 1988, although drug testing may not be required.[86]

Privacy claims likely are limited in many cases, considering that so many workers in the healthcare industry provide direct patient care and are thereby involved in safety-sensitive work. As such, the duty of care and responsibility owed a patient will invariably outweigh the privacy interests of a healthcare worker when the worker's responsibilities relate to the patient's welfare.[gg]

There are many different aspects of a testing program to consider. For example, drug and alcohol testing programs may provide that tests be conducted preemployment, on reasonable suspicion, postaccident, and/or on a random basis. Substance abuse policies should address such issues as who will be tested, what tests will be used, when testing will take place, the decision maker and the basis for the decision when reasonable suspicion testing

is involved, notification of employees and applicants, the consequences of a positive test, and safeguards for maintaining the confidentiality of testing information. As a result of the number and complexity of issues, employers are advised to obtain assistance of counsel when seeking to design and implement a substance abuse policy.

Environmental Issues

Materials handling practices at healthcare facilities can have an impact on patients, healthcare workers, and the surrounding community. Healthcare facilities face a number of environmental issues on a day-to-day basis, including medical, infectious, and hazardous waste, and wastewater discharge, all of which are governed by a variety of state and federal regulations. As with health and safety issues, involvement of counsel will assist in achieving and maintaining compliance.

■ Collective Bargaining and Protected Concerted Activities

Under the National Labor Relations Act of 1935 (NLRA), nonsupervisory private sector employees have the right to form, join, or assist labor organizations to bargain collectively and to engage in other protected, concerted activities.[87] This Congressional affirmation of rights ushered in a new era of union organizing. From the mid-1930s to 1958, the percentage of the private sector workforce represented by unions increased from approximately 14% to nearly 40%. In 2004, however, only about 8% of all employees in the private sector were represented by unions.[88] A variety of factors, including the change from a manufacturing- to a service-oriented economy, union corruption, increased efforts by management to oppose organizing, and the proliferation of laws designed to protect employees, contributed to this decline. Despite the relatively low levels of representation in the broader workplace, in recent years unions have dedicated significant resources to organizing employees in the healthcare industry.

The NLRA applies to nearly all private sector workplaces. Even though a physicians' practice may not have a union representing its employees, management should still be mindful of the NLRA. In addition to protecting employees' right to organize, the NLRA protects employees' right to engage in "concerted activities" for mutual aid or protection. Protected concerted activities are not limited to union organizing and strikes. Employee petitions, letter-writing campaigns, organized protests, or even comments on a Facebook page or other social media

---

gg. See, e.g., *American Federation of Government Employees, Local 2110 v. Derwinski,* 777 F. Supp. 1493 (Northern District of California 1991).

site, if undertaken with a view to discussing or improving the terms or conditions of employment, are activities arguably protected by the NLRA. Consequently, an employer that disciplines an employee for engaging in this type of conduct violates federal labor law. Such a violation is deemed an unfair labor practice.[hh]

Unfair Labor Practices

It is beyond the scope of this chapter to discuss all conduct that constitutes an unfair labor practice. Although unions also can commit unfair labor practices, this chapter focuses on the general prohibitions that apply to employers. An employer commits an unfair labor practice by doing any of the following:

- Interfering with, restraining, or coercing employees in their efforts to organize a union or to engage in other protected concerted activity
- Dominating or interfering with the formation or administration of a labor organization, or contributing to or supporting a labor organization[ii]
- Refusing to hire applicants, or terminating or otherwise discriminating against an employee because of the individual's support for, or membership in, a union
- Discharging or discriminating against an employee because he or she filed charges or provided testimony under the procedures of the NLRA
- Refusing to bargain collectively with a representative of its employees

Some general rules of conduct are obvious under these rules. For example, an employer cannot refuse to hire an applicant or cannot terminate an employee for being a union member or trying to organize a union in the workplace. Other rules are less intuitive. For example, the National Labor Relations Board (NLRB), with the approval of federal courts, has consistently held that an

employer may not prohibit its employees from discussing their wages in the workplace.[jj] Although it has been subject to much criticism and many past reversals, the current interpretation of the NLRA requires an employer to allow an employee to request and have a representative of his or her own choosing present during any interview or investigation that may lead to the employee's discipline or termination.[89] The representative must be a coworker, and contrary to prior interpretations of the NLRA, this right exists even if the employees do not have a union representing them in the workplace.

Employees' rights to engage in protected, concerted activity are not unchecked. Generally, employees cannot disparage an employer's product or services.[90] However, in the healthcare setting, at least one federal court found that two nurses engaged in protected, concerted activity when they were interviewed on television about their wages and staffing conditions at the hospital.[91]

In the context of labor organizing campaigns, an employer should anticipate that its conduct is likely to be scrutinized at a later date by the NLRB. Many labor law practitioners have reduced the NLRA's basic prohibitions in organizing campaigns to the helpful acronym, TIPS. An employer cannot Threaten or Interrogate its employees about union organizing or other protected concerted activity. An employer cannot Promise its employees any inducements (e.g., increased pay) to discourage interest in a union organizing effort. Nor can an employer spy or otherwise engage in any Surveillance of its employees' efforts to organize employees. Notwithstanding these rules, an employer has the right, as do its employees, to communicate its position on unions and union organizing and any facts relevant to that effort to its employees in a noncoercive, truthful manner.

Solicitation and Distribution

A common issue for employers, particularly in the context of an organizing campaign, is to what extent an employer may limit or govern employees' rights to solicit support for the union or other protected, concerted activity, or to distribute literature in the workplace. For most workplaces, the rules are fairly well settled. Lawful prohibitions for an employer include:

- Nonemployees generally can be prohibited from soliciting or distributing literature on the employer's property.
- Employees can be prohibited from soliciting other employees on employer property when the person

---

hh. The National Labor Relations Board, a five-member federal administrative agency, enforces and resolves disputes under the NLRA.

ii. The NLRA defines the term "labor organization" broadly and it includes, but is not limited to, a formally constituted union. An employer may commit an unfair labor practice by dominating or assisting any employee committee that exists for the purpose, in whole or in part, of dealing with employers concerning grievances, labor disputes, wages, rates of pay, hours of employment, or conditions of work. Employers have violated this provision by financing or forming employee committees. See *Grouse Mountain Assoc. II*, 333 NLRB No. 157 (2001). Congressional efforts to amend this portion of the statute have been unsuccessful.

jj. See, e.g., *Brockton Hosp. v. NLRB*, 294 F.3d 100 (D.C. Cir. 2002).

soliciting or being solicited is on working time. Working time does not include rest, meal, or other authorized breaks.

- Employees can be prohibited from distributing literature on employer property in nonworking areas during working time.
- Employees can be prohibited from distributing literature on employer property in working areas.

Many healthcare institutions, however, have facilities that are open to the public, and with their missions to care for sick or injured patients, special rules have emerged to govern solicitation and distribution issues in that setting. A healthcare facility may prohibit solicitation or distribution of materials by any employee at any time in immediate patient care areas of the facility. Immediate patient care areas include patient rooms, operating rooms, patient treatment areas, and corridors adjacent to those areas as well as elevators or stairways that are used substantially to transport patients.[kk]

On the other hand, a healthcare institution generally may ban distributions and solicitations in other areas only if necessary to avoid interference with the facility's operations or disturbance to patients.[92] For example, in a ruling upheld by a federal appellate court, the NLRB ruled that a hospital committed an unfair labor practice when it banned off-duty employees from distributing, at the hospital's front entrance, literature that addressed the alleged adverse impact on patient care resulting from the downsizing and restructuring of nursing staff.[92] The NLRB rejected the hospital's argument that the distribution of the literature, which allegedly contained "shocking and sensational headlines" and "horror stories" of patient injuries due to allegedly unsafe care at other healthcare institutions, constituted interference with the facility's operations and disturbance to its patients.[92]

For any solicitation and distribution policy to be valid, an employer must uniformly enforce the policy against all solicitation and distribution conduct, regardless of whether it is related to union activity. Courts have recognized, however, that permitting employee solicitations for charities such as the United Way or the Girl Scouts will not invalidate an otherwise broadly enforced nonsolicitation policy. Finally, a healthcare institution may have trouble enforcing bans on solicitation and distribution outside the building, particularly if the conduct is scheduled at times to coincide with shift changes.[93,94]

Electronic media have blurred the distinction between solicitation and distribution, and the law governing the

use of such media is beginning to emerge. An employee who sent to all employees an e-mail critical of a new vacation policy was found to have engaged in protected, concerted activity.[95] Similarly, an employer violated the NLRA by prohibiting an employee from displaying a union-related screen saver message on her computer that was seen by her coworkers.[96]

Organizing Rights

Until the 1970s, union organizing in the healthcare industry under the NLRA was not particularly widespread. Federal, state, and municipal hospitals are exempt from the NLRA's coverage, and until 1974 private nonprofit hospitals were not covered by the NLRA.[97] In 1974, however, Congress amended the NLRA to delete the exemption for nonprofit hospitals and to clarify the bargaining and strike obligations of employers in the healthcare industry. As a result, nonsupervisory employees of a healthcare institution may organize a union to represent them to bargain with their employer over the terms and conditions of their employment. The NLRA defines healthcare institutions as including "any hospital, convalescent hospital, health maintenance organization, health clinic, nursing home, extended-care facility, or other institution devoted to the care of sick, infirm, or aged persons."[98]

Under the NLRA, there are two ways for a union to gain the right to represent employees. First, an employer may voluntarily recognize a union as the majority representative of its employees. Second, if a union petitions the NLRB and can show support for the union among at least 30% of the employees in an appropriate unit, the NLRB will schedule an election among all the eligible employees in that unit to determine whether the union will represent those employees. If a majority of the employees voting in that election request that the union represent the employees for purposes of collective bargaining, then, absent any findings of election irregularities, the NLRB will certify the election results in favor of the union. Within certain parameters, an employer and its employees have the right to oppose the union's efforts to organize the employees.

One of the touchstones of the NLRA is that the NLRB will only certify a union as the representative of an appropriate unit for bargaining; that is, a group of employees with occupationally similar interests and concerns. For example, the NLRA provides that professional employees and nonprofessional employees may not be members of the same unit.[99]

Since 1935, the NLRB, through its quasi-judicial decision-making process, has developed general principles for units in a wide variety of industries. But in its 1974 amendments to the NLRA, Congress signaled to the

---

kk. See *Beth Israel Hospital v. NLRB*, 437 U.S. 483 (1978); see also *NLRB v. Baptist Hospital*, 442 U.S. 773 (1979).

NLRB that it should avoid the proliferation of bargaining units in the healthcare industry. In 1989, the NLRB responded by formally adopting a rule that established specific appropriate units for bargaining in acute care hospitals.[ll] Thus, in private acute care hospitals, the NLRB will conduct elections among employees seeking to be represented by a union petition only within one of these units.

Definition of Healthcare Institution Under the NLRA

The legislative history of the 1974 amendments to the NLRA links the definition of the term "healthcare institution" to the concept of "ongoing patient care":

> The scope of the application of the amendment is meant to include patient care situations and is not meant to include purely administrative health connected facilities. As an example, an insurance company specializing in medical coverage would not fall under the scope of these amendments, but would remain under general coverage of the act. An administrative facility or operation within a hospital, however, would be within the scope of the amendments as there would be a connection directly and indirectly with ongoing patient care. The crucial connection is the welfare of the patients and such connection would in certain cases be mere geographical proximity to ongoing patient care.[100]

Therefore, in its application of the healthcare amendments, the NLRB has distinguished between institutions directly involved in ongoing patient care and those it deems not directly involved. For example, in an early case applying the 1974 amendments to bargaining unit determinations, the NLRB determined that an independent, nonprofit blood bank, which served the needs of a number of area hospitals by recruiting blood donors and testing, processing, and distributing blood, was not a healthcare institution.[101] In another early case, the NLRB found that an employer that operated a diagnostic medical laboratory service that tested human blood, body fluid, and tissue for hospitals, clinics, nursing homes,

and individual doctors was not a healthcare institution within the meaning of the NLRA.[101] The NLRB determined that "the employer's operations is [sic] analogous to that of blood banks which the board has found not to be involved in patient care."[101,mm]

More recently, the NLRB again considered whether a blood bank constitutes a healthcare institution for unit determination purposes. In Syracuse Region Blood Center (SRBC),[102] the blood center at issue was the sole source of blood-related services for 38 hospitals in a 15-county area in central New York State, operating at a central facility, three fixed satellite sites, various mobile sites, and, to a limited degree, at hospitals. The blood center primarily performed homologous blood collections (i.e., from healthy donors), as well as autologous collections, donor pheresis (in which platelets or other components of the blood are retained by the bank for future use), patient pheresis (in which diseased or unwanted components of the blood are removed and the rest returned to the patient), and therapeutic phlebotomies (drawing blood for therapeutic purposes). The center's laboratories tested blood samples for blood type, antibodies, and diseases; performed laboratory work related to pheresis procedures; and performed 25 to 30 immunohematology consultations per month with hospitals or physicians seeking medical advice. The blood center's operations also included a bone marrow donor program and a tissue bank program.

The NLRB found that only two of the blood center's activities, patient pheresis and therapeutic phlebotomies, "indisputably involve patient care."[102] Although such activities made up only a small fraction of SRBC's overall operations (a combined total of 400 to 600 per year, in contrast with about 94,000 donor blood collections per year), the board found it sufficient to accord SRBC healthcare institution status, stating that "we find that [patient pheresis and therapeutic phlebotomies] are performed with sufficient regularity and in a sufficiently large number . . . that the employer is properly viewed to be devoted to the care of sick . . . persons" within the meaning of the NLRA.[102]

The board in Syracuse Region Blood Center summarily discounted the center's performance of laboratory services and its consultations with hospitals and physicians, as "[n]either of those functions is an indicator of health care institution status."[102(n.8)] The center's

---

ll. The eight units appropriate for acute care hospitals are registered nurses, physicians, all other professionals, technical employees, skilled maintenance employees, business-office clericals, guards, and all other nonprofessionals. Acute care hospitals are defined as those in which (1) the average length of patient stay is less than 30 days, or (2) more than 50% of all patients are admitted to units in which the average length of stay is less than 30 days.

---

mm. See also *Boston Medical Laboratory, Inc.*, 235 NLRB 1271, n.2 (1978) (concluding that "testing human medical specimens does not involve patient care"); *Center for Laboratory Medicine, Inc.*, 234 NLRB 387 (1978).

participation in bone marrow and tissue donor programs likewise provided no basis for the NLRB's decision, which rested solely on the activities that it deemed "indisputably" to involve the care of patients.[nn]

Special Issues in Organizing Campaigns

Supervisors have no authority to organize a union in the workplace because they are not covered by the NLRA. Among healthcare employers, the question of whether a particular group of employees are supervisors within the meaning of the NLRA has been a difficult issue. Employees with advanced education or training are not necessarily supervisors. Indeed, the NLRA provides for organizing among professional employees. Under the NLRA, a supervisor is any individual having authority, in the interest of the employer, to hire, transfer, suspend, lay off, recall, promote, discharge, assign, reward, or discipline other employees, or responsibility to direct them, or to adjust their grievances or effectively to recommend such action, if in connection with the foregoing the exercise of such authority is not of a merely routine or clerical nature, but requires the use of independent judgment.[103]

Defining whether a registered nurse is a supervisor is a fact-intensive issue, and litigation over that issue, particularly in the long-term healthcare industry, has been widespread.[oo] In acute care hospitals, registered nurses are often found not to be supervisors, but this generalization has exceptions, particularly for those nurses, such as in-charge nurses, who are involved in assigning work and managing other registered nurses.

Another issue of special interest has been whether interns and residents are "employees" under the NLRA. If so, then interns and residents have the right to organize unions and have the other protections afforded them under the federal labor law. The NLRB overturned 20 years of precedent by concluding that interns and residents—who are usually students as well—are covered by the NLRA.[104]

The applicability of the NLRA to employees of a contractor, such as a temporary services agency, may also prove nettlesome for employers in the healthcare industry, where the use of temporary workers is commonplace. In 2000, the NLRB, overturning its own precedent, determined that temporary workers may be included in the same bargaining unit with an employer's regular employees, even if the temporary agency and the employer do not consent to bargain as joint employers.[105] In *M.B. Sturgis Inc.*, the temporary workers performed the same work as the employer's employees, were subject to the same supervision, and were disciplined by the employer's supervisors (as opposed to the temporary agency's supervisors). The employer and the temporary agency were found to be joint employers of the temporary workers. The NLRB ruled, contrary to its prior decisional law, that where such a joint employer relationship exists between a temporary agency and a contracting employer, the NLRB may apply its established standards for determining whether all the relevant workers, irrespective of their particular employer, may be included in a single bargaining unit, notwithstanding that the employers may not consent to bargaining jointly with a union over terms and conditions of employment.[105]

Unless and until the courts review the NLRB's new interpretation of the NLRA as reflected in *M.B. Sturgis Inc.*, or the NLRB revisits its determination, the case will pose new and complicated challenges to healthcare employers. The decision will complicate the collective bargaining process for agencies and employers alike and may subject them to bargaining obligations and collective bargaining agreements covering employees over whom they may exercise very little control.

Private Recognition Agreements

Aside from NLRB-governed elections, there are other ways for employees and unions to persuade employees to select a union to represent them for purposes of collective bargaining. Unions have increasingly requested employers to agree to use private recognition agreements allowing employees to decide whether a union should represent their workforce. Private recognition agreements are being used with more frequency when a union already represents some portion of the employer's employees. In the healthcare industry, particularly in California, these agreements have become a more commonly used means of resolving issues of employee representation.

Private recognition agreements come in a wide variety; they are purely contractual arrangements between an employer and a union that govern the process by which employees decide whether a union should represent them. The hallmark of a private recognition agreement is that the parties decide not to use the NLRB election process. Some agreements are purely "card-check" agreements, whereby if a union presents signed authorization cards from a majority of the employees within a particular unit,

---

nn. Cf. *No. Suburban Blood Center v. NLRB*, 661 F.2d 632, 635 (7th Cir. 1981) (stating that "the crucial factor in the definition of health care institution is patient welfare" and rejecting the NLRB's view that patient care must physically occur at the facility to qualify it as a healthcare institution).

oo. See generally *NLRB v. Kentucky River Community Care*, 121 S. Ct. 1861 (2001).

the employer voluntarily agrees to recognize the union as the exclusive bargaining agent for the employees in that unit. Alternatively, the parties may agree to have an election that requires the employer to remain neutral in the campaign or grants the union certain access rights to share information with the employees.

Another common feature is an agreement that the parties will rely on arbitration to resolve disputes over unit definitions, voter eligibility, or conduct in violation of the parties' agreement. If a majority of the employees in an appropriate unit select a union to represent them, the employer agrees to recognize and begin bargaining in good faith with the union over terms and conditions of employment. Management and labor often disagree on the wisdom or fairness of private recognition agreements, but their increased use means employers must be prepared to deal with requests to use them.

Strikes and Picketing at Healthcare Institutions

A major purpose of Congress's 1974 amendments to the NLRA was "to minimize the potential for increased disruption of health care delivery resulting from increased labor activity by employees of health care institutions now that their activities were protected by the act."[106] Congress recognized that the traditional legal means employed by unions to bring pressure upon employers could cause disruptions and threats to health and safety in the healthcare industry if unchecked. Therefore, in addition to expanding the NLRA's coverage in the healthcare industry, the 1974 amendments also added Section 8(g) of the NLRA, which requires that a labor organization give 10 days' written notice "before engaging in any strike, picketing, or other concerted refusal to work at any health care institution. . . ."[107] Note, however, that only "healthcare institutions" are entitled to such notice.[pp]

Section 8(g)'s mandate applies to all picketing, regardless of the nature, character, or objectives of the picketing or the type of economic pressures generated.[108] Determining what activities require advance notice under Section 8(g) is a very fact-specific inquiry, but the NLRB has found it to extend beyond traditional ambulatory picketing and to include a union's mass[109] and a press conference conducted by a union outside a hospital entrance, accompanied by persons "milling around" the facility and holding signs regarding staffing levels.[110] On the other hand, in an advice memorandum, the general counsel of the NLRB opined that a large

number of union supporters' confrontational disruption and demonstration at a health fair held by a hospital on its own grounds was not "picketing" within the meaning of Section 8(g).[111]

Mergers and Effects on Bargaining

Given the proliferation of mergers and alliances in the healthcare industry, it is important for unionized institutions to be cognizant of their potential bargaining obligations with respect to mergers. The duty to bargain under the NLRA is limited to matters of "wages, hours, and other terms and conditions of employment. . . ."[112] There is no duty to bargain over management decisions that have an indirect and attenuated impact on the employment relationship and that are at the "core of entrepreneurial control."[113,114] Some management decisions involving the scope and direction of an enterprise are not primarily about conditions of employment, although the effect of the decisions necessarily may be to terminate employment. In such cases, although there may be no duty to bargain over a managerial decision, there is a duty to bargain about the results or effects of that decision.[113(at 677)] Bargaining over the effects of a decision must be conducted in a meaningful manner and at a meaningful time.[113(at 681–2)]

A decision to merge two unrelated corporate entities is not subject to a duty to bargain, but an employer may or may not have an obligation to bargain about the effects of a decision to merge.[115] Although there may be no duty to bargain about effects of a merger, there may still be a duty to provide information relevant to "effects bargaining." In general, an employer has "a duty to provide relevant information needed by a labor union for the proper performance of its duties as the employees' bargaining representative."[116] In one case, the NLRB found that two healthcare institutions had breached their duty to bargain in good faith by withholding information that a union had requested in connection with a planned merger. The union sought copies of documents explicating the merger's terms, plans for or information about proposed staffing changes at one hospital in consequence of the merger, and all documents pertaining to the hospitals' proposed corporate status within the merged group of facilities. The NLRB found the information to be relevant to the union's obligations, even though not directly linked to terms and conditions of employment. The Court of Appeals upheld the NLRB's determination, stating that "as long as a pending merger is sufficiently advanced, a union is entitled to request information shown by the totality of the circumstances to be relevant in order to prepare for effects bargaining."[117]

---

pp. See notes 97-103 and accompanying text.

Employment Eligibility Verification

Form I-9 Requirements

The primary immigration-related issue for all employers involves the verification of employees', including U.S. citizens', authorization to work in the United States. The Immigration Reform and Control Act of 1986 (IRCA), and its various amendments in 1990 and 1996, subject all employers and recruiters to civil and criminal penalties for knowingly hiring, recruiting or referring for a fee, or continuing to employ an unauthorized worker. IRCA attempts to balance the interests of prohibiting unauthorized employment of aliens and preventing discrimination against aliens and citizens alike. Performing their responsibilities under IRCA can be complicated and confusing for employers. Healthcare employers, which are often dependent on transient or less-skilled workers for a variety of tasks, receive and review more than their share of confusing documents, made all the more difficult by the often ready availability of fraudulent work-authorization and identity papers. The next few pages will touch on most of the important issues surrounding verification, especially in regard to the healthcare industry.

Employers and employees alike have responsibilities under IRCA, which prohibits an employer from knowingly hiring or continuing to employ an alien who does not have authorization for employment in the United States.[qq] An employer must screen each employee for identity and employment authorization. Every individual hired after November 6, 1986, must present evidence of employment authorization and identity to his or her employer. Every employer must examine and record this evidence on a Form I-9, which must be retained and made available upon request to the U.S. Citizenship and Immigration Services (USCIS) (formerly the Immigration and Naturalization Service) and other government agencies.

The first step in ensuring employment verification compliance is understanding who is and is not an "employee" who is subject to IRCA. Relevant exceptions for the healthcare industry include independent contractors. The regulations promulgated pursuant to IRCA define independent contractors as "individuals or entities who carry on independent business, contract to do a piece of work according to their own means and methods, and are subject to control only as to results."[118]

Thus, for example, individuals who provide services to a group of physicians, but who are employed by an agency contracted to provide such services to the group (such as a temp or employee leasing agency), are not considered employees of the physicians' group under IRCA.

Nevertheless, it should be noted that any person who enters into a contract, subcontract, or exchange to obtain the services of an alien knowing that the alien does not have authorization to perform the services is considered to have violated the employer sanctions provisions of IRCA.[119] For example, a hospital that contracts with a physical therapist as an independent contractor, knowing that he or she has an H-1B work authorization for another unrelated hospital, could be found to have violated IRCA.

Another class of individuals not considered to be employees are volunteers. Volunteers are individuals who provide their services without any compensation, including room and board, gifts, or other benefits.[120] A volunteer may receive certain benefits from the "employer," but the work arrangement must have been entered into without the expectation of compensation, and the benefit must not have been offered in exchange for the work.[121] Thus, a resident physician "moonlighting" in an ER is likely not a volunteer for I-9 purposes, and if that resident is a foreign national and does not have valid work authorization for the hospital, the hospital faces violations of both the verification and sanctions provisions of IRCA.

Employees have the affirmative duty under IRCA of proving both their identity and work eligibility.[122] At their time of hire, employees are required to complete the first section of the I-9 employment eligibility verification form. In addition, the employee must verify, under penalty of perjury, his or her status as a citizen or national of the United States, a lawful permanent resident, or an alien authorized to work in the United States. Failure to sign or date Section 1 of the I-9 is one of the most frequent mistakes made in completing the form. Ultimately, ensuring that the employee completes Section 1 fully is the employer's responsibility.

Section 1 of the I-9 form must be completed "at the time of hire," which is defined by the regulations as "the actual commencement of employment of an employee for wages or other remuneration."[123] The employee has three business days from the date of hire in which to present the documentation supporting the assertions in Section 1.[124] Upon reviewing these documents, the employer must immediately complete Section 2 of the I-9. If the employee cannot produce the actual documents within 3 days, then he or she may present a receipt showing application for a replacement document or a Form I-94 indicating either

qq. Employment is defined by the USCIS regulations as "any service or labor performed by an employee for an employer within the United States." 8 C.F.R. § 274a.1(h).

temporary evidence of permanent resident status or refugee status.[125] These are the only three situations in which a receipt can be accepted; a receipt is otherwise unacceptable.

In Section 2 of the I-9, the employer or its agent must attest under penalty of perjury that it has reviewed Section 1 and the documents required to attest to the accuracy of the responses. The I-9 form contains a list of the acceptable documents that an employee may present to the employer for inspection within 3 days of hire. If the individual is employed for less than 3 days, the documentation must be presented the day of hire. The employer is also required to note on the I-9 form the information disclosed in the documents and to sign and date the form.

Form I-9 contains three lists of documents from which the employee may choose to show identity and/ or employment authorization in order for the employer to complete Section 2. It is the employee's choice; the employer may not request or suggest any particular document. The employee may produce one document from List A that shows both identity and authorization to work in the United States or he or she may present one document from List B, establishing identity, and one from List C, showing employment authorization. The employee must produce originals, not copies, for the employer to review.[rr]

Although verification is very important, the employer always must be careful not to demand more or different documents than those necessary to comply with the verification requirements. An employer who demands more or different documents can be guilty of discrimination if it is proven that the demands were made with discriminatory intent. An employer cannot refuse to honor documents that on their face reasonably appear to be genuine and relate to the person presenting them. The employer may, but is not required to, photocopy and attach to the I-9 form the documentation presented by the employee.[126] Photocopies do not excuse failure to complete the form, however. If the employer decides to make copies, he should do so for all employees so as to avoid a charge of discrimination.

An employer of an individual who is a member of a collective bargaining unit and who is employed under a collective bargaining agreement between one or more unions and a multiemployer association may use an I-9 form completed within the past 3 years by a prior employer who is a member of the same association. This applies to persons hired 60 days or more after September 30, 1996, the effective date of the Illegal Immigration Reform and Immigrant Responsibility Act (IIRAIRA).

An employer is not required to verify eligibility for employment if the employee is not a new hire but is "continuing" his or her employment.[127] An employee is continuing his or her employment if at all times he or she has a "reasonable expectation of employment."[127] The USCIS regulations set out a number of situations in which employment is deemed to be continuing, such as during paid or unpaid leaves, strikes or labor disputes, and corporate reorganizations.[128]

Section 3 of the I-9 form is used when appropriate to update and reverify employment information. Employers are required to reverify employment eligibility when an employee's work authorization expires, and it is the employer's responsibility to maintain a system to prompt him or her to reverify employee information by the correct deadline.[129] The same rules regarding documents apply for reverification as for verification. If, at the time of updating and/or reverification, the employee's name has changed, then the employer must complete Section 3, Block A, of Form I-9. If an employee is rehired within 3 years of the date the I-9 was originally completed, and the employee is still eligible for employment on the same basis as indicated on the form, the employer would complete Section 3, Block B, and the signature block.[130]

If the employer needs to correct the I-9 form, the new information should be inserted, signed, and dated as of the time of the insertion. If the omission or mistake was in Section 1, the employee should also sign and date the correction. The form should never be backdated.

The employer must retain all I-9 forms, which are actually the property of the U.S. government. The employer is required to retain the I-9 forms for at least 3 years, or for 1 year after the employee's termination date, whichever is later.[131] I-9 forms should not be destroyed if the USCIS is in the process of investigating the employer. The employer must produce the forms at the request of the USCIS or other selected government entities; failure to do so is considered a violation of the Immigration and Nationality Act (INA).[132]

Failure to complete, correct, update, reverify, retain, or produce the I-9 form may result in a finding of a violation of the verification requirements. Employers may also face liability for failure to comply with the timeliness requirements (e.g., completion of the I-9 form within

---

rr. The actual document list is set out in the *Handbook for Employers M-274* (available from the USCIS website, http://www.uscis.gov). Employers may continue to reference the full list of documents on the current Lists A, B, and C in the handbook.

3 days of starting employment).[ss] Fines for paperwork violations occurring before September 29, 1999, are between $100 and $1000 for each individual for which a mistake or omission was made; fines for violations occurring on or after September 29, 1999, are between $110 and $1100.[133,134] In addition to imposing fines, the USCIS has the authority to require employers to take corrective action, such as education and posting notices.[135] Five factors are to be considered when setting the penalty: (1) the size of the employer's business, (2) the employer's good faith, (3) the seriousness of the violation, (4) whether the individual involved was an unauthorized alien, and (5) whether the employer has a history of previous violations.[134,tt] Additional factors may be considered, such as the ability of the employer to pay the proposed penalty.[136]

The IIRAIRA added an exemption for employers who have technical or procedural violations of the regulations. For technical or procedural failures to complete the form properly, if the employer made a good faith attempt to comply, the USCIS must explain the problem to the employer and allow 10 days for correction. If the failures are not corrected, penalties are imposed. The exemption does not relieve an employer who has engaged in "pattern and practice" of violations. This provision, added by the IIRAIRA, applies to failures occurring on or after September 30, 1996. Some examples of technical errors include failing to include an address or date on the form, accepting a List B document with a missing expiration date, or failing to date Section 2 of the form.

Substantive Violations of IRCA

Employers and recruiters are prohibited from knowingly hiring, recruiting or referring for a fee, or continuing to employ an unauthorized alien.[137] If the employer has attempted in good faith to comply with the employment verification requirements of IRCA, it has an affirmative defense against a violation finding, but that presumption can be rebutted if the USCIS can establish that the documents relied upon did not reasonably appear to be genuine. Employers are also prohibited from continuing to employ an unauthorized alien once his or her status is known.[138]

An employer's knowledge of the status of the unauthorized worker may be actual (evidenced by other employees or admissions of the employer's agents) or

constructive. The regulations define constructive knowledge as "knowledge which may fairly be inferred through notice of certain facts and circumstances which would lead a person, through the exercise of reasonable care, to know about a certain condition."[139]

Individuals or entities who knowingly employ unauthorized workers are subject to civil fines.[140-142] First-time violators for offenses that occurred prior to September 29, 1999, can be fined $250 to $2000 for each alien. The fine is between $2000 and $5000 for second offenders. After that, repeat offenders can be fined in the range of $3000 to $10,000 per alien for offenses occurring before September 29, 1999. For violations that occurred on or after September 29, 1999, the penalties are 10% higher in each category and range from $275 to $2200 for the first violation, $2200 to $5500 for the second violation, and $3300 to $11,000 for the third violation.

In addition to its regulations, the USCIS has set out guidelines for determining penalties within these ranges.[143] These guidelines provide for leniency for first-time violators and calculate fines starting at the statutory minimum with adjustments upward depending on aggravating factors. Fines for repeat violators start at the statutory maximum and work down accounting for mitigating factors. Criminal penalties (up to a $3000 fine for each unauthorized alien and 6 months imprisonment) may be imposed for pattern or practice violations.[144] The term "pattern or practice" covers "regular, repeated, and intentional activities" but does not include "isolated, sporadic, or accidental acts."[145]

In addition, it is a criminal violation for any person knowingly or in reckless disregard of the fact that the alien has come to, entered, or remains in the United States in violation of the law, to conceal, harbor, or shield from detection such alien in any such place, including any buildings or any means of transportation.[146] An employer may face criminal fines and/or imprisonment for up to 5 years for hiring 10 or more aliens that the employer knows were brought into the United States illegally in violation of the alien smuggling/criminal harboring provision.

Discrimination

The INA also contains antidiscrimination provisions that make it unlawful for persons or other entities (employers with four or more employees) from discriminating against an individual in hiring, discharging, recruiting, or referring for a fee because of national origin or citizenship status.[147] An employer cannot set different employment verification standards or require different groups of employees to present additional documentation, nor can it request that an employee present more or different documents than are required or refuse to accept a document that on its face

---

ss. *United States v. Peking Inc.*, 2 OCAHO 329 (June 18, 1991) (holding that an employer may not have an individual commence work prior to inspection of documents).

tt. See also 69 Interpreter Releases 253, 255–256 (Mar. 2, 1992).

appears genuine and related to the individual presenting it, if done for the purpose of discriminating against the individual.[148,uu] An employer cannot retaliate against an individual because he or she intends to file a charge or complaint, testify, or participate in any way in a proceeding under IRCA.[149] Moreover, an employer cannot refuse to accept a document or to hire an individual on the basis of a future expiration date on the document.

There are exceptions to the antidiscrimination provisions. For example, the provisions do not apply to employers with three or fewer employees.[150] In addition, the citizenship discrimination provisions do not apply to actions that are required in order to comply with any law, regulation, or executive order; required by any federal, state, or local government contract; or determined by the attorney general to be essential for an employer to do business with the federal, state, or local government.[151] The antidiscrimination provisions do not apply to national origin discrimination if the individual is covered by Section 703 of the Civil Rights Act of 1964.[152] On an individual basis, an employer may legally prefer a U.S. citizen or national over an alien with equal qualifications, but the qualifications of each must be equal.[153]

The antidiscrimination provisions are controversial because of their inherent conflict with the sanctions imposed against employers who hire unauthorized aliens. Balancing these two obligations can be burdensome to employers, who are prohibited from asking for different documents or more information, but are nevertheless subject to civil or criminal liability if they hire an unauthorized alien.[154]

The civil penalties for violations of the antidiscrimination provisions occurring prior to September 29, 1999, range from $250 to $2000 per person for a first offense, $2000 to $5000 for a second offense, and $3000 to $10,000 for a third offense. For offenses on or after September 29, 1999, the penalties increase by 10%: $275 to $2200 per person for the first violation; $2200 to $5500 for the second violation, and $3300 to $11,000 for the third violation. There are no criminal penalties for violations of the antidiscrimination provisions.

■ Conducting an Effective Internal Investigation

Employers in the healthcare industry, like those in virtually every other industry, face a burgeoning number of employee complaints and lawsuits alleging discrimination, harassment, financial improprieties, and other forms of alleged unlawful conduct in the workplace. In response—and as part of their continuous efforts to comply with increased federal and state regulation of workplace conduct—employers in the last decade drafted and disseminated to their workforce policies regarding equal employment opportunity, antidiscrimination, and workplace conduct. By the latter half of the decade, employers were, as never before, enforcing these policies by conducting internal investigations into employee complaints of misconduct.

For every action there is a reaction, and as employers increased their use of investigations, employees' lawyers responded by challenging the manner in which employers conducted their investigations. Employers began to see a new kind of legal claim—that they failed to conduct a proper investigation into the alleged misconduct. The difficult irony of this type of claim is that it has been made by the employee who raised the issue that resulted in the investigation and/or by the employee who was the subject of the investigation, depending on whichever individual was dissatisfied with the outcome.

Internal investigations have become an integral part of today's workplace. Effective investigations will often provide an employer with a successful defense to employment-related lawsuits. Conversely, an inadequate investigation may expose an employer to additional legal liability. For these reasons, it is critical that employers understand how to conduct effective internal investigations.

The Employer's Burden of Proof: What You Need and Do Not Need to Establish

Many employers fail to understand their "burden of proof" in conducting internal investigations, incorrectly fearing they have to prove "beyond a reasonable doubt" that the alleged misconduct occurred or did not occur. The real world does not work that way. Most employers lack the time and resources necessary to conduct the type of protracted and exhaustive fact-finding process that one associates with our judicial system. Fortunately, when reviewing employers' internal investigations in employment-related lawsuits, most courts do not impose on employers the same jurisprudential burdens of proof required in a court of law.

The standard of proof adopted by most courts can be paraphrased as follows: When reaching a decision in response to a workplace complaint of misconduct, the employer must make a good faith determination based on reasonable grounds that sufficient cause existed for its decision. The bottom line is that in order to take action against an employee for suspected misconduct, the employer need not be absolutely certain that the misconduct actually

---

uu. The IIRAIRA added the requirement that the request for more or different documents or refusal to accept proffered documents had to be done with the intent to discriminate.

occurred; the employer need only have acted in good faith and based on reasonable grounds.

What an Employer Must Do Before Conducting Any Investigation

The first step in conducting any investigation is to determine the most appropriate and effective method.[vv] It generally is advisable to contact competent legal counsel for assistance on this important threshold determination. It is important to make sure that the investigation is overseen and controlled by one person with competence, training, experience, and impartiality. Although it is sometimes necessary to have more than one person involved in the investigation (where, for instance, numerous interviews need to be conducted in a very short period of time), it is important to keep the investigation in as few hands as possible. This approach reduces the risk of inadvertent disclosure and aids in the ability to make consistent credibility assessments and factual findings.

Typically, the employer's human resources director should be responsible for assuring the integrity of the investigation process. A well-trained HR representative should conduct the investigation, collect the facts, draw conclusions, document the results, and make a recommendation to management. Management typically should be responsible for reviewing the recommendations of HR and making the decision to implement some or all of HR's recommendations. The investigation, when done properly, is an interactive, collaborative process between HR and management.

Initial Meeting with the Complaining Employee

The second step in the investigation generally is to meet with the complaining employee to determine whether an investigation is even necessary and, if so, to determine the nature and scope of that investigation. As with all investigative interviews, it is extremely important that the investigator take accurate and thorough notes during the initial meeting.

---

vv. In some cases, and for some employers, the investigation should be conducted by an outside counsel or other qualified professional. It is beyond the scope of this chapter to discuss investigations conducted by outside experts; suffice it to say that such investigations merit additional considerations, including (1) the possibility that federal and state law may afford certain employee notification rights not implicated by an investigation conducted strictly by the employer itself, and (2) the possibility that an investigation conducted by outside counsel may protect certain information under the attorney–client privilege and attorney work product doctrine.

In addition to identifying all of the relevant issues and assembling all of the relevant facts, the initial meeting should accomplish the following:

- Give the complaining employee confidence in the investigation process
- Emphasize the company's commitment to resolving the issues promptly and effectively
- Reassure the employee that the company does not tolerate retaliation against an employee who comes forward with a legitimate complaint, and invite him or her to let you know if he or she subsequently feels that he or she has been subjected to any retaliation
- Tell the employee that the company will limit the disclosure of information to those persons who have a legitimate business need to know (but do not promise confidentiality)
- Instruct the employee that he or she has a duty to keep the investigation and underlying issues confidential, and that the failure to do so may unduly affect the outcome of the investigation and result in discipline
- Make sure the employee understands that his or her continuing cooperation is necessary for a complete investigation and an effective resolution

If, after the initial meeting, the investigator determines that an investigation is warranted, the investigator should encourage (but not require) the complaining employee to provide a written summary of the issues and facts, and to identify all relevant documentation and witnesses. That will ensure that the investigator correctly understands all of the facts and issues raised and will avoid any misunderstandings later on. Regardless of whether the complaining employee provides a written summary, the investigator generally should give the employee a memo confirming the substance of the issues raised. Confirming the issues in writing will give the investigator and the complaining employee an opportunity to make sure all of the issues are clearly understood before starting the investigation.

Planning the Investigation

It is critical that the investigator organize and plan the nature and scope of the investigation before beginning to interview witnesses. Before interviewing anyone, therefore, consider whether there are any company policies or practices that apply to the situation. Identify and review all documents that may assist in conducting the investigation. If the company has a unionized workforce, consider whether the complaint implicates the collective bargaining agreement.

The investigator must give careful thought as to which employees should be interviewed. Cast too broad a net, and the investigator risks interviewing individuals to whom the existence and facts of the investigation should not be disclosed; cast too narrow a net, and he or she risks not interviewing individuals who may have valuable information. The obvious individuals include the complaining employee, the employee who is the subject of the investigation, percipient witnesses, and persons with relevant information and/or documents.

Give some thought to the order of the interviews. Sometimes there are strategic benefits to be gained by speaking with certain individuals before or after others. It is usually better to hold off on interviewing the peripheral players until after interviewing the key individuals, because it may be possible to conclude the investigation without even interviewing the peripheral players. A thoughtful ordering of witnesses may prevent unnecessary disclosure of information and lead to a more effective use of the company's resources.

Conducting the Investigation: Interviewing Witnesses

The effectiveness of an investigation will depend on how adept the investigator is at gathering the facts and then sifting through them to determine which ones are relevant and which ones are not. In most investigations the fact-gathering process is composed largely of interviewing witnesses, and it is critical that the investigator be well trained in the art of the interview. Preparation is the key.

Prepare a standard opening statement to use for each interview. The statement should address the concerns that the interviewee typically might have, such as the general subject of the investigation, what role the interviewee is playing in the investigation, how the information you receive from the interviewee will be used, whether the information will be kept confidential, and the possibility that the interviewee could be disciplined as a result of the investigation.

Outline the issues to be covered for each interview. Under each issue, list every fact that pertains to that issue. Under each fact leave room to write down the interviewee's response. Careful note taking is critical. Get down as many of the facts as possible during the interview, and complete the interview notes immediately after the conclusion of the interview.

Knowing how to ask a question is just as important as knowing what questions to ask. It is beyond the scope of this chapter to provide detailed pointers on effective interview questioning. However, the following are some issues that should be covered:

- Anticipate the questions likely to be asked by the interviewees and be ready with logical, reasonable responses.
- Be sensitive to the fact that being interviewed as part of an investigation can be stressful. (Putting the interviewee at ease also helps elicit information.)
- Stress that no conclusions will be reached until all of the facts are gathered and analyzed.
- Stress that information will be disseminated on a need-to-know basis only. (Again, do not promise confidentiality.)
- Stress that the interviewee has a strict duty to keep the investigation information confidential.
- Inform the interviewee that the company will not tolerate retaliation against employees who participate in an investigation.
- Explain that any employee who intentionally misdirects or interferes with an investigation will be subject to discipline.

Develop a standard closing:

- Ask the interviewee if there is anyone else he or she thinks should be interviewed.
- Review the interviewee's answers.
- Instruct the interviewee to contact you if he or she remembers or learns of additional information.
- Reemphasize the interviewee's obligation to maintain the confidentiality of the investigation.
- Answer any questions the person may have.
- Explain in general terms what will happen with the investigation from that point forward and when you expect to reach a determination.

When an Employee Asks to Have a Representative Attend the Interview: Weingarten Rights

Regardless of whether you have a unionized or union-free workforce, you need to be aware of your employees' Weingarten rights. First recognized by the U.S. Supreme Court in 1975 with respect to unionized employees only,[155] Weingarten rights entitle an employee under the NLRA to have a coworker present during an investigative interview that the employee reasonably believes may result in his or her being disciplined. In 2001, a federal court of appeals for the first time extended these Weingarten rights to nonunionized employees.[89]

Although it remains unclear whether other federal courts of appeal or the U.S. Supreme Court will adopt that extension of the law, nonunionized employers need to be aware of the possibility that Weingarten rights may apply to their workforce.

If an employee who reasonably believes that he or she may be disciplined in connection with an investigative interview requests the presence of a coworker in the interview, you must comply with that request in order to avoid the risk of having an unfair labor practices charge filed against you under the NLRA. If you are presented with a request to have a coworker present, you should decide among the following three options: (1) decline to proceed with the interview entirely; (2) proceed with the interview with the requested coworker present; or (3) represent to the employee that he or she will not be subjected to any discipline in connection with the investigation, thereby allowing you to proceed with the interview without the coworker being present.

Reaching a Conclusion and Making a Recommendation

After the investigator has conducted all of the necessary interviews and assembled all of the relevant facts, the investigator must analyze those facts and reach a conclusion as to what actually took place. Basic life experiences, common sense, and logic skills are required to do so. In determining what actually took place, examine the objective facts in order to reach a logical conclusion. Remember, it is permissible to be wrong in your conclusion—so long as you acted in good faith based on reasonable grounds.

After analyzing the facts and reaching a conclusion as to what happened, the investigator makes a recommendation to the appropriate member(s) of management regarding what, if any, action(s) should be taken. In formulating a recommendation, consider the following factors:

- Were any of the company's policies violated, and if so, was it a serious offense?
- What has the company done in the past in response to similar violations?
- How long has the employee who violated the policy been with the company, has he or she violated any other policies in the past, and what is his or her performance history?
- Are there any other circumstances that could affect your recommendation?
- What is your goal, and will the proposed course of action achieve that goal?

The investigator generally should conclude his investigation by compiling his or her findings, conclusions, and recommendations in an investigative report.

Implementing the Results of the Investigation

Management depends on the investigator to assist it in reaching an appropriate resolution of the issue. However, it ultimately must be a member of management who makes the decision as to what action to take and who will implement that action.

Management must make sure that the appropriate person follows up with the complaining employee to make sure he or she is properly informed of the investigation results. Management also must make sure that the appropriate person follows up with the accused employee, and describes the course and results of the investigation. The person who meets with the accused must be prepared to explain why the company reached the results it did. Anticipate the employee's questions and be prepared to answer them. Typically, the accused should be notified in writing of the results of the investigation. The memo is important, so it must be drafted carefully. Explain the issues that were raised, the steps that were taken, the conclusions that were drawn, the information on which those conclusions were based, and the actions being taken as a result. Encourage the employee to provide any additional information, and conclude by informing the employee whom to contact if he or she has any questions or additional information.

In most cases it is inappropriate to inform other employees about the results of the investigation. If you should be asked about the results by an employee who was interviewed in connection with the investigation, simply explain that the information is confidential and thank him or her for the assistance.

The Final Investigation File

At the conclusion of the investigation, a final investigation file should be assembled. The file should consist of whatever information needs to be kept for the company record. The file generally should show the key steps that were taken to investigate and respond to the issues raised, including the following:

- Written communications from the complaining employee and other witnesses/interviewees
- Issue confirmation memo to complaining employee
- Any interim action notifications
- Investigation report
- Results and notifications

- Notes and supporting documentation necessary to support key facts and conclusions in the investigation summary
- Communications with others that may be important to demonstrate the steps taken in the investigation

Only final copies of documents should be placed in the final investigation file. Drafts of the documentation listed should not be included in the file and should be destroyed if not inconsistent with the company's document retention policy. No other files containing investigation information should be kept. Human resources and management working files and notes should be reviewed to determine what is to be kept in the final investigation file and what is to be destroyed. Eliminate information stored on computers or disks.

The final investigation file should be marked as "need-to-know confidential," and access to the file should be limited accordingly.

Conclusion

The foregoing is a general outline of how to conduct an effective internal investigation. Obviously, the specific mechanics of any investigation will differ, depending on such variables as the nature of the issues raised, the person(s) raising them, and the size and structure of the organization. It is important, therefore, to contact employment counsel as soon as an employee complaint of misconduct is received so an investigation can be conducted in a manner well suited to the particular needs of the organization.

■ Employment Records and Record Keeping

In general, the goals of a records management system are to create and preserve records in compliance with the requirements of state, local, and federal law; preserve records in the event of litigation; create records to support personnel decisions; create and preserve records that will document rights that may be enforced at a later time (e.g., confidentiality and noncompete agreements); maintain a system that allows for efficient retrieval; and in general assist in effectively managing the workforce. Compliance always requires periodic follow-up to make sure that all staff handling employment records understand their responsibilities. Human resources should have a records retention policy that deals with all records created and maintained by the department.

Limiting Access

Personnel records should be available only on a need-to-know basis. Paper records should be kept in a limited number of locations in cabinets that can be locked and in offices that are locked at the end of the day. Computer records should be protected through limited access via password. When an employee who works with those records leaves the company, the ex-employee's password should be disabled immediately.

Segregating Records

To protect the privacy of employees, and to comply with statutory requirements, certain records must be kept separate from the employee's regular personnel file. In general, records relating to medical treatment and the employee's medical condition, as well as drug test results, must be segregated from other records. Additionally, attorney–client and work-product materials, such as attorney–client correspondence, notes of conversations with the company's attorney, and notes of internal conversations with respect to pending or threatened litigation, should be kept separate from the personnel file. At times it may be necessary to produce the file to third persons, such as a government agency, in response to a subpoena or in connection with ongoing litigation involving the institution. Segregating records in advance will prevent the harm that may occur in the too-often-seen scenario where the entire file is copied and produced to a third party without a careful review of its contents.

It is important to note that there are varying state laws relating to whether an employee may obtain access to his or her personnel file. Some states vest the employee with specific rights to inspect and copy the contents of the personnel file and may even provide deadlines as to when those tasks need to be accomplished. In those states, it is of particular importance that no privileged documents be included in the file.

Periodic Review of Forms and Records

The human resources department should conduct a periodic review of all forms to ensure compliance with state, federal, and local requirements, such as employment applications, FMLA forms, and I-9 forms. Not only should the form itself be reviewed, but also the manner in which staff are completing the forms should be scrutinized. For example, an audit should check to ensure that forms are signed when and where required, and that narratives such as employee reviews are grammatically correct and do not contain statements that are improper or that may give rise to liability.

Records Retention

A records retention program should balance the requirement to ensure compliance with all relevant laws with the business needs of the entity. The program contains two main components: a retention schedule, which specifies the length of time that records are to be kept, and procedures by which the program is implemented. The retention schedule should list every type of record maintained by human resources and the retention period for each record. In general, records must be maintained for at least the minimum period of time as set forth by statute, regulation, or general law.

Any destruction of records should follow a standard policy. Most importantly, as soon as the institution is made aware of pending or threatened litigation, there must be a mechanism in place to stop destruction of records that may relate to the litigation. If a court finds that an employer has adopted a destruction policy in bad faith for purposes of eliminating documents that may be used in anticipated litigation, that employer is subject to being sanctioned, and defense objectives may be seriously compromised. Even if documents routinely are destroyed pursuant to a record retention policy, and even if there is no pending litigation, the employer still may be required to maintain certain records if it knows that it will regularly be involved in a particular type of litigation, or if it knows that it has in the past and will in the future receive requests for certain documents on a routine basis through subpoena or otherwise, such as an audit by one or more governmental agencies.

The retention schedule and procedures should be reviewed annually so that the program can be revised to take into account changes in the records that the institution maintains, the changing needs of the institution, and any changes in the law. Further, vital records must be appropriately safeguarded, and provisions made for protection of records in case of a disaster. In many cases, the law may permit, and the entity may prefer, to store records electronically or on microfilm.

Special Issues Involving Electronic Mail

Electronic mail (e-mail) presents its own set of issues in creating and implementing a records retention policy. An e-mail is not simply the equivalent of a business record; rather, in practice it substitutes for hallway conversations, Post-it Notes, and informal memos, as well as being the repository of more formal documents. E-mail raises issues of particular concern in the area of employment law. Because e-mail is treated as an informal means of communication, and encourages informality and imprecision, it often results in the use of language that otherwise might not be expressed in the workplace.

Most e-mail messages are not of any long-term importance and should be deleted within a short period of time, preferably through an automatic system that deletes all messages that are more than a certain number of days old. Any messages that need to be retained can be transferred to a saved box or printed out and placed in a file.

E-mail is discoverable in litigation and is not protected from governmental agency investigations. It is particularly important, therefore, to devise and carefully monitor a policy that is sensitive to these potential concerns. As well, at the onset of a dispute or litigation, care should be taken to inform employees to preserve electronic records and evidence.

Particular Record-Keeping Requirements Under Federal Law

The following sections are a summary of some of the record-keeping requirements under various federal regulations dealing with labor and employment laws. In preparing a records retention schedule, each statute and regulation should be consulted and periodically reviewed for changes in the law.

Title VII, Civil Rights Act of 1964[156]

Employers must maintain employment records dealing with hiring, promotion, demotion, transfer, layoff or termination, rates of pay or other terms of compensation, and selection for training or apprenticeship. Records must be retained for 1 year from the date the record was created or the personnel action taken, whichever is later. If the employee is terminated involuntarily, the records must be kept for 1 year from the date of termination.

If a charge of discrimination is filed, all relevant personnel records must be preserved until final disposition of the charge. This obligation extends to preserving records relating not only to the charging party, but also to others holding similar positions and, in the case of a failure-to-hire charge, applications and tests of other applicants who applied for the same position.

Fair Labor Standards Act[157]

Employers are required to keep for 3 years all payroll records, collective bargaining agreements, trusts, and employment contracts, and to keep for 2 years all basic time and earnings cards showing daily starting and stopping times and wage rate tables.

Americans with Disabilities Act[158]

Medical records relating to disabilities must be maintained as confidential and kept separate from the main personnel file.

Family and Medical Leave Act[159]

In general, the record-keeping requirements for the FLSA apply. All records must be kept for 3 years and should include basic payroll and identifying employee data, dates of leave taken, hours of leave if taken in increments, and employee and employer notices of leave.

Records or documents relating to medical certifications, recertifications, or medical histories must be maintained as confidential medical records in separate files from the usual personnel files, and if the ADA is applicable, in conformance with ADA confidentiality requirements.

Age Discrimination in Employment Act[160]

The employer must maintain the following records for a period of 3 years: employee's name, address, date of birth, occupation, rate of pay, compensation earned each week, job applications, resumes, other forms of employment inquiry including records relating to failure or refusal to hire, promotion, demotion, transfer, selection for training, layoff, recall, or discharge; job orders submitted to any employment agency or labor organization for recruitment of personnel; and test papers disclosing the results of any employer-administered aptitude test considered by the employer in connection with any personnel action.

Equal Pay Act[161]

The employer must keep records that relate to payment of wages, wage rates, job evaluations, merit and incentive system, and seniority systems, including records of any practices that explain the basis for payment of wage differential, such as collective bargaining agreements. Records must be kept for at least 2 years.

Occupational Safety and Health Act[162]

The Occupational Safety and Health Administration has established a hazard communication rule. The purpose of the rule is to provide workers with information on hazardous chemicals that they may be exposed to in the workplace, so they can take steps to protect themselves. Under this rule, chemical manufacturers are required to review scientific information regarding chemicals produced or imported to determine if they are hazardous. For each such hazardous chemical, the manufacturer or importer must develop a material safety data sheet and appropriate warning labels. Finally, employers are required to develop a written hazard communication program and provide information and training to employees regarding the hazardous chemicals in the workplace.

Employers must prepare and retain records containing an analysis of the manufacturer's or importer's hazard determination procedures, a written hazard communication

program, and material safety data sheets pertaining to each chemical found at the employer's premises.

Immigration Reform and Control Act of 1986[163]

The employer must keep the completed Form I-9 for the longer of 3 years from the date of hire or 1 year after the date that the individual's employment is terminated. The employer is not required to make or keep copies of the supporting documentation, but may do so. USCIS investigators may inspect an employer's I-9 forms at any time. Department of Labor officials may also inspect I-9 forms; this usually arises in the course of a wage and hour audit.

Other Federal Laws

There are specific record-keeping requirements under a number of other labor and employment statutes, including requirements for federal affirmative action programs, the Employee Retirement Income and Security Act (ERISA), the Vietnam-Era Veterans Readjustment Assistance Act, the Rehabilitation Act of 1973, and Executive Order 11246.

Other Record-Keeping Requirements: State Laws

State laws often dictate record-keeping requirements for documents relating to workers' compensation, unemployment insurance, state wage and hour laws, employment contracts, and other employment agreements and policies, and similar documents.

References

1. 42 U.S.C. §§ 2000e, et seq.
2. 42 U.S.C. § 2000e(b).
3. Equal Pay Act of 1963, 29 U.S.C. §§ 206–209.
4. The Lilly Ledbetter Fair Pay Act of 2009, Pub L. No. 111-2, 123 Stat. 5 (2009) (codified in 29 U.S.C. and 42 U.S.C.).
5. *Faragher v. City of Boca Raton*, 118 S.Ct. 2275 (1998).
6. *Burlington Industries, Inc. v. Ellerth*, 118 S.Ct. 225 (1998).
7. Equal Employment Opportunity Commission. *Enforcement guidance: unlawful disparate treatment of workers with caregiving responsibilities.* EEOC Notice No. 915.002. October 10, 1995.
8. 42 U.S.C. §§ 12111–12117.
9. ADA Amendments Act of 2008 (ADAAA), 42 U.S.C. § 12101, et seq.
10. 42 U.S.C. § 12111.
11. 29 U.S.C. §§ 621, et seq.
12. 29 U.S.C. § 631(c).
13. 29 U.S.C. § 630(b).
14. N.Y.C. Admin. Code §§ 8–107, et seq.
15. S.F. Ordinance No. 433–94.
16. U.S. Department of Labor. Facts on executive order 11246—affirmative action. 2002. Accessed February 8, 2012, at http://www.dol.gov/compliance/laws/comp-eeo.htm
17. Fidell ER. Federal protection of private sector health and safety whistleblowers. *Administrative Law Journal.* Spring 1998:1, 2.
18. 31 U.S.C. §§ 3729–3733.

19. Kruchko J. *The Whistle Blower Protection Provision of the False Claims Act: advising government contractor clients and minimizing liability.* American Bar Association and National Association of Medicaid Fraud Control Units; 2001:7,8.
20. Krause JH. Medical error as false claim. *American Journal of Law and Medicine.* 2001;27.
21. N.Y. Labor Law § 741.
22. 15 U.S.C. §§ 1681, et seq.
23. Public Law 108-159, 111 Stat. 1952.
24. Public Law 108-159, § 611.
25. 29 U.S.C. §§ 2001–2009.
26. 29 U.S.C. § 2006.
27. 29 U.S.C. § 2006(d).
28. 29 U.S.C. § 2006(f).
29. 20 C.F.R. § 639.1.
30. 29 U.S.C. §§ 2102, 2103.
31. 29 U.S.C. § 2103.
32. *Tony and Susan Alamo Foundation v. Secretary of Labor,* 471 U.S. 290 (1985).
33. 29 U.S.C. § 206(a)(1).
34. 29 U.S.C. § 207.
35. 29 C.F.R. § 778.601.
36. 29 C.F.R. § 541.602.
37. 29 C.F.R. §§ 541.101, et seq.
38. 29 C.F.R. §§ 541.201, et seq.
39. 29 C.F.R. §§ 541.301, et seq.
40. *Fazekas v. Cleveland Clinic Foundation Health Care Ventures, Inc.,* 204 F.3d 673 (6th Cir. 2000).
41. United States Department of Labor. Wage and Hour Administrator's Opinion Letter. WH-266, WHM 99:1162 [BNA]; May 10, 1974.
42. Wage and Hour Administrator's Opinion Letter. WHM 99:8122-23 [BNA]; February 6, 1998.
43. 29 C.F.R. § 541.3(a)(4).
44. 29 C.F.R. § 791.2(a).
45. 29 C.F.R. § 791.2(b).
46. 29 U.S.C. § 2612.
47. 29 C.F.R. §§ 825, et seq.
48. 29 U.S.C. § 2601.
49. 29 C.F.R. §§ 825.100, et seq.
50. 29 U.S.C. § 2611(2).
51. 29 C.F.R. §§ 825.110, et seq.
52. 29 U.S.C. § 2612(a)(1).
53. 29 C.F.R. §§ 825.112, et seq.
54. 29 C.F.R. § 2612(e).
55. 29 C.F.R. §§ 825.208, 825.302, et seq.
56. 29 C.F.R. § 2613.
57. 29 C.F.R. §§ 825.305, et seq.
58. 29 C.F.R. § 825.301(c).
59. 29 C.F.R. § 2612(f).
60. 29 C.F.R. § 825.202.
61. 29 C.F.R. § 2612(b).
62. 29 C.F.R. §§ 825.203, et seq.
63. 29 C.F.R. § 2614(b).
64. 29 C.F.R. §§ 825.217, et seq.
65. Internal Revenue Code (IRC) § 501(c)(3).
66. 29 U.S.C. §1001, et seq.
67. Internal Revenue Service. General Counsel Memorandum 38283. February 15, 1980.
68. IRC § 401(k)(4)(B).
69. IRC § 403(b)(1)(A)(i).
70. Treasury Regulations § 1.403(b)-1(b)(1)(i).
71. Public Law No. 107-16.
72. Tax Reform Act of 1986, Public Law No. 99-514.
73. IRC § 457(a)–(e).
74. IRC § 457(f).
75. Employee Retirement Income Security Act § 3(1).
76. IRC §§ 79, 105, 106, 127, 129, 419, 419A & 4980B.
77. Employee Retirement Income Security Act §§ 101–111, 401–414, & 503.
78. Employee Retirement Income Security Act § 3(1).
79. Department of Labor Regulations § 2510.3–1(b)(1a).
80. Internal Revenue Service. General Counsel Memorandum 39616. October 16, 1986.
81. PLRs 702063, 9442031, 9629033, and 9722039.
82. 18 U.S.C. §§ 2510, et seq.
83. 15 U.S.C. §§ 1681, et seq.
84. Colgate Palmolive Co., 323 NLRB No. 82 (1997).
85. 29 U.S.C. §§ 651, et seq.
86. 41 U.S.C. §§ 8101, et seq.
87. 29 U.S.C. § 157.
88. U.S. Department of Labor, Bureau of Labor Statistics. Press release USDL 04-53. Union Members in 2003 January 21, 2004.
89. *Epilepsy Foundation of Northeast Ohio v. NLRB,* 268 F.3d 1095 (D.C. Cir. 2001), cert. denied, 122 S. Ct. 2356 (2002).
90. *NLRB v. IBEW Local 1229 (Jefferson Stan. Broadcasting),* 346 U.S. 464 (1953).
91. *Community Hospital of Roanoke Valley v. NLRB,* 538 F.2d 607 (4th Cir. 1976).
92. *Brockton Hosp. v. NLRB,* 294 F.3d 100 (D.C. Cir. 2002).
93. *Medical Center Hospital,* 244 NLRB 742 (1979).
94. *NLRB v. Presbyterian Medical Center,* 586 F.2d 165 (10th Cir. 1978).
95. *Timekeeping Systems,* 323 NLRB 244 (1997).
96. *St. Joseph's Hospital,* 337 NLRB No. 12 (2001).
97. *Damon Medical Laboratory Inc.,* 234 NLRB 333 (1978).
98. 29 U.S.C. § 152 (14).
99. 29 U.S.C. § 159(b).
100. 120 Congressional Record 13,559 (1974) (remarks of Sen. Taft).
101. *San Diego Blood Bank,* 219 NLRB 116 (1975).
102. 302 NLRB 72 (1991).
103. 29 U.S.C. § 152(11).
104. *Boston Med. Ctr.,* 330 NLRB No. 30 (1999).
105. *M.B. Sturgis Inc.,* 331 NLRB No. 173 (2000).
106. *No. Suburban Blood Center v. NLRB,* 661 F. 2d at 635 (citations omitted).
107. 29 U.S.C. § 158(g).
108. *District 1199 and Parkway Pavilion Healthcare,* 222 NLRB 212, enforc. den'd without opin., 556 F. 2d 558 (2d Cir. 1976).
109. *District 1199 and United Hospitals of Newark,* 232 NLRB 443 (1977).
110. *American Federation of Nurses, Local 535, SEIU and Kaiser Foundation Hosps.,* 313 NLRB 1201 (1994).
111. 1992 NLRB GCM LEXIS 91 (Western Medical Center, December 21, 1992).
112. 29 U.S.C. § 158(d).
113. *First National Maintenance Corp. v. NLRB,* 452 U.S. 666 (1981);
114. *Fibreboard Paper Products Corp. v. NLRB,* 379 U.S. 203 (1964).
115. *Providence Hospital and Mercy Hosp. v. NLRB,* 93 F. 3d 1012, 1018 (1st Cir. 1996).
116. *Detroit Edison Co. v. NLRB,* 440 US 301 (1979).
117. *Providence Hospital and Mercy Hospital v. NLRB,* 93 F. 3d at 1019.
118. 8 C.F.R. § 274a.1(j).

119. 8 C.F.R. § 274a.5.

120. 8 C.F.R. § 274a.1(c) & (f).

121. American Council for Nationalities Service. 66 Interpreter Releases 1173–74, 1188–89 (October 23, 1989).

122. INA § 274A(b)(2).

123. 8 C.F.R. § 274a.1(c).

124. 8 C.F.R. § 274a.2(b)(1)(ii).

125. 8 C.F.R. § 274a.2(b)(1)(vi).

126. 8 C.F.R. § 274a.2(b)(3).

127. 8 C.F.R. § 274a.2(b)(1)(viii).

128. 8 C.F.R. § 274a.2(b)(1)(viii)(A).

129. 8 C.F.R. § 274a.2(b)(1)(vii).

130. U.S. Citizenship and Immigration Service. Handbook for employers M-274. Accessed February 9, 2012, at http://www.uscis.gov

131. INA § 274A(b)(3)(B).

132. INA § 274A(b)(3).

133. INA § 274A(e)(5); 8 C.F.R. § 274a.10(b)(2).

134. INA § 274B(g)(2)(B)(v)-(vi).

135. 8 C.F.R. § 274a.10(b)(2).

136. *United States v. Morgan's Mexican & Lebanese Foods*, 8 OCAHO 1013 (1998).

137. INA § 274A(a)(1).

138. INA § 274A(a)(2).

139. 8 C.F.R. § 274a.1(l)(1).

140. INA § 274A(e)(4).

141. 8 C.F.R. § 274a.10(b)(1).

142. 28 C.F.R. § 68.52(c).

143. American Council for Nationalities Service. 69 Interpreter Releases 253, 255, App. II (March 2, 1992).

144. INA § 274A(f)(1).

145. 8 C.F.R. § 274a.1(k).

146. INA § 274.

147. INA § 274B.

148. INA § 274B(a)(6).

149. INA § 274B(a)(5).

150. INA § 274B(a)(2)(A).

151. INA § 274B(a)(2)(A) (citing INA § 274B(a)(2)(C)).

152. INA § 274B(a)(2)(B).

153. INA § 274B(a)(4).

154. INA § 274B(a)(6).

155. *NLRB v. J. Weingarten*, 420 U.S. 251 (1975).

156. 29 C.F.R. § 1602.14.

157. 29 C.F.R. Part 516.

158. 29 C.F.R. § 1630.14.

159. 29 C.F.R. Part 825.

160. 29 C.F.R. § 1627.2.

161. 29 C.F.R. § 1620.32.

162. 29 C.F.R.§ 1910.1200.

163. 8 C.F.R. § 274a.

Medical Practice Physician Compensation Plans

Bruce A. Johnson, JD, MPA

A medical practice's method of paying physicians for their professional and other services ranks as one of the most important issues affecting practice performance. Given that a medical practice is both a business and a collective of professionals, the adequacy of a practice's compensation arrangement is central to the success of the organization and its providers. This chapter reviews the principal issues and requirements related to effective medical practice compensation arrangements. It explores the context in which compensation plans operate, reviews the principal legal issues governing compensation, and explores alternative plan methodologies and other compensation-related issues.

■ Purpose and Rule of Compensation Plans

In its most fundamental sense, a medical practice's compensation plan involves a financial model that takes into consideration practice revenues and expenses in order to determine and pay compensation to physicians for their services. From a financial management perspective, key compensation plan considerations include how revenues and expenses are allocated, and effective financial management to ensure that sufficient funds are available to determine and pay compensation to the practice's physicians and other employees.

Yet experience demonstrates that compensation plans involve more than a series of mathematical calculations that yield a "paycheck" for physicians and other medical practice providers. From a broader perspective, a medical practice's physician compensation plan also serves as an important and clearly visible component of the practice's performance, incentive, and feedback system. As such, the plan may help to encourage or discourage, facilitate or undermine the medical practice's provider performance and success. A medical practice's compensation arrangement helps to encourage or discourage physician performance in furtherance of the organization's goals. The plan will serve as an important communication tool that expresses the types of activities the medical practice values, and it will help to reinforce the practice's culture. An effective compensation plan provides an essential foundation on which the success of the practice, as well as the professional satisfaction and success of its participating physicians, can be built.

Interplay of Reimbursement and Compensation Structures

Numerous factors may be creating the "perfect storm" to fundamentally realign the nation's physician practice infrastructure, including changes to the nation's healthcare payment and reimbursement systems. The federal Patient Protection and Affordable Care Act (PPACA) was signed into law on March 23, 2010. Among the PPACA's numerous policy objectives, the law seeks to test and ultimately reshape the Medicare reimbursement and payment systems by rewarding quality rather than volume. Under the law, various components of the U.S. Department of Health and Human Services are charged with implementing initiatives that focus on quality through quality- and value-based demonstration and pilot programs involving accountable care organizations, value-based purchasing, bundled payment projects, and numerous other initiatives. The law also sets forth a rough timeline over which the Medicare and Medicaid payment systems will be transformed.

Similar initiatives are under way in various states and/or sponsored by traditional insurance carriers and other purchasers or payors of healthcare services. In support of these initiatives, various organizations such as the Center for Healthcare Quality and Payment Reform have set forth their own road maps on how our healthcare delivery and payment systems can transition to systems involving "accountable care."[1]

As the reimbursement and payment structure moves toward an emphasis on quality and away from volume, the methods of physician compensation will also need to be aligned with the reimbursement structure.

Changing Context for Medical Practices

As the healthcare delivery and payment environments change, so do the defining characteristics of medical group practices. A "group practice" has a specific legal definition with legal implications, such as for purposes of satisfying the in-office ancillary services exception to the Stark law (as further discussed later in this chapter). Such requirements include that the group practice is a single entity with at least two member physicians who furnish substantially all of their patient care services through the group.

In contrast, the terms "medical group" and "medical practice" do not have specific legal definitions, but both have operational and practical definitions and attributes.

A "medical practice" is broadly defined as consisting of a group of physicians and other providers that may not necessarily view themselves as partners of a group but are involved in an overarching organizational structure. For example, physicians employed by a hospital may not view themselves as partners with the other physicians employed at the hospital, but they are all a part of the medical practice.

A "medical group" might be operationally defined as a group of physicians and other providers who furnish patient care to a population of patients, identify themselves as being involved with a single organization with a defined unified governance structure, and have largely shared values and a common culture.

Today, medical groups come in a variety of sizes and structures, including: (1) "traditional" physician-owned group practices, (2) independent practice association (IPA) or "network" model medical groups, (3) hospital/health system–affiliated medical groups, and (4) payor-affiliated groups.

In the traditional physician-owned group, the medical group practice usually consists of a partnership of physicians who have joined together to share the provision of patient services, practice operations, on-call burdens, and the like. Professional respect and financial responsibility are shared throughout the group, and commonly, there is some negotiated sharing of some or all of the practice's income and expenses.

In IPA and network model medical groups, physician groups participate in an IPA or network organization. In this structure, independent "traditional" medical group practices continue to exist, with each commonly having its own office, systems, and infrastructure—but the network still constitutes a medical group because its physicians share patients, a common governance structure in the context of the network, financial opportunities and risk, and at least some attributes of a common medical care culture.

Many hospital-affiliated medical groups use the hospital legal structure itself as the employing entity, such that no single legal platform has an exclusively physician practice orientation. Other hospital-affiliated medical groups may consist of multiple organizational and/or legal structures that comprise the medical group enterprise. In these models, most, if not all, of the tangible assets and financial risk associated with medical practice operations (e.g., facilities, equipment, nonphysician personnel, etc.) will be borne by the hospital/health system, although some of that risk will commonly be allocated to the hospital-affiliated medical group's physicians via the physician compensation structure.

In a payor-affiliated group, the physicians will commonly become direct employees of the health plan or an affiliated medical group legal entity. Physicians in these medical groups will sometimes own interests in a separate legal entity, but they will only rarely hold an ownership interest in the practice-related equipment or rights to payment for the services they furnish to patients.

Because there are various settings in which medical practice and third-party payment for medical services occur, different compensation structures are frequently used in one or more of these relationships and settings. What works in one situation may not necessarily work or be effective in another. Yet regardless of the setting, effective physician compensation plans tend to share a number of common characteristics.

Features of Effective Compensation Plans

Given the importance of compensation arrangements to a medical group's success, the ability to develop, implement, and manage an effective compensation plan is essential to effective practice management. Regrettably, there is no single compensation arrangement that is perfect or perfectly "fair." Each compensation plan is a reflection of the organization's particular mix of providers, goals, values, culture, history, traditions, reimbursement, environment, and other factors. Nonetheless, experience shows that effective compensation plans do tend to share a number of common features. Those plans that provide a solid (but frequently silent) framework for the practice's success typically contain at least the following key features:

- *Linkage to practice goals:* Effective compensation plans tend to help promote the overall goals of the medical practice organization and its individual physicians. Goals that are promoted either directly or indirectly through the plans commonly include:
  - Rewarding professional service production and work
  - Outreach activities
  - Enhancing patient and other "customer" satisfaction
  - Providing quality care
  - Other activities that are viewed as central to the practice's overall success
- *Reward work:* In today's challenging environment, the most successful plans focus on rewarding and encouraging "productive" work. This can be accomplished through direct measures such as the

inclusion of a strong productivity emphasis in the compensation structure, but also through structures that recognize the changing payment systems and the changing nature of different types of productive work. Successful medical practices ensure there is a close relationship between work levels and compensation, so that those who work harder and "smarter" in relation to external payment systems will generally receive more compensation.

- *Clarify performance expectations:* Effective compensation plans help to define and clarify the expectations a practice has for its physicians and other providers. For example, compensation plans that have a productivity component help to clarify how physicians are responsible and accountable for their own work levels. Plans that use equal share, guaranteed salaries, and similar methods commonly expect minimum levels of performance teamwork in the group as a whole. Today's compensation plans not only implicitly express certain core values and expectations related to physician performance, but also commonly provide a more explicit and specific definition of expectations related to minimum production and other performance levels, minimum work and access levels (e.g., weeks worked per year, days worked per week, and others), and other minimum performance standards.
- *Fiscally responsible:* Effective plans take into account the overall payment structure and the fiscal and financial condition of a practice. The plan ensures not only that practice physicians receive compensation for their services, but also that the practice has sufficient revenues to accommodate cash-flow needs, pay overhead expenses, and otherwise operate the practice as a sound business enterprise.
- *Recruit and retain physicians:* Physician decisions to join or depart from a practice are commonly based on many factors, typically including the expected level of compensation. Effective plans typically include the features already outlined, while also yielding bottom-line results that make the plan acceptable to individual physicians in order to promote recruitment and retention goals.
- *Clearly defined and consistently applied:* Effective plans are clearly defined—meaning that each plan is clearly expressed and uses objective measures (or, where required, narrowly defined and understood subjective criteria) to determine and pay compensation. Moreover, consistent application means that the plan encompasses an agreed-upon

set of rules and expectations that apply in a uniform and consistent manner.

- *Simple, understandable, and explainable:* Obviously, a plan must be understood in order to function as an effective performance feedback and incentive tool. Effective plans have relatively few methodological elements and can be easily traced, understood, and explained to others.

- *Open and transparent:* Only rarely is a "black box" compensation plan (i.e., one in which all decisions regarding compensation are hidden or vested in the discretion of a limited few) sustainable. In most settings, professionals require (and demand) information and transparency regarding how their compensation is calculated. Moreover, even in those settings where a committee determines compensation levels or a salary is negotiated, the process and recognition that this more subjective process is "how things are done" is itself widely understood.

- *Legally compliant:* As medicine is increasingly regulated, regulatory compliance is an essential element of an effective compensation arrangement. Compliance with applicable legal requirements such as the federal physician self-referral or Stark law, the antikickback law, laws and rules governing tax-exempt organizations, and others is essential for the medical practice and its providers.

■ Understanding the Context for Compensation Arrangements

Compensation and Culture

A medical practice's compensation plan will reflect, influence, and reinforce the practice's culture. As a result, changing a practice's compensation plan will also change the practice's culture, because the plan will create new incentives that are presumably more aligned with what the practice needs and values in a changing environment. Given the importance of the compensation plan to the promotion of practice goals and success, any modification to (or failure to address) the compensation plan risks undermining the practice's financial, business, and cultural foundation.

The types of compensation plans that may be effective for a particular practice will vary depending on the context, as will the implications associated with making changes to the compensation plan.

The Issue of Size

Although compensation is essential to every organization, the importance of an effective compensation plan is arguably heightened in a small group practice setting. For example, in a five-physician medical group practice that is physician-owned and operated, the departure of a physician due to an unacceptable compensation plan will typically have significant implications for the group's short- and long-term viability, and for the quality of life and other benefits that the group can offer to the physicians who remain. In contrast, the departure of a single physician from a much larger medical group practice will commonly have some financial and other implications for the group and its remaining physicians, but the impact may not be as severe because more individuals could assume the work of a departed colleague, plus such larger organizations typically have a corporate culture less likely to be impacted by the departure of a single individual. Likewise, in a larger group or entity that is not physician-owned, the direct financial impact may be further lessened.

Plan effectiveness is no less important to the short- and long-term viability of large medical groups. Even large medical groups tend to be composed of multiple practices or subgroups consisting of individual medical, surgical, and specialty service departments. Within each of these practice subgroups, the unique interpersonal and cultural dynamics that are more characteristic of smaller group practices will frequently be present. For example, the departure of a physician from a five-physician general surgery department in a medium to large group practice organization will have implications for both the group as a whole and the four surgeons who remain.

The size of the practice organization will commonly have implications for the type of compensation methodology used. Small groups commonly use compensation methods that pay closer attention to individual revenues and expenses. In a small group setting, individual physicians typically have a heightened interest in group and physician-specific financial statements, and take a more active role in the practice's overall management and financial performance.

Conversely, the more corporate culture and operating format in large groups are more likely to allow for the use of compensation arrangements that rely more heavily on base salary plus incentive or similar approaches. These methods tend to treat the large organization as a single economic unit with a single bottom line that must be managed, rather than as a collective of individual physicians functioning as separate economic units that happen to share the same organizational umbrella.

Single-Specialty and Multispecialty Practices

Compensation plans relate to practice culture, and that culture tends to be an expression of the practice's participants. If the providers are similar to each other, then the culture is more likely to be homogeneous. Thus, in single-specialty groups where all physicians have largely similar skill sets and have experienced similar residency, fellowship, and other training, the physicians will tend to be more alike than dissimilar. That similarity can provide a cultural foundation for the group that will enable the group's physicians to work through difficulties and compromise for the good of the organization because they share a common cultural background and perspective. It also frequently manifests itself in a practice compensation arrangement that promotes and supports sharing and teamwork.

Conversely, in a multispecialty setting where diversity of specialties and perspectives is the norm, the challenges with developing, implementing, and maintaining a single, uniform compensation plan increase significantly. The level of cultural similarity and cohesiveness among physicians is simply not the same in a multispecialty setting as in a single-specialty practice. Importantly, such cultural heterogeneity and diversity is also increasingly prevalent in single-specialty practices where subspecialization, revenue generation potential, and personal expectations regarding income levels vary from one physician to another. For example, orthopedics, cardiology, and other practices have their own forms of subspecialization and accompanying variations in earning potential. Today, formerly homogeneous single-specialty organizations are taking on the characteristics and challenges presented by the heterogeneity of multispecialty practices.

Private vs. Public Group Practice Settings

Through most of the last century, the vast majority of physician practices were privately owned and operated by physicians, rather than by hospitals, academic medical centers, or third-party investors. These "privately" physician-owned and -operated medical groups enjoyed the same characteristics of many other small businesses. Quality care, effective cost management, adequate productivity, and some level of entrepreneurial spirit provided the foundation for a successful private practice business model.

Increasingly, however, physicians and medical practices are affiliated with organizations that are not physician owned. Today, hospital-affiliated medical practices and groups are becoming the norm in many communities. Likewise, faculty practice plans affiliated with academic medical centers and teaching hospitals not only have the added complexity of being affiliated with tax-exempt charitable and educational organizations, but also must attempt to operate a successful business model while pursuing the academic environment's teaching, research, and service missions. Just as the diversity among providers creates its own challenges and complexities, the presence of multiple missions, multiple goals, and different values related to organizational objectives and success creates unique challenges when translated into compensation arrangements.

Group Practice vs. Employment Models

Compensation plans that operate in a physician-owned "group practice" setting consisting of a single entity that is primarily focused on the delivery of physician and related healthcare services commonly vary significantly from those involving direct employment relationships with a hospital or other organization. In a group practice setting, such as those existing in traditional physician-owned groups or in the constituent points of "network" medical groups involving separately organized medical groups, a core objective of the compensation plan is to consider the practice's revenues and expenses, and distribute available profit among practice physicians on an agreed-upon basis. The group provides the framework for the economic reality that all of the group's providers are "in it together" in economic and financial terms. If the group is financially successful, the providers, both individually and collectively, stand to receive additional compensation. Likewise, they feel the economic pain, both individually and as a group, if the practice experiences financial challenges.

Direct employment models such as those commonly used in hospital-affiliated and payor-affiliated medical groups, however, commonly create different financial and other relationships. Unless the compensation plan takes into account the overall financial viability of the organization or a particular subset of physicians and other employees in determining compensation, the basic nature of the employer–employee relationship between a physician and hospital, or between a physician and a payor organization, can be very different from that used in the more traditional physician-owned practice setting described earlier.

In an employment model, an individual physician's compensation may be determined by a direct one-on-one negotiation with the employer. In that context, the economic success or failure of other physicians within the same organization may have less direct implications for physician compensation and performance. As a result, the challenge in the context of compensation plan development is to promote group-wide accountability and financial performance, despite the reality of multiple employer–employee relationships between the organization and its providers.

■ Basic Plan Types

Compensation plans reflect and promote the unique culture of the medical group; as a result there are as many different types of compensation plans as there are groups. Nevertheless, close review reveals that the numerous plan methods may be classified into a number of broad types. Each type tends to adopt a particular financial or funds-flow model to the treatment of practice revenues and expenses, the importance of other incentives, and the determination of physician compensation. Thus, basic compensation models may be understood as falling along a continuum of models and plan types, with each taking a particular approach to medical practice finances. The continuum ranges from largely individualistic models, which treat each physician as a generally separate economic unit for compensation purposes, to team-oriented models in which the group's overall financial condition is the focus before the compensation is determined and paid. Between these two extremes are models that combine features of both approaches. These plan alternatives not only represent different approaches to compensations calculation, but also represent and support different medical practice cultures. A more detailed discussion of the continuum of plan types is provided in the following sections.

Individualistic Models

Individualistic compensation models tend to treat each physician in the medical group as largely his or her own separate economic unit for compensation plan purposes. In practical terms, the compensation plan allocates a portion of medical group revenues to each individual physician, then subtracts from those revenues specifically allocated expenses, resulting in the physician's compensation for services. Individualistic models, because of their approach to calculation, allow for issues and disputes to be raised relative to: (1) the appropriate method for allocating practice revenues, and (2) the appropriate allocation of practice overhead expenses.

Under individualistic models, practice revenues are commonly allocated among the group's physicians on a productivity basis in which a portion of practice revenues are credited to each physician based on individual professional service performance. As third-party payment systems evolve in the future, physician production and performance in such models also will need to evolve to recognize (and take into account) sources of practice income beyond those derived from pure fee-for-service production. This means that allocated revenues will include those derived from direct patient care, as well as funds paid by third-party payors under pay-for-performance (P4P)

systems, quality awards, care management stipends, and others. Performance will increasingly move beyond merely doing more medical procedures, to include other forms of productive work for which payment is made by third-party payors.

Physician production may be measured through any variety of means, including actual collections for professional services, percentage of gross or net charges, work relative value units (RVUs), and other methods. Production also will include funds obtained through other payments such as those limited to quality and value. Individualistic models also may include aspects of middle-ground models (described later in this chapter), such as equal share or similar allocation methods in connection with revenue allocation, as a means to promote teamwork and sharing.

A variety of overhead allocation methodologies is commonly used in practices using individualistic models, ranging from pure cost accounting methodologies in which the practice attempts to allocate overhead costs among individual physicians in a precise manner, to those that allocate practice operating costs in a negotiated manner. These negotiated expense allocation methods (e.g., 50% equal share, 50% variable/based on production) and other agreed-upon expense allocation methods seek to allocate overhead (and incentives) in a manner that is recognized as not based on resources utilized. They are crafted to achieve a reasonable and fair balance between resource use and accountability, but without the level of precision that is commonly expected from systems that use cost accounting–type methods. **Table 16-1** illustrates the financial funds flow used in a basic individualistic model assuming a hypothetical group of five physicians.[a]

Individualistic models are used in all types of medical groups and in all practice settings. They are frequently perceived as the most desirable and appropriate compensation structures in those practices in which there is significant variation among physicians in terms of production, specialization, work levels, goals, and related issues. Individualistic models are designed, by their nature, to make each individual physician responsible and accountable for his or her own production, performance, and share of practice overhead. Despite this, such models commonly result in significant attention to both the practice's revenue and overhead allocation methods, leading to the ever-present question of whether the practice's methodologies are fair.

---

a. Data presented in this table are provided to illustrate the financial funds flow or calculation methodology.

Table 16-1	Example: "Individualistic" Model				
	Dr. 1 ($)	Dr. 2 ($)	Dr. 3 ($)	Dr. 4 ($)	Dr. 5 ($)
Revenues					
Profits vs. receipts	458,723	562,738	425,262	672,819	598,726
Stark profits	12,342	12,342	12,342	12,342	12,342
Total allocated receipts	471,065	575,080	437,604	685,161	611,068
% of total	17%	21%	16%	25%	22%
Expenses					
Group overhead					
Fixed expenses	219,173	219,173	219,173	219,173	219,173
Variable expenses	68,681	83,847	63,803	99,896	89,094
Direct expenses	23,902	43,528	29,098	37,652	35,463
Total allocated expenses	311,757	346,548	312,024	356,722	343,730
Cash compensation	159,308	228,532	125,530	267,338	1,109,147

Team-Oriented Models

On the other end of the continuum of compensation models are what might be referred to as team-oriented models, which tend to treat the medical practice as a single economic unit for compensation purposes. The practice's revenues less the practice's expenses yields a pool of funding that is used to pay compensation to the physicians. Team-oriented methodologies recognize the practice's overhead expenses as a cost of doing business that must be borne by the organization, rather than being directly assessed as an expense against individual physicians. Moreover, in some models a portion of physician compensation (e.g., a base salary or other amount) is itself viewed as part of the practice overhead.

Within team-oriented models, variations of productivity and equal share may also be used. Thus, any number of methods for measuring work, production, and performance (e.g., collections from professional service charges, dollars per work RVU, combined production/equal share portions, quality of care, P4P, patient satisfaction, etc.) may be used to allocate funds within the compensation pool to determine individual physician compensation levels.

The utility of team-oriented models is that they have the potential to eliminate conflict over the allocation of practice expense. Team-oriented models work well in single-specialty practices and in other practices where there are not wide variations in physician work levels. Such models are also used in multispecialty groups, provided that physicians have work schedules within expected norms and have production that is generally within expected levels for the particular specialty.

Middle-Ground Models

Although individualistic and team-oriented compensation models represent the extremes on the continuum of compensation plans, the vast majority of medical practice compensation plans involve "middle-ground" models that combine aspects of both. In practical terms, middle-ground models typically combine individualistic approaches with methodological tools designed to promote teamwork and group orientation, along with measures that help to focus attention on cost of practice, quality, and other issues. Examples of common middle-ground models include base salary plus incentive models in which the base salary is guaranteed but the incentive component may be based on individual or group-oriented performance measures, quality P4P, or other performance measures.

For example, many hospital-affiliated compensation plans provide a base salary plus incentive plan that pays a reasonable base salary to physicians based on the faculty members' full-time equivalency (FTE). In order to receive incentive compensation, the physician may be paid based on an individualistic model in which medical practice revenues derived from the physician's work, and some or all of the practice's allocated expenses, are directly allocated to the physician. Some or all of any excess amount after these assessments will be allocated to the physician as incentive compensation. Under such models, the base salary effectively provides a minimum level of guaranteed compensation. The incentive component, however, incorporates individualistic approaches to determining the physician's compensation. Similar base plus incentive models are used in many academic medical practices including faculty practice plans.

Although only a minority of medical practices use a pure "equal share" approach, such models may reflect combinations of team-based and individualistic calculation methods. Under the simplest equal share model, funds in a compensation pool are allocated among group physicians on an equal share basis. A variation of this model involves the allocation of practice expenses on an equal share basis, coupled with an equal share/production-based approach to revenue allocation.

Dealing with Capitation

Capitated reimbursement systems, in which a physician or medical group is paid a fixed amount of reimbursement per member per month, are used less frequently by third-party payers to compensate physicians and medical groups than in the 1990s, at the height of managed care. Despite this, capitation remains an important reimbursement system in many communities, and full or partial capitation is likely to develop in the future. As a result, the issue of how to allocate the capitated funds and reward physicians for their professional services under the capitated system remains an important challenge to compensation systems.

Approaches to the treatment of capitated funds in the context of physician compensation systems tend to vary depending on the magnitude of capitation as a percentage of a medical practice's total patient care revenues. For those practices in which capitated funds comprise only a relatively slight portion of the practice or individual physician's revenues (e.g., less than 10–20% of total), the funds are typically treated much the same as all other funds for compensation purposes. That is, they may be allocated directly to a physician, then expenses subtracted to determine individual physician pay; the capitated dollars may be aggregated in determining all other practice profits; or they may be treated in another manner.

In practices in which capitated dollars comprise a significant portion of the practice revenues (e.g., 40% or more), the magnitude of the capitated dollar makes it essential that the practice focus on medical management. In these practices the compensation plan typically builds on information system capabilities that are used to allocate capitated dollars, or alternatively, the providers are paid a base salary with the incentive compensation based on performance in relation to managed-care goals.

In those practices where the intrusion of capitated reimbursement is somewhat substantial but still less than the dominant payment systems, the challenge of capitation is more significant. In these environments the capitated dollar is typically not so significant that it drives the pay plan and the incentives regarding resource utilization that underlie that plan. Practices in these environments use compensation models that combine a focus on production and productivity (for the noncapitated portion of the patient base) with an alternative approach for capitated patients. These models may also combine individualistic and team-based methods in the allocation of practice revenues.

For example, a relatively common approach to the allocation of capitated dollars involves distributing some portion of the capitated dollars directly to the patient's primary care physician, a portion based on patient visits to pay those physicians who actually provide the services to the patients, and the remaining portion based on some measure of outcomes—whether internally or externally generated. Similar approaches to the allocation of capitated revenues are sometimes used in specialty practices where the objective is to balance multiple values and incentives (e.g., equal share to promote teamwork, allocation based on work RVUs to reward complexity of service, and allocation based on patient visits to reward service).

The challenge in practice settings in which capitated systems do not constitute the dominant third-party payment arrangement is to balance conflicting incentives associated with more traditional fee-for-service medicine with those that are implicit and explicit in capitated and similar managed-care systems. As a result, the approach to the allocation of capitated and other funds paid under managed care (e.g., withhold pool rewards for clinical care, quality, etc.) tends to combine mechanisms focused on individual physician performance with those that also consider resource usage, teamwork, and other values.

The Role of Production and Productivity

A central theme in all of these models and virtually all compensation plans in successful medical groups is emphasis on production in determining and paying physician compensation. A key characteristic in the physician compensation models used in many better-performing medical groups is that there is close attention to production and work in the medical group's compensation plan. This emphasis is typically reflected not only in plan methodologies that adopt a pure or largely pure productivity method in determining and paying compensation, but also in medical practices that use a base salary component in compensation, because the base is frequently set with attention to production levels. Even in the case of practices that use an equal share approach to compensation, although production may not be measured through the economic or financial allocation model in these organizations, production still tends to be reflected in the overall practice culture. In these groups using equal share methods, a clear expectation of the group is that physicians will strive to work equally hard in meeting the group's patient care needs. The culture of production and productivity is expressed in the organization itself and its approach to doing business, rather than being directly manifested in the compensation plan.

Performance Expectations

An important component of effective compensation plans is the clarification of performance expectations. When working with professionals, it is typically difficult and often unpleasant to define specific expectations related to performance. Yet, with increasing diversity of individual goals, lifestyle preferences, work levels, and group size, medical groups frequently find it useful to clarify minimum performance levels expected of practice physicians. Consistent performance expectations related to access, service, and clinical practice are also more common as the delivery system moves toward systems of accountable care.

Performance expectations are frequently expressed in any number of key areas, and through multiple means. These include simple and objectively verifiable measures such as weeks worked per year, days of clinical service per week, on-call obligations, and levels of professional service productivity, which may be expressed in employment contracts or policies. Measures that focus on objectively verifiable requirements are typically easier to administer and more widely accepted as legitimate by practice physicians. More subjective measures such as participation in group administrative activities, outreach obligations, citizenship, professionalism, quality of care, and related issue areas also may be used to define and channel performance. These measures may also be expressed in contracts or policies, as well as in physician "compacts" or similar documents that focus on values, behaviors, and practice culture. Where subjective measures such as behavior, teamwork, and related issues are used, they are typically incorporated into compensation plans as only a relatively small portion of any physician's total pay.

As practices and their physicians become larger and more heterogeneous, with greater diversity of work levels, preferences, and individual physician goals, and as payment systems continue to change, the potential utility and importance of clearly defining performance expectations continues to increase. This is understandable because in the medical groups of the past that tended to be single-specialty and less diverse, the underlying practice culture would effectively define what was expected of physician performance. Because of increased diversity within the practice, those areas that may have once been implicitly articulated and defined must frequently be addressed in a more explicit manner.

■ Measuring Work and Allocating Costs

Every medical practice, regardless of its setting, has two basic factors that determine physician compensation: revenues and expenses or operating costs. Each compensation system deals with this fundamental financial equation to yield compensation levels for individual physicians. How these two variables are addressed is key to whether the compensation system is deemed to be fair or unfair. Obviously, the approach to revenue and cost allocation plays a significant role in the practice's level of harmony and success.

Measuring Work

In determining physician compensation, most physician compensation plans focus on services that physicians personally perform. Professional service collections (i.e., the fruits of each individual physician's own labor) frequently serve as the basis for measuring physician work. Four broad categories of measures are commonly used in medical practices:

- *Collections:* Actual cash received by the practice for professional or other services attributed to the activities of an individual physician.
- *Charges:* Gross or net (after contractual adjustments).
- *Work RVUs:* An objective measure of work and effort defined by Medicare or other programs that is used to determine and pay reimbursement to physicians and medical groups for services.
- *Hybrid measures:* These include point scales, time units, and similar methodologies.

Just as there is no perfect compensation plan, there is no completely perfect or correct method to measuring physician work.

Collections have the value and benefit of relating to something real—money actually received by the practice. Unlike charges, which can be set at any level, regardless of whether any reimbursement is actually received, collections reflect cash in hand that the practice has received for professional services. Collections are commonly allocated directly to individual physicians based on their personal service collection levels as part of the compensation formula, or used to allocate some or all of a larger compensation pool.

Charges represent the practice's "asking price" for professional and other healthcare services. Because third-party payers only rarely pay practices what they ask for, the list of charges, whether gross or net (after adjustments), is commonly viewed as having inherent inequities when applied in the context of a compensation plan. Nevertheless, every practice has a fee schedule, and physicians frequently feel that they have a general sense of the charges or asking price for various procedures. Moreover, because the practice determines the charge level, variations from one procedure to another may be perceived to be more objective and fair to the physicians because the practice has established the charge level through internal mechanisms.

When charges are used, they are commonly used to allocate a pool of total revenues (or potentially practice profits or a compensation pool) based on a percentage of production basis. That is, if an individual physician's total charges constitute 4% of the group's (or subset's) charges, that physician is allocated 4% of the total or a defined subset of revenues or a pool of funds available for compensation in the context of the compensation plan. In this manner the charges are used to merely allocate a defined pool based on an imperfect measure of work or effort.

As compared to other measures, gross charges—the asking price for a practice's services—are likely to be the least effective means of relating work or production to compensation, because the charges assigned to different services or procedures have little to no relationship to the actual payment. Some services may have a charge level set at 150% of the Medicare allowable, whereas others might have a charge level set at 300% (or some other percentage) of Medicare allowable—even though the practice may receive compensation equal to 110% of Medicare allowable for the particular services.

Some medical practices do continue to use gross or net charges as part of their compensation systems, but these are typically limited to those practices that have historically used such measures, as opposed to those that are developing a new compensation system. Those relatively few practices that use or adopt charges as part of the compensation arrangement tend to do so due to tradition or because of inadequate information systems or infrastructure that makes using other approaches (e.g., collections from professional services, work RVUs, etc.) difficult.

Work RVUs use a standard measure to determine and pay physician compensation. Most RVU-based compensation plans incorporate the Medicare Resource-Based

Relative Value Scale (RBRVS) that is also used by most other third-party payers as the basis for determining reimbursement for physician and other healthcare services. The RBRVS system was developed, in part, as a means to provide uniform payment for the same services, while taking into account variations in the cost of service provision in different parts of the country and other factors. RBRVS assigns RVUs to every Current Procedural Terminology (CPT) code for professional services for Medicare payment purposes. Three specific RVUs are assigned for each code:

1. An RVU for physician work
2. An RVU for practice expenses
3. An RVU for malpractice expenses

Many organizations elect to use work RVUs, in whole or in part, in their compensation plans because they arguably measure work in a more objective manner than charges, collections, or other methods. This is based on the reality that the RVUs for a single procedure (represented by a CPT code) will be the same regardless of the physician specialty or practice location. Thus, the use of work RVUs in the compensation plan allows an organization to reward work without regard to payer mix, reimbursement levels, or related issues. In essence, a standard ruler is used for purposes of measuring and awarding physician compensation.

Hybrid measures are used by a minority of practices to measure work and allocate revenues or a pool of compensation. These include home-grown measures based on time, practice-specific work values that are developed internally in a practice, point scales, or similar methodologies. They commonly allocate all or a defined subset of funds based on agreed-upon methodology. Thus, for example, many cardiology groups use homegrown methods such as time units or similar measures to allocate the pool of funds based on a percentage of time. Those physicians who worked harder as measured by the hybrid time units will receive a larger share of the compensation pool.

Allocating Costs

Looking at physician work deals with only one part of the financial equation. Practice expenses continue to be a fact of life and as such must also be addressed—either directly or indirectly—in the compensation system.

Compensation systems take different approaches to cost allocation. On the continuum of compensation plans, individualistic models allocate costs based on an agreed-upon methodology involving cost accounting or similar methods. In these methodologies the costs themselves are tracked within the practice, and cost allocation is an essential component of the compensation scheme.

Medical practices that use cost allocation methods, for example, commonly divide costs or expenses into broad categories: fixed costs (for such things as facilities and equipment), variable costs (that arguably vary based on resource utilization or production), and direct expense items that are typically consumed by, and allocated directly to, individual physicians.

Within these three broad categories there are as many cost allocation methods as there are compensation plans. Many groups allocate, for example, the fixed cost component on an equal share or percentage of time basis. Physicians who are working a full-time schedule will typically bear or be allocated a full-time or equal share portion of the fixed expenses. Conversely, physicians who work less than full time will sometimes be allocated a reduced share of the fixed expense category. Although such an approach is common, many medical groups also allocate the fixed component directly to all physicians in an equal manner, regardless of their time commitment or work levels, and the part-time physician bears a full-time share of the fixed expense items.

Variable expenses are commonly allocated on a fully variable or a combined fixed-variable cost basis. Thus, personnel costs, supplies, and the like may be allocated with a portion allocated equally, and the remaining portion allocated based on a percentage of production. This results in those physicians who have higher levels of production bearing a larger share of the practice's expenses.

Direct expenses are typically allocated directly to individual physicians. Direct expenses include professional liability insurance costs, continuing medical education (CME) expenses, physician-specific business expenses, and the like. Some groups also allocate the physician's personal support personnel, whether a medical assistant, a physician assistant, or another provider, as a cost that is allocated directly to the physician. Because the physician most commonly receives the credit for the extender's work and performance, the physician also commonly bears the associated risk and expense.

Although it is commonly perceived that there is a "correct" or a "fair" approach to cost allocation, experience reveals that only rarely will two organizations allocate costs in precisely the same manner. Indeed, a survey of compensation plans used in better-performing medical groups revealed that apart from expense items that are commonly allocated on a direct basis, other broad expense items such as supplies and services, administrative costs, personnel, rent, and the like may be allocated among physicians in a practice using any number of methods.

Although there may not be a correct or inherently fair methodology for cost allocation, the cost allocation issue nevertheless provides the basis for substantial levels of negotiation (and potential conflict) in any medical practice. This conflict may be manifested most evidently in multispecialty practices where the perceived resource consumption differences between primary care and specialist physicians are most acute. As a result, compensation plans with complex cost allocation methodologies are more common in small, medium, or even some large multispecialty groups than in their more cohesive single-specialty practices.

In the multispecialty setting, disputes and perceptions regarding overhead may occur between primary care physicians with more intensive office-based practices, and medical and surgical specialist physicians whose procedurally oriented practices require them to spend more time in hospitals and other settings where no direct overhead cost is (arguably) incurred. Yet as referenced previously, even single-specialty practices have their own multispecialty characteristics. For example, cardiology groups may experience cost allocation disputes between invasive, interventional, noninvasive, and electrophysiology physicians. Likewise, orthopedic groups sometimes have conflicts between the general orthopedists, spine surgeons, joint replacement specialists, hand surgeons, and others. In such instances, a common perception is that time away from the practice (i.e., time in the hospital performing surgeries) involves relatively lower levels of resource usage that should yield lower overhead costs and higher levels of compensation.

Not every organization specifically allocates costs as discussed here. Individualistic and middle-ground models use a methodology that determines physician compensation on a negotiated rather than precise basis, and these compensation structures typically include some allocation of costs.

Team-based models generally seek to stay away from direct cost allocation, and instead view the cost of practice as a cost of doing business. The compensation plan focuses on allocating the compensation pool, and frequently practice expenses include a portion of physician compensation in the form of a base salary. Yet even team-based models are not immune from the type of conflict that can undermine a compensation plan and a group's cohesiveness. Although practice expenses are not directly allocated or charged to individual physicians under many such models, physicians commonly still have perceptions of their relative overhead rates despite the absence of direct cost allocation methods. By illustration, the physician who knows he or she produced $1 million yet receives $400,000 in compensation almost inevitably perceives that he or she has experienced an overhead rate of 60 percent—regardless of whether the practice has allocated $600,000 of costs or overhead to the physician as part of the compensation plan.

Other Measures

In addition to the basic model involving consideration of work and/or revenues and expenses, many practices use other more intangible or subjective measures to determine at least a portion of physician compensation. These frequently focus on issues of patient satisfaction, quality, subgroup-level financial or other performance, administrative services, and others. Such methods are most common in large organizations, as well as in tax-exempt or hospital-affiliated practice enterprises. Although feasible, small group practices frequently experience challenges in using subjective measures to allocate and reward compensation because they tend to view themselves more as partnerships than as corporations. Physicians in a 5-member, 10-member, or even larger group practice may experience queasiness in making subjective or even arguably objective judgments regarding their colleagues' performance or worth based on patient satisfaction, quality, or similar criteria.

On the other hand, more subjective factors are commonly used to allocate a portion of compensation in larger, more established organizations, including hospitals and others. In such organizations, compensation committees, quality review boards, objective patient satisfaction scores in relation to targeted levels of performance, and similar measures are used to assess performance and award compensation.

Likewise, measures focusing on group-level financial or other performance will typically provide for the allocation of defined dollar amounts (commonly based on a percentage of base salary or the like) for performance in relation to defined targets or goals. Such targets and goals may include financial performance as well as performance based on outreach targets, patient access standards, increased patient visit volumes, or the like. Performance is frequently evaluated by reference to agreed-upon criteria, and the group or subgroup as a whole and its individual participants receive a defined level of compensation based on their performance in relation to the target.

In the face of changing payment and reimbursement systems, many established medical groups are working to transition from their current compensation practices that base compensation largely or entirely on physician levels of production, to those that consider quality and other metrics in determining and paying compensation. By illustration, many large, well-respected clinics and medical groups compensate their physicians using a pure-production compensation model (in which the physician receives additional compensation for each unit of work), or by using a fixed salary, where the salary itself is based on physician production. However, to transition the compensation structures, many such organizations have developed a strategy to incrementally move to a compensation plan consisting of a base salary plus incentive components, with the incentive components including compensation that will be awarded based on performance in relation to individual and group or "team"-oriented targets. Such plans will commonly reward individual physicians when they meet a defined target for patient access. Other incentives may consider physician-specific continuity of care or physician-specific patient satisfaction scores. In each case, a predefined incentive award may be evaluated and awarded on an annual or semi-annual basis.

Likewise, to help promote the team orientation that is likely to be required under emerging systems of accountable care, many organizations are also awarding a portion of total potential compensation based on performance in relation to location- or department-wide targets regarding patient access or other variables. Patient access will commonly be measured by the availability of department-wide next available appointments, and the department will receive an incentive payment for meeting a defined target. As the use of the patient-centered medical home (PCMH) approach to healthcare delivery is adopted and used, many medical groups will base a portion of available incentive compensation on whether a particular practice site or location achieves defined levels of the PCMH performance, thereby joining the site's providers together in furtherance of a shared goal.

Overall, many compensation structures will likely migrate over the next few years, changing from systems focusing entirely on productivity and cost management to those designed to focus provider attention on access, quality, value, teamwork, and other variables.

Plan Methods and the Importance of Context

As consistent with the underlying theme of this chapter, the context in which the compensation plan operates plays a large role in the nature of the plan. Plans that are found in small, privately owned medical practices are frequently dramatically different from those used in large, integrated delivery systems—although the methodologies share common characteristics. Smaller groups, whether in privately owned and operated medical practices or in hospital-affiliated or academic practice models comprising individual divisions or departments, frequently involve individualistic compensation models. Yet small medical group settings also use team-based models that allocate available revenues or profit on an agreed-upon basis including based on an equal share, percentage of production, or combined methodology.

Many hospital-affiliated and academic practice models use "base plus incentive" systems, a variation of a team-based model discussed previously. Base plus incentive systems will pay individual clinicians a defined base salary based on specialty, years of practice, historic production, and other factors. The base salary frequently comprises only a subset of the estimated total compensation, with the additional or "incentive" component determined by other factors. Market data such as surveys from the Medical Group Management Association (MGMA), the American Medical Group Association (AMGA), and other sources are frequently used to establish base salary levels based on physician specialties, work levels, seniority, academic rank, and other factors.

Hospital-affiliated and academic medical groups also commonly use production-based compensation methods that expressly consider or mimic practice overhead costs associated with differing levels of production. Many hospital-affiliated medical groups use a defined dollar amount per work RVU to determine and pay compensation to the organization's physician employees. Thus, for example, the organization may determine that the median level of compensation per work RVU based on a composite of MGMA, AMGA, and other measures may equal $40 per work RVU. Individual physicians will be paid this or a slightly adjusted amount for every work RVU they personally perform.

The strength of such methodologies is that they reward physicians for their work without regard to external payment levels, payer mix, or related factors. Likewise, the linkage to market data provides a level of internal and external validity to the dollar amount paid per work RVU. As with any system, however, the primary challenge with such a method stems from setting the dollar-per-work-RVU conversion factor at an acceptable level, while also ensuring that the organization has sufficient revenues to pay the compensation due. Hospitals and small and large medical group practices have experienced the challenge of agreeing to pay compensation at a level that cannot be supported financially.

An additional variation of the basic dollars per work RVU model uses a graduated dollar amount per work RVU, with different dollar amounts paid based on varying levels of productivity. Moreover, instead of linking the dollar amount per work RVU to reported MGMA, AMGA, or similar values, many methods use a calculation approach to determine a starting point conversion factor for physician compensation; that is, median compensation levels as measured by market are divided by median work RVUs to determine the calculated level of compensation per work RVU at the median level of production. In essence, the common theme is that median work levels should yield median compensation.

Importantly, methods such as those just described assume there is some correlation among work levels, overhead rates, and compensation. A physician whose production would place him or her at the twenty-fifth percentile as measured by MGMA or other market data would produce lower levels of revenues and would typically have a higher overhead rate (expressed as a percentage of total revenues produced) than a colleague producing at the fiftieth or seventy-fifth percentile. Because the largest portion of medical practice costs are fixed (typically in the range of 60–80%), physicians with lower production levels will, under such plans, effectively need to cover their operating costs before receiving additional amounts in compensation. Thus, under these RVU methodologies, a graduated scale is used to pay increasing dollar amounts per work RVU that are themselves linked to physician production.

Aside from these basic methodologies, a multitude of other methods and configurations are used in medical group compensation plans. These include compensation methods that combine equal share and production measures, and methods that combine different approaches to measuring work or production such as team-based models that allocate a portion of the total compensation pool based on percentage of work RVUs, on an equal share basis, and a portion based on collections. Such models may also include a cost allocation component that is layered on top of the revenue allocation method.

There is no perfect compensation plan, only alternative compensation plans that are more or less imperfect for a particular set of physicians at a particular point in time. The challenge in crafting the appropriate compensation plan for a particular medical group and context is to craft a plan that reasonably promotes the practice's goals, while also maintaining a reasonable level of physician satisfaction with the arrangement. The methodological tools outlined earlier, whether they involve methods of measuring work or allocating revenues, tracking expenses, promoting individual and team responsibility, or other goals, are merely methodological tools akin to chess pieces to be used in crafting the arrangement that will work for a particular group of providers, in a particular setting, at a particular point in time.

Noncompensation Issues with Compensation Plan Implications

A consistent theme throughout this chapter is the importance of nonfinancial factors on physician compensation. Group size, group dynamics, organizational setting, and the like play an important role in compensation methodologies. Likewise, whether an organization is small or large, whether it is privately owned or publicly affiliated in the form of a hospital employment, hospital-affiliated, or academic practice setting, also influences the type of methodology that can be used.

Apart from these broad contextual issues, other issues also arise in the context of compensation plan development, implementation, and ongoing operations. These noncompensation issues have very real implications.

Practice Buy-In and Buy-Out Arrangements

The first noncompensation issue with compensation plan implications relates to practice buy-in and buy-out arrangements. Historically, physicians and physician practices were based on a partnership model. Physicians who joined a practice were required to pay an amount of money, directly through out-of-pocket outlays, indirectly through salary deductions, or through both methods, to buy their way into the practice. Once the buy-in was completed, the new partner or shareholder physician enjoyed all the fruits of ownership in the enterprise, including equal participation in the compensation plan.

Today many physician-owned medical groups use practice buy-in approaches similar to those in other professional service firms. New physicians will typically work in an associate status for 1 to 2 years, or another defined period of time. Associate status provides an opportunity for the new physician to build a practice base, and allows the group's partner physicians to evaluate the new physician's clinical competence and ultimately determine whether the associate should become an owner. New physicians are frequently expected to meet certain work-related targets before partnership is considered, related to revenue generation, clinical competence, and the like. They also may provide a slight but reasonable return on investment to the practice and its existing owners, either in financial terms or in other ways, such as work that is shifted to the new physician and opportunities that the new physician creates for the practice.

New owners must also commonly meet certain financial obligations related to buy-in in physician-owned medical groups. Most small medical practices use one of two basic buy-in valuation methods. In an increasing

number of practices, the buy-in amount is set in advance at a predefined "token" or other reasonable value (for example, in the $1,000 to $50,000 range). In these practices the new partner is viewed as being valuable because of the additional contribution to overhead, work, call coverage, and other value they bring, apart from any potential direct monetary value that they provide to the practice's existing owners.

Other physician-owned practices use a defined methodology to determine the buy-in value, typically based on the value of the practice's fixed assets (e.g., furniture and equipment) and accounts receivable (A/R). In these cases the buy-in amount is calculated via a set formula to define the purchase price of the stock (i.e., depreciated book value of the practice's tangible assets, net of liabilities, excluding A/R or goodwill, divided by the number of physicians who will be owners after the transaction has occurred). An additional value based on a defined share of A/R (for example, A/R generated by the physician or a share of the total practice A/R, adjusted for expected collections) may also be defined and assessed as part of the buy-in arrangement. The asset being paid for via the A/R calculation may be referred to using any number of names, but in bottom line terms, it represents income forgone that is part of the total buy-in package. Practices using these more specific valuation methods arguably still have fair arrangements because the same method has been used in the past, and will be used in the future.

Buy-in arrangements in physician-owned medical groups have compensation-related implications because they (and buy-out arrangements discussed later) affect the amount of compensation to be received by the new partner physician, or by those physicians who remain after the departure of a physician via practice buy-out. Because buy-in arrangements define the price that must be paid to join a private, physician-owned practice, the payment of that price may decrease the level of compensation otherwise available to a physician during the time he or she joins a practice, with potential implications for recruitment, retention, and physician willingness to join the practice and become an owner.

Moreover, the approach to buy-in will typically be linked to the approach to compensation, specifically how the practice treats the funds that were generated by the new owner physician during his or her status as an associate. Under a pure productivity-based model, for example, the new partner may need to start from scratch in terms of generating accounts receivable that will pay the physician's compensation during the initial months as an owner. Alternatively, the compensation plan may provide credit for the A/R generated while the physician worked as an associate, but not provide full credit for A/R in the context of deferred compensation arrangements paid on departure if the physician has only been with the practice a relatively short period of time (typically 3 to 5 years) as of the date of departure. The challenge is to develop buy-in arrangements that meet the practice's and new physician's perceived views of fairness, while also promoting the physician-owned practice's recruitment and retention goals.

The flip side of buy-in arrangements, the buy-out mechanism, frequently mirrors the buy-in in certain respects. Practices that use the token stock buy-in method (such as a flat stock purchase price of $10,000) may return the token when the physician leaves active practice. Likewise, those that define the stock purchase value based on the value of fixed assets commonly use the same or a similar valuation method at the time of buy-out. Those that require the physician to purchase a share of A/R (either through direct cash outlays or salary deferrals, or indirectly via the operation of the group's compensation plan) provide for the payment of a portion of A/R on termination of employment via a deferred compensation/severance or similar arrangement. The calculation methods of the buy-in and buy-out event should generally be the same, even though the dollar values paid may differ because they occur at different points in time.

As with practice buy-in arrangements, the approach to buy-out can also have implications for compensation, recruitment, and retention in the practice. Buy-out arrangements that provide a large payout to departing physicians (e.g., for practice goodwill or some other measure that goes beyond the physician's personal production) can undermine the compensation levels of those who remain. Moreover, expensive buy-outs that must be made to multiple physicians over an extended period of time and, in the process, decrease the remaining physicians' compensation levels, when coupled with practice buy-in obligations for more junior physicians, can create an environment in which physician recruitment and retention is undermined.

Of course, the buy-in and buy-out discussion focuses on the existing arrangement with physician-owned medical groups, in which new physician employees can become true owners of the practice. In other medical group settings, notably hospital-affiliated medical groups, true buy-in structures that involve payments in exchange for ownership interests are typically not used. Nonetheless, some, but not all, hospital-affiliated compensation models will use surrogate buy-in type arrangements that ensure new physicians do not receive the same amount of compensation as more senior physicians. These systems typically provide for different compensation during a 1- to 2-year "associate" period, after which the physician will migrate to an "established" physician compensation plan.

Practice Transition

Practice transition issues relate to the desires of physicians at different points in their career to change or slow down their practice for one reason or another. Transition has historically referred to desires by senior physicians to work part-time or reduced time, or have reduced (or no) call schedule. Today, transitional issues arise with a broader complement of physicians, both male and female, seeking time away from practice to raise children, to care for elderly parents, or simply to enjoy a less rigorous practice style and lifestyle.

The challenge with transition arrangements is the delicate balance required to both fulfill the transitioning physician's goals and to keep the medical practice viable. In financial terms, the physician in a transition mode generally must accept a lower level of compensation for the opportunity of a nontraditional practice. This reduced compensation level will be expressed in a number of ways, such as an equal allocation of overhead costs (which reduces take-home pay due to generally lower levels of production by the physician in transition), or in some instances a wholly separate and different compensation plan. Transitioning physicians are frequently placed on a nonpartner or special compensation arrangement that recognizes that their practice is not the same as their full-time colleagues'. Challenges and conflict occur, however, when the transitioning physician's compensation plan, coupled with lifestyle opportunities, is perceived to be more beneficial than that enjoyed by full-time physicians—but without the associated costs.

The reality of a transition event is that it generally results in at least some net transfer of work from the physician engaged in the transition to those who remain. For that reason, many practices develop consistent policies that consider, and attempt to balance, the transitioning physician's and group's needs. In doing so they wrestle with and address key questions such as:

- Minimum level of time commitment required for a physician to remain an employee and/or a partner in the practice
- Whether a transitional practice model is a right or a privilege
- Number of physicians who can be in a transitional practice at one time
- Prerequisites and time limits associated with a transitional work arrangement

- The cost of the transition opportunity in terms of overhead or reduced compensation
- The transition arrangement's impact on the physician's other rights and opportunities including governance and decision making in the practice

Overall, buy/sell and transition arrangements tend to relate to three key issues—work, power, and money—which must be maintained in balance in the medical practice's unique business and social context:

- Individual physician and group views of the amount and type of effort individual physicians contribute to the organization. Specifically, whether those seeking to become practice partners or seeking to modify their practice are contributing to the group at acceptable levels, and how the addition of a new physician or the transition of an established physician would affect the practice and its other providers negatively
- The formal and informal means of physician influence and control over the practice's future
- The financial implications of a buy/sell or transition arrangement on an individual physician, other physicians, and the medical practice as a whole

Although other issues may influence perceptions of what's right and fair, experience shows that these three must be understood and addressed in crafting any effective buy-in, buy-out, or transition solution. Accordingly, the practical objectives of effective buy-in, buy-out, and transition arrangements include:

- Crafting a reasonable approach to buy-in that can be met by the physician whose long-term participation in the practice is desired
- Providing a fair deal while also ensuring that the buy-out event doesn't sabotage the practice's future success by the arrangement provided to the departing physician
- Assuring that the practice, the transitioning physician, and the physicians who remain obtain a fair deal in any transition arrangement

On-Call Obligations

The third major noncompensation issue with compensation implications relates to on-call obligations and desires by individual physicians to reduce their on-call schedules. A reduction in call may be in the form of a reduced number of days on call or an outright elimination of on-call obligations.

As with many issues, the importance of the on-call termination or reduction varies from one medical practice to another, and from specialty to specialty. Certain specialties (e.g., dermatology, allergy) typically have relatively limited on-call obligations in the form of required night and weekend emergency service requirements. On the other hand, other practice specialties (e.g., internal medicine, cardiology, general surgery, OB/GYN, orthopedics) have more significant on-call obligations, meaning that the physicians have a far greater likelihood of being called to attend to emergency requirements. For physicians in these specialties, a reduction in call or a termination in on-call duties is viewed as a significant benefit to one physician, while imposing additional obligations on other physicians in the practice.

Group size also has implications for the magnitude of any change in the on-call obligations. Regardless of whether the medical practice consists of a small number of individual physicians or exists in a larger group but shares calls among several different relatively small call groups, any change in the number of "bodies" to assume the on-call obligations will have a direct effect on the quality of life of those physicians who continue to assume the group's on-call duties. By illustration, a reduction from five to four physicians in a surgical group or department taking on-call obligations results in a 25% increase in the total number of days on call for the four physicians who continue to take on-call obligations.

Medical practices adopt many different approaches to on-call obligations. Some require physicians to continue taking call regardless of their tenure, age, or other issues. Call obligation is viewed as an ongoing obligation and minimum performance expectation of every physician in the practice.

Other groups elect to eliminate call without financial cost on the occurrence of certain events or based on defined criteria. Such criteria typically include physician age, years of service with the group, and length of time during which the physician can continue to practice in the group, but not take full on-call obligations.

Some groups reduce, but do not eliminate, on-call obligations, therefore making on-call service more palatable. This can be in the form of requiring nights but no weekends, fewer days on call, or related approaches.

Some medical groups assign a monetary value to the obligation to take call and link that to the compensation that is otherwise earned and paid by the physician. This may be in the form of negative incentives such as an outright reduction in the amount of compensation that is otherwise earned by the individual physician. For example, groups or subsets of physicians who provide for an equal share or base salary component to their compensation plan reduce that equal share or base salary component by some agreed-upon level (e.g., 25–35%). The physician benefiting from the reduced call obligation receives less compensation. That reduced compensation is, in turn, allocated to the practice's remaining physicians who have assumed the on-call obligation.

Other practices attempt to craft changes to call more in the form of a positive incentive. The groups set aside a specific pool of funds that is used to pay physicians for their on-call obligations. Under this approach, the group pays each physician for the work that he or she does, and those who elect to reduce or terminate call will simply not participate in the on-call pool.

The majority of groups combine one or more of these techniques to come up with a reduced or terminated on-call policy. Groups might require, for example, that physicians may only terminate call on achieving a specific age (e.g., age 55, 60, or 65 years). Only those physicians who have achieved this specific age and required years of service with the group or predecessor organizations would be eligible for the reduced or terminated call obligations (e.g., 25 years with the practice). Until those two criteria are met, on-call obligation is mandatory. These groups also assess a financial penalty on those physicians who meet these criteria and elect to cease or reduce their on-call obligations.

Overall, the issues related to buy-in/buy-out, physician transition, on-call, and related obligations and opportunities have important implications for a medical practice's compensation arrangement. These issues are rarely determinative of the methodology. Yet as physician demographics in the practice change, practice diversity increases, and other cultural and relational factors come into play, these issues will frequently take center stage and have a significant implication for the compensation methodology and physician satisfaction with the compensation plan.

Administrative Services

A final compensation-related issue involves compensation for administrative services undertaken by physicians. The approach taken by medical groups to such issues varies dramatically. In small practices some level of responsibility for administrative services is typically expected of all physicians. It is viewed as a reality of working in a small-practice setting.

As practices increase in size they typically elect to focus their administrative activities by retaining nonphysician professionals, and in many instances, by appointing a physician to assume a more active leadership role. In these instances the question of compensation for the physician's administrative services gains importance.

In most cases the adage that "you get what you pay for" applies in a medical practice, just as in other settings. Professionals can be expected to devote some level of work for the good of the group, but as the time commitment, level of responsibility and engagement, and other features associated with administrative service increase, demands and expectations for compensated administrative service also increase.

Practices that pay for administrative service determine pay levels based on any number of methods. Some practices pay all physicians a defined "token" for attending meetings such as board meetings or special committee meetings that demand additional time and/or responsibilities. The token will typically be taken from the practice's other funds available for compensation, and as such, will reward those who provide service while decreasing (typically only slightly) the funds otherwise available for payment through the practice's compensation plan.

Other practices assign dollar values to certain important administrative and leadership positions that are assumed by physicians. Thus, a practice's president, medical director, or other position has a defined stipend to be paid to the physician who occupies the position.

In practices sufficiently large that a full-time or largely full-time administrative role is needed, the practices tend to determine a base salary arrangement for administrative activities.

The practical objective of administrative compensation is typically to provide a fair level of compensation for a physician's administrative services. In most instances, however, the amount of compensation is less than could otherwise be earned by the physician in an active practice. Thus, the approach to setting pay levels is based on what is fair and reasonable, rather than based on an opportunity cost.

■ Legal Considerations

Various legal prohibitions affect physician compensation arrangements. Not surprisingly, the specific legal issues that affect any compensation plan depend on context—specifically, the context of where the employment relationship lies: in a privately owned and operated physician group, or in a more public practice setting such as a hospital-affiliated medical practice, an academic faculty practice plan, or similar setting.

Although the potential range of legal issues is enormous, the primary legal restrictions include restrictions imposed by the federal physician self-referral or Stark law, the Medicare antikickback law, the Civil Monetary

Penalties statute, and those statutes applicable to tax-exempt organizations.

The Stark Law

The federal physician self-referral or Stark law generally prohibits physicians from making referrals of certain "designated health services" to organizations with which the physician has a financial relationship.[2] Specifically, under the Stark law a physician cannot make a referral to an entity for the furnishing of designated health services, which may be payable by Medicare or Medicaid, if the physician (or an immediate family member of the physician) has a financial relationship with the entity, unless an exception under the law applies.

Claims to Medicare for services furnished in violation of the law are denied and repayment is required. The law also provides for fines under certain circumstances, and physicians and organizations that violate the Stark law also can be excluded from participating in the Medicare and Medicaid programs. If all required elements are present to trigger the Stark law's application to a physician's financial and referral relationship, an exception under the Stark law must be fully complied with to avoid penalties.

The law was originally enacted in 1989, and then expanded in 1991. Final regulations implementing the expanded Stark law were published in three phases: Phase I (January 4, 2001), Phase II (March 26, 2004), and Phase III (September 5, 2007). Rules governing Stark are continually modified through incremental changes that are published via annual updates to the Medicare physician fee schedule. The law and the regulations are together referred to as the Stark law. Included in the regulations is guidance related to physician compensation arrangements, including the law's application to compensation arrangements in group practices.

Major implications of the Stark law in the context of medical group and hospital-affiliated compensation arrangements include the following:

- Various services provided by medical practices, hospitals, and other organizations are defined as designated health services that are subject to the Stark law prohibitions. These include laboratory, radiology and other imaging services, outpatient prescription drugs, and inpatient and outpatient hospital services. Therefore, an exception to the Stark law must be identified and relied on to allow physicians to make referrals to various organizations including the physicians' employer medical practice, hospitals, and other organizations for such services.

- Private practice and certain hospital-affiliated medical groups can rely on the Stark law's exception for in-office ancillary services. An essential requirement for meeting the terms of this exception is that the medical group practice qualify as a bona fide group practice for purposes of the Stark law, which imposes specific requirements on the compensation methodology that may be used in the group practice. Such a qualification can enable the group to provide laboratory, x-ray, outpatient prescription drugs, and other designated health services through the group practice, and retain revenues from those services to pay the group practice's operating expenses, physician compensation, and other costs. This is the primary exception relied upon to permit traditional, physician-owned medical groups to furnish and receive payment for Medicare-payable ancillary services.

- The Stark law also affects the compensation plan methodologies that can be used in bona fide employment contexts involving physicians and hospitals and other medical practices. Here, too, the primary concern is that no compensation may be paid based on the volume or value of referrals for designated health services, and further, only certain forms of productivity or other bonuses may be provided as part of the compensation plan. In addition, the compensation under a bona fide employment arrangement must be consistent with fair market value and commercially reasonable.

Assuming that a group practice qualifies as a bona fide group practice for Stark law purposes, compensation arrangements for group practice physicians must be structured to comply with the Stark law. The result is that the group can furnish designated health services and retain revenues and income from those services—whether those services consist of clinical laboratory services, radiology services, outpatient prescription drugs, or other services provided through the group practice. The group practice may also pool and allocate those revenues (either gross revenues or net of expenses) within the group practice as part of the group's physician compensation plan, provided that the pooling and distribution methodology complies with the Stark law requirement that the distribution not be based on the volume or value of the physician's referrals (plus other applicable requirements).

The Stark law also affects the compensation arrangements with group physicians, regardless of whether the group independently furnishes designated health services (i.e., through the group itself) or whether such services are furnished by a hospital or health system. Specifically, the Stark law and associated regulations prohibit the payment of any compensation based on the volume or value of the employed physicians' referrals (or other business generated between the parties). In this instance the referrals would include referrals for designated health services including inpatient and outpatient hospital services, clinical laboratory services, outpatient prescription drugs, or other services that are defined as designated health services under the law.

Even if physician compensation arrangements involving tax-exempt hospitals comply with the requirements of the Stark law, the ultimate level of compensation received by each physician would still be subject to the requirements of reasonableness under applicable tax-exempt organization rules, as discussed in a later section.

The Antikickback Law

The second primary legal restriction applicable to physician compensation arrangements, such as those found in the group, is provided under the federal antikickback statute.[3] In general, this law prohibits the payment of any remuneration—essentially anything of value—in exchange for physician referrals.

Specific "safe harbor" restrictions are provided under the antikickback law for compensation paid to employees of a medical group practice or other organization. Other safe harbor provisions are frequently relied on to allow for other financial transactions between a physician and other organization (e.g., medical director agreements with hospitals). In all cases, hallmarks of a legally compliant compensation relationship include the existence of written agreements (e.g., contraction documents) governing the contractual relationship, a contractual term of at least 1 year, and that the level of compensation paid under the agreement is consistent with fair market value (along with other more specific requirements). Compliance with a safe harbor under the antikickback statute is optional; failure to strictly comply with a safe harbor does not mean that the law has been violated.

Civil Monetary Penalties

The Civil Monetary Penalties statute prohibits a hospital from knowingly making a payment or other incentives to physicians to reduce or limit items or services furnished to Medicare or Medicaid beneficiaries, and prohibits a physician from knowingly accepting such payment. Concerns may arise in compensation arrangements that could be interpreted to require or encourage physicians to reduce care to patients, such as "gain-share" savings compensation or similar programs. These arrangements must be carefully crafted to include limits to ensure that all patients receive all medically and necessary items and services covered by the Medicare program, and the quality of patient care services is not impacted adversely as a result of the program.

The Office of Inspector General (OIG) has issued several advisory opinions approving of hospitals' gain-sharing arrangements with physician organizations. These arrangements contained many different cost and quality measures designed to change participating physicians' operating room and laboratory practices to curb the inappropriate use or waste of medical supplies, such as limiting the use of certain surgical supplies and devices to an as-needed basis, opening packaged items only as needed during a procedure, and substituting less costly items where substitutions would have no appreciable clinical significance. In reviewing and considering safeguards in gain-sharing arrangements, the OIG considered many factors, including the transparency and accountability of the specific cost-saving actions and resulting savings, the existence of credible medical support for the position that implementation of the recommendations would not adversely affect patient care, and whether the distribution of profits from the program sufficiently mitigates any incentive for an individual participating physician to generate disproportionate cost savings.

Importantly, the Civil Monetary Penalties statute also has potential application to shared savings and similar programs likely to be considered and implemented under the PPACA health reform program. When a hospital makes a payment to a physician and links that payment to the physician's care, then the law needs to be considered and addressed.

Tax-Exempt Issues

Provisions of the Internal Revenue Code (IRC) governing tax-exempt organizations impose restrictions on both the amount of compensation and the methodology used by tax-exempt organizations, such as most of the nation's hospitals, to determine and pay compensation to their physician employees. IRC section 501(c)(3) provides that hospitals can generally obtain and maintain tax-exempt status so long as they operate exclusively for religious, charitable, or educational purposes, "no part of the net earnings of which inures to the benefit of any private shareholder or individual."[4] These requirements have been construed to prohibit hospitals from paying excessive compensation to "insiders" including physicians, hospital management, and others. They have further implications for the manner in which compensation is determined and paid—the plan methodology.

Until 1996, organizations that violated the requirements of IRC section 501(c)(3) risked losing their tax-exempt status—although such a drastic remedy was only rarely imposed. In 1996, however, Congress enacted IRC section 4958—typically referred to as the intermediate sanctions legislation—which provides for an "intermediate" remedy to the revocation of an organization's tax-exempt status. The intermediate sanctions law imposes taxes on persons who are influential to tax-exempt enterprises and who either benefit from or approve transactions that are not consistent with fair market value. Specifically, section 4958 provides for the imposition of personal excise taxes on "disqualified persons" (DPs) who benefit from "excess benefit transactions." Taxes may also be defined and imposed on the organization managers who approve those transactions under certain circumstances.

An excess benefit transaction occurs when an exempt organization provides an economic benefit to a DP and receives less than the value of the benefit in return. Transactions that are reasonable and consistent with fair market value will not constitute excess benefit transactions. The most common form of excess benefit transaction involves unreasonable compensation for services, but excess benefit transactions can also involve exchanges of property. Excess benefit transactions can result from direct or indirect dealings between a tax-exempt organization and a DP, including through intermediary entities.

Certain persons are automatically deemed to have substantial influence over the exempt organization and, as such, will be deemed to be disqualified persons: voting members of the governing body; persons holding a position comparable to that of president, CEO, COO, CFO, or treasurer; and certain others.

For persons not falling into one of those categories, including most physicians who have financial relationships with an exempt organization, a "facts and circumstances" test is used to determine whether the person has substantial influence over the exempt enterprise. Factors that tend to suggest substantial influence over the affairs of the exempt organization include:

- The person's compensation is primarily based on activities of the organization that the person controls.
- The person has or shares substantial budgetary authority (i.e., authority to determine a substantial portion of the organization's capital expenditures, operating budget, or employee compensation).
- The person has substantial management authority (i.e., the person manages a discrete segment of the organization that is a substantial portion of the

activities, assets, income, or expenses of the organization as a whole).
- The person owns a controlling interest in an entity that is itself a DP.
- The person is a nonprofit organization controlled by one or more DPs.

These facts, either individually or in combination, will contribute to a classification as a DP under the facts and circumstances test.

Compliance with both IRC section 501(c)(3) and the intermediate sanctions legislation (section 4958) requires, as a practical matter, that compensation levels paid to physicians must be "reasonable" and consistent with fair market value. Compensation for this purpose includes all items of compensation including salary, fees, bonuses, severance payments, vested and earned deferred compensation, and other benefits.

Despite statutory and regulatory requirements that compensation must be reasonable and consistent with fair market value, there is no definitive measure of the "reasonableness" of compensation. Rather, what is reasonable compensation is defined as the amount that would ordinarily be paid for like services, by like organizations, in like circumstances. The determination of whether a particular level of compensation is reasonable rests on consideration of the facts and circumstances surrounding the transaction and the compensation arrangement. Certain factual criteria are relevant to the question of reasonableness including whether the compensation was agreed to in an arms-length transaction, and whether the compensation is generally consistent with what others in the marketplace would earn for their services.

The requirement that compensation must be reasonable does not require physicians and other persons who are associated with tax-exempt organizations to receive less than their colleagues in the nonexempt world; nor must they donate their services to the exempt enterprise. Instead, industry standards and the operation of the market are the only real measure of reasonableness, and salary surveys such as those conducted by the MGMA and AMGA are frequently used to provide evidence of comparability and to help determine the reasonableness of compensation.

In addition to the question of reasonableness, various Internal Revenue Service (IRS) materials offer guidance that provides the foundation for the development of acceptable compensation methodologies in the context of tax-exempt organizations. Compensation plans used by tax-exempt hospitals are typically different than those used in a private practice setting. Guidance from the IRS has consistently prohibited compensation based on a distribution of net income from the exempt organization. Further, compensation methodologies that serve as disguised dividends or other devices to distribute the profits of the exempt enterprise or that convert the essential nature of the tax-exempt organization into a joint venture are prohibited.

Because of these provisions, compensation arrangements used with physicians in tax-exempt organizations must be crafted to comply with applicable tax-exempt organization rules and requirements. Simply put, a tax-exempt hospital can't collect the money, pay the bills other than physician compensation, and pay what's left over (if any) to a hospital's physician employees. The IRS is interested not only in the amount of compensation paid, but also how that compensation is determined and paid.

In general, incentive compensation arrangements that have been approved by the IRS for use in hospital and other tax-exempt settings include the following safeguards:

- An arm's-length contractual relationship exists between the tax-exempt organization and the physician or other party.
- The incentive payment serves a real and discernible business purpose of the exempt organization; for example, the incentive compensation arrangement helps to promote the exempt organization's charitable mission in furnishing healthcare services to members of the community.
- The amount of compensation is not dependent principally on incoming revenue of the exempt organization, but rather, on the accomplishment of the objectives of the compensation contract (e.g., seeing patients regardless of ability to pay).
- A review of actual operating results reveals no evidence of abuse or unwarranted benefits (i.e., the compensation that was paid was not unreasonable in amount).
- The presence of a ceiling or reasonable maximum so as to avoid the possibility of a windfall benefit to the service provider based on factors bearing no direct relationship to the level of service provided

In light of this list, various methodological and process safeguards are typically imposed in compensation plan methodologies to help promote both the reasonableness of compensation levels and the compensation methodology itself. Revenue procedure 97-13 dealing with tax-exempt bonds also imposes certain requirements that inform physician compensation arrangements with tax-exempt hospitals and other exempt organizations. Under revenue procedure 97-13, a compensation transaction generally falls within a recognized safe harbor if the amount of compensation is reasonable for the services rendered, with no compensation based in whole or in part on a share of the net profits from the operation of the exempt facility.

Arrangements that are generally not treated as net profits arrangements include the payment of compensation based on:

- A percentage of gross or adjusted gross revenues (net of bad debt, adjustments, etc.), or a percentage of expenses from a facility, but not both.
- A capitation fee or a per-unit fee (i.e., based on RVUs).
- Payment of a productivity reward equal to a stated dollar amount based on increases or decreases in gross revenues (or adjusted revenues) and reductions in total expenses—but not both—in any annual period during the term of the contract. Such an arrangement generally does not cause the compensation to be based on a share of net profits.

Provisions of the intermediate sanctions legislation as well as an increased emphasis on compliance activities have led to steps in the process of determining the compensation levels to be paid by tax-exempt hospitals and other organizations to their affiliated physicians. Perhaps the most important step involves the use of outside experts to independently assess and sign off on compensation levels; such activities can provide a rebuttable presumption that the compensation levels are, in fact, reasonable. Under the intermediate sanctions law and associated regulations, compensation payments will benefit from a "rebuttable presumption" that the transaction terms are reasonable and consistent with fair market value if:

- The transaction is approved in advance by an authorized body with no conflict of interest in the transaction, such as a board, committee, or other party authorized under state law to approve the transaction on the exempt organization's behalf
- The authorized body obtained and relied on "appropriate data as to comparability" prior to making its decision
- The authorized body adequately documented the basis for its decision concurrent with the determination

Once the rebuttable presumption is established, the IRS can only show that the transaction is not reasonable or is inconsistent with fair market value by demonstrating that the comparability data were unreliable or improper.

Therefore, abiding by the process to establish the rebuttable presumption can be of substantial benefit to both managers and DPs.

The authorized body must review appropriate data as to comparability in its decisions. Importantly, court decisions confirm that the data must be closely comparable to the exact type of transaction or arrangement, and take the specific features of the deal into account. For compensation deals, acceptable comparability data include data regarding compensation paid by other similar organizations (both tax-exempt and for-profit) for comparable positions, independent compensation surveys, independent appraisals, and actual written offers from similar institutions that are competing for a DP's services. If the authorized body determines that reasonable compensation is higher or lower than the range of comparable data obtained, the authorized body must document the basis for its decision.

Establishing the rebuttable presumption is important to both the managers who approve a transaction and the DPs who benefit from a transaction. Under the intermediate sanction rules, so long as a manager's participation in an excess benefit transaction is not willful and was due to reasonable cause, the managers will benefit from the presumption of reasonableness even if they are ultimately deemed to be wrong in an enforcement context. This means that the managers can effectively eliminate their own potential liability in their capacity as organizational managers by establishing the rebuttable presumption. But DPs can also garner benefits from the process used to establish the rebuttable presumption.

The four legal prohibitions referenced in this section serve as the major framework for physician compensation arrangements. A common theme through all of these provisions is the requirement that compensation received by physicians and others must be reasonable and consistent with fair market value.

Additional requirements that are related specifically to one or more of those legal prohibitions shape the compensation arrangements and specific compensation methodologies. For example, designated health services could presumably be provided through a medical practice organized as a group practice while still complying with the Stark law, although compensation arrangements within the group practice would nevertheless need to be structured to ensure that compensation was not paid based on the volume or value of physician referrals. If the group practice is affiliated with a hospital, additional compliance safeguards related to the antikickback law and tax-exempt organization requirements would also apply.

Compliance Strategies

Because of the various legal issues affecting physician compensation arrangements, a sound compliance strategy is required in connection with the development, implementation, and management of any physician compensation plan. Particular compliance issues that must be kept in mind vary depending on the context. Private practice medical groups that are physician-owned or owned by for-profit entities generally need to consider the requirements of the federal physician self-referral or Stark law and the antikickback statute. Those practices that are affiliated with a hospital or an academic medical center, including faculty practice plans and others, need to also pay attention to laws and rules governing tax-exempt organizations, including IRC section 501(c)(3) and the intermediate sanctions rules provided in section 4958.

Importantly, a central theme to several of these legal doctrines relates to the concept of fair market value; that is, one or more exceptions under the Stark law (i.e., the employment exception, the personal services exception, and others) require that compensation terms must be consistent with fair market value. Likewise, safe harbors under the antikickback statute also impose a fair market value standard.

Both the Stark and antikickback laws generally require that fair market value is equal to the value in an arm's-length transaction consistent with general market value. The value is the same as that for general commercial purposes, not adjusted to include additional value that one or both parties may attribute to the referral of business.

Tax-exempt organizations also require fair market value and reasonableness determinations. In the tax-exempt organization context, however, there is arguably some greater flexibility in the range of fair market value for physician services. The charitable purpose of the exempt organization may enable the organization to have slightly greater flexibility in providing compensation levels because the organization is meeting community needs. From the standpoint of intermediate sanctions requirements, fair market value is defined as the price at which a willing buyer and seller would agree, neither acting under any compulsion to agree and both having a reasonable knowledge of relevant facts.

Standards of fair market value are not the same in all cases and under every legal doctrine. Indeed, the OIG has indicated that, in connection with compliance with the antikickback safe harbors, the tax-exempt organization compliance standards are not necessarily relevant to safe harbor compliance. Moreover, the OIG has indicated that the value of referrals must be excluded from fair market value determinations. Thus, the definition of fair market value in the eyes of the OIG is not the same as the typical commercial definition where an ability to make referrals and ongoing business relationships would generally be viewed as relevant to the assessment. Similar standards are imposed under the Stark law regulations.

From a compliance perspective, the difference in fair market value standards does not necessarily mean that an assessment of fair market value provided in one context is of no value in another. That is, in promoting compliance and promoting the reasonableness and fair market value of compensation levels in the context of an audit or litigation, any assessment of reasonableness and fair market value is likely to be better than no assessment whatsoever.

In promoting compliance with Stark, antikickback, and other legal requirements, it is important to pay close attention not only to ultimate results (i.e., the total amount of compensation earned and paid in a particular context), but also the process that was used to get to that compensation level . Arm's-length negotiations and relationships where both parties are actively engaged in the bargaining process are critical to compliance. Coupled with these are standards related to the amounts paid by similar organizations for similar services. This second factor leads to the use of market data such as that published by the MGMA, AMGA, and other services for each practice specialty. These data are used in reasonableness assessments conducted to obtain the rebuttable presumption of reasonableness under the intermediate sanctions rules provided in section 4958 of the IRC, and in internal and external assessments of fair market value designed to promote compliance with the Stark law, the antikickback law, and others.

Understanding Market Data

All sources providing market data have their own limitations. For example, data from the MGMA physician compensation and production survey are based on a survey of MGMA medical practices. These typically include a relatively large number of single-specialty practices and smaller practice organizations. In contrast, the AMGA compensation survey deals mainly with relatively large, privately owned, hospital-affiliated and academic faculty practice plans. The differences in the culture, operating format, revenue sources, and other features of these organizations manifest themselves in the compensation and production data.

The market data generally represent a distribution of data from the responding practices and participating physicians. MGMA, AMGA, and other survey data have some level of bias in that they are derived only from member

or participating practices that elect to participate in the organization self-report surveys. This is in contrast to a scientifically selected, statistically valid, random sample of medical practices and/or their physicians.

In reviewing the data, attention to various statistics is important. The size of the sample is the threshold requirement for assessing the quality of the underlying data. Few measures of central tendency will be used in assessing or evaluating the data. The mean or average represents the measure of central location. The mean is generally not the best measure of central tendency due to the ability for the mean to be skewed by extreme (high or low) values.

The median is also a measure of central tendency representing the midpoint in a set of data. Because the midpoint lies directly in the middle of all of the observed values, the median serves as a better measure of central tendency. Finally, the standard deviation represents the measure of dispersion around the mean within a particular data set. The standard deviation provides information regarding the magnitude of dispersion or variance around the mean.

In a normal distribution of data, the mean and the median are at, or close to, the same point; that is, in a normal distribution, there is a strong correlation between the mean and the median, suggesting that the midpoint in the data range is also at or about the same level as the actual average. In most instances, however, the survey data provided by the MGMA, AMGA, and other organizations is skewed to the right. This means that the mean is typically higher than the median, primarily due to the incidence of extreme values at the higher end of the compensation scale.

Using Market Data

In addition to understanding the distribution of typical survey data, reasonableness, and fair market value assessments, a number of other factors related to commercially available market data must also be kept in mind. First, the survey definitions for particular values are essential to understand. For example, gross charges are limited to those from professional services (excluding charges for ancillary services such as laboratory, x-ray, and other technical components such as drugs).

Importantly, because the MGMA and other data sets reflect various tables or "cuts" of the data, different physicians and/or practices are represented in each particular cut. Because of this, different tables in the MGMA and other data do not necessarily compute; that is, production at the median level as measured by gross charges or work RVUs may or may not yield median compensation levels. Likewise, multiplying the median number of RVUs for a particular specialty as reflected in the MGMA data by the medical level of compensation per work RVU generally does not yield median compensation levels. This is because the different tables represent different cuts of the data. It is, therefore, inappropriate to assume or expect a direct one-to-one correlation from one table to another.

Likewise, a study of MGMA data suggests that even if we understand a physician's particular level of production, that production may yield differing levels of compensation in a particular medical group. This is due, at least in part, to the operation of the physician compensation plan. Thus, although one might expect median production to generally yield median levels of compensation, a review of the data suggests that median production typically yields a level of compensation that surrounds a relatively broad range below and above the median value.

Similarly, the data suggest that as production increases, the range of compensation paid to a physician at the same or similar level of production tends to widen. Based on a review of family practice, general surgery, cardiology, and other practice specialties represented in MGMA data, there is a common range of pay between the twentieth and eightieth percentiles of productivity for most specialties. Specialist physicians at the highest level of productivity exhibit the widest range of compensation. Thus, for those specialists with the highest levels of production, the physicians may have relatively low or extremely high levels of compensation. This variation is most likely due to the compensation plan used in the particular medical practice. For example, practices that base compensation almost entirely on productivity will typically yield a higher level of compensation for those physicians producing at the highest levels. On the other hand, those that include a base salary or equal share component would typically yield significantly lower levels of compensation for those physicians producing at the highest levels. Based on the review of MGMA data, the overall range of compensation paid is typically lowest for primary care specialties.

Promoting Compliance

To promote a compensation plan's compliance with the legal requirements discussed in the previous sections, close attention to detail is required. Because of the importance and potential sanctions under the Stark law, structuring to comply with the Stark law is essential to compliance. Using Stark as the starting point, the medical practice must rely on a specific exception or exceptions in connection with the compensation arrangement. Those exceptions have implications for the particular methodology that can be used, and the compliance issues that might arise. For example, the Stark law's in-office ancillary

services exception allows for the payment of overall profit shares or productivity bonuses to physicians in a medical group practice. The in-office ancillary services exception imposes a wide variety of specific requirements that must be met in order for a medical practice to rely on this exception. This exception will only be available in true group practice settings. Thus, privately owned and operated as well as hospital-affiliated medical practices and many faculty practice plans can rely on this exception.

Other arrangements will rely on other exceptions to the Stark law. For example, hospital-affiliated employment relationships will most commonly rely on the Stark law's exception for employment. This exception imposes different standards and requirements, related to productivity bonuses, than are available in a group practice context. Specifically, under the in-office ancillary services exception, the medical group can, in fact, collect and allocate revenues and profits from ancillary services across members of the group practice. Likewise, physicians can also receive productivity bonuses that include credit for services that are furnished "incident to" the physicians' personally performed professional services.

The Stark law's employment exception, on the other hand, allows for productivity bonuses, but only with respect to a physician's personally performed services. Thus, in the hospital employment or other employment context in which the Stark law's employment exception is being relied on, only production credit can be provided for personally performed services, and no credit may be provided for services that are "incident to" the physicians' services.

Apart from being clear on the identification of the particular Stark law exception, steps to promote legal compliance require close attention to other key factors and process variables designed to promote compliance with applicable legal requirements, including those imposed on tax-exempt organizations. Key process steps include:

- Documenting the process used and ensuring that arm's-length negotiations are present in the determination of compensation levels
- Where appropriate, obtaining a fair market value assessment in appropriate context through an internal or independent valuation process
- Assuring that the fair market value assessment is appropriately focused and considers, where appropriate, all relevant legal standards, including those applicable to Stark, antikickback, and tax-exempt organization requirements
- Assuring that all specific requirements of the Stark law exception, including those related to

compensation system methods, productivity bonuses, and the like, are met

- Monitoring arrangements that are in place over time but are renewed or modified to assure complete performance and to update fair market value assessments

- Ensuring that effective legal counsel with specialized expertise reviews the compensation methodology, including funds flow and documentation, to assure that fair market value and other determinations are appropriate and updated over time

Importantly, enforcement actions related to perceived legal violations tend to arise as a result of claims or complaints made by insiders to a medical practice organization, as opposed to focused enforcement initiatives. Disgruntled former employees are among the most potent sources of compensation-related compliance complaints.

In addition to maintaining an effective compliance program to identify problems and address issues raised by employees and others, medical practices should maintain appropriate documentation to demonstrate the appropriateness of the compensation system in the event of an audit or review. Such documentation is mandated by the Stark law in the case of the in-office ancillary services exception. Documentation should optimally include not only the compensation plan narrative, but also funds flow and other information that can be tracked retrospectively to demonstrate compliance. Appropriate records are also important in the exempt organization context. These records can demonstrate the arm's-length nature of an underlying transaction, as well as internally or externally generated assessments of reasonableness and fair market value. To comply with the rebuttable presumption of reasonableness under the intermediate sanctions rule, tax-exempt organizations must also follow a strictly defined process for the review and approval of compensation levels for certain insiders or disqualified persons to the organization.

■ Developing and Changing Compensation Plans

Due to the importance of physician compensation to a medical practice's success, it goes without saying that changes and adjustments to a compensation plan can have potentially far-reaching implications. Modifications to a plan that undermine physician morale and motivation can undermine the financial success of the organization as a whole, not to mention the job security of the

organization's leadership. Likewise, compensation plans used for hospital-employed and similar settings that are crafted to meet physician preferences and goals without attention to underlying financial conditions can yield massive losses and financial shortfalls, thus undermining the fiscal and financial viability of the entire enterprise. For these and other reasons, activities to develop, modify, and implement physician compensation plans in any practice setting are of critical importance.

Active involvement in the plan development process is essential for a successful plan to be developed that will help achieve the organization's goals related to performance—financial and otherwise. Modifications to any physician compensation plan require a basic level of "cultural readiness" for the new plan. Because a compensation plan constitutes a silent framework that underlies the organization as a whole, decisions to change the compensation model "for the heck of it" are not advised. Rather, perceptions by key players in the organization that change is required for one reason or another should be present before a plan is changed. These perceptions might be from individual physicians who perceive the plan to be unfair for a particular reason. Such perceptions might also be held by the leadership of the organization, who perceive that the compensation plan results in an excessive financial drain on the enterprise, that physician performance is not at expected levels, or that the plan has, or results in, other problems. Overall, any desire or move to change a compensation plan must be based on a base level of cultural readiness and a perception that the current plan is not working for one reason or another.

Assuming the decision has been made to modify or develop a new plan, the process is as important as the outcome. Because a compensation plan is essential to promoting a medical practice's goals, starting with those goals and objectives as the framework provides a solid foundation for plan development. Clearly identifying, for example, that increased levels of productivity and individual physician production are needed and essential, physician recruitment and retention challenges are occurring, or that other issues need to be addressed is important to ensuring that the model is developed based on guiding principles, rather than financial outcome.

Once plan goals have been identified, issues and concerns related to modifications of the plan (i.e., the perceived unintended and negative consequences that could arise from charges) should also be placed on the table. These factors provide useful information to help assess reality and maintain perspective. For example, many physicians consider any decrease in compensation to be unacceptable. Others reject any required increase in work levels in order to maintain compensation levels or to obtain additional compensation. Such statements may illustrate unrealistic views in today's environment. The identification of such views can help define the key issues and concerns that influence the plan development process, while also helping to assess whether physician views are realistic in practical terms.

Compensation plan development should occur through a process in which physicians are active participants and have an ability to express their opinions about the compensation plan development process and its outcome. Such participation is important, if not essential, to physician buy-in for the ultimate plan.

Most plan development activities involve the services of a compensation committee that works with the practice administrator or external consultant to define the compensation plan's goals, explore potential plan architectures, and assess and modify the plan that is ultimately developed. Only late in the plan's development will actual numbers be shared with committee members in order to evaluate the plan's implications for individual physician compensation levels. Sharing numbers late in the process rather than early on is essential because objectivity regarding the plan's outcome can be lost once data showing projected compensation levels under a proposed model are shared.

Although many issues have compensation plan implications (e.g., buy-in, buy-out, transition, and on-call obligations), it is typically best to address such issues outside of the basic compensation plan development process. This is because such issues tend to affect only a small subset of the medical group's physicians. Allowing such issues to take center stage allows the unique exception to define the process. Given that the success of the medical practice depends on the services of the physicians who have a full-time practice, defining the plan that works for those physicians (who generally constitute the vast majority of the physicians in the organization) is essential before moving on to address special requirements that affect only a minority.

An essential consideration for most compensation plans is the means and timing by which the medical practice will transition from the current plan to a new plan that is developed through a compensation plan development process. In most instances, a necessary ingredient to promote physician buy-in of any new plan is to ensure that the physicians understand the new plan, while also providing the physicians whose performance (and compensation) will inevitably be impacted by the new plan with a reasonable opportunity to adjust their professional and personal performance in a way that will provide for reasonable financial rewards.

The reality of any change to a compensation system is that the mere act of changing the "rules" governing the determination and payment of compensation will inevitably mean that some physicians will receive more compensation and others will receive less. The objective of the compensation plan transition process is to define a timeline over which the new plan will be implemented, and during which the physicians will be able to understand the new plan and make necessary adjustments. The transition time period is also designed to allow the medical practice to create the necessary infrastructure, data and reporting systems, and the like to implement a new plan.

The need for a structured transition process is particularly important as medical practices develop compensation structures that will help the organization migrate into changing payment systems and accountable care. Although future payment systems may involve an increased focus on quality and value, the data and other systems in most medical practices are typically not equipped to address the needs of the new system. Therefore, the compensation plan transition process may need to include a defined time period over which new systems, measures, reports, and so on are developed and used to provide the necessary infrastructure for a desired compensation structure.

Lastly, despite a medical practice's best efforts to develop a new compensation plan that will be sustainable in the long term, perhaps the only constant in medical practice today is the constant of change. Only rarely can compensation plans be maintained without modification or complete change over time. It is not unexpected for a compensation methodology to change every 3 to 5 years. The need to change is due to a wide variety of internal and external factors such as practice demographics, the complement of physician specialties, revenues from ancillary services, and others. External factors that are typically beyond the organization's control include the underlying reimbursement and contracting environment including payment methodologies (fee for service, capitation, or the like), the number of physicians completing fellowship or residency training in a particular specialty during a single year, recruitment challenges, and other factors.

Of course, some compensation plans will simply outlive their usefulness for one reason or another. Such plans may be viewed to be unacceptable for financial, behavioral, and other reasons. The combination of all of these factors and others can lead to a conclusion that today's compensation plan no longer meets the medical practice's needs. The outcome of that realization may be an active process to modify the compensation plan to develop something better, or at a minimum, a structured review process to reevaluate the plan, consider incremental changes, or confirm that the plan is the best that can be used at this particular point in time.

■ Conclusion

The physician compensation plan is an essential component of every medical practice's overall physician incentive and feedback mechanism. Far more than merely a financial model for allocating revenues and expenses and determining physician paychecks, the compensation plan often represents the most visible component of the practice's feedback and performance monitoring system. A compensation plan that is perceived to be fair by rewarding work and commitment to the practice by appropriate levels of compensation can serve as a silent framework for the medical practice's operation. On the other hand, a compensation plan that is viewed by many of the practice's physicians as a demotivator and generally unfair can undermine the practice's viability.

Only rarely is a medical compensation plan viewed by physicians in the practice as the best or the most important reason for participation in the enterprise. Yet a plan that does not meet basic requirements for the group and its physicians can be a significant hindrance to medical practice success.

Experience suggests that there is no perfect compensation plan. Moreover, experience suggests that the best compensation plan for a particular practice is most likely the one that makes every physician at least a little bit unhappy.*

References

1. Miller HD. *Transitioning to accountable care: Incremental payment reforms to support higher quality, more affordable health care.*
2. 42 U.S.C. § 1395nn.
3. 42 U.S.C. § 1³20a-7b(b).
4. 26 U.S.C. § 501(c)(3).

* The author wishes to thank Sera Chong, Associate, Polsinelli Shughart, P.C., Denver, Colorado, for her assistance in preparing this chapter.

Regulatory and Design Issues for an Effective Physician Practice Compliance Program

Michael R. Costa, JD, MPH
John M. McKelway, JD
Jennifer Itzkoff, JD

Just as immunizations are given to patients to prevent them from becoming ill, physician practices may view the implementation of a voluntary compliance program as comparable to a form of preventative medicine for the practice.

—OIG Physician Guidance[1]

Medicare and Medicaid fraud and abuse continue to remain a top priority for the government. The Health Insurance Portability and Accountability Act of 1996 (HIPAA)[2] gave the Office of Inspector General (OIG) of the U.S. Department of Health and Human Services (HHS) an ongoing, substantial budget increase to continue prosecuting instances of unscrupulous billing practices. The U.S. Department of Justice has assigned hundreds of prosecutors and the FBI has engaged hundreds of new agents to focus specifically on healthcare fraud and abuse. In addition to federal enforcement activities and regulations, states are seeking to coordinate their activities in the area with the federal government and have their own self-referral, antikickback, and false claims acts and regulations. In response to the government's pressures, and seeing an opportunity to challenge claims, private insurers have increased their investigations and scrutiny of providers as well. Along with this governmental and private insurer activity, many patients and other individuals are aware of the OIG Fraud and Abuse Hotline, and qui tam (whistleblower) actions are increasingly being brought by private individuals hoping to get a percentage of the government's recovery. The oft-repeated statement, "It's not a question of whether a physician's practice will be audited, but simply a question of when," may in fact hold a measure of validity.

In fiscal year 2010, the federal government recovered a record $4 billion from health fraud cases.[3] As a result of these activities, as well as prior-year judgments, settlements, and administrative impositions, the federal government collected more than $1.3 billion.[4] More than $1 billion of the funds collected and disbursed in 2002 were returned to the Medicare Trust Fund.[3] An additional $42.8 million were recovered as the federal share of Medicaid restitution.[3] At the time, this was the largest return to the government since the inception of the program. In addition, federal prosecutors filed 445 criminal indictments in healthcare fraud cases in 2002, and a total of 465 defendants were convicted for healthcare fraud–related crimes.[3] There were also 1746 civil matters pending and 188 civil cases filed in 2002.[3] HHS excluded 3756 individuals and entities from participating in the Medicare and Medicaid programs or other federally sponsored healthcare programs, most as a result of licensure revocations.[3] This record number of exclusion actions was the result of collaborations with state Medicaid Fraud Control Units (MFCUs) and state licensure boards.

In light of the seriousness of fraud and abuse offenses, substantial increases in the size of many physician practices, ongoing enforcement activity, and associated criminal and civil penalties, physicians need to continue their compliance efforts to ensure that they are abiding by all relevant state and federal laws governing fraud and abuse-related violations. Voluntarily developed and implemented compliance plans can be an effective tool in preventing, monitoring, and correcting civil and criminal violations. An effective physician practice compliance plan provides internal controls: (1) to promote adherence to the applicable law and program and health plan requirements; (2) to prevent violations; and (3) to detect problems that have already occurred so they can be addressed before they worsen. Another advantage to having an effective physician practice compliance plan is that it provides evidence that any mistakes made by a physician or his or her practice were inadvertent. Most importantly, a physician practice compliance plan needs to be viewed as an ongoing project. Put another way, such a plan cannot be effective unless it is revisited on a regular basis.

■ Summary of Fraud and Abuse Laws

There are a number of overlapping federal and state statutes relating to healthcare fraud and abuse. From a physician's perspective, the following is a summary of the criminal, civil, and administrative statutes most commonly used to prosecute healthcare fraud and abuse.

Federal Criminal Statutes

A variety of criminal statutes are often used by the federal government to prosecute healthcare fraud. The next several sections describe some of the most common.

Health Care Fraud (18 U.S.C. § 1347)

It is a crime to knowingly and willfully execute (or attempt to execute) a scheme to defraud any healthcare benefit program, or to obtain money or property from a healthcare benefit program, through a false representation. This law applies not only to federal healthcare programs, but also to most other types of healthcare benefit programs, such as commercial health insurance plans. Conduct that frequently gives rise to liability includes the following:

- Billing for services never provided to patients
- Upcoding: billing for more extensive services than were actually rendered
- Falsely certifying that services were medically necessary (On every HCFA 1500 claim form, a physician must certify that the services rendered were medically necessary for the health of the beneficiary.)
- Unbundling: billing for each component of the service instead of billing an all-inclusive code
- Billing for noncovered services as if covered
- Flagrant and persistent overutilization of medical services with little or no regard for results, the patient's ailments, condition, or medical needs
- Consistent use of improper or inappropriate billing codes, such as billing for the same level of service or diagnosis code irrespective of the services rendered in the individual case

The following are three common examples of healthcare fraud:

- A physician intentionally billed Medicare for treatments that he never actually rendered for the purpose of fraudulently obtaining Medicare payments.
- A psychiatrist billed Medicare, Medicaid, TRICARE, and private insurers for psychiatric services that were provided by her nurses rather than herself.
- A physician intentionally upcoded the level of service rendered to patients to increase Medicare payments.

False Statements Relating to Health Care Matters (18 U.S.C. § 1035)

It is a crime to knowingly and willfully falsify or conceal a material fact; make any materially false statement; or use any materially false, fictitious, or fraudulent writing or document in connection with the delivery of or payment for healthcare benefits, items, or services. An example would be a physician who certified on a claim form that he performed laser surgery on a Medicare beneficiary when he knew that the surgery was not actually performed on the patient.

Theft and Embezzlement in Connection with Health Care Benefit Program (18 U.S.C. § 669)

It is a crime to knowingly and willfully embezzle, steal, or intentionally misapply any assets of a healthcare benefit program. An example of conduct punishable under this statute would be a physician office manager who knowingly embezzles money from the practice's bank account that includes reimbursement received from the Medicare program.

False Claims Act (18 U.S.C. § 287)

The False Claims Act is one of the primary tools used by the federal government to prosecute fraudulent billing practices under Medicare and Medicaid. The statute prohibits the presenting of a claim to the United States that the claimant knows to be "false, fictitious, or fraudulent." The range of conduct punishable under the False Claims Act is extremely broad and includes: (1) billing for services that were not rendered; (2) filing claims for services billed at inflated rates; and (3) filing for services that were not medically necessary.

Mail and Wire Fraud (18 U.S.C. §§1341 and 1343)

Correspondence with Medicare and Medicaid generally involves the use of the mails and electronic wiring systems, so parties engaged in submitting false claims to the government frequently fall subject to prosecution under the mail and wire fraud statutes. Specifically, government programs and private providers invariably utilize the mails to send or receive payments, explanation of benefit forms, and other related documents.

Similarly, providers often submit claims to the government through electronic wire systems. Consequently, these two statutes, which prohibit the use of the mails or the wires to further "scheme" or defraud, are often applied against parties submitting false claims.

The mail and wire fraud statutes cover the entire range of fraudulent conduct punishable under the Health Care Fraud and False Claims Acts. Examples provided by the OIG include the following:

- A physician knowingly and repeatedly submits electronic claims to the Medicare carrier for office visits that she did not actually provide to Medicare beneficiaries with the intent to obtain payments from Medicare for services never performed.
- A neurologist knowingly submits claims for tests that were not reasonable and necessary and intentionally upcoded office visits and electrocardiograms to Medicare.

Medicare and Medicaid Patient Protection Act of 1987 (42 U.S.C. § 1320a-7b(a))

This statute proscribes six specific types of conduct, including the making of false statements, the concealment of information with intent to induce improper payments, improperly converting federal payments, and submitting claims for services provided by unlicensed individuals. This section's most commonly enforced provision

prohibits individuals from "knowingly and willfully mak[ing] or caus[ing] to be made any false statement or representation of a material fact in any application for any benefit or payment under [the Medicare or Medicaid programs]." Claims containing any false statements regarding material facts are actionable under this provision, so many activities beyond the blatant billing for unrendered services may lead to violations. Other prohibited conduct under this provision includes misrepresenting services actually rendered (e.g., upcoding) and falsely certifying that certain services were medically necessary.

Obstruction of Criminal Investigations of Health Care Offenses (18 U.S.C. § 1518)

This statute is frequently used during a healthcare fraud investigation by the government. The statute prohibits the obstruction of a criminal investigation in any material way, such as by failing to produce subpoenaed records, destroying or altering records, or attempting to influence the testimony of an employee questioned by government investigators. Examples include the following:

- A physician instructs his employees to tell OIG investigators that he personally performs all treatments when, in fact, medical technicians do the majority of the treatment and the doctor is rarely present in the office.
- A physician under investigation by the FBI for reported fraudulent billings alters her patient records in an attempt to cover up the improprieties.
- A physician intentionally fails to produce certain records during an investigation because they could incriminate him.

Antikickback Statute (42 U.S.C. §1320a-7(b))

The federal antikickback statute provides criminal and civil penalties for certain business arrangements that are influenced by the referral of patients for healthcare services covered by a federal healthcare program, such as Medicare and Medicaid. Specifically, the antikickback law prohibits the knowing and willful solicitation, receipt, offer, or payment of any remuneration (which includes payments and anything else of value) whether direct or indirect, overt or covert, in cash or in kind, in return for referring an individual for any item or service covered by a federal healthcare program, or purchasing, leasing, ordering or arranging for, or recommending or arranging for the purchase, lease, or ordering of any item or service paid for (in whole or in part) under a federal healthcare program.

The general purpose of this statute is to prohibit anyone from paying or accepting a payment in exchange for referring a patient for services that might be covered by the Medicare and Medicaid programs. Generally, a physician cannot give gifts or anything of value in order to induce referrals of patients to his or her practice. Furthermore, the opposite is also true: a physician cannot accept gifts or things of value from a vendor, such as a medical laboratory, in order to do business with that vendor. Of interest to physicians is the fact that many standard recruitment incentives offered by hospitals to physicians may constitute illegal remuneration. A list of suspected incentives includes:

- Free or discounted office space or equipment
- Free or discounted billing, nursing, or other staff services
- Free training for a physician's office staff
- Income guarantees
- Low-interest or interest-free loans, including "forgiven" loans
- Payments for physician services that involve few substantive duties or exceed fair market value
- Payment for physician continuing medical education courses, or travel and expense payments to attend conferences

Safe Harbor Regulations. Because the literal wording of the antikickback statute prohibits a number of transactions generally believed to be necessary or beneficial to the healthcare industry, Congress authorized the creation of a number of "safe harbors" that permit conduct prohibited under this act. The following are some of the items covered by the safe harbor regulations:

- Payments reflecting returns on investment in connection with investments in certain business entities
- Payments made in connection with space or equipment rental arrangements
- Personal services and management contracts (e.g., medical director contracts or other independent contractor arrangements)
- Sale of a physician practice
- Referral services
- Practitioner recruitment
- Ambulatory surgical centers
- Referral agreements for specialty services

A physician entering into an arrangement involving any of these practices, or where there is the potential for the referral of patients for services, should consult with a competent healthcare attorney.

State Criminal Laws

In addition to the various federal laws that may apply, numerous state laws can also impact physician practices.

For instance, many states also have an antikickback statute that is similar to the federal statute with one typical major exception: the state statutes usually have no "intent" requirement. States also have false healthcare claims statutes that prohibit the submission of fraudulent bills to private health insurers and other healthcare organizations. Additionally, such statutes often prohibit the solicitation or receipt or any "bribe or rebate" in connection with a private healthcare entity. Apart from criminal prosecution, the health insurer is authorized to bring a civil action to recover the full amount inappropriately paid, together with attorneys' fees and the costs of investigation. In some circumstances, state prosecutors may also charge individuals suspected of healthcare fraud and abuse with larceny and the making of false statements in a statement verified under penalties of perjury.

Civil and Administrative Statutes

Like their criminal counterparts, state and federal civil and administrative statutes must also be carefully taken into consideration when putting together an effective physician practice compliance program.

Federal False Claims Act

The civil False Claims Act (FCA) is the law most often used to bring a civil case against a healthcare provider for the submission of false claims to a federal healthcare program, including Medicare or Medicaid. As a result of its penalty provisions, the FCA represents one of the most powerful enforcement tools the federal government has at its disposal in connection with healthcare fraud. Under the FCA, any person or entity knowingly making a false claim to the government (i.e., to Medicare or Medicaid) is liable for mandatory civil penalties and fines. The mere filing of a false claim that is never paid triggers liability under the FCA. Each individual false claim submitted to Medicare or Medicaid gives rise to potential penalties between $5500 and $11,000, coupled with treble damages for the amounts paid by the government. Consequently, each false line item claimed can result in thousands of dollars of liability. In cases where providers submit significant numbers of claims (e.g., hospitals or laboratories), total exposure to liability may amount to millions of dollars. Often, the government merely has to brandish the amount of potential liability under the FCA to leverage settlements with providers who would be financially crippled if found guilty. To establish liability under the FCA, the government must establish the following: (1) the provider presented or caused to be presented to an agent of the United States a claim for payment, (2) the claim was false or fraudulent, and (3) the defendant knew that the claim was false or fraudulent. Importantly, the knowledge requirement for liability under the civil FCA is lower than under the criminal statute.

The civil FCA defines "knowing" and "knowingly" as either actual knowledge, deliberate ignorance, or the "reckless disregard of the truth or falsity of the information." As a result, a physician does not have to deliberately intend to defraud the government to be liable. Liability can be imposed on a provider who has deliberately or recklessly chosen to ignore the truth or falsity of the information on a claim submitted for payment, when the provider knows, or has noticed, that information may be false. An example of deliberate ignorance would be a physician who ignores provider update bulletins and thus does not inform his or her staff of changes in the Medicare billing guidelines or does not update his or her billing system in accordance with said changes. When claims for nonreimbursable services are submitted as a result, the FCA has been violated. An example of reckless disregard would be a physician who assigns the billing function to an untrained office person without inquiring whether the employee has the requisite knowledge and training to accurately file such claims. At the same time, physicians are not subject to criminal, civil, or administrative penalties for innocent mistakes or errors, or even negligence. Specifically, the Department of Justice has stated that where billing errors, honest mistakes, or negligence result in improper claims the provider may be asked to return the funds, but without penalties. Indeed, in the Compliance Program Guidance for Individual and Small Physician Practices, the OIG states the following:

> Even ethical physicians (and their staffs) make billing mistakes and errors through inadvertence or negligence. When physicians discover that their billing errors, honest mistakes, or negligence result in erroneous claims, the physician practice should return the funds erroneously claimed, but without penalties. In other words, absent a violation of a civil, criminal, or administrative law, erroneous claims result only in the return of funds claimed in error.

The following are some examples provided by the OIG of conduct that violates the FCA:

- A physician submitted claims to Medicare and Medicaid representing that she had personally performed certain services when, in reality, the services were performed by a nonphysician and they were not reimbursable under the federal healthcare programs.

- A cardiologist intentionally upcoded office visits and angioplasty consultations that were submitted for payment to Medicare.
- A podiatrist knowingly submitted claims to the Medicare and Medicaid programs for nonroutine surgical procedures when he actually performed routine, noncovered services such as the cutting and trimming of toenails and the removal of corns and calluses.

Federal Physician Self-Referral Prohibitions (The Stark Law)

The Stark prohibitions are designed to prevent physicians from fraudulently making money from the patients they treat. The Stark law prohibits a physician from referring a Medicare or Medicaid patient for "designated health services" in which the physician (or immediate family member) has an ownership or investment interest or compensation relationship. In practice, the prohibitions have caused grave uncertainty for physicians and providers of healthcare services as they struggle to respond to the market forces that have reshaped the healthcare industry over the past few years.

In 1993, Congress enacted "Stark II." This law expanded the referral and billing prohibitions to Medicaid, as well as added 10 additional "designated health services" as follows:

- Physical therapy services
- Occupational therapy services
- Radiology services, including magnetic resonance imaging, computerized axial tomography scans, and ultrasound services
- Radiation therapy services and supplies
- Durable medical equipment and supplies
- Parenteral and enteral nutrients, equipment, and supplies
- Prosthetics and orthotics
- Home health services and supplies
- Outpatient prescription drugs
- Inpatient and outpatient hospital services

For the purpose of the Stark law, the term "referral" is defined as an item or service for which payment may be made by Medicare or Medicaid. In the event a patient obtains an item or service from an entity in which the physician or family member has a financial relationship, the Stark law is violated unless one of the statutory or regulatory exceptions apply. Examples of violations of the Stark law include the following:

- A physician works in a medical clinic and also owns a freestanding laboratory located in the same city. The physician referred all orders for laboratory tests on her patients to the laboratory she owned.

- A physician agreed to serve as the medical director of a home health agency (HHA) for which he was paid a sum substantially above the fair market value for his services. In return, he routinely referred his Medicare and Medicaid patients to the HHA for home health services.
- A physician received a monthly stipend of $500 from a local hospital to assist him in meeting practice expenses. The doctor performed no specific services for the stipend and had no obligation to repay the hospital. The doctor referred patients to the hospital for inpatient surgery.

Unlike the antikickback statute, which is a statute separate and apart from the Stark law, an intent to violate the Stark law is not required for penalties to be imposed. The Stark law is entirely objective and is a "zero tolerance" statute. Thus, knowledge of the scope and application of the Stark law is crucial to avoid sanctions. It is beyond the scope of this chapter to discuss the Stark law and the various statutory and regulatory exceptions in any detail. However, if a physician or an immediate family member has a financial interest in one of the "designated health services," such physician should seek legal advice about the arrangement, because the penalties under the law are severe. A physician can be subject to a civil monetary penalty of up to $15,000 per claim for each prohibited service and exclusion from the Medicare and Medicaid programs.

Civil Sanctions, Fines, and Exclusions

There are additional, noncriminal sanctions that may result from criminal liability or may be separately imposed for nonconforming conduct. Generally, civil (noncriminal) sanctions include civil monetary penalties and exclusion from participation in the Medicare and Medicaid programs. Civil monetary penalties, in addition to criminal penalties, can be imposed for violations of the fraud and abuse laws. Civil monetary penalties of up to $10,000 per item or service, plus an assessment of up to three times the amount claimed for each such item or service, may be imposed on any provider who knowingly presents or causes to be presented a claim for Medicare or Medicaid reimbursement that: (1) is for an item or service that the person knows or should know was not provided as claimed; (2) is for an item or service and the person knows or should know the claim is false or fraudulent; or (3) is presented for a physician's service by a person who knows or should know that the individual who furnished

the service was not properly licensed as a physician or is a physician who falsely claimed to the patient that he or she is specialty certified by a medical specialty board.

Exclusions

Exclusions can result from a conviction for healthcare fraud or other impermissible conduct. If a physician is excluded from the Medicare or Medicaid programs, it means that no Medicare or Medicaid payments will be made for any services rendered by that physician. The OIG has the authority to exclude physicians and other healthcare providers from the Medicare and Medicaid programs. There are two categories of exclusion: mandatory and permissive.

Mandatory Exclusion. Individuals or entities convicted of any of the following crimes must be excluded from participation in Medicare and Medicaid for a minimum of 5 years:

- A criminal offense related to the delivery of an item or service under Medicare or Medicaid
- A criminal offense under federal or state law relating to the neglect or abuse of a patient in connection with the delivery of a healthcare item or service
- A felony under federal or state law relating to fraud, theft, embezzlement, breach of fiduciary responsibility, or other financial misconduct against a healthcare program financed by any federal, state, or local government agency
- A felony under federal or state law relating to the unlawful manufacture, distribution, prescription, or dispensing of a controlled substance

Permissive Exclusion. There are a number of grounds for which the OIG has discretion to exclude a physician from the Medicare and Medicaid programs for a minimum of 3 years. The following list is not all-inclusive, but includes some of the most frequently used grounds for permissive exclusion:

- Misdemeanor convictions relating to healthcare fraud
- Convictions relating to fraud in programs other than those dealing with healthcare
- Convictions for obstructing an investigation
- Misdemeanor convictions for controlled substance violations
- License revocations or suspensions
- Fraud, kickbacks, and other prohibited activities
- Submitting claims for unnecessary or substandard services
- Submitting false or improper claims

- Exclusion or suspension from any other federal or state healthcare program
- Defaulting on a health education loan or scholarship obligation
- Entities controlled by an individual who is subject to mandatory exclusion
- Failure to disclose required information
- Failure to grant immediate access to a fraud investigator
- Failure to take corrective action

State Administrative and Licensing Consequences

Physicians who have been convicted of larceny, fraud, or any other crime in connection with the billing of state Medicaid programs are not permitted to participate as Medicaid providers. In most cases, state Medicaid agencies have the discretion to terminate or exclude physicians who work in a close professional association with providers convicted of a program-related offense. Most professional licensing boards, including local boards of registration in medicine, are empowered to discipline licensees based solely on the fact that the licensee has been convicted of a crime. Further, anything that may be characterized as "misconduct" may be the foundation of a complaint and disciplinary action. Healthcare fraud allegations that either have resulted in a criminal conviction or have been settled civilly may therefore form the basis of a licensing board's investigation or a professional society's disciplinary proceedings.

Fraud Alerts

Beginning in 1989, the OIG began to issue "special fraud alerts" designed to inform the healthcare industry about conduct that potentially violates fraud and abuse laws. The following is a brief summary of the special fraud alerts that impact the physician community:

- *Special Fraud Alert on Routine Waiver of Copayments or Deductibles:* In May 1991, the OIG issued an alert to advise the healthcare industry that it would be investigating providers, such as physicians, who are paid on the basis of charges and routinely waive (do not bill) Medicare deductibles and copayment charges to beneficiaries for services and items covered by the Medicare program. The OIG opined that such systemic conduct results in false claims, violations of the antikickback statute, and excessive utilization of services and items paid for by Medicare.
- *Special Fraud Alert on Hospital Incentives to Referring Physicians:* In May 1992, the OIG identified suspect arrangements between hospitals and

physicians involving incentives to physicians to refer patients to the hospital. These include incentives that reduce physicians' professional expenses (discounted office space or free staff services) or increase physician revenue (hospital payment each time the physician refers a patient to the hospital).
- *Special Fraud Alert on Arrangements for the Provision of Clinical Lab Services:* In October 1994, the OIG discussed how certain arrangements between physicians or other healthcare providers and outside clinical laboratories to which they refer patient specimens may implicate the antikickback statute. The alert notes arrangements involving phlebotomists from a laboratory placed in a physician's office may implicate the statute if additional services are rendered for the physician. Other situations mentioned include discounts for referrals, waiver of charges to managed-care patients, free pickup and disposal of biohazardous waste products, and free testing for healthcare providers, their families, and their employees.
- *Special Fraud Alert on Home Health Fraud:* In June 1995, the OIG identified suspect kickback arrangements initiated by home health providers with physicians, beneficiaries, hospitals, and rest homes in return for referrals, fraud in annual cost reports, false billing practices, and claims for services not rendered. Suspect arrangements for referrals include offering free services and disguising referral fees as salaries by paying for services not rendered or in excess of fair market value, among others.
- *Physician Liability for Certifications in the Provision of Medical Equipment and Supplies and Home Health Services:* In January 1999, the OIG issued this alert to make physicians more aware of the significance of certifications of medical necessity for durable medical equipment or home healthcare and how they could contribute to fraud and abuse and overutilization of healthcare services. The alert gives examples of inappropriate certifications that the OIG's investigations uncovered, such as a physician knowingly signing a number of forms falsely representing that services are medically necessary in order to qualify the patient for home health services, a physician falsely certifying that a patient is confined to the home and qualifies for home health services, and a physician signing a stack of blank Certificates of Medical Necessity (CMNs) to be completed with false information in support of fraudulent claims for the equipment, among others. The alert is also careful to say that physicians are not personally liable for erroneous claims due to mistakes, inadvertence, or simple negligence.

- *Special Fraud Alert on Rental of Space in Physician Offices by Persons or Entities to Which Physicians Refer:* Issued in February 2000, this alert identifies arrangements for physician office rental space that may possibly be disguised as kickbacks to induce referrals. These arrangements include comprehensive outpatient rehabilitation facilities (CORFs) that provide physical and occupational therapy and speech or language pathology services in physicians' and other practitioners' offices; mobile diagnostic equipment suppliers who perform diagnostic-related tests in physicians' offices; and suppliers of durable medical equipment, prosthetics, orthotics, and supplies that set up "consignment closets" for their supplies in physicians' offices. The OIG focuses on three features of suspect rental arrangements: (1) the appropriateness of rental agreements (e.g., whether payment of rental has traditionally been provided for free or for a nominal charge), (2) the rental amounts (e.g., in excess of fair market value based on certain factors), and (3) "time and space considerations" (e.g., unreasonable or unnecessary for a commercially reasonable business purpose of the supplier–tenant). The OIG also gives specific guidance as to how rental calculations may be made for appropriate time and space considerations. Lastly, the alert "strongly recommend[s] that parties to rental agreements between physicians and suppliers to whom the physicians refer or for which physicians otherwise generate business make every effort to comply with the space rental safe harbor to the antikickback statute. . . ."

■ Identified Physician Compliance Risk Areas

As mentioned earlier, the OIG published a federal notice seeking information and recommendations for developing its formal guidance for individual and group physician practices on September 8, 1999. In its Compliance Program Guidance, the OIG identified specific "risk areas" that it focuses on during investigations of physicians. These are discussed in the following sections.

Coding and Billing

The OIG reports that the following risk areas associated with billing have been among the most frequent subjects of investigations and audits:

- *Billing for items or services not rendered or not provided as claimed:* For example, an ophthalmologist

billed for laser surgery he did not perform. As one element of proof, he did not even have laser equipment or access to such equipment at the place of service designated on the claim form as where he performed the surgery.
- *Submitting claims for equipment, medical supplies, and services that are not reasonable and necessary:* This involves seeking reimbursement for a service that is not warranted by a patient's documented medical condition.
- *Double billing resulting in duplicate payment:* Double billing occurs when a physician bills for the same item or service more than once. Although duplicate billing can occur due to simple error, the knowing submission of duplicate claims, which is sometimes evidenced by systematic or repeated double billing, can result in liability.
- *Billing for noncovered services as if covered:* For example, a physician bills Medicare using a covered office visit code when the actual service was a noncovered annual physical. Physician practices should remember that "necessary" does not always constitute "covered," and that this example is a misrepresentation of services to the federal healthcare programs.
- *Knowing misuse of provider identification numbers that results in improper billing:* An example of this is when the practice bills for a service performed by Dr. B, who has not yet been issued a Medicare provider number, using Dr. A's Medicare provider number. Physician practices need to bill using the correct Medicare provider number, even if that means delaying billing until the physician receives his or her provider number.
- *Unbundling comprehensive procedure codes:* Unbundling is the practice of a physician billing for multiple components of a service that must be included in a single fee. For example, if dressings and instruments are included in a fee for a minor procedure, the provider may not also bill separately for the dressings and instruments.
- *Failure to properly use coding modifiers:* A modifier, as defined by the *Current Procedural Terminology (CPT)* manual, provides the means by which a physician practice can indicate when a service or procedure that has been performed has been altered by some specific circumstance but not changed in its definition or code.
- *Clustering:* This is the practice of coding and charging one or two middle levels of service codes exclusively, under the philosophy that some will be higher, some lower, and the charges will average

out over an extended period. In reality, this over-charges some patients while undercharging others.

- *Upcoding the level of service provided:* Upcoding is billing for a more expensive service than the one actually performed. For example, Dr. X intentionally bills at a higher reimbursement code than what she actually renders to the patient.

Reasonable and Necessary Services

The OIG recognizes that physicians should be able to order any tests, including screening tests, they believe are appropriate for the treatment of their patients. However, a physician practice should be aware that Medicare will only pay for services that meet the Medicare definition of reasonable and necessary "for the diagnosis or treatment of illness or injury or to improve the functioning of a malformed body member."[4]

Documentation

Timely, accurate, and complete documentation is important to clinical patient care. This same documentation serves a second function when a bill is submitted for payment, namely, as verification that the bill is accurate as submitted. The following are some guidelines identified by the OIG to ensure accurate medical record documentation:

- The medical record should be complete and legible.
- The documentation of each patient encounter should include the reason for the encounter; any relevant history; physical examination findings; prior diagnostic test results; assessment, clinical impression, or diagnosis; plan of care; and date and legible identity of the observer.
- If not documented, the rationale for ordering diagnostic and other ancillary services should be easily inferred by an independent reviewer or third party who has appropriate medical training.
- CPT and *International Classification of Diseases*, 9th edition, Clinical Modifications (ICD-9-CM) codes used for claims submission should be supported by documentation and the medical record.
- Appropriate health risk factors should be identified. The patient's progress, his or her response to and any changes in treatment, and any revision in diagnosis must be documented.

HCFA 1500 Form

Another documentation area for physician practices to monitor closely is the proper completion of the HCFA 1500 form. The OIG opines that the following

practices will help ensure the form has been properly completed:

- Link the diagnosis code with the reason for the visit or service.
- Use modifiers appropriately.
- Provide Medicare with all information about a beneficiary's other insurance coverage under the Medicare Secondary Payer (MSP) policy if the practice is aware of a beneficiary's additional coverage.

Improper Inducements, Kickbacks, and Self-Referrals

As discussed earlier, the antikickback statute and Stark law provide criminal penalties for individuals and entities that knowingly offer, pay, solicit, or receive bribes or kickbacks or other remuneration in order to induce business reimbursable by federal healthcare programs. The laws also prohibit a physician from making a referral to an entity with which the physician or any member of the physician's immediate family has a financial relationship if the referral is for the furnishing of designated health services. Civil penalties, exclusion from participation in the federal healthcare programs, and civil FCA liability may also result from a violation of these prohibitions.

In addition to developing standards and procedures to address arrangements with other healthcare providers and suppliers, physician practices should also consider implementing measures to avoid offering inappropriate inducements to patients. Examples of such inducements include routinely waiving coinsurance or deductible amounts without a good faith determination that the patient is in financial need or failing to make reasonable efforts to collect the cost-sharing amount. In the OIG Special Fraud Alert "Routine Waiver of Medicare Part B Co-Payments/Deductibles" (May 1991), the OIG describes several reasons why routine waivers of these cost-sharing amounts pose concerns. The alert sets forth the circumstances under which it may be appropriate to waive these amounts.

■ The Physician Practice Compliance Program

Issues exist as to whether the physician practice compliance plan can be developed affordably and where and how to begin. As to costs, the OIG's view as expressed in its published compliance program guidance is that although it may require significant additional resources or reallocation of existing resources to implement an effective compliance program, the long-term benefits of implementing the program significantly outweigh the costs. However, the fact remains that, although much of the same effort must be engaged in by a physician practice as by a large institution or healthcare business in developing a compliance plan, a physician practice, depending on its size, may be less able to bear the associated expenses. This is especially true in this healthcare market of decreasing reimbursement and increasing costs.

Although there are certain minimum common elements to a physician practice compliance plan, there is no one right way to develop the plan. Instead what is important is that the plan is effective in meeting the goals of training, prevention, detection, and correction. Plans must be tailored to the particular practice and its specific issues. The plan should not be a "cookie cutter" document, and should be designed in an effective fashion so as to promote, as opposed to discourage, implementation.

In formulating the plan, it is crucial to consider the practicality and reasonableness of the processes that are being established. If the processes are not practical and reasonable, there is a higher likelihood that what is set forth in the plan will not entirely be implemented. This eventuality, in some respects, is worse than not having a plan. Thus, it is better to develop a narrowly tailored plan that can be implemented than a more expansive "full-blown" plan, which largely remains unimplemented and on the shelf. An unimplemented plan can be considered a sham and potentially used against a physician under investigation.

The lynchpin of a plan is its effectiveness in preventing errors in coding and billing, and the first step in developing a compliance plan is the baseline audit. Issues with respect to this first step include whether a practice can conduct its own audit. Also, if an outside consultant is engaged, the practice must determine what would be an appropriate process and scope for such an audit.

In addition to the baseline audit, the plan should contain the following minimum elements:

- The establishment of specific standards, rules, and procedures that are reasonably capable of reducing the prospect of wrongdoing by the organization's employees and agents in connection with the billing of third-party payers and other areas of regulatory risks
- The appointment of a trustworthy and empowered compliance officer to oversee the overall compliance efforts
- Training and education sessions and dissemination of information in order to ensure effective communication of standards, rules, and procedures

- Initial and ongoing auditing and monitoring designed to detect improper billing activities and other areas of regulatory risk, including a reporting system that permits employees and agents to report improper conduct without fear of retribution
- A commitment to enforcement of the compliance program through appropriate disciplinary measures, and the establishment of processes to investigate reports and enforce the program and to take corrective action

According to the OIG, an "effective" compliance program contains at least seven basic components, discussed in the following sections.

Conducting Internal Monitoring and Auditing

According to the OIG, an ongoing evaluation process is important to a successful compliance plan, and beginning with an audit of your practice is an excellent way to determine what, if any, problem areas exist. Once determined, you can then focus on the risk areas associated with those problems. The OIG suggests there are two types of reviews that can be performed as part of your evaluation: (1) a standards and procedures review, and (2) a claims submission audit.

The OIG compliance program does not elaborate on specific standards and procedures. Instead, it recommends that an individual or individuals in the physician practice should be charged with the responsibility of periodically reviewing the practice's standards and procedures to determine if they are complete and current. If not, they should be updated to include changes in the government regulations that are relied on by physicians and insurers, such as changes in CPT and ICD-9-CM codes.

In addition to the standards and procedures involved, the OIG recommends that bills and medical records be reviewed for compliance with applicable coding, billing, and documentation requirements. Further, each physician practice needs to determine whether to review claims retrospectively or concurrently with the claims submission.

The OIG believes there are many ways to conduct a baseline or starting audit. In the program it recommends that claims for services that were submitted and paid during the initial 3 months—after implementation of an education and training program—be examined, in order to give a physician practice a benchmark against which to measure future compliance effectiveness. Following the initial or baseline audit, periodic audits should be conducted at least once each year to ensure that the compliance program is being followed. Due to the limited resources of some group physician practices, the OIG recommends that, at a minimum, physicians should conduct a review of claims that have been reimbursed by federal health programs.

It is important to remember that the OIG considers one of the most important components of a successful physician compliance audit protocol to be an appropriate response when the physician practice identifies a problem. The response can be as straightforward as a timely repayment with an appropriate explanation to Medicare or the appropriate payer from which the overpayment was received. In others, the physician practice may want to consult with a coding and billing expert to determine the best course of action. Although there is no "best" response, timely action is required.

Implementing Compliance and Practice Standards

After a physician identifies his or her practice's risk areas, the next step is to develop a method for dealing with those risk areas through the practice's standards and procedures—a central component of any compliance program.

The OIG recommends that a physician focus first on risk areas most likely to arise in his or her particular practice. Further, and in order "to assist physician practices in performing this initial assessment,"[6] the OIG has developed a list of four potential risk areas affecting physician practices: coding and billing; reasonable and necessary services; documentation; and improper inducements, kickbacks, and self-referrals. As discussed in the previous section, there are nine coding and billing practices that have been the most frequent subjects of investigations and audits by the OIG. Yet, having stated the OIG's areas of concern, it provides little guidance on what specific steps to take for coding and billing other than (1) written standards and procedures should ensure that coding and billing are based on medical record documentation, and (2) the coder or the physician should review all rejected claims pertaining to diagnosis and procedure codes.

With regard to reasonable and necessary services, the OIG is again more definitional than practically helpful. Here the OIG refers to the Medicare definition of reasonable and necessary—"for the diagnosis or treatment of illness or injury or to improve the functioning of a malformed body member."[4] In this section of the program, the OIG states the obvious in that Medicare will only pay for services that meet the Medicare definition of reasonable and necessary. It does go on, however, to state what may not be so obvious: "A physician practice

can bill in order to receive a denial for services, but only if the denial is needed for reimbursement from the secondary payer."[4]

The OIG recommends that physicians focus on two specific types of documentation: medical record documentation and the HCFA 1500 form. As mentioned earlier, medical record documentation can serve two functions—clinical patient care and verification that the bill is accurate as submitted. To make sure the 1500 form is properly completed, HCFA emphasizes three points: link the diagnosis code with the reason for the visit or service, use modifiers appropriately, and provide Medicare with all information about a beneficiary's other insurance coverage, if the practice is aware of a beneficiary's additional coverage.

Last, the OIG concludes that a physician practice would be well-advised to have standards and procedures that encourage compliance with the antikickback statute and the physician self-referral law. Again, it does not list specific standards and procedures, but its main areas of concern: financial arrangements with outside entities to whom the practice may refer federal program business, joint ventures with suppliers of goods and services to the practice, consulting contracts or medical directorships, office and equipment leases, and gifts or gratuities of more than nominal value.

Designating a Compliance Officer or Contact

In this section of the program, the OIG is careful to restate that "the resource constraints of physician practices make it so that it is often impossible to designate one person to be in charge of compliance functions."[7] Therefore, the OIG concludes that in lieu of having a designated compliance officer, the physician practice could instead describe in its standards and procedures the compliance functions for which designated employees, known as "compliance contacts," would be responsible.

For example, one person could be responsible for preparing written standards and procedures; another could be responsible for conducting or arranging for periodic audits and ensuring that billing questions are answered. Another possibility is that one individual could serve as compliance officer for more than one entity. In addition, the physician practice could outsource all or part of the functions of a compliance officer to a third-party consultant.

Whether the compliance person is located on the inside or the outside, he or she should oversee the implementation and monitoring of a compliance program; establish periodic audits; periodically revise the compliance program in light of changes in the practice, changes in the law, or changes in the standards of government and private-payer health plans; develop and implement a training program that focuses on the components of the compliance program; ensure that the OIG's "List of Excluded Individuals and Entities" has been checked with respect to all employees, medical staff, and independent contractors; and investigate any report or allegation concerning possible unethical or improper business practices.

Conducting Appropriate Training and Education

According to the OIG, education is the logical next step after problems have been identified and the practice has designated a person to oversee training. In the program, the OIG identifies three basic steps for setting up educational objectives: determine who needs training (both in coding and billing and in compliance); determine the type of training that best suits the practice's needs (seminars, in-service training, self-study); and determine when and how often education is needed and how much each person should receive. In addition, a physician practice should strive for two goals when conducting compliance training: All employees will receive training on how to perform their jobs in compliance with the standards of the practice and any applicable regulations, and each employee will understand that compliance is a condition of continued employment. Training should emphasize that following the standards and procedures will not get a practice employee in trouble, but violating the standards and procedures may subject the employee to disciplinary measures.

The OIG understands that most physician practices do not employ a professional coder and that the physician is often primarily responsible for all coding and billing. However, when a third-party billing company is involved, the physician is encouraged to work with the billing company to ensure that documentation is adequate for the billing company to submit accurate claims on behalf of the physician. This appears to be an invitation to participate in billing accuracy. However, the physician compliance plan, and the OIG's clear encouragement to get involved in the practice's billings, still seem to be an excellent entrée to discussing billing practices with management companies or billing companies. Again, it would be difficult for the OIG not to get involved if a management company or a billing company would not discuss its billing for a client's physician services. Not to do so would be an obstruction to physicians who are attempting to establish a compliance program under OIG directives.

Responding Appropriately to Detected Offenses and Developing Corrective Action

In OIG's opinion, violations of a physician practice's compliance program, significant failures to comply with applicable federal or state law, and other types of misconduct threaten a practice's status as a reliable, honest, and trustworthy provider of healthcare. Therefore, when a practice determines it has detected a possible violation, the next step is to develop a corrective action plan and determine how to respond to the problem.

The OIG's "voluntary" compliance guidelines strongly suggest that the physician "take decisive steps to correct the problem" and "such steps may involve a corrective action plan, the return of any overpayments, a report to the government, and/or a referral to law enforcement authorities."[7] One suggestion given is for the physician to develop his or her own set of monitors and warning indicators, which might include significant changes in the number or types of claim rejections and reductions; correspondence from the carriers and insurers challenging the medical necessity or validity of claims; illogical patterns or unusual changes in the pattern of CPT, Healthcare Common Procedure Coding System (HCPCS), or ICD-9 code utilizations; and high volumes of unusual charge or payment adjustment transactions.

Physician practices that detect violations could analyze the situation to determine whether a flaw in their compliance program failed to anticipate the detected problem, or whether the compliance program's procedures failed to prevent the violation. In any event, it is prudent, according to the OIG, even absent the detection of any violations, for physicians to periodically review and modify their compliance programs.

Developing Open Lines of Communication

In this section of the guidelines, the OIG emphasizes that the nature of a small physician practice dictates that open lines of communication and information exchanges are a "must," but need to be conducted through a less formalized process than that which has been envisioned by prior OIG guidance.

For group physician practices, the OIG concludes that a meaningful and open communication system can include:

- Requiring employees to report conduct that a reasonable person would believe to be erroneous or fraudulent.
- Creating a user-friendly process such as an anonymous drop box.
- A statement that failure to report erroneous or fraudulent conduct is a violation of the compliance program.

- If a billing company is used, communicating with the billing company's compliance officer or contact staff to coordinate billing and compliance activities.
- Using a process that maintains the anonymity of the persons involved in the reported conduct.
- Declaring that there will be no retribution for reporting conduct that a reasonable person acting in good faith would have believed to be erroneous or fraudulent. Yet, it also needs to make clear that there may be a point at which the individual's identity may become known or may have to be revealed in certain instances.

Enforcing Disciplinary Standards Through Well-Publicized Guidelines

Finally, the last step a physician practice may wish to take, in the OIG's opinion, is to incorporate measures into its practice to ensure that practice employees understand the consequences if they behave in a noncompliant manner. In the OIG's view, an effective physician practice compliance program includes procedures for enforcing and disciplining individuals who violate the practice's compliance or other practice standards. Along these lines, the OIG recommends that a physician practice's enforcement and disciplinary mechanisms ensure that violations will result in consistent and appropriate sanctions, including the possibility of termination, but at the same time be flexible enough to account for mitigating or aggravating circumstances.

Disciplinary actions, if any, could include oral warnings, written reprimands, probation, demotion, temporary suspension, termination, restitution of damages, and referral for criminal prosecution. The OIG strongly recommends that any communication resulting in the finding of noncompliant conduct be documented in the compliance files by including the date of incident, name of the reporting party, name of the person responsible for taking action, and follow-up action taken. Another suggestion is for physician practices to conduct checks to make sure all current and potential practice employees are not listed on the OIG lists of individuals excluded from participation in federal healthcare or government procurement programs.

Formal Integration of the Compliance Program

Each physician group practice has its own structure and mode of operation. The strengths and weaknesses of the group practice's structure and operations must be assessed for compliance readiness. Based on that assessment, a compliance plan must be customized in accordance with government expectations for the group practice. Off-the-shelf plans are insufficient to meet the practice's needs if they are not adequately and appropriately tailored for the group practice. The plan must be customized to the size of the group practice, and take into account the types of services provided, the practice's organization and reporting structures, and applicable governmental regulations.

The compliance program should address all operational areas of the group practice and be administered by a compliance officer who reports directly to the chief executive officer or medical director on compliance matters. The group practice should also have in place a compliance committee to oversee the development and implementation of the plan. The committee and compliance officer's activities should build on existing policies. Billing and reimbursement operations along with other financial planning and budgeting practices are typically the focus of compliance efforts. In addition, integrating compliance efforts in several other key areas such as human resources, patient rights protection, quality and performance improvement programs, and medical records management can greatly enhance the effectiveness of the group practice's programs for compliance with reimbursement rules and antikickback and antifraud statutes and regulations.

Compliance Counsel

Before embarking on developing and integrating a compliance plan, a group practice should seek and identify its compliance counsel and other compliance advisors. The attorney that a group practice uses for compliance issues should be not be the same as the one used for routine legal matters. Group practices seeking to implement an integrated, effective compliance program will most likely need to engage the services of experienced compliance professionals on at least an interim basis. The initial risk assessment for most group practices should be confidentially performed by an outside compliance expert. Ongoing compliance programs that are developed and delivered in house can be greatly augmented by these same types of experts. Group practices should look for experienced organizations that will provide the group practice, alone or in concert, comprehensive advisory services that include educational programs, training program design and delivery, hotline support, hotline training, compliance risk assessment, and research data and regulatory updates on compliance issues.

In seeking competent legal counsel and compliance consultant(s), group practices will want to look for counsel and consultants that match the needs of the practice. Although many healthcare lawyers and consultants have expertise in one or more specific areas of healthcare issues, it is important that a group practice engage those that best serve the group practice's compliance requirements. In seeking the right match, a practice may wish to use the following guide:

1. *Conduct a search (similar to the request for proposals [RFP] process used for most vendors):* Although this may not be as formal a process as the typical RFP, preparation is critical. Determine what legal expertise would be most important and helpful to the group practice, and try to match that expertise with the potential counsel or consultant candidates. The group practice should be looking for an attorney or consultant, not necessarily a law or consulting firm. The group practice will want to know that, when a need arises, it will be assisted by the person it selected, and not have to rely on "someone" in the firm to help in a given situation. In preparing the RFP, the group practice should determine the following:

   a. What healthcare disciplines are most closely associated with the group practice? Some examples are:
      - Primary care
      - Specialty practice areas
      - Radiology
      - Home health
      - Ambulatory surgery centers
      - Clinical diagnostics
      - Outpatient services
   b. What types of issues or concerns are likely to raise compliance issues for the group practice? Some examples are:
      - Antikickback issues
      - Coding-related concerns
      - Provider contracts (e.g., hospital–physician relationships, joint ventures, medical equipment partnerships)
      - Medical staff concerns
      - Patient care concerns
      - Potential false claims
      - Billing system issues
      - Stark concerns
   c. What other legal counsel resources are currently utilized by or available to the group practice? For example:
      - Does the group practice have in-house counsel available to assist in routine matters?
      - Does the group practice have designated "corporate counsel" (e.g., outside law firms)

that is used to provide routine legal assistance? If so, is that counsel routinely involved in advising the organization on the types of matters that could be the focus of compliance investigations (e.g., joint ventures, physician contracts, compensation arrangements, vendor agreements)?
      - Does the group practice have the ability to access counsel (either in-house counsel or outside attorneys) at the discretion of the compliance officer?

2. *Seek referrals from other compliance officers:* Ask for recommendations about possible attorneys from other compliance officers in the area (or healthcare associations).

   a. Ask whether the compliance officer uses separate compliance counsel. If so, what is that attorney's specific healthcare expertise?
   b. Does the attorney also act as counsel to the healthcare organization in any other capacity? If so, what is it? What kind of compliance matters did the attorney handle?

3. *Personally interview candidates:* The compliance officer should meet with potential advisors at the group practice, tell them exactly what the hospital is looking for (based on the analysis of the information above), and obtain the following information:

   a. Other group practice clients and how the attorney or consultant provides them with compliance-related counsel.
   b. Attorney's or consultant's specific background and expertise, particularly in those areas of compliance risk most important to the group practice organization, as well as the name and availability of the attorney or consultant who will handle the group practice's issues. Assurances that "the firm has people experienced in that area" are insufficient.
   c. The attorney's or consultant's fee schedule and hourly billing rate, and whether he or she requires a retainer.
   d. How frequently the attorney or consultant bills (e.g., monthly, quarterly, semiannually). The group practice should require that each bill be thoroughly itemized.

Financial Operations
Billing

The group practice needs to conduct regular internal and periodic independent audits of its billing processes.

The group practice must also ensure that coders and their supervisors receive specific and certified training. The starting point for implementation of a compliance plan is the OIG's latest work plan. The OIG work plan comes out at the beginning of each calendar year and focuses on the major issues that will be reviewed at group practices across the country. The following payment and reimbursement areas have been consistently included in the work plans and should be addressed in the compliance plan:

- Laboratory
- Ambulatory surgery
- Emergency department
- End stage renal dialysis
- Home health
- DRG creep
- Medical necessity: physician documentation
- Cost reporting (reserve cost reports)
- Rehabilitation services
- "Take home" drugs
- Self-administered drugs
- Stark regulations
- Pharmacy
- Central supply

Again, it is important to note that a fully implemented compliance plan requires ongoing auditing. Audits are best conducted by independent review organizations with the intent of ensuring that all policies and procedures that are in the compliance plan are being adhered to on a daily basis. The audits should ensure identification of systemic billing errors. The source of many errors in group practices can be traced to misinformed and ill-educated third-party payers. The group practice should ask

> . . . an independent review organization that specializes in third-party reimbursement to design and execute a plan that identifies the flagrant, negligent, malicious, and systemic errors for the area under review. Results of ongoing systems tests, audits, and corrective actions should be reported to the compliance officer with trends and analyses reported directly to the group practice's internal management or board of directors. That type of compliance plan implementation will demonstrate the initiative and seriousness that a group practice places on its compliance plan. In the event an investigation takes place at your facility, these areas that have been regularly tested by an independent review organization will provide evidence that the group practice has taken the appropriate steps to implement a meaningful compliance plan.

Billing and claims operations systems should be reviewed and procedures for claims submission adopted to ensure that:

- All physician services are properly documented.
- All claims accurately reflect the services provided and documented.
- Only true, properly documented services claims are submitted.
- The integrity of medical records and documentation is maintained—late entries, corrections, and margin entries are correctly authenticated, flagged, and explained.
- Claims are submitted only for those services for which there exists proper documentation that remains available for audit.

In addition to supporting the reasonableness and medical necessity of services billed to Medicare, physician and clinical documentation must comply with CMS's current evaluation and management (E&M) documentation guidelines. Group practices should consider using preformatted forms that include prompts for required information and allow for ease and accuracy of billing audits. Computerized and voice-activated note-taking programs should be constructed so that continuation or submission depends on completing the record according to the E&M standard. Systems should be put in place to prevent "delinquent" records from arriving at the billing department to be corrected. For example, radiology and other diagnostic services require a signed physician's order. The signed order must also include the diagnosis and reason for the test. Registration for these services should not permit patients to receive services without proper documentation on hand. The billing department should obtain an order from the physician with the relevant information before performing the test. Scheduling should be adjusted to accommodate these requirements. Outpatient services require more specific information than physicians routinely include. "Routine laboratory tests" or tests ordered to "rule out" various conditions are not appropriate without additional specific information.

Financial Arrangements

Each financial arrangement entered into by the group practice needs to be scrutinized to determine whether it violates any of the prohibitions against kickbacks or self-referrals. Furthermore, Medicare conditions of participation that address the group practice's plan and budget require that all contracts, joint venture agreements, and other financial arrangements comply with applicable federal, state, and local laws. The compliance officer should ensure that counsel has reviewed present arrangements and enter into only those arrangements that meet muster. Pursuant to the compliance committee's recommendation and a resolution by the board of directors, each contract involving a threshold dollar amount should be required to be reviewed and approved by counsel before execution.

In an age of cost cutting and a need to reconcile lower reimbursement rates with increased service and supply costs, group practices often seek to leverage their purchasing power and take advantage of volume discounts. This becomes a compliance issue under Medicare Part A if the discounts are not accurately reported to regulatory authorities and, for those who file them, not accurately reflected on billing records. It also becomes a Medicare Part B compliance issue if the group practice fails to maintain current lists of each supply or service for which participating physicians generate a bill and the actual prices for those items. Under managed-care programs, the list price may not be as meaningful as it once was, but Medicare's CPT codes include the HCPCS codes assigned to them and form the basis for Medicare billings for outpatient services. The chargemaster must be continually maintained and serviced to ensure that CPT codes are accurately added and deleted so Medicare is not erroneously charged for noncovered items or items that are integral to room or procedure charges.

The federal government has exempted qualified group purchasing arrangements and certain discount programs from antikickback prohibitions. HHS and the OIG have stated:

> Safe harbors relating to discounts, employees and group purchasing organizations are specifically required by statute. The discount exception was intended to encourage price competition that benefits the Medicare and Medicaid programs. The proposed discount provision was limited in application to reductions in the amount a seller charges for a good or service to the buyer. The discount could take the form of a specified price break, or the inclusion of an extra quantity of the item purchased "at no extra charge." We did not propose to protect many kinds of marketing incentive programs such as cash rebates, free goods or services, redeemable coupons, or credits.

Human Resources and Staffing Practices
The group practice should ensure that the human resources department is adequately trained on the compliance plan and the code of conduct. It is essential that

the human resources staff understand that adherence to both is a condition of employment. The group practice compliance team, counsel, and human resources department need to compile a policy that informs employees and potential employees that background checks will be conducted. The policy should outline the extent of the investigations based on job responsibilities. The policy should be included in recruitment packages as well as the employee handbook. New applicants should complete a detailed initial application that includes an acknowledgment of and permission for the hospital or practice to conduct a background check. At a minimum, all practitioners need to be screened to determine whether they have been excluded from the Medicare program. Other state debarment databanks must also be queried. In accordance with hospitals' credentialing requirements (with which group practices must comply), each applicant must have his or her licenses and other relevant credentials verified. Truthfulness and completeness in the application (including the content of resumes) must be clearly delineated as a condition of employment. The group practice should conduct criminal checks and more intense scrutiny for positions of higher authority and for those employees who will work in areas of high vulnerability. In accordance with applicable laws and labor agreements, employees should be notified that retention or promotion will be contingent upon satisfactory background checks.

Human resources departments should also tailor exit interviews to elicit information concerning compliance problems. Those interviews serves two purposes. First, they elicit intelligence that should be reported to and acted upon by the compliance team. Second, they permit the hospital to identify employees who knew about compliance or Medicare violations but chose not to take action or report until their departure. The exit interviewer should ask the departing employees if they took any documents with them, copied any documents, or provided any documents to persons outside of the group practice.

Quality Improvement Initiatives
Part and parcel of a compliance plan is regular monitoring, auditing, and analysis to ensure that the plan is being followed. Regular, ongoing, and visible auditing of compliance activities of individual departments should be a key component of an overall performance improvement program. As described earlier in this chapter, the follow-up to information gleaned from this process, of course, is of paramount importance. Medicare conditions of participation require the group practice to have in place programs that document taking effective remedial action for noncompliance.

The group practice can use survey techniques, sampling methods, and other protocols to establish trends and deviations for established norms. Using on-site visits, surveys, interviews, examination of written directives from various departments, and trend analyses, the compliance team should be able to detect problems in the area of impermissible referrals, kickbacks, and coding. The compliance team should have enough information to determine why deviations occur and take prompt remedial action with additional monitoring to ensure that the intervention was effective. If the analysis reveals a delay in detecting problems, the compliance plan should be altered accordingly.

Moreover, the compliance program itself should adopt continuous quality improvement or performance improvement principles to monitor and improve its effectiveness. Those improvement activities should be measured against valid benchmark policies and practices for compliance programs. The compliance program is only as good as its implementation on a regular and consistent basis. The group practice compliance team should also be involved in the retention of auditors, such as accountants hired by the group practice to perform independent review functions. The compliance officer should inform the independent reviewers in writing of the content of the group practice's code of conduct and its compliance plan. In addition, the retention of the reviewers should be contingent upon their actions being consistent with those policies. The group practice should implement appropriate follow-up to ensure that the activities of the auditors are consistent with the compliance plan without interfering with the independent nature of their activities.

Each department should be surveyed periodically to determine its compliance health. Employees should be surveyed to determine their general awareness of compliance and knowledge about specific features of it, such as who the compliance officer is, how to access the compliance hotline, whether the group practice provides information concerning compliance, and whether supervisors encourage staff to report problems.

The compliance staff should evaluate itself concerning knowledge of and access to the federal regulations, annual training in current compliance matters, and the effectiveness of the incorporation of compliance into the group practice's in-service training program.

The CEO and senior executives need to be included in compliance training and assessment. Those executives should be able to state whether the organization has a standard code of conduct with which all members must comply, whether the governing body has issued a corporate compliance resolution, and whether the organization has adopted written procedures for investigating potential fraud. The senior leadership should know:

- When the code of conduct was last reviewed and updated
- To whom the compliance officer reports
- How the practice reduces the risk of hiring and retaining employees likely to break the law
- How compliance efforts measure against other initiatives and training requirements
- What significant trends are noted in hotline calls
- What the group practice's greatest areas of risk are
- How the organization stops violations, once discovered, from recurring

Compliance Training

The introductory compliance training should be tailored to address issues most relevant to the group practice. There are commercially available products that provide self-paced, computer-assisted learning aimed at ensuring that all personnel on all shifts receive validated training. Certain programs, such as those provided by Health Care Compliance Strategies, provide specific modules directed at the compliance obligation of physicians, nonphysician clinical staff, and administrative staff. Other organizations, such as the Council of Ethical Organizations, provide compliance officer training and certification, specific hotline management training, and compliance training concerning billing and coding issues. The initial training should be followed up at least annually to reinforce learning and to demonstrate by repetition and perseverance the group practice's commitment to compliance.

The Group Practice Compliance Plan Within an Organized Delivery System

It is important to remember that a group practice compliance plan is part of the overall compliance efforts of an organized delivery system. Such delivery systems often include inpatient and outpatient services, long-term care, home health care, assisted living, hospital settings, and many more. Therefore, any group practice compliance plan must be designed commensurate with those compliance activities undertaken by such other entities within the system. Ensuring consistency is vital not only for overall compliance efforts, but also for administrative simplicity in training and routine auditing and monitoring.

The group practice is a critical component of any organized healthcare delivery system, so compliance efforts are often modified as necessary in accordance with the needs of other components within the system. For instance, as discussed previously, group practices face vast billing and regulatory restrictions that often require much compliance planning. Often such billing and regulatory issues are also faced by other entities within the system, and their solutions can easily be adapted.

■ Conclusion

Reducing the potential for inaccurate billing practices and creating a climate of compliance with the law are the primary reasons for implementing and maintaining a compliance plan. It is far less expensive to develop a compliance program to prevent mistakes from being made than to defend a Medicare postpayment audit based on a statistical sampling of paid claims that can result in a demand for repayment of an extrapolated amount of money. At the same time, the process of developing a compliance program allows the involved physicians to better understand how the practice is actually operating. In fact, the development of a compliance program is more akin to the implementation of an overall risk management program for the practice.

Physicians practicing in today's complex and highly regulated environment must realize that compliance means more than simply adopting a boilerplate document labeled "compliance plan." The key to an effective compliance plan is for the practice to establish a culture of ethical behavior and compliance.

Employees must understand that every member of the practice, from physicians to billing personnel and clerical staff, is expected to behave legally and ethically at all times.

The OIG's physician compliance program guidelines are sobering and may be viewed as a "pain" by most. However, the program guidelines should be reviewed and utilized in a practical and realistic manner. As stated by the OIG, "physician practices may view the implementation of a voluntary compliance program as comparable to a form of preventative medicine for the practice." [8] Moreover, sometimes patients need to be reminded to keep taking their medicine.

References

1. Office of Inspector General. OIG Compliance Program for Individual and Small Group Physician Practices. Notice. (65 FR 59434, Thursday, Oct. 5, 2000).
2. Health Insurance Portability and Accountability Act of 1996 (HIPAA). Public Law 104-191.
3. U.S. Department of Justice. Press release Health Care Fraud Prevention and Enforcement Efforts Recover Record $4 Billion; New Affordable Care Act Tools Will Help Fight Fraud. January 24, 2011. Accessed February 7, 2012 <http://www.justice.gov/opa/pr/2011/January/11-asg-094.html>
4. 42 U.S.C. 1395y(a)(1)(A).
5. *See supra,* note 1, pg. 59438.
6. Ibid. at 59441.
7. Ibid. at 59443.
8. Ibid. at 59435.

CHAPTER

18

Implementing and Operating a Physician Practice Compliance Program

Lawrence F. Wolper, MBA, FACMPE

Planning and implementing a compliance plan and program have far greater operational implications to physician organizations than are apparent in much of the literature. Before implementing a compliance plan and program, broad organizational and operational issues should be considered by the individual physician, physician group practice, or physician organization (e.g., management services organization, independent practice association [IPA], faculty practice plan, large network, or group practice). Succinctly stated, the question is: Can individual physicians, small physician practices, or even larger physician organizations plan, implement, and operate successful compliance programs within their current organizational and operating structures, corporate cultures, management styles, and historical manners of doing business, or do some of these organizational matters need to be addressed and possibly changed before a plan can succeed? Over the years since the inception of compliance regulations, most practices have had compliance plans created, largely by attorneys, and many have implemented certain aspects of their plans, but how many compliance plans are actually operating on an everyday basis as initially planned, or, conversely, how many are

relegated to written documents that are filed or reside on a bookshelf?

Before proceeding further with this discussion, it is important to note that for the purposes of the Office of Inspector General's (OIG's) compliance plan guidelines and programs, the term "physician" is defined as "(1) a doctor of medicine or osteopathy; (2) a doctor of dental surgery or of dental medicine; (3) a podiatrist; (4) an optometrist; or (5) a chiropractor, all of whom must be appropriately licensed by the state."[1]

It is clear from the OIG Compliance Program for Individual and Small Group Physician Practices that the intent of a compliance plan and program is to install a *working system* to reduce or eliminate abusive and fraudulent practices, not only relating to billing and collections, but also, eventually, to other areas of business risk. The OIG appears to be sympathetic to the limited resources of small practices and individual physicians: "The guidance provides great flexibility as to how a physician practice could implement compliance efforts in a manner that fits with the practice's existing opportunities and resources."[2] Significantly, the OIG has loosened the requirement that physician practices implement all seven of the basic components of an effective compliance program derived from the federal sentencing guidelines and listed in previous guidances as necessary for other types of healthcare providers. The OIG acknowledges that full implementation of all components may not be feasible for smaller physician practices, and that a practice can begin by identifying risk areas that, based on the practice's history, would benefit from closer scrutiny as well as specific policies, monitoring, and training. But, nonetheless, the plan is intended to be operational.

Although sympathetic to the limitations faced by smaller groups, "The OIG believes that written policies and procedures can be helpful to all physician practices, regardless of size and capability."[1] The OIG also appears to suggest a more detailed and comprehensive standard for larger practices: "By contrast, larger practices . . . can use both this guidance [i.e., the recent guidelines for individual physicians and small group practices] and the Third-Party Medical Billing Company Compliance Program Guidance."[1]

In response to the broad range of compliance plans that may be required for physician groups and the current trend toward the emergence of larger practices via merger and acquisition, the scope of this chapter encompasses not only an exploration of the elements of a compliance plan and program, but also the organizational, operational, and managerial challenges that physicians and practice managers are likely to face, and do experience, when planning and implementing a compliance program. It is important to note that sections of this chapter (e.g., auditing and monitoring) present standards and principles that are not OIG requirements or recommendations, although in using terms such as "independence," "objectivity," and "internal controls" one must suspect that the OIG had in mind some of the matters discussed in this chapter.

This chapter is organized into the following topics:

- The compliance plan within the context of a physician practice
- The elements of compliance plans and programs
- A planning and implementation work plan

The Compliance Plan Within the Context of a Physician Practice

Collectively, the federal sentencing guidelines and the OIG Compliance Program for Individual and Small Group Physician Practices refer to procedures that are not necessarily incorporated into the *daily* operations of many physician organizations, regardless of size or organizational setting. For example, they refer to auditing, monitoring, internal controls, sampling, due diligence, and standards of organizational and employee behavior. Even though most practices may currently have written plans, have an identified compliance officer, and have implemented some other elements suggested by the OIG, one wonders how many practices have plans that actually are anchored in everyday operations.

The OIG recommendation that a compliance plan include internal auditing to focus on high-risk billing and coding issues[1] necessitates the implementation of a range of organizational and operational changes. This holds true for smaller practices that may select only a simple random sample of a small number of charts per provider or federal payer, but is even more important for larger physician practices that will select larger samples and should use established audit and sampling guidelines.

In addition, OIG compliance guidance refers to *responsibility*, *authority*, and *lines of communication* (e.g., when defining the role of the compliance officer). These elements are not always clearly defined in physician practices because of the frequent duality of management roles between physicians and lay practice managers, as well as other factors that differentiate physician practices and physician organizations from organizations in other industries. One of the more recent challenges resulting from the increase in practices with hundreds of physicians is the modification of compliance plans that were created for smaller practices. More important, however, is the consistent operational initiation of more robust compliance plans, and the routine use of the plans. Lines of communication in recently merged practices, perhaps with different operating cultures and lines of authority, may interrupt the daily attention to the compliance plan. Although the OIG compliance guidance does not address these issues directly, they are nonetheless important to the creation of a compliance program and the effectiveness of the compliance officer's or contact's position, regardless of the size of the practice.

Planning and implementing a compliance plan and program should begin with an understanding of the organizational contexts into which these plans will be placed, and what managerial and operational changes may be required to accommodate these programs and ensure that they are effective and dynamic over time. This section addresses a range of management and organizational functions necessary for implementing a compliance plan.

Delegation, Responsibility, and Authority

Management involves working with and delegating functional tasks and responsibilities to other people in an organization to achieve the objectives of the organization. "Responsibility" is defined as a duty or activity that has to be accomplished. A high degree of delegation of responsibility and decision making in a physician practice implies that many employees, particularly at senior levels, do not require constant oversight. Generally, in larger and more complex organizations, the need to delegate responsibility is greater. Delegation allows senior staff more time to accomplish tasks that are consistent with their level of experience, education, and areas of direct responsibility. "Authority" is defined as the power to act on someone else's behalf. The delegation of responsibility should be accompanied by the granting of a concomitant amount of authority to carry out the delegated tasks. Authority also involves the ability to make decisions, often independent of a superior in the organization.

In physician practices, responsibility and authority are not always delegated in parity with one another. Physicians, primarily because they have been medically trained in an apprenticeship setting, generally are comfortable delegating medical tasks to other physicians and clinical personnel, because they assume that individuals who also have been medically trained are capable of a range of clinical tasks. On the other hand, physician leaders often have less experience and comfort with delegating business tasks to lay personnel. Because the nature of medicine and physician practice has both medical service and business elements, it is likely there always will be an overlap in roles between physicians and lay management, even in small groups. This is dissimilar to organizations in most other industries. This overlap in roles—and often the related managerial tensions—tends to increase as the following practice characteristics or combinations of these characteristics increase:

- Practice size (numbers of physicians, other providers, and lay staff)
- Hierarchical complexity
- Range of clinical services offered
- Degree of organizational decentralization
- Involvement in medical education and research

The most notable organizational settings that are an example of all of these characteristics, and in which there are particular challenges to implementing and managing a compliance plan and program, are faculty practice plans, the emerging large practices that often are located at multiple sites, and practices that are partnerships wherein most partners want a say in what is going on in the practice. In these settings, lines of communication, responsibility, and internal controls can become obscured. For example, if a faculty plan or emerging large group is decentralized along departmental and clinical or specialty lines, delegation of responsibility and authority from upper levels of management to lower levels, as well as laterally, can become difficult. It is not unusual in many faculty plans, as well as large multispecialty groups, for an imbalance to exist between the responsibility and the authority delegated to management, with the authority being more resident in positions held by physicians.

If the amount of authority delegated is not commensurate with the level of responsibility, the ability to execute the tasks necessary to achieve the goals of the organization is hampered. Therefore, to implement and *operate* a compliance plan and program, the individuals with delegated responsibility for the entire program (e.g., the full- or part-time compliance officer or contact) or for components of the program (e.g., auditors, receptionists, billers, or collectors) also must be given a requisite amount of authority.

When considering the functions of a compliance officer, larger practices may wish to turn to the Compliance Program Guidance for Third-Party Medical Billing Companies, which identifies that the organization "should designate a compliance officer (and/or a compliance committee) to serve as the focal point for compliance activities. This responsibility may be the individual's sole duty or added to other management functions depending upon the size and resources of the organization, and complexity of the task." The Guidance stresses that it is critical to the success of the program that the compliance officer have "appropriate authority," be a high-level official in the organization, and have "direct" access to the organization's governing body (in a smaller practice, shareholders), all other senior management, and legal counsel.[3]

Carrying out these themes in larger physician practices, physician organizations, and faculty practice plans may require that the compliance officer and related compliance functions be centralized, while including the assistance and input of departmental chairpersons and managers. Direct access to the governing body suggests that these individuals should have enough authority to accomplish their responsibilities without being pressured or influenced by physician clinical department heads.

In its Compliance Guidance for Individual and Small Group Physician Practices, the OIG takes a more relaxed view of delegation related to the compliance officer or contact for small practices. Unlike the guidelines for billing companies, small practices may designate more than one employee with compliance-monitoring responsibility, and these individuals can be called compliance contacts. The OIG also suggests that a compliance officer can serve that role for more than one practice, or a practice may outsource that function to an outside person. The OIG notes that care should be exercised in making the decision regarding the manner in which the organization fills the role of compliance officer.

For small practices, the issue of independence and potential conflicts of interest can become problematic if assigning compliance roles to an office manager or billing staff, or indeed anyone whose regular responsibilities are activities that represent an area of risk for the practice. The OIG recommendation could, for example, lead to a supervisor auditing the correctness and adequacy of his or her own billing, as well as that of the doctor(s) for whom he or she works. This may be a very difficult task in a small, closely held practice. It generally would require added oversight from the physician, who, because it is his or her records and billings that are being audited, may not be entirely independent either. Further, reliable auditing results require not only a knowledge of correct billing and coding, but also an awareness of correct auditing approaches. In small practices, billing staff may not have the requisite knowledge. An alternative may be to outsource the auditing function, which the OIG recognizes as an acceptable solution.

Planning, Controlling, Evaluation, and Feedback

Planning, controlling, evaluation, and feedback are important to the success of all organizations, and they are at the core of effective *operating* compliance programs. They are referred to in OIG compliance guidelines for billing companies and laboratories, in the federal sentencing guidelines, and in the OIG Compliance Program for Individual and Small Group Physician Practices. The three elements of management in any organization are planning, controlling, and conducting evaluation and feedback. Although systems for planning, controlling, and conducting evaluation and feedback cannot completely eliminate fraud, abuse, or waste, the existence of these controls can provide a reasonable mechanism to better ensure that these types of exposures are reduced over a period of time.

These three components of management form a continuous cycle, and they are important to the implementation of a compliance plan and program within a physician practice. It is only in recent years that physician practices have evolved from a "cottage" industry to a consolidating, corporately oriented industry. Therefore, these elements, as a continuous cycle, generally are not present in physician practices, regardless of size or organizational complexity. Therefore, the implementation of a compliance program is likely to require that one or more of these elements be put in place. This may be easier said than done.

A discussion of this management cycle (i.e., planning, controlling, and conducting evaluation and feedback) and the tasks within each of these three components can provide the basis for many physician practices to plan and implement a compliance program. As mentioned earlier, these elements are identified in the seven basic compliance plan steps.

Strategic, Long-Term, and Operational Planning

There are three levels of planning: strategic, long-term, and operational. *Strategic planning* typically has a 5-year analytical horizon. This level of planning includes market research; analysis of competition, market needs, and trends; assessment of opportunities and market threats; and evaluation of the strengths and weaknesses of the organization. Strategic planning answers the two-part question, "What businesses do we want to be in, and how do we want to conduct those businesses?" The outcome of these analyses clarifies the broad goals of the organization for the next 5 years. Goals are defined as long-range aims for a specific time period. Some of these goals are articulated in an organization's mission statement, corporate bylaws, codes of ethics, and other statements of corporate vision. Objectives stem from goals, and they are defined as specific results that are expected within a time period, usually by the end of a budget cycle (typically 1 year).

Therefore, the commitment to compliance planning and a compliance program, as well as to the ongoing process of reducing and eliminating fraudulent, abusive, and wasteful corporate practices, ideally should stem from the strategic plan of a practice. It is not a government assumption that all groups have a strategic plan, and it is possible to make the commitment to compliance goals without having a written strategic plan in place, but it is easier to execute compliance goals if they also can be stated in strategic terms along with other long-term goals that may support the achievement of compliance planning.

For example, a compliance plan should require that new employees be properly screened and reference checks be conducted to determine if individuals have a record of prior offenses related to fraudulent or abusive practices. It also should require that position descriptions be drafted and regularly updated for employees engaged in the compliance process (as well as all other employees). If these functions have not occurred in a physician practice, or have been performed in too informal a manner, another strategic goal that supports compliance planning and ongoing programs would be to implement a more formal human resources function internally, or to outsource it.

Long-term planning has a shorter time horizon than strategic planning, typically not less than 1 year and no more than 4 years. It answers more detailed questions about how to execute the broad strategic goals of the organization, and it includes the identification of financial and performance objectives, as well as the human and physical resources that may be necessary to accomplish the strategic plan.

Operational planning has the shortest time frame—typically less than a year—but it can be broken down into shorter intervals such as months or days. Operational planning encompasses assignment of tasks to designated personnel, required budgets, and production timetables.

Controlling

The second stage in the three-stage management cycle is management or internal control. In the Field Work Standards for Performance Audits that are used by federal auditors, the comptroller general of the United States defines management control in its fourth field work standard as the "organization, methods, and procedures adopted by management to ensure that its goals are met."[4] Management controls include systems for measuring, reporting, and monitoring program performance. These field work standards include four categories of management controls, the following two of which are directly applicable to controls in a physician practice:

- *Program operations:* "Controls over program operations include policies and procedures that management has implemented that reasonably ensure that a program meets its objectives."[5]
- *Validity and reliability of data:* "Controls over the validity and reliability of data include policies and procedures that management has implemented to reasonably ensure that valid and reliable data are obtained, maintained, and fairly disclosed."[5]

Applied to physician practices, the latter would include controls over the information used by physician practices, physician organizations, and physician billing computer systems to bill and collect for services rendered to patients. The application of these types of controls extends beyond the billing system because demographic and insurance information derives from the activities of appointment schedulers, registration personnel, and insurance companies. The absence of data validity and reliability controls, particularly in the appointment scheduling and registration subsystems of a practice's billing and collection process, can lead to incorrect billing at the least, the over- or undercollection of copayments and deductibles, or patterns of not collecting copayments or deductibles. Each is an area of risk.

Management texts define internal controls in a similar manner. Management controls are those policies and procedures that:

- Ensure the efficient and effective use of resources
- Involve the development of standards for employee performance
- Design work plans for the implementation and monitoring of internal programs
- Institute methods for motivating employees and appraising their performance
- Solve operational problems, coach, and counsel

In most organizations, many, if not all, of these functions involve human resources management or a human resources department. The human resources management function in many physician practices is informal, or does not exist. Therefore, in implementing a compliance plan, many practices need to assess the degree to which they use effective human resources management.

Effective internal control over the billing and collection functions in small and large practices generally requires the creation and maintenance of internal operating policies and procedures. Related to the billing and collection cycle only, these policies and procedures should, at a minimum, encompass appointment scheduling, patient registration, insurance, data input, patient checkout, and collection. In practices that outsource computerized billing, vendor manuals provide only one component of this requirement. They are supplemental and generally pertain only to the computer system. They should be used in conjunction with policies and procedures manuals that are specific to the practice and its major operating systems.

Evaluation and Feedback

Evaluation and feedback, the third and last phase of the management cycle, involves both qualitative and quantitative methods for assessing whether the procedures and controls that have been established have resulted in the achievement of the program's goals. It leads to the beginning of the planning phase of the management process.

Methods for assessing the achievement of a program's goals can include analysis of budget outcomes, statistical analysis of the performance criteria that were established early in the management cycle, surveys of senior executives and employees, and retrospective audits. The evaluation and feedback phase of the management cycle is very important because it determines whether modifications need to be made in the planning and controlling phases to better ensure the achievement of the organization's strategic and long-term goals. If plans need to be modified, added, or deleted, the evaluation and feedback phase provides the information and analyses for management to make these decisions. If controls in one or more segments of a practice's procedures or policies are weak and need to be tightened in order to increase the probability of detecting unacceptable practices, it is the evaluation and feedback phase that provides the information to management to make these changes.

The OIG recognizes that the establishment and effectiveness of a compliance plan and program evolve over a period of time, and perhaps, particularly in smaller groups, initially focus only on matters related to accurate and proper billing. The evaluation and feedback mechanism ensures that the compliance process in small or large physician practices remains dynamic, current with changes in regulatory change, and in keeping with the unique characteristics of each physician practice.

In most industries, large organizations obtain annual audits by accounting firms that are in accordance with generally accepted accounting principles (GAAP). Many of these types of audits also include a separate management letter, in which the accounting firm can identify weaknesses in operations, internal controls, and other matters that could increase the risk of embezzlement, improper handling of financial information, the security of and accuracy of information, and other matters. Few physician practices, even larger ones, obtain a full independent audit, and many continue to use a less in-depth preparation of annual financial statements called a compilation. Empirically, it can be concluded that it is rare that a practice would also obtain a management letter. Therefore, unless through more informal methods, the practice may never become aware of weaknesses in its own operations, financial management, internal controls, and other aspects of the practice that could adversely affect the organization.

Human Resources Management

Particularly for larger group practices, compliance plans and programs should include the following:

▪ Position descriptions for all employee categories that are involved in compliance (presumably for all position categories)

▪ Evaluation of employees and performance feedback periodically

▪ Employee sanctioning for those who do not adhere to the practice's ethical guidelines or policies and procedures related to the compliance plan

▪ Conformance to applicable labor, wage, and salary and other federal (e.g., Occupational Safety and Health Act) and state laws

▪ Methods to communicate with and receive communications from employees

▪ Recruitment and screening of prospective employees and checking of their references

▪ Compliance training for new and existing employees

Even if effectively used, these functions are not foolproof. Bad hires will occur, as will unidentifiable but adverse employee activities. The government is looking for reasonable and diligent efforts in the recruiting process, the employee evaluation mechanism, training, and other human resources management functions that can reinforce high ethical standards and reduce the possibility of illegal behavior.

Most, if not all, of the preceding functional tasks involve human resources management. Except for larger medical practices with established human resources management departments, many of these functions may not be in place or exist at all. In smaller practices, they may be handled informally. Human resources management, whether resident in a department within a larger practice or performed informally or outsourced in smaller practices, typically encompasses the following six functions:[6]

1. Human resources planning
   - Job analysis and job descriptions
   - Staffing levels
   - Staffing plans and policies and workforce objectives
   - Job evaluation
   - Wage and salary administration and merit and compensation planning
2. Employment
   - Identifying sources to recruit new candidates
   - Interviewing, testing, and performing reference checks of prospective candidates
   - Maintaining records and turnover statistics
3. Induction and orientation
   - Design of staff orientation programs
   - Processing of benefits
   - Performance of follow-up within probationary period

4. Training and development
   - Design and implementation of skills training and management development programs
   - Administration of tuition refund programs
5. Employee training and development
   - Design and administration of performance evaluation program
   - Training of management in management and motivational skills
   - Design and coordination of employee communication methods and programs
   - Administration of employee newsletter
6. Health and safety
   - Physical examinations
   - Occupational Safety and Health Administration (OSHA) requirements

The question that needs to be asked is, "Does this physician practice have these functions in place, informally or formally?" If the answer generally is unfavorable, a practice implementing a compliance plan should consider which other functions need to be put in place.

To reiterate, the seven basic steps outlined by the OIG contain many principles and functions that are related to human resources management. Most can be accomplished through an existing human resources management department, can be delegated to appropriate personnel in smaller practices, or can be outsourced. Because of the range of functions that involve expertise in human resources management, it is important for practice managers and physicians to ensure that these tasks are monitored and evaluated, particularly in practices with a limited number of personnel or whose personnel lack the requisite expertise.

Management Styles, Corporate Culture, and Compliance

In small or large groups, an underlying purpose of compliance activities is to create a culture within the organization that engenders the prevention, identification, and resolution of behaviors that are inconsistent with federal and state law, private insurer program requirements, and the practice's ethical and business policies. These goals and related policies should originate at the governing body level of the practice or, in smaller groups, with the physician owners. As stated earlier, they should be articulated in strategic plans, corporate bylaws, policies and procedures, and other corporate documents. Small practices should have bylaws and other corporate

documents in which to infuse these communications. Moreover, they should be reinforced by the actions and attitudes of the physicians in the practice, as well as senior management, on a uniform and consistent basis so as to engender an attitude among all employees that there is zero tolerance for behaviors that are inconsistent with the practice's compliance policies.

The creation of an organizational culture is easier said than done; it requires time, conscious effort, and commitment of capital. In smaller practices, the culture often is a function of the personalities and management and medical styles of the key physicians. In larger integrated practices, corporate culture is influenced more by the attitudes and actions of the governing body, medical director, and senior management as well as the ongoing management decisions that support the cultural vision of the practice. In decentralized but organized physician practices and faculty plans, corporate culture arises from the governing board, medical director, and senior management. It also is dependent on departmental managers and physician chairpersons to reinforce the corporate culture. In larger, more complex types of practice settings, the physician clinical department chairs, particularly in large, dominant clinical departments, can create a departmental culture that is not necessarily in harmony with the corporate culture. In these situations, the role of the medical director is even more important.

Culture, therefore, is changeable over time as the priorities of a practice evolve and the medical and managerial leadership changes. Because of the relationship between corporate culture and management style, as it pertains to compliance plans, an overview of major management theories may be useful.

Management Practices

Even in the smallest of organizations and physician practices, there is a relationship between the manner in which individuals (including physicians) manage and the establishment of corporate culture. Each of the management practices discussed in this section has a certain type of management style or attitude, and each may have a different impact on the ease of implementing a compliance plan and motivating employees and physicians to embrace it.

During the mid-1800s through the early 1900s, the classical school of management first attempted to apply scientific approaches to management. Frederick W. Taylor, who is often referred to as the father of scientific management (as opposed to modern personnel administration), was among the first to introduce scientific principles to increase the efficiency of workers.

The efforts of Taylor and other classicists were directed specifically at worker efficiency—learning the correct way to perform a task, or series of tasks, as determined by experts such as engineers, scientists, and managers in the field. Work was broken down into a series of standardized tasks, each of which was designed to produce the most efficient process. Taylor claimed that hidden waste in an organization and the resulting cost was a function of worker inefficiency. He believed that workers needed to be won over and led by management, and he was firmly committed to the principle that management was the only force that determined the nature of the work process and the workplace. Won over and led certainly describes a particularly autocratic and centralized style with no focus on workers or their needs. This style in a physician practice would not likely create an environment conducive to compliance plans.

Whereas the classical school concentrated on work tasks performed by employees, the behavioral school of the late 1800s to 1950s stressed that sound management arises from an understanding of workers and what motivates them to work efficiently. This acknowledgment created very different, more democratic management styles that were worker inclusive. The genesis of this assertion was an outgrowth of the well-known Hawthorne experiments conducted by the social scientists Elton Mayo and F. J. Roethlisberger.[7] These experiments greatly influenced the modern human relations movement in organizations and had a significant impact on our understanding of human behavior in the work environment. During these experiments, Mayo and his colleagues changed certain physical aspects of the work environment, such as lighting. They found that regardless of the intensity of the lighting, or any other changes in the work setting, worker productivity was enhanced. Mayo and associates discovered that the employees were responding not to the researchers' changes to the work setting, but rather to the fact that the workplace was more enjoyable. This stemmed from the workers' belief that they were taking part in an important experiment and felt a common identity and sense of belonging with the other participating employees. These factors, which related to the relationships among employees and individual employee psychology, were thus called human relations factors. In summary, these researchers observed that employees tended to cluster in informal groups in order to fill voids in their lives in the workplace that arose from an absence of management attention to their basic need for cooperation and comradeship.

Rensis Likert and Daniel Katz later identified that managers play a very important role in the success of an organization. Managers who were employee focused, were cooperative and reasonable, and used a democratic management style were more likely to be successful than those who focused primarily on production.[8]

A. H. Maslow's work added to our understanding of the needs and motivations of workers. He identified five sets of goals or basic worker needs: psychological, safety, love, esteem, and self-actualization. Maslow further found that these needs not only were related to one another, but also were arranged in a hierarchy of importance. Maslow posited that when a lower-level need was fairly well satisfied, the next higher need in the hierarchy emerged.[8] Other behavioral researchers and managers to this day see the worker as having perpetual needs that are both personal and social. These needs suggest that employees want to satisfy, through their work, their need for security, independence, participation, and growth.

Applying the principles of Maslow and other behavioral scientists, Japanese industrialists innovated quality circles in the 1970s. The outcomes include enhanced self-images of workers, increased quality, improved worker morale, and greater managerial ability. This approach to the worker, the work environment, and management style is what underlies successful human resources management in hospitals and physician practices around the country.

In implementing some or all of the core principles stated in the seven basic elements, most of which require employee cooperation and "buy-in" to the compliance plan, the physicians and managers in both small and large practices should consider what type of management style and culture they have in place. It would appear that the closer their management style is to the findings of Maslow and the others who followed his tenets, the more fertile will be the environment for compliance planning and effective management in general. Because physician practices continue to evolve from small independent workplaces to larger, more corporate settings, physicians and management need to be attentive to human resources management, management style, and corporate culture. The principles that arise from the work of Maslow and others point to the hazards of operating a physician practice, large or small, in an autocratic manner.

Many physician practices are high-volume, high-stress settings in which physicians and staff can be overburdened. It may appear easier in these settings to use an autocratic, production-oriented style, but this approach tends to demotivate employees. The behaviorist approach tends to engender a team concept that is more conducive to maintaining high morale.

■ The Elements of Compliance Plans and Programs

The previous section places the compliance plan and program into the broader context of general management, operations, organization, and internal controls. One could argue that if physician practices employed the elements that are discussed later in this section, they would already have a significant portion of the framework for a compliance plan in place and operating on an ongoing basis. This argument generally would be correct; all the practice would need to do is to infuse a set of guidelines that were specific to the seven basic elements. However, even in today's consolidating practice environment and with the emergence of much larger and multi-office settings, many may still not employ the types of organizational, managerial, or formal human resources management practices that one would find in most other types of organizations.

A discussion of the managerial and operational implications of implementing a compliance plan should facilitate understanding of the areas physician practices may need to address in implementing any or all of the seven basic components of a compliance program.

Evaluating the Size of a Practice

The OIG guidance for physician practices targets individual physicians and small group physician practices, and recommends that practice size and resources be considered in designing an appropriate compliance program. The OIG also suggests that larger physician practices may wish to refer to, and adopt, as is applicable, elements of the more comprehensive guidelines for third-party billing companies. However, the OIG does not offer suggestions regarding what distinguishes a small from a large physician practice. This poses little difficulty to obviously large practices such as faculty practice plans, IPAs, and other physician organizations, but what of the majority of the other practices in the country? How do they determine whether they are small, moderate, or large for the purpose of designing and implementing a compliance program?

Regardless of the lack of guidance from the OIG, there are certain operational and financial characteristics that reliably can be considered in determining relative practice size. Some are quantitative, whereas others relate more to operational or organizational characteristics. It is important to note that for most practices a single criterion will not define a practice as small or large. However, when using a few criteria, a practice is likely to come to a reasonable decision about its relative size. Using many

criteria, a few key determinants to size that a practice may wish to consider are as follows (nonhospital-owned multispecialty groups are used as examples, but similar information is available in the cited publication for major single-specialty practices):

- *Total practice revenues:* A broad financial determinant of size is revenues generated per year, expressed as either total practice revenues or revenues per physician. A practice may wish to use the Medical Group Management Association's *Cost Survey* (published annually based on prior years' data) to determine its relative revenue size.
- *Medicare receipts:* The number of receipt dollars collected by a practice from Medicare also indicates relative practice size. In addition, it can be used by a practice to determine how substantial it is in terms of the magnitude of payments made to it by the Medicare program, which may relate to audit risk. (Note that the relationship between Medicare payments made to a practice and the risk of being audited is conjecture.) A practice may also wish to analyze its own percentage of Medicare charges and revenues from total collections.
- *Operational expenses:* The level of operating expenses of a practice can be an indicator of practice size and complexity because payroll costs are typically a majority of total operating expenses. Further, practices with multiple offices and more complex organizational structures generally will sustain larger overhead obligations.
- *Number of physicians and support staff:* The number of physicians and nonphysicians in a practice is a strong indicator of practice size. However, care should be exercised in using these criteria because in certain specialties a few physicians and staff are capable of generating substantial revenues. The practice might then qualify as large in terms of revenues, but not necessarily on the basis of expense levels.
- *Organizational complexity:* Does the practice have more than one office? If so, how many satellite offices are there? The number of satellite offices is an indicator of organizational complexity and relative size.

Another consideration in determining organizational complexity is the nature of the governing body of the practice. A board of directors that meets regularly or having regular partnership meetings is more common in larger physician practices and physician organizations.

If, in considering all of the preceding factors, a practice generally skews toward the higher percentiles in the

Cost Survey, it may conclude that it contains many elements of a larger practice. If so, it should consider implementing all seven components of an effective compliance program, as well as integrating other aspects of the OIG guidance for third-party billing companies.

The Basic Components of an Effective Compliance Program

Although the essence of the basic elements in the federal sentencing guidelines can be found in all of the OIG compliance guidances, the manner in which the OIG has applied the elements (i.e., examples of what measures can be taken to comply with the seven elements) varies between the guidelines directed to billing companies and those issued for individual doctors and small group practices. For example, the most recent guidelines directed at individual physicians and small group practices appear to apply some of the principles more broadly in recognition of the organizational differences between small practices and typically larger organizations such as billing companies.

The differences between the guidelines for billing companies and those for individual physicians and small group practices appear most noticeable in the requirements for policies and procedures manuals, the suggestion that a compliance officer be identified, the recommendations for internal audits and related sample sizes, the assessment of areas of risk, the communication methods for reporting alleged wrongdoing, and the training requirements. In these categories, the OIG occasionally recommends less formal, less costly approaches that are tailored to the resources of individual and small physician group practices. On the other hand, the OIG appears to feel that certain compliance components (such as written standards and procedures and auditing) should be implemented regardless of organizational size or type.

However, the OIG compliance guidance for physician practices does not give any definitive indication about which specific component will be deemed acceptable for a partially implemented compliance program or provide a standard measure of staff or financial resources to indicate when the OIG would expect a practice to fully implement all seven components. Large practices need to implement a detailed and complete compliance structure, similar to the one outlined in other OIG guidances and in particular, the Third-Party Medical Billing Company Guidance. Individual and small practices may choose to implement a compliance program only partially, targeting the areas of risk identified in internal auditing or as part of a progression toward full implementation of a compliance program. The following section presents all seven elements to address the management issues involved in each, so as to cover the full range of implementation options for physician practices, regardless of size and resources.

1. *Standards of conduct and policies and procedures:* Standards of conduct and policies and procedures for employees should be developed that include a commitment to compliance by the physician practice and its senior management. The standards should function as a guideline that provides detail regarding the intent to reduce or eliminate the possibility of wrongdoing. The standards should promote integrity, objectivity, and trust and be supported by the board, senior management, and staff. Standards and procedures should be reasonably capable of reducing the prospect of criminal conduct.

2. *Designation of a compliance officer:* A compliance officer should be hired or designated who is a high-level individual, has overall responsibility for the program, and has the responsibility and authority to ensure that the program is consistently enforced and monitored, evaluated, and modified so that it conforms to changes in regulations. This individual must have direct access to the uppermost levels of management and to the governing board. The compliance officer must have the authority to review all documents and materials that are relevant to compliance activities. He or she must have the authority to review contracts and obligations that may contain referral and payment provisions that could violate statutory or regulatory requirements. It is important to note that due care should be exercised to prevent authority from being delegated to those with an inclination to engage in illegal activities. Screening should be reasonable and diligent.

3. *Conducting effective training:* An educational and training program should be designed and implemented that ensures an understanding of compliance requirements and internal policies and procedures. The program can be provided internally or by outside professional organizations. Initial training should include a review of the company's standards of conduct; employees should sign an attestation that they have a knowledge of and commitment to those standards. Training also should include billing and coding matters, as well as summarize fraud and abuse statutes.

4. *Effective lines of communication:* Effective mechanisms should be developed that will allow employees and other agents, in good faith, to report known or suspected misconduct without fear of reprisal. The OIG suggests a confidential hotline, e-mail, and drop box in the practice, although other mechanisms can be used.

5. *Auditing and monitoring:* Auditing and monitoring mechanisms should be developed that can reasonably detect criminal conduct by employees and other agents. The courts have carefully scrutinized these auditing mechanisms when determining how effective a compliance plan has been. It is important that these mechanisms be designed and used properly. Documentation of audit processes and findings should be detailed.

   At a minimum, these audits and reviews should "be designed to address the billing company's compliance with laws governing kickback arrangements, coding practices, claim submission, and reimbursement and marketing."[9] Techniques that can be considered include testing billing and coding staff on their knowledge of reimbursement criteria, checking personnel records to determine whether any individuals who have been reprimanded for compliance issues in the past are among those currently engaged in improper conduct, distributing questionnaires to solicit impressions of employees and staff, and performing trend analysis or longitudinal studies that seek to identify deviations over a given period.[10]

   The reviewers should possess the qualifications and experience necessary to identify potential issues with regard to the subject matter being reviewed, be objective and independent of line management, and have access to audit and healthcare resources and to relevant personnel and areas of operation.[10]

6. *Establishing disciplinary guidelines:* Disciplinary guidelines and penalties should be developed that consistently and uniformly define actions that will be taken when an individual commits an offense, fails to detect and/or report an offense, or makes a bad faith report that offenses are, or have been, occurring.

7. *Responding to detected offenses and developing corrective action initiatives:* Documented corrective action should be taken in response to identified weaknesses in compliance standards and procedures. This documentation should include any changes that need to be made to the compliance plan that are designed to prevent any future offenses of the same kind.

■ Managerial Implications of Implementing the Compliance Plan

The operational implications of implementing a compliance plan in any size practice actually extend beyond the basic compliance elements. In fact, many of the elements, as implemented (even in their most simple form and in the smallest practices), may represent features and functions that have never existed in physician practices or do exist, but in basic forms. For example, auditing and monitoring to detect breaches in compliance (and the rectification of those breaches) is, perhaps, the most distant from the organizational fabric of most practices. On the other hand, it is one of the more important of the OIG guidelines. Auditing is a high-risk and difficult function if done properly, even if the practice is small and conforms to the recent guidelines for individual physicians and small practices. If an audit, even one involving a small sample, is conducted poorly or by individuals without the requisite knowledge and experience, it may lead to greater liability.

Many of the seven basic elements involve human resources management functions that may never have existed, or may not exist in a formal manner. Even though the OIG provides for less formal compliance approaches for smaller practices, certain human resources approaches need to be in place to conform to the OIG guidelines. For example, does the practice have personnel manuals or operations manuals that include requirements and mechanisms to reference-check prospective employees, and does it have written annual employee performance evaluations that tie performance to compensation and promotions? Does the practice have internal management controls designed to identify and reduce billing and coding errors, as well as feedback mechanisms to convey changes in billing and coding so that they are no longer being performed incorrectly? If the practice does have these types of controls in place, does it discipline or terminate employees who do not adhere to exemplary compliance standards or, conversely, have written procedures in which employees are rewarded for exemplary performance? Each practice needs to answer these and related questions to determine how it might need to modify existing operations, augment human resources, and implement new procedures and internal controls.

The operational and organizational implications of implementing a compliance plan and program generally can be categorized into two areas of management: (1) those that relate to general management functions, and (2) those that involve human resources management functions. As shown in **Table 18-1**, there are 12 functions that fall within these two categories. All originate from the seven basic elements.

General Management Functions

This section discusses basic management functions that are common to all organizations. In order for a compliance plan to really be integrated into the fabric of an organization, and for the Compliance Plan to "take life" it should be integrated into the functions that govern almost all organizations in most industries.

Review and Upkeep of Corporate Documents, Mission Statement, and Codes of Ethics

The compliance plan should begin with a statement of commitment from the governing board or shareholders (i.e., in a smaller practice) that underscores their intent that the practice and its employees exhibit a code of conduct that is consistent with preventing, identifying, and reducing or eliminating wrongdoing. These principles, infused into the practice's mission statement, applicable policies and procedures, and other corporate documents,

Table 18-1	Compliance Plan and Program: Organizational Functions
General Management Functions	
Corporate documents, mission statement, and code of ethics	
Operating policies and procedures	
Assessment of risk	
Internal auditing	
Communication and reporting systems	
Investigation of wrongdoing	
Program assessment and evaluation	
Human Resources Management Functions	
Organizational design, responsibility, authority, and delegation	
Training	
Personnel policies and procedures	
Personnel discipline, enforcement of policies, and terminations	
Position descriptions	

should be simply written, easily comprehended, and accessible to employees. New employees should be given the code of ethics and mission statement, be allowed a reasonable amount of time to read them, and be asked to sign a statement that they have read and understand the code of ethics and intend to diligently adhere to its provisions. It is important to note that these policy statements need not be overly detailed; they should not describe overarching ideals unless the practice intends to initiate and enforce them. Crafting goals that a practice cannot reasonably achieve can lead to demotivated employees and an ineffective compliance plan. There should be periodic updates of the mission statement and code of ethics designed to incorporate exogenous change (e.g., regulations) and internal change within the practice (e.g., new risk factors).

It is important to emphasize here that the OIG compliance guidance for small and individual physician practices does not include the development of a code of conduct in the seven basic elements of an effective program, contrary to guidances the OIG has released thus far for other types of healthcare providers. Larger physician practices that have the resources to implement a full compliance program following the elements contained in the Compliance Program Guidance for Third-Party Medical Billing Companies should likely include a code of conduct in their program. Although the OIG does not recommend a code of conduct for smaller practices as part of its compliance initiative, a code of conduct can provide an easy-to-develop tool that lays a framework for more-specific compliance efforts.

Operating Policies and Procedures

Fundamental to the operating structure of any organization is the establishment of operating policies and procedures that govern what employees do in an organization and how they go about doing it. Procedures set forth the correct and efficient way to perform operational tasks, including the use of internal controls that are designed to detect and correct errors or deviations from established procedures. Applicable policies and procedures in the practice should be reviewed to determine whether they are sufficient to comply with compliance standards. Where necessary, they should be revised or newly written. Policies and procedures, as noted in the audit section later in this chapter, also provide the standards against which an auditor will review a practice. The policies and procedures should be simply written and understandable.

On-the-job training is not uncommon in physician practices. There are both advantages and disadvantages inherent in this. One major disadvantage is that the same individual may not train all new employees (because of personnel turnover, dependence on part-time individuals, and so forth). Therefore, that which is taught may be someone's interpretation of how to perform certain tasks. The existence of a written procedure manual presents an opportunity to have a resource that will define the manner in which functions should be performed. Therefore, it should be made part of the initial training of all new employees. Procedure and policy manuals are dynamic documents and, as such, should always be changed to accommodate modifications in operations, external requirements, new technologies, and other factors that affect what is done in an organization.

A word of caution is in order. The manuals a billing company gives to a practice when automating its billing systems define the manner in which the automated billing system should be used. They can affect certain operational processes, but they should not be used in lieu of having operational manuals for the entire practice. According to the OIG, the practice should, however, periodically review the sections of the billing systems manuals that describe the manner in which coding edits are used.

Assessment of Risk

The assessment of risk is an important factor in determining the scope of a compliance program. Although the area of billing and collections is an acceptable beginning point, a compliance program should go beyond the prevention, detection, and correction of Medicare and Medicaid billing and coding irregularities, including compliance with regulations regarding antikickback and anticompetitive behavior, OSHA, and other requirements. As will be discussed further in this chapter, the assessment of an organization's risks also is important for defining the scope of internal audits.

As discussed earlier, the OIG has identified a number of risk areas that should be considered for small and larger practices. Organizational status and organizational structure also should be considered in determining risk. Practices that are part of multiprovider systems need to consider their relationships with the hospital system and other physicians in relation to Stark law prohibitions against self-referrals, free or below-market cost of space or equipment rentals, or other benefits they may obtain. Likewise, a practice that is part of a large physician network or management service organization (MSO), or one that has expanded significantly as a result of merger or acquisition, should consider whether it has additional risks. If these are potential risks, the practice should consider a legal audit of contracts.

Practices that use multiple offices (this does not have to be a large practice) may have higher risks related to having weak internal controls or the inconsistent application of correct billing and coding standards. Practices with many physicians within specific specialties may have a higher risk related to not uniformly applying billing and coding standards. Surgical specialty practices may not have as much concern with coding for evaluation and management (E&M) services as would a multispecialty group. On the other hand, there are many surgical specialty practices that derive a great deal of their revenues from E&M services. This only serves to underscore how important it is to define the practice's risks before designing the scope of the compliance plan.

In summary, it is important that the practice place the greatest compliance efforts on those areas that may represent the most significant risk. In addition, if a compliance plan has too great a scope, it places the practice in the position of possibly not being able to satisfy all plan goals.

Internal Auditing

As stated earlier, internal auditing (sometimes referred to as performance or operational auditing) is one of the key components in a compliance plan and program, whether in a small or large practice. In order to be done well, and to produce reliable information, requisite knowledge of the audit process, proper sample selection, and experience are necessary. Improperly conducted audits can place a practice at greater liability. Therefore, audits should be properly scoped, and they should be supervised by competent individuals who are independent and objective. Audits can, and usually are, retrospective. They also can be concurrent, in which case they perform more of a monitoring function.

Because of the importance of the audit function within the compliance plan, as well as the expectation that an audit should extend beyond billing and coding matters, this subject will be explored in greater detail. This discussion is not intended to establish a higher standard than the OIG may require, but rather to acquaint the reader with key principles that underlie sound auditing. If all of these principles cannot be adhered to initially, they provide a series of goals toward which a practice can evolve as its compliance plan matures.

There are various types of audits. Most individuals are aware of financial audits, which are an independent and objective assessment designed to provide reasonable assurance that the information presented in the financial statements of an organization do not contain material misstatements regarding the operating results of the organization and that the financial statements have been prepared in accordance with. Accounting firm professionals with expertise in the financial audit function generally conduct financial audits. The American Institute of Certified Public Accountants (AICPA) promulgates comparatively strict accounting and auditing guidelines (generally accepted auditing standards) that govern financial audits. Government audit standards closely follow those of the AICPA.

Operational (performance and compliance) audits are independent, objective, and systematic examinations of evidence for the purpose of providing an assessment of the performance of an organization, a unit within an organization, a function, or a program in order to improve accountability, efficiency and effectiveness, internal controls, profit, and decision making. These audits encompass:

- Assessments of financial performance
- Use of human and other organizational resources (i.e., appropriateness of staffing levels)
- Compliance with laws that affect the organization
- Policies, procedures, and internal controls
- Management structure and internal communications

Performance audits can be broad and encompass all of the preceding and more, or they can be very targeted at specific organizational units, functions, procedures, or personnel in an organization. Often, a baseline or annual comprehensive audit will reveal areas of concern or weakness, but before conclusions can be reached, more specific and intensified audits may be necessary. Frequently, a comprehensive performance audit will reveal areas of weakness in systems and controls or other factors that should be of concern to management. These should be rectified and thereafter reviewed in more targeted audits.

Prior to beginning periodic (minimally annual) audits, the OIG suggests performing a baseline audit. A baseline audit should consist of all of the following; annual audits thereafter should consist of the first two items listed.

- *Operational (performance audit):* As previously identified, this type of audit generally consists of a review of all major operating systems (scheduling, registration, billing and collections practices, checkout and payment, medical records filing, general ledger and accounting, physician and nonphysician staffing levels, marketing and practice-building activities, and financial analyses). It also would include a review of coding and documentation (*Current Procedural Terminology* and

International Classification of Diseases) for appropriateness and compliance with regulations and guidelines. In addition, it would include a review of medical record documentation to determine whether the documentation supported the codes that were used.
- *Legal review:* This is a review of all contracts, such as space rentals; equipment leases; co-ownership/shareholder contracts with institutional or physician providers; and any arrangements, formal or otherwise, wherein a practice receives payment from a supplier, vendor, or the like.
- *Other compliance areas:* This is a review of the practice's compliance with OSHA, the Clinical Laboratory Improvement Act (CLIA), and so forth.

In performing an audit, the following factors are essential:

Auditor Independence. Whether government or AICPA guidelines are followed, it is apparent that the principles of independence and objectivity should be considered when contemplating compliance audits in a physician practice setting. Therefore, a further review of the meaning of these principles seems warranted.

Government auditors use four general standards[11] to describe independence, three of which relate more directly to the auditor's role in physician practice organizational settings. Although these standards for independence and objectivity relate to financial auditing, in principle they apply to all types of auditing. In reality, the last thing a practice wants is to have its audit results invalidated by the government because the practice's auditor was not independent or objective.

The first government principle states that the auditor (internal or external) and audit staff (i.e., the organization conducting the audit) should possess adequate professional proficiency for the tasks required. The second principle states, "In all matters relating to the audit work, the audit organization and the individual auditors, whether government or public, should be free from personal and external impairments to independence, should be organizationally independent, and should maintain an independent attitude and appearance."[12] This standard "places responsibility on each auditor and the audit organization to maintain independence so that opinions, conclusions, judgments, and recommendations will be impartial and will be viewed as impartial by knowledgeable third parties."[13]

There are three general classes of impairments to an auditor's independence—personal, external, and organizational. Personal and external impairments will be discussed because of their relevance to physician practices. Personal impairments can include[14]:

- Official, professional, personal, or financial relationships that might cause an auditor to limit the scope of the review, to limit disclosure, or to weaken or slant findings in any way
- Preconceived ideas toward individuals, groups, organizations, or objectives of a program that could bias the audit
- Previous responsibility for decision making or managing an entity that would affect current operations of the entity or program being audited
- Biases, including those induced by political or social conscience

In a physician practice setting these may include situations in which a compliance auditor may have an ownership interest in a business entity owned by the practice (e.g., an ambulatory surgery center or billing company), may be a close friend or relative of a physician in the practice, may previously have worked in the department being audited, or may have worked closely with one or more of the physicians being audited (e.g., a nurse or technician). In any of these situations, the auditor and the audit results may be in question because of the actual or perceived impairment of the auditor. In large practices that may hire a compliance officer who will conduct the audits, these issues may be of less concern. Practices, large or small, that identify someone from within, however, should consider these issues. In small practices in which compliance personnel have responsibility for many functions, it is important that the compliance officer not be someone whose independence is impaired by virtue of the other functions for which he or she is responsible.

The second principle relates to external impairments. These involve impairments to the auditor's independence and ability to have complete freedom to make judgments. They include, but are not limited to, "external interference or influence that improperly or imprudently limits or modifies the scope of an audit, limits the selection or application of audit procedures, appears to overrule or influence the auditor's judgment, or that influences the auditor's continued employment for reasons other than competency."[15]

The third principle is organizational independence. The OIG refers to this when stating, in numerous of its compliance guidelines, that the compliance officer should have access to senior management and the board. This principle also states that the auditor should be sufficiently removed from the political pressures that arise from within the organization. If the auditor is an employee,

one might speculate that an organizational impairment may arise from inside the organization if, for example, the physicians being audited have an opportunity to review their medical record documentation prior to the auditor having access to it, or if the physicians try to modify the scope of the audit. This clearly would be a situation in which the authority of the auditor, and his or her ability to be independent, would be compromised. Another organizational impairment might occur if the physicians who are potentially affected by an auditor's report of findings have an opportunity to review and change the report prior to its issuance.

Auditor Objectivity. The AICPA defines objectivity as "a state of mind, a quality that lends value. It is the distinguishing feature of a professional. The principle of objectivity imposes the obligation to be impartial, intellectually honest, and free of conflicts of interest."[16] Objectivity is theoretically uniformly applicable to any organization regardless of size or ownership. However, physician practices generally are closely held businesses in which physicians often have a direct and dominant influence over the management and operations of the practice. In most respects this is no different from small businesses in other industries except for the fact that the product or service of a physician practice, namely medical or surgical services, perhaps requires that a physician play a role in the management of the practice, certainly in those issues that are clinical in nature. The conventional relationship between a board and management does not exist, as in most industries. Therefore, a tension can arise from the duality of management responsibility in many physician practices.

How this duality affects the compliance officer and his or her objectivity (and independence) is a matter that warrants consideration when assigning responsibility to an individual. In turn, it is something about which physicians should be aware once the audit function is in place.

Other Factors Relating to Auditing. Performance auditing, and indeed compliance auditing, should use accepted standards so that the findings and recommendations are not compromised or invalidated. The following five field work standards for performance audits are noteworthy:

1. *Work is to be adequately planned.* The scope and objectives of an audit should be clearly defined, as well as the audit, sampling, and other methodologies. Methodologies should be used to provide sufficient, competent, and relevant evidence to achieve the objectives of the audit.

Methodology includes not only the nature of the auditors' procedures, but also their extent (e.g., sample size). The plan should consider the internal controls that exist (or do not exist) in the organization, the results of prior audits and management reports, legal and regulatory requirements, and other factors that can affect the audit.[17]

2. *Staff are to be properly supervised.* Staff who are conducting an audit should be supervised by a senior staff person, and should understand the scope and purpose of the audit.[18]

3. *When laws, regulations, and other compliance requirements are significant to audit objectives, auditors should design the audit to provide reasonable assurance of compliance with them.* In all performance audits, auditors should be alert to situations or transactions that could be indicative of illegal acts or abuse.[19]

4. *Auditors should obtain an understanding of management controls that are relevant to the audit.* Management controls are the plan of organization, methods, and procedures that are adopted by management to ensure that goals are met. They include processes for planning, organizing, directing, and controlling operations, and they use systems for measuring, reporting, and monitoring organizational performance.[20] If the auditor believes that management controls are weak, particularly those that affect the reliability of information, then the scope of the audit should be expanded. As practices get larger, it can be expected that auditors will be more obliged to conduct expanded audits.

5. *Sufficient, competent, and relevant evidence is to be obtained to afford a reasonable basis for auditors' findings and conclusions.* Evidence is categorized as physical, documentary, testimonial, and analytical.[21] A record of auditors' field work should be retained in the form of working papers. As stated earlier, most practices do not obtain full financial audits, and even fewer have a management letter issued. "Working papers serve three purposes: they provide the principal support for the auditors' report, aid the auditors in conducting and supervising the audit, and allow others to review the audit's quality. Working papers should contain sufficient information to enable an experienced auditor having no previous connection with the audit to ascertain from them the evidence that supports the auditors' significant conclusions and judgments."[22]

Communication and Reporting Systems

Communication and reporting systems should be available so that employees can report compliance problems. Confidentiality should be maintained, but it is important that employees be aware that it is not being guaranteed. How this is accomplished in a physician practice is a matter of choice, and the methods for communication and reporting that already may exist in the practice play a role. Practices may use a hotline, a designated answering machine, or a suggestion box in a central location. Employees should be encouraged to identify their name and telephone number should someone need to contact them for additional information, and they should be made aware that the practice will not retaliate for information made in good faith.

All reports should be entered into a secured computer data file. They should be subjected to a preliminary inquiry designed to determine whether more comprehensive investigation is required. A summary of the results of the preliminary inquiry also should be logged. If the results of the preliminary inquiry demonstrate that a comprehensive investigation is appropriate, that investigation should be planned and implemented expeditiously. Investigations also can arise from audit findings.

Investigation of Wrongdoing

If the compliance officer determines in a preliminary review of a confidentially submitted employee complaint that an investigation is required, the process is similar to an audit. Investigations should conform to the audit principles discussed earlier (i.e., planning, scope, collection of evidence, documentation in working papers). Investigations should be conducted with the input of counsel throughout the process, and they may require the assistance of others in the practice or outside professionals. Interviewing technique is very important in an investigation, particularly if the person being interviewed is suspected of a crime. In these circumstances, it may be useful to have an additional person attend the meeting.

The compliance officer should provide investigative summaries and recommendations to the compliance committee of the board, and to the board when applicable. On a quarterly basis, the compliance committee should summarize all pertinent compliance activities and results (e.g., audits, investigations) to the full board.

Program Assessment and Evaluation

The impact of the compliance program should be assessed on an annual basis, and findings should be used to make modifications to the program. However, acute weakness in the compliance plan and program, particularly in the neophyte years, should be rectified on a concurrent basis. As discussed previously in this chapter, evaluation and feedback make up one of three critical phases of good management in general. Therefore, the assessment of the compliance program hopefully will be part of an existing and productive feedback process. The compliance officer should prepare an annual report for management and the board that provides documentation relating to the activities that have occurred during the year, summarizes audit and investigative efforts and actions that were taken, and makes suggestions for change (as required) in the compliance plan and specifically changes that have or will be made to comply with applicable regulations. The documentation, when possible, should refer to the seven basic elements in a compliance program. It should be reasonably, but not overly, detailed. Counsel should review the report in draft form to assess whether the action to disclose and correct the reported problems is sufficient to demonstrate that the program is effective.

Assessment of program effectiveness also can be solicited via group interviews with employees and physicians and through surveys. It is important to include questions that assess whether employees and physicians are aware of the program, the reporting mechanisms, and other features of the compliance plan. If there are new employees who can be interviewed, they often can provide a barometer for how visible the compliance program is and whether employee training is effective in familiarizing new employees with the practice.

Human Resources Management Functions

Formal human resources management departments are not typical in physician practices. Often, the functions consistent with human resources management are shared by a number of employees in a practice, are the responsibility of the practice manager, or are not in place at all. As stated earlier, many of the organizational implications of the seven steps involve functions that traditionally are considered human resources management. This section will discuss those functions.

Organizational Design, Responsibility, Authority, and Delegation

The best-conceived compliance program will have little chance of success if installed in a practice in which the lines of authority and communication are unclear or conflict. Likewise, if personnel responsibilities are not well defined and delegation is haphazard, these factors will interfere with program effectiveness. In a well-run practice

all of these organizational elements must be defined and clear. The chain of command should be apparent, communication should be upwardly and downwardly effective, and responsibility and authority should be delegated in a balanced manner.

The compliance plan should be supported by the governing board or, in smaller groups, the physician shareholders. In large practices that can economically justify recruiting a compliance officer, that individual should have access to the board and the chief executive officer and report to one or the other. As discussed earlier, the compliance officer should not have impaired independence or objectivity.

Training

Education and training can assume many forms. Regulations change frequently, government fraud and abuse alerts are regularly issued, and many other compliance-related issues change. Therefore, education and training should include updates on internal changes that have been made to the practice's compliance programs. Ideally, training begins with the establishment of a budgeted number of dollars for the purpose of internal and external education. Larger practices may wish to budget for the preparation and presentation of seminars and workshops conducted by their own staff. Smaller practices that do not have a formal budget can earmark a specific number of dollars for external staff and physician compliance training. The compliance officer should organize this effort.

As part of an annual planning process, external seminars and workshops should be identified and prospectively scheduled for attendance. Obtaining continuing education credits provides an added incentive to employees. Participants, including physicians from the practice, should be identified to attend. Attendees should be selected to attend educational seminars that are consistent with their organizational roles (e.g., billers should attend seminars relating to billing and coding issues, an OSHA supervisor should attend OSHA seminars, and so forth). Attendance at compliance workshops should be noted in annual (or more frequent) evaluations. Those who attend outside seminars should be asked to prepare presentations for their colleagues on what they learned.

Other materials such as cassette tapes, CDs, and manuals are useful for education. In smaller practices these forms of internal education might be more economically feasible than outside education. Newsletters, printed regulatory updates, booklets, and other compliance material should be routed to appropriate staff with a check-off box in which each person reading the material can acknowledge that it was read. Internal management meetings should discuss the practice's policies and procedures related to compliance and proper billing. On a periodic basis the compliance officer should make presentations to the board to keep members abreast of compliance and regulatory changes.

Personnel Policies and Procedures

All policies and procedures should be reviewed, and modifications should be made, as required, to incorporate components of the compliance plan. They should include the following:

- Policies and procedures related to enforcement and discipline (how wrongdoing was identified, documentation of billing errors, and corrective action that has been taken)
- Policies and procedures related to rectifying wrongdoing
- Policies and procedures to avoid the recurrence of wrongdoing, to identify the preventive steps that will be taken, and to document the training that will occur to remedy similar problems in the future

All policies and procedures (whether operating or personnel) should be easy to read and comprehend, not overly detailed, and designed to foster the application of judgment. Personnel policies and procedures should include, at a minimum, the following topical areas:

- Standards of employee conduct
- Disciplining personnel
- Termination
- Recruiting personnel and obtaining references (includes verification of licensure and other credentials and a check for prior government sanctions)
- Retrospective and concurrent performance evaluations
- Confidentiality relating to employee disclosure of knowledge related to wrongdoing

Employee annual evaluation forms should include performance criteria related to the employee's contributions to the compliance process and to upholding exemplary ethics. In addition, supervisors should be evaluated based on their contributions to upholding the compliance process.

Personnel Discipline, Enforcement of Policies, and Terminations

Enforcement is another critical element in compliance plans and programs for at least two reasons. First, if there is no enforcement of the program, then the government will not consider it effective. Second, and more operationally

important, if employees conclude that there is no enforcement of the policies and procedures related to preventing, detecting, and remedying wrongdoing, then they will not be motivated to uphold the principles of the program. The most available method of enforcement is the written annual employee performance evaluation. Employees exhibiting behavior contrary to the compliance plan should receive adverse write-ups in their annual evaluations. If the behavior is adverse but can be rectified, then a memorandum should be placed in their personnel file at the time of the infraction. In addition, problem employees can be moved to a quarterly performance review until their behavior changes positively, or until enough documentation of adverse behavior exists to support their termination. Employees who support the program should receive positive evaluations.

In cases of documented and serious instances of wrongdoing, employees should be warned or suspended from their responsibilities. In certain instances, immediate termination may be justifiable, particularly for repeat offenses. If criminal behavior is involved, the practice should be prepared to involve law enforcement after first seeking the opinion of counsel.

The discipline or punishment should parallel the infraction. The practice is ill advised to terminate an employee for an innocent first mistake. It should refer this employee for more training and implement additional supervision. Continued, but intermittent, errors of the same or similar type should receive more serious disciplinary response. Repeated (i.e., chronic) problems, or those in which the behavior is extremely serious or criminal, may require termination. Counsel should be sought in these situations.

It is important to document all enforcement and disciplinary decisions and actions in the employee's personnel file. Although no two noncompliance problems are necessarily the same, the practice should endeavor to apply its policies uniformly and fairly in order to preserve the credibility of the compliance officer and the compliance program, as well as to avoid wrongful dismissal and other labor law concerns.

Review and Upkeep of Position Descriptions

Position descriptions are the crux of recruiting, wage and salary administration, performance evaluation, authority, responsibility, delegation, and communication. All of these elements of management are affected by or influence the success of a compliance program. A compliance program not only requires the creation of a position description for the compliance officer (or modification of the position description of the employee who will perform this function part time), but also necessitates modifications to the position descriptions of all employees who will be responsible for adherence to compliance standards (compliance contacts).

The position description for the compliance officer, for example, should encompass:

- Designing, implementing, and modifying the compliance plan and program
- Hiring or internally using other staff to administer the compliance program
- Ensuring (possibly with the human resources manager or credentialing supervisor) that all clinicians have current licenses and required certifications
- Developing and overseeing educational and training programs
- Designing, participating in, and coordinating compliance audits
- Establishing communications systems for employees to report compliance concerns
- Investigating alleged wrongdoing and taking (or causing to be taken) disciplinary action
- Evaluating the impact of the compliance program
- Preparing reports to senior management and the board (or shareholders in smaller practices) periodically (at least annually)

Patten and colleagues suggest the use of eight principles as a guide to writing a position description[23]:

1. Arrange job duties in logical order. If a definite work cycle exists, duties may be described in chronological order. When work cycles are irregular, more important duties should be listed first, followed by less important duties.
2. State separate duties clearly and concisely without going into such detail that the description resembles motion analysis.
3. Start each section with an active functional verb in the present tense.
4. Use quantitative words where possible.
5. Use specific words where possible.
6. Avoid proprietary names that might make the description obsolete when equipment changes occur.
7. Determine or estimate the percentage of time spent on each activity, and indicate whether the duties are regular or occasional.
8. Limit use of the word "may" with regard to certain duties.

Job descriptions also can include in the heading a definition of the position (e.g., the chief executive officer), to whom the person reports (e.g., the board), and the staff members reporting to the person (e.g., all billing staff).

A Planning and Implementation Work Plan

The design, implementation, and operation of a written compliance plan are likely to require an appreciable amount of time and resources. To ensure that the compliance program eventually extends beyond compliance with billing and coding guidelines (the government's initial intent) and remains an ongoing, dynamic process, human resources such as physicians, management, outside professionals in practice and organizational consulting, coding experts, and attorneys may be necessary.

The general work plan that follows contains suggestions that should be further tailored to the specific needs of the practice. Where applicable, the work plan identifies alternatives for both small and large practices; however, it is important to remember that no one compliance plan is a universal fit for all practices, and it is not certain how the OIG defines small or large practice. The work plan is not exhaustive in detail, because its purpose is to outline a broad approach that the user can supplement with task detail. In defining a starting point, the work plan assumes that a practice knows little about the federal compliance plan guidelines and is literally starting at the beginning. It is important to note that since the original legislation, practice size has increased significantly, as have hospital-owned physician practices. Therefore, it is anticipated that many of the following tasks now apply to a large number of practices.

Tasks should be committed to a Gantt chart. These types of task and check-off lists identify the tasks and subtasks that are required to accomplish a particular project or program; assign tasks to individuals with responsibility for those tasks; and estimate the number of calendar days, weeks, or months that may be necessary for implementation. The Gantt chart is not only a planning tool, but also a monitoring tool that can be used to assess progress against a predetermined set of timed goals and over a long time period.

Sample Compliance Plan and Program Work Plan

All italicized text applies to small practices.

Phase I: Initial Compliance Planning and Fact Finding

Task 1: Board of Directors (Physician or Physician Shareholders) Express an Interest in Compliance Planning.

- *Subtask 1.1:* Form an ad hoc committee. The board preliminarily assigns fact-finding responsibility to an ad hoc committee of the board. The committee members are the president of the practice, the physician chair of the quality assurance subcommittee of the board, the chief executive officer (CEO), and the chief financial officer of the practice. The committee is asked to attend appropriate seminars, workshops, and so forth and to seek professional advice in order to develop a knowledge base that can be presented to the board in writing and in an oral presentation in 6 weeks. (*The president of the practice assigns this task to a shareholder who has been involved in billing and coding matters and to the practice manager. They are asked to present their findings in 8 weeks.*)

- *Subtask 1.2:* Develop knowledge regarding compliance. Research and develop an inventory of presentations and workshops that are devoted to compliance plans, and identify professionals who may be available to speak about compliance plans.

- *Subtask 1.3:* Conduct research and develop reports for the board (*shareholders*).

Task 2: Hold a Meeting of the Board of Directors (*Shareholders*) to Hear Presentations and to Vote.

- *Subtask 2.1:* Present ad hoc committee findings to the board. Presentations are made to the board (*shareholders*), and a recommendation is made to proceed with the development of a compliance plan and program. A budget is presented as part of the findings of the report.

- *Subtask 2.2:* Conduct a board vote. Board members (*shareholders*) vote to accept the recommendations to proceed with the development of a compliance plan and to hire a compliance officer. Vote is taken and passed. The ad hoc committee is dissolved, and the board votes to create a permanent compliance subcommittee of the board. The compliance officer is to report to the CEO. Responsibility and authority are given to the compliance committee to design and implement the plan and to seek the board's input as appropriate. (*Shareholders vote favorably and establish a working committee to develop a compliance plan. The two members remain the same, and the practice manager is assigned the part-time role of compliance officer. The compliance officer is asked to develop a budget for planning and implementing a compliance plan so that a "make vs. buy" decision can be made due to the practice's limited internal resources.*)

Task 3: Develop Compliance Planning Work Plan. The compliance committee asks the CEO to develop a written work plan to ensure that the process of planning

and implementing the plan proceeds smoothly and on time. It is assumed that the practice will keep the function of compliance planning internal, except, perhaps, to have a baseline audit performed by an outside company. (*The practice manager develops an informal work plan.*)

Task 4: "Make vs. Buy" Decision.

- *Subtask 4.1:* Solicit proposals from outside professionals. Although they think they will internalize the compliance planning function, the large group practice solicits proposals from outside consultants. Proposals are solicited from attorneys to conduct a legal audit of rental agreements, lease contracts with equipment vendors, and so forth. Proposals also are solicited from consultants to conduct a billing and coding audit and to develop a compliance plan and program after the baseline billing audit is conducted.

- *Subtask 4.2:* Make a decision relative to make vs. buy. The costs to internalize the compliance function are equal to the costs to have this function performed by outside professionals. Therefore, the practice elects to internalize the function in order to control costs as well as the process. (*Costs to develop the plan internally [hire a senior billing supervisor, as well as the practice manager's time] are less than the cost of using external professional support. Nonetheless, shareholders decide to expend the funds for outside assistance because they are concerned that the process might divert too much internal human resources time and might interfere with operations and increase billing and other errors. The high costs associated with outside professional services are determined to be largely a one-time expense that will allow the practice to internalize the majority of the compliance program functions in the future.*)

Task 5: Design Position Descriptions and Recruit Compliance Officer.

- *Subtask 5.1:* Design position descriptions. Reporting relationships are contemplated, and there are two apparent options: the compliance officer can report directly to the CEO of the practice and be a member of the compliance committee of the board, or the compliance officer can report directly to the compliance committee of the board, specifically the chair of that committee. The latter approach is not inconsistent with many other industries that use internal audits. The intent underlying this approach is that the board desires to assess all levels of the organization and to keep the audit function totally independent of management. However, the former option is selected because it is determined that reporting to the CEO will facilitate the resolution of compliance problems that are identified. The human resources department designs the position description and obtains approval from the CEO. The position description is inclusive of, but not limited to, the following:

- Defines the role to plan and implement the compliance plan inclusive of policies and procedures
- Develops and plans both internal and external educational and training programs for each category of personnel and tries to obtain continuing education credits for employees
- Designs and coordinates internal audits in accordance with applicable standards for auditing and sampling
- Establishes a mechanism for employees to report suspected violations confidentially and to evaluate those reports preliminarily
- Works with the CEO and other senior managers and physicians to evaluate internal controls continuously and to modify them as required
- Implements disciplinary measures directly or through administrative channels
- Evaluates the compliance plan annually (at a minimum) and identifies areas for change

Subtask 5.2: Hire/internally recruit compliance officer. A compliance officer is hired with significant compliance and internal auditing capability. The hiring is contingent on a check of references. The human resources department conducts the reference check and administers a personality test to the compliance officer. (*The practice assigns this responsibility to the practice manager on a part-time basis and increases that person's salary. The practice manager, for compliance issues, will report to a designated physician.*)

Task 6: Develop a Code of Ethics.

Subtask 6.1: Design a code of ethics and incorporate it into corporate documents. The compliance officer drafts a code of ethics, which is reviewed by the CEO and other members of the compliance committee. It is submitted, as a draft, to members of the board for their informal input. Modifications are made. The final code of ethics is submitted to the board and adopted. Then, the code of ethics is added to appropriate corporate documents and to the practice's mission statement. The new

mission statement is posted in employee areas and patient waiting rooms and is incorporated into the personnel manual and new employee orientation process. The compliance officer designs a mechanism to periodically review and update the code. (*The practice manager drafts a code of ethics and the shareholders approve it. It is added to the practice's general operations manual. New employees are given an operations manual to review when hired, and periodically they attend workshops on manual provisions. The manual is periodically reviewed by the practice manager. A performance question is added to the annual employee evaluation form related to the degree to which the employee cooperates with the principles of the compliance plan.*)

Task 7: Identify Areas of Risk in the Practice. The reports are thoroughly reviewed with particular emphasis on the risks noted. The risks are categorized as follows:

- Risks related to billing and collections
  - Upcoding
  - Internal controls relating to billing information
  - Billing for services not rendered
  - Inappropriate balance billing
  - Appropriateness of E&M coding
  - Discounts and professional courtesy write-offs
  - Routine waiver of copayments
  - Improper "incident to" billings
  - Failure to refund credit balances promptly to patients or insurers
  - Billing for services rendered by unqualified, uncertified, or unlicensed personnel
  - Failure to periodically review the billing software of the practice's automated physician billing company
  - Coding without documentation or making assumptions about the appropriate CPT or diagnosis code in the absence of (or due to inadequate) medical record documentation in instances where someone other than the physician defines the code to be used
  - Improperly altering existing medical records
- Operational, organizational, and legal risks:
  - The number of office sites, physicians, and employees may increase control risks.
  - Prior Medicare investigations may increase the practice's risks.
  - The practice's specialty may put it at a higher risk (*same for a smaller practice*).
  - Compliance with federal or state regulations such as self-referral, antitrust, and antikickback,

particularly for practices that are part of multiprovider systems in which they may rent space and equipment from a hospital or other providers.

- Compliance with CLIA, the Americans with Disabilities Act, and OSHA, as applicable. *(Smaller practices may not face many of these risks. Types of risks that may relate to smaller practices include a lack of or laxness in applying internal controls over billing and other data.)*

Task 8: Conduct Baseline Audit.

- *Subtask 8.1:* Have a baseline audit conducted by outside professionals. An outside consultant conducts a baseline billing and operations audit. This audit is designed to independently and objectively assess the policies, procedures, work flow, data accuracy and reliability, staffing levels, billing practices, and internal controls of the practice. It includes a review of a sample of bills for coding correctness and medical records for documentation appropriateness. Counsel conducts a legal audit of all employee contracts, physician contracts, rental and lease agreements, employee and physician compensation methods, and so forth. It also assesses compliance with federal and state laws (OSHA, antitrust, CLIA). Other consultants assess other areas of compliance, as necessary. *(The same audits are conducted for the small practice.)*
- *Subtask 8.2:* Receive baseline audit results. The consultants issue their reports to the compliance officer and members of the compliance committee. The reports outline weaknesses in internal systems, policies and procedures, internal controls, staffing levels, coding and billing practices, areas of operational risk, and so forth. Although they do not identify any wrongdoing, they do outline new policies and procedures that should be used in the future to report these types of problems internally (and possibly externally on the advice of counsel), to rectify those problems, and to incorporate methods to assess the effectiveness of the changes. This includes, but is not limited to, changes in policies and procedures, disciplinary measures including termination, documentation of investigations that were completed and identification of the corrective action taken, and changes in the curriculum of staff education to integrate new findings.

Phase II: Implementation

Task 9: Create an Implementation Team. To implement the applicable changes suggested in the baseline audit, and to begin to design and implement the compliance plan, the compliance officer creates an ad hoc committee of physicians, managers, and supervisors. The committee largely consists of middle managers and existing supervisors in the practice. They meet on a monthly basis. Committee members are assigned specific recommendations with a specific timeframe within which implementation must occur, based on the milestones in the Gantt chart. *(The practice manager or compliance officer is charged with the responsibility for implementing the findings and recommendations of the consultants. In smaller practices it requires less effort because there is greater hands-on control of the process, but limited resources result in implementation taking longer.)*

Task 10: Revise Position Descriptions.

- *Subtask 10.1:* Review position descriptions. All employee and physician position descriptions are reviewed. Where applicable, they are modified to reflect commitment to compliance and to assign responsibility for functions related to compliance. *(The smaller practice never has maintained position descriptions. The practice manager prepares position descriptions for all personnel, factoring in responsibilities for compliance. The practice manager obtains the approval of shareholders.)*
- *Subtask 10.2:* Modify position descriptions as required. Modified position descriptions are forwarded to the employees who now have responsibility for compliance. They are asked to sign a statement acknowledging that they are aware of these new responsibilities.

Task 11: Review and Modify Operating Policies and Procedures. All policies and procedures (e.g., billing and collections, appointment scheduling, registration, personnel) are reviewed and modified as required. The policies and procedures address, at a minimum, the following:

- *Enforcement and discipline (personnel policies):* How wrongdoing will be identified, how billing errors will be documented, and how corrective action will be taken.
- *Rectifying wrongdoing (billing and collections and other operating areas of a practice):* Procedures to avoid recurrence, identify preventive steps that will be taken, and document training that will occur to remedy problems in the future. Related to billing and information development processes, the practice should have written internal control procedures. *(Most, if not all, of the preceding apply to the smaller practice because it does not have the range of written*

policies and procedures of the larger practice. It is too cumbersome to begin to write new policies and procedures manuals in the short term [this will be designated as a long-term project]. In lieu of expanding its existing general policies and procedures manual, the small practice decides to document changes and additions to policies and procedures in the minutes of its periodic meetings of shareholders.)

Task 12: Review and Revise Personnel Policies and Procedures. All policies and procedures should be easy to read and to comprehend, not overly detailed, and designed to foster the application of judgment. Personnel policies and procedures relate to:

- Standards of employee conduct
- Disciplining personnel and uniformity thereof
- Termination
- Recruitment and obtaining references (verification of licensure and other credentials; existence of prior government sanctions; signed acknowledgments from new employees that they have read the code, were given an opportunity to ask questions, and understand it)
- Retrospective and concurrent performance evaluations
- Confidentiality relating to employee disclosure of knowledge related to wrongdoing
- Employee annual evaluation forms (which now include performance criteria related to employee contributions to the compliance process and to upholding exemplary ethics; supervisors now will be evaluated on their contributions to upholding the compliance process)
- Review of all existing and prospective contracts with physicians and outside provider organizations (to ensure they are not out of compliance; perform with CEO)

Task 13: Develop Internal Audit Processes. Of all the implied requirements in the seven basic elements, periodic audits represent perhaps the greatest challenge to physician practices both large and small. Auditing is generally not a function performed in most practices because it requires expertise that falls beyond the technical and experiential base of most professionals in practice management, and is high risk if not conducted properly.

The purpose of this task is to design and implement a reasonable audit process performed by internal staff or by qualified external auditors. This decision depends on the human resources capacity of the practice and its financial resources. Auditing is a high-risk area in general, and

must be conducted properly and consistently. Individuals with requisite training in the audit process, with a keen appreciation of confidentiality, and with independence and objectivity should conduct audits.

Although an external baseline audit is suggested by the OIG, internal auditing should be made an integral part of a compliance plan. A broad annual audit should occur (see Task 8), and periodic audits, often targeted, should occur throughout the year.

- *Subtask 13.1:* Define the scope of the audit. When defining the scope of the audit, the following should be considered at a minimum: size of practice; baseline audit findings (did the baseline audit reveal any significant areas of weakness that need to be rechecked, did it suggest the need to implement certain controls, policies, or procedures that need to be tested for the first time?); prior audit history (have there been any prior Health Care Financing Administration [HCFA] or OIG audits?); areas of billing risk based on the practice's specialty; number of offices, staff, and physicians; the degree of employee turnover in operationally critical functions; new or updated automated billing systems; and prior internal audits or reports rendered by management or outside consultants. It is important to note that future audits should consider the findings and recommendations of all historical audits and that the scope of a current audit includes verification that prior recommendations have been implemented and are operating satisfactorily. This type of continuity and due diligence are what the OIG generally looks for, and are consistent with accepted professional auditing practices. The scope of the audit also would define whether the auditors are targeting only billing and collection issues, or if the scope is broader and includes operational functions (scheduling, registration, internal controls, etc.), compliance with other federal and state regulations, contracts, and so forth.

- *Subtask 13.2:* Determine sample size. Sample size and type (e.g., random or targeted, retroactive or concurrent) are determined in accordance with the scope and frequency of the audit. Sampling techniques should be selected. Larger groups may wish to refer to the OIG rules relating to large practices, and other audit and sampling guidelines (e.g., AICPA audit guidelines). *(The guidelines for individual physicians and small group physician practices suggest there is no set formula for how large a sample should be, but acknowledges that larger samples better ensure confidence in the findings. The OIG's basic guide is 2 to 5 medical records per insurer, or 5 to 10 medical records per physician for each audit.)*

■ *Subtask 13.3:* Develop an audit work plan. The work plan is the guide used by the compliance officer or audit team to conduct the audit. It stems from the scope of the audit, and it provides a detailed checklist of the functions that need to occur during the audit, what is being audited, documentation requirements, and reporting needs.

■ *Subtask 13.4:* Select the sample. This effort generally includes the applicable medical records or portions thereof, explanations of medical benefits (EOBs) for those medical records, and billing and collection activity reports for the transactions being audited from the practice's billing system. If the audit scope encompasses more than billing and collections, other internal documents will be sought. When conducting an operational (i.e., performance) audit, the policies and procedures of the organization become the first guideline against which the auditors will hold the organization accountable. Then, further operational standards are applied to determine whether there are reasonable policies, procedures, and internal controls in place to prevent and detect wrongdoing.

■ *Subtask 13.5:* Conduct the audit (field work). Field work must be adequately supervised by the compliance officer or other competent individual. It is best that the auditors be independent and objective so that their findings are credible. Audit planners are referred to the Comptroller General Field Work Standards for Conducting Performance Audits that are used by government auditors, as well as the AICPA standards that are used by accountants in financial auditing and consultants in performance audits. The field work generally will consist of reviews and analyses of charge tickets, medical record documentation, and computer records; interviews with staff and, sometimes, patients; certain tests for internal controls; and observations. If the audit extends beyond billings and collections, the field work will review original source documents (e.g., contracts, policies, and procedures) and include interviews. An important field work standard concerns the collection of evidence (i.e., documentation):

Sufficient, competent, and relevant evidence is to be obtained to afford a reasonable basis for the auditors' findings and conclusions. A record of the auditors' work should be obtained in the form of

working papers. Working papers should contain sufficient information to enable an experienced auditor having no previous connection with the audit to ascertain from them the evidence that supports the auditors' significant conclusions and judgments.[24]

The text relating to working papers in the previous quote identifies one of the more important contributors to successful auditing: the ability of an experienced auditor having no previous connection with the audit to ascertain from the working papers what the primary auditors' evidence was in support of their conclusions and judgments. (*Smaller practices can narrow the scope and sample size of audits and increase their frequency in order to reduce the internal staff time required. Alternatively, they may retain outside staff to conduct periodic audits. To the extent possible, they should adhere to the principles of auditing discussed herein, particularly related to ensuring independence and objectivity, developing an audit plan, obtaining evidence, and documenting findings in working papers.*)

■ *Subtask 13.6:* Write the audit report. The audit report should identify the scope of the audit, major findings and recommendations, and suggested follow-up. It should be written by the compliance officer and submitted to the compliance committee of the board, and follow-up resolutions should be made by this committee. Follow-up should be assigned to specific individuals in the practice, and periodic checks made thereafter to ensure conformity. Recommendations also can call for follow-up audits that are more targeted to specific physicians, practice office sites, procedure codes, or operational units within the practice. (*The practice manager should submit findings and recommendations from the audit [whether developed internally or by outside professionals] to the shareholders of the practice.*)

■ *Subtask 13.7:* Involve legal counsel. The practice may wish to share sensitive information with counsel to determine further strategies regarding the manner in which that information should be presented. Counsel can assist in determining whether certain findings warrant reporting to the government.

Task 14: Establish Internal Communications and Reporting Systems. This task refers to establishing internal methods that would allow employees to confidentially communicate wrongdoing that they perceive. It can include a hotline, drop box, designated telephone answering machine, or standardized form to be submitted to the compliance officer. All communications should be entered into a central logbook or a secured computer database. It is important that employees be given assurances of confidentiality; however, guarantees cannot be extended because employees may need to be queried in the future if the investigation yields confirming results requiring further action or reporting. *(Recent guidelines for individual physicians and group practices suggest that an effective open-door policy or a drop box are sufficient in smaller practices.)*

- *Subtask 14.1:* Conduct a preliminary inquiry. A reasonable preliminary inquiry is conducted regarding reported wrongdoing. This inquiry should determine whether no further action is required or further analysis and inquiry are warranted.
- *Subtask 14.2:* Conduct a full investigation (see Task 15). If the findings are suggestive of wrongdoing or behavior that is inconsistent with the practice's code of ethics, a full investigation may be appropriate.
- *Subtask 14.3:* Report sensitive findings to counsel, if required. This action is designed to address significant areas of concern and to develop appropriate courses of action.
- *Subtask 14.4:* Document. All steps, relevant information, findings, and corrective action (if employed) should be documented.

Task 15: Conduct a Full Investigation. Based on reasonable preliminary investigations (Task 14), the compliance officer may have reason to conduct, or have conducted, a full investigation. A full investigation is similar in process to an audit. It may be more targeted based on the employee's report or the findings of an audit.

- *Subtask 15.1:* Define the scope of the investigation. In an investigation, the scope is likely to be more targeted than in an audit. The investigator should be mindful, however, not to limit the scope such that important evidence or related wrongdoing (similar to the specific complaint that triggered the review) is overlooked.
- *Subtask 15.2:* Determine the sample size (if appropriate in an investigation). Sample size and type are determined in accordance with the scope and the frequency of the audit. Sampling techniques should be selected.
- *Subtask 15.3:* Develop an investigation work plan. The work plan is the guide used by the compliance officer or team to conduct the investigation. It stems from the scope of the investigation and provides a detailed checklist of the functions that need

to occur during the investigation, what is being investigated, documentation requirements, and reporting needs.

- *Subtask 15.4:* Select the sample. The sample generally includes the applicable medical records or portions thereof, EOBs for those medical records, and billing and collection activity reports for the transactions being investigated from the practice's billing system. If the scope encompasses more than billing and collections, other internal documents will be sought.
- *Subtask 15.5:* Conduct the investigation (field work). Field work must be adequately supervised by the compliance officer or other competent individual. It is best that the investigators be independent and objective so that their findings are credible. The field work generally will consist of review and analysis of charge tickets, medical record documentation, and computer records; interviews (staff and, sometimes, patients); tests for internal controls; and observation. If the investigation extends beyond billings and collections, it will include a review of original source documents (e.g., contracts, policies, and procedures) and interviews. When conducting an investigation, the policies and procedures of the organization become the first guidelines against which investigators assess alleged wrongdoing because they should be reflective of current billing, coding, and collection requirements. If alleged wrongdoing is found, further operational standards will be applied to determine if there are reasonable policies, procedures, and internal controls in place to prevent and detect future wrongdoing. As with audits, the collection of evidence (i.e., documentation) is paramount (see the Subtask 13.5 discussion of working papers). An important field work standard concerns the collection of evidence (i.e., documentation).

Sufficient, competent, and relevant evidence is to be obtained to afford a reasonable basis for the auditors' findings and conclusions. A record of the auditors' work should be obtained in the form of working papers. Working papers should contain sufficient information to enable an experienced auditor having no previous connection with the audit to ascertain from them the evidence that supports the auditors' significant conclusions and judgments.[25]

(Smaller practices can narrow the scope and sample size of investigations and increase their frequency in order to reduce the time required of internal staff. Alternatively, they may retain outside staff to conduct periodic investigations.)

- *Subtask 15.6:* Write the investigation report. The report should identify the scope of the investigation, major findings and recommendations, and suggested follow-up. It should be written by the compliance officer and submitted to the compliance committee of the board, and follow-up resolutions should be made by the committee.
- *Subtask 15.7:* Involve legal counsel. The practice may wish to share certain information with counsel to determine further strategies and whether certain findings warrant reporting to the government. If refunds are necessary, they should be made promptly, typically within 60 days. *(The practice manager should submit findings and recommendations from the investigation [whether developed internally or by outside professionals] to the shareholders of the practice.)*

Task 16: Enforce and Remedy Wrongdoing. Policies and procedures for enforcing and remedying wrongdoing are in place. On the basis of audits, investigations, or performance evaluations that reveal personnel that persistently do not cooperate with the code of ethics or compliance plan, steps should be taken. Those steps should uniformly align with the established policies and procedures of the practice. Operational changes should be put in place promptly as well. All actions, whether related to personnel or changes in the operations of the practice, should be documented. *(Same applies to the smaller practice.)*

Enforcement can include counseling employees and physicians regarding improper or illegal practices, probation or suspension if there were prior warnings, and terminations. The employee evaluation should be made part of the enforcement process. If employees are evaluated annually, it should be documented in the yearly review. If an employee already has received an annual review, it is appropriate to place a memorandum to the personnel record in the employee's file. Conducting more frequent performance reviews after an employee has been counseled is not inappropriate.

Task 17: Report to the Compliance Committee *(Shareholders)*. The compliance committee should meet periodically to report and discuss audit and investigation findings, enforcement, and disciplinary action that may have been taken, and any operational changes that may have been implemented to reduce wrongdoing. The committee also should report any changes in operations that may be necessary to reduce wrongdoing or improper behavior, improve employee and physician awareness of compliance requirements, and increase education related to compliance. *(The practice manager should meet periodically with key staff who are involved in the compliance program to report major findings and to suggest ongoing changes in the compliance program.)*

Periodically, perhaps on a quarterly basis, the compliance officer *(practice manager)* should submit a written report to the board of directors *(shareholders)* that outlines the activities that have occurred during the prior period. It also should report any recommendations that should be incorporated into future audits designed to determine whether there is compliance with new regulations and guidelines or if there were weaknesses that were detected (and rectified) that need to be rechecked through audit technique.

The compliance officer *(practice manager)* may wish to speak to counsel prior to discussing certain matters with the board *(or with shareholders at a meeting)*, or have counsel at meetings at which sensitive matters may be discussed.

Task 18: Educate and Train. Education and training can assume many forms. Regulations change frequently, government fraud and abuse alerts are issued regularly, and many other compliance issues change. In addition, although the OIG acknowledges that practices *(particularly smaller ones)* may begin their compliance program to target only billing and coding irregularities, the OIG expects that practices will expand their compliance programs over the years. Therefore, education and training should include updates on internal changes that have been made to the practice's compliance programs.

- *Subtask 18.1:* Prepare a budget for education. Allot a budgeted number of dollars for the purpose of internal and external education. Larger practices may wish to budget for the preparation and presentation of seminars and workshops conducted by their own staff. The compliance officer should organize this effort.
- *Subtask 18.2:* Identify seminars and workshops prospectively. As part of an annual planning process, external seminars and workshops should be identified and scheduled for attendance. Obtaining continuing education credits provides an added incentive to employees.
- *Subtask 18.3:* Identify attendees. Attendees, including physicians from the practice, should be identified. They should be selected to attend educational seminars that are consistent with their organizational roles (e.g., billers should attend seminars relating to billing and coding issues, an OSHA supervisor should attend OSHA seminars, and

so forth). Attendance at compliance workshops should be noted in annual evaluations. In addition, those who attend outside seminars should be asked to prepare presentations for their colleagues based on what they learned.

- *Subtask 18.4:* Identify and acquire other materials. Other materials such as disks and manuals should be purchased and used routinely, especially for new employees.

- *Subtask 18.5:* Disseminate information internally. Compliance information should be distributed internally and at periodic office staff meetings. Internal management meetings should discuss the practice's policies and procedures related to compliance and proper billing. Minutes of meetings should be kept. Newsletters, printed updates, booklets, and other compliance material should be routed to appropriate staff with a check-off box in which each person receiving the material can acknowledge reading it.

- *Subtask 18.6:* Give educational presentations to the board. On a periodic basis the compliance officer should conduct presentations to the board in order to keep members abreast of compliance and regulatory changes. (*The practice manager should keep shareholders abreast of changes in compliance requirements for economic reasons. Small practices may elect to make more use of update newsletters, CDs and computer programs, booklets, and internal meetings to learn and communicate new information. If the practice sends a representative to an outside seminar, then that individual should be responsible for bringing back pertinent information and presenting it to all personnel and, when applicable, to the physicians.*)

Phase III: Evaluation and Feedback

Task 19: Evaluate the Compliance Plan and Program Annually. The compliance plan and program should be analyzed on an annual basis and changes made as required. Changes made to conform to new external requirements should be documented. The practice can conduct internal surveys and interviews to determine if changes need to be made to aspects of the compliance plan. (*The practice manager should prepare a report describing the accomplishments of the program, any disciplinary actions that have been taken, and suggested changes to the plan and program.*)

Task 20: Prepare an Annual Report to the Board (*Shareholders*). The compliance committee and compliance

officer should prepare and present an annual report to the board of directors. The board should consider any recommended changes to the compliance plan, code of ethics, and policies and procedures.

The CEO should conduct an annual performance evaluation of the compliance officer's impact on the compliance plan and the degree to which the level of compliance has been enhanced. (*The practice manager should present the annual report at an annual meeting of the shareholders. Any suggested changes to the compliance plan should be discussed and voted on. Appropriate discussion should be committed to the minutes of the meeting.*)[*]

References

1. Office of Inspector General. OIG compliance program for individual and small group physician practices. Accessed at http://www.hhs.gov/oig/
2. Office of Inspector General. *News release: Inspector general issues voluntary compliance program guidance for physician practices.* Washington, DC: Author; 2000.
3. Office of Inspector General. 1998. Compliance Program Guidance for Third-Party Medical Billing Companies. 13 (63 Fed. Reg. 70138).
4. Government Accounting Office/Office of the Comptroller General. *Field work standards for performance audits 10.* Washington, DC: Author; September 1994.
5. Government Accounting Office/Office of the Comptroller General. *Field work standards for performance audits 11.* Washington, DC: Author; September 1994.
6. Metzger N. Human resources management. In: Wolper LF, ed. *Health care administration: planning, implementing, and managing organized delivery systems.* New York: Aspen; 1999:282–284.
7. Wolper LF. *Implementing a physician organization.* American Medical Association; 1996:13–5.
8. Likert R, Katz D. *Motivation: the core of management.* American Management Association; 1953:3–25.
9. Office of Inspector General. *Compliance program guidance for third-party medical billing companies 20.* Washington, DC: Author; 1998.
10. Office of Inspector General. *Compliance program guidance for third-party medical billing companies 21.* Washington, DC: Author; 1998.
11. Comptroller General of the United States. General standards. In: *Government auditing standards.* Washington, DC: Author; 1994.
12. Comptroller General of the United States. General standards. In: *Government auditing standards.* Washington, DC: Author; 1994:Section 3.11 at 3.
13. Comptroller General of the United States. General standards. In: *Government Auditing Standards.* Washington, DC: Author; 1994:Section 3.12 at 3.
14. Comptroller General of the United States. General standards. In: *Government auditing standards.* Washington, DC: Author; 1994:Section 3.16 at 4, 5.
15. Comptroller General of the United States. General standards. In: *Government Auditing Standards.* Washington, DC: Author; 1994:Section 3.17 at 5.

---

[*] This now-revised chapter originally appeared in Aspen Publishers' *Physician Compliance Resource Manual* (www.aspenpublishers.com). Reprinted with permission.

16. American Institute of Certified Public Accountants. *Code of professional conduct.* 1999:Section 55, Article IV at 1.

17. Comptroller General of the United States. Field work standards for performance audits. In: *Government auditing standards.* Washington, DC: Author; 1994:Section 6.2 at 1.

18. Comptroller General of the United States. Field work standards for performance audits. In: *Government auditing standards.* Washington, DC: Author; June 1994:Section 6.22 at 7.

19. Comptroller General of the United States. Field work standards for performance audits. In: *Government auditing standards.* Washington, DC: Author; June 1994:Section 6.26 at 7.

20. Comptroller General of the United States. Field work standards for performance audits. In: *Government auditing standards.* Washington, DC: Author; June 1994:Section 6.39 at 10.

21. Comptroller General of the United States. Field work standards for performance audits. In: *Government auditing standards.* Washington, DC: Author; June 1994:Section 6.47 at 13.

22. Comptroller General of the United States. Field work standards for performance audits. In: *Government auditing standards.* Washington, DC: Author; June 1994:Section 6.46 at 12.

23. Patten et al. *Job evaluation: text and cases 93–94.* 3rd ed. Homewood, IL: Richard D. Irwin; 1964.

24. Comptroller General of the United States. Field work standards for conducting performance audits. In: *Government auditing standards.* Washington, DC: Author; June 1994:Section 6.46 at 12.

Tax-Qualified Retirement Plans and Fringe Benefits

Richard A. Naegele, BA, MA, JD
Kelly Ann VanDenHaute, BS, JD

This chapter is divided into two parts. Part 1 focuses on tax-qualified retirement plans that can be adopted by physician groups and other medical employers to provide tax-advantaged retirement benefits for physicians and other employees. Part 2 reviews some of the requirements and advantages of cafeteria plans and other employer-provided fringe benefit plans permitted under the Internal Revenue Code.

◼ Tax-Qualified Retirement Plans

This section provides brief summaries of 12 different types of retirement plans available to physician organizations and other employers. Factors such as the size and profitability of the physician group in conjunction with the goals and objectives of the physician employees will be important in determining which type of retirement plan is appropriate for a given employer.

Tax-qualified retirement plans serve many important functions for physicians including forced savings, providing an independent source of wealth apart from the value of the practice, protection of assets from potential creditor

claims, and, of course, accumulation of sufficient assets for retirement. In addition to providing these and other advantages, qualified retirement plans have been vastly improved by recent changes in law. Qualified plans can now be structured to provide large benefits for physicians and other key employees at a minimal cost for benefits for rank-and-file employees.

Arguably, the two most important functions of qualified retirement plans are providing employee benefits and acting as tax shelters. As a general rule, the tax shelter aspect is emphasized in smaller plans and employee benefits are emphasized in larger plans. Both features are present in all plans, however, and should be recognized when designing a plan. Even in a plan designed primarily as a tax shelter for physicians and other key employees, the funding of benefits for rank-and-file employees should not be viewed in a negative light. Participation in a retirement plan should always be presented to employees in a positive manner and can be used to encourage employee loyalty and longevity and thereby reduce employee dissatisfaction and turnover. Thus, participation by non-key employees engenders a more cohesive staff and can reduce employee training and turnover costs. Employers should remember that proper and positive communication to employees is the key to employee appreciation of retirement plans and other fringe benefits.

Tax Advantages of Qualified Plans

Tax-qualified retirement plans provide several tax advantages for employers and employees. First, employer contributions are deductible in the year made. Contributions are deductible if made prior to the due date for the corporate tax return, including extensions.[1] Second, participants are taxed only when they receive payments from the trust.[2] Third, the retirement trust is tax-exempt and the trust funds accumulate income tax free.[3] Additionally, Social Security taxes are paid neither on employer contributions to tax-qualified retirement plans nor on distributions to participants from such plans. Federal Insurance Contributions Act (FICA) and Federal Unemployment Tax Act (FUTA) are paid on employee elective deferrals (e.g., employee contributions to a 401(k) or 403(b) plan).

Because the various taxes on compensation (federal, state, and local taxes plus FICA/Medicare) for a physician employee can total nearly 50%, tax-qualified retirement plan benefits may, in effect, be provided with 50-cent dollars. For example, a physician employee receives 100% of a $50,000 contribution to a qualified retirement plan but, after the payment of taxes, could receive as little as 50% of the same $50,000 paid directly to the physician as compensation.

A comparison to nonqualified deferred compensation plans highlights the tax advantages of qualified plans. A nonqualified deferred compensation plan is an unfunded, unsecured promise to pay benefits at a future date. Contributions to a nonqualified plan are deductible by the employer only in the year that the employee picks up the benefit in income. Thus, for a taxable employer, there is no tax-free or tax-deferred growth. Although nonqualified plans may be informally funded, the employee/beneficiary is, at best, an unsecured general creditor of the employer and the benefits are subject to claims by the employer's creditors.

Types of Qualified Plans

Appendix 19-1 at the end of this chapter provides a comparison of five types of retirement plans and a summary of certain retirement plan limitations. Appendix 19-2 lists some of the contribution and funding limits applicable to such plans.

Profit-Sharing Plan

Profit-sharing plans are the most flexible of all qualified plans. The employer is not obligated to make contributions to the plan, but each year it can elect to contribute any amount between 0% and 25% of the annual compensation of the covered employees. The level of employer contributions may be determined each year by the employer or by a contribution formula written into the plan.

For all defined contribution plans, the maximum annual additions (which include employer contributions, forfeitures, and employee contributions) under Internal Revenue Code (IRC) Section 415(c) for each year is the lesser of 100% of compensation or $40,000 (adjusted, $50,000 for 2012). Thus, contributions and forfeitures allocated on behalf of each participant cannot exceed these limitations.

The IRS requires that contributions to a profit-sharing plan be recurring and substantial. Although an employer does not have to make contributions every year, the employer's contributions must be more than single or occasional.[4] In Revenue Ruling 80-146, the Internal Revenue Service stated that a plan may be considered to be terminated if no contributions have been made to the plan for five consecutive plan years.

Section 401(k) Plan

A Section 401(k) cash or deferred compensation plan is a type of profit-sharing plan under which employees may elect to defer a portion of their compensation to the plan. An individual could defer a maximum of $17,000 to a 401(k) plan in 2011. Employees who have attained age 50 are permitted to defer additional "catch-up" contributions. (For 2012 this was $5,500.) Thus, the total deferrals for an employee age 50 or older in 2012 was $22,500.

In addition to satisfying the requirements applicable to a regular profit-sharing plan, a 401(k) plan must also satisfy the average deferral percentage (ADP) test for each plan year.[5] The ADP consists of two alternative tests that measure the deferral of income of eligible highly compensated employees (HCEs) in comparison to the deferral of all other eligible employees. Under one limit, the ADP for HCEs is limited to 125% of the ADP for the eligible nonhighly compensated employees (NHCEs). Under the second limit, the ADP for HCEs is limited to the lesser of 200% of the ADP for the eligible NHCEs or the ADP for the eligible NHCEs plus two percentage points. An HCE is generally an employee who either is a 5% or greater owner (in either the current or the prior year) of the employer or earned $110,000 (adjusted) or more from the employer (in the prior year).[6] An NHCE is any employee who is not an HCE.

Safe Harbor 401(k) Plan[7]

A safe harbor 401(k) plan satisfies the nondiscrimination rules (the ADP test) if it meets the following requirements: (1) a notice requirement, and (2) one of two contribution requirements. The notice requirement is met if each employee eligible to participate in the plan is given written notice (prior to the plan year) of his or her rights and obligations under the plan. The notice must be given between 30 and 90 days before the beginning of each plan year.

The contribution requirement under the safe harbor may be satisfied by an employer-matching contribution by using the basic formula. The basic formula is satisfied if the employer provides a matching contribution on behalf of each NHCE of (1) 100% of the employee's elective contributions up to 3% of compensation and (2) 50% of the employee's elective contributions to the extent that they exceed 3% (but not 5%) of the employee's compensation (e.g., the employee must defer 5% of compensation to receive a 4% employer matching contribution). The contribution requirements may also be met by an enhanced formula providing a match that is at least equal to the amount of the match that would be made under the basic formula. A match of 100% of the first 4% deferred is an acceptable enhanced formula (e.g., the employee must defer 4% of compensation to receive a 4% employer match). The employer matching safe harbor contributions must be nonforfeitable and subject to the restrictions on withdrawals that apply to elective deferrals.

In lieu of a matching contribution, the employer may contribute a nonelective contribution of at least 3% of an employee's compensation to a defined contribution plan on behalf of each NHCE who is eligible to participate in the plan, regardless of whether the employee makes an elective contribution. A plan must specify the formula requirement (the matching contribution or the nonelective contributions). As a general rule, a plan may not rely on the safe harbor unless the plan document reflects such requirements before the first day of the plan year.

Plans may not rely on the safe harbor for a plan year unless the plan year is 12 months long. For a new plan, however (other than a successor plan) the first plan year may be less than 12 months, but must be at least 3 months. A new plan for a newly established employer may be less than the 3-month minimum. A plan is a successor plan if 50% or more of the eligible employees for the first plan year were eligible under another 401(k) plan of the employer in the prior year.[8]

A profit-sharing plan can be amended to add safe harbor 401(k) features up to 3 months before the end of the plan year as long as the plan is not a successor plan (as defined in the previous paragraph), the cash or deferred elections begin not less than 3 months prior to the end of the plan year, and the other safe harbor requirements are otherwise satisfied for the period during which deferral elections are permitted.[9]

Compensation:	$50,000	$100,000	$245,000
	x .04	x .04	x .04
Match:	$2,000	$4,000	$9,800
Deferral:	$16,500	$16,500	$16,500
Subtotal:	$18,500	$20,500	$26,300
Catch-Up (Age 50):	$5,500	$5,500	$5,500
Total:	$24,000	$26,000	$31,800

Figure 19-1 Safe harbor 401(k) example (2011)

Figure 19-1 shows the levels of benefits available to employees at various levels of compensation. The employer cost to provide the benefits in this example is limited to a maximum of 4% of the compensation of covered employees. Employer profit-sharing contributions can also be made to the plan to increase the level of benefits to employees.

Money Purchase Pension Plan
In this type of defined contribution plan, contributions to the plan are fixed, but the benefits are not. Contributions are based on a fixed percentage of annual compensation for all plan participants. Thus, under a 10% of compensation money purchase plan, an employee earning $170,000 would receive a $17,000 contribution, and an employee earning $10,000 would receive a $1,000 contribution.

As with all defined contribution plans, the benefits ultimately paid to a participant will depend on the size of the annual contributions, the number of years contributions are made before retirement, and investment gains and losses. Forfeitures may be used to reduce employer contributions or to increase benefits under the plan.[10] The employer can deduct contributions to a money purchase plan up to the total of all annual additions for all participants; for 2012, this was the lesser of 100% of compensation or $50,000 for each participant. However, the maximum deduction is 25% of the total compensation of all eligible participants.

Stock Bonus Plan
A stock bonus plan is similar to a profit-sharing plan, except that contributions and distributions are generally made in stock. The regulations define a stock bonus plan as "a plan established and maintained by an employer to provide benefits similar to those of a profit-sharing plan, except that contributions by the employer are not necessarily dependent upon profits and the benefits are distributable in stock of the employer company." Treasury Reg. section 1.401.1(a)(2)(iii). Similar to a profit-sharing plan, there must be a definite predetermined formula

allocating contributions among the participants. There is no requirement for having a formula for determining the amount of contributions.

Distributions from a stock bonus plan can be made in cash at the participant's option. With respect to securities that are not traded on an open market, the participant must be given a put option to have the securities repurchased by the employer. An employee stock ownership plan (ESOP) is a leveraged stock bonus plan in which the plan secures a loan to purchase the securities of the employer.

Cross-Tested Profit-Sharing Plan[11]
(New Comparability Plans)

A cross-tested profit-sharing plan is a plan under which the contribution percentage formula for one category of participants is greater than the contribution percentage formula for other categories of participants. To satisfy the nondiscrimination requirements of the IRC Section 401(a)(4) general test, participants are put into different "rate groups" and the rate groups are tested separately for nondiscrimination.

To determine rate groups, a cross-tested profit-sharing plan expresses each participant's allocation of employer contributions and forfeitures as an equivalent benefit rate at the plan's normal retirement age rather than as an allocation rate. When equivalent benefit rates are used, the method is referred to as "cross-testing" because it analyzes the benefit at normal retirement age (e.g., age 62) that would be generated from the allocation as if the plan were a defined benefit plan. Thus, whereas most defined contribution plans are tested for nondiscrimination based on the allocation of contributions and defined benefit plans are tested based on projected future benefits, cross-tested plans are defined contribution plans that are tested for nondiscrimination based on projected benefits.

U.S. Treasury regulations prescribe that cross-tested plans need (1) broadly available allocation rates that increase as an employee ages or accumulates additional service or (2) to satisfy a minimum gateway with different allocation rates so that the percentage of pay allocation for HCEs is no more than three times the percentage of pay allocation for NHCEs (safe harbor of 5% for NHCEs).[12,a] The U.S. Treasury regulations also contain a 7 1/2% of compensation cap on any contribution that may be required under the rules applicable to defined benefit/defined contribution combination plans.

Under a cross-tested plan, it may be possible for a physician employer to structure a plan to provide for the maximum benefit (e.g., $50,000 for 2012) for physician

employees while providing benefits of as little as 5% of compensation to nonphysician employees. It is also possible to structure a plan with several different rate groups and to provide different levels of benefits to different groups of employees.

Defined Benefit Pension Plan

Under a defined benefit plan, the level of benefits is fixed and contributions are determined by an actuary to provide adequate funding to furnish those benefits at retirement. Contributions to a defined benefit plan are mandatory, although some flexibility can be built into the plan. In the context of a closely held business, the primary issue is determining how much the key employees want to shelter from taxes. The benefit formula is then, in effect, prepared in reverse to accomplish the goal of sheltering a specific amount of money. An example of a benefit formula is 3% of compensation times years of service. Under such a formula, an employee retiring with 20 years of service would be entitled to a life annuity with annual benefits equal to 60% of the employee's average annual compensation.

The maximum benefit (expressed in the form of a single life annuity) that can be funded is the lesser of $160,000 (adjusted, $200,000 for 2012) or 100% of an employee's annual compensation for the three highest consecutive years of service.[13] The $200,000 amount is reduced for benefit payments commencing prior to age 62 and increased for benefit payments commencing after age 65. Benefits for participants with fewer than 10 years of participation under the plan must be proportionately reduced. It is important to note that a professional corporation defined benefit plan covering 26 or more employees may be subject to coverage by the Pension Benefit Guaranty Corporation (PBGC), which would entail additional costs for the employer.

A defined benefit plan may be considered by an organization employing physicians if the physician employees desire to receive retirement plan contributions exceeding the defined contribution limits of $50,000 (adjusted) per year. Under a defined benefit plan, a physician or other employee age 55 or older could accrue benefits in excess of $200,000 per year. Defined benefit plans are age-weighted and, therefore, older employees generally accrue greater benefits in a given year than younger employees. Additionally, benefits under a defined benefit plan are fixed by the benefit formula under the plan and contributions to the plan by the employer are mandatory each year.

Cash Balance Plan

A cash balance plan is a type of defined benefit plan that defines an employee's benefit as the amount credited to a hypothetical account. The account receives allocations

---

a. Effective the first day of the plan year commencing after December 31, 2001.

(usually expressed as a percentage of pay) as the employee works. The account is also credited with interest adjustments until it is paid to the employee. Thus, a cash balance plan is a type of defined benefit plan that expresses an employee's benefit in a manner similar to a defined contribution plan.

A cash balance plan is different from a defined contribution plan in that, as a defined benefit plan, a cash balance plan defines an employee's retirement benefit by a formula, and the employee's retirement benefit does not depend on either the employer's contributions to the plan or the investment performance of the plan's assets, as it would in a defined contribution plan. The employee's benefit under a cash balance plan is based on a hypothetical account guaranteed by the plan rather than a true individual account under a defined contribution plan.

A cash balance plan is different from other defined benefit plans in that a cash balance plan defines an employee's benefit as the amount credited to an account; in contrast, other defined benefit plans typically define an employee's benefit as a series of monthly payments. An accrued benefit is the portion of an employee's normal retirement benefit that he or she has earned at a given point in his or her career. Under a cash balance plan, the accrued benefit is often expressed as the employee's hypothetical account balance. For example, an employee might receive an allocation equal to 4% of pay each year he or she works, and the employee's account might be credited with interest at 5%, compounded annually, until it is paid.

For a physician employer, a cash balance plan can provide greater stability in the level of annual benefit accruals than a traditional defined benefit plan, and still permit the increased levels of funding permitted by a defined benefit plan. Additionally, a cash balance plan can be designed to provide more consistent levels of benefits between older and younger employees than can be achieved under traditional defined benefit formulas.

Section 403(b) Plan

A Section 403(b) plan, also known as a tax-sheltered annuity (TSA) plan, is a retirement plan for employees of public schools, employees of tax-exempt organizations, and certain ministers. The plan is referred to as a 403(b) plan because it is established pursuant to Section 403(b) of the Internal Revenue Code. Any "eligible employee" can participate in a 403(b) plan. Eligible employees include employees of tax-exempt organizations established under Section 501(c)(3) of the Internal Revenue Code, employees of public school systems who are involved in the day-to-day operations of a school, employees of cooperative

hospital service organizations, and certain ministers.[14,b] Therefore, a 403(b) plan may be available as a retirement plan for physicians and other employees of tax-exempt employers such as hospitals and universities.

Contributions may be made to 403(b) accounts through elective deferrals made under a salary reduction agreement, nonelective contributions made by the employer, and after-tax contributions. Section 403(b) plans are subject to the same contribution limits as defined contribution plans. The limit on elective deferrals for a 403(b) plan through a salary reduction agreement is the same as the limit for 401(k) plans ($17,000 for 2012, plus a "catch-up" contribution of $5,500 for individuals age 50 or older).[15] The limit on total contributions for 2012 was $50,000 (adjusted by cost of living).

The basic nondiscrimination requirements that apply to qualified retirement plans also apply to 403(b) plans with respect to nonelective contributions and matching contributions of the employer.[16] For elective deferrals under a salary reduction agreement, a separate nondiscrimination rule applies. If any employee of the employer sponsoring the 403(b) plan can make elective deferral referrals, the plan is discriminatory unless the opportunity to make elective deferrals of more than $200 is available to all employees on a basis that does not discriminate in favor of highly compensated employees.[17] Basically, any employee with compensation from the employer of at least $200 per year must be permitted to make elective deferrals to a 403(b) plan adopted by the employer.

Participants in a 403(b) plan cannot invest in individual stocks. Instead, their choices are: (1) an annuity contract, which is a contract provided through an insurance company; (2) a custodial account, which is an account invested in mutual funds; or (3) a retirement income account set up for church employees.[18] The assets of a 403(b) plan are generally held in a custodial account (unlike other retirement plans, in which assets are held in a trust), so at least one federal court of appeals has questioned whether 403(b) accounts are entitled to the protection from creditor claims afforded to other tax-qualified retirement plans.

Generally, a distribution cannot be made from a 403(b) account until the employee: (1) reaches age 59 1/2; (2) has a severance from employment; (3) dies; (4) becomes disabled; or (5) in the case of a salary reduction contribution, encounters financial hardship.[19] Required minimum distributions from a 403(b) plan must be received by April 1 of the calendar year following the later of the calendar year in which a plan participant becomes 70 1/2 or the calendar year in which the plan participant

---

b. See also IRS Publication 571.

retires.[20] Generally, a plan participant can roll over tax free all or any part of a distribution from a 403(b) plan to a traditional IRA or an eligible retirement plan.[21]

Other Retirement Plans

Section 457 Plan

IRC Section 457 governs the tax treatment of all nonqualified deferred compensation plans maintained by state or local governments or tax-qualified organizations. Any amount of compensation deferred by an employee or independent contractor under an eligible deferred compensation plan of a state or local government or a tax-exempt organization is includible in income for federal tax purposes only for the taxable year in which such compensation is paid or otherwise made available to such individual.[22]

An eligible deferred compensation plan under Section 457 is a plan that meets the following requirements:

- The plan provides that only individuals who perform service for the employer may be participants.
- The plan is established and maintained by a state, political subdivision of a state, or agency, or instrumentality of a state or political subdivision of a state, or any other organization (other than a governmental unit) exempt from federal tax.
- The maximum amount that may be deferred under the plan for a taxable year shall not exceed the applicable dollar amount ($17,000 for 2012, adjusted).
- Compensation may be deferred for any calendar month only if an agreement providing for such deferral has been entered into before the beginning of such month.
- Amounts may not be made available to participants or beneficiaries earlier than the calendar year in which the participant attains age 59 1/2, the participant separates from service with the employer, or the participant is faced with an unforeseeable emergency.
- The plan meets the minimum distribution requirements of IRC Section 401(a)(9) (e.g., distributions must commence not later than age 70 1/2).
- All amounts of compensation deferred under the plan, all property and rights purchased with such amounts, and all income attributable to such amounts, property, or rights shall remain solely the property and rights of the employer, subject to the claims of the employer's general creditors.[23]

One important issue to note is that under the Economic and Growth and Tax Relief Reconciliation Act of 2001 (EGTRRA), an individual is no longer required to coordinate the maximum annual deferral amount for a 457(b) plan (i.e., an eligible plan) with contributions made to a 401(k) or 403(b) plan. Therefore, a physician or other employee can defer the maximum applicable dollar amount to each plan. For example, in 2012 an employee could defer $17,000 in a 403(b) or 401(k) plan and also defer an additional $17,000 in a 457(b) plan.

If a plan does not meet the statutory definition of an eligible deferred compensation plan, the amounts held are not deferred for tax purposes and instead are taxable to the individual in the year the amounts are no longer subject to a "substantial risk of forfeiture."[24] The rights of a person to compensation are subject to a substantial risk of forfeiture if that person's rights to such compensation are conditioned upon the future performance of substantial services. Therefore, once an individual has performed all services necessary to receive payment at any point in the future, the deferred amount is taxed as compensation to the individual.

Simplified Employee Pensions (SEPs)[25]

A SEP is an individual retirement account that is employer-funded and can accept an expanded rate of contributions. An employer's annual contribution to a SEP on behalf of each employee is limited to the lesser of (1) 25% of the employee's compensation (not reduced for employee contributions to the SEP), or (2) $50,000 (for 2012).

The employer must contribute to the SEP on behalf of each employee who: (1) has attained age 21, (2) has performed service for the employer for at least 3 of the immediately preceding 5 years, and (3) has performed service for the employer during the year for which the contribution is made (regardless of whether the employee is still employed by the employer at the end of such year) and has received at least $550 (adjusted for cost of living) in compensation for such year. Nonresident aliens with no income from U.S. sources and employees covered by a collective bargaining agreement with whom retirement benefits have been the subject of good faith bargaining may be excluded from participation.[26]

Withdrawals from a SEP must be permitted. Therefore, employer contributions cannot be conditioned on their retention in the plan and withdrawals cannot be prohibited.[25] Contributions by an employer may not discriminate in favor of highly compensated employees and must bear a uniform relationship to compensation (excluding compensation in excess of $250,000, adjusted).[27] Contributions must also be made to SEPs on behalf of employees who have attained age 70 1/2.[28]

Salary Reduction Simplified Employee Pensions (SARSEPs).[29] A SARSEP may be maintained by an employer who did not have more than 25 employees who were eligible to participate at any time during the preceding taxable year. Employees may elect to receive cash or make elective deferrals to a SARSEP. The elective deferrals are subject to the same $17,000 (indexed) limit applicable to 401(k) plans and are aggregated with 401(k) elective deferrals for the purposes of such limit. FICA and FUTA must be withheld from employee elective deferrals to SARSEPs. Employee elective deferrals are available only if at least 50% of the eligible employees elect to make such deferrals. Additionally, the deferral percentage for each HCE cannot be more than 125% of the average deferral percentage for NHCEs.[30]

Employers have not been permitted to establish SARSEPs since 1996. SARSEPs established prior to 1997 may continue to receive contributions under the pre-1997 rules. Employees hired after 1996 may participate in SARSEPs established before 1997.[30]

It is important to note that a SEP is a type of employer-sponsored IRA and is not a tax-qualified plan under IRC Section 401(a). SEPs do not enjoy the protection from creditor claims afforded to tax-qualified retirement plans. Therefore, although SEPs have fewer administrative requirements than qualified plans and are not required to file the annual Form 5500 report with the U.S. Department of Labor, they are generally not a good choice for physician employees due to a possible lack of creditor protection outside of bankruptcy.

Savings Incentive Match Plan for Employees (SIMPLE) Individual Retirement Account (IRA)[31]

Employers with 100 or fewer employees who received at least $5,000 in compensation in the preceding year may adopt a SIMPLE plan if they do not maintain another qualified plan (i.e., a qualified plan, a SEP, or a 403(b)). An employer may not maintain a plan in which any employee receives an allocation of contributions or an increase in accrued benefits for plan years beginning or ending in that calendar year. However, an employer may adopt and maintain a SIMPLE IRA for noncollectively bargained employees even if it maintains a qualified plan for collectively bargained employees.[32] Employees may contribute by salary reduction up to $11,500 (for 2012, adjusted for cost of living) of compensation per year (up to 100% of earned income or compensation). Catch-up contributions are available for individuals who have attained age 50 (catch-up contribution of $2,500 were allowed for 2012 [adjusted for cost of living]).

Employers must satisfy one of two contribution formulas. Under the first contribution formula, an employer matches 100% of employee salary reduction contributions up to 3% of compensation. Under the second contribution formula, an employer may elect to make a nonelective contribution of 2% of compensation for each eligible employee who has earned at least $5000 of compensation from the employer during the year. Both employer and employee contributions are 100% vested at all times.

Employees may participate in a SIMPLE plan if they: (1) received at least $5,000 in compensation from the employer during any two preceding years, and (2) are reasonably expected to receive at least $5,000 in compensation during the year. Employees who are covered under a collective bargaining agreement and certain nonresident aliens may be excluded from participation. Elective deferrals to SIMPLE IRAs are subject to the overall $17,000 (adjusted) limit on elective deferrals to retirement plans under IRC Section 402(g). The Section 402(g) limit is a cumulative limitation applying to all elective deferrals by an individual in a given year made under Sections 401(k), 403(b), 408(k) (SARSEPs), and 408(p) (SIMPLEs).[33]

Eligible employees may elect to make elective deferrals during the 60-day period before the beginning of the year (or before the employee becomes eligible to participate). A plan may also allow a participant to modify salary reduction contribution percentages during the year.

An employer must contribute elective deferrals to the employee's account not later than 30 days after the last day of the month for which the contributions are made. Employer contributions must be made by the due date for the employer tax return (plus extensions) for the year on behalf of which the contributions are made. Employees who withdraw contributions during the 2-year period beginning on the date they first commenced participation in the SIMPLE plan will be assessed a 25% additional tax.[34]

It is important to note that a SIMPLE IRA is a type of employer-sponsored IRA and is not a tax-qualified plan under IRC Section 401(a). A SIMPLE IRA does not enjoy the protection from creditor claims afforded to tax-qualified retirement plans. The possible lack of creditor protection (outside of bankruptcy) and the lower limitations imposed on contributions to SIMPLEs generally more than offset the advantages of reduced administration and make SIMPLEs a poor choice for a retirement plan for a physician employer.

Protection of Qualified Plan Assets from Creditors

One of the often overlooked benefits of tax-qualified retirement plans is the protection of the plan assets from the claims of creditors of either the employer or the plan participant/employee. This section provides a brief discussion of the creditor protection rules.

ERISA and Internal Revenue Code Nonalienation Provisions

The Employee Retirement Income Security Act (ERISA) Section 206(d)[35] and Internal Revenue Code (IRC) Section 401(a)(13) state that qualified plans must contain provisions prohibiting the assignment or alienation of plan benefits. With the exception of qualified domestic relations orders[36] and federal tax levies and judgments,[37] a participant's benefits under a tax-qualified plan are generally insulated from creditors' claims. The antialienation rules of ERISA and the IRC also include three additional exceptions to offset a participant's benefits under a plan where the participant has breached a fiduciary duty or committed a crime against the plan and is ordered to repay the plan by a criminal or civil judgment or consent decree.[38]

General Creditors of the Sponsoring Employer

The general creditors of a corporation or other sponsoring employer cannot reach the assets contained in such employer's qualified retirement plan. The statutory rationale is that a qualified retirement plan is established for the exclusive benefit of the employees and their beneficiaries.[39] Furthermore, the terms of the trust must be such as to make it impossible, prior to the satisfaction of all liabilities to the employees and their beneficiaries, for any part of the funds to be diverted to purposes other than the exclusive benefit of the employees and their beneficiaries.[40] Because the employer does not have any significant rights with respect to the trust assets, its creditors have no rights regarding the trust assets.

The Bankruptcy Abuse Prevention and Consumer Protection Act of 2005

The Bankruptcy Abuse Prevention and Consumer Protection Act of 2005 (BAPCPA) made significant changes in bankruptcy rules and added specific protections for tax-qualified retirement plans and IRAs. BAPCPA is effective for bankruptcy petitions filed on or after October 17, 2005.

BAPCPA exempts retirement plan assets from a debtor's bankruptcy estate if such assets are held by a tax-qualified retirement plan, a Section 403(b) plan, a Section 457 plan, or an IRA (including traditional IRAs, Roth IRAs, SEPs, and SIMPLEs). The retirement plan exemption applies regardless of whether the debtor elects the federal or state bankruptcy exemptions.

The exemption for IRAs is limited to $1 million. However, the $1 million limit does not apply to employer-sponsored IRAs (e.g., SEPs or SIMPLEs). Additionally,

rollovers into IRAs from qualified plans are also exempt from the $1 million limit.

BAPCPA exempts assets in retirement plans that satisfy the applicable requirements of the Internal Revenue Code. A retirement plan is deemed to be qualified under BAPCPA if it has received a favorable determination letter from the IRS. If the plan has not received a favorable determination letter, the debtor must demonstrate that: (1) neither the IRS nor a court has made a determination that the plan is not qualified, and (2) (a) the plan is in substantial compliance with the Internal Revenue Code, or (b) the plan is not in substantial compliance but the debtor is not materially responsible for the failure.

In summary, under BAPCPA, qualified plan, SEP, and SIMPLE assets are protected with no dollar limitation. IRAs and Roth IRAs are protected to $1 million; however, rollover assets in an IRA are not subject to the $1 million limit. The 2005 Bankruptcy Act only applies to assets in bankruptcy. One must look to state law for protection of IRA assets in state law actions (e.g., garnishment).

Owner-Only Plans Are at Risk Outside of Bankruptcy

In *Yates v. Hendon*, 124 S.Ct. 1130 (U.S. Sup. Ct. 2004), the U.S. Supreme Court noted that Department of Labor Advisory Opinion 99-04A interprets 29 CFR §2510.3-3 to mean that the statutory term "employee benefit plan" does not include a plan whose only participants are the owner and his or her spouse, but does include a plan that covers as participants one or more common-law employees, in addition to the self-employed individuals. The Supreme Court noted that "[t]his agency view ... merits the Judiciary's respectful consideration."

In *Lowenschuss v. Selnick*, 117 F.3d 673 (9th Cir. 1999), the Ninth Circuit held that:

> An employee pension benefit plan that had been properly established and maintained pursuant to ERISA can lose its ERISA-qualified status for bankruptcy purposes through the mere attrition of non-owner participants where it covered only the owner-employee at the time of the bankruptcy filing.

The 2005 Bankruptcy Act appears to draw no distinction between owner-only plans and other qualified plans with respect to bankruptcy exemption. Such plans may, however, be at risk outside of bankruptcy.

403(b) Plans May Not Be Protected Outside of Bankruptcy

The U.S. Sixth Circuit Court of Appeals held in *Rhiel v. Adams*, No. 03-8011 (6th Cir. December 10, 2003) that only assets that are held "in a trust" are excludable from property of the bankruptcy estate by 11 U.S.C. §541(c)(2).

The Bankruptcy Court for the Southern District of Ohio held that the 403(b) plans (for the husband and wife) were "ERISA-qualified" as contemplated by the Supreme Court in *Patterson v. Shumate*. As such, they were not the property of the (bankruptcy) estate, and were not subject to administration by the (bankruptcy) trustee.

The Sixth Circuit reversed the Bankruptcy Court and remanded the case for further proceedings based on the fact that the debtors had not shown that the Section 541(c)(2) "in a trust" language had been satisfied. The Sixth Circuit held that only assets of an ERISA plan held in a trust would be excluded from the bankruptcy estate and that assets in a custodial account may not be excluded.

The 2005 Bankruptcy Act specifically protects 403(b) plans and does not distinguish between trust and custodial accounts. It is unclear how the Sixth Circuit will interpret its decision in *Rhiel* outside of bankruptcy.

ERISA and Bankruptcy Protections After Distribution from Retirement Plan

In *Hoult v. Hoult*, No. 02-2128 (U.S. First Circuit Court of Appeals, 2004), the U.S. Court of Appeals for the First Circuit held that the antialienation provisions of ERISA and the IRC do not restrict the alienation of pension benefits that have already been distributed to plan participants or beneficiaries. Once the benefits have been distributed from the plan, a creditor's rights are enforceable against the beneficiary, but not against the plan itself.

BAPCPA provides limited postbankruptcy protection for distributions of retirement plan assets to plan participants. "Eligible rollover distributions" retain their exempt status after they are distributed.[41] It is unclear whether such distributions are protected for more than 60 days if they are not rolled over to an IRA or another qualified plan. Required minimum distributions and hardship distributions are not protected because they are not eligible rollover distributions.

Creditor Protection for IRAs and Other Non-ERISA Plans Outside of Bankruptcy

IRAs, SEPs, SIMPLE IRAs, government plans, and most church plans are not covered under the nonalienation provisions of either ERISA or the IRC and, therefore, a participant's benefits under such plans are subject to creditors' claims outside of bankruptcy unless protected under state law.[42]

As stated earlier, the 2005 Bankruptcy Act protects IRA assets up to $1 million. SEPs, SIMPLEs, and rollover assets are protected in excess of the $1 million limit. State law with respect to the protection of IRA assets still applies for purposes of state law actions (e.g., garnishment). Appendix 3 at the end of this chapter provides a state-by-state analysis of IRAs as exempt property outside of bankruptcy.

Participant Direction of Plan Investments[43]

Defined contribution plans can provide for direction of investment by individual plan participants.[43,44] If a plan satisfies the requirements of ERISA Section 404(c), plan fiduciaries have some protection from fiduciary responsibility for the investment of retirement plan assets where plan participants direct the investment of their plan accounts.

U.S. Department of Labor Regulations prescribe extensive requirements to qualify as an ERISA Section 404(c) plan. In order to satisfy ERISA Section 404(c), a plan must permit each participant to: (1) choose from a broad range of investment alternatives with at least three diversified investment choices (called "core alternatives") with materially different risk/return characteristics (e.g., a stock mutual fund, a bond fund, and a balanced fund); (2) give investment instructions (e.g., make new investment elections and transfer current balances) at least once every 3 months and possibly more often if appropriate in light of the market volatility of the investment alternatives; (3) diversify investments both generally and within investment categories; and (4) receive current information from the plan that enables participants to make informed investment decisions.[c]

Participant Loans[45]

Plan loans to participants must bear a reasonable rate of interest, be adequately secured, provide a reasonable repayment schedule, and be made available on a nondiscriminatory basis.[46] Loans must be repaid within 5 years unless used for acquisition of a participant's personal residence.[47] Level amortization is required with at least quarterly payments over the term of a loan. A loan will be treated as a taxable distribution if it exceeds the lesser of (1) $50,000 or (2) the greater of $10,000 or 50% of the participant's vested accrued benefit.[47] The $50,000 limit is reduced by the highest outstanding loan balance during the 1-year period prior to the loan. Treasury regulations permit a grace period before a loan will be declared to be

---

c. DOL Advisory Opinion 2003-11A (9/18/2003) states that mutual fund "profiles" can be used to satisfy the requirements that a fiduciary provide a prospectus for each mutual fund either immediately before or immediately following a participant's investment in the fund.

in default and the outstanding balance on the loan will be deemed to be distributed from the plan. The grace period cannot extend beyond the last day of the calendar quarter following the calendar quarter in which the required installment was due.[48]

Summary

In summary, employer-sponsored retirement plans provide the best way for physician employees to accumulate significant wealth. By contributing pretax dollars into a tax-exempt trust protected from the claims of potential creditors, physician employers provide their physician employees with the best possible employee benefit. The forced savings aspect of tax-qualified retirement plans should not be overlooked and should be considered one of the key benefits of such plans. Studies have shown that it is much easier for physicians and other employees to save for retirement through employer-sponsored plans as opposed to trying to save on their own. Although less than 10% of eligible individuals contribute on their own to IRAs, 70% of eligible employees contribute to employer-sponsored 401(k) plans when presented with the opportunity to do so. Thus, employer-sponsored retirement plans provide a valuable employee benefit and help physicians and other employees save money for retirement.

■ Cafeteria Plans, Employee Fringe Benefits, and COBRA

The key to the employer-provided fringe benefit plans reviewed in this chapter is that such plans are tax-advantaged and funded on a tax-deductible or pretax basis by employers and/or employees. It is important for physician groups and other medical employers to provide health insurance and other fringe benefits to physicians and other employees. Such benefits are often viewed by employers as a necessary component of employment, and employers want and need to provide fringe benefits to employees to promote job satisfaction and encourage employee retention. This chapter also provides a summary of the COBRA group health plan continuation coverage requirements.

A chart summarizing some of the eligibility and coverage requirements for several employer-provided fringe benefit plans is provided in **Appendix 19-4** at the end of this chapter.

IRC Section 125 Cafeteria Plans

A cafeteria plan is an employer fringe benefit plan that permits participating employees to choose from two or more benefits consisting of cash and qualified benefits.

The cafeteria plan must offer both a cash benefit and at least one qualified benefit. A plan that offers only two qualified benefits or only two cash benefits is not a cafeteria plan. The cash may result from contributions by the employer to the plan, or may be the result of a voluntary salary reduction by the employee.

Qualified Benefits

A benefit is qualified if it does not defer the receipt of compensation and is excluded from gross income by an express provision of another section of the IRC. Qualified benefits include medical disability insurance, accident/health insurance, group-term life insurance (up to $50,000), dependent care assistance, group legal coverage, and 401(k) cash or deferred arrangements. Qualified benefits *cannot* include[49]:

- Contributions to a medical savings account under IRC Section 106(b)
- Scholarship and fellowship grants excludable under IRC Section 117
- Qualified educational assistance excludable under IRC Section 127
- Fringe benefits excludable under IRC Section 132 (de minimis fringes, no-additional-cost service fringes, employee discounts, working condition fringes)
- Any product that is advertised, marketed, or offered as long-term care insurance [IRC Section 125(f)]
- Deferred compensation under IRC Section 125(d)(2)
- Meals and lodging under IRC Section 119

Benefits do not lose qualified status merely because they are included in income solely due to violations of nondiscrimination rules (discussed later in this section) affecting the underlying benefits.[50]

Plan Participants

Participation in a cafeteria plan must be limited to employees.[51] Former employees are treated as employees, but self-employed individuals, as defined in IRC Section 401(c), are not. Although former employees are generally treated as employees, a cafeteria plan may not be established predominantly for their benefit. Further, only employees may have the right to elect benefits under the plan, although the plan may provide benefits for the spouse and beneficiaries of an employee who is a participant.[52] Eligibility to participate in a cafeteria plan may include up to 3 years of service. Participation commences not later than the first day of the first plan year after eligibility requirements are met.[53]

Although a spouse and dependents may benefit from the plan, they are not active participants in the plan.

Upon the death of the employee, the spouse may be given a right to elect coverage. However, the surviving spouse is not treated as an active participant merely because the surviving spouse makes such an election.[54]

Plan Contributions

The cafeteria plan may be financed with employer contributions, as well as after-tax employee contributions. In addition, the employer and employee may enter into a salary-reduction agreement under which the employee's salary is reduced by a given amount and the employer agrees to contribute an equal amount to the cafeteria plan for the employee's benefit. The contribution is treated as the employer's contribution if the employee had not actually or constructively received the salary payment when the salary-reduction agreement was entered into.[55] Therefore, the employee is allowed to make a contribution with pretax dollars.

Taxation of Employees

In order for a qualified benefit to be received tax-free by an employee under a cafeteria plan, the benefit must meet all the requirements of the specific IRC section that gives the benefit tax-free status. IRC Section 125 suspends application of the constructive receipt rules for benefits that are otherwise not taxable. It does not create new tax-exempt benefits.[56] However, benefits treated as cash are fully taxable.

Electing Benefits

An employee must elect nontaxable benefits under an IRC Section 125 cafeteria plan before the alternative cash benefit becomes currently available to him or her. Otherwise, the employee will be taxed as if he or she had received the cash benefits.[57] A benefit is currently available to a plan participant if the participant is free to receive the benefit currently or if he or she could receive it by making an election or by giving a notice of intent to receive the benefit. However, a benefit is not currently available if there is a substantial limitation or restriction on the participant's receipt of the benefit.[58] A participant who has elected a benefit under the plan and has started to receive the benefit may not generally revoke the election during the period of coverage (i.e., the plan year), even if the revocation only applies to future benefits.[59]

A cafeteria plan may, on a reasonable and consistent basis, automatically adjust all effective participants' elective contributions for health plans if (1) the cost of a health plan provided by an independent third-party provider under a cafeteria plan changes and (2) under the terms of the cafeteria plan employees are required to make a corresponding change in their premium payments.

Alternatively, if the premium increases significantly, a cafeteria plan may permit participants to (1) make a corresponding change in their premium payments or (2) revoke their elections and, in lieu thereof, to receive, on a prospective basis, similar coverage under another health plan.[60] For dependent care assistance, election changes may not be made due to a change in cost if the provider is a relative of the employee.[61]

A cafeteria plan will not fail to satisfy Section 125 if it changes the employee's election to provide coverage for a child if a judgment, decree, or order resulting from a divorce, legal separation, annulment, or change in custody requires coverage for a child under the employee's plan. An employee is also permitted to make an election change to cancel coverage for such a child if the order requires the spouse, former spouse, or other individual to provide coverage for the child and that coverage is, in fact, provided.

If an employee, spouse, or dependent who is enrolled in an accident or health plan of the employer becomes entitled to coverage under Medicare or Medicaid (Part a or Part b of Title XVII of the Social Security Act, or Title XIX of the Social Security Act), the cafeteria plan may permit the employee to make a prospective election change to cancel or reduce coverage of that employee, spouse, or dependent under the accident or health plan. In addition, if an employee, spouse, or dependent who has been entitled to such coverage under Medicare or Medicaid loses all eligibility for such coverage, the cafeteria plan may permit the employee to make a prospective election to commence or increase coverage of that employee, spouse, or dependent under the accident or health plan.

If coverage under a plan is significantly curtailed or ceases during a period of coverage, the cafeteria plan may permit affected employees to revoke their elections under the plan. In that case, each affected employee may make a new election on a prospective basis for coverage under another benefit package option providing similar coverage. Coverage under an accident or health plan is significantly curtailed only if there is an overall reduction in coverage provided to participants under the plan so as to constitute reduced coverage to participants generally.[61] Further, if during a period of coverage a plan adds a new benefit package option or other coverage option (or eliminates an existing benefit package option or other coverage option), the cafeteria plan may permit affected employees to elect the newly added option (or elect another option if an option has been eliminated) prospectively on a pretax basis and make corresponding election changes with respect to other benefit package options providing similar coverage.[61]

A participant may revoke a benefit election and make a new election during a period of coverage if the change is caused by, and consistent with, a change in the participant's family status. Examples of such changes are marriage or divorce; death of the spouse or a dependent; birth or adoption of a child; change in residence of an employee, spouse, or dependent; the employee or his or her spouse switching from full-time to part-time status (or part-time to full-time); the employee or spouse taking an unpaid leave of absence; a significant change in the health coverage of the employee or employee's spouse attributable to the spouse's employment; and the termination (or commencement) of a spouse's employment. Additionally, an employee who separates from service may terminate benefits. Also, the plan may terminate the benefits of an employee during a period of coverage if the employee fails to make the required premium payments.[61]

FICA and FUTA Tax

Payments under a cafeteria plan are excluded from the definition of "wages" subject to FICA and FUTA tax, if they are otherwise excluded from such wages and it is reasonable to believe that under IRC Section 125 they would not be treated as constructively received.[62]

Deferral of Compensation

A cafeteria plan may not include any plan that provides for the deferral of compensation.[63] Nor may it allow employees to carry over unused elective contributions for plan benefits from one plan year to the next. Such a carry-forward is treated as a deferral of compensation. Also, a plan may not allow participants to use contributions for one plan year to purchase benefits that will be supplied in a later year.[64] However, reasonable premium rebates or policy dividends paid with respect to benefits provided under a cafeteria plan do not defer compensation if they are paid within 12 months of the close of the plan year.[65] IRS Notice 2005-42 permits a grace period immediately following the end of each plan year during which unused benefits or contributions remaining at the end of the plan year may be paid or reimbursed to plan participants for qualified benefit expenses incurred during the grace period. Expenses for qualified benefits incurred during the grace period may be paid or reimbursed from benefits or contributions remaining unused at the end of the immediately preceding plan year. The grace period must not extend beyond the fifteenth day of the third calendar month after the end of the immediately preceding plan year to which it relates (i.e., "the 2 and 1/2 month rule").

Vacation Days

A cafeteria plan may allow employees to receive additional or fewer paid vacation days than the employer otherwise provides. However, an elective vacation provision may not be used to defer compensation. If a plan allows a participant to be paid in cash for unused elective vacation days, the payment must be made before the end of the plan year and before the end of the employer's taxable year to which the elective contributions relate. Allowing employees to exchange vacation days in the current plan year for payments in the next plan year would not be a disqualifying deferral of compensation.[66] A participant is deemed to use his or her nonelective vacation days before his or her elective vacation days.[67]

> *Example:* Employer A provides all its employees with 1 week of paid vacation each calendar year. Employer A establishes a calendar year cafeteria plan under which each participant may choose to forgo cash or another benefit for any calendar year in exchange for one additional week of paid vacation during the year. If the employee elects the optional week of vacation and fails to use it during the calendar year, the value of the unused week may be paid to the employee in cash before the end of the year. However, the week may not be carried over to the next calendar year, and its value may not be cashed out or used for any other purpose during the next calendar year.

Qualified Cash or Deferred Arrangement

Although a cafeteria plan cannot include plans providing for deferred compensation, it can include a profit-sharing or stock bonus plan that has a qualified cash or deferred arrangement under IRC Section 401(k). Amounts contributed under the employee's election are treated as nontaxable benefits for cafeteria plan purposes.[68] After-tax employee contributions under a defined contribution plan, subject to the nondiscrimination rules of IRC Section 401(m), are also allowed. Furthermore, employer matching contributions may be made with respect to before-tax or after-tax employee contributions.[69]

Formal Plan Requirements

The written cafeteria plan document must contain:

- A description of each benefit available under the plan including the periods of coverage (need not be self-contained; the description may be incorporated by reference [e.g., group legal plans, dependent care plans])
- The plan rules governing participation
- Procedures by which employees make elections under the plan (specified period during which elections are made, the extent to which such elections

are irrevocable, and the period in which such elections are effective)

- The manner in which employer contributions are made under the plan
- The plan year
- The maximum amount of employer contributions available for any participant

The plan document must also describe the maximum amount of elective contributions available to any employee. This may be done by stating the maximum dollar amount or the maximum percentage of compensation that may be contributed as the elective contributions by employees or by stating the method for determining the maximum amount or percentage.[70]

As a practical point, employers may wish to maintain separate written plans for benefits offered under cafeteria plans. An employer may wish to offer the benefits to employees outside of the plan or the same benefits may be offered in two or more plans. Moreover, cafeteria plans may avoid being subject to ERISA if each substantive benefit in the cafeteria plan is contained in a separate written plan satisfying ERISA. Additionally, certain benefits (e.g., group legal services, uninsured medical expense reimbursements, and dependent care service) are required to be set forth in separate written plans. If the cafeteria plan is subject to ERISA, the plan must name the fiduciaries and comply with ERISA.

Flexible Spending Arrangements

A flexible spending arrangement (FSA) is an employee benefit program that reimburses employees for certain expenses they incur and under which the maximum amount of reimbursement for a period of coverage is not substantially greater than the total premiums paid. The flexible spending arrangement rules apply if the maximum reimbursement is less than five times the premium.[71] The Patient Protection and Affordable Care Act of 2010 imposes a $2,500 limit on annual salary reduction contributions to health FSAs offered under cafeteria plans, effective for taxable years beginning after December 31, 2012.[72] The $2,500 amount is indexed for inflation for taxable years beginning after December 31, 2013.

Special rules are applied to health plans that are FSAs in order to prevent them from being used as devices for avoiding the restrictions on the deduction of personal medical expenses. This deduction applies for medical expenditures in excess of 7.5% of the individual's adjusted gross income. Health FSAs must be bona fide health plans and not separate, employee-by-employee health expense reimbursement accounts that operate like employee-funded defined contribution plans. A health FSA must

qualify as an accident or health plan under IRC Sections 105 and 106. In particular, health FSAs must exhibit the risk-shifting and risk-contribution characteristics of insurance, and payments must be made specifically to reimburse participants for medical expenses incurred previously during the period of coverage.[73] The employee's risk can be controlled by limiting the maximum salary reduction and healthcare spending account reimbursement to a relatively low amount (e.g. $500) or by establishing a year of service requirement for eligibility.

The maximum amount of reimbursement under a health FSA must be available at all times during the period of coverage. It cannot depend on the extent to which the participant has paid the required premiums for the period. Nor may the schedule for premium payments during the period of coverage be based on the rate or amount of claims already incurred during the period. The period of coverage for a health FSA must be 12 months or, in the case of a short plan year, the entire short year.[74]

A health FSA can only reimburse medical expenses as defined in IRC Section 213. It may not treat participants' premium payments for other health coverage as reimbursable expenses. To obtain reimbursement, the participant must provide the health FSA with a written statement from an independent third party stating the amount of the medical expense incurred. The participant must also provide a written statement that the expense is not reimbursable under any other health plan. The medical expenses must have been incurred during the participant's period of plan coverage. The time when the medical expense is billed or paid is not relevant.[75] As a result of the Patient Protection and Affordable Care Act of 2010, health FSAs can only reimburse medicines and drugs other than insulin if the medicine or drug is prescribed (determined without regard to whether a prescription is necessary to acquire the drug).[76]

If a health FSA has an experience gain (forfeitures) for a year of coverage, the gain may be used to reduce the next year's premiums or may be returned to the premium payers. The experience gain must be allocated on a reasonable uniform basis that is not related to the claims experience of individual participants.[77] FSAs providing dependent care assistance are subject to rules similar to those for health FSAs, except that the requirement of uniform coverage throughout the coverage period does not apply.[78]

Nondiscrimination Rules

The nondiscrimination rules are designed to encourage cafeteria plans to provide adequate benefits to rank-and-file employees.[79] If a cafeteria plan meets the other requirements of IRC Section 125, but fails to comply with the nondiscrimination rules, the benefits received by rank-and-file employees are protected by cafeteria plan rules. However, benefits received by highly compensated participants or key employees may be included in income.[80]

The cafeteria plan rules do not apply to any benefit of a highly compensated participant that is attributable to a plan year in which the plan discriminates in favor of highly compensated individuals as to eligibility to participate, or in favor of highly compensated participants as to contributions or benefits.[81] A "highly compensated individual or participant" is not the same as a "highly compensated individual" under IRC Section 414(q). For purposes of IRC Section 125, "highly compensated participants" and "highly compensated individuals" mean plan participants and individuals who are: (1) officers, (2) greater than 5% (voting or valuation) shareholders, (3) highly compensated, or (4) spouses or dependents of any persons in 1–3.[82]

Any benefit taxable because of violation of the nondiscrimination rules is treated as received or accrued in the tax year in which the plan year ends.[83] If the cafeteria plan is discriminatory in favor of highly compensated employees, a highly compensated employee is taxed on the maximum taxable benefits that such employee could have selected for the plan year.[84]

A plan is considered to have nondiscriminatory coverage if it benefits a class of employees that the IRS determines is not discriminatory in favor of highly compensated employees. Such a plan must not require more than three consecutive years of employment for plan participation, and the employment requirement for each employee must be the same. Further, the plan must permit otherwise eligible employees to begin participation no later than the first day of the plan year beginning after the completion of three consecutive years of employment.[85]

Health benefits under a cafeteria plan will not be considered to be discriminatory if: (1) total contributions for each participant include either an amount equal to 100% of the cost of health benefit coverage under the plan of the majority or of similarly situated highly compensated participants, or an amount equal to or greater than 75% of the cost of health benefit coverage of the similarly situated participant who has the highest cost health benefit coverage under the plan; and (2) contributions or benefits exceeding those amounts bear a uniform relationship to compensation.[86]

If statutory nontaxable benefits provided to key employees under the plan exceed 25% of the total of such benefits provided to all employees under the plan, tax-favored treatment will not apply to any benefit of a key

employee. "Statutory nontaxable benefits" in this context do not include group-term life insurance in excess of $50,000 or benefits that are normally taxable but permitted by regulations. "Key employee" is defined in IRC Section 416(i)(1). Any benefit taxable because of violation of the discrimination rule is treated as received or accrued in the tax year in which the plan year ends.[87]

A plan is not discriminatory if it is maintained under an agreement that the IRS finds to be a collective bargaining agreement.[88] Also, for purposes of the nondiscrimination tests, all employees of a commonly controlled group of businesses or of an "affiliated service group" are treated as employed by a single employer.[89]

Effect of the Family and Medical Leave Act on the Operation of Cafeteria Plans

Under the U.S. Treasury Regulations at Section 1.125-3, an employee taking Family and Medical Leave Act (FMLA) leave may revoke an existing election of group health plan coverage under the cafeteria plan. Additionally, the employee must be permitted to choose to be reinstated (under the same terms) in the group health plan coverage provided under the cafeteria plan upon returning from FMLA leave.[90]

While on FMLA leave, an employee is entitled to continue group health plan coverage whether or not provided under the cafeteria plan. The employee is responsible for continuing to make the premium payments. The cafeteria plan may, on a nondiscriminatory basis, offer one or more of the following payment options to an employee who continues group health plan coverage while on unpaid leave:

- *The prepay option:* Under the prepay option, the cafeteria plan may permit an employee to pay, prior to commencement of the FMLA leave, the amounts due during the FMLA leave period. These contributions may be made on a pretax salary reduction basis.

- *The pay-as-you-go option:* This option is generally made available on an after-tax basis. These payments are due (by the premium due date) during the FMLA leave period.

- *The catch-up option:* The employer and employee may agree to allow the premiums to be paid after the FMLA leave period is over. Under this provision, the employer and employee must agree in advance of the FMLA leave period that: (1) the employee will continue health coverage during the FMLA leave period; (2) the employer will assume responsibility for advancing payments of the employee's premiums during the FMLA leave period; and (3) these advanced amounts must be paid by the employee when the employee returns from the FMLA leave.

Contributions under this option may be made on a pretax salary reduction basis when the employee returns from the FMLA leave.[91]

Please note that these provisions do not apply if the employee is on paid FMLA leave.[92] It is also important to realize that FMLA does not require employers to maintain an employee on nonhealth benefits (e.g., life insurance) during the leave period.[93]

Simple Cafeteria Plans[94]

One intent of the new healthcare reform legislation is to encourage small employers to provide health insurance coverage benefits to their employees, particularly on a tax-free basis. To accomplish this goal, for years beginning after December 31, 2010, the law provides eligible small employers with the ability to offer a "simple cafeteria plan" under which a safe harbor from the nondiscrimination requirements generally applicable to cafeteria plans is provided. Additionally, small employers are provided a safe harbor from the nondiscrimination requirements applicable to certain qualified benefits offered under the plan. For purposes of the simple cafeteria plan provisions, a small employer is defined as an employer that employed an average of 100 or fewer employees on business days during either of the two preceding tax years.

Under a traditional cafeteria plan, an employer may offer employees a choice of either certain qualified benefits or cash. If an employee selects any of the qualified benefits offered, the value of such benefits is not includible in his or her income. Despite its advantages, however, a cafeteria plan is subject to strict rules whereby it may not discriminate in favor of highly compensated participants. A failure to satisfy these nondiscrimination rules results in the inclusion of the qualified benefits in the highly compensated participant's income.

Conversely, under the new healthcare reform, a simple cafeteria plan provides small employers with a safe harbor from these nondiscrimination requirements applicable to cafeteria plans and certain qualified benefits offered under the plan. Under this safe harbor, an eligible employer offering a simple cafeteria plan and certain qualified benefits offered under it will be treated as meeting any applicable nondiscrimination requirements during such year, provided certain requirements are met.

First, under a simple cafeteria plan, an employer must make a contribution to provide qualified benefits under the plan on behalf of each qualified nonhighly compensated employee eligible to participate in the plan, regardless of whether such employee makes a salary reduction contribution, in an amount equal to: (1) a uniform percentage of not less than 2% of the employee's compensation for the plan year, or (2) an amount not less than the lesser of 6% of the employee's compensation for the plan year or twice the amount of the salary reduction contributions of each qualified employee.

Second, all employees with at least 1,000 hours of service for the preceding plan year must be eligible to participate in the plan (with certain exceptions), and each eligible employee must be given the opportunity to elect any qualified benefit offered under the plan subject to the terms and conditions applicable to all participants.

Essentially, like the increasingly popular safe harbor 401(k) plan, the simple cafeteria plan's safe harbor allows a small employer to avoid complex nondiscrimination rules. With relatively minimal required contributions and a broadening of eligibility for the plan, this new healthcare reform tool may be a great asset to eligible small employers.

Employee Fringe Benefit Qualification and Nondiscrimination Rules

Group-Term Life Insurance

Under IRC Section 79, an employer can provide up to $50,000 of group-term life insurance to employees tax-free. Coverage exceeding $50,000 is included in an employee's income, not at actual cost but at the favorable rates provided in Regulation Section 1.79-3(d)(2). The $50,000 threshold refers to the life insurance coverage amount, not to an employee's earned income; therefore, the fact that an employee earns less than $50,000 is irrelevant.[d]

Employees may be excluded from a plan if: (1) such employees have not completed 3 years of service; (2) they are part-time (customary employment of less than 20 hours per week) or seasonal employees (customary employment of not more than 5 months per year); (3) they are nonresident aliens who receive no U.S. income from the employer; or (4) they are covered by a collective bargaining agreement in which benefits provided under the plan were subject to good faith bargaining.[95] A plan is not discriminatory as to eligibility to participate if one of the following four tests is satisfied: (1) at least 70% of all employees receive benefits under the plan; (2) at least 85% of all employees participating in the plan are not key employees; (3) the plan benefits employees under a classification set up by the employer that the IRS determines does not discriminate in favor of key employees; or (4) the plan is part of a cafeteria plan satisfying IRC Section 125 requirements.[96]

If a group-term life insurance plan discriminates in favor of key employees with respect to either benefits

---

d. Robert Charles Fohrmeister, T.C. Memo 1997-159.

provided or eligibility to participate, then the key employees will report as income the higher of the actual premium paid by the employer or the amount from the table found in the regulations for all coverage provided by the employer. Plan benefits are discriminatory unless all benefits available to key employees are also available to all other participants—provided, however, that there is no discrimination merely because the insurance provided each participant bears a uniform relationship to compensation.

The nondiscrimination rules do not apply to church plans maintained for church employees. The terms "church plan" and "church employee" are defined in IRC Sections 414(e)(1) and (3). A church plan must be established and maintained by a church or association of churches exempt from tax under IRC Section 501(c)(3)—provided, however, that the term "church employee" does not include any employee of an educational entity above the secondary school level (other than a school for religious training) and it does not include an employee of a hospital, a medical school, a medical research institution, or another charity with similar exempt purposes. Therefore, physician employees of a hospital or educational institution controlled by a church would not be considered to be church employees and would be subject to the nondiscrimination rules.

Additional requirements apply with group-term life insurance provided to less than 10 full-time employees of the employer throughout the calendar year. In such groups, the insurance must be provided to all full-time employees of the employer or to all full-time employees who provide evidence of insurability that is satisfactory to the insurer.[97] The amount of the insurance provided can be uniform for all employees regardless of compensation (e.g., $10,000 of life insurance for all employees) or based on compensation. If based on compensation, the insurance must be computed as a uniform percentage of compensation or on a basis of "coverage brackets" established by the insurer. No coverage bracket may be more than 2 1/2 times the next lower bracket, and the lowest bracket must be at least 10% of the highest bracket.[98] The evidence of insurability concerning eligibility for coverage or the amount is limited to a medical questionnaire completed by the employee that does not require a physical examination.[99] In applying these rules, employees may be excluded if they are denied insurance because they are part-time or fail to complete a waiting period not to exceed 6 months.[100]

The cost of group-term life insurance that is includable in the gross income of the employee is considered "wages" subject to Social Security tax.[101] Generally, only the cost of life insurance coverage in excess of $50,000 will be subject to Social Security tax. The employer is required to report amounts includable in the wages of current employees on the W-2. The employer may treat the wages as though paid on any basis so long as they are treated as paid at least once each year.[102] The employer is not subject to the withholding requirements, but must file an information return for each calendar year. Currently, the Form W-2 satisfies this requirement.[103]

Group-term life insurance coverage up to $2,000 for an employee's spouse or other dependent is excludable from gross income as a de minimis fringe benefit under IRC Section 132(e). Because benefits excludable under IRC Section 132 may not be provided under a cafeteria plan, the group-term life insurance coverage of the spouse or dependent may not be offered under a cafeteria plan.[104]

Accident and Health Plans

Prior to the Patient Protection and Affordable Care Act of 2010, only employers that maintained *self-insured* medical plans were subject to the nondiscrimination tests in IRC Section 105(h). However, effective for plan years beginning on or after September 23, 2010, most employers that maintain insured medical plans will also be subject to the nondiscrimination test in IRC Section 105(h) upon the issuance of form guidance on the matter.[105]

Employees may be excluded from such plans if: (1) the employees have not completed 3 years of service; (2) the employees are under age 25; (3) they are part-time (less than 35 hours per week) or seasonal employees (less than 9 months per year); (4) they are covered by a collective bargaining agreement if health and accident benefits were the subject of good faith bargaining; or (5) they are nonresident alien employees who receive no U.S. income from the employer.[106]

A plan is not discriminatory as to eligibility to participate if one of the following tests is satisfied: (1) 70% or more of all employees receive benefits under the plan; (2) 80% or more of all eligible employees receive benefits under the plan if at least 70% of all employees are eligible; or (3) the plan benefits employees under a classification set up by the employer that is determined by the IRS not to discriminate in favor of highly compensated individuals (e.g., a "fair cross-section").[107] A discriminatory plan will require highly compensated individuals to take "excess reimbursements" into income. Highly compensated individuals include the five highest paid officers, the more than 10% owners, and the highest paid 25% of all employees (other than excludable employees who are not participants).[108]

The amount that is treated as excess reimbursement depends on whether the plan is discriminatory as to eligibility to participate or as to benefits offered under the plan. If a plan provides discriminatory benefits (benefits available to highly compensated individuals that are not available to all other plan participants), then the entire amount of the benefit is an excess reimbursement. A plan discriminates in favor of highly compensated employees as to benefits unless all benefits provided for highly compensated employees and their dependents are also provided for all other participants and their dependents.[109] If a plan provides discriminatory coverage (benefits are the same for all participants, but the plan discriminates in eligibility to participate), then the excess reimbursement is determined by multiplying a highly compensated individual's reimbursement by a fraction where the numerator is the amount of benefits received by all highly compensated individuals during the plan year and the denominator is the total amount of benefits received by all plan participants during the year.

Dependent Care Assistance Programs[110]
Under an IRC Section 129 dependent care assistance program, employees generally receive tax-free dependent care assistance up to $5,000 annually. The contributions and benefits under the plan cannot discriminate in favor of HCEs[e] or their dependents. In addition, the dependent care assistance program must benefit a class of employees that the IRS determines does not discriminate in favor of HCEs. Employees may be excluded from a plan if such employees have not reached age 21 and completed 1 year of service, or if such employees are in a unit of employees covered by a collective bargaining agreement if dependent care benefits were the subject of good faith bargaining.[111]

Dependent care assistance plans must satisfy a nondiscrimination "average benefits test." This test requires that the average benefit provided to NHCEs be at least 55% of the benefits provided to HCEs. If the benefits are provided through a salary reduction plan, this test may disregard any employee whose compensation is less than $25,000. Although there is no statutory code section specifically authorizing the 55% test to be limited to a line of business basis, the legislative history states that the 55% average benefit test was to be performed on a separate line of business basis.[112] In addition to the average benefits test, no more than 25% of the dependent care assistance benefits paid during the year may be provided to 5% (or more) owners (or their spouses or dependents).[113] Benefits provided under a discriminatory

dependent care assistance plan will be taxable income to the HCEs participating in the plan. NHCEs will continue to exclude benefits from taxable income.

The expenses must be incurred for either: (1) a dependent under the age of 15 or (2) a spouse or other dependent of the employee who is physically or mentally incapable of caring for him- or herself.[114] An individual is considered to be physically or mentally incapable of caring for him- or herself if, because of the mental or physical defect, the individual is "incapable of caring for his hygienic or nutritional needs or requires full-time attention of another person for his own safety or the safety of others."[114] The mere fact that the individual is unable to engage in substantial gainful activity or to perform the normal household functions of a homemaker or care for minor children is not sufficient. A person's status as a qualified dependent is determined on a day-to-day basis. Thus, for example, if a dependent turns 15 on July 1, the expenses incurred after July 1 will not be treated as employment-related expenses. Generally, by January 31 of each year, the employer must give the participating employee a written statement showing the amount of expenses paid or incurred for that employee during the preceding calendar year.[115]

Educational Assistance Programs[116]
An educational assistance plan under IRC Section 127 enables an employee to receive up to $5,250 tax-free annually for use on qualifying educational expenses. The only employees excludable from a plan are those who are covered under a collective bargaining agreement, provided that educational assistance benefits were bargained for in good faith. The nondiscrimination rules of IRC Section 127 provide that no more than 5% of the educational expenses paid under the plan during a plan year may benefit 5% (or more) owners, their spouses, and their dependents. The plan must be written and be for the exclusive benefit of employees, and the employer may not allow employees to choose between educational assistance and other taxable pay.

Other Employee Fringe Benefits
Under IRC Section 132, no-additional-cost services, qualified employee discounts, and employee eating facilities meeting certain requirements are nontaxable fringe benefits. HCEs may exclude these benefits only if such benefits are provided in a nondiscriminatory manner.

COBRA Group Health Plan Continuation Coverage Under IRC Section 4980b
COBRA is a Federal law stemming from ERISA, the Internal Revenue Code and the Public Health Service

---

e. As defined in IRC §414(q).

Act ("PHSA"). The COBRA provisions of the Code apply to group health plans of private-sector employers, while the COBRA provisions of the PHSA apply to the group health plans of state and local governments.

Overview and Affected Plans

Group health plans must give each qualified beneficiary who would lose coverage under the plan as a result of a qualifying event the right to elect, within the election period, continued coverage under the plan. Continued coverage means that the coverage must be identical to the coverage provided to similarly situated beneficiaries under the plan with respect to whom a qualifying event has not occurred. If the coverage is modified for a group of similarly situated beneficiaries, then the same modification must be made for all qualified beneficiaries under the plan. Employers with fewer than 20 employees on a typical business day during the preceding calendar year are exempt from the continuation coverage regulations. There may, however, be similar state law requirements for employers with less than 20 employees.

A "qualified beneficiary" is defined as the spouse or dependent child (including a newborn, adopted child, or child placed for adoption at the time of the qualifying event or at any time during the COBRA coverage) of the covered employee on the date before the qualifying event for that employee. In the case of employment termination or reduction in the hours of the covered employee resulting in loss of coverage, the term "qualified beneficiary" includes the covered employee.

A chart summarizing the COBRA requirements is available in **Appendix 19-5** of this chapter.

Qualifying Events

A qualifying event is any of the following events that, but for the continuation coverage required under these rules, would result in the loss of coverage of a qualified beneficiary. They are as follows:

- The death of the covered employee
- The employment termination (other than in the case of gross misconduct) or reduction of hours of the covered employee's employment
- The divorce or legal separation of the covered employee from the employee's spouse
- The covered employee becoming entitled to benefits under the Social Security Act Title XVIII
- A dependent child ceasing to be a dependent child under the generally applicable definitions of the plan
- A bankruptcy proceeding commencing on or after July 1, 1986, with respect to the employer from whose employment the covered employee retired at any time

Period of Coverage

The period of required coverage begins on the date of the qualifying event and ends on the earliest of the following: (1) 18 months after termination of employment (except in the case of discharge for gross misconduct) or reduction in hours of the covered employee's employment, except in the case of a bankruptcy proceeding with respect to the employer; or (2) if within 18 months after such termination or reduction in hours of covered employment, the covered employee dies, becomes divorced or legally separated, becomes entitled to benefits under Social Security Act Title XVIII, or ceases to be a dependent child of the employee, then the covered period is 36 months after such termination or reduction in hours of covered employment. Coverage is extended for up to a maximum of 29 months for certain employees who are disabled at the time of a qualifying event or become disabled during the first 60 days of COBRA coverage.

Notwithstanding these rules, eligibility for coverage will cease on:

- The date the employer ceases to provide any group health plan to any employee
- The date when coverage ceases because of failure by the beneficiary to make a timely premium payment (generally considered timely if payment is made within 30 days after the due date)
- The date when the qualified beneficiary becomes covered under any other group health plan (that does not contain any exclusion or limitation with respect to any pre-existing condition, or if such plan does contain an exclusion or limitation with respect to pre-existing conditions, when the qualified beneficiary is not subject to the exclusion or limitation due to the application of the Health Insurance Portability and Accountability Act of 1996) or in the case of a qualified beneficiary other than a retiree, the spouse of the covered employee, the dependent child of the employee, or the surviving spouse of the covered employee, the date on which he or she becomes entitled to benefits under Social Security Act Title XVIII.

Effective for post-1989 qualifying events, a qualified beneficiary who becomes covered under a new employer's plan will be permitted to continue coverage on the prior plan if the new employer's plan does not cover pre-existing conditions of that qualified beneficiary.

Premium Payments

The plan may require the payment of a premium from the beneficiary for the period of continued coverage, but in no event can the payment exceed 102% of the regular premium. A payment can be made in monthly installments. If an election is made after the qualifying event, the plan can permit payment for continuation coverage during the period preceding the election to be made within 45 days of the date of the election. For a disabled qualified beneficiary extending the 18-month continuation coverage to 29 months, the premium for the additional 11 months continuation beyond the 18-month coverage may not exceed 150% of the regular premium.

No Requirement of Insurability
The coverage may not be conditioned upon, or discriminate because of, a lack of evidence of insurability.

Election Period
The election period: (1) begins on the date of the qualifying event, (2) which is of at least 60 days in duration, and (3) ends on the later of 60 days after the qualifying event or 60 days after the qualified beneficiary receives notice as provided for under the notice requirements. A qualified beneficiary who, during the election period, voluntarily waives COBRA can revoke the waiver at any time prior to the end of the election period. However, if the waiver is revoked, coverage need not be provided retroactively.[117]

Notice Requirement
Written notice of the rights of the covered employee and his or her spouse must be provided to the employee at the time coverage begins. The employer must notify the plan administrator of: (1) the death of the covered employee, (2) the termination (except by reason of gross misconduct) or reduction of hours of the covered employee's employment, (3) the covered employee becoming entitled to benefits under Social Security Act Title XVIII, or (4) a bankruptcy proceeding within 30 days of the date of the event. The covered employee or qualified beneficiary must notify the plan administrator of the divorce or legal separation of the covered employee from the spouse or a dependent child ceasing to be a dependent child under the generally applicable definitions of the plan.

The plan administrator will notify the qualified beneficiary (e.g., the former spouse or child) in the case of the events described above where the covered employee or qualified beneficiary notifies the plan administrator of such beneficiary's rights under this subsection. Notification of a qualified beneficiary's rights must be given within 14 days of the plan administrator receiving notice from either the employer or employee, whichever is applicable.

Penalties and Noncompliance
Failure to satisfy the healthcare continuation rules results in an excise tax equal to $100 per day for each qualified beneficiary not receiving an option to continue coverage during the noncompliance period. For purposes of determining the amount of the excise tax, if there is more than one qualified beneficiary in the same family, the maximum amount of the excise tax with respect to such family is $200 per day. The noncompliance period starts on the date the failure first occurs and ends on the earlier of: (1) the date the failure is corrected, or (2) 6 months after the last date on which the employer could have been required to provide such continuation coverage to the qualified beneficiary, determined without regard to whether the qualified beneficiary paid any required premium. The excise tax does not apply if a failure was due to reasonable cause and not to willful neglect, provided the failure is corrected within the first 30 days of the noncompliance.

A special audit rule applies despite the 30-day grace period or reasonable diligence rule. Under the audit rule, where a failure with respect to a qualified beneficiary is not corrected by the date a notice of examination of income tax liability is sent to the employer and the failure took place or continued during the period under examination, the excise tax will not be less than the smaller of $2,500 or the amount of the excise tax computed without regard to the reasonable diligence exception and 30-day grace period rule. Further, if the failure is more than de minimis with respect to the employer (or multi-employer plan), then the dollar amount is $15,000. The maximum penalty for failure to provide coverage due to reasonable cause and not willful neglect is the lesser of: (1) 10% of the total amount paid or incurred by the employer (or predecessor employer) during the preceding tax year for the employer's group health plans, or (2) $500,000. A failure to comply with continued health coverage rules is considered corrected if (1) the rules are retroactively satisfied to the extent possible and (2) the qualified beneficiary is put in the same position that he or she would have been in but for the failure.

Summary
Group health plans and other fringe benefits are valuable benefits that can be provided to physicians and other employees by physician employers on a tax-advantaged basis. In some cases, it is possible to provide tiers of benefits with different levels of benefits for different groups of employees. In conjunction with tax-qualified retirement plans, employer-provided fringe benefits permit employers to provide benefits that are deductible to the employer but not taxable to physicians and other employees. In this way employers can provide employees with benefits that are more valuable to the employees than additional compensation.

Appendices

Table 19-1 Comparison of Types of Tax-Qualified Retirement Plans

Plan Elements	Profit-Sharing	401(k)	Cross-Tested Profit-Sharing	Money Purchase Pension	Defined Benefit	Comments
1. Contributions:						
(a) Employer: Mandatory	No	No	No	Yes	Yes	Generally, employer contributions for profit-sharing and 401(k) plans are discretionary.
(b) Employer: Discretionary	Yes	Yes	Yes	No	No	Contributions for profit-sharing and 401(k) plans can range from 0–25% of aggregate eligible compensation.
(c) Employee: Pretax	No	Yes	No	No	No	Generally, elective deferrals for 401(k) were limited to the lesser of 100% of compensation or $17,000 for 2012. Nondiscrimination testing limits elective deferrals for HCEs to a multiple of the NHCEs' elective deferrals.
(d) Employee: After Tax	Yes	Yes	Yes	Yes	Yes	Subject to nondiscrimination testing.
(e) Employer: Matching	Yes	Yes	No	No	No	Employer may proportionately match employee elective deferrals or after-tax contributions, subject to nondiscrimination testing.
2. Overall Limitation on Contribution Based on Eligible Compensation:						
(a) On Employer Contribution (§404)	25%	25%	25%	25%	Limitations based on benefits, not on contributions	Limitation does not include employee elective deferral contributions.
(b) On Allocation to Each Employee (§415)*	Lesser of 100% of comp. or $50,000 for 2012	Lesser of 100% of comp. or $50,000 for 2012	Lesser of 100% of comp. or $50,000 for 2012	Lesser of 100% of comp. or $50,000 for 2012	Annual benefit limit is lesser of 100% of comp. or $200,000 for 2012	Limitation aggregates employer contributions, matching contributions, employee contributions, and forfeitures.

* Profit-Sharing, 401(k), cross-tested profit-sharing, and money purchase pension plans are all classified as defined contribution plans and are subject to many of the same restrictions.

Table 19-1 Comparison of Types of Tax-Qualified Retirement Plans (continued)

Plan Elements	Profit-Sharing	401(k)	Cross-Tested Profit-Sharing	Money Purchase Pension	Defined Benefit	Comments
3. Eligibility to Participate Maximum Restrictions:						
Age	21 years	21 years	21 years	21 years	21 years	Additional exclusion available for employees covered by a collective bargaining agreement. Any additional exclusion of employees is subject to nondiscriminatory coverage and participation testing.
Service	2 years	1 year	2 years	2 years	2 years	
4. Maximum Vesting Schedules of Employer Contributions:**						Employee contributions and elective deferrals are always fully vested. Employer matching contribution can be subject to vesting schedule.
(a) If 1 Year of Service	5 year cliff 7 year graded	5 year cliff 7 year graded	5 year cliff 7 year graded	5 year cliff 7 year graded	5 year cliff 7 year graded	
Top-Heavy Matching Contribution (eff. 2002) All Defined Contribution Plans (eff. 2007)***	3 year cliff 6 year graded	3 year cliff 6 year graded	3 year cliff 6 year graded	3 year cliff 6 year graded	3 year cliff 6 year graded	
(b) If 2 Years of Service	2 year cliff	N/A	2 year cliff	2 year cliff	2 year cliff	
5. Participant Loans	Yes	Yes	Yes	Yes	Yes	Optional plan provision. Generally, a loan cannot exceed the lesser of $50,000 or 50% of participant vested benefit. Loan is generally repaid by monthly or quarterly payments over 5-year term at market interest.

**See Summary of Vesting Schedules

***The top-heavy schedules (3 year cliff or 6 year graded) are the maximum vesting schedules for all defined contribution plan contributions made on or after the first day of the 2007 plan year.

(continues)

Table 19-1 Comparison of Types of Tax-Qualified Retirement Plans (continued)

Summary of Vesting Schedules

Vesting Schedule	Immediate	2-Year Cliff	3-Year Cliff	5-Year Cliff	6-Year Graded	7-Year Graded
Year 1	100%				0	0
2		100%			20	0
3			100%		40	20
4					60	40
5				100%	80	60
6					100%	80
7						100%

Plan Elements	Profit-Sharing	401(k)	Cross-Tested Profit-Sharing	Money Purchase Pension	Defined Benefit	Comments
6. Distribution of Vested Benefits Upon:	Death	Death	Death	Death	Death	
	Disability	Disability	Disability	Disability	Disability	
	Retirement	Retirement	Retirement	Retirement	Retirement	
	Employment termination	Employment termination	Employment termination	Employment termination	Employment termination	
7. In-Service Distributions	Yes	Hardship Age 59 1/2	Yes	Only upon attainment of plan's normal retirement age or age 62	Only upon attainment of plan's normal retirement age or age 62	Profit-sharing plans may permit in-service distributions as an optional provision. IRS regulations define the events qualifying for hardship distributions from 401(k) plans. Hardship distributions are limited to participant elective deferrals. In-service distributions from all plans must commence at age 70 1/2.
8. Benefits Subject to PBGC Coverage	No	No	No	No	Yes	
9. Participant Individual Accounts	Yes	Yes	Yes	Yes	No	

Table 19-1 Comparison of Types of Tax-Qualified Retirement Plans (continued)

Plan Elements	Profit-Sharing	401(k)	Cross-Tested Profit-Sharing	Money Purchase Pension	Defined Benefit	Comments
10. Plan Benefit at Retirement or Other Termination of Employment	Vested account balance (employer and employee contributions, forfeitures, and investment gains and losses)	Vested account balance	Vested account balance	Vested account balance	Vested accrued benefit based on plan benefit formula	Maximum annual benefit from defined benefit plan is lesser of 100% of average compensation or $195,000 (adjusted by cost of living).
11. Plan Contributions/ Benefits Weighted in Favor of Older and/or Long Service Employees	No	No	Yes	No	Yes	Contributions under a defined contribution plan (other than a cross-tested profit-sharing or a target benefit plan) are generally allocated based on a participant's compensation, without regard to age or service (e.g., a 50-year-old employee with 20 years of service and a 30-year-old employee with 5 years of service will receive the same contribution if they have the same compensation). Cross-tested and target benefit plans take the participant's age into account and test contributions for nondiscrimination purposes based on future projected benefits.
12. Level of Benefits Paid to Participants Is Affected by Plan's Investment Performance	Yes	Yes	Yes	Yes	No	In a defined contribution plan, income, expenses, gains, and losses with respect to plan investments affect the value of the participants' individual accounts. In a defined benefit plan, investment income and the like affect the funding standard account only—not the ultimate amount of benefits paid to an individual participant.

Table 19-2	**Retirement Plan Dollar and Percentage Limits**					
	2007 ($)	**2008 ($)**	**2009 ($)**	**2010 ($)**	**2011 ($)**	**2012 ($)**
Annual compensation for plan purposes (for plan years beginning in calendar year) 401(a)(17)	225,000 indexed in 5,000 increments	230,000	245,000	245,000	245,000	250,000
Defined benefit plan, basic limit (for limitation years ending in calendar year) 415(b)	180,000 indexed in 5,000 increments	185,000	195,000	195,000	195,000	200,000
Defined contribution plan, basic limit (for limitation years ending in calendar year) 415(c)	45,000 indexed in 1,000 increments	46,000	49,000	49,000	49,000	50,000
401(k) / 403(b) plan, elective deferrals (for taxable years beginning in calendar year) 402(g)	15,500 indexed in 500 increments	15,500	16,500	16,500	16,500	17,000
457 plan, elective deferrals (for taxable years beginning in calendar year)	15,500 indexed in 500 increments	15,500	16,500	16,500	16,500	17,000
401(k) / 403(b) / 457, catch-up deferrals (for taxable years beginning in calendar year) (Age 50+) 414(v)	5,000 indexed in 500 increments	5,000	5,500	5,500	5,500	5,500
SIMPLE plan, elective deferrals (for calendar years) 408(p)	10,500 indexed in 500 increments	10,500	11,500	11,500	11,500	11,500
SIMPLE plan, catch-up deferrals (for taxable years beginning in calendar year) (Age 50+) 408(p)	2,500 indexed in 500 increments	2,500	2,500	2,500	2,500	2,500
Defined contribution plan §415 percentage of compensation contribution limit 415(c)	100% of compensation					
Profit sharing plan §404 percentage of compensation deduction limit	25% of compensation					
Elective deferrals	Do not count against §404 deduction limits					
SEP contribution / deduction limit 408(k)	25% of compensation					
IRA contribution limit 408(a)	4,000	5,000	5,000	5,000	5,000	5,000
IRA catch-up contribution (Age 50+)	1,000	1,000	1,000	1,000	1,000	1,000
Highly Compensated Employee 414(q)	100,000	105,000	110,000	110,000	110,000	115,000
SEP Coverage 408(p)	500	500	550	550	550	550
FICA Covered Compensation	97,500	102,000	106,800	106,800	106,800	110,100
PBGC Maximum Monthly Insured Benefit			4,500	4,500	4,500	

Table 19-3	State-By-State Analysis of Individual Retirement Accounts as Exempt Property*			
State	State Statute	IRA Exempt	Roth IRA Exempt	Special Statutory Provisions
Alabama	Ala. Code §19-3-1(b)	Yes	No	
Alaska	Alaska Stat. §09.38.017	Yes	Yes	The exemption does not apply to amounts contributed within 120 days before the debtor files for bankruptcy.
Arizona	Ariz. Rev. Stat. Ann. §33-1126(B)	Yes	Yes	The exemption does not apply to a claim by an alternate payee under a QDRO. The interest of an alternate payee is exempt from claims by creditors of the alternate payee. The exemption does not apply to amounts contributed within 120 days before a debtor files for bankruptcy.
Arkansas	Ark. Code Ann. §16-66-220	Yes	Yes	A bankruptcy court held that the creditor exemption for IRAs violates the Arkansas Constitution—at least with respect to contract claims.
California	Cal. Code of Civ. Proc. §704.115	No	No	IRAs are exempt only to the extent necessary to provide for the support of the judgment debtor when the judgment debtor retires and for the support of the spouse and dependents of the judgment debtor, taking into account all resources that are likely to be available for the support of the judgment debtor when the judgment debtor retires.
Colorado	Colo. Rev. Stat. §13-54-102	Yes	Yes	Any retirement benefit or payment is subject to attachment or levy in satisfaction of a judgment taken for arrears in child support; any pension or retirement benefit is also subject to attachment or levy in satisfaction of a judgment awarded for a felonious killing.
Connecticut	Conn. Gen. Stat. §52-321a	Yes	Yes	
Delaware	Del. Code Ann. Tit. 10, §4915	Yes	Yes	An IRA is not exempt from a claim made pursuant to Title 13 of the Delaware Code, which pertains to domestic relations order.
Florida	Fla. Stat. Ann. §222.21	Yes	Yes	An IRA is not exempt from claim of an alternate payee under a QDRO or claims of a surviving spouse pursuant to an order determining the amount of elective share and contribution.
Georgia	Ga. Code Ann. §44-13-100	No	No	IRAs are exempt only to the extent necessary for the support of the debtor and any dependent.
Hawaii	Haw. Rev. Stat. §651-124	Yes	Yes	The exemption does not apply to contributions made to a plan or arrangement within 3 years before the date a civil action is initiated against the debtor.
Idaho	Idaho Code §55-1011	Yes	Yes	The exemption only applies for claims of judgment creditors of the beneficiary or participant arising out of a negligent or otherwise wrongful act or omission of the beneficiary or participant resulting in money damages to the judgment creditor.
Illinois	Ill. Rev. Stat. Ch. 735, Para. 5/12-1006	Yes	Yes	

(continues)

Table 19-3 **State-By-State Analysis of Individual Retirement Accounts as Exempt Property* (continued)**

State	State Statute	IRA Exempt	Roth IRA Exempt	Special Statutory Provisions
Indiana	Ind. Code §34-55-10-2	Yes	Yes	
Iowa	Iowa Code §627.6	Yes	Yes	
Kansas	Kan. Stat. Ann. §60-2308	Yes	Yes	
Kentucky**	Ky. Rev. Stat. Ann. §427.150(2)(f)	Yes	Yes	The exemption does not apply to any amounts contributed to an IRA if the contribution occurred within 120 days before the debtor filed for bankruptcy. The exemption also does not apply to the right or interest of a person in an IRA to the extent that right or interest is subject to a court order for payment of maintenance or child support.
Louisiana	La. Rev. Stat. Ann. Sects. 20-33(1) and 13-3881(D)	Yes	Yes	No contribution to an IRA is exempt if made less than one calendar year from the date of filing bankruptcy, whether voluntary or involuntary, or the date writs of seizure are filed against the account. The exemption also does not apply to liabilities for alimony and child support.
Maine	Me. Rev. Stat. Ann. Tit. 14, §4422(13) (E)	No	No	IRAs are exempt only to the extent reasonably necessary for the support of the debtor and any dependent.
Maryland	Md. Code Ann. Cts. & Jud. Proc. §11-504(h)	Yes	Yes	IRAs are exempt from any and all claims of creditors of the beneficiary or participant other than claims by the Department of Health and Mental Hygiene.
Massachusetts	Mass. Gen. L.Ch. 235, §34A	Yes	Yes	The exemption does not apply to an order of court concerning divorce, separate maintenance, or child support, or an order of court requiring an individual convicted of a crime to satisfy a monetary penalty or to make restitution, or sums deposited in a plan in excess of 7% of the total income of the individual within 5 years of the individual's declaration of bankruptcy or entry of judgment.
Michigan**	Mich. Comp. Laws 600.6023	Yes	Yes	The exemption does not apply to amounts contributed to an individual retirement account or individual retirement annuity if the contribution occurs within 120 days before the debtor files for bankruptcy. The exemption also does not apply to an order of the domestic relations court.
Minnesota	Minn. Stat. §550.37	Yes	Yes	Exempt to a present value of $30,000 and additional amounts reasonably necessary to support the debtor, spouse, or dependents.
Mississippi	Miss. Code Ann. §85-3-1	Yes	No	
Missouri	Mo. Rev. Stat. §513.430	Yes	Yes	If proceedings under Title 11 of U.S. Code are commenced by or against the debtor, no amount of funds shall be exempt in such proceedings under any plan or trust that is fraudulent as defined in §456.630 of the Missouri Code, and for the period such person participated within 3 years prior to the commencement of such proceedings.
Montana	Mont. Code Ann. §31-2-106(3)	Yes	No	The exemption excludes that portion of contributions made by the individual within 1 year before the filing of the petition of bankruptcy that exceeds 15% of the gross income of the individual for that 1-year period.

Table 19-3	State-By-State Analysis of Individual Retirement Accounts as Exempt Property* (continued)			

State	State Statute	IRA Exempt	Roth IRA Exempt	Special Statutory Provisions
Nebraska	Neb. Rev. Stat. §25-1563.01	No	No	The debtor's right to receive IRAs and Roth IRAs is exempt to the extent reasonably necessary for the support of the debtor and any dependent of the debtor.
Nevada	Nev. Rev. Stat. §21.090(1)(r)	Yes	No	The exemption is limited to $500,000 in present value held in an IRA that conforms with §408.
New Hampshire	N.H. Tit. 52 §511:2	Yes	Yes	Exemption only applies to extensions of credit and debts arising after January 1, 1999.
New Jersey	N.J. Stat. Ann. 25:2-1(b)	Yes	Yes	
New Mexico	N.M. Stat. Ann. §42-10-1, §42-10-2	Yes	Yes	A retirement fund of a person supporting him- or herself or another person is exempt from receivers or trustees in bankruptcy or other insolvency proceedings, fines, attachment, execution, or foreclosure by a judgment creditor.
New York	N.Y. Civ. Prac. L. and R. §5205(c)	Yes	Yes	Additions to IRAs are not exempt from judgments if contributions were made after a date that is 90 days before the interposition of the claim on which the judgment was entered.
North Carolina	N.C. Gen. Stat. §1C-1601(a)(9)	Yes	Yes	
North Dakota	N.D. Cent. Code §28-22-03.1(3)	Yes	Yes	The account must have been in effect for a period of at least 1 year. Each individual account is exempt to a limit of up to $100,000 per account, with an aggregate limitation of $200,000 for all accounts. The dollar limit does not apply to the extent the debtor can prove the property is reasonably necessary for the support of the debtor, spouse, or dependents.
Ohio**	Ohio Rev. Code Ann. §2329.66(A)(10)	Yes	Yes	SEPs and SIMPLE IRAs are not exempt.
Oklahoma	Okla. Stat. Tit. 31, §1(A)(20)	Yes	Yes	
Oregon	OR. Rev. Stat. 18.358	Yes	Yes	
Pennsylvania	42 PA. Cons. Stat. §8124	Yes	Yes	The exemption does not apply to amounts contributed to the retirement fund in excess of $15,000 within 1 year before the debtor filed for bankruptcy.
Rhode Island	R.I. Gen. Laws §9-26-4	Yes	Yes	The exemption does not apply to an order of court pursuant to a judgment of divorce or separate maintenance, or an order of court concerning child support.
South Carolina	S.C. Code Ann. §15-41-30	No	No	The debtor's right to receive IRAs and Roth IRAs is exempt to the extent reasonably necessary for the support of the debtor and any dependent of the debtor.
South Dakota	S.D. Cod. Laws 43-45-16; 43-45-17	Yes	Yes	Exempts "certain retirement benefits" up to $1 million. Cites §401(a)(13) of the IRC (Tax-Qualified Plan Non-Alienation Provision). Subject to the right of the State of South Dakota and its political subdivisions to collect any amount owed to them.

(continues)

Table 19-3	State-By-State Analysis of Individual Retirement Accounts as Exempt Property* (continued)			
State	**State Statute**	**IRA Exempt**	**Roth IRA Exempt**	**Special Statutory Provisions**
Tennessee**	Tenn. Code Ann. §26-2-105	Yes	Yes	
Texas	Tex. Prop. Code Ann. §42.0021	Yes	Yes	
Utah	Utah Code Ann. §78-23-5(1)	Yes	Yes	The exemption does not apply to amounts contributed or benefits accrued by or on behalf of a debtor within 1 year before the debtor files for bankruptcy.
Vermont	Vt. Stat. Ann. Tit. 12 §2740(16)	Yes	Yes	Nondeductible traditional IRA contributions plus earnings are not exempt.
Virginia	Va. Code Ann. §34-34	Yes	Yes	Exempt from creditor process to the same extent permitted under federal bankruptcy law. An IRA is not exempt from a claim of child or spousal support obligations.
Washington	Wash. Rev. Code §6.15.020	Yes	Yes	
West Virginia	W.Va. Code §38-10-4	Yes	No	
Wisconsin	Wis. Stat. §815.18(3)(j)	Yes	Yes	The exemption does not apply to an order of court concerning child support, family support or maintenance, or any judgments of annulment, divorce, or legal separation.
Wyoming	Wyo. Stat. §1-20-110	No	No	

* Under the Bankruptcy Abuse Prevention and Consumer Protection Act of 2005 (BAPCPA), qualified plan, SEP, and SIMPLE assets are protected with no dollar limitation. IRAs and Roth IRAs are protected to $1,000,000. However, rollover assets in an IRA are not subject to the $1,000,000 limit BAPCPA only applies to assets in bankruptcy. One must look to state law for protection of IRA assets in state law (*e.g.*, garnishment) actions or other creditor claims outside of bankruptcy.
** Kentucky, Michigan, Ohio, and Tennessee: The U.S. Court of Appeals for the Sixth Circuit ruled in *Lampkins v. Golden*, 2002 U.S. App. LEXIS 900, 2002-1 USTC par. 50,216 (6th Cir. 2002) that a Michigan statute exempting SEPs and IRAs from creditor claims was preempted by ERISA. The decision appears, however, to be limited to SEPs and SIMPLE IRAs.

Table 19-4 **Comparison of Tax-Qualified Fringe Benefit Plans**

Plan Elements	Group Term Life Insurance IRC §79	Dependent Care Assistance IRC §129	Educational Assistance IRC §127	Health Insurance IRC §§105 & 106	Health Benefits IRC §105(h)
1. Excludable Employees:					
(a) Service Less Than…	3 Years	1 Year	None	Any	3 Years
(b) Union Coverage	Yes	Yes	Yes	Yes	Yes
(c) Part-Time or Seasonal	Yes (20 hours per week/5 months per year)	No	No	Yes	Yes (25–35 hours per week/9 months per year)
(d) Under Age …	None	21 Years	None	Any	25 Years
2. Discrimination Testing:	(a) 70% of all employees; or (b) 85% of participants are not key employees. Plus special rules for employers with less than 10 employees.	Average benefits to NHCEs are at least 55% of HCE benefits and no more than 25% of total benefits go to 5% owners, their spouses, and dependents.	No more than 5% of the total benefits paid to 5% owners, their spouse, and dependents.	N/A	(a) 70% or more of all employees receive benefits; or (b) 80% of eligible employees receive benefits if 70% of all employees are eligible.
3. Penalty for Discrimination as to:					
(a) Benefits	Key employees receive no exclusion; key employees include in income the higher of actual premium or table amount in regulations.	HCEs take entire benefit into income.	HCEs take benefits into income.	N/A	HCEs take into income the excess reimbursements they receive over the NHCEs' benefits.
(b) Coverage	Key employees receive no exclusion; key employees include in income the higher of actual premium or table amount in regulations.			N/A	HCEs take into income a portion of their reimbursement multiplied by a ratio in which all HCE reimbursements bear to total benefits paid under the plan.
4. Maximum Tax-Free Benefit If Plan Nondiscriminatory:	$50,000 term life insurance policy	$5,000	$5,250	N/A	N/A

Table 19-5	Key Ages for Social Security and Retirement Plans
Age 49 and Younger	Individuals covered under 401(k) plans could contribute up to $17,000 in 2012
Age 50	Employees age 50 or older may make catch-up contributions. These employees could contribute an additional $5,500 into a 401(k) plan in 2012 for a total of $22,500.
Age 55	If the employee terminates employment from his or her employer after attaining his or her fifty-fifth birthday, he or she can begin to take penalty-free distributions from the employer's 401(k) plan or other tax-qualified retirement plan at this age. Distributions from tax-qualified retirement plans are still taxed as ordinary income, but the additional 10% tax on distributions prior to age 59 1/2 will not apply.
Age 59 1/2	IRA withdrawals are permitted without penalty and are taxed as ordinary income. 401(k) plans may also permit in-service withdrawals (by current employees) at age 59 1/2.
Age 62	Social Security begins, but benefits will be reduced by 25% to 35% if benefits are received at age 62. If the beneficiary also continues to work while receiving Social Security benefits prior to full retirement age, his or her Social Security benefits will be reduced by 50 cents for each dollar earned above $14,640 in 2012.
Age 65	Medicare eligibility begins. Beneficiaries may sign up for Medicare Part B during a 7-month window that begins 3 months before the month of their sixty-fifth birthday and ends 3 months after such month. It is important to sign up for Medicare Part B promptly because the monthly premium increases 10% for each 12-month period in which a person was eligible for Medicare Part B but did not enroll. If the beneficiary or spouse is still employed and covered by a group health plan after age 65, he or she has 6 months to enroll in Medicare Part B after that person leaves the job before the penalty kicks in.
Age 66	This is the year that individuals born between 1943 and 1954 are eligible to receive full Social Security retirement benefits. For those born between 1955 and 1959, the full retirement age gradually increases from age 66 and 2 months to 66 and 10 months. The month a person reaches his or her full retirement age, Social Security benefits are no longer reduced if he or she continues to earn income from working.
Age 67	For those born in 1960 or later, the age at which they can receive full Social Security retirement benefits is age 67.
Age 70	Social Security benefits will increase by 8% for each year a person delays receiving benefits up until age 70. After age 70 there is no additional incentive to delay collecting Social Security benefits.
Age 70 1/2	At age 70 1/2, individuals must begin to receive required minimum distributions from IRAs and, in most cases, employer retirement plans. Non-5% owners in employer-sponsored retirement plans may delay distributions until the later of age 70 1/2 or the date of their actual retirement. The amount of the required minimum distribution is calculated by dividing the balance of the IRA and employer-sponsored retirement plan accounts by the person's life expectancy as determined by Treasury Regulations under the Uniform Distribution Table. Individuals who fail to receive the required minimum distributions are assessed a 50% penalty on the amount that should have been distributed. For 2009 only, required minimum distributions could be skipped without penalty.

Table 19-6	COBRA Continuation Coverage Requirements COBRA IRC §4980B
What the law does	Requires an employer to provide an employee or his or her covered dependents with the option to extend group coverage under health insurance plans and contracts for any participant who would otherwise lose coverage for virtually *any* reason.
Which employers must comply	Employers with 20 or more employees in the preceding year; government and church plans are exempt.
Which individuals have continuation coverage under the law?	Each "qualified beneficiary" is covered by the law. Qualified beneficiaries are those individuals covered by the plan (even for 1 day) who are: 1. Widowed spouses and dependent children 2. Employees (and their spouses and dependent children) who have been terminated (voluntarily, except for gross misconduct) or have had their hours reduced 3. Divorced or separated spouses and their legal dependents 4. Medicare-ineligible spouses and their dependent children 5. Dependent children no longer meeting the plan's definition of dependent children

What is the duration of continuation coverage?	1. Coverage for 18 months from termination date for employees or 18 months from date hours are reduced below plan eligibility.
	 2. Coverage for 29 months if employee is disabled at time of termination or reduction of hours or during 18-month continuation coverage period.
	 3 Coverage for 36 months for:
	   (a) Widowed spouse and dependent children
	   (b) Divorced or legally separated spouse and dependent children
	   (c) Medicare-ineligible spouse
	   (d) Dependent children who no longer meet plan's eligibility
	 4. Coverage by another group health plan will terminate COBRA coverage during the continuation coverage period only if the new plan does not contain a preexisting condition exclusion or limitation that applies to the qualified beneficiary.

Employee contribution to cost of coverage	Employer may require the employee or qualified beneficiary to pay up to 102% of the cost to the employer for identical coverage for similar individuals covered by the employer-paid plan. Qualified beneficiary may elect to pay contribution monthly. For disabled employees, employer may charge 150% of premium for the nineteenth through twenty-ninth months of coverage.
Employer notification requirements	1. Notice must be given to every covered employee and his or her spouse at the time the law takes effect. 2. New employee and his or her spouse must get notice when coverage commences. 3. Notice must be given within 14 days to every qualified beneficiary when they actually become eligible for continuation coverage, and the option to continue coverage must last at least 60 days after the latter of the eligibility date or notification date.

References

1. IRC §404(a).
2. IRC. §402(a).
3. IRC §501(a).
4. Treas. Reg. §1.401-1(b)(2).
5. IRC §401(k)(3)(A).
6. IRC §414(q).
7. IRC §401(k)(12); IRS Notice 98-52; IRS Notice 2000-3.
8. IRS Notice 98-1.
9. IRS Notice 2000-3.
10. IRC §401(a)(8).
11. 26 CFR §1.401(a)(4)-8(b); Rev. Rul. 2001-30.
12. Treasury Regulation Section 1.401(a)(4)-8(b).
13. IRC §415(b).
14. IRC §403(b)(1)(A).
15. IRC §402(g).
16. IRC §403(b)(12)(A)(i).
17. IRC §403(b)(12)(A)(ii).
18. IRC §§403(b)(1), 403(b)(7), 403(b)(9).
19. IRC §403(b)(11).
20. Treas. Reg. §1.403(b)-3, Q & A-1.
21. IRC §§403(b)(8), 402(c).
22. IRC §457(a).
23. IRC §457(b).
24. IRC §457(f).
25. IRC §408(k).
26. IRC §408(k)(2). Prop. Regs. §1.408-7(d) and §1.219-3(b)(2).
27. IRC §408(k)(3)(C).
28. IRC §219(b)(2).
29. IRC §408(k)(6).
30. IRC §408(k)(6)(C).
31. IRC §408(p).
32. IRC §408(p)(2)(D)(I), as amended by the 1998 Act.
33. IRC §402(g)(3).
34. IRC §72(t).
35. 29 USC §1056(d)(1).
36. IRC §414(p).
37. Treas. Reg. §1.401(A)-13(B)(2).
38. IRC §401(a)(13)(C) and (D); ERISA §206(d)(4) and (5).
39. Code §401(a)(1); Treas. Reg. §1.401-1(b).
40. Code §401(a)(2); Treas. Reg. §1.401-2.
41. 11 USC §522(b)(4)(D).
42. ERISA §§4(b) and 201; IRC §401(a); 29 CFR §2510.3-2(d).
43. ERISA §404(c).
44. 29 CFR §2550.404c-1.
45. IRC §72(p); IRC §4975(d)(1); ERISA §408(b)(1).
46. IRC §4975(d)(1); ERISA §408(b)(1).
47. IRC §72(p).
48. Reg. §1.72(p)-1, Q&A-10(a).
49. Prop. Reg. §1.125-2, Q. and A.-4d.
50. Prop. Reg. §1.125-2, Q. and A.-4(a)(2)(iii).
51. IRC §125(d)(1)(A).
52. Prop. Reg. §1.125-1, Q. and A.-4.
53. IRC §125(g)(3)(B).
54. Reg. §1.125-1 Q. and A.-4.
55. Prop. Reg. §1.125-1, Q. and A.-5 and 6.
56. Prop. Reg. §1.125-1, Q. and A.-16.
57. Prop. Reg. §1.125-2, Q. and A.-2.
58. Prop. Reg. §1.125-1, Q. and A.-14.
59. Prop. Reg. §1.125-2, Q. and A.-6.
60. Prop. Reg. §1.125-2, Q. and A.-6(b).
61. Reg. §1.125-4.
62. IRC §3121(a)(5)(G), IRC §3306(b)(5)(G).
63. IRC §125(d)(2)(A).
64. Prop. Reg. §1.125-2, Q. and A.-5(a).
65. Prop. Reg. §1.125-2, Q. and A.-5(b).
66. Prop. Reg. §1.125-2, Q. and A.-5(c).
67. Prop. Reg. §1.125-2 Q. and A.05(c)(2).
68. IRC §125(d)(2)(B).
69. Prop. Reg. §1.125-2, Q. and A.-4(c).
70. Prop. Reg. §1.125-1, Q. and A.-3; Prop. Reg. §1.125-2, Q. and A.-3.
71. Prop. Reg. §1.125-2, Q. and A.-7(c).
72. IRC §125(i), as amended by PPACA Pub. L. No. 111-148 (2010) and HCERA, Pub. L. No. 111-152 (2010).
73. Prop. Reg. §1.125-2, Q. and A.-7(a).
74. Prop. Reg. §1.125-2, Q. and A.-7(b)(2) and (3).
75. Prop. Reg. §1.125-2, Q. and A.-7(b)(5) and (6).
76. IRC §106(f), as added by PPACA, Pub. L. No. 111-148 (2010).
77. Prop. Reg. §1.125-2, Q. and A.-7(b)(7).
78. Prop. Reg. §1.125-2, Q. and A.-7(b)(8).
79. IRC §125(b).
80. Prop. Reg. §1.125-1, Q. and A.-10.
81. IRC §125(b)(1).
82. IRC §125(e).
83. IRC §125(b)(3).
84. Prop. Reg. §1.125.1, Q. and A.-11.
85. IRC §125(g)(3).
86. IRC §125g(2).
87. IRC §125(b)(2) and (3).
88. IRC §125(g)(1).
89. IRC §125(g)(4).
90. Reg. §1.125-3, Q. and A.-1.
91. Reg. §1.125-3, Q. and A.-3.
92. Reg. §1.125-3, Q. and A.-4.
93. Reg. §1.125-3, Q. and A.-7.
94. Code 5105(b), as amended by Reconciliation Act Section 1004(d).
95. IRC §79(d)(3)(B).
96. IRC §79(d)(3)(A).
97. Reg. §1.79-1(c)(2)(i).
98. Reg. §1.79-1(c)(2)(ii); Rev. Rul. 80-220.
99. Reg. §1.79-(c)(2)(iii).
100. Reg. §1.79-1(c)(4).
101. IRC §3121(a)(2).
102. IRS Notice 88-82.
103. IRC §6052; Reg. §1.6052-1(a).
104. Temp. Reg. §1.125-2T, Q. and A.-1(a).
105. PHSA §2716, as added and amended by PPACA, Pub. L. No. 111–148 (2010).
106. Reg. §1.105-11(c)(2)(iii).
107. Reg. §1.105-11(c)(2)(ii).
108. IRC §105(h)(5).
109. Reg. §1.105-11(c)(3).
110. IRC §129.
111. IRC §129(d)(9).
112. IRC §129(d)(8).
113. IRC §129(d)(4).
114. Reg. §1.44A-1(b)(4).
115. IRC §129(d)(7).
116. IRC §127.
117. Reg. §54.498B-6, Q. and A.-4.

Medical Malpractice: An Explanation and Analysis

Chris Morrison, Esq.
Julie M. Brightwell, BSN, JD, CPHRM
Dan Bucsko, MBA, MHA, FACHE, CMPE, CPHRM
Susan Shephard, MSN, CPHRM
Darrell Ranum, JD, CPHRM

Despite a physician's best efforts, he or she may become a defendant in a medical malpractice lawsuit. Medical malpractice has received a great deal of attention. Rising medical malpractice premiums have brought this cause of action to the fore, and have spurred efforts to reform medical malpractice in the United States, at both the state and federal level. However, despite this attention, there have not been nearly as much public discussion of what the cause of action itself entails, and the ramifications it has for physicians who find themselves in the middle of a malpractice lawsuit. This chapter broadly discusses what the medical malpractice cause of action involves, from both a theoretical perspective and a practical perspective; its consequences for the physician; insurance issues; and reform.

The Cause of Action for Medical Malpractices

Medical malpractice essentially is a cause of action for negligence, which generally is an action for the failure to act with reasonable care. As part of a medical malpractice action, a plaintiff must prove four specific elements: (1) the physician owed a duty of care to the plaintiff; (2) the physician breached that duty of care; (3) the plaintiff suffered injuries; and (4) the physician's breach of duty was the cause of the plaintiff's injuries. Although all of these factors are important, the two that place the actions of the physician under the closest scrutiny are whether a duty was owed to the plaintiff and whether the care rendered was in accordance with the prevailing professional standard of care for physicians.

In the medical malpractice context, whether the physician owes a duty to the plaintiff depends on the formation of the physician–patient relationship, which is technically a legal issue but depends highly on the specific facts of a given case. Once the physician–patient relationship is established, the physician has a certain duty to the patient, which is typically expressed as providing medical services in accordance with the prevailing professional "standard of care." The standard of care is the touchstone of most medical malpractice actions. The physician must be shown to have fallen short of the standard of care to establish a breach of duty. Next, the plaintiff must show that the breach of the duty owed to him or her as a patient caused harm. Finally, the plaintiff is required to prove the amount of damages, although certain types of damages are not subject to the same mathematical or economic calculus as others.

■ The Physician–Patient Relationship

If a physician has no duty to a given individual, then that individual cannot have a cause of action against a physician for malpractice. A physician's duty to a patient first arises at the formation of the physician–patient relationship, and ends when the relationship is terminated. The termination of the physician–patient relationship has its own set of pitfalls, including a physician's improper termination of the physician–patient relationship.

Formation of the Physician–Patient Relationship

Formation of the physician–patient relationship is a crucial issue, and is particularly important because of how medical malpractice actions typically name defendants. The plaintiff in a medical malpractice action will frequently cast a "dragnet" with the complaint, naming as many potential defendants as possible and containing as many theories of liability as possible in the hope that at least one of the people or entities named will either settle to get out of the case early or will actually be the party responsible for the malpractice, if there is any. A physician might be named because of one of the following circumstances: a brief conversation with another physician, being the physician on the on-call roster at the time of the alleged malpractice, or otherwise being incidentally involved in a given case. However, without the existence of a physician–patient relationship, a physician cannot legitimately be held liable for an injury suffered by a patient due to alleged malpractice.

The formation of the physician–patient relationship is also a subject of particular concern to on-call physicians, or physicians who are contacted on an informal basis for a quick professional opinion or suggestion about a patient's condition or a particular course of action. There are physicians who have expressed and demonstrated reluctance to answer pages or phone calls that they know are from an emergency room or hospital floor, for fear that by answering that page or call, they are exposing themselves to liability for anything that might happen to the patient before they get there. In other cases, even physicians who are not on call are reluctant to give informal advice to a colleague, for fear that they will be held liable if something happens to go wrong in the course of the patient's care.

The formation of the physician–patient relationship is a legal issue, but is highly dependent on the facts of a given case. In general, the physician–patient relationship is a consensual relationship in which the patient knowingly seeks the physician's assistance and in which the physician knowingly accepts the person as a patient. A consensual relationship can be found to exist where a physician contacts another physician on behalf of the patient, or where a physician accepts a referral of a patient, the reasoning being that the consent of the patient to the service provided by the second physician is implied.

The formation of a physician–patient relationship frequently depends on the degree and nature of the physician's involvement. Simply being on call, or even giving general advice regarding a medical condition or course of treatment, will not necessarily be enough to establish a physician–patient relationship for the purpose of affixing liability for medical malpractice. There are cases that state explicitly that simply being on call in itself is not sufficient to establish a physician–patient relationship for the purpose of medical malpractice liability. For example, in a Michigan case, a resident in the emergency room of a hospital contacted the ear, nose, and throat specialist (ENT) who was on call.[1] The ENT informed the resident that he didn't feel well, could not come in to see the patient, and to contact another physician to see that patient. The patient later filed a medical malpractice action that named, among other defendants, the on-call ENT. The court found that the patient could not maintain a malpractice lawsuit against the ENT because no physician–patient relationship had been formed. There are other cases in which the courts found no physician–patient relationship, such as when an emergency room physician contacted an on-call physician who did not come in to the hospital,[a] or when he or she received general advice and recommendations from the on-call physician or other physicians.[b]

On the other hand, there are cases in which consultations that the physician believed or contended to be merely "informal" were found to give rise to a physician–patient relationship sufficient to support the duty of care to the patient, or were at least found to present a sufficient

---

a. This is certainly not meant as a recommendation to refuse to come in when on call. Under federal law, physicians who fail to respond to call in the context of an emergency may be subject to civil monetary penalties up to $50,000, as well as exclusion from the Medicare, Medicaid, and other publicly funded health programs. See 42 U.S.C. § 1395dd(d)(1)(B), (C). Failing to take call can also result in action against a physician's privileges by the medical staff or the hospital's board.

b. See, e.g., *Irvin v. Smith* (S.Ct.Kan. 2001) 31 P.3d 934.

basis in fact for a jury to determine that such a relationship existed between the physician and the patient. For example, in one such case a cardiologist consulted with an emergency room physician on a patient presenting with severe chest pain.[2] The cardiologist was not the on-call cardiologist for the emergency room at that time. However, he briefly discussed the patient's case with an emergency room physician, during which time he was presented with the patient's clinical history and results of her physical examination, reviewed the EKG results of the patient, and made certain conclusions regarding course of treatment and appropriateness of discharge.

The cardiologist contended that this consultation was merely informal, and therefore he had no duty of care to the patient. However, the court determined that these facts established a physician–patient relationship between the cardiologist and the patient, even though there was no direct relationship between the cardiologist and the patient. The court noted that the cardiologist was in a unique position to prevent future harm to the patient because of knowledge and experience superior to that of the emergency room physician insofar as the diagnosis of a heart condition was concerned, and paid particular attention to the degree of involvement in the case. The court stated that this was not an informal exchange of information where one physician was acting merely as a resource for another. Rather, this was a situation where the treating physician was not in a position to accept or reject the advice of the cardiologist; he subordinated his judgment to that of the cardiologist in determining diagnosis, treatment, and disposition, and clearly relied on the cardiologist's advice. Under these circumstances, the court concluded that the cardiologist owed the patient a duty of care in rendering medical advice regarding the patient's diagnosis and treatment.

In another case, a court found there was evidence that could support a jury finding that a physician–patient relationship existed, again without a direct relationship and under the assertion that the consultation was "informal."[3] In this case, a cardiologist was assessing a patient with two blocked coronary arteries. An angiogram had been performed on the patient, but the cardiologist was not trained to read angiograms, nor did he perform angioplasty as part of his practice. The angiogram was ultimately submitted to two interventional cardiologists who reviewed the angiogram and who transmitted a message back to the cardiologist that the patient was a candidate for angioplasty. The patient was scheduled for angioplasty and died during the procedure.

In defending the lawsuit that followed, the two interventional cardiologists argued in part that they had no physician–patient relationship with the decedent, and therefore owed him no duty of care. However, the court found that there were genuine issues of fact as to whether the interventional cardiologists had been asked to render a service for the patient by interpreting test results (i.e., the angiogram), and determining the suitability of angioplasty to be performed on the patient. The court also mentioned the fact that the interventional cardiologists had an in-person conference with the patient's cardiologist to review the patient's history and decide on the appropriateness of the procedure. Therefore, there was enough evidence for a jury to reasonably conclude that the interventional cardiologists in the case had a physician–patient relationship that imposed a duty of care on them.

The formation of the physician–patient relationship depends on the degree and manner of involvement a physician has with a patient's case. On the one hand, merely being on call or being asked for general advice does not seem to support the formation of this relationship. However, when a physician undertakes to direct the care of a patient, then the establishment of the relationship seems fairly clear. Nevertheless, unless the facts clearly demonstrate that the physician never formed a relationship with a patient that imposed a duty on the physician, this will typically be decided by the jury. If a consultation goes beyond a mere "informal" exchange of information, then a physician–patient relationship may be found to exist.

Termination of the Physician–Patient Relationship

A patient or physician may want to end the physician–patient relationship for a variety of reasons. The most obvious, and hopefully the most common, is because the need for the relationship is now over. However, physicians often have other reasons for desiring to terminate their relationship with a patient, such as nonpayment, noncompliance, disruptive behavior, or personality conflict issues. A physician might also terminate a patient from his or her practice because that physician is no longer a contracted provider with that patient's HMO, or the patient is dropped from his or her insurance plan. Whatever the case may be, termination of the physician–patient relationship must generally have certain characteristics to make sure that: (1) the relationship has in fact been terminated, thus ending any continued duty to the patient as a physician, and (2) that a cause of action for abandonment of the patient does not arise.

In general, once the physician–patient relationship is established, the relationship continues until it is ended by the consent of the parties, is revoked by the dismissal of the physician, the physician's services are no longer needed, or the physician withdraws from the case.[c] A physician must give proper notice to the patient, and afford the patient the opportunity to procure other medical attendance.[d] Failure to do so may result in abandoning the patient. The physician should consult with an attorney and/or their medical professional liability carrier to understand what notice time is required in their state and also to receive guidance on the content of the letter and mailing procedures. Abandonment can be defined as the termination of the professional relationship between the physician and patient at an unreasonable time or without affording the patient the opportunity to procure an equally qualified replacement.[e]

Whether abandonment has taken place is a factual issue. For example, in one Michigan case, a patient was admitted for a cerclage when the physician told the patient he was not going to perform the procedure because the patient had filed a lawsuit against another physician.[f] The patient obtained the procedure from another physician 4 days later, but miscarried. In a somewhat less inflammatory case, a California court found that the termination of a patient from a medical practice while still in need of medical care, accompanied by a 2-week lapse between termination and securing medical care with another group practice, was sufficient to create a triable issue of fact as to whether the patient had been given ample time to retain other physicians.[g] In contrast, an Oklahoma court decided there was no factual support for an abandonment claim when a physician told a patient he would no longer treat her, but referred her to another physician that same day, gave the patient the names of several doctors in the relevant practice area, and even contacted them for her.[4,h]

---

c. See *Tierney v. Univ. of Mich. Regents* (Mich.Ct.App. 2003) 669 N.W.2d 575.

d. See *Church v. Perales* (Tenn.Ct.App. 2000) 39 S.W.3d 149.

e. See *Haidak v. Corso* (D.C.Ct.App. 2004) 841 A.2d 316.

f. Tierney, supra.

g. See *Scripps Clinic v. Superior Court of San Diego County* (2003) 108 Cal. App.4th 917.

h. Although more of a risk-management issue, physicians can minimize the risk of liability for abandonment by having (and following) clearly defined policies designed to give patients sufficient notice of termination of the relationship, adequate time to secure care from another physician, and even some degree of assistance with finding another physician. The American Medical Association has published what it considers appropriate steps to take in terminating the physician–patient relationship, available at http://www.ama-assn.org

■ The Standard of Care

The standard of care is a critical aspect of a medical malpractice action. Without proving the relevant standard of care, and that a physician failed to conduct him- or herself consistent with the standard of care, a malpractice action should fail, with only a few exceptions. The definition of the standard of care can vary, but generally reflects the concept of what an objectively reasonable physician in a similar situation would do, as explained further in the following section. The standard of care is almost always required to be established by expert testimony, except in a few cases where it is obvious to a person of reasonable experience what the standard of care is (such as cases of leaving surgical instruments inside a patient). The problem with the standard of care is that although it is typically meant to be an objective standard, it is frequently finessed into a subjective standard (i.e., what another physician would have done or believes should have been done differently than the physician who initially treated the patient, rather than what a similarly situated physician reasonably should have done).

Defining the Standard of Care

The standard of care may be defined as that which a reasonable and prudent member of the medical profession would undertake under the same or similar circumstances.[5] Another definition of the standard of care is that level of care, skill, and treatment which, in light of all relevant surrounding circumstances, is recognized as acceptable and appropriate by reasonably prudent similar healthcare providers.[6] The standard of care has also been defined as exercising the degree of care, diligence, and skill ordinarily possessed and exercised by a minimally competent and reasonably diligent, skillful, careful, and prudent physician in that physician's field of practice.

This standard is meant to be objective. In other words, the standard of care is supposed to depend on what a reasonable physician would have done under similar circumstances. Whether the physician in question took a course of action that he or she believed to be reasonable, or was in accordance with that physician's best judgment, is irrelevant to the standard of care. A physician may be genuinely convinced that a patient had a particular diagnosis or that a particular course of treatment was appropriate and carried out properly, but this does not mean that the course of action was what a reasonable and prudent member of their profession would have done under the same or similar circumstances. Additionally, another physician's subjective preferences or a mere difference of opinion is not necessarily indicative of the standard of care, although it is frequently advanced as such in the course of expert testimony.

Establishing the Standard of Care

The standard of care must almost always be established through the testimony of expert witnesses. There are exceptions to this rule where the malpractice is so obvious that the existence of medical malpractice can by determined by the jurors' common knowledge or experience.[i] Such cases might include wrong-site surgery or leaving surgical instruments inside a patient.[7] The rest of the time, however, the plaintiff must provide expert testimony to establish the standard of care and to show that the physician failed to meet the standard of care. These experts are typically other physicians from the same field of practice, and must meet certain criteria established by state law before they may testify as expert witnesses.

Qualifications and requirements for expert witnesses can vary. If the opinion is as to the standard of care, then the testifying expert must also be substantially familiar with the applicable standard of care for the specific care at issue at the time of the alleged breach; practice in the same subspecialty or a subspecialty with a substantially similar standard of care; and, in the event the defendant physician is board-certified, be certified by the same or a similar board. There are exceptions that may apply if the physician provided care outside his or her specialty, or if the court finds that the expert possesses sufficient training, experience, and knowledge to provide the testimony.

Other states can be more general or more particular in their qualifications and requirements for experts in medical malpractice cases. Nevada statute says simply that expert medical testimony in a case involving alleged medical negligence may only be given "by a provider of medical care who practices or had practiced in an area that is substantially similar to the type of practice engaged in at the time of the alleged negligence."[8] Obviously this is quite broad, and places a great amount of discretion with the judge to decide who may properly testify as an expert witness. Other states, such as Florida, are much more particular, setting forth specific criteria depending on whether the subject of the suit is a specialist, a general practitioner, neither a specialist nor a general practitioner, or an emergency room physician, and requiring specific amounts and types of experience.[j]

Although expert witnesses have to be able through education, training, and experience to testify as to certain matters in a medical malpractice case, there is no requirement that the witness be an "expert" in the general sense. An expert witness need not be the recognized authority on a particular procedure or in a particular specialty. In fact, the expert does not even need to be preeminent in his or her field of practice, or even be that good a doctor. As a strategic matter, attorneys on both sides will try to get experts with impressive credentials, because juries will generally review those credentials and decide who has more credibility in the "battle of the experts." However, such qualifications are not required, and not always pursued. This can be a frustrating experience for a physician who is being told that he or she failed to meet the standard of care by someone who may have less experience, or may not have gone to a medical school of equal prestige or quality.

Additionally, although expert testimony is supposed to address the theoretically objective issue of the standard of care, it can often substitute the subjective for the objective. Because medical malpractice actions are truly an exercise in 20-20 hindsight, the testimony will typically be applied to the standard of care in place at the time the care was delivered. In other words, the standard of care testimony will often be crafted around the facts of the particular case, as opposed to a standard articulated in advance and the facts compared thereafter. The testimony regarding standard of care has great potential for including the preferences and biases of the individual giving the testimony. Although an expert might not couch it in explicit terms, testimony as to the breach of the standard of care will often be about what the expert witness would have done differently, or what could have been done better. This is not necessarily consonant with the principle of the standard of care, which is supposed to be an objective determination of what a reasonably prudent similar physician would have done in like circumstances. During the course of a deposition or a trial, if the attorney is doing his or her job, the attorney will challenge and reduce the credibility of the expert's opinion, and try to show where the opinion relies on personal preference or bias, rather than the standard of care. Nevertheless, although expert testimony is typically required, and is supposed to provide evidence of an objective standard of care, there are subjective aspects that are inherent in having an individual person with his or her own set of training and experiences testify about the propriety of another physician's conduct.

The Locality Rule

Some states apply the locality rule in addition to other qualifications to determine if an expert witness will be allowed to testify. The locality rule says that an expert testifying against a physician has to practice or otherwise have

i. See *Valcin v. Public Health Trust* (Fla.Dist.Ct.App.1984) 473 So.2d 1297.
j. See, e.g., Fla. Stat. Section 766.

experience in the same or similar locality or community as the physician who is alleged to have committed malpractice. The logic underlying this rule is to prevent unfair comparisons between the standard of care in communities where resources and facilities might vastly differ.[k] The locality rule generally has not been applied to specialists, for which a great deal of standardization has taken place through board certification entities, and has been diluted or overruled in some jurisdictions. As medical knowledge and training have become more standardized, and communications technology has advanced, the locality rule has become of less relevance than in the past.

Hospital Bylaws, Policies, and Industry Standards

Although expert testimony is typically required to establish the standard of care, as well as its breach, there are other sources used as evidence of the standard of care. Items such as hospital bylaws,[l] state health regulations,[m] national standards,[n] other organizational bylaws,[o] internal manuals,[9] and professional society guidance[p] can be considered as evidence of the standard of care, and consequently as evidence of a breach of the standard of care. Such evidence is typically not considered to be sufficient in and of itself to establish the applicable standard of care, but it can be used for that purpose in connection with expert testimony.[q] These kinds of documents are particularly prominent in cases involving board-certified physicians, for whom their respective board authorities may have issued clinical practice guidelines or other material that may be relevant to the standard of care.

■ Breaching the Standard of Care

Without a breach of the physician's duty of care to the patient, the patient cannot recover damages. The breach of the standard of care will be the subject of expert testimony, just like the standard of care itself, and typically will be testified about by the same expert witnesses. The issue of

k. See *Birchfield v. Texarkana Memorial Hospital* (S.Ct.Tex. 1987) 747 S.W.2d 361.
l. See *Gathings v. Muscadin* (Ill.Ct.App. 2001) 743 N.E.2d 659.
m. See *Hernandez v. Nueces County Medical Society Community Blood Bank* (Tex.Ct.App. 1989) 779 S.W.2d 867.
n. Ibid.
o. Ibid.
p. See *Davenport v. Ephraim McDowell Memorial Hospital, Inc.* (Ky.Ct.App. 1989) 769 S.W.2d 56.
q. See, e.g., *Boland v. Garber* (S.Ct.Minn. 1977) 257 N.W.2d 384. (Hospital rules are admissible as evidence of standard of care in the community, but are not conclusive on the issue of negligence.)

breach is a comparison of the physician's actions against the objective standard of care that applied in that situation.

Theoretically, the mere existence of a medical injury does not create a presumption or inference of negligence against the healthcare provider. Under the law, a physician is not a warrantor of the outcome of a procedure or course of treatment. The plaintiff may argue that because there was an injury, there must have been malpractice. This is flawed logic, but is nevertheless a reality of a medical malpractice action and must be kept in mind. Additionally, in cases that present highly sympathetic plaintiffs, such as cases of injured children or any type of catastrophic injury, such as paralysis, juries may be more inclined to award damages to the plaintiff, simply because they conclude that the plaintiff needs to be taken care of monetarily, not necessarily because of any fault on the part of the physician.

Allegations for Breaches of the Standard of Care

Some common theories of medical malpractice include the failure to diagnose, failure to treat, failure to treat properly, and failure to refer or obtain a consult. There are almost innumerable variations of the facts that will be cited in support of a claim for failure to diagnose in breach of the standard of care: symptoms were misinterpreted; tests should have been ordered but weren't; tests were ordered but they were the wrong tests; the right tests were ordered, but they were misread; the tests were read correctly, but the wrong diagnosis was reached; the right diagnosis was reached, but in an untimely manner; and so on. Failure to obtain an appropriate medical history often accompanies failure to diagnose.

Causes of action based on treatment issues can follow a similar pattern of reasoning. The condition was diagnosed, but never treated; the condition was treated, but the treatment was negligently performed; the condition was treated, but a different treatment should have been applied; the condition was treated appropriately but ineffectively, and another course of treatment should have been substituted; the correct course of treatment was properly applied, but follow-up was inadequate. Another theory of failure to treat is that the physician masked the patient's symptoms with pain medication instead of providing "real" treatment.

The failure to call a specialty consult or make a specialty referral is yet another theory that bridges both diagnosis and treatment theories. The types of allegations might be that the patient should have been evaluated by a surgeon, but the consult or referral wasn't made; the physician was inexperienced in diagnosing or treating a particular disease or illness, and should have called a consult or referred to a specialist; or that the patient's symptoms or diagnosis were within the exclusive purview of a specialist. Not involving a specialist would have to be a breach of the standard of care in order to be properly actionable.

Theories of falling below the standard of care form the foundation of the plaintiff's case. Not adequately counseling a patient on preventive measures, such as diet and exercise, can be the subject of a lawsuit, as can failing to send a patient to a facility that does more of a particular type of test or procedure, and thus would be better at obtaining information. Other theories may involve the failure to provide genetic counseling or testing to pregnant patients, resulting in the birth of a defective child (although not every state allows this as a cause of action), or even discussing the pros and cons of certain testing or treatment rather than just ordering the test or insisting on the course of treatment. Although some theories of malpractice may not yet have a track record of success, plaintiffs' lawyers do continue to develop new and innovative ways to succeed with their cases.

■ Causation

A breach of the standard of care alone is insufficient to hold a physician liable for medical malpractice. One of the essential elements of the cause of action for medical malpractice is that the breach of the standard of care caused the patient's injuries. Although there are many nuances to the issue of causation, certain aspects are particularly important. Causation has to be established by a preponderance of the evidence (this is discussed in more detail in the section addressing burden of proof at trial), and is typically supplied through appropriate expert testimony. Testimony about causation has to be more than surmise, conjecture, or guesswork. For causation to be established, there must be testimony indicating that there is a reasonable medical probability or reasonable medical certainty that the course of action caused the plaintiff's injuries, or that a different course of action would have avoided the plaintiff's injuries. Causation has to be more than merely possible, it has to be probable. Therefore, even if plaintiffs can prove a breach, they should not be able to prevail in a medical malpractice case if they cannot demonstrate that the breach caused the injury.

■ Liability for the Actions of Others
Vicarious Liability
Vicarious liability is a legal doctrine that says a principal is liable for the negligence of an agent of that principal, when that agent is acting on the principal's behalf and within the scope of his or her duties as the agent of the principal. A principal can be a person or an entity, such as a professional association or other corporation. Agency can be actual, meaning there is a principal that explicitly authorizes another individual to act on the principal's behalf. It can also be apparent, in which a principal takes some kind of action that leads another person to reasonably believe that an individual is acting on that principal's behalf, and the person acts according to that reasonable belief. The plaintiff in a lawsuit will typically have to prove one of these two theories of agency to hold a person or entity liable for the actions of the alleged agent.

Vicarious liability will frequently be applied in cases involving hospital residents and "captive" specialties, such as emergency medicine and radiology. However, vicarious liability is also applied against professional associations or group practices. It is not uncommon to find a physician named as a defendant, along with the physician's group practice, professional association, ambulatory surgical center, or other such entity. Professional associations or group practices may have (or at least are thought to have) deeper pockets than any one individual physician, and therefore will likely be named on the malpractice complaint. This is one of the reasons why physicians typically, or at least should, have a liability insurance policy that covers their group in addition to any policy they carry for personal liability. Vicarious liability can also apply to hold a physician or physician group liable for the negligence of an employed healthcare professional, such as a physician's assistant, nurse practitioner, registered nurse, and the like. Thus, the employing entity is well-advised to have an insurance policy in place sufficient to cover any potential negligence by its employees, including nonphysicians.

Captain of the Ship/Borrowed Servant
Legal doctrines known as the "borrowed servant" or "captain of the ship" exist in some states, which can expose a physician to liability for the negligence of other healthcare professionals, even if those healthcare professionals are not the employees of the physician or the physicians' group or professional association.[r] This doctrine typically is applied in surgical cases, in which the operating room personnel are often employees or contractors of the hospital. The theory behind this doctrine is that the surgeon, as the controlling person in the operating room, has the ultimate responsibility for the care of the patient, and has a nondelegable duty to ensure that proper care is given in all circumstances. Thus, even though the surgeon performing the operation may not directly commit any

---

r. See, e.g., *Vargas v. Dulzaides* (Fla.Dist.Ct.App. 1988) 520 So.2d 306; *Thomas Intermedics Orthopedics* (1996) 47 Cal. App.4th 957; *Starcher v. Byrne* (S.Ct.Miss.1997) 687 So.2d 737; *Szabo v. Bryn Mawr Hospital* (Pa.Super.Ct. 1994) 638 A.2d 1004.

negligent acts, the surgeon may sometimes be held liable for the other practitioners assisting in the operation.

The borrowed servant doctrine is slightly different from the captain of the ship theory, but the end result can be the same. Under the borrowed servant doctrine, a "servant"—more contemporarily called an agent or employee—in the general employment of one person, who is temporarily loaned to another person to do that person's work, becomes during that period of time the servant of the borrower, although he or she remains in the general employment of the lender. The borrower of the employee then becomes, for the purposes of vicarious liability, the employer of that employee to the exclusion of the lender. The application of the rule depends on the question of whose work is being performed, and it must appear that the servant is under the borrower's exclusive control and direction as to the work in progress.

The borrowed servant doctrine has both offensive and defensive application. A plaintiff may allege that certain individuals were the borrowed servants of a physician during an operation, for example, in order to hold the physician liable for any negligence of those individuals. This might or might not be alleged at the same time as a claim for vicarious liability against the hospital, as an alternate theory of liability. However, the borrowed servant doctrine is also a way for hospitals potentially to avoid vicarious liability for the negligence of their employees. In some cases, a hospital may raise this doctrine as a defense against liability. Using this defense can strain relations with the physician and medical staff in general, and thus a hospital that is a codefendant with a physician may be reluctant to raise it. Nevertheless, it is a possibility during the course of a malpractice action.

Negligent Hiring or Credentialing

This cause of action is often seen in the same complaint as a medical malpractice action. Many states recognize the doctrine of corporate negligence, meaning that a corporation can be liable for failing to act with due care. In the case of organizations that provide healthcare, due care may include the appropriate credentialing, hiring, and retention of appropriately skilled healthcare practitioners.[s] This action typically is raised against hospitals, but can be raised against other corporations, including outpatient surgical facilities.[10] Negligent hiring or credentialing is based on the premise that the entity that hires or otherwise allows a physician to practice medicine on its behalf or within its four walls has a duty to act

reasonably in the determination to allow that individual to practice. The failure to do so may expose the organization to liability.

Joint and Several Liability

Joint and several liability is a longstanding legal doctrine that says when there are multiple individuals whose negligence all contributed to the plaintiff's injuries, each one of the individuals is entirely liable to the plaintiff for the wrongful conduct of the others when they cannot or will not pay their share of the plaintiff's damages.[t] In other words, under this doctrine, Defendant A may only be marginally responsible for the injuries suffered by the plaintiff, but if Defendants B, C, and D don't have any money, or refuse to pay, the plaintiff can collect the entirety of the damages from Defendant A. The logic underlying such a doctrine is to make sure that plaintiffs are fully compensated for their injuries, even if it comes from someone who does not have the greatest fault. This doctrine is usually tempered by a cause of action for contribution, under which the defendant that had to pay more than his or her fair share can sue the other defendants to recover the other defendants' share of liability that he or she had to pay.

The potential unfairness to defendants that arises from a strict application of the doctrine of joint and several liability has given rise to some degree of reform. Joint and several liability has, in some states, been limited at least with respect to noneconomic damages. In general, these reforms provide that the extent of joint and several liability will be limited based on the defendant's percentage of fault.

■ Damages

There are two basic types of damages typically involved in a medical malpractice action: economic and noneconomic. Economic damages are those damages that are generally a quantifiable economic loss. Economic damages include such things as past and future medical expenses, past and future lost wages, and loss of earning capacity. Past medical expenses and lost wages are easy enough to quantify. However, future damages attributed to alleged malpractice are generally the subject of expert testimony. Vocational rehabilitation specialists, life-care planners, and economists typically will be involved in reviewing and providing testimony as to the individual's earning capacity, future medical expenses, and the like. The economist typically takes figures provided by the

---

s. See *Thompson v. Nason Hosp.* (S.Ct.Penn. 1991) 591 A.2d 703; *Insinga v. LaBella* (S.Ct.Fla. 1989) 543 So.2d 209.

t. This is admittedly an oversimplification of the doctrine of joint and several liability.

life-care planner, representing the various medical and other expenses that will be incurred over time, projects the total cost into the future, and then reduces the number to present value (i.e., the sum of money in current dollars that, assuming certain interest, market performance, and inflation factors, will provide the amount needed to pay for the patient's economic damages).

Noneconomic damages are entirely different. These are nonquantifiable damages that a patient may recover for such things as present and future physical pain and suffering, present and future mental suffering, and loss of capacity for the enjoyment of life. These damages are controversial because they are not subject to quantification, and depend largely on the patient's subjective experience and the sympathy of the jury. Sometimes expert testimony is offered from psychiatrists, psychologists, and other mental or emotional health specialists to discuss the distress the plaintiff has experienced. Because these types of damages cannot be measured objectively, and because of the concern that such damages are frequently excessive, many states have proposed or imposed caps on noneconomic damages.

Punitive damages are technically a type of noneconomic damages, but should not be confused with what is typically meant by noneconomic damages. Punitive damages are designed to punish wrongdoing and deter future misconduct, rather than to compensate the plaintiff for economic or noneconomic harm. Before a plaintiff may recover punitive damages, he or she must prove a level of misconduct greater than mere negligence in following the standard of care. Punitive damages are typically reserved for cases that demonstrate intentional misconduct or gross negligence on the part of the physician. One definition of *intentional misconduct* is that the defendant had actual knowledge of the wrongfulness of the conduct and the high probability that injury or damage to the claimant would result and, despite that knowledge, intentionally pursued that course of conduct, resulting in injury or damage. *Gross negligence* has been defined as the defendant's conduct having been so reckless or wanting in care that it constituted a conscious disregard or indifference to the life, safety, or rights of persons exposed to such conduct. It is important to note that, depending on state law, punitive damages may or may not be covered by insurance.

Frivolous Lawsuits

It would be a rare case in which a physician being sued for malpractice did not believe the lawsuit to be frivolous. Whether a lawsuit is considered frivolous in the eyes of the courts is another issue. However, there is growing interest

in what remedies a physician may have if he or she has been wrongfully named in a lawsuit, or the lawsuit is otherwise found to be without merit. There are two common legal mechanisms for a physician to potentially recover a portion of his or her losses resulting from being improperly sued. The first is statutory attorney fee provisions, and the second is the cause of action for malicious prosecution.

Many states provide for awards of attorneys' fees and expenses to individuals that have been sued without substantial justification, frivolously, or in bad faith.[u] However, the individual seeking such an award has to demonstrate to the court that the cause of action was without a reasonable basis in law or in fact. This can be a difficult proposition in medical malpractice actions, which are driven by expert opinion. If reasonable minds can differ as to the existence of a basis for the action, then an award under these types of provisions will be difficult to obtain. This can be even more difficult in states that have a presuit certification requirement, in which an expert witness has to certify that the defendants deviated from the standard of care before a suit can even be brought. Unless the certification is completely unwarranted, showing that the litigation that followed was without basis can be a difficult proposition.

The second possible avenue of recovery for an improper lawsuit is through the cause of action for malicious prosecution. The elements of malicious prosecution are generally as follows: (1) the institution or continuation of original judicial proceedings; (2) by or at the instance of the (current) defendants; (3) the termination of such proceeding in the (current) plaintiff's favor; (4) malice in instituting the proceedings; (5) want of probable cause for the proceedings; and (6) suffering damages as a result of the action or prosecution complained of.[v] Prevailing in a cause of action for malicious prosecution is even more difficult than receiving attorneys' fees and expenses under the statutory provisions previously mentioned. Not only does the suit have to be without reasonable basis, but there also must be a finding of malice on the part of the person bringing the initial lawsuit, which is a requirement generally not found in the attorneys' fee provisions discussed earlier. Malice in this context does not necessarily mean ill will or spite, but rather that the initial proceeding was brought for a purpose other than properly recovering

u. See, e.g., Ala. Stat. Section 12-19-272; Fla. Stat. Section 57.105; Cal. Code of Civ. Proc. Section 128.5; A.R.S Section 12-349. This list is not exhaustive.

v. See *Alpha Gulf Coast, Inc. v. Jackson* (S.Ct.Miss. 2001) 801 So.2d 709; *Alamo Rent-A-Car, Inc. v. Mancusi* (S.Ct.Fla. 1994) 632 So.2d 1352.

damages for injuries sustained through the fault of the physician. Malice can be inferred from the circumstances of the case, such as the lack of probable cause, gross negligence in bringing the action, and so forth. Malice, as well as lack of probable cause, can be difficult to prove when medical malpractice cases are about matters of opinion, and especially when the certification of an expert was obtained prior to suit. It would have to be very clear that the initial lawsuit was so devoid of merit that the only purpose had to be an improper one.

The Role of Insurance

No discussion of medical malpractice would be complete without addressing medical malpractice insurance. Many states require that physicians obtain malpractice insurance as a condition of practice. Most physicians obtain medical malpractice insurance regardless of a requirement to do so to protect themselves from the potentially devastating financial consequences of a medical malpractice suit. It is important to understand some of the basic characteristics of medical malpractice insurance policies, and the significance they have for the course of a malpractice lawsuit or other such proceeding against a physician.

Insurance policies offered to physicians for medical malpractice liability are generally "claims made" policies rather than "occurrence" policies. Under an occurrence-based policy, the physician is afforded coverage for events of malpractice that occur while the policy is in effect. This means, for example, that if the coverage period for the policy is January 1, 2004, through December 31, 2004, and the physician commits an act during that period that becomes the subject of a malpractice suit in March 2005, then the physician is covered under the policy.

Under a claims-made policy, insurance coverage applies only to claims against the policy made by patients during the coverage period. This type of insurance gives carriers greater predictability in terms of loss experience, but it can create problems for physicians if they find themselves changing insurance carriers, for whatever reason: change in employment, bankruptcy of current insurer, unacceptably high premiums, and so on. Because of the nature of claims-made policies, a physician may not be covered for an alleged incident of malpractice that occurred during the life of the policy, but for which no claim was made until after the policy expired or terminated. This can be addressed to some degree through the purchase of "tail coverage," which extends the reporting period of the underlying insurance policy. However, tail coverage is usually very expensive, and on occasion there may be time limits on the reporting period.

There is also a growing interest in the possibility of "going bare" (i.e., practicing without any medical malpractice insurance at all). This has become popular with some physicians for whom medical malpractice premiums have become a disproportionately large part of overhead expenses. Some groups of physicians, such as OB/GYNs—for whom malpractice premiums have become especially expensive—have arranged for one or two physicians in the group to be covered by malpractice insurance. Those physicians are the only physicians in the practice who deliver babies; the remainder of the group members limit their practice to lower-risk endeavors and may have more limited insurance coverage.

Although going bare can seem appealing to physicians whose malpractice premiums are consuming significant portions of their income, it is not without risk. By not carrying insurance the physician is potentially placing his or her professional and personal assets at risk. Without careful and comprehensive asset-protection planning by a qualified attorney, one lawsuit can wipe away a career's worth of financial gain. Declaring bankruptcy may not necessarily be a sure thing, and bankruptcy itself can have adverse consequences. Second, malpractice policies not only provide indemnity (payment to the plaintiff), they generally provide for the cost of defending a malpractice lawsuit. Thus, unless the physician has a separate policy for legal fees, the cost of defending a malpractice lawsuit would come out of the physician's pocket.

Another drawback to going bare is that, in states such as Florida, the physician is required to put the licensing authority on notice that he or she is going bare, and is guaranteeing that up to a certain amount of a medical malpractice settlement or judgment will be paid. If that amount isn't paid, the physician's license is subject to suspension as well as further discipline, which can have far-reaching effects, especially if a physician is licensed in or seeks to become licensed in additional states.

Finally, medical malpractice insurance is frequently required by managed-care organizations, hospitals, ambulatory surgical centers, and other entities with which physicians often need to have relationships in order to maintain a viable practice. Thus, if a physician is considering going bare, it is essential for that physician to seek out competent legal advice to determine whether it is lawful in the state in which he or she practices and if any conditions are placed on going bare by state law, and to discuss proper asset-protection planning.

Notice of Claims

Before insurance carriers are obligated to defend a particular claim, the insured must usually give notice of the claim to the insurer. The purpose for notice is to give the insurer the opportunity to investigate the claim and protect itself from fraudulent or exorbitant claims, as well as to decide on whether the carrier wishes to settle or defend the claim.[11] Depending on the state, notice provisions may be prescribed either by statute or by the insurance policy itself. For example, in California the insured is required to tender notice of the injury or accident claim within 20 days of the event.[12] Some policies might contain language that an insured is to "immediately" or "as soon as possible" inform the insurer of the claim. Both Pennsylvania and Florida have interpreted such language to mean that notice must be given within a reasonable time, depending on the circumstances of the case.[13] Once the insurance carrier has received notice, Nevada requires that the carrier acknowledge receipt of the insured's claim within 20 days.[14]

Other states require strict compliance with notice provisions; otherwise the insurer need not assume liability on the policy for that claim.[15] This is contrary to the policy of some jurisdictions, which permit the insured's substantial compliance with the respective notice conditions in circumstances that render it unreasonable for the insured to comply with the notice provisions, and where the insured can show that he or she had made a good-faith effort to comply with the provisions.[16] If the insured meets the substantial-compliance analysis, then to avoid liability, the insurer must show that the delay or the failure of the insured to meet the notice provisions caused prejudice to the insurer.[17]

Duty to Defend

Once proper notice has been given to the insurance carrier, the insurer will be obligated to assume the defense of the insured for that claim. This duty to defend is contractual in nature.[w] If the insurance contract is unclear or ambiguous as to whether a duty to defend exists, then the contract is usually interpreted against the carrier, and the court finds such a duty.[x] The duty to defend bestows on the insurer complete control over the defense and may include the unilateral right to make all necessary decisions, including settlement and selection of counsel.[18] If the policy has a "consent to settle" clause, the carrier must obtain the insured's consent prior to settlement. The insured's consent may also be required by state law. If a duty to defend has been established, the question then concerns the types of claims that the insurer is required to

defend. Some jurisdictions require that the carrier defend not only those claims that fall within the scope of the policy, but also those that may fall outside the policy.[19] Thus, the insurance carrier must rely on the allegations of the complaint to determine whether the claim falls or potentially falls within the policy. This is also known as the "complaint-allegation rule."[y] It is not unusual for states to provide that if the complaint alleges facts demonstrating numerous grounds for liability, the carrier not only is obligated to defend those claims that are covered by the policy, but also is obligated to defend the entire suit.[20] In at least one jurisdiction, California, the carrier must also defend the uncovered claim(s), until the carrier can produce undeniable evidence of the defense cost of the uncovered claim(s).[21]

The duration of the duty to defend varies from state to state, and may even extend into appellate proceedings. In some states, the duty to defend continues as long as the plaintiff asserts claims that fall within the scope of the insurance policy.[22] In other states, the duty to defend continues until: (1) there has been a judgment or settlement in the underlying action; (2) the insurer has received a final judgment in its favor in an action for declaratory relief; (3) the policy limits have been paid by a primary insurer in a case in which excess coverage exists and it would be unreasonable for the primary insurer to bear the entire cost of the defense (in such a situation, the excess insurer would be liable for the further costs of defense); or (4) the insured explicitly consents to the insurer's withdrawal from the defense.[23] The duty to defend can continue through appeal, even on claims that have been dismissed.[24] It can also extend to appealing adverse judgments, if good-faith grounds exist to do so.[25] It has also been held that if the insurance contract is ambiguous as to whether the insurer is to provide post-trial remedies (i.e., appeal), then the insurer has the duty to prosecute an appeal for the insured.[26]

Insurers may be subject to liability if they breach the policy by withdrawing before the duty to defend has ended. Breach of the insurance contract can result in an insurer's liability to reimburse the insured for: (1) the amount that was designated for injuries to third persons, and (2) all necessary costs and expenses incurred by the insured in defending the action.[27] In some cases, the insured may not only recover monies payable to third parties and the expenses incurred in defending the action, but also expenses for an appeal if the grounds for an appeal are reasonable.[28]

---

w. See *National Sav. Ins. Co. v. Gaskins* (Tex.Ct.Civ.App. 1978) 572 S.W.2d 573, 576.

x. See *Cadwallader v. New Amsterdam Casualty Co.* (1959) 396 Pa. 582.

y. See *National Union Fire Ins. Co. v. Merchants Fast Motors Lines* (S.Ct.Tex. 1997) 939 S.W.2d 139, 142.

Bad Faith

In dealing with the insured and deciding on whether to settle the claim, the insurer must act in "good faith." Some courts have characterized good faith as more than a simple showing of sincerity, but it demands an honest, objective evaluation of the case in order to best determine the advisability of a settlement.[29] Moreover, bad faith is described as a frivolous or an unfounded refusal to pay policy proceeds, the result of a breach of a known duty (i.e., good faith and fair dealing) through some motive of self-interest or ill will.[30] A breach of good faith also has been described as conduct that violates standards of decency, fairness, or reasonableness.[31]

In favoring the rights of the insured, states may impose on the insurer the duty to approach a settlement as if the policy did not contain coverage limits, and demand that the insurer give equal consideration to the insured's financial obligation and exposure as well as its own.[32] Other states demand that the insurer, in handling the defense of the claims of the insured, exercise a degree of care and diligence as a person of ordinary care and prudence would do in the management of his or her own business.[33] The insurer's good-faith duty may also include advising the insured of settlement opportunities, advising about the probable outcome of litigation, warning of the possibility of an excess judgment, and informing the insured of any steps he or she might take to avoid the same.[33] In any event, states generally stress a policy that respects the rights of the insured when the insurer is handling his or her claim.

Insurance companies may have an affirmative duty to settle imposed on them. Such a duty might, for example, require the insurer to settle claims within policy limits when there is a substantial likelihood of recovery in excess of those limits, to protect the insured from exposure to excess liability.[34] If the insurer has incontrovertible proof that the claim is valid, then it has the responsibility to effect a settlement, including the initiation of settlement negotiations and making good-faith settlement offers.[35] In other jurisdictions, the insurer does not have to settle a claim when a judgment against the insured may exceed the amount of coverage under the policy, but may decline to settle if it finds the chance of nonliability to be real and substantial, and that the decision to litigate instead of settle the case was one made in earnest.[29,36] Thus, to establish an act of bad faith, one might have to demonstrate that: (1) the insurer lacked a reasonable basis for denying coverage, and (2) the insurer knew or recklessly disregarded its lack of reasonable basis.[37] The scope of this duty and what constitutes bad faith in executing this duty varies from state to state.

An insurer will be found to have acted in bad faith if it violates its duty to settle or other obligations requiring good faith. In such a circumstance, the insurer may be exposed to different types of liability. Such liability may include known and foreseeable compensatory damages incurred by the insured.[38] If an insurer breached its good-faith requirement in settling the claim, the insurer may be liable for the entire judgment amount, including amounts that are in excess of the policy.[z] Depending on the jurisdiction, punitive damages may also be available, if the insurer has acted with malice, gross negligence, or reckless disregard for the rights of the insured[39] for a showing of malice, fraud, or oppression.[aa]

In summary, insured physicians should know and understand the respective rights and obligations of both their insurers and themselves. Physicians who do not know what their rights are with respect to their insurers are at a disadvantage.

■ The Litigation and Trial Process

Physicians tend to be wary of lawyers, even their own. A physician may believe a lawyer is encouraging a patient to sue them for medical malpractice, or that their own lawyer works for the insurance company, not them. Although this attitude can be understandable, it can also impair the ability of an attorney to represent the physician to the best of his or her ability. If there are any concerns about a conflict of interest, those should be addressed and resolved immediately, as well as any other concerns about legal representation. Otherwise, lack of trust can lead to holding back information from the attorney, not providing information on time to the attorney, and not cooperating with the attorney during the course of the lawsuit. All of these can significantly strain the relationship with the attorney, and harm a physician's case. If there are doubts about the attorney's competence or the manner in which he or she is handling the case, then the insurance carrier should be contacted about assigning different counsel. Again, these are things that should be taken care of sooner rather than later, so there can be full cooperation and no mistrust.

The Initiation of a Medical Malpractice Lawsuit

A medical malpractice suit may begin in one of two ways. In states that require presuit investigation or notice prior

---

z. See *G.A. Stowers Furniture Co. v. Am. Indem. Co.*, 15 S.W.2d 544 (Comm. App. 1929); *Hamilton v. Maryland Casualty Co.* (2002) 27 Cal.4th 718, 728; *Thomas v. Lumbermens Mut. Cas. Co.* (Fla.Dist.Ct.App. 1982) 424 So.2d 36.

aa. See *Crisci v. Security Ins. Co.* (1967) 66 Cal.2d 654, 661.

to the filing of a lawsuit, a physician may receive a letter from a plaintiff's lawyer informing the doctor that they are initiating presuit investigation as a precursor to filing a lawsuit, a letter indicating that a suit is going to be filed, or both. If there is no presuit process, or the process requires only the written certification of another physician that the standard of care was breached, then the process will likely begin with the service of a complaint. At this point, the physician needs to put his or her insurance carrier on notice in order to trigger coverage and cause assignment of counsel.

The Presuit Screening Process

As part of past efforts to reform the medical malpractice system, various states have required potential medical malpractice plaintiffs to consult with an expert and obtain an opinion as a condition of bringing suit. In some cases, this requirement is satisfied by the plaintiff's attorney's certification that he or she has consulted an expert, and based on that consultation a reasonable basis exists for bringing suit. In other cases, an actual expert report or affidavit indicating that a reasonable basis exists for bringing suit must be furnished either prior to or within a specified period of time after commencing the lawsuit. An informal presuit investigation process may be required prior to filing suit. Some plaintiffs must also provide advance notice to a physician prior to commencing a lawsuit against that physician.

Although presuit investigation and certification procedures are meant to curb frivolous or baseless medical malpractice actions, these procedures do not always have the desired effect. In the experience of many physicians and defense attorneys, presuit procedures turn out to be mere formalities that are not particularly effective in weeding out frivolous cases. It is not difficult to find experts whose business is producing presuit affidavits for a fee, and it is not uncommon to see the same names repeatedly appearing on these affidavits or certifications. Additionally, because the presuit process is generally geared to the determination of a "reasonable basis" for suit or for some possible indication that malpractice took place, rather than the overall merit of the suit and its probability of success, the process is not necessarily designed to screen out marginal cases.

Complaint

It is important to act promptly on receiving a complaint. Ignoring a complaint won't make it go away. Ignoring it long enough can, however, result in a default being entered against the physician, and the possibility of judgment being entered without a trial. The complaint will contain standard language defining the parties, the court's jurisdiction over the matter, and the appropriateness of venue in that court. The complaint also will set forth the facts that the plaintiff believes support the claims for medical malpractice, and the damages they have allegedly suffered. Physicians do not have a great deal of involvement in answering the complaint, particularly if the allegations are worded very generally. The more factual detail involved, the more a physician may be involved with his or her attorney in the process of answering the complaint.

Discovery

Once the suit has been answered, there is a period during which discovery takes place, which is when the parties engage in fact-gathering in anticipation of trial. In general, discovery is a mutual obligation designed to prevent surprises at trial. This provides the parties with the opportunity to obtain records and other information from the other side, so that there is the opportunity to evaluate the legitimacy and strength of the case. Discovery can be abused, however, by repeated requests for the same information, requesting information that is of no relevance to the cause of action, or making extremely broad, burdensome, or needlessly voluminous requests. Discovery also is not supposed to be used as part of a "fishing expedition" into the records of another (i.e., being used in connection with a pretextual complaint in the hope of finding some wrongdoing, or going so far beyond the issues at hand that the requests themselves have no purpose other than to find some wrongdoing without a basis for searching).

There are basic types of discovery requests that are used in a medical malpractice case, specifically requests for production and interrogatories. Responses to these discovery requests are subject to deadlines. Requests for production are used to obtain documentary and other physical evidence. This might include medical records, office policies, phone records, sign-in sheets, consult notes, and any other documentation or physical evidence that might be relevant to the case. Although the request goes to the attorney, the physician or the physician's designee (such as an office manager) must spend time locating the requested documents and providing them in a timely fashion. The failure to comply timely with discovery, unless the attorney has raised objections to the discovery requests or received an extension, can result in sanctions, such as having to pay the opposing party's attorneys' fees incurred if they go to court to require the response to discovery.

Interrogatories are questions designed to obtain facts relevant to the case at hand. In cases involving personal injury, such as a medical malpractice case, interrogatories may be standardized. They may ask for such information from the physician as educational and professional background, access to medical literature, experience with addressing the same type of medical cases as the plaintiff's, and information regarding the underlying facts of the case. Ultimately, the defense attorney will provide the answers to the opposing party, but he or she will typically work with the physician on drafting answers to the interrogatories.

The most disruptive and most stressful aspect of discovery to the physician may be the physician's deposition. A deposition is sworn oral testimony given in response to questioning by the opposing party's attorney, and which is transcribed word for word by a court reporter. It is extremely important to be well prepared for a deposition. This point cannot be emphasized enough. The physician giving the deposition has to realize that statements made in a deposition establish the basis for the litigation and trial process. Inconsistencies and mistakes can and will be used at trial to undermine credibility. Saying the wrong thing or giving the wrong answer can severely undermine the defense of the case. Attorneys and the physician must prepare diligently for deposition; the facts of the case should be fully understood as well as all relevant medical record information. The attorney should provide adequate time to prepare for a deposition.

There is no substitute for thorough and effective preparation by the physician's defense lawyer, and the following comments are no exception. However, there are a few key things to know about a deposition. The physician needs to know the medical records, and any other records that relate to the plaintiff, as completely as possible. Testimony that is inconsistent with or contradicts an entry in the medical record gives the plaintiff's attorney the ability to undermine the physician's credibility. In the minds of a jury, lack of credibility or a lack of mastery over the facts can easily translate into lack of competence.

It also is important to know that a deposition is not confessional; it is not collegial; it is not a peer review or an academic learning experience. The attorney taking the deposition is trying to affix blame, and the physician is the object of that blame. Carefully thought-out responses that remain consistent throughout the course of the deposition are very important, and it is important that responses are designed to make the course of action the physician took sound as reasonable and appropriate as possible. Emotional control is extremely important as well, especially if the deposition is videotaped.

Answer only the questions that are asked, and be sure of the question before it is answered. Sometimes what the question asks and what the individual hearing the question thinks is being asked are two entirely different things. If

there is any uncertainty about what the question means, the attorney asking the question should be asked to repeat or rephrase. It also is important to listen to the questions in order to avoid the trap of giving a different answer to the same question that has been packaged in a different way. This is a common tool used to create inconsistency in testimony, and needs to be watched for carefully.

This is hardly a complete list, but it points out some of the important aspects of giving deposition testimony. Knowing the information is obviously vital, but it is only the first step. How the information is packaged and delivered, as well as how the physician handles him- or herself, are also very important to the deposition process, as well as trial testimony.

■ Trial

Trial lawyers will spend substantial numbers of hours reviewing evidence, preparing opening statements, preparing their witness examinations, preparing their witnesses to testify, preparing closing arguments, preparing objections, preparing jury instructions, and preparing themselves mentally for the trial ahead. Nothing is left to chance unless it is absolutely necessary. "Surprise" witnesses, "surprise" evidence, seat-of-the-pants questioning, and extemporaneous speaking are not, or at least should not be, prevailing characteristics of an actual trial. Although attorneys certainly have to be aware of the dynamics of the trial—how the jury is reacting, how witnesses are conducting themselves, how the judge is responding—and adjust accordingly, it is done mostly with alternate strategies or contingency plans contemplated in advance, based on the discovery that was conducted in the many months beforehand.

General Sequence of Events

The plaintiff has the burden of proving his or her case at trial. The plaintiff's attorney typically gives an opening statement about what the facts that are going to be presented will show to the jury. The plaintiff's side then presents its witnesses, including its experts. The plaintiff often testifies, if able, as does anyone else who may have relevant testimony. The plaintiff may have issued subpoenas to various individuals that require them to appear and testify. In some cases, these could include the employees of a physician or a physician group. The defense has the opportunity to cross-examine each witness.

Once the plaintiff is finished putting on its case, the defense then typically gives its opening statement and presents its evidence in opposition to the plaintiff's case. When both sides are finished, the respective attorneys for the parties make a closing argument that summarizes the evidence and tells the jury what conclusions it should reach from the evidence. The judge then gives instructions to the jury as to the law that applies to the case, and how it should govern the jury's deliberations. The jury renders a verdict, which is read into the record. The jury is dismissed, and court is adjourned. This process can take days or even weeks to complete.

Respective Roles of Judge and Jury

In general terms, the judge is the ultimate arbiter of the law in a courtroom. He or she makes all the decisions about who may testify, whether certain evidence will be allowed or excluded, whether to sustain (allow) or overrule (not allow) objections made by attorneys, and whether at the close of the plaintiff's case the trial should even continue.[bb] Judges have very broad discretion as to these matters, and are generally not overturned by appellate courts unless it is shown that the judge abused his or her discretion or made a clear error of law, and that it prejudiced the losing party in some significant way.

Juries, on the other hand, are the ultimate arbiters of the facts. They are the ones who have to decide whether the preponderance of the evidence weighs in favor of the plaintiff or the defendant. They are the ones who have to be convinced that one side or the other should prevail based on the testimony and other evidence presented before them.

Medical malpractice cases present a special challenge, because they can deal with complicated medical issues, on which reasonable physicians can and do disagree, even with the benefit of an entire career's worth of knowledge and experience. The jury has only a few days or so, depending on the length of the trial, to grasp the medical jargon and issues raised in the case. Thus, the facts and the medical opinions have to be broken down in such a way that an average layperson can be sufficiently educated on a discrete set of medical issues to make a reasoned decision about the case at hand. This education must be carefully handled; it can't be done in a patronizing or condescending manner, or the result can be alienating the jury. Also, jurors are only human. They make mistakes, they get confused, they misunderstand things, and they have emotions that can be manipulated. There are many other significant aspects to jury involvement in a medical malpractice trial, and various methods used to educate and persuade a jury.

Burden of Proof

At a medical malpractice trial, the plaintiff has the burden of proving his or her case by a "preponderance of the evidence." Preponderance of the evidence is the burden of proof for basically all civil causes of action. This burden of proof may be defined as the "greater weight of the evidence; superior evidentiary weight that, though not sufficient to free the mind wholly from all reasonable doubt, is still sufficient to incline a fair and impartial mind to one side of the issue than the other."[40] Stated another way, preponderance of the evidence is proof that leads the trier of fact to find that the existence of a contested fact is more probable than its nonexistence.[41] This means that the plaintiff must provide evidence showing it is more likely than not that his or her claims are true.

The key elements of a medical malpractice case are established by expert witness testimony. Expert witnesses must be able to testify to a degree of reasonable medical certainty or probability that the alleged breach of the standard of care caused the plaintiff's injuries.[cc]

An expert's testimony cannot be based on assumptions about the case that are without a basis in fact. Additionally, opinions that rest on guess, surmise, or conjecture, or lack a reasoned explanation, are insufficient.[42] For example, a physician's expert testimony that if certain events came together, a retractor left in a patient could have been a cause for the growth of bacteria, and that it "just sort of makes sense" that the infection spread to another site in the patient's body without any explanation, was insufficient to establish causation.[42] Likewise, a physician's expert testimony that if the patient had a particular injury (torn rotator cuff, in this case), it should have been repaired primarily and the patient would probably have recovered well, was found (along with other similar statements) to be too speculative, equivocal, and conclusory to sustain issues of causation of the patient's injuries, or of the standard of care.[43] Cases that do not have an adequate factual basis to support the allegations are usually dismissed prior to trial. If the plaintiff does not

---

bb. Although not discussed in detail here, if the plaintiff has put on his or her case, and it is clear that there are no facts on which a reasonable jury could render a verdict in favor of the plaintiff, then the defense may move for and the judge may possibly grant a motion for a directed verdict. In those circumstances, a directed verdict is essentially a finding for the defendants without the defense having to put on its case or for the jury to render a verdict. The specific requirements for the substance of these motions, and when they may be raised, are subject to the rules of civil procedure for each state.

cc. See, e.g., *Ochoa v. Pacific Gas and Elec. Co.* (1998) 61 Cal.App.4th 1480; *Zwiren v. Thompson* (S.Ct.Ga. 2003) 578 S.E.2d 862.

bear the burden of proof when presenting their evidence at trial, the case is subject to dismissal upon a motion by the defendant, at the conclusion of the plaintiff's case.

Appeal

The rules of civil procedure provide for post-trial motions to address trial errors that result in an adverse outcome. One option is to appeal the case on matters of law. Each state has its own rules of appellate procedure, setting forth the requirements for the appellate process. An appeal is a limited review of trial court rulings of certain findings or events that took place during the trial that the appealing party argues were incorrect. It is not an opportunity to try the case over again. Appellate courts do not reexamine the facts that were presented. They review the record of the trial and the briefs of the parties, and listen to the argument of counsel. They do not receive evidence, listen to witnesses testify, or make judgments about the credibility of witnesses. Their only role is to determine whether the law was correctly applied at trial.

The appellate court reviews the trial court proceedings to determine if there was substantial evidence to support the findings, but does not substitute its own judgment for the jury's. Simply because the evidence could have supported a different conclusion than that reached by the jury, or reasonable minds could differ as to the significance and meaning of certain evidence, is not a legitimate basis for disturbing the findings of fact.[44]

A party might also appeal the rulings of the judge during the course of the trial, such as limiting the number of witnesses that could testify, allowing certain evidence over objection, or excluding other evidence that the party thought should have been admitted. These are matters traditionally left within the discretion of the trial judge, and that discretion is very broad. Appellate courts will not disturb a discretionary action taken by a trial judge unless it can be shown that the judge abused that discretion.[45] This can mean that the appellate court is persuaded that the trial court's decision is clearly against the logic and effect of the circumstances before the court.[46] The abuse-of-discretion standard has even stronger variations, such as one court's articulation that abuse of discretion is found only if an unprejudiced person, considering the facts on which the trial court acted, would say that there was no excuse for the ruling made.[47] For example, the exclusion of the sole expert relied on by a party because of an erroneous view of his qualifications has been held to be an abuse of discretion.[48] If an expert's opinion on causation would (if credited by the jury) provide legally sufficient support for a finding in the plaintiff's favor on the issue of causation, it would be an abuse of discretion to strike that testimony.[43] On the other hand, allowing a previously undisclosed witness to testify might not constitute an abuse of discretion, depending on the circumstances.[49]

Even if the appellate court determines that the judge abused his or her discretion or otherwise made an error, that mistake or error may still not constitute grounds for reversal. Appellate courts generally recognize the harmless error doctrine. This doctrine essentially states that an error at the trial court level will not be overturned if the error is harmless (i.e., did not affect or would not affect the outcome, or it was not reasonably probable that the appealing party would have obtained a more favorable result otherwise).[50] For example, a court's exclusion of expert witness testimony, even assuming such exclusion was error, has been found harmless when it would have been essentially duplicative of testimony given by other expert witnesses.[51] On the other hand, in a case involving a plaintiff allegedly injured by a ventilator malfunction or disconnection, a trial court's erroneous admission of a nurse training manual that described generally the mental trauma of vent dependency was found to be harmful error.[52] The court reasoned that the introduction of what it characterized as a highly emotional and irrelevant document must have colored the jury's interpretation of the evidence, and thus could not have been harmless error.

Appeals can have strategic value after a trial has taken place. For example, a jury may render a verdict that awards a plaintiff damages in excess of the defendant's policy limits. The defendant may plan to appeal that verdict, which is usually a laborious and time-consuming process. In exchange for the defendant waiving the right to appeal, the plaintiff may agree to settle for an amount less than the award, rather than go through the appellate process. Even if the verdict was within limits, but at a level the defense thought was excessive or without clear support, an appeal can be used as leverage to negotiate a post-trial settlement. Thus, although successfully appealing a verdict can be difficult, the mere fact of a meritorious appeal can spur negotiations between the parties to settle for a reduced amount.

Consequences of a Medical Malpractice Action

A medical malpractice suit has consequences beyond monetary liability. Liability from a medical malpractice action can affect a physician's insurance premium rates and insurability. In states that have insurance requirements, this can be devastating for a physician's practice.

Payments for medical malpractice made on behalf of a physician and other medical practitioners must be reported to the National Practitioner Data Bank (NPDB), where hospitals that conduct credentialing and peer review will access the information. Events leading to allegations of medical malpractice may prompt internal hospital peer reviews or state medical board inquiries.

Effect on Insurance

A medical malpractice suit can affect both the cost of insurance and the insurability of a physician. Current insurers know about settlements or judgments because they pay the claims. Prospective insurers typically ask for a past claims history, along with settlement and judgment amounts. Based on an assessment of past claims, insurance companies determine whether to accept physicians as new policyholders. Policies may be canceled for existing policyholders if an analysis of a physician's claims reveal practices that are substandard or are difficult to defend. When insurance companies nonrenew policyholders, new insurance may be difficult to obtain.[dd]

National Practitioner Data Bank and Other Databases

Federal law requires that each entity, including an insurance company that makes payment on behalf of a physician, must report information regarding the payment and the circumstances of the payment. This report is made to the National Practitioner Data Bank (NPDB), which is provided for by federal regulation to receive and maintain these reports. The term "medical malpractice action or claim" broadly includes a written claim or demand for payment based on a healthcare provider's furnishing (or failure to furnish) healthcare services, and includes the filing of a cause of action, based on the law of tort, brought in any court of any state or the United States seeking monetary damages. The filing of a lawsuit is not required to trigger these reporting requirements; a written demand is sufficient. The payment only has to be reported if it is for the benefit of an individual practitioner or practitioners.

Reports of malpractice payments are to be made not only by insurance companies, but also by other entities that might make payments on behalf of individual practitioners. Such entities might include a professional

corporation or professional association of practitioners that makes a payment to settle a malpractice claim for the benefit of one of its physicians. However, individual subjects are not required to report payments they make for their own benefit to the NPDB. Reports of malpractice payments must contain certain information, including the amount of payment, whether the payment was for a settlement or a judgment, and a description of the acts or omissions and injuries or illnesses on which the action or claim was based. These reports are confidential, and access is limited to only those parties or entities that are listed in the applicable regulations. Hospitals are obligated to request information regarding practitioners from the NPDB under certain circumstances. Certain individuals and their attorneys may have access to NPDB information regarding a practitioner in connection with a medical malpractice action, but only if a hospital is named and evidence is provided that the hospital failed to request information regarding a practitioner as required by law. The information may be used solely with respect to litigation resulting from the action or claim against the hospital.

In addition to the NPDB, insurance companies and other entities are required to report medical malpractice payments to the appropriate state licensing board, board of medical examiners, or similar state licensing body. This requirement is imposed not only by federal law, but also states often require physicians to report payments in satisfaction of medical malpractice settlements or judgments to their licensing board. A malpractice payment is frequently made publicly available by the state board, and is often easily accessible via the Internet. The failure to report these payments as required under state law can be grounds for discipline by the state licensing agency.

State Licensure Board Actions

A medical malpractice lawsuit is not the only legal action that might be taken when someone makes allegations of malpractice against a physician. It is possible that the patient or another person would report the same allegations of malpractice to the physician's licensing board. If someone makes a complaint to the physician's state licensing board, the board may begin an investigation into the allegations of substandard care. In most states, the failure to practice medicine with reasonable skill and safety, or failing to practice in accordance with the prevailing professional standard of care, constitutes a basis for discipline against the physician's license.

A board can also start such proceedings on its own. Such a proceeding might begin on the board's receipt of a report of a malpractice settlement or judgment. The consequences of the board finding that a physician failed

dd. Reports of physicians moving to other states because of high malpractice insurance premiums can be found in various news sources, including the following article: "Malpractice Insurance Rates Send Doctors Fleeing to Colo.," *Denver Post*, March 4, 2004.

to meet the standard of care can result in disciplinary actions, including reprimand, monetary penalties, suspension, or probation, and if the case is egregious enough, revocation of the license.

Hospital Privileges

A medical malpractice action can have an adverse effect on a physician's hospital privileges as well. A history of medical malpractice settlements or judgments is available to hospitals through the NPDB, which they receive as part of the credentialing process. If a physician has a significant history of medical malpractice actions, the hospital may consider the risk of liability to itself, for potential vicarious liability and for negligent credentialing, to be too high and deny privileges on that basis. Additionally, if the physician is a party to a medical malpractice lawsuit, a hospital may investigate the matter on its own if it happened inside the hospital, and potentially begin proceedings under the medical staff bylaws or the hospital bylaws, depending on the facts of the case.

Intangible Consequences

Although a malpractice suit has clear professional and monetary consequences, the effect on the physician personally can be profound. Being sued is stressful, especially for physicians who have dedicated their careers to helping people overcome injury, illness, and disease. It is very difficult not to personalize a medical malpractice suit, and equally difficult to control feelings of anger and anxiety, of insult and effrontery. The stress on the physician is very real and needs to be addressed, rather than ignored, for the sake of the physician's well-being.

■ Legislative Attempts to Address Medical Liability

The following two examples illustrate attempts by state and federal legislators to address an uncontrolled tort system.

The Medical Injury Compensation Reform Act (MICRA)

Periodically, the medical malpractice insurance industry experiences premium pricing fluctuations. In the 1970s and early 1980s, many states were concerned about the rising costs of medical malpractice and the effect or potential effect they would have on patient care. Many states enacted various types of reform, but the reform most often cited by both opponents and proponents of such reform is the Medical Injury Compensation Reform Act (MICRA), which California enacted in 1975.

MICRA included multiple legal reforms for medical malpractice causes of action. In particular, MICRA limited joint and several liability for physicians as to noneconomic damages. Also, the collateral source rule was changed to allow evidence of certain benefits to be admitted at trial to reduce the award to the plaintiff. At the same time, the source of those benefits was prohibited from exercising any rights of indemnity or subrogation to recover those benefits, ensuring that the plaintiff was made whole for his or her injuries. The centerpiece of MICRA was a limit on noneconomic damages in medical malpractice cases. In California, these damages are capped at $250,000. The damages cap has survived challenges to its constitutionality, unlike in other states whose attempts to cap noneconomic damages were overturned by their courts.

The HEALTH Act

In 2002, federal legislation was introduced into the House of Representatives that contained broad tort reform language. Called the Help Efficient, Accessible, Low-cost, Timely Healthcare (HEALTH) Act of 2002, this legislation focused primarily on reform in the area of medical malpractice. The legislation itself contained Congressional findings that the civil justice system is adversely affecting patient access to healthcare services, better patient care, and cost-efficient healthcare. It states that the healthcare liability system is a costly and ineffective mechanism for resolving claims of healthcare liability and compensating injured patients, and is a deterrent to the sharing of information among healthcare professionals, which impedes efforts to improve patient safety and quality of care. To the end of addressing these concerns, the HEALTH Act offered reform in the following areas: statutes of limitation,[ee] noneconomic and punitive damages, joint and several liability, contingency fee arrangements,[ff] the collateral source rule, and periodic payment of judgments.

---

ee. The statute of limitations refers to the time period within which a plaintiff must bring a lawsuit. Absent special circumstances, suits brought after the statute of limitations has expired will be barred.

ff. Most plaintiffs' attorneys take medical malpractice cases on a contingency fee basis, meaning that they get paid based on a percentage of the award, if any. Because contingency fees can be somewhere around 40% of the award or settlement, and the attorney's court costs are typically deducted from the award or settlement first, the attorney can end up taking home more than the plaintiff. It also creates a direct personal financial incentive in the case that some might argue presents a conflict of interest with the client in some situations. These are some of the arguments that are made in support of reducing the amount that can be extracted as a contingency fee.

The HEALTH Act provided for unlimited recovery of all economic damages. It defined economic damages as objectively verifiable monetary losses incurred as a result of the provision of, use of, or payment for (or failure to provide, use, or pay for) healthcare services or medical products, such as past and future medical expenses, loss of past and future earnings, cost of obtaining domestic services, loss of employment, and loss of business or employment opportunities. In catastrophic cases, these damages could obviously be very high. Additionally, it could be argued that many of the costs defined as non-economic damages are included in this broad definition of economic damages. For example, pain management, psychiatric counseling, medication, and other such expenses should still be recoverable under this language.

The HEALTH Act sought to limit the recovery of noneconomic damages to a maximum of $250,000, regardless of the number of parties against whom an action was brought or the number of separate claims or actions brought with respect to the same occurrence. The HEALTH Act defined noneconomic damages as damages for physical and emotional pain, suffering, inconvenience, physical impairment, mental anguish, disfigurement, loss of enjoyment of life, loss of society and companionship, loss of consortium (other than loss of domestic service), hedonic damages, injury to reputation, and all other non-pecuniary losses of any kind or nature.

The damages-limitation language was somewhat ambiguous as to what constituted economic or noneconomic damages. For example, a patient may experience or develop intractable pain as a result of a medical injury. Pain is recognized as a legitimate medical phenomenon. Treatment in the form of pain management, with the associated office visit fees, medications, and other expenses, would constitute medical expenses that would be compensable as economic damages. The cap on noneconomic damages would include "physical and emotional pain," limiting the damages available to compensate for pain and suffering.

Another important aspect of the HEALTH Act was nationwide reform of the collateral source rule, which, in some states, provides that an individual's award for medical malpractice may not be reduced by the amount of payments from collateral sources such as health insurance or public benefits. The HEALTH Act would have specifically permitted any party in a lawsuit to introduce evidence of collateral source benefits. Such benefits would include any amount paid or reasonably likely to be paid in the future to or on behalf of the claimant, or any service, product, or other benefit provided or reasonably likely to be provided in the future to or on behalf of the claimant as a result of the injury or wrongful death.

The purpose behind such a provision is to prevent a "double recovery" or windfall to a medical malpractice plaintiff by making the physician pay for expenses already reimbursed by insurance or another payer source. One of the arguments against such a reform is that it shifts the burden for compensating a victim of malpractice from the practitioner who committed the malpractice to the patient's insurer, or to the state if the patient receives public health benefits. It also has been argued that this would leave malpractice victims potentially undercompensated, because their insurers could recoup from them the amounts paid as benefits from their settlement or jury award.

There are other important aspects of the HEALTH Act not discussed here. However, the HEALTH Act essentially federalizes reforms that have already been enacted in certain states. It also embodies an approach to reform based on leaving the current system generally intact, but changing certain discrete aspects of that system.

■ Conclusion

As mentioned at the beginning of this chapter, medical malpractice is based on the theory of tort law that requires a plaintiff to prove four elements. Unless the plaintiff can show that the (1) physician owed a duty of care to the plaintiff; (2) the physician breached that duty of care; (3) the plaintiff suffered injuries; and (4) the physician's breach of duty was the cause of the plaintiff's injuries, the plaintiff will not be successful. To demonstrate a breach of a duty, plaintiffs rely on experts and other resources to describe the standard of care for reasonably prudent physicians in the same or similar circumstances.

The legal system provides a forum for aggrieved patients to seek remedies from their physicians when those patients believe they have been harmed by the action or inaction of their physician. The system has limitations, but frequently provides for fair resolution of medical malpractice disputes.

References
1. *Oja v. Kin* (Mich.Ct.App. 1998) 581 N.W.2d 739.
2. *Diggs v. Arizona Cardiologists, Ltd.* (Ariz.Ct.App. 2000) 8 P.3d 386.
3. *Bovara v. St. Francis Hosp.* (Ill.Ct.App. 1998) 700 N.E.2d 143.
4. *Sparks v. Hicks* (S.Ct.Okla. 1996) 912 P.2d 331.
5. *Snow v. Bond* (S.Ct.Tex. 1969) 438 S.W.2d 549.
6. Fla. Stat. Section 766.102(1).
7. *Reynolds v. Burt* (Fla.Dist.Ct.App. 1978) 359 So.2d 50.
8. Nev. Rev. Stat. Section 41A.100.2.
9. *Moyer v. Reynolds* (Fla.Dist.Ct.App. 2001) 780 So.2d 205.
10. *Oven v. Pascucci* (2000) 46 Pa.D.&C.4th 506.

11. *Sterling State Bank v. Virginia Surety Co.* (S.Ct.Minn. 1969) 173 N.W. 2d 342, 346.

12. Cal. Ins. Code § 551.

13. *Hargrave v. Fidelity Mut.Life Ins. Co.* (Pa.Super.Ct. 1961) 175 A.2d 912; *Laster v. United States Fidelity & Guar. Co.* (Fla.Dist.Ct.App. 1974) 293 So.2d 83, 86.

14. Nev. Admin. Code Ch. 686A, § 665.

15. *Milton v. Preferred Risk Ins. Co.*(Tex.Ct.Civ.App. 1974) 511 S.W.2d 83, 85.

16. *Brakeman v. Potomac Ins. Co.* (S.Ct.Pa. 1977) 371 A.2d 193; *Continental Casualty Co. v. Shoffstall* (Fla.Dist.Ct.App. 1967) 198 So.2d 654, 656.

17. *Tiedtke v. Fidelity & Casualty Co.* (S.Ct.Fla. 1969) 222 So.2d 206.

18. 5-152 Florida Torts § 152.30.

19. *Reinsurance Ass'n v. Timmer* (Minn.Ct.App. 2002) 641 N.W.2d 302; *Texas Prop. & Cas. Ins Guar. Assoc. v. Southwest Aggregates* (Tex.Ct.App. 1998) 982 S.W.2d 600, 607; *Jostens, Inc. v. Mission Insurance Co.* (S.Ct.Minn. 1986) 387 N.W.2d 161, 165; *Cadwallader v. New Amsterdam Casualty Co.* (1959) 396 Pa. 582; *First Am. Title Ins. Co. v. National Union Fire Ins. Co.* (Fla.Dist.Ct.App. 1997) 695 So.2d 475, 476.

20. *Baron Oil Co. v. Nationwide Mut. Fire Ins.* (Fla.Dist.Ct.App. 1985) 470 So.2d 810, 813-814; *Jostens, Inc. v. Mission Insurance Co.* (S.Ct. Minn. 1986), 387 N.W.2d 161, 165.

21. *Gray v. Zurich Ins. Co.* (1966) 65 Cal.2d 263.

22. *Baron Oil Co. v. Nationwide Mut. Fire Ins.* (Fla.Dist.Ct.App. 1985) 470 So.2d 810, 813–814; *Woida v. North Star Mut. Ins. Co.* (S.Ct. Minn. 1981) 306 N.W.2d 570, 574; *Travelers Ins. Co. v. Volentine* (Tex.Ct.Civ.App.1979) 578 S.W.2d 501, 505; *Moeller v. American Guar. & Liab. Ins. Co.* (S.Ct.Miss. 1996) 707 So.2d 1062.

23. 6-82 California Torts § 82.11.

24. *Meadowbrook v. Tower Ins. Co.* (S.Ct.Minn. 1997) 559 N.W.2d 411, 416–417.

25. *Aetna Ins. v. Borrell-Bigby Electric Co.* (Fla.Dist.Ct.App. 1989) 541 So.2d.139, 141.

26. *American Cyanamid Co. v. American Home Assurance Co.* (1994) 30 Cal. App.4th 969, 975–980.

27. *Mannheimer Bros. v. Kansas Cas. & Sur. Co.* (1921) 149 Minn. 482; *Travelers Ins. Co. v. Chicago Bridge & Iron Co.* (Tex.Ct.Civ.App. 1969) 442 S.W.2d 888, 900.

28. *Buss v. Superior Court* (1997) 16 Cal.4th 35, 55–56.

29. *United States Fire Ins. Co. v. Royal Ins. Co.* (3d Cir. 1985)759 F.2d 306.

30. 33 Duq. L. Rev. 351 citing *Polselli v. Nationwide Ins. Co.*, 23 F.3d 247, 751 (3d Cir. 1994).

31. *Cenac v. Murry* (S.Ct.Miss. 1992) 609 So.2d 1257, 1272.

32. *Short v. Dairyland* (S.Ct.Minn. 1983) 334 N.W.2d 384; *Bell v. Commercial Ins. Co.*, 280 Fed.2d 514 (3d Cir. 1960).

33. *Boston Old Colony Ins. Co. v. Gutierrez* (S.Ct.Fla. 1980) 386 So.2d 783.

34. *Kransco v. American Empire Surplus Lines Ins. Co.* (2000) 23 Cal.4th 390.

35. *American Fire & Casualty Co. v. Davis* (Fla.Dist.Ct.App. 1962), 146 So.2d 615, 617–618.

36. *Bell v. Commercial Ins. Co.*, 280 F.2d 514 (3d Cir.1960).

37. *Adamski v. Allstate Ins. Co.* (Pa.Super.Ct 1999) 738 A.2d 1033.

38. *The Birth Center v. St. Paul Cos., Inc.* (2001) 567 Pa. 386.

39. *Aetna Casualty & Surety Co. v. Day* (S.Ct.Miss. 1986) 487 So.2d 830.

40. Garner B (ed.). *Black's law dictionary* (7th ed.). West Group; 1999:1201.

41. *Johnson v. Wyoming* (S.Ct.Wyo. 2001) 23 P.3d 32.

42. *Jennings v. Palomar Pomerado Health Systems, Inc.* (2003) 114 Cal. App. 4th 1108.

43. *Walker v. Corley* (2003) Tex. App. LEXIS 7580 (unpublished).

44. *RAD-Razorback Ltd. Partnership v. B.G. Cooney Co.* (S.Ct.Ark. 1986) 713 S.W.2d 462; *Tinagero v. Phillips* (Conn.Ct.App. 1989) 559 A.2d 234; *Contel Systems Corp. v. Gores* (Mich.Ct.App. 1990) 455 N.W.2d 398.

45. *In re Cynthia A.* (Conn.Ct.App. 1986) 514 A.2d 360.

46. *Daub v. Daub* (Ind.Ct.App.1994) 629 N.E.2d 873.

47. *People v. Snider* (Mich.Ct.App. 2000) 608 N.W.2d 502.

48. *Brown v. Colm* (1974) 11 Cal.3d 639.

49. *Dunlap v. Dash* (2004) Mich. App. LEXIS 567.

50. *Vasquez v. Rocco* (S.Ct.Conn. 2003) 836 A.2d 1158; *Parris v. Sands* (1993) 21 Cal.App.4th 187.

51. *Parris v. Sands* (1993) 21 Cal.App.4th 187.

52. *Florida Patient's Compensation Fund v. Von Stetina* (S.Ct.Fla. 1985) 474 So.2d 783.

53. Beider P, Hagen S. *Limiting tort liability for medical malpractice*. Washington, DC: Congressional Budget Office; January 8, 2004.

Facility Design and Planning for Physician-Based Group Practices

Richard Sprow, AIA
Sonya Dufner, FASID
Christian F. Bormann, AIA, NCARB, LEED AP
Jason Harper, AIA, LEED AP
John Rodenbeck, AIA, NCARB, LEED AP BD+C

The intent of this chapter is to outline some of the key issues and steps involved in establishing physician-based group practices and in building new facilities for them. This framework of information is intended to assist those considering establishing a group practice in decision making about facilities that will directly impact operations and finances for the life of the organization. The goal is to provide the consumer of specialized healthcare design consultant services with a better understanding of the design process and to establish useful guidelines for the design of efficient group practice space, whether to fit out a new space or to construct a new building. These group practice facilities may be freestanding, jointly owned (hospital and doctors), surgery centers, imaging centers, health and wellness facilities, doctors' offices, urgent care centers, or the like.

Today's physician-based group practices are rapidly evolving from simple doctors' offices to more sophisticated and comprehensive healthcare facilities that can offer nearly all the services of a hospital. The management of group practices has become increasingly complicated, with the pressures of ever-changing insurance payment and reimbursement systems. Although a large majority of U.S. physicians practice individually or in small groups, a growing trend is the consolidation into ever-larger group practices. Another option that many are considering is partnering under the umbrella and brand of a larger health system for management and facility support. Growth in the use of electronic medical records, as well as the increasing complexity and cost of medical equipment, has steadily increased the capital costs of establishing group practices. Recently enacted healthcare reform legislation is putting increased pressure on hospital-based healthcare systems to consolidate physician practices under their management umbrella. The establishment by hospital-based medical systems of accountable care organizations and the movement towards a "medical home" model of care in anticipation of healthcare reform are leading to increasing consolidation. All of these pressures are leading many physicians to consider joining larger group practices, merging their established practice with other groups, or joining a health system that can provide logistical support and access to capital.

The Basics of Architectural Design Services

The essential criterion that separates inpatient hospitals from outpatient care centers is the overnight stay of the patient. Otherwise, the two facility types can be quite similar. Before a discussion about the planning and design of group practices, it is first necessary to become familiar with how professional architectural services are obtained and delivered.

The planning and construction decisions for a healthcare facility, whether it is an inpatient acute care facility or an outpatient ambulatory facility, are complex; the assistance of trained and licensed professionals to advise the owner or operator of the new facility is essential. A physician-based group practice facility project could include a new building, a renovation, or interior design of existing constructed space. Each of these options requires a slightly different planning approach. To begin the design process for a new healthcare facility, the owner needs to hire the services of a professional architect. The architect has the special skills and training to help the owner define and quantify their functional needs.

Architects

In the United States, architects are professionals trained in building design and renovation, and are licensed by each state. The terms "architect" and "registered architect" are legally protected, because of their responsibility to protect public health and safety by creating code-compliant facilities. Some architects are general practitioners, whereas others specialize in certain facility types such as healthcare facilities. When a project involves significant construction, a building permit with an architect's seal is required on the drawings before construction can begin.

Interior Designers

Interior designers are professionals specifically trained to plan and design interior spaces, including space planning and renovations. Although some states license interior designers and their training is similar to that of architects, they are not generally able to be legally responsible for new buildings or major renovations that involve structural work. Although architects may also deliver interior design services, interior designers are trained more specifically in the creation of interior space and the use of furnishings, finishes, and lighting. A project is most successful when both architects and interior designers collaborate. Although many may consider themselves to have good taste when it comes to interior design or decorating, the particular value of hiring experienced and trained interior designers for a healthcare interior fit-out project should not be underestimated. An architect or an interior designer with experience in healthcare facilities can provide a design that maximizes efficiency, minimizes operational costs, responds to the needs of staff, and enhances the experience of patients, while avoiding costly pitfalls.

The interior designer works closely with the architect and the design team, and for the renovation of interior space often leads the design effort. The interior designer may develop the program and may create the interior space design and concept, including the overall plan layout with partitions and all surfaces, ceilings, lighting, and furnishings. Part of this responsibility includes the selection and specification of all finish materials and built-in furnishings. Sometimes the scope of work for an interior designer includes furniture, accessories such as window treatments, signage, and artwork.

Consulting Engineers

A new healthcare facility project almost always requires the additional design expertise of various engineering disciplines such as mechanical, electrical, plumbing, and fire protection engineers. If the project is a new building or an addition to an existing building, it will also require structural engineers to design the structural system and civil engineers to design the site on which the building is situated. Some architectural firms include these engineering disciplines (referred to as architectural/engineering or A/E firms); others hire these additional design experts as subconsultants to their own firm. Engineering firms also can be contracted directly to the owner in cases that do not involve architectural or interior design work. Typically, however, the architect is contracted directly to the owner for the complete design of a facility, and contracts out whatever additional expertise is required. This way, the architect is contractually responsible for the total coordination of all the work of the various disciplines.

Building Systems Engineers

In the simplest of terms, building systems engineers are responsible for the design and specification of the working parts of the facility and infrastructure: heating, air conditioning, lighting, electrical systems, plumbing, and fire protection. These engineers work closely with the architect and interior designer, coordinating system layout and design with the architectural layout. Depending on the size and scope of the project, they may be assisted by specialized subconsultants in areas such as information technology, data networks, audiovisual, vibration control, specialized lighting design, acoustic design, and communication systems.

Structural Engineers

Structural engineers are responsible for the design and calculation of the supporting structure and foundations for a building or for a renovation, based on the architectural design. Design considerations such as seismic requirements are often a critical part of their work. The structural engineer also evaluates and designs how to support very heavy equipment or systems such as overhead surgical lights, MRIs, CTs, or high-density storage systems.

Site/Civil Engineers

Civil engineers design and plan all the work outside a building's walls, such as site grading, paving, drainage, underground site utilities, site lighting, and of course, parking and access roads. They may also handle special design elements such as flood hydrology or traffic studies. Depending on the project's scope, they may also work with landscape architects to design exterior spaces and other specialized consultants such as traffic engineers or parking structure designers.

Medical Equipment Planners

Because few healthcare facilities have the staff to devote to planning the detailed equipment needs of a major facility project, a medical equipment planning consultant can help to select, specify, purchase, and install medical equipment. This can be especially critical in early design stages, when the design team needs equipment information for coordination before the owner has typically begun to consider these details. This coordination of the space planning necessary to accommodate major equipment, as well as the proper design of all required infrastructure needed to serve and operate it, is crucial to the success of any healthcare facility.

Furniture Vendors, Planners, and Suppliers

Furniture dealers provide and install furnishings and furniture systems based on the interior designer's design and specifications. From detailed quotations through warehousing, delivery, and setup, they can be hired to relieve the owner of many of the details of furniture coordination.

Commissioning Agents

Specialized consultants can assist an owner with moving and organizing the start-up of a new facility. Such consultants are usually included only as part of very large projects. They can be responsible for planning and purchasing moving services, coordinating with furniture dealers, or adjusting and testing building systems before occupancy. Hiring a mechanical system commissioning agent can be a crucial step in ensuring that complex systems are operating properly and efficiently after construction is complete, minimizing any potential operating issues after the installing contractor has left the project. They also can assist in training the owner's staff in all aspects of operation of the new system. In high-performance, energy-efficient "green-building" designs, ensuring proper operations through a commissioning process led by an experienced commissioning agent is necessary to ensure that the performance of the mechanical systems meets expectations as promised.

Miscellaneous Specialty Consultants

Depending on the complexity of the project, the architect may need to bring in additional specialized expertise to address more specific aspects of the design solution, including acoustics, building and systems vibrations, information technology, security systems, vertical circulation (elevators), signage, and even artwork.

■ Beginning the Project

Establishing the Parameters of the Project

Before proceeding with the design of a new building or fit-out project, it is important to properly establish the parameters of the project. How big does it need to be? How much space is required? Where will the project be located? Is the site being considered for the project appropriate and adequate? Is adequate infrastructure available to serve the project area? These questions are not simple and should be considered carefully prior to making real estate decisions or proceeding with the project.

Selecting a Design Team

The selection of the design team needs to be based on trust and comfort, because it will be a long-term relationship lasting months or years, with significant long-term financial implications. Achieving this relationship requires a clear two-way flow of information. This information includes the owner's programmatic requirements, budget, and constraints for the group practice facility, as well as the design team's knowledge and approach to the project. The best owner/designer relationships include a trusted advisory role for the design consultant, rather than having the designer dictate solutions. When the owner consults the design professionals in all decision making that could impact the facility, the design professionals can properly advise the owner regarding the implications of such decisions. As a consultant acting for the owner, the design professional can translate goals and needs into a specific design solution, but is not in a position to guarantee schedule, cost, or the final outcome of construction, which he or she does not control.

As when selecting any other service professional, referral sources are a starting point for making an informed choice of a designer or architect. Professional organizations such as the American Institute of Architects (AIA), American Society for Healthcare Engineering (ASHE), American Society of Interior Designers (ASID), and International Interior Design Association (IIDA) have both local and national databases of member firms organized by type of expertise. An Internet search using these and other directory sources can identify professionals with specific types of experience, rather than just a geographic listing. Firm information including previous project examples is often available on the Web to help identify firms with a style and approach that may align with a particular project's needs.

Preparing a Request for Proposal

Selecting a design team for a major facility project, such as a physician-based group practice facility, is an important decision with long-term implications, and should be done in an informed businesslike way, not simply by reacting to recommendations or brochure presentations. Prior to issuing a request for proposal (RFP), the owner may opt to prequalify firms by sending out a request for qualifications (RFQ) to select firms. In this way, the owner can determine which architecture/interior design firms have the best qualifications for the particular project before engaging in a proposal process. The RFQ typically asks for qualifications, background, and basic firm information, but does not request a formal fee proposal. Once firms have been narrowed down based on the RFQs, the owner can move on to RFPs.

The RFP is the key to an organized selection of design professionals. It can be used to obtain parallel responses from potential architects to a set of critical questions. The RFP is a very important document because the quality, thoroughness, and accuracy of the architect's proposal depends in large part on the quality and content of the RFP.

The most basic requirement of the RFP is a clear description of the project and its parameters, including its anticipated size, the anticipated project constriction budget, the required scope of design services, and the key schedule milestone dates. Will the project be a new building or a renovation? Will it include interior design services and selection of furnishings and equipment? How many square feet (or square meters) of space are involved? Does the owner have a master plan or a detailed program of space needs for the facility, or is that to be part of the consultant's work scope? Are there specific time or budget constraints that will impact services to be provided or limit potential design solutions? The information is

specific. Sometimes it makes sense for the owners to hire an architect to help them write the RFP.

Besides outlining the extent of professional services needed, the RFP should include a clear statement of the expected criteria that the owner will use to select the successful design team. In a typical approach, design firms are asked to first submit qualifications describing their experience on similar projects, resumes of specific staff that would work on the projects, and their general approach. After the owner reviews and evaluates these capabilities, only the best-qualified firms (the "short list") are asked to make more detailed technical proposals, including a detailed work plan, schedule, and fee proposal. Some or all of these firms may then be interviewed. To get the clearest responses, it is useful to explain whether the final selection will be based on experience, owner–architect chemistry, approach, fee proposed, or some combination of these factors.

The Architect's Proposal

Upon receipt of the Owners' Request for Proposal for the project, the Architect will prepare a detailed proposal including the scope of services to be provided, their proposed fees, and design schedule. Based on their understanding of the detailed scope of services required for the project, gleaned from the information provided in the RFP, the Architect will assemble the professional staff with appropriate skills for the project. This is done concurrently with preparation of a project schedule because experience level relates directly to the time required to accomplish a task. The most experienced and senior staff are normally responsible for the overall leadership and management of a project as well as setting the overall design strategy that best aligns with the owner's goals and objectives. Their level of experience and expertise typically enables them to address effectively the specific needs of the client and arrive at successful solutions efficiently, quickly, and most economically.

Selecting Consultants

Although some architecture and design firms have in-house engineers on staff, many do not. Depending on the services available from the architect's firm, additional consultants may be needed to complete the design of the new facility. It is typically the architect's responsibility to obtain whatever additional consulting services are required for the project by subcontracting to specialty consultants and including them on the design team. The subconsultants' fees are added to the architect's fees.

The Interview Process

Upon receipt of the architect's proposals in response to the RFP, the owner should schedule a series of interviews with the prospective design teams that they are considering hiring to design the project. For the owner of the facility, the point of interviews with the prospective design team is to test the interpersonal chemistry and professional responsiveness of the short-listed design firms and to learn something about their approach to the specific assignment. There is little benefit in simply having a personal presentation of the firm's generic experience and background or asking for design solutions from the design team without the opportunity for them to really understand the needs of the project first. Successful design solutions require engagement and interaction with the owner and the owner's staff, not just a striking architectural image. An effective way to achieve this goal is with structured interviews with the design firm and an agenda of items to be discussed. Interviews can normally be accomplished in 45 to 60 minutes, including time for questions and discussion. Often members of the interview group will ask similar questions of each presenter, to gauge their relative strengths. The interview process is in and of itself an educational process for the owner, which enables him or her to see the differences between design teams and their approaches to the project.

Key Interview Questions

Firms invited for interviews should be given an agenda in advance, with a request to introduce the specific team members to carry out this assignment; a discussion of the key planning, design, budget, and schedule issues that the team thinks will drive the direction of the project; and a discussion of singular examples of the firm's previous work that best highlight these issues. The goal of the interview is to assess which design team would be the best to work with, how knowledgeable they are about related project issues, and their level of interest and commitment to the project. Because the design team usually will not have had access to all of the facility's information about the project or a chance to work with the healthcare facility's team to discuss issues and develop alternatives prior to the interview, the interview generally does not include a design solution. The goal is to select a professional advisor with confidence, not to choose the most attractive idea at such an early stage. Some sample interview questions should be focused on the project's goals, but more general questions should be included to allow discussion. The following are some examples of appropriate questions:

- What is the experience of the proposed specific individuals with similar projects?
- Clarify the roles of the individuals on the team. For example:
  - Who will be the prime contact on a day-to-day basis?
  - Who is in charge from the consultant side?
  - What specialized consultants (such as engineers, lighting designers, and medical equipment planners) are proposed?
- How are the firm's financial resources, stability, staff resources, and facilities?
- Is the design firm's location convenient to the facility's team for frequent interaction?
- What is the firm's approach to this project, including key ideas to be considered in design?
- Do you have an understanding of local codes and the construction market?
- What is your design philosophy, style, and approach?
- Do you have similar project experience, with references?
- Please describe the scope of services proposed, with work plan and design schedule.
- Please supply examples of the architectural design aesthetic of your other work.

Determining the Scope of Work

On the macro level, the overall project schedule summarizes the major steps to a project, starting with the initial response to an RFP, through design, construction, owner occupancy of the new space, and perhaps even a postoccupancy evaluation. On the micro level, a more detailed, well-constructed project schedule becomes a work plan for the project. It takes into account all individual and sequential tasks involved in producing a design, and the scheduled duration for each task. The architect is usually responsible for establishing and maintaining the design portion of the project schedule and clearly communicating this timeline of events to the owner and the entire design team. The tasks on this master schedule are given time durations, for which hours and, subsequently, fees can be assigned. Of particular importance to the owner are the key decision milestones and the expected time commitment of the owner and the staff, so that the healthcare facility can plan this into its work schedule.

Architects' Design Fees

Negotiation of professional fees should be a separate process, after the interview to select the preferred firm, because fees are essentially dictated by staff time needed for the project. The discussion should focus on the right fee for the specific team, scope of services, and work plan discussed and needed by the group practice for the project. Professional firms in a given market region have generally similar labor and overhead costs, and in general ought to be similar in their fees. A very low fee compared to the others usually indicates the use of less staff time or of less experienced staff rather than the senior presenters who may have made such a good impression at the interview.

Architectural fees for professional planning and design services represent the amount of time and associated expense required for the professional(s) to provide the contracted services, plus a reasonable margin for profit. In architectural design and planning, the physical "deliverable" is traditionally the articulation of design solutions in the form of drawings and specifications. In addition, depending on the level of contracted services, the project may require design concepts to be developed and explained in a written narrative as well as with diagrams, graphics, photographs, notes, material samples, and presentations. Depending on the unique needs of the project, the practice, together with the architect, can determine what medium might be best to represent the practice's goals for its particular needs.

There are several different methods by which the design professional may determine the fees required to design the project, and each requires several initial steps to determine the total cost for a professional team to provide the required services. The design professional assesses the complexity of the problem in terms of a design solution, and tallies all the requirements, totals their value in terms of billable rates of professional staff, estimates reimbursable expenses, and includes a profit margin. The total is normally the fee for service.

Types of Fee Structures

The architect and the owner can engage in an agreement for services based on a variety of compensation structures. The following are a few of the more common fee structures:

- *Fixed fees:* This is perhaps the most common form of compensation agreement between a healthcare facility and the architect. A fixed fee is a total compensation figure, often referred to as a lump sum, inclusive of all services the architect and all required consultants agree to provide the owner. Reimbursable expenses, discussed later in this section, are usually in addition to this fixed fee.
- *Hourly fees:* As the name implies, an hourly fee arrangement means for each hour the architect works on the project, he or she is compensated within the limits of the agreed-on maximum fee limit. Sometimes this is referred to as working on a "time-and-materials" or a "timecard project" basis because it costs the healthcare facility the direct expense of the professionals' time and expenses for producing the work. There is often a maximum

limit, or "upset," to an hourly fee, thereby giving the architect some budgetary limits. Usually hourly fee arrangements are better suited for smaller consulting or limited planning services in which the architect or designer is kept on a retainer basis for services as they are needed.

- *Other fee structures:* There can be as many different types of fee structures as there are unique needs of clients. The exact structure depends on how the office suite will be constructed, furnished, leased, or subleased, and what time constraints there are for the construction schedule. These agreements typically are used more by developers, design–build teams, and construction managers; they are not the typical fee-for-service arrangement that architects use.

Project-Related Expenses

In addition to the professional fees paid directly to professional staff, other expenses incurred in the process of delivering the design services usually include:

- Plotting, printing, and reproducing drawings and documents
- Overnight mail and courier services
- Travel costs for the design team in connection with the project (airfare, train fare, rental car, etc.)
- Subsistence allowance for meals when traveling
- Three-dimensional models and materials required to build physical models
- Other miscellaneous items as negotiated between the architect and owner

The architect is typically entitled to be reimbursed for these expenses. Depending on the size of the project and the extent of the accounting paperwork required by the architect, sometimes the architect charges a nominal fee for accounting management of all of the expenses as well those of his or her design subconsultants, usually in the range of 5–10% of the expense total.

Understanding the many steps involved in determining a fee is important to a healthcare facility because its members are often involved in the fee negotiations with the architect. Knowing some of the complexities of the architect's work, or at least the many considerations that go into a fee calculation, helps explain the rationale behind the fee, and therefore takes some of the mystery out of the fee negotiation. Once the overall project schedule is established, all the tasks have been identified, the design team has been selected, and the consultant team has been assembled, the architect can then calculate the required fee to deliver the project. A basic method by which the architect may begin to calculate the fee is to determine the hours required by each professional on his or her team to deliver the scope of work required of the project. Then the billable rates for each professional can be added up, an anticipated amount can be added for expenses, and an overhead factor for a reasonable profit can be added.

Architectural/design firms should provide a list of their hourly billable rates for each level of professional in their employ. Billable rates normally include the actual hourly rate the employee earns based on salary, plus the firm's overall overhead expenses, which include the employee's benefits, cost of their office, equipment, utilities, and the general costs of doing business. Once the hours have been determined, the total dollar value for each of these categories becomes the overall fee. If required, the architect will break down the fee into each of these categories to show how it was calculated. An example of a simple fee tabulation is summarized in **Table 21-1**. This calculation assumes a project team for a hypothetical, small project.

The fee is calculated and negotiated based on as specific a scope of work as possible. If the scope of the work changes, which means work is either added or subtracted, normally an adjustment is made to the professional fees. When the scope changes, the owner and architect should review the agreed-on fees and make adjustments as appropriate to fairly compensate the design team for the services they have provided or must yet provide.

Table 21-1 Sample Project Team with Billable Rates for Fee Determination

Staff	Hours	Billable Rate ($)	Subtotal Fee ($)
Principal in charge	40	200	8,000
Senior designer	60	150	9,000
Project architect	120	110	13,200
Junior staff	200	75	15,000
Subtotal			45,200
Engineering consultant fees			20,000
Direct expenses (estimate)			5,000
Subtotal			25,000
Total professional fees			70,200
Anticipated reimbursable expense budget			12,000

Professional Service Fees

The conventional method of fee determination is a basic, direct, illustrative example of precisely where each required element falls into the overall fee. However, this is only one method. Other methods for fee calculation are used throughout the architectural industry, some of which are shorthand approaches for coming up with a fee that is generally in the same range as the analytical steps outlined in the previous section.

Cost of Construction Method. One approach architects sometimes use to determine fees, and that the healthcare center can use to compare fees, is to charge a fee based on a percentage of the anticipated cost of construction for the project. If a project construction budget is $5 million, for example, a design fee could potentially be 5–10% of the cost of construction, depending on regional economic factors that affect the cost of construction and the complexity of the project. For example, an administrative office suite or exam room suite is easier to design (i.e., might require less time and fees) than an endoscopy practice that requires a special ceiling structure for lights, high-output ventilation systems, medical gases, and more durable and expensive finish materials. This method of fee calculation is sometimes used to determine an order-of-magnitude fee for budgeting purposes, but in general, is less accurate than the analytical approach previously outlined.

Cost per Drawing Sheet Fee Calculation. It was once common practice to determine a fee for a project by determining the total number of drawing sheets required for the construction documents and assigning a set number of work hours per sheet. This number of hours was amalgamated from years of experience and would include a percentage of time for design, coordination, and actual drawing. This method was more effective when architectural drafting was all done by hand. Now that the architectural and design profession is predominantly computerized and drawings are mostly done electronically, the hours per sheet method is not an accurate assessment tool. Sharing and reusing electronic information leads to improved efficiencies and saved time; however, sometimes the time savings are offset by the additional time required to manage the computer drafting systems and vast libraries of electronic information.

Getting the Project Started

Once the owner or administration of the healthcare facility hires a design firm, they need to understand the steps in the design process. With a planning and design team on board, the facility's first need is to clearly define the mission and goals of the project: What are you trying to achieve? This needs to be discussed at the first working session. Budget limitations, approval processes, schedule constraints, functional needs, internal political issues, and broader issues such as brand identity are ideas to consider when defining goals for the project. A well-prepared RFP would include much of this project background information, as discussed in the previous section. The parameters of a successful project include a clear and agreed-upon direction from the start, and a sharing of that direction among the team that is composed of healthcare facility members and design consultants. It is important to have shared goals and a common definition of a successful project, in terms of design, image, function, budget, schedule, and quality, before beginning a design solution.

There are traditional well-defined "phases" of architectural design that start with general design concepts and then gradually add layers of design specificity until the project is completely defined, described, and detailed in drawings and specifications. It is important to know what these phases are because designers use them frequently as a matter of shorthand, and each has fairly well-defined parameters and definitions. These will be discussed in the following sections.

Architectural Programming

The architectural program defines functional and space needs and ideally the quality and character of the space that will be accommodated in the project. At a minimum, it is a listing of required rooms and their sizes, but properly used, the program can be an important planning tool to explore organizational and operational assumptions. Wherever possible, it should be quantified in terms of function and clearly define such items as:

- How many patient records need to be stored in the file room?
- How many patient visits will each provider handle each day?
- How many clerical staff will work in the billing office?
- How many visitors will accompany each patient?
- What will be the hours of operation?

The discussions leading to answers for such questions can often be facilitated by the design professional, who specializes in the "what if" questions that can lead to design insights and creative solutions. Planning a space to accommodate several functions can potentially reduce total space needed and improve flexibility. For example, smaller private offices and more shared conference and consult spaces can reduce the amount of space that remains unused at any given time. It is unrealistic to expect every space to be used all the time. An efficiency factor of 80% use of typical exam rooms, for example, is a reasonable

goal. The use of specialized procedure or diagnostic rooms will often be much lower, due to more complicated room cleaning, setup, and turnaround times.

Programs set out as a spreadsheet can also serve as a preliminary budgeting tool to track staff needs, equipment, and cost of space based on typical unit costs. The balance of space by type can be adjusted and the cost impact considered. In addition, the correlation between practice volume and space needs can be seen. For example, if each exam room can serve 10 to 12 daily patient visits, or 2,500 to 3,700 per year (depending on hours of operation, procedure time, and days worked), it is possible to see the point at which a six-exam-room suite will become overtaxed, and eight rooms will be needed in order to handle the anticipated patient volume.

In order to understand space in buildings and how it is calculated, it is important to understand a few key definitions. Programming classifies space in three categories:

- *Net square footage (nsf):* The actual space within a specific room or work area. (A simple analogy to remember this is the net area of a room is the space that could get carpet.)
- *Departmental gross square footage (dgsf):* Includes the nsf plus the circulation space between rooms, such as corridors, stairs, and housekeeping space, as well as building construction components like interior partitions and columns. The dgsf is measured from the exterior windows inward. The dgsf is calculated with a multiplier that ranges from 1.4 to 1.7 times the nsf.
- *Building gross square footage (bgsf):* Includes the dgsf plus the area occupied by the overall building construction, such as thickness of exterior walls, mechanical shafts, egress stairways, and elevator shafts.

Key to the programming phase is that the design team, as well as the owner, uses a rigorous analytical process and avoids anecdotal statements regarding space needs, such as the amount of space one has now, or had in some previous practice, or simply a fixed number of rooms per provider. The point at which planning decisions have the greatest leverage in terms of cost savings for the life of the facility is when they can be tested and adapted as the space program is developed. The cost of a facility is primarily dependent on the size of the facility, as defined by the program, and the resulting construction and amount of infrastructure required. This infrastructure includes the building structure and enclosure and its heating, air-conditioning, electrical, and plumbing requirements. Many requirements are dictated by local building codes or health department regulations based on the overall size and purpose of the facility.

Table 21-2 is an example of an architectural space program. The basis of the entire design is derived from the architectural program, so it is a very important piece of the process. The architectural program should be finalized and correlated to a construction budget before design begins. Ideally, all key decision makers will sign off on the final program. This final signed-off program will then be the agreed-to basis upon which the project will be designed, with the sign-off representing approval to commence design. Changes made by the owner to the

Table 21-2	Generic Program—Orthopedic Center			
Area/Function	Qty	SF Each	Total	Comments
Entry	1	100	100	Vestibule
Waiting	1	300	300	For 10–15
Business office	1	180	180	2 workstations. Check-in/check-out
Nurse station	1	100	100	Counter. Medicine cabinet
Exam room	4	100	400	
Cast room	1	150	150	No plaster—storage along 1 wall
Radiology room	1	200	200	Use patient toilet
Processing	1	30	30	Rapid processor
Control	1	30	30	
Dressing	1	55	55	Size for handicapped
Patient toilet	2	55	110	Size for handicapped
Doctor office	2	125	250	Potential second doctor
Doctor view/chart	1	100	100	1 per doctor
Education/credit/counseling	1	100	100	
Staff lounge	1	100	100	
Staff toilet	1	55	55	Size for handicapped
Storage	1	50	50	
Soiled hold	1	50	50	
Wheelchair storage	1	40	40	
P.T. reception	1	150	150	2 people
P.T. waiting	1	250	250	For 10–12
P.T. toilet	2	55	110	Size for handicapped
P.T. office	2	80	160	
Exercise	1	1000	1000	Open area
Modality	1	300	300	4 stations—open area
P.T. equipment/wheelchair	1	60	60	
Janitor closet	1	30	30	
Mechanical	1	130	130	
Total Net Square Feet			4590	
Net-to-gross factor			1.4	
Total Gross Square Feet			6426	

Planning Assumptions
- Orthopedic Center including offices and physical therapy, occupational health, and sports medicine
- Parking: 10 spaces/doctor plus parking for physical therapy
- Needs to be handicapped accessible

program after design commences may have a drastic effect on the design process and will likely lead to additional design fees being necessary.

Schematic Design (SD) Phase

With agreement on program needs as defined in the architectural space program, schematic or preliminary concepts are developed to fit the program plans and the site. This early phase is the time to test the program fit by considering basic stacking of functions, if it is a multifloor structure, and horizontal adjacencies of the program elements, as well as to establish the basic design concept. Schematic drawings are normally made to scale, but sometimes show walls on drawings as only a single line, often without the detail of doors and other construction. (See **Figure 21-1**.) The point of this step is to establish an understanding of the size, layout, design intent, and physical scope of the project. Conceptual interior or exterior designs are often discussed, but require considerable design development.

If the project is a new building, then schematic design is more extensive because it involves development of the architectural concept for the building, as well as proposed engineering systems for infrastructure, structural framing, and site work. A preliminary order-of-magnitude cost estimate can be made based on the final program and the schematic design. The entire package should be presented to the healthcare facility's decision-making group for approval before proceeding further. A physical sign-off on the documents by the various representatives of the practice is a useful technique to get everyone focused on the importance of this phase and ready to commit to the approved design. Once the design has progressed, it is more difficult and expensive to go back to the issues of how many rooms, how much space, and what planning adjacencies are required.

Design Development (DD) Phase

With owner approval of the schematic design and the SD budget, the design team leads the process of making more detailed design decisions, room by room, system by system. Working closely with the ambulatory care center's team and facility users, the designers review the features and requirements for each element of the facility design in preparation for making detailed construction drawings. This is the point in the design process where furnishings, cabinetry, medical equipment, computer and communication systems, and interior finishes all need to be discussed in detail. Items that are not identified and recorded here, even including apparently minor items such as special electrical outlets, telephone and data locations, special hardware needs, or specific finishes, will not appear in the final construction documents and will thus not be included in contractor bids. Adding these items into the

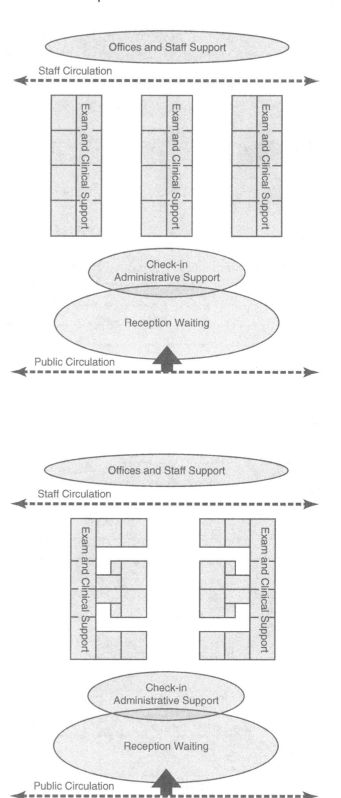

Figure 21-1 Planning concept diagrams.

design later will be at a much higher cost. Room data sheets, such as the one in **Table 21-3**, are a method architects use to collect this important and detailed information from the owner to incorporate into the design.

Table 21-3 Generic Room Data Sheet

Project Information		RDS	Approvals	Date
Project Name:	General Hospital Medical Office Building	☑ Initial		
Project Number:		☐ Interim		
Department:	Orthopedic Center	☐ Final		
Room Name:	Staff Break Room	☐ Revisions		
Room No.	1003			

Walls	Floor	Base	Ceilings
☑ GWB (painted)	☑ VCT	☑ Vinyl	☑ ACT 2x2
☐ Ceramic Tile (full ht.)	☐ Sheet Vinyl	☐ Rubber	☐ ACT 2x4
☐ Ceramic Tile (wainscoting)	☐ Carpet (broadloom)	☐ Ceramic Tile	☐ GWB
☐ Fabric	☐ Carpet (tiles)	☐ Carpet	☐ Mylar/Vinyl Clean Tile
☐ Vinyl	☐ Ceramic Tile	☐ Other (specify)	☐ GWB w/ACT adhered
☐ Other (Specify)	☐ Epoxy Terrazzo	☐ Other (specify)	☐ Special
Notes:	☐ Wood	☐ Other (specify)	☐ Other (Specify)
	☐ Wood Simulation	Notes:	☐ Other (Specify)
	☐ Other (specify)		Notes:

Electrical Items	Power	Communications/Data	Lighting Fixtures
☑ Clock	☑ General	☑ Telephone	☑ Fluorescent 232
☐ E/T Clock	☐ Life Safety	☐ Intercom	☐ Fluorescent 234
☑ TV	☐ Emergency	☑ Nurse Call	☐ Pendant Fixtures
☐ CCTV	☐ Ground Jack	☐ Emergency Code	☑ Under Cabinet Task Lights
☐ Duplex	☐ GFI	☐ Dictation	☐ Reading Light
☐ Other	☐ Other	☐ Paging	☐ Over Bed Light
Notes:	Notes:	☐ Fax	☐ Exam-ceiling mtd
		☐ Computer	☐ Night Light
		☑ Other	☐ Other (Specify)
		Notes: Dishwasher and garbage disposal	Notes:

HVAC	Gases		Plumbing		Environment Conditions
☐ Air Change Requirements	☐ Comp Air	QTY:	☑ Sink	QTY: 1	☐ Acoustical Trtmt
☐ Exhaust	☐ Oxygen	QTY:	☐ Toilet - HC	QTY:	☑ Daylight Req.
☐ Temp. Range:	☐ Vacuum	QTY:	☐ Shower	QTY:	☐ Radiation Shldg.
☐ Humidity Range:	☐ Nitrogen	QTY:	☐ Urinal	QTY:	☐ RF Shielding
☐ Negative Pressure	☐ Nitrous Oxide	QTY:	☐ Tub	QTY:	☐ Leaded Glass
☐ Positive Pressure	☐ Evac.	QTY:	☐ Flush Rim Sk	QTY:	☐ Special:
☐ WAGE	☐ Natural Gas	QTY:	☐ Floor Drain	QTY:	Notes:
☐ Other:	☐ Notes:		☐ Bed Pan Washer		
	☐		☑ Other		
			Notes: Dishwasher		

Fire Protection	Casework	Structural Issues	Special Requirements
☐ Alarm	☑ Base Cabinet	☐ Floor Loading	☐ Handrails
☐ Sprinkler Heads	☑ Wall Cabinet	☐ Floor Mtd Equip.	☐ Wall Protection
☐ Exiting Signage	☐ Desk	☐ Ceiling Mtd Equip.	☐ Corner Guards
☑ Smoke Detector	☐ Base Cb. W/Sink	☐ Vibration Isolation	☐ Bed Locator
☐ Heat Detector	☐ Pedestal	☐ Slab Depression	☐ Bumperguards
☐ Other	☐ Custom	☐ Addtn'l Ceiling Structure	☐ Combo Handrail/Bumper
Notes:	☐ Metal	☐ Addtn'l Floor Structure	Notes:
	☐ P-lam	☐ Coordinate Ductwork	
	Notes:	Notes:	

This is also the stage where input from the healthcare facility is essential, including such information as a highly detailed medical and office equipment list with catalog sheets, sizes, clearances, and utility requirements. For comparison, in the schematic design phase, a cardiology exam room might be identified as a stress test room and sized accordingly, but at the design development phase the actual make and model of the treadmill, its voltage requirements, and its computer system all need to be determined in order for the design to include the space and services required. Design development is the time to explore the detailed look of the facility too, with three-dimensional drawings, renderings, or physical or electronic models of key interior and exterior spaces, samples of proposed materials, and preliminary studies of construction details.

The product of the DD phase will be both drawings and a written outline specification that describes most of the products, fixtures, and materials to be used in the construction. In general, the overall project scope of work and definition of the major architectural and engineering systems must be clearly defined. From the DD package of drawings and written specifications, a detailed cost estimate should be prepared for approval. Although previous unit cost estimates may have been prepared by the design team or a contractor for the schematic design at little cost, the design development estimate should be a detailed professional estimate by an independent construction cost-estimating consultant or a construction manager retained to provide what's called preconstruction services. Architects and engineers generally do not have the firsthand experience with construction costs that is required at this phase. The best interest of the healthcare facility at this point is a realistic and conservative estimate by a qualified cost estimator, plus provision of both design and construction cost contingencies to allow for the unknown.

Ideally, after the design development estimate is completed, the facility's architect and estimator should meet to review cost and schedule assumptions and discuss alternatives and possible savings. Once again, at the end of the DD phase, a specific sign-off and approval from all members of the healthcare facility team are highly recommended.

Construction Document (CD) Phase

Construction documents, sometimes called "working drawings," describe in detail the final project required by the healthcare facility. The drawings and written specifications form the basis of the bid price by contractors. The specifications, or project manual, describe in writing the specific materials, workmanship, and systems to be used and how they will be used. The detailed drawings, specifications, and other documents used for bidding by contractors are the "blueprints" that are the basis for building the facility. These documents are of critical importance. If something is not included in the bid documents, it will not be in the bid price and will not be included in the construction of the finished facility, except at extra cost. Design requirements and features that may have been discussed with the design team or thought to be promised at some point along the way need to be indicated explicitly in the construction documents; otherwise, they will not be included. The design team often implements a series of quality-control checks throughout the CD phase to ensure all the details have been thoroughly worked out and shown on the drawings.

Construction Administration (CA) Phase

Once a contractor or construction manager has been selected, either through low bid or by negotiation, the design team typically assists the healthcare facility in working with the contractor. Early in the construction phase, they request and review for approval a detailed construction schedule and a detailed breakdown of construction costs. In addition, the contractor submits samples of the actual materials selected by the design team, catalog copies of products to be used, and shop drawings prepared by subcontractors for items they will fabricate such as cabinetry and windows.

During the construction process, representatives from the design team observe and advise the healthcare facility team on progress, usually attending periodic owner–architect–contractor meetings that are led by the contractor. The design team reviews all of these various submittals for compliance with the design drawings and specifications and provides comments back to the contractor. As an important protection, architects are often asked to sign off on contractor payment requests to confirm the extent of progress and the presence of construction materials on-site.

At substantial completion of the work, the architect will assist the owners in final inspections and prepare a written "punch list" of deficiencies that the contractor needs to correct. Sometimes more extensive on-site services by the design team are available as an option, such as detailed inspections or full-time on-site representatives—all at additional cost. In any case, it is important to understand that the designer is legally prevented from directing the actual construction work itself and can act only as an agent reporting to and advising the healthcare facility.

■ Sustainable Building and LEED

Sustainable building practices increase the efficiency by which building projects use resources while reducing impacts on the environment and human health. These so called "green practices" are achieved through efficient use of water, energy, and other natural resources, in addition to paying attention to reduced waste, pollution, and environmental degradation. The healthcare sector is the second most energy-intensive user in the United States, and with energy costs going up, it is worthwhile to aggressively consider investing in greater energy efficiency with the added benefit of reducing the facility's potentially environmental impacts. In an era when energy costs are increasing dramatically and societal concerns turn toward global warming, conservation of resources, and recycling, having a facility that is responsive to those societal concerns may be in the best interests of the healthcare facility and its employees. In addition to environmental concerns for energy and natural resource consumption and conservation, green design also takes into consideration construction materials that are harmful to the environment and directly to human health. Polyvinyl chloride, or PVC, typically found throughout healthcare facilities, exposes people to chemicals and fumes from cleaning products that are harmful to human health. New, greener products are becoming available to replace these potentially harmful materials.

The Leadership in Energy and Environmental Design (LEED) Green Building Rating System is a third-party certification program created by the U.S. Green Building Council (USGBC) that is a benchmark for the design and construction of sustainable buildings, communities, and developments. LEED is a nationally recognized tool for measuring overall sustainable performance in five categories: sustainable site development, water savings, energy efficiency, materials selection, and indoor environmental quality. An integrated design process is essential to the successful development of a sustainable project. Sustainable design strategies should be linked to the specific client goals and values, leading to the broader pursuit of design excellence.

There is a growing awareness of these concerns among design professionals, and an accreditation program through LEED has emerged for those who demonstrate understanding of sustainable processes, systems, and design, as well as proficiency in applying sustainable design approaches. Many sustainable design strategies are just part of good, responsible design by well-trained architects, such as siting a building to maximize its solar orientation for optimum solar heat gain in the winter and minimized solar heat gain in the summer. This might also translate into treating the exterior elevations of the building differently to optimize the solar, heat, light, and wind conditions, such as low-emissivity glass on windows, or adding passive solar shades to exterior elevations. Sustainable design measures such as these are simple and add little or no cost to the construction, but can have dramatic effects on the energy required to heat and cool the building.

Some sustainable strategies, such as incorporating a combined heating and power system or using captured rainwater from the site for sewage conveyance, for example, are more complicated and require specialized expertise to implement. Measures such as these, while adding construction costs to the building, eventually pay for themselves and yield savings over the life of the building. As owners increase their awareness of sustainable design practices, the construction industry will become more accustomed to building ecologically responsible designs. In turn, more recycled materials and sustainable products will emerge and reach the market, and it will be easier and more affordable to build sustainably designed buildings. Utility companies and government agencies have become avid supporters of buildings that have reduced energy demands, and many of them offer grants and financial or tax incentives to owners to implement energy-saving systems in their buildings.

As community-based businesses relying on serving the community, healthcare facilities and physician practices may be expected to be part of a healthy, ecologically responsible facility. They will be expected, therefore, above all other facilities, to provide a healthy, nonharmful environment in which to provide medicine. Achievement of LEED certification can help demonstrate that the practice and business value these concerns and are responsible members of the community they serve.

■ Construction Services

Once the healthcare team has a design solution for its new facility(ies), it needs to hire a builder to construct the architect's design. A common misperception by those unfamiliar with the design and construction process is that the architect builds the project. The architect is trained to design the project, not actually construct it. There are different types of builders and approaches to building. The following sections discuss some of the more common builder types.

General Contractors

Typical contractors provide building services based on bids from detailed construction documents developed by the architect. Usually the general contractor will handle basic building shell work directly but will subcontract specialized trade construction, such as mechanical, plumbing, electrical services, or site work to other, more specialized tradespeople.

Construction Managers

More than a contractor, a construction manager (CM) is equipped to provide fee-based supervision, scheduling, and direction of the construction process. Depending on the facility's needs, these services may include preconstruction cost estimating and construction planning services. The CM may provide some construction services directly or may subcontract some or all of the work. Through negotiation, the CM may be asked to provide a fixed price for the project at any stage of design, called a guaranteed maximum price (GMP) contract, which by definition includes substantial design and construction contingencies.

Subcontractors

Trade contractors, usually working under the direction of a general contractor or CM, provide specific construction services, such as plumbing or electrical work, with bids based on detailed construction documents prepared by the architect. It is usually up to the general contractor or CM to schedule and coordinate their work, again based on the material prepared by the architect.

Design/Build Contractors

In order to meet some facilities' needs for a simplified, single source of responsibility, design/build (D/B) contractors provide construction management and design services as one package, usually through subcontractors. Architectural services, interior design, and engineering services are provided and directed by the D/B firm. The features of this approach are negotiated price and quality. When the D/B firm is responsible for a fixed price and content, it is also responsible for the design and quality decisions needed to meet that price.

■ Construction Delivery Methods

There is a variety of approaches a business can use to construct its clinical space. The best choice depends on how the healthcare facility wants to finance construction.

Design/Bid/Build: The Traditional Approach

In the traditional model for building projects, the owner selects all team members for both the design and construction components. Architects, interior designers, and other consultants are selected and hired by the owner. Once the owner hires these consultants, he or she must manage all of them and the process. After a design and its construction documents have been developed by this team, and the design is complete, the final construction cost is fixed by multiple contractor bids on these specific design documents. The contractor bids are analyzed, and generally the lowest bid that includes all of the specified scope of work is accepted. Because all of the team members work directly for the owner, the project's design quality is determined by practice members, who approve the final design. Depending on the experience of the team and the clarity of the owner's goals, the result can be a slow but more transparent process. In the end, all decisions are approved by the owner, who also pays all of the costs of the project.

Design/Build Method

A contrasting approach is one in which a contractor assembles and controls all the members of a completely integrated team of designers and builders. The contractor offers to provide a facility to meet the group practice's stated needs, essentially as a "package deal," and to be the single point of contact to simplify the process. In this approach the owner relinquishes some control of the design team, and to some extent the control over project quality, but has the benefit of having to deal with only one entity, the design/build contractor. The package price is fixed by negotiation at any stage of design and can be a lump sum or "cost plus with savings returned" arrangement. To meet the agreed price, the contractor retains the design team, directs design choices, and sets the overall quality of the project. The design/build method is not as transparent to the owner as the design/bid/build process because many of the design decisions are made internally between the contractor and the design team. If needs are clear and decisions can be made easily, this can be a faster process, but at the cost of reduced owner input and control.

■ The Quality of the Interior Environment

The group practice administrator needs to be aware of some of the more technical details that will be handled directly by the design team, but require input and decisions by the administrator and facility users, such as final materials and finish selections.

Interior Materials and Finishes

The selection of materials and visible finishes is an important part of reducing operating costs and representing the desired brand identity of the group practice. The look and feel of the built space should convey and reinforce the desired image or branding characteristics of the practice, whether the image desired is traditional, conservative, modern, cutting edge, comforting, warm, reassuring, clearly organized, or technologically advanced. The choice of materials can also be a tradeoff between durability and flexibility, and first cost versus life-cycle cost. Lighter materials, such as drywall construction and acoustical tile ceilings, offer a high degree of flexibility and are relatively easy to change or replace when needed—even if finish materials are more elaborate, such as wood paneling or special finishes. Heavier construction, such as masonry, plaster, and terrazzo, is considerably more durable but more difficult to change and sometimes impossible to reuse when functional needs change.

The choice of finish materials is a balance between the desired appearance and the realities of maintenance. Commercial facilities such as hotels and stores often plan for more extensive continued cleaning and maintenance and more frequent replacements of damaged material than is typical for medical practices. Delicate or easily soiled materials that are not well maintained are less attractive than simpler materials that can be kept clean and presentable. Designers generally are well aware of the limitations and maintenance needs of materials, but must be apprised of the anticipated cleaning and maintenance services in order to select the appropriate materials.

Maintenance Issues

Commercial-grade carpet and upholstery fabrics are designed to be easy to maintain and durable, even when subjected to heavy wear, but will still require prompt attention to spills and stains. If the facility operator or maintenance service contractor is not able to provide this level of attention, more durable materials should be considered.

In areas subject to spills and bodily fluids, water-repellant and waterproof, resilient, and easily cleaned materials are recommended. In addition to a careful choice of materials, the space-planning process also needs to consider convenient space for housekeeping and maintenance equipment. Equipment such as vacuums and floor polishers should be stored near the point of use.

In addition to cleaning, consider the maintenance issues of items such as lamp replacements for light fixtures, design of ventilation and plumbing systems to minimize ongoing maintenance, and the durability of surfaces and their ease of repair. Painted walls and doors are easily damaged, but can be repainted with little effort and expense. Wall covering is more durable than paint, but when it gets damaged it costs more to repair or replace.

Wood surfaces can be scratched and scarred, but also sanded and refinished. Plastic laminate, once chipped, cannot be repaired and must be replaced. Finishes and materials should be carefully selected to provide the desired high-quality appearance in select areas of the office suite, and more durable, lower-maintenance materials in the more utilitarian, heavy work spaces. Particularly challenging is a space that is both for patients and requires a high degree of durability and maintainability such as an exam room. Here the choice of materials involves weighing both patient appeal and long-term durability.

Millwork and Casework

A common feature of most medical spaces is the standard use of built-in cabinetry (architectural millwork or casework), which can become a large cost item. Millwork is generally custom-made for a facility and might include special paneling, woodwork, reception desks, or custom doors. Casework, by comparison, is composed of a system of premanufactured modular cabinetry components and counters, which may be selected from a vendor's standard sizes.

Millwork can be custom constructed of many materials. The most commonly used finish materials for custom millwork cabinetry are solid wood, wood veneer, and plastic laminate. Glass and metal components can be incorporated into custom designs. Counters can be made of plastic laminate, solid surface (such as Corian), stone, or other materials, depending on the design intent, desired durability, and whether the counter will come in contact with water. Casework, by contrast, is most often made of plastic laminate on particleboard, but can also be made of wood or metal.

Because millwork and casework are both expensive and space-consuming, one approach for the group practice administrator is to start out with little or no casework and add it only as needed for specific uses. Although many areas such as exam rooms do require work counters, sinks, and storage, the amount of casework needed may be less than expected. Current standards, for example, require sinks accessible to the physically challenged with no storage below, so the traditional sink base cabinet is often replaced by an apron panel to conceal plumbing, while allowing access for maintenance. Alternatively, a wall-hung sink with no cabinet below can be used. Wall space is needed above and around sinks for accessories such as soap and towel dispensers, sharps disposal containers, and glove dispensers.

Some practices may choose to use mobile carts for supply storage instead of built-in cabinets. Mobile carts can be a flexible way to restock supplies and provide a mobile work surface in an exam or treatment space. Sometimes spaces are more flexible and optimized when less is built in and storage functions are accommodated using mobile carts. Below-counter storage is typically underutilized because it is not convenient or ergonomic to use for frequently needed items. It sometimes results in the unnecessary and expensive hoarding of supplies, simply because the space is available. Where substantial storage is needed, as in procedure rooms, clean supply rooms, or workrooms, highly adaptable and mobile storage systems can be more effective than the usual casework or built-in shelves.

Lighting

Natural lighting is often preferred by patients and staff for all the positive effects it offers to one's psychological outlook and mood. Whenever access to natural light cannot be achieved, artificial lighting and how it is designed becomes an important factor. The proper design of lighting affects both the function and the ambiance of any well-designed space. Specialized lighting may be needed in certain procedure areas, but often portable lamps are as effective as more expensive built-in lights. Large-scale procedure or surgical lights require specific structural design to provide heavy-duty mountings above the ceiling. In exam and general areas, current designs often use inexpensive direct/indirect fluorescent lighting in lay-in acoustic tile ceilings, which creates attractive lighting while still providing a high level of light. Consideration should be given to what the patient sees when looking up at the ceiling during an exam. Providing lighting fixtures with shielded lamps in such situations is appropriate. Additional task lighting under upper storage cabinets or above a hand-washing sink may also be welcoming. In waiting and public areas, lower levels and indirect light may be more appropriate. Low-voltage halogen lighting is useful for accents, displays, or artwork.

Plumbing Fixtures

Some medical areas may have specific requirements for hands-free fixtures at hand-washing locations where invasive procedures are performed and sterile environments are required. These special fixtures can be either wrist blades or infrared electronic faucet controls. Foot or knee controls tend to have higher maintenance and cleaning issues and are usually avoided. Details such as faucet spout heights, size and depth of sinks, and special equipment requirements all need to be coordinated between users and designers. Sinks in specialized areas, such as where plaster work is done and in darkrooms, may need specific traps to screen out plaster or chemicals.

Wall-mounted plumbing fixtures are typically easier to clean around but require provision of steel carrier frames inside the walls during construction. Floor-mounted fixtures are simpler but may require more effort to clean.

Physical Settings for Group Practices

The types and complexities of healthcare services that can be delivered outside a licensed hospital setting are regulated by building codes in effect for the site selected and the local state department of health that has jurisdiction for that area. Basic medical services administered to patients in a typical business day, and thereby not requiring any kind of overnight hospitalization or accommodations, can normally be provided in a building type that is classified as, and designed as, office space. More complex outpatient treatments that might require sedation usually must be done in a facility classified as an ambulatory healthcare center. The physical difference is subtle and pertains primarily to fire and life safety codes, travel distances, and whether patients are capable of self-preservation, or are sedated or completely anesthetized for a procedure. Construction codes require ambulatory care centers to allow for but limit the number of anesthetized patients in the facility at any one time. Ambulatory care centers can have extensive diagnostic and treatment services within them, much like hospitals; however, the specific services they provide are limited by their hours of operation and inability to accommodate overnight patients. For example, if the group practice includes an ambulatory surgery center, the surgical procedures provided will have to be limited to those patients can recover from without being admitted overnight.

The Programmatic Needs of a Physician-Based Group Practice

Once the organizational and operational structure of the facility has been determined, the programming requirements can begin to be assessed. Programming is both an analytical and a conceptual process by which the functional and operational goals of the business are identified, defined, and quantified. Some of the space requirements are derived from mathematical calculations using guidelines for utilization and volume projections; others are based on the unique operational and staffing needs of the practice. This is one of the more important and complicated steps in the process because all design and budgeting parameters henceforth are derived from the program. Therefore, it is important to understand some of the key aspects of the complex process architects refer to as "programming."

Projecting Programming Needs

Facility planning for medical practices or clinics was once comparatively simple and formulaic. It was generally the rule that each physician would occupy a private office used for patient consultation and after-hours work, with one or more adjoining examination rooms. Highly productive physicians or nurse practitioners in certain specialties might have three or four exam rooms in their cluster of space. Office and exam space was often a function of rank or seniority and did not necessarily have any direct correlation to patient visit volume. The procedures that could be done in the office were comparatively minor, and it was impractical and too costly to have extensive diagnostic testing or imaging equipment beyond basic laboratory analyzers and x-ray capabilities.

The changing organization and economics of healthcare have made the highly efficient use of facilities much more critical, and accepted healthcare facility planning benchmark standards have evolved in the industry. These new standards reflect both a volume-driven programming method and the collective experience of major healthcare organizations.

Instead of planning for the number of rooms based on old rules of thumb or anecdotal needs by individual practitioners, planning now starts with the idea that medical practice involves specific procedures that each have a well-defined space need. When strategically grouped together in a group practice facility, a more comprehensive array of integrated services can be provided. Exam rooms, consulting rooms, testing areas, and procedure spaces each have specific equipment needs and minimum space requirements for their functions, often defined by regulation or clinical guidelines and protocols. Exam rooms, for example, are generally required to have a minimum clear floor area of 80 square feet (7.43 square meters), including space for an exam table, hand-washing sink, and writing surface, at a minimum. As more equipment and technology are added to assist with care over time, and as more specialized types of exam rooms are included in the program, the corresponding size of the common exam room can grow to 120 to 135 square feet.

Volume-Based Programming

Volume-based programming takes into account the estimated practice volume and typical procedure times, which can vary substantially among different specialties.

For example, to accommodate a projected 20,000 annual patient visits, key assumptions might be hours of operation (e.g., 5 days per week, 10 hours per day), typical visit time in the exam room (e.g., 30 minutes), and percentage of utilization for each room, to allow for patient turnover, cleaning, and staff downtime (e.g., 60%). With that set of beginning assumptions to test, the number of rooms needed would be:

- 5 days × 10 hours × 50 weeks/yr = 2,500 hours available per room per year.
- Utilization at 60% of available hours = 1,500 utilized hours per year per room.
- At 30 minutes per use, each room could accommodate 3,000 annual visits.
- 20,000 target annual visits/3,000 = 6.66 rooms, or rounded, 7 exam rooms.
- With 250 working days per year, each room would average eleven 30-minute visits per day if utilized at 60%.

Although physicians may see 15 or 20 patients per session in bursts of activity, many academic medical centers find that actual visits average only six to eight per day, due to irregular patient scheduling, low utilization on certain afternoons, reduced operating hours, or use of exam rooms for nonessential purposes such as patient counseling or education, which could be done elsewhere in nonmedical spaces. Before creating more specialized and expensive space, attention to operational issues can help to ensure that the best use is made of capital investments.

Similar methods can be used to project space needs for other patient contact areas and for the support and staff work space required. Once the model is developed, different assumptions (Saturday hours, better utilization, faster visits, more volume) can be easily tested and their impact on space needs clearly seen. The basic model also assumes a fairly even flow of patients spread throughout the day. Block scheduling (having all patients report to the office at 9 AM or 1 PM, for example) and allowable waiting time have a direct impact on the number of rooms needed to accommodate peaks of patient flow. So does the decision to provide certain specialized services, such as EKG testing or nutrition counseling, only at certain times.

Programming Benchmark Standards

In its simplest and most logical terms, effective programming requires that you work through a projection of realistic space and facility needs based on the unique organization and operations of the practice. The following typical guidelines for very efficient primary care practices have been defined:

- 1.1 to 1.5 square feet of gross practice space per HMO member served
- Three to four annual patient visits per gross square foot (33–44 visits per square meter)
- 2,500 gross square feet per full-time care provider or physician
- 4,000 minimum annual visits per full-time provider (about 16 per day)
- Two to three exam spaces per full-time provider (usually for consultation also), depending on specialty
- Staff support of one RN per team and one medical assistant per two providers
- Six to eight exam room visits/day for academic medical centers

Modular Planning for Optimum Flexibility

Using modular space planning to allow for operational flexibility is another key in determining space needs. Because most group practices have a number of individual providers or specialists who work at different times and may have very different patient volumes, the most efficient facilities allow for flexible use of medical practice spaces at different times in order to optimize efficiency. If generic clinical spaces are provided and organized for varying uses, high-volume services such as internal medicine or cardiology might use four rooms for six half-day sessions per week, whereas a specialty such as dermatology might use one half-day session for a number of shorter patient visits.

Efficient planning also should consider the need for basic small examination rooms, where most patient visits can be done, versus the need for a smaller number of larger procedure rooms to accommodate more specific treatments or equipment. Using procedure space for routine exam visits is both less intimate for patients and an inefficient use of space and equipment. Physician consult space needs to be provided, either as a defined area within the exam room or as a nearby shared space. The economic need for higher efficiency and physician productivity makes the more traditional use of a dedicated office/consult before or after the exam visit a luxury of both time and space.

Office Space Planning Trends

Office size standards in all industries have been trending toward smaller spaces in response to cost pressures, leading to more efficient configurations for office areas. The traditional secretarial and private office spaces, furnished with large desks and credenzas with files, have

given way to flexible modular clerical workstations, which provide more work surface and storage in a more ergonomically designed environment. Open or private offices with wall-mounted furniture systems and larger multifunction conference areas and spaces for collaboration are typical spaces needed to support the interactive and collaborative way some clinicians practice today. All work spaces should be sized for computers and their accessories, such as printers and flat screens, with multiple data and telephone connections at each location for printers, scanners, and the like.

Scheduled Use of Rooms

To make the most efficient use of valuable space, the inclusion of shared-use room such as conference rooms, which can be scheduled by multiple users, and shared support areas such as file rooms, work areas, and staff break rooms are an ongoing trend. "Hoteling" and shared-use offices are often provided for staff that may be at one location only part-time. Each standardized work cubicle or private office should have data and telephone connections to accommodate laptop computers, plus basic work and temporary file space. Typical net space allocations for office areas are:

Clerical workstation with computer and file storage	48 sq ft (6 × 8)
Clinical workstation with computer, storage, and guest chair	64 sq ft (8 × 8)
Private office with work space, files, and guest chair	110 sq ft (10 × 11)
Senior staff office with work and meeting areas	150–180 sq ft (10 × 15+)
Executive office with sofa, conference, and work areas	180–240 sq ft (10 × 18+)

■ Operational Considerations

Although the inner operations of any particular group practice will be unique to that business, there are typically strong similarities between practices in how patients flow through, and what clinical and support functions are required. A thorough understanding by the designer of the operational needs and optimal work flow that the group practice wishes to achieve will inform both the programmatic space needs of the facility and the layout of various functional spaces required.

Patient Flow and Program Spaces

Space planning or layout design for group-practice facilities starts with an analysis and understanding of the desired and most efficient patient circulation and staff work flow and its impact on adjacencies and design choices. Breaking down and describing the detailed operational flow of staff, materials, and patients desired by the practice will help the designer to understand how to optimize functional adjacencies and efficiently plan the group practice.

The following sections describe a number of typical functions located in a group practice.

Patient/Public Entrance

The way that patients access and approach the practice should be visible, clear, and welcoming. Adequate parking should be provided; proximity to public transportation increases the accessibility of the practice to the public. The entrance space sets the image of the group practice and is the first area the patient experiences. Clear signage, a convenient way of getting from the street to the front door, and a gracious entry are welcoming and hospitable to patients and families and help provide a positive encounter. Simple architectural details such as a window or glass wall next to the entrance door provide visibility and help patients to confirm they are in the right place and that the practice is open.

Establishing a brand identity is a consideration for many group practices as they market their services and compete for patient business within their healthcare markets. Planning decisions can either reinforce or subvert the positive image of the practice to the general public. Careful consideration should be given to the image and attractiveness of the design of the main entrance area in order to reinforce the identity of the group practice. The use of an identifying and colorful graphic logo, carefully coordinated with the architectural and interior design, can also go a long way toward establishing the identity of the group practice in the eyes of the public.

Reception

The reception area is the public's first impression upon entering and says a lot about the practice. The receptionist should have clear visibility of the door, allowing him or her to visually acknowledge the patient's arrival. The goal should be to allow a personal welcome from a caring member of the practice, not a window in a wall with a bell to call for assistance. Planners and designers need to consider this first encounter and design to make it a positive experience in a professional setting. Signage should be positive and friendly and kept to a minimum. Signs stressing procedural rules and payment terms are not as welcoming and ideally should not be posted inside the initial encounter space. Reception counters need to be low enough to accommodate a person in a wheelchair, and should be as open and welcoming as possible. The patient and family

often enter with many questions and are looking for positive reinforcement. The design emphasis should be placed on creating opportunities to engage with patients, rather than on shielding the staff from them and screening off working areas. The quality of the material choices utilized at the entrance and reception areas can convey a visual sense of reassurance and professional quality.

Waiting Area

Once acknowledged, patients and their accompanying family members need a welcoming space with comfortable seating. Even though waiting time is typically and ideally limited, comfort of the seating area should be emphasized. This can help calm an otherwise anxious patient who may have a health issue on his or her mind. The seating itself needs to meet the needs of people who may be older, frail, and probably not feeling well and who may need assistance in getting up or sitting down. For the elderly and infirm, seat height needs to be high, generally at least 18 inches, and seats need to be fairly firm, with fixed arms that can help someone settle into or rise out of a chair. Low, soft seating or chairs that can tip or tilt are very difficult for some people to use and can be uncomfortable. A mix of movable individual armchairs and small two-seat sofas offers a choice to patients and their families as well as an inviting appearance. Arranging the seating in smaller-scale groupings can break down the scale of larger waiting areas and brings to mind a more comfortable residential-scale seating arrangement. Two-seat sofas are ideal for two people or a parent and a child. Larger sofas tend to become the territory of only one or two persons and reduce the overall seating capacity of the room. Consider providing a variety of seating venues, such as café tables and chairs, or a library table, in addition to the traditional armchairs and sofas, in order to provide greater choice to the public and to reduce the tendency of larger waiting areas to have a "bus station" feel. Appropriate lighting levels and quality furniture that can be moved for small family groups make the space friendly, professional, and ultimately flexible.

Coat storage should be provided in the waiting room and should be both convenient and reasonably secure. For practices with business-oriented patients or long waiting times for accompanying family, such as in an oncology practice or a treatment facility, a commonly seen amenity is a work counter with electrical outlets for laptop computers, charging cell phones, Internet access, and often a small pantry or coffee hospitality bar. Computer access is ideal for a patient to fill out medical history online, to access patient educational materials, or to look at upcoming clinic-related activities and programs.

Whether to provide a television in the waiting area is a common question and depends on the image and character of the practice. Generally pediatric practices require several TVs and video game areas for different age groups, but adult practices may find TVs to be intrusive. The design goal, as with the whole issue of waiting room style, is to match the expectations and comfort level of the target patient market, or to provide a choice of smaller spaces in which to wait.

Appointments and Scheduling

Every practice needs a conveniently located appointment desk in order to see patients on the way out of the office in a natural flow. This area should be distinct from the reception area, even if only at the other end of the same work counter, and should be provided with acoustical separation. Departing patients need to be accommodated promptly, without waiting while new arrivals have an extended conversation with the receptionist. Like the reception area, this function needs to accommodate wheelchair patients with a low counter area and convenient work space. Unlike the reception area, this function often requires some privacy to discuss billing instructions, insurance coverage, financial matters, and follow-up appointments.

Billing and Payments

Although routine payment arrangements can be processed at the appointment desk, often more privacy is needed to discuss payment arrangements with the patient or family. A small private office adjacent to the accounting area works well, with entrances from the patient corridor and from within the office suite. Acoustical privacy should be incorporated into the design of this area.

Medical Records

Although computerized recordkeeping is now part of almost every group practice, the idea of paperless offices has proven to be a challenge. Patient records accumulate a variety of paperwork, including that generated from internal procedures, a variety of related records such as lab test results and diagnostic images, as well as records from other providers outside the practice. Most large practices have found open-shelf filing to be the most flexible and efficient method. Records storage space needs to be estimated based on average file size, volume of patients, and length of time records must be held in active storage before being archived elsewhere. Filing space is estimated based on typical folder thickness, which may be 1 inch for common practices or more for specialized, long-term care. Open-shelf files more than seven shelves high can only be accessed with a step device or ladder, which creates a limit on shelf height. Open library-type shelving requires aisle space.

High-density shelving systems are also available. Shelving units in these systems roll to create aisles only as needed and require less overall space. However, the greater density of these systems can create a greater than normal structural load that must be considered, especially when located on upper floors of a building, and structural upgrades to the floor might be required. File space should be conveniently and centrally located adjacent to the admitting and billing areas of the practice.

Staff Services
Staff Entrance

In even the smallest practice, if space allows, there should be a separate staff and physician entrance, not readily visible to patients. Patients who are waiting for their appointments are not likely to understand the normal comings and goings of staff during the day, especially if the physicians have to visit their patients in the hospital. Staff should have their own discreet entrance. The staff entrance should be designed and located with consideration for security, both for the office and for staff entering and leaving. Good visibility, good lighting, and easy access to the street are all elements to consider.

Staff Break/Multipurpose Room

Because much of the staff may remain on-site all day, a dedicated staff break room should be provided, especially if the practice has evening hours with little opportunity for the staff to leave the office suite for breaks or meals. The staff break room is a mixed-use space, providing not just a location for staff to take breaks and have meals, but also a common area where staff can gather socially or check e-mail, or even a venue for vendor presentations, all of which should occur out of patient sight. It should ideally be provided with natural light and a view so that staff can truly get away and relax during their breaks. With kitchen facilities, as well as tables and chairs, the staff room can serve multiple purposes and may be the only area available that can accommodate a large staff meeting. Consideration should also be given to lockers or other storage areas for personal items such as coats, uniforms, purses, and shoes for staff members who may not have their own offices but need to secure their personal items.

Staff Work Areas

The staff members who support the clinical activities of the practice need individual work areas located close to the patient care areas of the practice in order to minimize their travel distance. Each location should provide needed supplies and computer work space, with the ability to sit down and record patient information. In most ambulatory care settings, decentralized workstations within each clinical pod or cluster are needed, rather than a central nurse station or office arrangement typically seen in hospitals. Work spaces should be designed ergonomically for maximum comfort. Thoughtful planning of work spaces and their convenient adjacency to patient areas can help to minimize staffing needs by allowing staff in one location to supervise several patient areas at once.

Clinical Areas
Exam Rooms
The examination room is the most basic outpatient planning unit. Almost all physician practice patient interactions occur within the exam room: interviews, consultations, examinations, minor treatments and procedures, follow-up, blood draws, and taking of vital signs. The overall throughput productivity and capacity of a practice come down to how well the exam room is utilized; it's the basic building block of the business. The design of the exam room demands careful consideration and attention to detail. Well-designed exam rooms can pay dividends in both patient perceptions and operational efficiency.

Although typically modest in size, exam rooms have three discrete and overlapping zones: the family zone, the physician documentation/work zone, and the patient exam zone. Patient and family space is the first requirement, with some privacy for changing clothes and provisions for seating for any accompanying family members. The Mayo Clinic, for example, has developed a standard exam room that provides a built-in sofa for family seating, which can accommodate a varying number of people and provides a welcoming, noninstitutional look to the room. Clothing hooks, shelves for clean gowns, and privacy curtains are all useful, depending on patient type and the proposed use of the room.

A place for the physician to write or dictate notes should be located in a separate zone within this room, preferably arranged to allow the physician to be face to face with the patient while charting. The charting area often requires a computer workstation, sometimes with a printer, plus telephone, paper and supply storage, reference literature or pamphlets, chairs for the patient and a family member, and an office chair or stool for the physician. New technologies such as smart phones and portable tablet computers offer new ways to enter, access, and manage patient data and can offer space savings and greater convenience.

Examination space should be arranged with recognition that many physicians are trained to work from the right-hand side of the patient, with the patient's head to their left. The physician should be able to stand at the table, out of the swing of the door. The patient's lower body should be oriented away from the door, to provide extra privacy, especially in rooms used for gynecological exams. The feeling of privacy is very important in the patient's perception of the quality of the service provided. In some layouts, cubicle curtains can help define the patient territory. An alternative in very small rooms is to reverse the door swing to shield views, by having the door open toward the table rather than to swing against the wall as would be typical.

The exam table may be fixed or adjustable, powered or manual, but should be standardized throughout the practice as much as possible. Wall-mounted diagnostic instrument sets, with oto/ophthalmoscope and blood pressure cuff, if used, are often located on the wall behind the exam table, with a nearby electrical outlet for the rechargeable battery. Fluorescent room lighting is usually adequate, but some specialties may require portable or fixed procedure lights. Careful consideration for the specification and stocking of warmer color temperature fluorescent lamping is important in the perception of the quality of fluorescent lighting used in group practice spaces. Variable light levels can be achieved through switching arrangements or dimmable lighting. This may be desirable in certain clinical situations such as ultrasound rooms.

For maximum provider productivity and interchangeable use of rooms, highly efficient designs include one room type, with all exam rooms essentially the same, from general layout down to the location of supplies and details of the rooms. Having identical rooms may be more useful over the long term than the construction economy of having left- and right-handed rooms to allow sink plumbing to be shared, because standardization of physical components for frequent tasks helps to minimize operational variables, resulting in increased efficiencies. In other words, if the alcohol and cotton swabs are in the same drawers in every exam room, then the staff will spend less time looking for these items over the course of the day. All of the rooms should have doors and exam tables in the same relationship, and all should have equal work spaces and storage areas, and similar finishes, wherever possible.

Designers should work closely with the physician group on the development of the design for the exam room. This is the room where they will spend most of their working hours over the years and generate most of their practice income. For larger projects, it is often helpful to construct a full-size exam room mock-up early in the process, in order to fine-tune the design of this most important room.

Nurse Work Space

The nurse or assistant work area usually serves a group of exam/procedure rooms, and often a communication or visual signal system is used to keep the process moving. Some practices use systems of colored lights or signage flags outside exam rooms to indicate to nurses and physicians when patients are in the room or ready for a specific procedure. The work area needs a computer, telephone, fax machine, and printer, because staff cannot easily leave to go to a central location for this equipment. Storage for medications and clean supplies should be provided very close to the work area.

Procedure Rooms

In addition to basic exam rooms, a practice often includes larger rooms for special purposes, such as minor surgery, endoscopy, or orthopedics. Determining space and planning needs for these rooms starts with considering what equipment will be used. Will procedures require a typical exam table, a procedure stretcher, or a special unit, such as an ENT/dental chair? Is specialized procedure lighting required, and if so, will it be portable, ceiling-mounted, or wall-mounted? Is it a specialized medical equipment item or part of the general lighting provided in the building? Sinks and storage cabinets may be needed. For some rooms a specific location, type, and size of sink may be needed, such as a scrub sink with special hands-free controls. Special finishes, such as provisions for wet areas, seamless flooring, washable walls, or a cleanable ceiling may be needed. Some rooms, such as endoscopy suites, may require specific storage cabinets for items such as long scopes and carrying cases; they also may have very specific size and construction requirements and need adjoining utility and cleanup spaces, with specialized equipment.

Diagnostic Imaging Suites

Diagnostic imaging is part of many practices and has its own set of very specific space-planning considerations, starting with patient waiting and dressing areas and gowned waiting space.

Diagnostic Imaging. Digital imaging has rapidly become the technology of choice for almost all types of diagnostic imaging, because it offers great flexibility, allows remote sharing of images, and eliminates darkrooms and reduces film or image file space. Typical modalities include radiography, fluoroscopy, chest x-ray, and mammography. Processing and reading areas are required, whether or not a digital system is used. This central technician work area includes digital film printers, an x-ray processor for film, view boxes for films, and picture archiving and communication system (PACS) terminals for viewing digitized images.

For all of these imaging functions, radiation shielding design issues include lead-lined wall partitions and doors, and leaded glass view windows. The thickness and extent of shielding required is based on a calculation by a consulting radiation physicist, usually retained by the group practice. Detailed design of the imaging rooms relies on specific layouts provided by the equipment vendor for use by the design team; equipment is installed only after the general construction work is complete.

Computed Tomography (CT) Scan. Similar to other diagnostic imaging rooms, computerized tomography (CT) scanners have unique planning requirements. Space and planning issues include the large size of the gantry and table unit, its weight, and its orientation. Patients on the table are positioned in the doughnut-shaped gantry for an x-ray cross-section of their body, so it is important for the technician in the adjoining control room to be able to look down the bore of the machine, to keep the patient in sight. Access to the unit for servicing requires space around it, and a separate adjoining room is usually required to house the electronics cabinets for the equipment. A dedicated refrigeration unit provides additional cooling for the gantry. Lead shielding is required because x-ray radiation is used. The lead shielding is based on specific radiation physicist calculations.

Magnetic Resonance Imaging (MRI). Magnetic resonance imaging (MRI) machines combine radio waves in a strong magnetic field to produce cross-sectional images that can show more detail of soft tissue than other imaging methods. Although no x-rays are used, and lead shielding is not required, the special nature of these units requires both radio frequency (RF) shielding to screen out other signals and often magnetic shielding to contain the strong magnetic field. The heart of the system is a very large and heavy doughnut-shaped, superconductive electromagnet that is cooled internally with liquid helium.

The magnetic field, even while contained within the room, presents special dangers from loose ferrous metal objects. The strength of the magnetic field can erase magnetic media, such as credit cards and ID badges. Safety protocols impose specific space-planning requirements for safety zones around the unit, which are under the control of the technical staff and can exclude dangerous, noncompatible objects and equipment. Within the safety zone, all equipment and construction must be nonferrous, including items such as stretchers, tools, and oxygen tanks. If the MRI system is turned off ("quenched") suddenly, the helium can absorb the heat and boil off as a gas and must therefore be vented through a large vent pipe to a safe area outside the building. Because of the weight of the magnet, often about 7 tons, and its sensitivity to vibration, it requires special structural engineering design and a structural analysis of how to move it into and out of the space. Exterior access must be considered for the future, when outdated equipment will need to be replaced; many layouts provide removable wall or roof panels to accommodate this. Like the CT suite, the MRI requires an adjacent control room and electronic equipment room, plus its own patient holding and stretcher transfer spaces within the controlled zone.

Ultrasound. Unlike other common imaging modalities, ultrasound diagnostic or procedure/biopsy rooms use portable equipment and require no room shielding. The equipment itself is a large, bulky cart, which needs to be positioned alongside an exam table. A work space in the same room is needed for technician charting, and the room needs to be large enough to accommodate seated family members.

Special Testing Suites

Doppler Ultrasound for Echocardiology. Similar to ultrasound technology often used for prenatal testing, Doppler ultrasound uses large but portable equipment for post-stroke testing. Results are monitored on video and often videotaped for review later.

Stress Testing/Treadmills. In addition to a treadmill, space is needed for the computer system and EKG that monitors the patient's response and charts the result. In the same room, a work counter and exam table are needed. The treadmill itself is a heavy-duty, commercial-grade type that may require special electrical service.

Nuclear Medicine

Nuclear studies use radioactive isotopes and monitor their absorption and distribution within the body by placing the patient in a large gamma camera, similar in size to an x-ray machine. Depending on the type and amount of isotope to be used, lead shielding of the room may be required. Nearby space is needed for a "hot lab," where isotopes are stored and prepared; a "hot injection" area, where isotopes are administered to patients; and a gowned waiting area for patients who have been injected. These areas may also need to be shielded, and the hot lab itself needs special finishes and equipment, such as stainless steel counters and lead-lined storage cabinets.

Laboratories

Advances in automated clinical laboratory equipment, such as chemistry analyzers, have allowed laboratories to be faster and more automated, and to employ fewer people and thus be less costly. Remote centralized laboratories are the most cost-efficient, because they can also be linked to the group practice and provide a digital medical record. Instead of the traditional chemistry lab look, the facility is now a flexible environment for larger electronic instruments, with flexible utilities and supply storage instead of lab workbenches and cabinets.

■ Planning Typologies and the Clinical Environment

Programmatic and operational needs will vary among the practices within a large group practice. Here are some sample questions that demonstrate some of the operational variability that could be present within a group practice:

- Will the group practice have a central patient reception/information desk in a main lobby for all patients as well as decentralized departmental-specific reception desks to receive patients at individual clinical departments? Will waiting, registration, and other administrative functions also be centralized or decentralized?
- Are any clinical services affiliated with functions at an acute care facility? If so, how might the functions provide coordinated and convenient service to the patient?
- What are the hours of operation for the entire center? Do they vary for specific clinical services within the practice? Will the clinical program require late evening hours? For example, if the group practice includes an ambulatory surgery program component, will two staff shifts be required in order to receive preoperative patients in the early morning, yet remain open so that afternoon surgical cases can recover without the patient needing to be admitted to an acute care facility for recovery?
- Logistically, will the group practice purchase and receive supplies centrally that will then be distributed by a paid staff? Or will individual supplies be purchased, tracked, and received by individual practices within the larger group practice?
- How many access points to the facility are needed? How many exit points? Will there be a dedicated patient discharge lobby for patients recovering from surgery and waiting for transportation home? What are the security implications from the access points?
- Are there any electronic systems that will help move patients through the facility, such as electronic appointment making?
- Are any medical education or teaching components anticipated?

■ Will the group practice be connected to an acute care hospital? If so, will there be dedicated connection corridors to allow supplies and services to flow between the hospital and group practice suite as well as corridors for patient flow? If not, will the group practice be near an acute care facility? How will patient transportation be handled between the two if the ambulatory care center requires acute care backup?

These are just a few samples of the in-depth questions that need to be asked when structuring the physical typology of a group practice. Questions such as these help determine how the practice will operate and how the various clinical, administrative, and support functions will interact and coordinate.

Patient Registration: Centralized Versus Decentralized

Perhaps one of the more perplexing and challenging operational considerations to handle effectively in a large group practice center is that of centralized or decentralized administrative functions. The group practice should ideally function as a coordinated and integrated system of ambulatory clinical services, much like a hospital, but without the inpatient bed component. Ideally, the administrative systems are integrated and coordinated so that the patient experience is convenient, simple, well-coordinated, and efficient. The larger the group practice gets, the more challenging this becomes, especially if the practice is on multiple floors of a building. One method to ensure complete coordination of the patient experience throughout the facility and, in fact, throughout the system, is to carefully construct the administrative interaction points in order to keep the flow of patients consistent, simple, and steady.

A centralized patient registration/check-in/check-out/payment/financial counseling/scheduling function for a group practice with diverse medical components requires a large number of administrative staff to provide all of these services in a coordinated, efficient way. The check-in process normally requires patients to provide updated background information, their detailed medical history, verification of their insurance coverage, any required copayments, and other information upon entering the practice. If all patients must go through this process, adequate staff must be provided to keep up with the flow to avoid a patient flow logjam. This can require substantial space that must be adequately programmed and designed.

If all the multiple services and practice components make use of the centralized administrative receiving and check-out points, instead of duplicating this function within each practice area, space can be saved and the number of overhead full-time employee positions can be minimized. This can also help to make the overall group practice more operationally efficient and increase total patient throughput. An effective way to ensure that all of the miscellaneous administrative functions that a patient/visitor must experience during their visit to the group practice are accounted for is through the use of a flow chart diagram. Each step and each potential procedural scenario for the patient can be anticipated using this method, in order to ensure that space and staff are planned in a way that facilitates a smooth, uninterrupted, and linear flow. A patient-focused approach ensures that the group practice is geared toward the patient as the customer. Convenience for the patient is emphasized whenever possible, with services either brought to the patient or collocated so that the patient can complete all of the various administrative functions required in one location and in one simple sequence.

Arranging Clinical Spaces

There are various methods for arranging clinical spaces in an outpatient setting, each in response to operational models as well as personal preferences and the desired ambiance of the practice. The most common and basic planning unit for group practices is the common exam room. As mentioned earlier, exam rooms range in size from a small code minimum of 80 square feet up to 135 square feet. A room's size depends on the type of practice that will use it and the processes and equipment the room is to accommodate. The following sections review a few ways to organize exam rooms and their support functions.

Finger Corridors

A basic, flexible, and efficient layout for exam rooms is the finger corridor. In this arrangement, parallel corridors of exam rooms are arranged next to each other. Generally the waiting and administrative functions are located at the front of the department, and the finger corridors extend away from the administrative areas. This provides visibility down the corridors towards the exam room doors and, if utilized, the room status indicator lights or flags projecting slightly from the walls, indicating whether the room is in use. A band of support functions, physician offices, or internal administrative functions is normally located toward the far end of the exam room corridors.

This "layering" of spaces allows for a transition of spaces from public to semipublic to private. Locating exterior windows at the end of the corridors is an effective way to allow natural daylight into the clinical corridors, providing a sense of daytime orientation.

The real advantage of the exam room finger corridor configuration is that it allows for the efficient utilization of exam rooms. If volumes require, exam rooms in adjacent corridors can be used for spillover volume without having to change staffing. In addition, when modular room sizes are used, the plan can be readily converted for use by other practice types or even as office space with little remodeling required.

Exam Room Pods

Another arrangement of exam rooms is the cluster or "pod" whereby four to eight exam rooms are clustered around a dedicated sub-waiting room and staff support functions. Each pod is normally accessed by a single door, creating a suite. Each pod has a direct connection to the public zone (patient waiting and reception) and staff work areas (private offices, specialized procedure and diagnostic testing areas), and clean and soiled work areas. The pod concept lends itself to teams of clinicians who operate out of a pod or two and who have their own dedicated nursing or technician staff, as well as administrative staff, all working within the exam room pod. A practice group could schedule, for example, 2.5 modules for five half-day sessions per week. This approach can simplify group practice scheduling and help to maximize the use of space over time, allowing for the greatest possible patient throughput per exam room.

Although a pod configuration may allow for a more intimate and private setting for patient care, it also tends to separate the clinical and administrative staff and can result in the duplication of services, thus creating some level of inefficiency. In addition, the exam room pod configuration can limit visibility from a central location, preventing staff from seeing whether the exam rooms are occupied or need service. The pod configuration may not provide the needed flexibility to adjust to volume variations as well as a finger corridor arrangement, and sometimes requires the staffing of an adjacent pod of exam rooms even when only one patient is being served.

Ballroom

A variation on the exam room cluster or pod is the ballroom model, which can be used when all the exam rooms for a particular medical specialty are collocated and wrapped around the perimeter of a shared waiting room. This model is a self-contained ambulatory department

and can include reception/registration, waiting seating, public toilets, and clinical support space, although support functions are usually not accessible from the waiting areas. Although this model provides clinical autonomy for the specialty and allows visibility of the exam rooms for managing patient flow, it does not provide for privacy in and out of the exam rooms. This type of configuration is more commonly found in the planning of emergency departments, where the visibility and movement of patients of all types through the clinical space based on an unpredictable intake is the priority.

■ Shared Support Functions

A well-planned and efficient group practice might want to consider having shared support functions, similar to the shared administrative functions of a centralized reception area. These shared support functions include the staff lounge/break room, staff conference room, staff multi-purpose room/library, staff locker rooms, showers, and toilets, as well as larger subdividable conference rooms. Conference/classroom functions can be reserved via a shared scheduling mechanism. When these spaces are combined and shared, they can be larger and can offer more amenities for more people. This model is in contrast to having decentralized and dedicated staff break rooms and locker rooms closer to each department.

■ The Clinical Neighborhood Model

As group practices become larger and more sophisticated and provide more hospital-like services, they are increasingly as functional as full-service hospitals, minus the overnight patient capability, which is restricted by code. With more specialized clinical components, multiple patient access points throughout the facility may be necessary. Practices also can use their size to become increasingly more integrated, in order to optimize clinical and operational efficiencies. A one-stop healthcare approach, with fewer access points for specialized care, can be more patient-friendly and simpler. The clinical neighborhood model has emerged as an option for larger group practices.

This model groups clinical services by disease, with the simple objective of collocating all the related services that a patient suffering from a particular illness or condition might need throughout their path to wellness. For example, instead of having separate clinical departments for orthopedics, physical and/or occupational therapy, spine and back care, hand surgery, and imaging, each with its own support functions and "front door," the clinical neighborhood model groups all these related and similar services into the "musculoskeletal neighborhood." Now a patient with any one of these ailments can go to the musculoskeletal neighborhood and receive all the clinical consultation, treatment, and care they might need within the neighborhood.

The neighborhood model can incorporate the use of shared support functions, as well as centralized reception and check-in functions. This model is particularly effective when the group practice is affiliated with an academic medical center because additional specialties can be incorporated into the continuum of care of the neighborhood, and clinical research can be conducted on a broader set of related disciplines.

■ Planning for Growth and Change

Group practice facilities, even more so than hospitals, are faced with a lack of data for reliable long-term planning. Although changing patient demographics, including the aging of the population, can be predicted to some extent, changing practice approaches, new technology, and new ways of paying for services make predicting the future difficult. The impact of recent healthcare reform is also yet to be seen. Often the only safe assumption is that over the life of the facility the practice will evolve, but in ways that cannot be predicted with certainty. Changes in technology and reimbursement cause frequent changes in facilities, as services and specialty staff are added or discontinued, and as the patterns of patient flow change. Because the group practice's physicians can never really know with certainty what lies ahead, the best planning response is one that incorporates flexibility at reasonable cost, rather than a plan that exactly reflects the practice as it exists now. Assume that staff, operations, and equipment will change, and plan accordingly.

Flexible planning for future change starts with floor area size; larger, rectilinear floors are easier to configure in different ways than unusual shapes or narrow wings. Higher floor-to-floor heights offer more flexibility for changing building services such as air conditioning. Lay-in acoustical tile ceilings are common, largely because they provide a high degree of flexibility as compared to more fixed architectural ceilings. Electrical and data/telecommunications services can be routed through the flexible ceiling. Multiple vertical risers are needed throughout the space to provide some level of flexibility in the future location of plumbing fixtures.

Sometimes a flexible planning approach is to provide standard rooms of similar sizes, each similarly equipped, so that exam rooms can serve different specialties as needed, and office, consult, exam, and procedure functions can be interchanged later. The challenge for the design team is to look beyond current practice so that a new facility can offer flexibility to accommodate future changes and other potential arrangements rather than simply reflect the old model.

■ Codes and Guidelines for Healthcare Facilities

Guidelines for Design and Construction of Hospital and Health Care Facilities

One of the most comprehensive and easily accessible references for medical facility requirements is the publication *Guidelines for Design and Construction of Hospital and Health Care Facilities* (Guidelines), produced by the Facilities Guidelines Institute with assistance from the American Institute of Architects and the U.S. Department of Health and Human Services (HHS). HHS finances and regulates medical practice. As the latest edition of the general standards first published by the federal government in 1947, the Guidelines have become the established minimum national standard for medical facilities. As a guideline, not a prescriptive code, it is one of the reference standards for organizations such as the Health Care Financing Authority (HCFA), which provides Medicare and Medicaid funding for services, and JCAHO, which accredits hospital-based services. Many, but not all, states have adopted a specific edition of the Guidelines as their state code for health facilities. It is important to point out that the Guidelines outline minimal standards for safety and operations, not optimum planning parameters. In different sections, the Guidelines publication sets out requirements for primary care and ambulatory care services, as well as hospital, nursing home, rehabilitation, and mental health facilities. In some cases, private practice facilities may not be required to meet the Guidelines. However, facilities such as those in which Medicaid or Medicare patients will be seen will fall under federal jurisdiction and must be designed to meet the requirements of the Guidelines.

Local Health Codes

Practice managers and designers must be familiar with health codes in effect where they are located, which may also include city, county, and/or state codes. Some of these codes are oriented more to the operational requirements for medical practice, and some have specific physical requirements (such as minimum room sizes, locations for hand-washing sinks, or limitations on exiting and safety requirements). Often, local codes will cross-reference national standards such as the Guidelines, the Life Safety Code (NFPA 101) published by the National Fire Protection Association, and the Americans with Disabilities Act (ADA) which prescribes accessibility requirements for those with disabilities. The design team should be familiar with what the local codes require. Some states or jurisdictions also have their own codes for accessibility, which may exceed the requirements of ADA.

Building Codes: Business Use

Each locality also has its own regulations for building construction and use, which must be met along with the health-related codes. Building functions are often designated by use groups, each with a range of permitted functions or services. In most areas, basic group medical practice functions fall under a "business" use, assuming no patients are kept overnight and none (or a specified minimum number) are incapacitated by use of anesthetics or other means. More extensive services would fall under ambulatory care or outpatient hospital or institutional use, with more stringent standards for construction and fire protection needing to be met. An important factor to analyze in this regard is the special requirements imposed if ambulatory care services are provided by a hospital or licensed entity at an off-site location. In some cases, to be reimbursed as hospital-provided services, the facilities need to meet the higher standard for hospital outpatient services, which may require more specialized air conditioning, ventilation, fire protection, or emergency power requirements than are typically found in a business-use facility.

Health and Safety Issues

Medical facility space planning includes an awareness of health issues that could affect patients and staff. In addition to the basic safety regulations, most notably the Life Safety Code (National Fire Protection Agency, NFPA101), other environmental regulations include Occupational Safety and Health Administration (OSHA) workplace requirements and the removal of hazardous materials. Renovation of existing facilities may require a specialized hazardous materials consultant to survey and test for the presence of hazardous items such as lead paint or asbestos-containing materials that may not be visible or apparent. If found, these materials all require a specific treatment plan, which could range from permanent encapsulation in a covering material to removal under highly controlled conditions and disposal in a hazardous materials landfill. The removal process requires temporary enclosures, special air handling, and the use of licensed contractors to remove materials according to a plan approved by local authorities having jurisdiction.

When construction of an office suite takes place adjacent to other suites, or renovation is done inside an office suite, careful precautions must be taken to isolate and control construction dust, debris, and whenever possible, noise. Often a contractor will wall off a construction area with temporary partitions or wrap the area in heavy plastic to curtain dust and dirt. If there are no operable windows in the office suite, a mechanical system is used to move and filter all the interior air. Containing the dust is important so that it doesn't get caught up in the ventilation system and potentially recirculate throughout the suite.

Accommodating Disabilities

Access for disabled users is required by the Americans with Disabilities Act (ADA), which is a civil rights law rather than a code or regulation. The ADA requires that facilities make provisions to accommodate both patients and staff who may be disabled and allows those users to sue the facility owner if access is not provided. Designers are generally familiar with the details required to comply with the ADA. The effect of this set of regulations has been to require more space in healthcare facilities. Corridors are wider, there is more space around doors, accessible toilets and showers are more generous, and rooms become larger to allow for wheelchair access. Small, tight plans with narrow passages and sliding doors are no longer allowed. Simpler, smoother-flowing plans with more generous space are required. Changes in floor levels require more space for ramps or wheelchair lifts, and even a step or two up to a staff work area requires a ramp and railing. Sections of counters and reception desks and windows are lower, whereas sinks and other items may be higher to allow for wheelchair access under the sink. Doors are wider and may require power operators. All of these changes are generally an improvement, but many require more space and additional cost to implement.

■ Time, Cost, and Quality

All facilities' design and construction decisions have an impact on time (to design and construct), cost (capital, operations, and maintenance), and quality (durability and image). The preferred solution is a balance of these issues. Shortening construction time limits material choices and leads to increased labor costs to meet deadlines; higher design quality and better materials often (but not always) tend to increase first costs and may or may not reduce future maintenance costs.

In considering the cost and quality issues of traditional methods versus a design/build arrangement, there is an important link between the decision-making role and the final cost and quality. One of the realities of the design and construction process is that in the end, the facility owner is the only party who will pay for the result, in terms of both capital and maintenance, regardless of the form of contract used. Making a designer or builder responsible for meeting a set cost requires making them the final arbiters of overall quality; trying to enforce a promise of high quality in one area will lead to less visible cuts in others, if the overall cost is fixed. As the representative of the healthcare facility, the administrator should be looking for a clearly articulated balance of cost and quality for decision making, not a reliance on assumptions, promises, and guarantees.

The two most immediate concerns for the practice manager undertaking a facility project are control of the cost and time for the project. Because design and construction time is largely a reflection of the complexity of the project and the clarity of the process, the budget is the key starting point for establishing a plan and using it as a tool for maintaining control.

Budget

Casual discussion often involves the budget as a general statement, but it is critical for the healthcare facility to define terms and be very specific, because the "construction budget" often referred to by team members is in fact only a small part of the total eventual cost of the facility project. Although the construction cost is clearly the cost of constructing the design, consider also the other elements required:

- Land acquisition cost includes both the purchase price of the land for a new building or the purchase of an existing building for renovation and also all of the associated real estate transaction costs, such as broker fees, boundary survey, transfer taxes, closing costs, and the like.
- Soft costs are the costs incurred by the owner of the project, such as leasing costs; legal fees; local and state government application and approval fees; taxes; fees for consultants, brokers, and advisors; and the internal labor and overhead costs of the facility-planning effort itself. An important component of this item can be salary costs for the healthcare facility staff who are spending time organizing and managing the project, which should properly be considered part of its cost.
- Fees will be required for the design team (architect, interior designer, consulting engineers) as well as other potential consultants: elevator design, signage, furniture, artwork, materials handling,

data network, equipment planning, space programming, and many others.

- Equipment cost includes both the medical equipment needed to operate the facility (such as exam tables, x-ray equipment, instruments, and supplies) and the general office equipment (copy machines, computer system, telephone system, maintenance equipment).
- Furnishings are the loose items that are not equipment—not only desks and chairs, but also office accessories, plants, artwork, wastebaskets, and shelving. If not selected by the medical equipment consultant or interior designer, all of this will require the practice staff's time to select, specify, purchase, receive, assemble, and put in place.
- Testing costs include information that may be needed for the design team, depending on the site, such as site topographic survey, subsurface investigations and geotechnical consulting, hazardous material surveys (and remediation costs), air- and water-quality testing, hydrology studies in flood areas, and quality testing during construction for materials such as concrete and welded steel.
- Moving costs include not only packing, shipping, and unpacking, but also consulting fees to help plan a complicated move. If phased occupancy is needed, moving costs might also include temporary swing space or temporary utility services.

Construction Cost Factors

When professional estimators or construction managers offer projected construction costs, they take into account a number of factors beyond simply the design shown in the documents provided to them, including the following:

- The size of the project can impact overall costs. A small project will still have contractor mobilization, overhead expenses, and site general conditions (such as protection, cleanup, and temporary office space) that must be applied to the project. These costs are not related to the area constructed but rather to the length of time the construction goes on. For a large project, these costs are a lower proportion of the total cost.
- The quality level of the project, besides being reflected in the cost of materials, also has other implications. The use of costly or unusual materials or systems requires more supervision time and probably more rework to correct errors in the field. Very high standards of workmanship, if required

by the designer, can also increase overall costs for supervision and coordination. Are sprinkler heads required to be centered in ceiling tiles exactly, or not? These quality assumptions invite the contractor to budget more effort.

- The complexity of planning and design is reflected in the contractor's assumptions about productivity and the time needed to build the project. Relatively simple, independent, or repetitive identical components are easier to build than complex assemblies of many different items. A freestanding, easily accessible project site is easier and less costly to build than one with limited contractor access and restricted work hours.
- The phasing of the project can multiply cost assumptions, because each construction phase needs more supervision and requires trade contractors, such as electricians and plumbers, to return several times. Each distinct phase requires inspections and approvals before moving on to the next.
- Schedule flexibility also impacts overall cost. Are there outside schedule constraints and specific dates by which things must be complete? Is timing of the work limited, for example, to only weekends or after hours?
- Access and staging also complicate the process. Work in existing buildings requires dust-control partitions, security, protection of elevators, and accommodating existing users' schedules. Difficult or complex access from truck-loading areas, or temporary staging of materials in some other area, add to costs. Construction work in congested urban areas tends to be more expensive due to lack of space for receiving and staging construction materials.

Financing Group Practice Facilities

Group practice facilities are usually financed under some form of developer model, with either an external developer providing some or all of the services or the group itself acting as developer. Even when the facility is associated with a large healthcare provider, the provider will often look to a developer for the financing in order to preserve its own resources for other programs, typically in acute care.

When an external developer is involved, it can function either in a traditional developer role or in a build/operate role. In the former, the developer will secure project financing, develop the building, and then lease the facility to the group. In the build/operate model, the developer retains a more active long-term role, operating the facility on behalf of the group. This could be just operating the physical plant, but more often includes provision of some functional services, such as reception and the like. There are many developers who have established a specialty in the ambulatory care center and medical facility field for this very reason.

The advantage of having a developer in the project, whether traditional or build/operate, is that it can deal with many of the complexities around development and finance and free the group to focus on healthcare delivery. The main disadvantage is that the developer needs to be rewarded for its contribution, and in the longer term the costs to the group can be higher.

When a group acts as its own developer, it must bring the same level of expertise to the table as an independent developer. There is significantly more to developing an ambulatory care center facility than a conventional office development, and the practice has to be well versed in these issues if it is to act as its own developer. In order to secure financing, it will need access to both bank and private equity funds, because bank or conventional loan financing is usually not sufficient to cover all costs. Because of the risks associated with the income streams for medical providers, the lending institutions typically will require significant levels of equity, or at-risk, funds in the project. Private equity funds will often be available, quite possibly from group members, but establishing appropriate terms and rewards can be challenging, and having group members as investors in the property, often at different proportions to their membership in the group, can lead to long-term conflicts if the structures are not well defined.

In order to secure the funding, the group will need to have appropriate income models both reflecting anticipated revenue and addressing income risks due to changing reimbursement patterns over time; competition from other providers, including major healthcare providers, who are increasingly using market dominance to develop satellite group facilities; changing patient demographics; and the like. All of these areas require expertise that may not reside with the group members. If, however, the group can provide these, either internally or through the use of consultants, the risks and rewards can be higher.

For groups that act as their own developer, the sources of financing will vary greatly over time; bank or institutional loans will usually be a significant source, but not all banks or institutions will fund medical projects at any given time. Costs and levels of equity investment or risk coverage will vary among institutions, and a lot of research will be required to find the best financing for a given project. Private equity investors are much more difficult to find without strong connections in the equity market. There is a danger that the group could make a poor selection, in either cost or relationship, in its eagerness to secure private equity funding. Typically, other financing is not available to group practices. Major providers can be faced with antitrust or tax issues if they fund facilities, and bond financing is rarely open to such practices.

■ Planning Your New Facility

Before you begin to plan and design a new office space, an overall strategy is needed to serve as a roadmap for facility development. It is imperative for the architect to know the strategic plan and understand the vision of the organization in order to help guide the decision-making process with the best interest of the group practice in mind.

Ideally, a strategic plan exists and simply needs to be confirmed. The plan should define how the organization intends to function and grow, relative to both external and internal factors. External factors include demographics, patient types, competition, and reimbursement structures; internal factors are relative to an analysis of strengths and weaknesses in the services and operations.

The group practice should carefully consider how to improve and prepare the organization for the future. Due to rising demand and facility costs, operational efficiency is a key consideration. What can be done to improve client service? Are there gaps in clinic schedules, or can

hours of operation be extended? A building program will not solve operational problems, but it can help serve as a catalyst for change, and it can be designed to support the organization's practice model.

It is important to carefully consider who will attend the design meetings and how these chosen few will communicate with the rest of the practice. It is impractical for all members of the practice to be involved directly with the design process, but everyone should feel they are participants. Those who attend design meetings need to be the voice of all staff, representing a cross-section of people who work in the practice. Who has the experience and skills to manage the design process and also has the trust of their counterparts in the practice? Those persons attending meetings should be consistent throughout the project and do their best to attend all of the design and planning meetings with the design team.

Commitment to a design project takes time but can be very rewarding for a group practice. As consumers of healthcare services become savvier, one of the ways a group practice can promote itself is through the design. The design of the facility can help to identify a feeling of professionalism; it can make staff feel supported and patients feel welcome and cared for. An excellent source of information on how built environments can support healthcare is the Center for Health Design (http://www.healthdesign.org), which is a nonprofit organization working to demonstrate that using evidence-based design in hospitals and healthcare facilities can improve the quality of healthcare.

Index

CPSIA information can be obtained
at www.ICGtesting.com
Printed in the USA
JSHW042235250722
28526JS00004B/73